# Male Infertility and Sexual Dysfunction

**Springer**
*New York*
*Berlin*
*Heidelberg*
*Barcelona*
*Budapest*
*Hong Kong*
*London*
*Milan*
*Paris*
*Santa Clara*
*Singapore*
*Tokyo*

Wayne J.G. Hellstrom

Editor

# Male Infertility and Sexual Dysfunction

With 236 Illustrations, 38 in Full Color

**Compliments of**

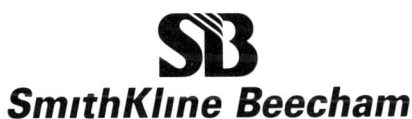

**SmithKline Beecham**

*Pharmaceuticals*

**distributor of**

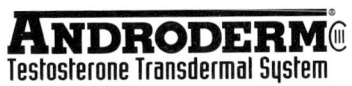

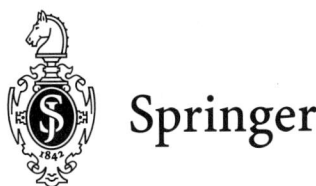 Springer

Wayne J.G. Hellstrom
Associate Professor of Urology
Chief, Section of Andrology and Male Infertility
Department of Urology
Tulane University School of Medicine
1430 Tulane Avenue SL 42
New Orleans, LA 70112-2699, USA

Library of Congress Cataloging-in-Publication Data
Male infertility and sexual dysfunction/Wayne J.G. Hellstrom,
    editor.
        p.    cm.
    Includes bibliographical references and index.
    ISBN 0-387-94859-7 (hardcover: alk. paper)
    1. Andrology.  2. Infertility, Male.  3. Impotence.
I. Hellstrom, Wayne J.G.
    [DNLM: 1. Infertility, Male.  2. Sex Disorders.  WJ 709 M24532
    1997]
RC875.M35   1997
616.6′9–dc20                                     96-32477

Printed on acid-free paper.

Production coordinated by Chernow Editorial Services, Inc., and managed by Natalie Johnson; manufacturing supervised by Jeffrey Taub.
Typeset by Best-set Typesetter Ltd., Hong Kong.
Printed and bound by Maple-Vail Book Manufacturing Group, York, PA.
Printed in the United States of America.

9 8 7 6 5 4 3 2 1

ISBN 0-387-94859-7 Springer-Verlag New York Berlin Heidelberg   SPIN 10547038

*This book is dedicated to Blackwell B. Evans, Sr., M.D., who was a friend, an inspiration, and a mentor in urology; and to my family—John Erik, Joshua, Kyle, and Gina—for their continuing support.*

# Foreword

This comprehensive volume fills a need for information on current methods of diagnosis and new means of treatment of both male infertility and sexual dysfunction. These fields have expanded so rapidly that for practicing physicians it has become somewhat impossible to keep up with the latest advances merely by reading the journals. Here, the editor-in-chief has assembled a first-rate crew of experts from around the world and assigned topics in their areas of expertise. The resulting chapters range from basic principles and tests to newest diagnostic and therapeutic methods. Each chapter is limited to a discussion of a specific aspect of andrology. This focus on specific disorders allows the reader to quickly secure the diagnostic tools and a plan for treatment.

Although andrology has become a specialty of its own, general practitioners and general urologists still diagnose and treat the majority of these patients. Thus, they need a source of practical, current information on which to base their management. In addition, the information laid out in this text will suggest what problems should be referred to the specialist.

This is a book to keep at hand in the office or clinic for ready reference when a patient is seen with a complaint of infertility or impotency.

*Frank Hinman, Jr., M.D., F.A.C.S., F.A.A.P., F.R.C.S. (Hon.)*
University of California School of Medicine
San Francisco, California

# Preface

Infertility is more common than most would imagine. One in seven couples will have difficulty conceiving during their reproductive lives, and the male factor is implicated as the cause in up to 50% of these cases. The landmark birth of Denise Brown by in vitro fertilization in 1978 was matched in significance in 1992 by the introduction of intracytoplasmic sperm injection (ICSI) in humans. Although ICSI is now a mainstream topic in discussions about assisted reproductive techniques, it needs to be considered as an adjunct in the treatment of male infertility. To treat only the sperm and not do a complete history and physical examination as we were taught in medical school is unconscionable. The field of male infertility crosses more than one discipline, with a knowledge of urology, endocrinology, immunology, and even gynecology needed for the physician to address many of the common clinical presentations. Infertility may well be the presentation of a serious medical condition, and the emotional and financial impact on the couple undergoing any assisted reproductive technique should never be underestimated.

Male sexual dysfunction, like male infertility, is receiving greater public attention. According to recent estimates, between 20 and 30 million American men suffer from some degree of sexual dysfunction. Comparative figures generally apply worldwide. Surprisingly, only a small proportion of men experiencing impotence have undergone evaluation or received treatment, often because of either their own reluctance or their physician's lack of comfort in dealing with the subject of sexuality. Some critics have commented that with the prevailing level of managed care and the introduction of effective oral medications, the necessity for knowing about the mechanics and psychogenics of male sexual dysfunction is no longer required. Nothing can be further from the truth. Despite the logic of goal-directed therapy, most patients are dissatisfied with this form of care. And, for the inquisitive physician, a knowledge of the underlying mechanisms of causation and prevention is intellectually fulfilling and a driving force for improved patient care. In no way has the introduction of oral agents for treatment of impotence brought an end to the necessity of investigation. New knowledge, unforeseen complications, and innovative treatment lie ahead.

These projections and anticipations are significant and worthy of our attention. To this end, *Male Infertility and Sexual Dysfunction* combines discussions of the latest advances in basic research with the recent innovations in the disciplines of male infertility and sexual dysfunction.

Similar to the progress witnessed in other academic domains, the field of andrology continues to evolve, perhaps at an even more rapid pace than certain other areas of medicine. Nonetheless, it would be impossible to discuss every issue in andrology in a single volume, and it would be unlikely that a single individual could comprehensively cover all the latest developments in every specific area. For this reason, select international authorities have contributed in-depth coverage of their areas of expertise.

Part I begins with a discussion of male infertility and continues to the basic sciences, office evaluation, laboratory and imaging techniques, use of testicular biopsy, and the basic information that an andrologist should have about the female partner. Next is a group of specialized chapters dealing with immunologic infertility, genital inflammation, and reactive oxygen species, followed by clinically applicable chapters on medical management, sperm processing, and surgical techniques that aid or ensure the union of healthy gametes. Adolescent andrology and future concerns about genetics and gonadotoxicity are included in this section on male infertility.

Part II reflects a more diverse format in coverage of sexual dysfunction. The basics of office evaluation, androgen insufficiency, and duplex and nocturnal penile tumescence (NPT) studies are covered. Attention is then given to more abstract subjects on neurotransmission, penile neurology, premature ejaculation, and psychogenic impotence. Finally, the medical, noninvasive, and surgical techniques are detailed.

The study of andrology is indeed a moving target. The dogma of today will be the history of tomorrow. The goal of this volume is to provide a base of current knowledge and set standards of clinical care to assist andrology researchers and clinicians of today. These will in turn lay the foundations for the discoveries of tomorrow.

I would like to take this opportunity to thank June Banks Evans, Ann Morcos, and Michon Breisacher Shinn for their tireless efforts and invaluable support in collecting, correcting, and processing the many manuscripts that went into this volume. My sincere appreciation to Raju Thomas, M.D., for his continued support and to Esther Gumpert and Anne Fossella at Springer-Verlag for their professional guidance and good cheer through all phases of the writing of this book.

Wayne J.G. Hellstrom

# Contents

# Contributors

*R. John Aitken, Ph.D.*, MRC Reproductive Biology Unit, Edinburgh EH3 9EW, UK

*Stanley E. Althof, Ph.D.*, Department of Urology, School of Medicine, Case Western Reserve University, Beachwood, OH 44122, USA

*Neil Baum, M.D.*, 3525 Prytania Street, New Orleans, LA 70115, USA

*Arnold M. Belker, M.D.*, Department of Urology, Division of Surgery, School of Medicine, University of Louisville, Louisville, KY 40292, USA

*Alexandru E. Benet, M.D.*, Department of Urology, Montefiore Medical Center, Bronx, NY 10467, USA

*Gregory A. Broderick, M.D.*, Department of Urology, Hospital of the University of Pennsylvania, Philadelphia, PA 19104, USA

*Wesley W. Bryan, M.D.*, Department of Urology, Tulane University School of Medicine, New Orleans, LA 70112-2699, USA

*Seck L. Chan, M.D.*, Pan Pacific Urology, San Francisco, CA 94115, USA

*P. Ronald Clisham, M.D.*, Department of Obstetrics and Gynecology, Tulane University School of Medicine, New Orleans, LA 70112-2699, USA

*Glenn R. Cunningham, M.D.*, Department of Medicine and Research Development, Baylor College of Medicine, Veterans Affairs Medical Center, Houston, TX 77030-4298, USA

*Paul C. Doherty, Ph.D.*, VIVUS, Inc., 545 Middlefield Road, Menlo Park, CA 94025, USA

*Erma Z. Drobnis, Ph.D.*, Fertility Laboratories, University of Missouri-Columbia, Columbia, MO 65203, USA

*Julia A. Drose, B.A., R.D.M.S., R.D.C.S.*, Department of Radiology, University of Colorado Health Sciences Center, Denver, CO 80262, USA

*Lev Elterman, M.D.*, Department of Urology, Rush-Presbyterian-St. Luke's Medical Center, Chicago, IL 60612, USA

*David A. Gilbert, M.D.*, Department of Plastic Surgery, Eastern Virginia Medical School, Norfolk, VA 23510, USA

*Sarah K. Girardi, M.D.*, Department of Urology, New York Hospital-Cornell University Medical Center, New York, NY 10021, USA

*Irwin Goldstein, M.D.*, Department of Urology, Boston University School of Medicine, Boston, MA 02118, USA

*Marc Goldstein, M.D.*, Department of Urology, New York Hospital-Cornell University Medical Center, New York, NY 10021, USA

*Nestor F. Gonzalez-Cadavid, Ph.D.*, Department of Surgery, Division of Urology, School of Medicine, University of California at Los Angeles, Harbor-UCLA Medical Center, Torrance, CA 90509, USA

*John E. Gould, M.D., Ph.D.*, Department of Urology, School of Medicine, University of California at Davis, Sacramento, CA 95817, USA

*Jeremy P.W. Heaton, M.D.*, Department of Urology, Queen's University, Kingston General Hospital, Kingston, Ontario K7L 2N6, Canada

*Wayne J.G. Hellstrom, M.D.*, Department of Urology, Section of Andrology and Male Infertility Tulane University School of Medicine, New Orleans, LA 70112-2699, USA

*Frank Hinman, Jr., M.D.*, Department of Urology, University of California at San Francisco San Francisco, CA 94143-0738, USA

*Max Hirshkowitz, Ph.D.*, Veterans Affairs Medical Center, Department of Research and Psychiatry, Houston, TX 77030, USA

*Gerald H. Jordan, M.D.*, Department of Urology, Eastern Virginia Medical School, Norfolk, VA 23510, USA

*Klaus Peter Juenemann, M.D.*, Department of Urology, Faculty of Clinical Medicine of the University of Heidelberg, Mannheim, D-68135, Germany

*Laurance A. Levine, M.D.*, Rush-Presbyterian-St. Luke's Medical Center, Chicago, IL 60612, USA

*Stephen B. Levine, M.D.*, Department of Psychiatry, Center for Marital and Sexual Health, School of Medicine, Case Western Reserve University, Beachwood, OH 44122, USA

*Ronald W. Lewis, M.D.*, Department of Surgery, Section of Urology, Medical College of Georgia, Augusta, GA 30912-4050, USA

*Tom F. Lue, M.D.*, Department of Urology, University of California at San Francisco, San Francisco, CA 94143-0738, USA

*Martina Manning, M.D.*, Department of Urology, Faculty of Clinical Medicine of the University of Heidelberg, Mannheim, D-68135, Germany

*Joel L. Marmar, M.D.*, Division of Urology, Robert Wood Johnson Medical School and Division of Urology, Cooper Hospital Medical Center, Camden, NJ 08103, USA

*R. Dale McClure, M.D.*, Virginia Mason Medical Center, Seattle, WA 98111, USA

*Randall B. Meacham, M.D.*, Department of Urology, University of Colorado Health Sciences Center, Denver, CO 80262, USA

*Brett C. Mellinger, M.D.*, Department of Clinical Urology, Albert Einstein College of Medicine, Yeshiva University, Mineola, NY 11501, USA

*Arnold Melman, M.D.*, Henry and Lucy Moses Hospital Division, Montefiore Medical Center, Bronx, NY 10467, USA

*David F. Mobley, M.D.*, Section of Urology, Memorial Hospital, Houston, TX 77024-2414, USA

*Manoj Monga, M.D.*, Department of Urology, Tulane University School of Medicine, New Orleans, LA 70131-2699, USA

*Alvaro Morales, M.D.*, Department of Urology, Queen's University, Kingston General Hospital, Kingston, Ontario K7L 2V7, Canada

*John J. Mulcahy, M.D., Ph.D.*, Department of Urology, Indiana University Medical Center, Indianapolis, IN 46202, USA

*John Mulhall, M.D., Ph.D.*, Department of Urology, Boston University Medical Center, Boston, MA 02118, USA

*Durwood E. Neal, Jr., M.D.*, Division of Urology, University of Texas Medical Branch, Galveston, TX 77550-0540, USA

*Robert D. Oates, M.D.*, Department of Urology, Boston University Medical Center, Boston, MA 02118, USA

*Dana A. Ohl, M.D.*, Section of Urology, University of Michigan Medical Center, Ann Arbor, MI 48109-0330, USA

*James W. Overstreet, M.D., Ph.D.*, Departments of Obstetrics and Gynecology, Division of Reproductive Biology, University of California at Davis, Davis, CA 95616, USA

*Osvaldo F. Padron, M.D.*, Department of Urology, Section of Male Infertility, The Cleveland Clinic Foundation, Cleveland, OH 44195, USA

*Farhad Parivar, M.D.*, Department of Urology, University of California at San Francisco, San Francisco, CA 94143-0738, USA

*Jon L. Pryor, M.D.*, Department of Urologic Surgery, University of Minnesota, Minneapolis, MN 55455, USA

*Jacob Rajfer, M.D.*, Division of Urology, University of California at Los Angeles, Harbor-UCLA Medical Center, Torrance, CA 90509, USA

*Gloria Richard-Davis, M.D.*, Department of Obstetrics and Gynecology, Tulane University School of Medicine, New Orleans, LA 70112-2699, USA

*Kenneth P. Roberts, Ph.D.*, Departments of Urologic Surgery, Cell Biology, and Neuroanatomy, University of Minnesota, Minneapolis, MN 55455, USA

*Peter N. Schlegel, M.D.*, Department of Urology, New York Hospital-Cornell University Medical Center, New York, NY 10021, USA

*Steven M. Schlossberg, M.D.*, Departments of Urology and Anatomy, Eastern Virginia Medical School, Norfolk, VA 23510, USA

*Allen D. Seftel, M.D.*, Department of Urology and Reproductive Biology, School of Medicine, Case Western Reserve University, Cleveland, OH 44106-5046, USA

*Ira D. Sharlip, M.D.*, 2100 Webster Street, San Francisco, CA 94115, USA

*Suresh C. Sikka, M.S., Ph.D.*, Departments of Urology and Pharmacology, Tulane University School of Medicine, New Orleans, LA 70112-2699, USA

*Rebecca Z. Sokol, M.D.*, School of Medicine and Obstetrics and Gynecology, University of Southern California, Los Angeles, CA 90033, USA

*Jens Sonksen*, Department of Surgery, Section of Urology, Visiting Research Investigator, University of Michigan Medical School, Ann Arbor, MI 48109-0330, USA

*Claudio Telöken, M.D.*, Department of Urology, Federal Cien. Medicas and ISCMPA, Porto Alegre, RS 90480-003, Brazil

*Anthony J. Thomas, Jr., M.D.*, Department of Urology, Section of Male Infertility, The Cleveland Clinic Foundation, Cleveland, OH 44195, USA

*Eric Wespes, M.D.*, Service d'Urologie, Hôpital Erasme, Brussels, 1070, Belgium

*Steven K. Wilson, M.D.*, 2010 Chestnut Street, Van Buren, AK 72956, USA

*Armand Zini, M.D.*, Department of Urology, New York Hospital-Cornell University Medical Center, New York, NY 10021, USA

# 1
# Anatomy and Physiology of the Male Reproductive System

Kenneth P. Roberts and Jon L. Pryor

From the hypothalamo-pituitary-testicular axis to the sexual accessory glands, a complex, coordinated system provides reproductive and sexual functioning for the male. Breakdown of this coordinated system is responsible for infertility in approximately 7.5% of all males as well as for 20 million men in the United States who suffer from erectile dysfunction. An understanding of the anatomy and physiology of the reproductive and sexual systems is the basis for treating these problems.

## Testicle

### Anatomy

The layers covering the testis and their derivations, beginning superficially, are as follows:

1. skin
2. dartos fascia—continuation of Scarpa's fascia over the scrotum
3. external spermatic fascia—derived from external oblique aponeurosis
4. cremasteric muscle/fascia—derived from internal oblique muscle/fascia
5. internal spermatic fascia—derived from transversalis fascia
6. tunica vaginalis—remnant of the abdominal peritoneum

The tunica vaginalis is the remnant of the processus vaginalis, a portion of the abdominal peritoneum that evaginates through the body wall via the inguinal canal during the third month of gestation. The testis projects into the abdominal peritoneum from behind as it descends into the scrotum around the time of birth. This development explains the two layers of tunica vaginalis around the testis—the outer parietal layer and an inner visceral layer closely apposed to the testis. Normally, there is a small amount of fluid between the visceral and parietal layers; a hydrocele is an excessive accumulation of fluid between these layers. In rare cases, the tunica vaginalis remains continuous with the abdominal peritoneum, a condition that can also result in a hydrocele or indirect inguinal hernia.

The testes receive their blood supply from the testicular arteries, the cremasteric arteries, and deferential arteries (Fig. 1.1). The bilateral testicular arteries are the primary blood supply of the testes. They arise from the abdominal aorta, just inferior to the origin of the renal arteries, and course in the retroperitoneum toward the pelvis. Midway between their origin and the iliac crest, the testicular arteries cross over the ureters and pass laterally into the pelvis, reaching the spermatic cord at the level of the internal inguinal ring. The arteries then pass through the inguinal canal, as a component of the spermatic cord, and into the scrotum to the testes. The cremasteric arteries, also referred to as the external spermatic arteries, are branches of the inferior epigastric artery and originate as branches of the external iliac arteries. The deferential arteries are branches of the internal iliac arteries. The deferential arteries traverse much of the length of the vas deferens

# Venous

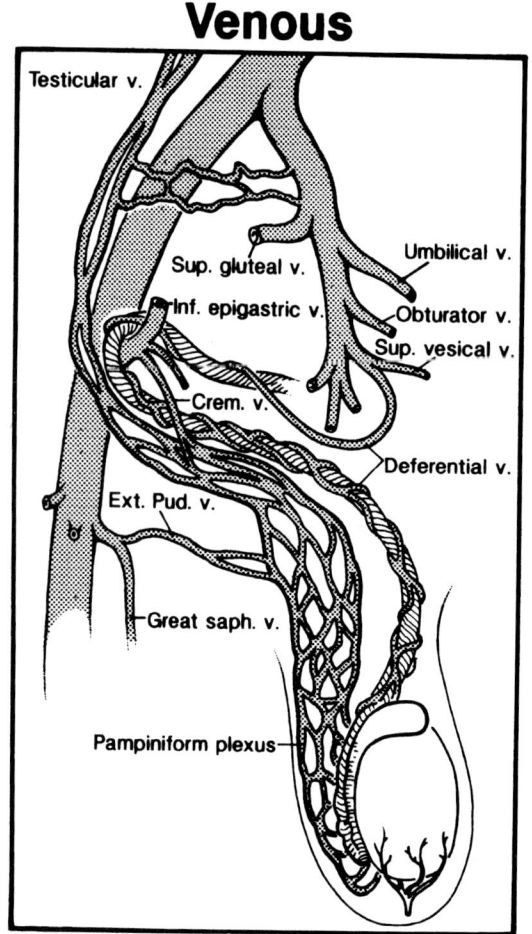

# Arterial

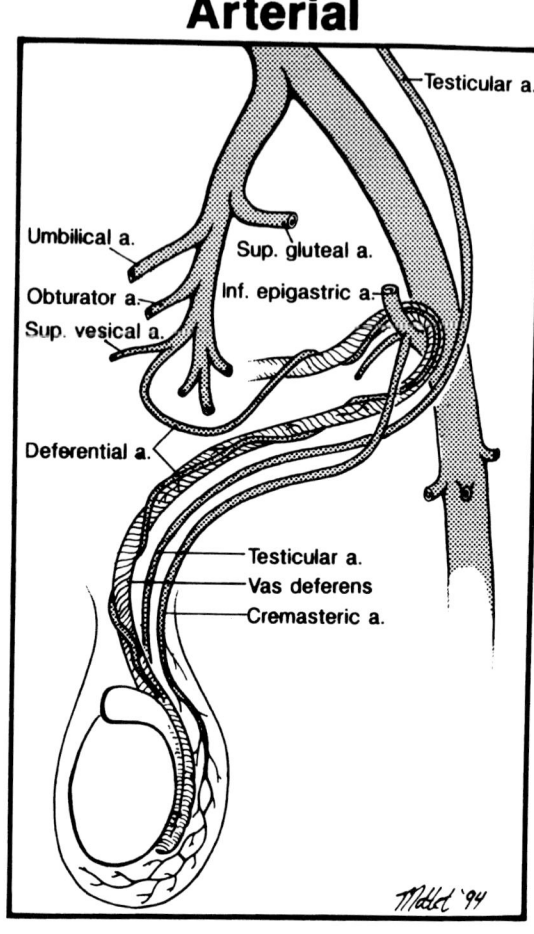

FIGURE 1.1. The venous (left) and arterial (right) anatomy of the testis.

and supply it with blood. The cremasteric and deferential arteries also access the ipsilateral testis via the spermatic cord. Although the testicular arteries are the primary blood supply to the testis, there is sufficient anastomotic communication among all three arteries so that any one artery can often be obliterated without loss of adequate blood supply to the testis.[1,2]

The intratesticular arterial anatomy is somewhat variable, but conforms to a general pattern that is clinically important (Fig. 1.1). The testicular artery pierces the tunica albuginea at the posterior aspect of the superior pole, courses down to the inferior pole, and then ascends along the anterior surface, just under the tunica albuginea, giving off several branches that course into the testicular parenchyma. The

highest density of surface arteries is contained in the anterior, medial, and lateral surfaces of the inferior pole, and the lowest density is found in the medial and lateral aspects of the superior pole.[3] To prevent iatrogenic injury to the testis, these superficial arterial branches should be considered when performing a testis biopsy or when tethering the inferior pole of the testis during orchiopexy.[4]

The venous anatomy of the testis is a particularly important feature of the male reproductive tract. The veins emerging from the testis form a dense network of intercommunicating branches known as the pampiniform plexus (Fig. 1.1), which extends through the scrotum and into the spermatic cord. The arteries supplying the testis pass through this plexus of veins en route to the testis. The venous blood (33°C) cools the arterial blood at abdominal temperature (37°C) by a countercurrent heat exchange mechanism. After traversing the inguinal canal, the venous plexus disperses into veins that follow the arterial supply of the testis. The right testicular vein empties into the inferior vena cava. In contrast, the left testicular vein normally enters the left renal vein.

There are three anatomical features of the left testicular vein that are implicated in the etiology of the predominantly left-sided varicocele. First, the left testicular vein is longer than the right testicular vein, which supposedly causes increased hydrostatic pressure in the left compared with the right testicular vein. Second, the left renal vein courses anteriorly to the abdominal aorta and posteriorly to the superior mesenteric artery, and is therefore predisposed to compression. This compression, referred to as the "nutcracker effect," will raise the pressure in the left renal vein and, as a consequence, in the left testicular vein. Third, some autopsy studies have shown valves to be absent more frequently (40%) in the left testicular vein compared with the right (3%), allowing renal vein blood to reflux more frequently into the left testicular vein.[5] Because these anatomical features are much more common than the occurrence of a varicocele, not one of them can be considered as the sole cause of a varicocele. However, these unique anatomical features of the left testicular vein may contribute to the increased frequency of a left-sided as opposed to a right-sided or bilateral varicocele.

Classic dissections in several species have shown that the autonomic nerve supply to the testis is derived from the spermatic plexus, which is composed of nerve fibers originating at vertebral levels T10-L1.[6] Later work has suggested that the superior spermatic nerve carries these nerve fibers along the course of the spermatic vessels to the testis.[7,8] This pattern of innervation accounts for the clinical observation of referred testicular pain to the lower thoracic and upper lumbar regions and vice versa. Presently, studies using retrograde axonal tracings have shown that the primary innervation of the rat testis is supplied by the major pelvic ganglia and pelvic accessory ganglia, with only a minor

component from the spermatic plexus.[9] These issues raise the question of whether a similar neuroanatomy may be present in the human.

The testis itself is composed of seminiferous tubules, the site of germ cell production (Fig. 1.2). The seminiferous tubules are contained within septa formed by projections of the tunica albuginea radiating inward from the anterior aspect of the testis. The septa converge on the mediastinum testis, a fibrous mass at the posterior aspect of the testis that supports structures (e.g., blood vessels, efferent ducts) entering and exiting the testis. The seminiferous tubules are looped tubules continuous at their ends with the rete testis, a network of collecting tubes in the mediastinum that forms a manifold for collecting the spermatozoa produced by the seminiferous tubules. The rete testis is connected to the efferent ducts that provide a connecting conduit for sperm transport to the epididymis.

## Physiology

The testis has two primary functions: (1) to produce mature spermatozoa within the seminiferous tubules, and (2) to produce testosterone from Leydig cells within the interstitium of the testis.

### The Seminiferous Tubule

The seminiferous tubule is made up primarily of Sertoli cells, germ cells, and peritubular myoid cells (Fig. 1.3). The Sertoli cell is a nondividing somatic cell of epithelial origin that forms the wall of the tubule. The Sertoli cell extends from the basement membrane at the periphery of the tubule. Tight junctional complexes between adjacent Sertoli cells form an effective barrier to the passage of macromolecules from lymph, in the interstitial space, to the lumen of the tubule. Thus, tight junctional complexes divide the seminiferous tubule into two separate compartments: (1) the adluminal compartment, consisting of that portion of the seminiferous tubule internal to the tight junctions; and (2) the basal compartment, consisting of that portion of the seminiferous tubule external to the tight junctions. The germ cells proliferate and differentiate into spermatozoa within the wall of the seminiferous tubule. Each germ cell develops in intimate association with the Sertoli cell, surrounded by the Sertoli cell plasma membrane. The seminiferous tubule is surrounded by a layer of peritubular myoid cells that are responsible for transport of mature germ cells toward the epididymis by peristalsis of the tubule. These cells have also been shown to have a regulatory effect on Sertoli cell function by producing paracrine factors that stimulate Sertoli cell–secreted protein synthesis.

## Spermatogenesis

Spermatogonia, the immature germ cells, reside along the basement membrane of the seminiferous tubule in the basal compartment. These cells undergo several mitotic divisions to generate a large population of cells that will enter the meiotic prophase as primary spermatocytes. The mitotic divisions also continually replenish the stem cell population to allow the indefinite production of spermatozoa. The first mitotic cell divisions take place in the fetal tes-

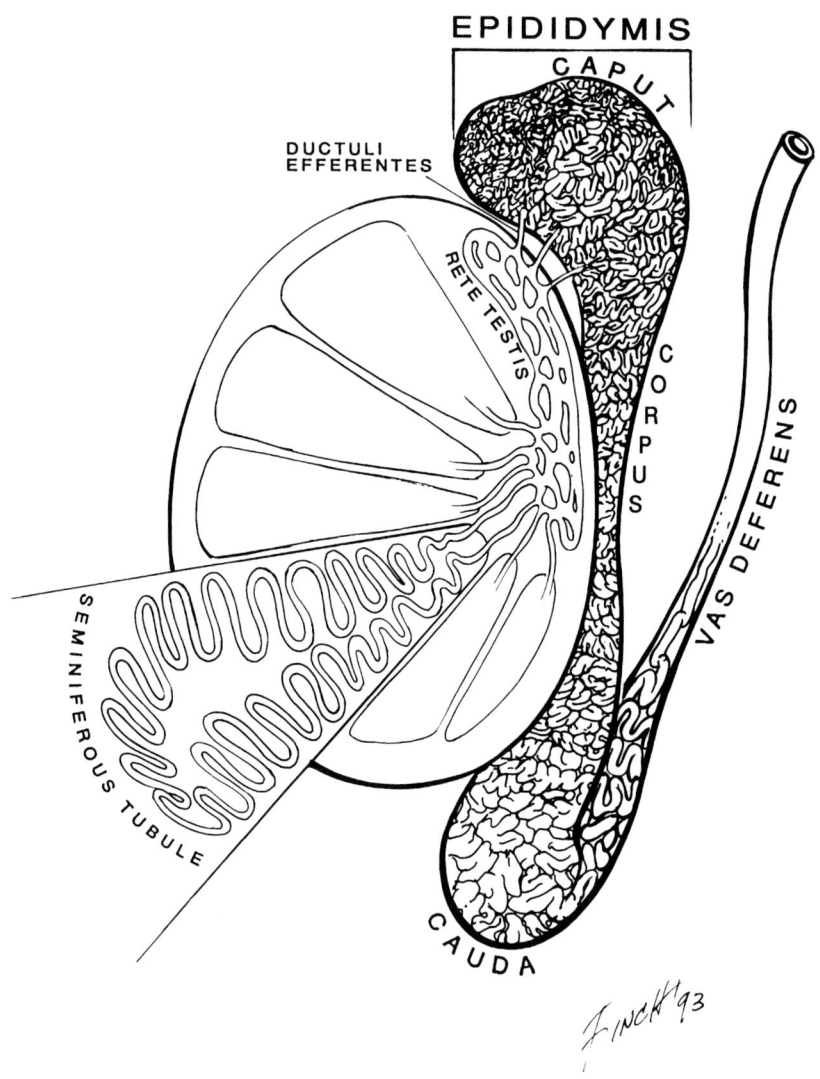

FIGURE 1.2. The testis and epididymis. The epididymis is located posterolateral to the testis. Four to 12 ductuli efferentes serve as a conduit between the rete testis and the initial portion of the caput epididymis.

tis, generating the spermatogonia and primary spermatocytes that are present in the testis at birth. There is no further development of germ cells until adolescence when, with the onset of puberty, there is a rise in serum gonadotropin and androgen levels, signaling the testis to continue with production of germ cells.

Meiosis comprises two cell divisions following replication of the chromosomes, generating haploid germ cells at the conclusion. The prophase of the first meiotic division is long and is subdivided into five stages: (1) leptotene, (2) zygotene, (3) pachytene, (4) diplotene, and (5) diakinesis (Fig. 1.4). In the leptotene stage, the chromosomes, which at this stage are each composed of two sister chromatids, are evident as thin filaments that attach themselves to the nuclear envelope. In the zygotene stage, the two sets (one paternal and one maternal) of 23 homologous chromosomes pair and form trilaminar structures known as "synaptonemal complexes." In the pachytene stage, DNA is

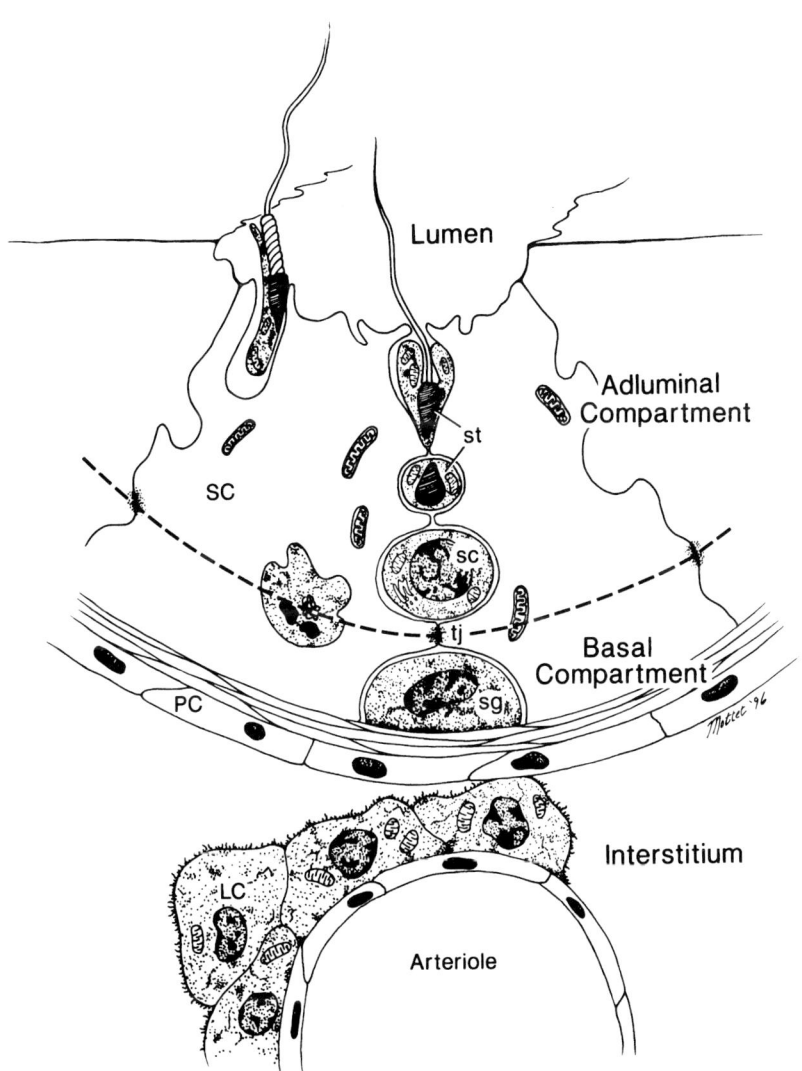

FIGURE 1.3. The seminiferous tubule and the interstitium of the testis. Tight junctional (tj) complexes between adjacent Sertoli cells form a barrier impermeable to macromolecules and functionally divide the wall of the seminiferous tubule into adluminal and basal compartments. Cell types pictured include Leydig cell (LC), Sertoli cell (SC), spermatogonia (sg), spermatocyte (sc), and spermatid (st).

# MEIOSIS I

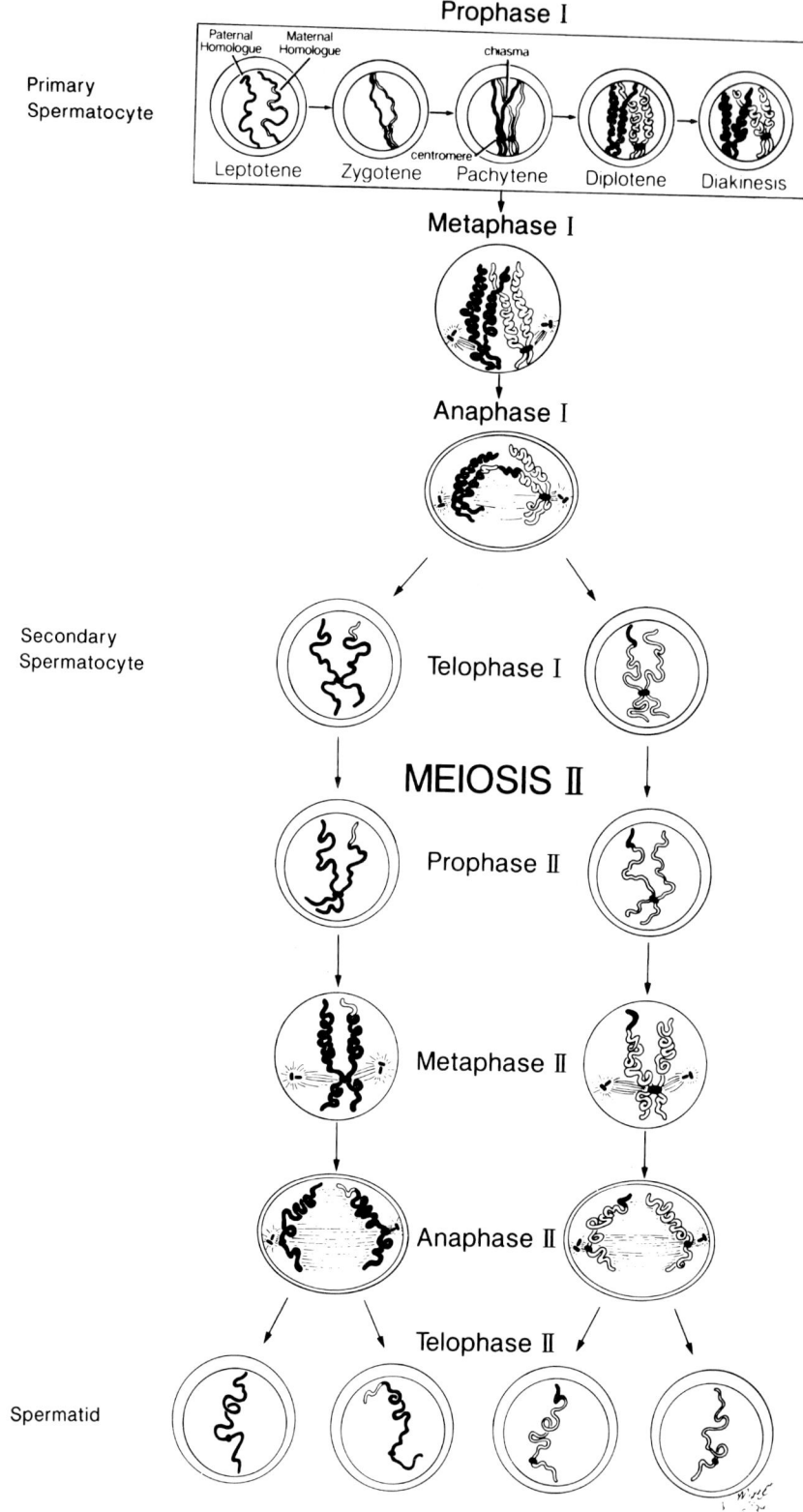

Prophase I

Primary
Spermatocyte

Paternal    Maternal
Homologue  Homologue

chasma

centromere

Leptotene    Zygotene    Pachytene    Diplotene    Diakinesis

Metaphase I

Anaphase I

Secondary
Spermatocyte

Telophase I

## MEIOSIS II

Prophase II

Metaphase II

Anaphase II

Telophase II

Spermatid

exchanged between homologous chromosomes, the transfer being mediated by the synaptonemal complex in a large recombinant nodule. The pachytene stage lasts 16 days in a human. In the diplotene stage, the chromosomes separate in a process called dysnapsis, and areas where there was exchange of genetic material are clearly seen as connecting sites called chiasmata. In the final stage of diakinesis, the chromosomes condense. The cells then proceed through metaphase, where the chromosome pairs align at the equatorial plate, and anaphase, where the paired chromosomes move to opposite poles of the cell. This separation of chromosomes is different from mitosis: in meiosis the two copies of maternal or paternal chromatids segregate to each daughter cell, whereas in mitosis each pair of sister chromatids separates and moves to opposite poles. During telophase, the final stage of the first meiotic division, cytokinesis occurs and two daughter cells result.

Interestingly, cytokinesis (the separation of cytoplasm during cell division) is incomplete in germ cell division, and all the germ cells derived from a common spermatogonium remain in a syncytium (connected by cytoplasmic bridges) until the mature germ cells are released at spermiation. This syncytial arrangement presumably allows cohorts of germ cells to communicate efficiently and to coordinate their synchronous development. The daughter cells at the completion of the first meiotic division are termed secondary spermatocytes. There is a very short interphase between the first and second meiotic division, as no DNA synthesis occurs. Almost immediately, the process of the second division begins, and the secondary spermatocytes progress from prophase through telophase. This second division closely resembles mitosis, where there is separation of the sister chromatids along the centromere. At the end of the second meiotic division, each secondary

spermatocyte has divided, and the daughter cells, now called spermatids, each contain a haploid genome. Thus, at the end of meiosis one primary spermatocyte has divided twice to give rise to four spermatids. The two primary purposes of meiosis have been accomplished: (1) the generation of the haploid cell type by the reduction division, and (2) the generation of genetic variation by exchanging segments of homologous chromosomes and the random separation of maternal/paternal chromosomes.

The early spermatids are round cells that bear no resemblance to the mature spermatozoa. Spermatids undergo the unique process of differentiation, called spermiogenesis, to transform into the elongated flagellar cells capable of motility (Fig. 1.5). This transformation includes the development of the acrosome, the condensation of the nuclear chromatin, shedding of excess cytoplasm, and the development of the tail (flagellum). The acrosome is a large vesicle formed from the Golgi apparatus that contains the hydrolytic enzymes necessary for the penetration of the zona pellucida of the egg. The nucleus of the spermatid elongates, as the nuclear DNA is tightly packaged to minimize the nuclear volume. The flagellum forms at the lower pole of the elongating spermatid, opposite the acrosome. The mitochondria coalesce at the proximal portion of the flagellum, forming the mitochondrial sheath and generating the energy required for motility. As germ cells progress through spermiogenesis, they move toward the lumen of the seminiferous tubule, and upon completion of spermiogenesis, mature spermatozoa are released into the lumen of the tubule. The release of the mature germ cell is known as spermiation. The entire process of spermatogenesis in the human, from spermatogonia through spermiation, takes approximately 72 days.

Because of the exponential proliferation of germ cells during spermatogenesis, the germ

---

FIGURE 1.4. The division of spermatocytes by meiosis, as described in the text. Each chromosome is composed of two sister chromatids in the leptotene stage, but the two sister chromatids are closely apposed at this stage and are, therefore, difficult to differentiate from each other until the pachytene stage of the first prophase. (From: Pryor, J.L. "What are the unique chromosomal events leading to the formation of a haploid male germ cell". In: Robaire, B., Pryor, J.L., and Trasler, J.M. Handbook of Andrology, Lawrence, Allen Press, 1995, with permission from the American Society of Andrology.)

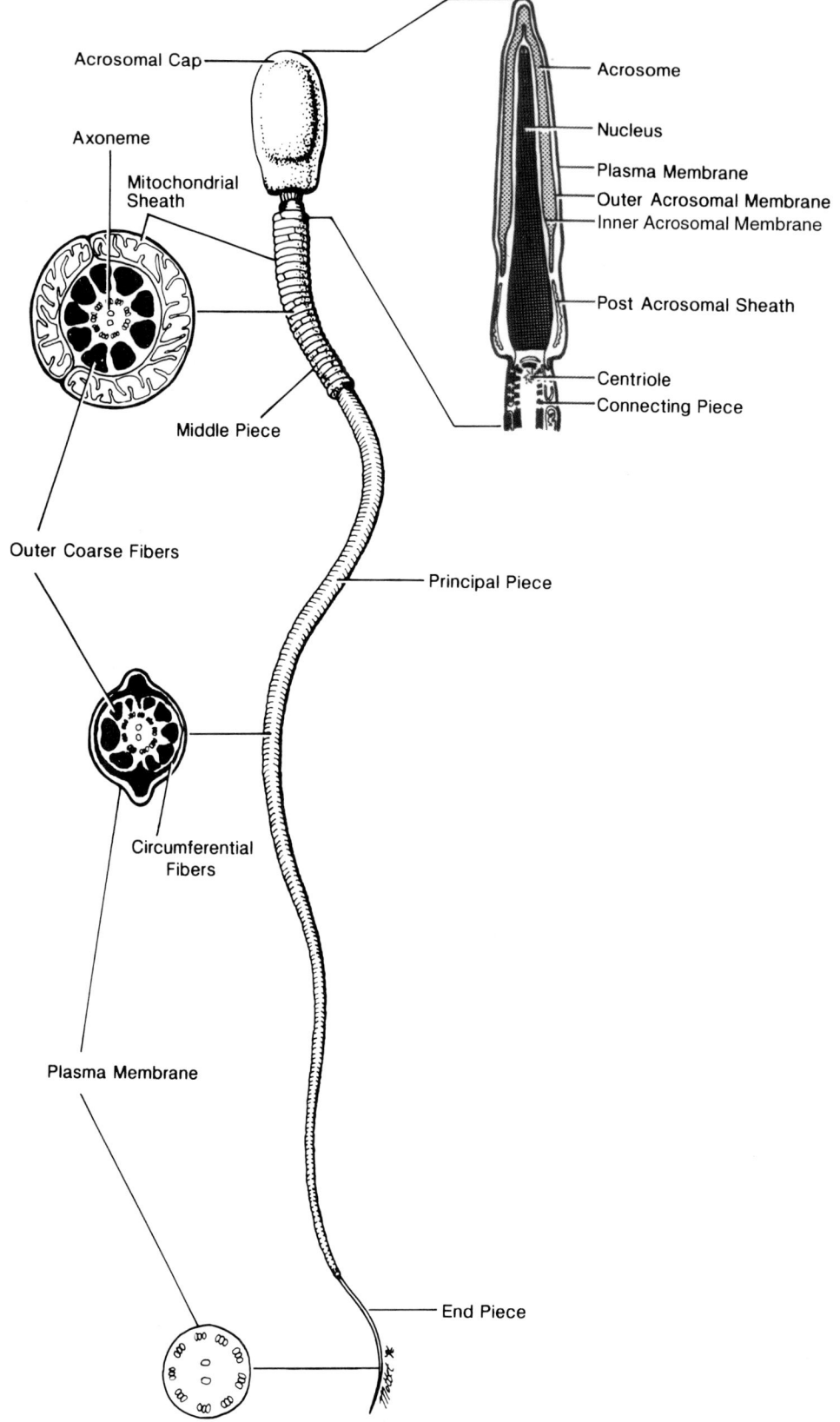

FIGURE 1.5. The structural features of the mature human sperm.

cell population accounts for the majority of the testicular volume. Thus, the loss of germ cells will, in most cases, result in a decrease in testicular volume.[10] In many cases the decrease in volume will be proportional to the extent of germ cell loss. This fact underscores the clinical importance of carefully assessing testicular volume in patients complaining of testis-related problems as a noninvasive indicator of spermatogenesis.

## The Sertoli Cell

Germ cell development from primary spermatocyte through spermatozoa takes place in the adluminal compartment of the seminiferous tubule, beyond the tight junctional complexes. The composition of the luminal fluid in this compartment is composed primarily of Sertoli cell secretions. It is this fact, combined with the close physical association of the germ cells with the Sertoli cells, that has led to the concept of the Sertoli cell as the "nurse cell" of the tubule, facilitating the maturation of the meiotic and postmeiotic germ cells. The Sertoli cell has several distinct functions in support of spermatogenesis. First, the Sertoli cell provides physical support for germ cells, providing a scaffold upon which the germ cells develop and move toward the lumen of the tubule. Second, the Sertoli cells form the blood-testis barrier by virtue of the tight junctions that exist between adjacent Sertoli cells (Fig. 1.3). This barrier is required to isolate the meiotic and postmeiotic germ cells from the interstitial lymph and to maintain the integrity of the unique environment required for germ cell development. Third, Sertoli cells define the environment in which the germ cells mature. Sertoli cells provide this environment by supplying nutritional factors for germ cell metabolism (e.g., lactate), secreting proteins, and other factors required for germ cell maturation (e.g., transferrin), and secreting paracrine factors that provide cell-to-cell signaling between germ cells and Sertoli cells (e.g., activin). Fourth, Sertoli cells phagocytose the excess germ cell cytoplasm that is sloughed in the form of a residual body prior to spermiation.

Because germ cell development is dependent on proper Sertoli cell function, some attempt has been made to measure Sertoli cell–secreted products in patients with infertility as an indirect indicator of Sertoli cell function (or dysfunction). Among the Sertoli cell markers that have proved useful for such studies are transferrin and inhibin. Inhibin is a Sertoli cell–specific product that is present at low, but measurable, levels in the serum.[11] Although serum transferrin does not reflect Sertoli cell function, transferrin can be measured in seminal plasma as a marker of Sertoli cell function.[12] The ability to monitor Sertoli cell function will improve as more Sertoli cell–specific molecules become available.

## Endocrine and Paracrine Requirements of Spermatogenesis

The initiation and maintenance of spermatogenesis in the human require the synergistic actions of follicle-stimulating hormone (FSH) (a gonadotropin secreted by the pituitary) and testosterone (the primary androgen produced by the testicular Leydig cells). Although germ cells are dependent on these hormones, the germ cells do not possess receptors for either FSH or testosterone and, consequently, cannot respond directly to these hormones.[13–15] However, Sertoli cells possess receptors for both FSH and testosterone. Thus, because Sertoli cells directly communicate with the meiotic and postmeiotic germ cells, the actions of FSH and testosterone on germ cells are thought to be mediated by the Sertoli cells. The endocrine-regulated gene products that are required for germ cell development and produced by the Sertoli cells are largely unknown. However, Sertoli cells synthesize several paracrine factors (molecules that promote cell-to-cell communication within a tissue) such as inhibin, activin, and müllerian-inhibiting hormone (also known as müllerian-inhibiting substance [MIS], or müllerian-inhibiting factor [MIF]). These and other paracrine factors may be important in mediating the endocrine signals from the Sertoli cells to the germ cells.

There are other paracrine interactions in the testis that are undoubtedly important for proper testis function and spermatogenesis. The germ cells communicate with the Sertoli cells by producing their own paracrine factors.

For instance, spermatids have been shown to secrete basic fibroblast growth factor (bFGF), which stimulates the production of secreted proteins by Sertoli cells.[16] The peritubular myoid cells produce PmodS, in response to androgen stimulation by Leydig cells, which stimulates Sertoli cell function.[17] Note that even testosterone is a "paracrine" factor when acting within the testis.

Abnormal spermatogenesis is often associated with a decline in Sertoli cell function. For instance, a dysfunctional Sertoli cell can adversely affect germ cell production as well as have decreased inhibin production, resulting in clinically elevated FSH levels. Alternatively, abnormal germ cells can adversely affect Sertoli cells, which, in turn, can lead to a decrease in inhibin levels and an elevated FSH level. Given the intimate interactions between germ cells and Sertoli cells, the primary defect in cases of abnormal spermatogenesis can be either Sertoli cell or germ cell dysfunction.

# Epididymis and Vas Deferens

## Anatomy

### Epididymis

The epididymis is the site of sperm maturation and storage. It is derived, along with the vas deferens and the seminal vesicles, from the mesonephric (wolffian) duct. The mesonephric duct makes contact with the tubules of the developing rete testis via the epigenital tubules. The epigenital tubules eventually form the 4 to 12 ductuli efferentes that connect the epididymis to the rete testis. The mesonephric duct in the region of the epigenital tubules becomes convoluted and develops to form the epididymis, a single convoluted tubule through which the testicular sperm must pass.

For descriptive purposes, the epididymis is divided into three major regions: (1) caput, (2) corpus, and (3) cauda (Fig. 1.2). The caput epididymis, also known as the head or globus major, overlies the upper pole of the testis. The first part of the caput epididymis is referred to as the proximal segment. The cauda epididymis, also known as the tail or globus minor, lies

at the inferior pole and is continuous with the vas deferens. The intervening region is referred to as the corpus or body of the epididymis and is only loosely attached to the testis. Sperm mature as they traverse the caput and corpus regions of the epididymis and are stored in the cauda epididymides.

The epididymis is surrounded by the visceral layer of the tunica vaginalis in all but its posterior aspect. Because the corpus is loosely attached to the testis, the tunica vaginalis in this region forms a sinus or cleft between the lateral surface of the testis and the epididymis. The lateral location of this epididymal-testicular cleft is useful intraoperatively to establish the normal (untwisted) position of the testis. The vascular supply of the epididymis is extensive and somewhat variable in its detail.[18] The epididymal artery, a branch of the testicular artery originating at a variable distance above the epididymis, supplies the caput epididymis and courses along the body of the epididymis to the cauda epididymis where it anastomoses with the vasal artery. The epididymal artery also forms anastomotic communications with the cremasteric artery and the subtunical portion of the testicular artery via small branches that pierce the tunica albuginea. Thus, the epididymis is supplied with blood from an extensive arterial plexus, originating from the same arteries that supply the testis.

The venous drainage of the epididymis varies in its detail but also follows a general pattern.[18] In most cases, the veins of the caput and proximal corpus communicate directly with the veins of the pampiniform plexus. The veins arising from the cauda and distal corpus regions form the marginal vein of the epididymis that normally communicates with the vasal vein. Variations of this general pattern of venous drainage are not unusual.

### Vas Deferens

The vas deferens is a thick, muscular tube that carries sperm from the cauda epididymis to the ejaculatory ducts in the prostate. The first part of the vas deferens, originating at the cauda epididymis, is tortuous and is referred to as the *convoluted portion*. The vas deferens courses superiorly, along the back of the epididymis, passes through the inguinal canal with the testicular artery and veins, and enters the pelvis at the level of the internal inguinal ring. From this point, the vas deferens courses posteriomedially, over the junction of the ureters with the bladder, passing behind the bladder from above and entering the prostate in an inferiomedial direction. As the vas deferens approaches the prostate, adjacent to the seminal vesicle, it becomes dilated. This portion of the vas deferens is called the ampulla. Thus, the vas deferens provides continuity of the testis with the secondary reproductive structures (i.e., prostate and seminal vesicles) within the pelvis.

The vas deferens, like the epididymis and seminal vesicle, is derived from the mesonephric ducts. The common embryological origin is of clinical importance in that absence of the vas deferens may also indicate absence of the epididymis and seminal vesicle.

The vas deferens receives its blood supply from the deferential artery. This artery arises as a branch from the umbilical artery, itself a branch of the internal iliac artery, and is accompanied by the deferential vein. Although the deferential vein passes through the spermatic cord along with the testicular veins, it does not contribute significantly to the pampiniform plexus.[19]

## Physiology

There are three primary functions of the epididymis: (1) it is responsible for the maturation of infertile testicular sperm to fertile mature sperm, (2) it acts as a peristaltic conduit for the active transport of sperm from the testis to the vas deferens, and (3) it serves as a storage site for mature sperm.

Upon leaving the testis, sperm are nonmotile and, in general, are unable to fertilize the egg through natural means. Maturational changes that endow sperm with the capability to become motile and fertilize take place as sperm transit the epididymis en route to the vas deferens.[20,21] However, the condensed nucleus of sperm is transcriptionally inactive (i.e., no genes are being expressed), and there is very little, if any, translation (i.e., protein synthesis)

in the epididymal spermatozoon. Thus, the maturation of sperm does not occur by transcription and translation within the germ cell but is carried out by default in the microenvironment of sperm as they transit the epididymis. Experimental data from animal and human studies show that sperm undergo maturational changes that can be documented in many cases as changes that occur to the protein composition on the sperm surface. The regional expression of many different genes and secretion of region-specific proteins and other compounds in the epididymis suggest a linear maturational mechanism for sperm as they transit this organ.[22] In addition, many region-specific epididymal products are regulated by androgens and other testicular factors.[23] In this respect, the maturation of sperm in the epididymis, as well as production of sperm in the testis, is dependent on androgen stimulation.

The function of the epididymis as an organ for sperm maturation has been questioned in recent years. Pregnancy can result from bypassing most of the epididymis by anastomosing the vas deferens to the caput epididymis during a vasoepididymostomy or bypassing the epididymis entirely by anastomosing the vas deferens to the ductuli efferentes, but this does not mitigate the role of the epididymis in sperm maturation. Overall, there is less of a chance for pregnancy when the vas is attached to the caput as opposed to when it is attached to the cauda epididymis, and it is possible that the vas deferens itself may contribute to the maturation of the spermatozoa in such surgically altered patients.[20]

The transit time of the sperm in the human epididymis averages 12 days but is highly variable, with some sperm progressing through the epididymis in as few as 2 days.[24,25]

The cauda epididymis stores approximately 52% of the epididymal reserves.[25] However, both the storage capacity and the ability to maintain viability in the cauda epididymis appear to be less in the human than in other mammals. The sperm storage capacity of the human cauda epididymis has been questioned by data showing that the sperm number in the ejaculate after vasoepididyostomy, which effectively removes the cauda epididymis, is sometimes within the normal range.[26] In regard to viability, the motility of sperm in the human decreases faster as the time between ejaculations (i.e., abstinence) increases than it does in other mammalian species, suggesting the human cauda is not as effective in preserving motility as it is in other species.[20] The high number of sperm in the first ejaculate after vasectomy suggests that the vas deferens may significantly contribute to sperm storage in the human.[20] Because the vas deferens is probably not as capable of preserving sperm viability as the cauda epididymis, the significant storage capacity of the vas deferens may explain the suboptimal retention of sperm viability in the human.[27] Understanding the limits of sperm storage by the human epididymis and vas deferens has significant clinical implications when researchers determine the optimal abstinence period for semen collection or timed intercourse; an abstinence period too short may deplete the limited storage capacity in the human and result in low sperm count, whereas an abstinence period too long may decrease sperm viability.

# Seminal Vesicles and Prostate

## Anatomy

### Seminal Vesicles

The seminal vesicles are glands, approximately 5 cm in length, that arise as extensive outpocketings of the mesonephric ducts at the level of the prostate. Thus, these glands also share common embryological origins with the vas deferens and the epididymis. They occupy a location lateral to the vas deferens, at the posterior and inferior aspect of the bladder. The seminal vesicles are secretory glands and contribute the majority of the volume of the ejaculate. The secretions of the seminal vesicles combine with the contents of the vas deferens as both come together at the prostate.

The seminal vesicles receive blood from branches of the bilateral prostatic arteries, before these arteries divide into the urethral and capsular branches. The venous return of the seminal vesicles is via the prostatic plexus to the internal iliac veins.

### Prostate

Like the seminal vesicles, the prostate is an organ unique to the male reproductive tract, and it contributes secretions to the ejaculate. The prostate arises as buds from the primitive posterior urethra and penetrates the surrounding mesenchyme. The primitive buds give rise to tubules that develop into separate lobes: (1) the large right and left lateral lobes, (2) the middle lobe, and (3) the very small anterior and posterior lobes. The lobes are composed of ductules lined with secretory epithelium that drain through the converging tubules into the prostatic urethra. Although the lobes develop independently, there is no apparent gross or morphologic distinction between the lobes in the mature prostate gland.

A recent anatomical description of the prostate has been developed by McNeal,[28] which distinguishes prostatic zones based on morphologic features derived from systematic sectioning of the adult prostate (Fig. 1.6). The prostatic urethra is the reference structure for this anatomical system, with regions of the prostate named in relation to it. The anterior zone of the prostate is fibromuscular and contributes a sphincteric action on the urethra. The posterior part of the prostate is divided into a peripheral zone and a central zone. These two regions, which essentially lie in the coronal plane defined by the distal prostatic urethra, compose the bulk of the glandular prostate, with the peripheral zone being about three times larger than the central zone. The central zone surrounds the ejaculatory ducts as they traverse the prostate from the level of the entry of the vas deferens to the verumontanum. The peripheral zone lies primarily inferior to the central zone, and its ducts enter the urethra distal to those of the central zone. The peripheral zone is of particular clinical significance, because this is the primary site of prostatic neoplasms. The area anterior to the central zone and lateral to the proximal prostatic urethra is the transition zone, which makes up only about 5% of the normal prostate gland. Although histologically identical to the peripheral zone, the transition zone is not disposed to the formation of neoplasms. However, it is the primary site

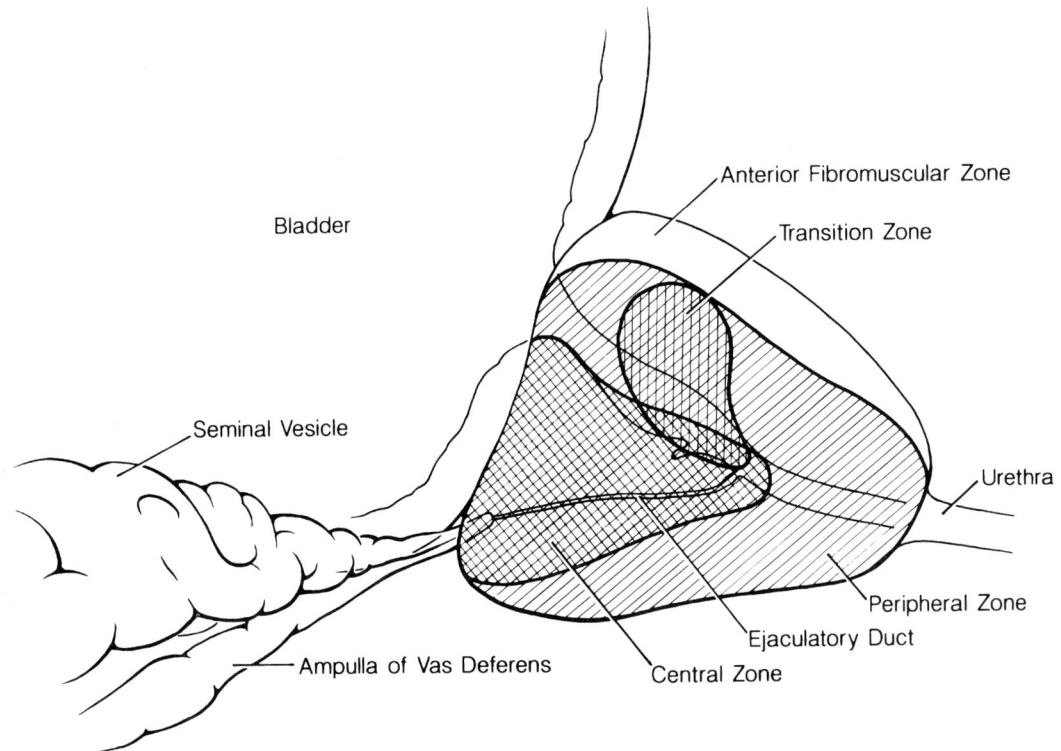

FIGURE 1.6. Sagittal view of McNeal's zonal anatomy of the prostate. Notice that the urethra forms a 35° anterior angulation at the level of the mid-prostate that divides the urethra into a proximal and distal segment of approximate equal length. The verumontanum is entirely within the distal segment. The glandular tissue makes up two thirds of the pros- tate, whereas the fibromuscular structures make up one third. The two primary regions of the glandular prostate are the peripheral zone, which makes up 75% of the glandular tissue, and the central zone, which makes up 25% of the glandular prostate. The central zone surrounds the ejaculatory ducts as they course through the prostate.

for the formation of benign prostatic hyperplasia (BPH).

The prostate derives its arterial supply from bilateral prostatic arteries, which are themselves derived from the union of the inferior vesicle artery and the middle rectal artery on each side of the pelvis. The middle rectal and inferior vesicle arteries are branches of the anterior division of the internal iliac arteries. The prostatic artery divides into a capsular branch and urethral branch. The urethral branches penetrate the prostate superiorly, close to the bladder neck, and traverse the prostate on either side of the urethra, giving blood to the periurethral portion of the prostate. The capsular branches course along the exterior aspect of the prostatic capsule and supply the outer por-

tion of the prostate. Venous return from the prostate is via the prostatic venous plexus, located just under the fibrous capsule of the prostate gland. This plexus also receives blood from the base of the bladder and the deep dorsal vein of the penis. The prostatic venous plexus drains into the internal iliac veins.

The autonomic innervation to the prostate, as well as to the other pelvic organs and the penis, is derived from the pelvic plexus. Sympathetic nerve fibers to the pelvic plexus originate from the thoracolumbar segments T10-L2 and parasympathetic fibers from the sacral segments, S2-S3.[29] Prominent nerve ganglia are situated at the junction of the prostate and seminal vesicles. From these ganglia, nerve fibers course along the lateral aspect of the seminal vesicles, extend inward toward the bladder neck, and descend along the postero-lateral aspect of the prostate toward the apex.[30] These latter nerve fibers contain the autonomic supply to the penis and can be spared during radical prostatectomy to avoid subsequent impotence.[31] Autonomic nerve fibers penetrate the prostate, primarily into the glandular tissue of the peripheral and central zones, with some of the nerves penetrating the substance of the prostate along the ejaculatory ducts. The sympathetic innervation is thought to be responsible for emission of secretory products from both the prostate and seminal vesicles.

## Physiology

The primary purpose of the seminal vesicles and prostate, often referred to as the sexual accessory glands, is to provide a fluid environment for sperm. Approximately 95% of an ejaculate is made up of a fluid from the sexual accessory glands, and less than 5% is made up of sperm cells. The seminal vesicles contribute the greatest proportion of the fluid to an ejaculate. Some of the primary factors secreted by the seminal vesicle include phosphorylcholine, ascorbic acid, flavin, prostaglandins, fructose, and clotting factors. The exact role of these substances in fertilization is not well understood. The prostaglandins, known to relax the myometrium of the uterus and cervical muscle in the female, may participate in sperm transport. Fructose is thought to be an energy source for sperm, and the lack of fructose in an ejaculate indicates blocked ejaculatory ducts or absent or atrophic seminal vesicles. Clotting factors from the seminal vesicle are responsible for the clotting of the ejaculate. If an ejaculate is very fluid and does not form a coagulum, then this is another physical finding of blocked, absent, or atrophic seminal vesicles.

The prostate is a 20-g musculoglandular organ that secretes the second highest proportion of fluid (approximately 0.5 ml) to the ejaculate. Factors secreted by the prostate gland include citric acid, acid and alkaline phosphatases, plasminogen activator, lactate dehydrogenase (LDH), amylase, albumin, β-glucuronidase, polyamines (e.g., spermine, spermidine, and putrescine), and various proteases, as well as calcium, magnesium, and zinc. Approximately 10 minutes after an ejaculate coagulates, it begins to liquefy. There are several proteolytic enzymes—including plasminogen activator, seminin, and prostatic-specific antigen (PSA)—that may be responsible for lysis of the coagulum and thus liquefaction of the ejaculate.

The growth of the prostate is under the control of androgens. The free portion of testosterone diffuses across the cell membrane of prostatic cells where it is reduced by the enzyme 5α-reductase to the more potent androgen, dihydrotestosterone (DHT). DHT binds to an androgen receptor where it is translocated into the nucleus and binds to DNA at androgen-responsive elements (AREs). The AREs regulate the expression of androgen-responsive genes. By blocking the reduction of testosterone to DHT with a 5α-reductase inhibitor, such as finasteride, many of the secretions and functions of the prostate will quiesce. The components of the stromal compartment, including the extracellular matrix, are also involved in prostate growth.

The paired bulbourethral glands situated in the urogenital diaphragm secrete approximately 0.2 ml of fluid in an ejaculate. Although the first part of an ejaculate is primarily sperm and fluid from the prostate, and the second part of an ejaculate comes primarily from the seminal vesicles, there is significant intermixing of fluids in the ejaculate so that motile sperm are also present in the later part of an ejaculate. Therefore, a split ejaculate is rarely diagnostic in the evaluation or treatment of the infertile male.

# Penis

## Anatomy

The penis is typically divided into three anatomic parts: (1) the body, (2) the glans, and (3) the root. The body is the cylindrical external portion that is itself composed of three parts: the corpus spongiosum through which the urethra passes and the bilateral corpora cavernosa, the erectile bodies of the penis. Within the corpora cavernosa is spongy tissue that consists of endothelial-lined smooth muscle spaces called sinusoids. The glans penis is the distal expansion of the corpus spongiosum. The root of the penis is in the superficial perineal space and thus is not visible externally. The root is made up of the proximal corpora, which diverge as they approach the perineum, forming the crura of the penis. The crura adhere to the ramus of the ischium, ending at the ischial tuberosity. Proximally the corpus spongiosum dilates, forming the bulbous penis. The corpus spongiosum and the two corpora cavernosa are each surrounded by a fibroelastic covering, the tunica albuginea. The tunica albuginea forms a septum with small perforations between the two closely apposed corpora cavernosa that allows blood from one corpus to permeate the contralateral corpus, which explains why medication injected into one corpus affects the contralateral corpus. The crura are surrounded by the ischiocavernosus muscle, and the bulbus penis is surrounded by the bulbospongiosus muscle, which contributes to the clonic contractions of these structures during ejaculation. A thick layer of connective tissue, referred to as Buck's fascia, surrounds the corpus spongiosum and corpora cavernosa in a figure-eight fashion. Superficial to Buck's fascia is the dartos, followed by skin. The body of the penis is supported by two suspensory ligaments: (1) the fundiform ligament (a continuation of the linea alba), and (2) the more proximal (deeper) suspensory ligament that attaches to the pubic ramus and merges with the tunica albuginea of the penis. The normal anatomic position of the penis is in the erect state; thus, the ventral penis is the surface with the corpus spongiosum and the urethra, and the corpora cavernosa and dorsal neurovascular bundle are dorsal (posterior).

The blood supply to the penis is derived primarily from the internal pudendal artery, a branch of the anterior division of the internal iliac artery (Fig. 1.7). However, there is tremendous variation in the arterial supply to the penis, with a high incidence of an accessory pudendal artery that commonly arises from vesical and obturator arteries.[32] The internal pudendal artery becomes the common penile artery that branches to give rise to the bulbourethral, cavernous, and dorsal arteries (Fig. 1.7). The bulbourethral arteries give blood supply to the bulb of the penis with branches to the corpus spongiosum. The cavernous arteries course centrally through each corpora, giving off numerous helicine arteries that supply blood to the sinusoids of the corpora cavernosa, and are the primary arteries responsible for erections. The dorsal arteries course along the dorsal surface to the glans penis.

There are three main routes of venous drainage of the penis: (1) the superficial dorsal vein, (2) the deep dorsal vein, and (3) the cavernous vein. The superficial dorsal vein is visible external to Buck's fascia and drains most of the penile skin into the great saphenous vein. Venous blood from the sinus spaces of the corpora cavernosa drain into venules on the undersurface of the tunica albuginea. Blood from these subtunical venules exits the tunica albuginea via the emissary veins which, in turn, drain into the circumflex veins. Emissary veins from the dorsal surface of the penis and the circumflex veins primarily drain into the deep dorsal vein, which empties into the periprostatic (retropubic) venous plexus. Thus, the deep dorsal vein drains the glans penis as well as the distal corpora cavernosa and corpus spongiosum. Finally, the emissary veins from the proximal corpora cavernosa and crura empty medially into the cavernous and crural veins, respectively. These veins join with urethral (bulbar) veins from the proximal corpus spongiosum to form the internal pudendal vein. There is also an anastomosis between the cavernous veins and the periprostatic plexus.[33] Both the periprostatic and internal pudendal veins ultimately drain into the internal iliac veins.

Most of the sensation of the penis is via the dorsal penile nerve, a branch of the internal pudendal nerve. The somatic portion of the pudendal nerve also innervates the bulbospongiosus and ischiocavernosus muscles, which contract during ejaculation. Nerve supply responsible for erections is the parasympathetic autonomic system via the pelvic plexus (S2-S4), also referred to as the nervi erigentes. The nervi erigentes course along the posterolateral

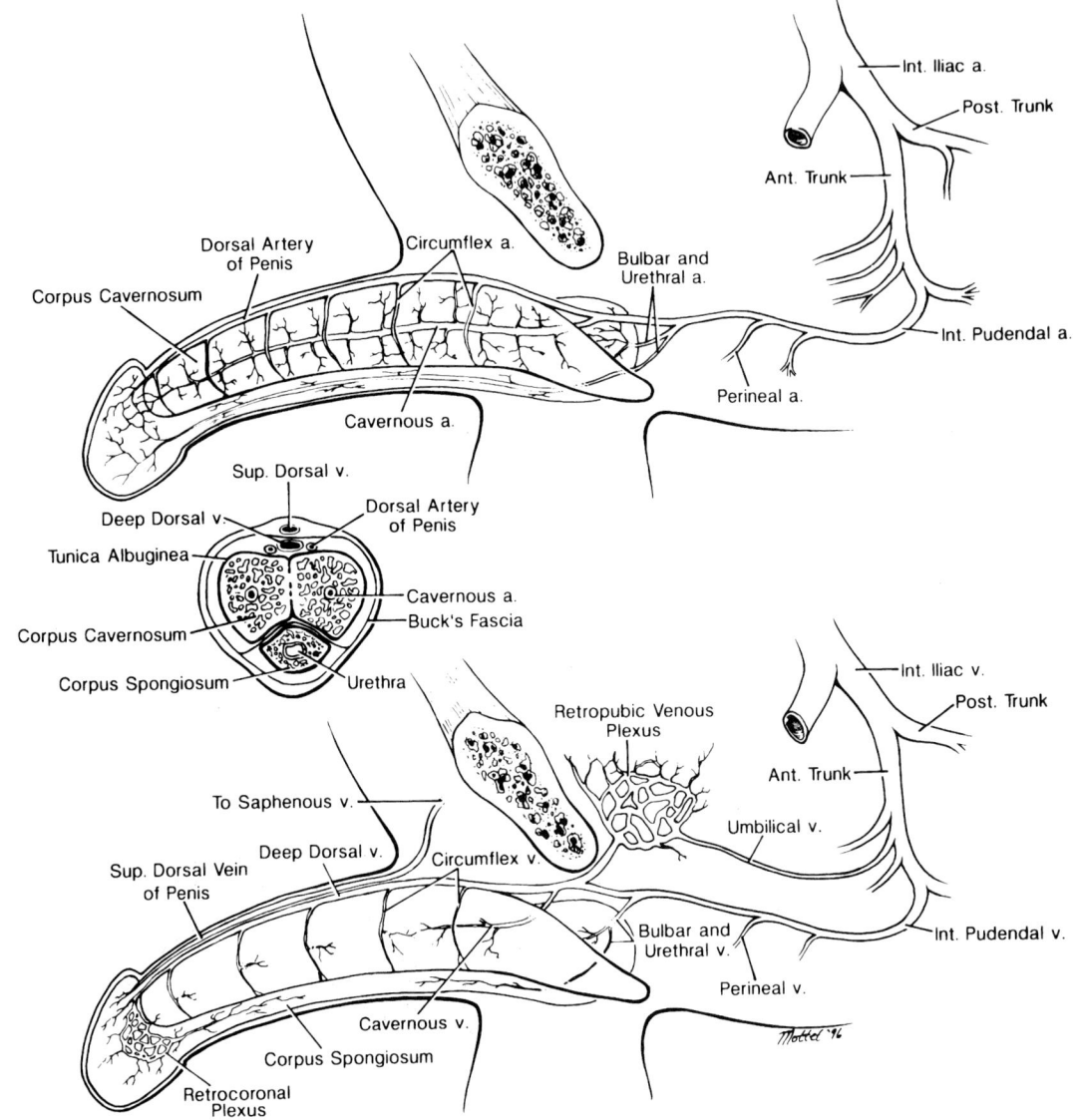

FIGURE 1.7. The arterial (top), cross-sectional (middle), and venous (bottom) anatomy of the penis.

prostate adjacent to the rectum and run toward the apex of the prostate and lateral to the membranous urethra where they penetrate the corpus cavernosum.

## Physiology

Understanding of the physiology of erections has been greatly advanced by Virag's[34] observation that the smooth-muscle relaxant papaverine causes erections when injected directly into the corpora cavernosa. Similar results were demonstrated by Brindley[35] with the injection of the α-adrenergic blocking agent phenoxybenzamine into the corpora cavernosa. These findings clearly demonstrate the importance of dilatation of the trabeculae and penile arteries in producing an erection.

When the penis is flaccid, the sinusoids of the corpora cavernosa are under chronic sympathetic stimulation and are constricted. However, with neurostimulation these sinusoidal spaces relax, causing increased arterial blood flow to the penis and filling the trabecular spaces with blood.[36] The expanded sinusoidal spaces compress the subtunical venules and pinch off the emissary veins, thus significantly impeding the outflow of blood.

As previously stated, the primary neural innervation to produce an erection is parasympathetic via the nervi erigentes. Recently, however, nitric oxide (NO) has been shown to be the noncholinergic, nonadrenergic neurotransmitter responsible for erections. Nitric oxide synthase, which produces NO from L-arginine, has been localized to the autonomic nerves of the penis.[37] NO causes relaxation of vascular and trabecular smooth muscle in the corpora by increasing the synthesis of the second messenger cyclic guanosine monophosphate (cGMP) in the smooth muscle cells.[38,39] The recent elucidation of this neural stimulatory pathway controlling erectile function may lead to new pharmacologic interventions for the treatment of erectile dysfunction.

# Hypothalamo-Pituitary-Testicular Axis

## Anatomy

The three endocrine organs required for spermatogenesis are the hypothalamus, the pituitary body, and the testis (Fig. 1.8). The hypothalamus is located in the lower aspect of the third ventricle of the brain. The pituitary body is located in the hypophysial fossa, inferior to the hypothalamus, is connected to the hypothalamus by the pituitary stock, and is divided into anterior and posterior lobes. The posterior lobe is known as the neurohypophysis and is stimulated by neurons from the hypothalamus. The anterior lobe, also known as the adenohypophysis, communicates with the hypothalamus via the portal blood system and is stimulated by neuropeptides released by the hypothalamus into the portal bloodstream.

## Physiology

The hypothalamus synthesizes and releases, in a pulsatile fashion, the decapeptide gonadotropin-releasing hormone (GnRH) into the portal system. GnRH stimulates cells in the anterior pituitary to synthesize and release the glycoprotein hormones' follicle-stimulating hormone (FSH) and luteinizing hormone (LH). FSH acts on the Sertoli cells, the only cells known to express the FSH receptor in the male, and LH is responsible for stimulating production of testosterone from the Leydig cells in the interstitium of the testis (Fig. 1.8). Measurement of LH, FSH, and testosterone in the blood of normal men shows episodic peaks of approximately 90-minute intervals, reflecting the pulsatile release of GnRH from the hypothalamus.[40] Testosterone produced by the Leydig cells feeds back to the pituitary and hypothalamus to downregulate LH secretion. Testosterone is also readily converted to estrogen by aromatase in the testis and peripheral tissues and has an inhibitory effect on LH secretion by the pituitary.[41,42] Stimulation of the Sertoli cell by FSH results in production of inhibin, which feeds back to the pituitary in a negative fashion, thus decreasing FSH production. Inhibin and testosterone feedback at the pituitary and hypothalamus complete this endocrine loop (Fig. 1.8).

The pulsatile release of GnRH is required for the release of FSH and LH. A GnRH agonist given in a constant, nonpulsatile fashion will downregulate the GnRH receptor, and LH, FSH, and subsequent testosterone secretion will be suppressed.[43] This mechanism of testosterone suppression is exploited clinically as a strategy for ablating testosterone in men with androgen-responsive prostate cancer.[44] Under normal circumstances, serum testosterone levels fluctuate, with peaks in the morning and nadirs in the evening. Therefore, levels should be reassayed at different times during the day if an inappropriately abnormal level is obtained.

### Mechanism of Hormone Action

FSH and LH are glycoprotein hormones composed of two disulfide-linked polypeptides, alpha ($\alpha$) and beta ($\beta$). The $\alpha$ subunit is identical in both hormones, whereas FSH and LH have unique $\beta$ subunits. It is the $\beta$ subunit that endows the hormone with its receptor specificity and, as a result, cell specificity. The $\alpha$ subunit is

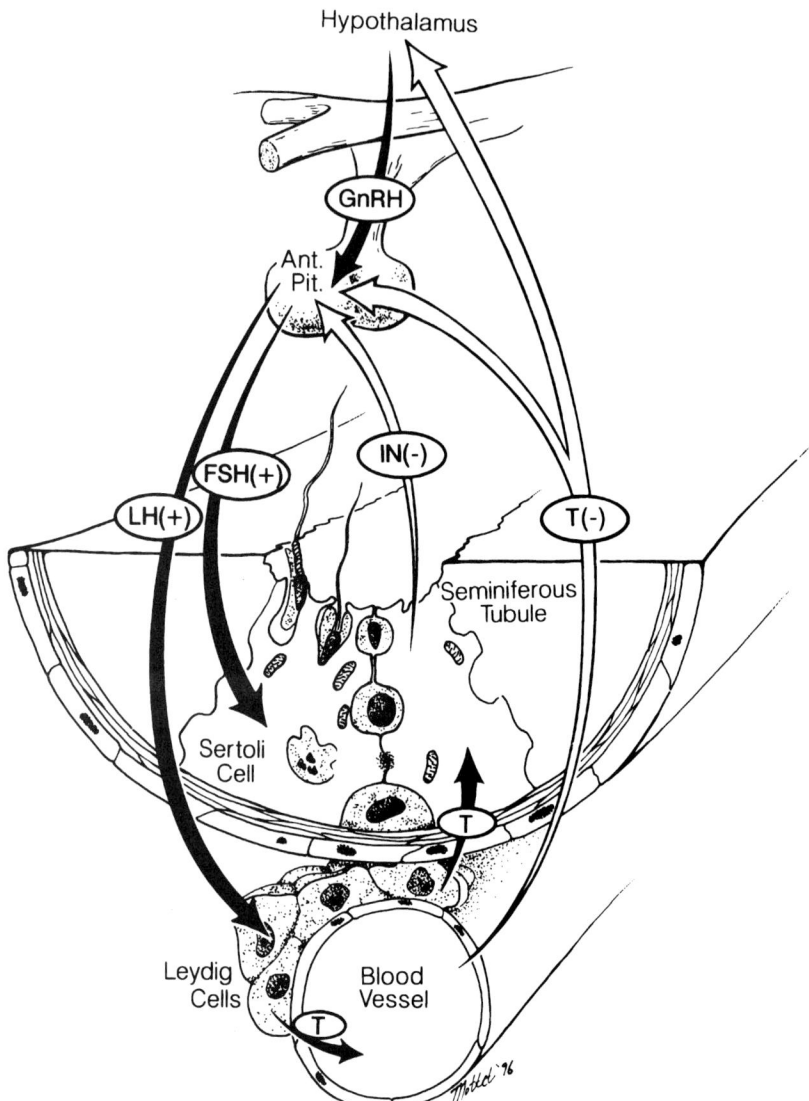

FIGURE 1.8. The hypothalamo-pituitary-testicular axis. The anterior pituitary (Ant. Pit.) releases luteinizing hormone (LH) and follicle-stimulating hormone (FSH) in response to gonadotropin-releasing hormone (GnRH) stimulation from the hypo-thalamus. FSH has a stimulatory effect on Sertoli cells and LH stimulates testosterone production by Leydig cells. LH, and to a lesser extent FSH, is downregulated by testosterone. FSH is downregulated by inhibin (IN) produced by Sertoli cells.

responsible for eliciting the cellular response. The receptors for FSH and LH are transmembrane proteins that have an extracellular hormone binding domain coupled to guanine nucleotide binding proteins (G-proteins) intracellularly (Fig. 1.9). When the hormone ligand (i.e., FSH or LH) binds to the receptor, a complex is formed with adenylate cyclase to stimulate cyclic adenosine monophosphate (cAMP) production from adenosine triphosphate (ATP). Cyclic AMP stimulates protein phosphorylation, resulting in a cascade of intracellular events that leads to the physiologic action of these hormones (Fig. 1.9). Although cAMP/protein kinase A pathway is the most well understood mechanism by which gonadotropins act, there is evidence that these hormones stimulate target cells via other signaling pathways as well.[45]

Androgens act via the nuclear androgen receptor. The androgen receptor is a ligand activated transcription factor that actively regulates gene transcription after binding to testosterone or dihydrotestosterone (DHT). Androgen binding results in a conformational change in the receptor that endows it with the ability to bind to specific DNA sequences, called androgen response elements (AREs), in the regulatory region of androgen regulated genes. The binding of the activated androgen receptor then influences, either positively or negatively, the expression of the target gene (Fig. 1.9). In the prostate and seminal vesicles,

androgen action results in growth of the glands and in increased secretory activity. In the testis, testosterone acts to drive spermatogenesis. The pubertal maturation of male sexual organs and the development of secondary sexual characteristics are also androgen dependent.

It is important to remember that testosterone can be enzymatically converted to DHT or 17β-estradiol ($E_2$) in one enzymatic step. DHT is a more potent androgen with a higher affinity for the AR than testosterone (T), whereas $E_2$ acts via the estrogen receptor (ER) and typically has antagonistic effects to androgen. Thus, T is a prohormone for both DHT and $E_2$, and the biologic effect of T will often depend on the conversion of T to $E_2$ or DHT.

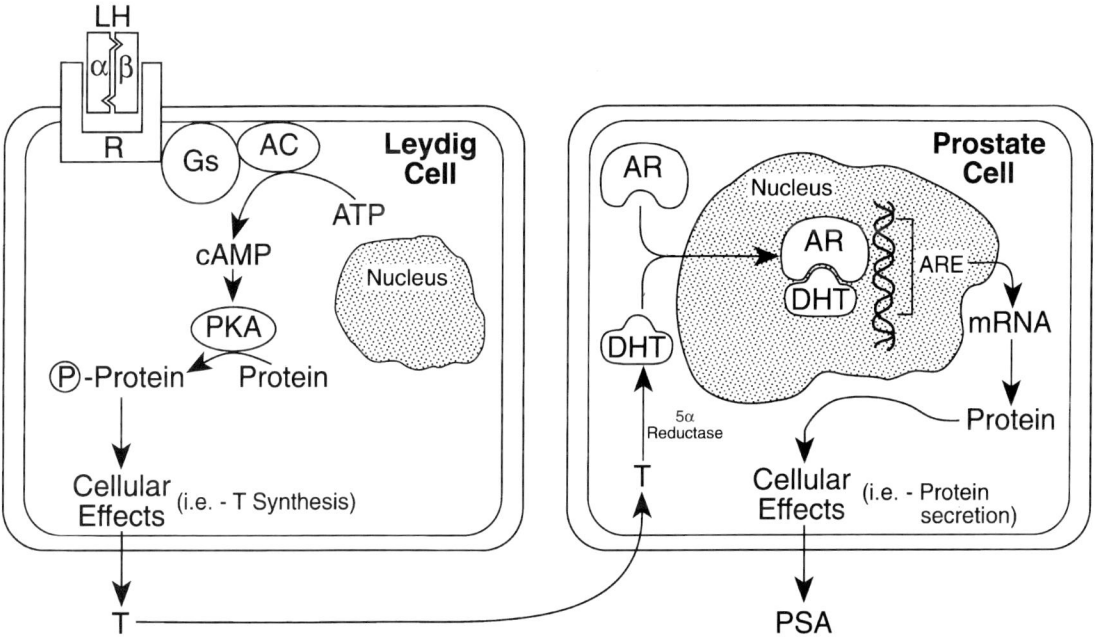

FIGURE 1.9. Mechanism of action of gonadotropins and androgen is illustrated by the interaction of Leydig cells and prostatic epithelial cells, respectively. LH, a glycoprotein hormone comprised of α and β subunits, binds to its receptor (R) on the surface of the Leydig cell causing activation of adenylate cyclase (AC) via a stimulatory G protein (Gs). Adenylate cyclase converts ATP to cyclic AMP (cAMP), which activates protein kinase A (PKA) causing the phosphorylation of key regulatory proteins and resulting in a functional response, tes-

tosterone biosynthesis. Testosterone enters the prostatic cell by passive diffusion where it is converted to 5α-dihydrotestosterone (DHT), a more potent androgen, by the converting enzyme 5α-reductase. DHT binds to the androgen receptor (AR). This complex binds to the androgen response element (ARE) found in androgen-responsive genes, and facilitates the transcription of these genes. The new gene products reflect androgen-regulated functions of the cell such as the production of prostate-specific antigen (PSA).

# Conclusion

The high incidence of health problems that involve the reproductive and sexual systems largely accounts for the significant amount of basic research in these areas. This has led to specific clinical advances, most notably in the treatment of benign prostatic hypertrophy with alpha blockers, nerve-sparing radical prostatectomies, and intracavernous pharmacotherapy for the treatment of erectile dysfunction. In other areas, like reproduction, technological advances like micromanipulation of sperm seem to be far ahead of our understanding the pathophysiology of infertility. Micromanipulation can often result in a pregnancy for a couple with infertility, but not until we advance our understanding of the basic science of reproduction will we be able to specifically identify those who will need and benefit the most from this new therapy. Therefore, to successfully treat patients, and do so in a cost-effective and efficient manner, requires not only further research in the reproductive system, but also that clinicians stay abreast of the advances that should follow.

# References

1. Kormano M, Nordmark L. Angiography of the testicular artery: III. Testis and epididymis analyzed with a magnification technique. *Acta Radiol Diagn.* 1977; 18:625–633.
2. Lee LM, Johnson HW, McLoughlin MG. Microdissection and radiographic studies of the arterial vasculature of the human testes. *J Pediatr Surg* 1984; 19:297–301.
3. Jarow JP. Intratesticular arterial anatomy. *J Androl* 1990; 11:255–259.
4. Jarow JP. Clinical significance of intratesticular arterial anatomy. *J Urol* 1991; 145:777–779.
5. Ahlberg NE, Bartley O, Chidekel N. Right and left gonadal veins: anatomical and statistical study. *Acta Radiol* 1966; 4:593–601.
6. Langley JN, Anderson HK. The innervation of the pelvic and adjoining viscera. *J Physiol* 1986; 20:372–406.
7. Mitchell GAG. The innervation of the kidney, ureter, testicle and epididymis. *J Anat* 1935; 70:10–32.
8. Kuntz A, Morris RE. Components and distribution of the spermatic nerves and the nerves of the vas deferens. *J Comp Neurol* 1946; 85:33–44.
9. Rauchenwald M, Steers WD, Desjardins C. Efferent innervation of the rat testis. *Biol Reprod* 1995; 52:1136–1143.
10. Johnson L, Petty CS, Neaves WB. A comparative study of daily sperm production and testicular composition in humans and rats. *Biol Reprod* 1980; 22:1233–1243.
11. Plymate SR, Paulsen CA, McLachlan RI. Relationship of serum inhibin levels to serum follicle stimulating hormone and sperm production in normal men and men with varicoceles. *Endocrinology* 1992; 74:859–864.
12. Yoshida K-I, Nakame Y, Uchijima Y. Seminal plasma transferrin concentration in normozoospermic fertile men and oligozoospermic men associated with varicocele. *Int J Fertil* 1988; 33:432–436.
13. Anthony CT, Kovacs WJ, Skinner MK. Analysis of the androgen receptor in isolated testicular cell types with a microassay that uses an affinity ligand. *Endocrinology* 1989; 125:2628–2635.
14. Sar M, Lubahn DB, French FS, et al. Immunohistochemical localization of the androgen receptor in rat and human tissues. *Endocrinology* 1990; 127:3180–3186.
15. Heckert LL, Griswold MD. Expression of follicle-stimulating hormone receptor mRNA in rat testes and Sertoli cells. *Mol Endocrinol* 1991; 5:670–677.
16. Hans LS, Sylverter SR, Kim KH, et al. Basic fibroblast growth factor is a testicular germ cell product which may regulate Sertoli cell function. *Mol Endocrinol* 1993; 7:889–897.
17. Skinner MK. Cell-cell interactions in the testis. *Endocr Rev* 1991; 12:45–77.
18. MacMillan EW. The blood supply of the epididymis in man. *Br J Urol* 1954; 26:60–71.
19. Wishahi MM. Anatomy of the spermatic venous plexus (pampiniform plexus) in men with and without varicocele: intraoperative venographic study. *J Urol* 1992; 147:1285–1289.
20. Bedford JM. The status and the state of the human epididymis. *Hum Reprod* 1994; 9:2187–2199.
21. Amann RP, Hammerstedt RH, Veeramachaneni DNR. The epididymis and sperm maturation: a perspective. *Reprod Fertil Dev* 1993; 5:361–381.
22. Garrett SH, Garrett JE, Douglass J. In situ histochemical analysis of region-specific gene expression in the adult rat epididymis. *Mol Reprod Dev* 1991; 30:1–17.

23. Cornwall GA, Hann SR. Specialized gene expression in the epididymis. *J Androl* 1995; 16:379–383.
24. Rowley M, Teshima JF, Heller LL. Duration of transit of spermatozoa through the human male ductular system. *Fertil Steril* 1970; 21:390–396.
25. Amann RP, Howards SS. Daily spermatozoal production and epididymal spermatozoal reserves of the human male. *J Urol* 1980; 124:211–215.
26. Schoysman RJ, Bedford JM. The role of the human epididymis in sperm maturation and sperm storage as reflected in the consequences of epididymovasostomy. *Fertil Steril* 1986; 46:293–299.
27. Freund M, Davis JE. Disappearance rate of spermatozoa from the ejaculate following vasectomy. *Fertil Steril* 1989; 20:163–170.
28. McNeal JE. The zonal anatomy of the prostate. *Prostate* 1981; 2:35–49.
29. Lepor H, Gregerman M, Crosby R, et al. Precise localization of the autonomic nerves from the pelvic plexus to the corpora cavernosa: a detailed anatomical study of the adult male pelvis. *J Urol* 1985; 133:207–212.
30. Higgins JRA, Gosling JA. Studies on the structure and intrinsic innervation of the normal human prostate. *Prostate (Suppl)* 1989; 2:5–16.
31. Quinlan DM, Epstein JI, Carter BS, et al. Sexual function following radical prostatectomy: influence of preservation of neurovascular bundles. *J Urol* 1991; 145:998–1002.
32. Breza J, Aboseif SR, Orvis BR, et al. Detailed anatomy of penile neurovascular structures: surgical significance. *J Urol* 1989; 141:437–443.
33. Aboseif SR, Breza J, Lue TF, et al. Penile venous drainage in erectile dysfunction. Anatomical, radiological and functional considerations. *Br J Urol* 1989; 64:183–190.
34. Virag R. Intracavernous injection of papaverine for erectile failure. *Lancet* 1982; 2:938.
35. Brindley GS. Cavernosal alpha blockage: a new technique for investigating and treating penile impotence. *Br J Psychiatry* 1983; 143:332–337.
36. Lue TF, Hricak H, Marich KW, et al. Evaluation of arteriogenic impotence with intracorporal injection of papaverine and the duplex ultrasound scanner. *Semin Urol* 1985; 3:43–48.
37. Burnett AL, Tillman SL, Chang TSK, et al. Immunohistochemical localization of nitric oxide synthase in the autonomic innervation of the human penis. *J Urol* 1993; 150:73–76.
38. Burnett AL. Role of nitric oxide in the physiology of erection. *Biol Reprod* 1995; 52:485–489.
39. Ignarro LJ, Bush PA, Buga GM, et al. Nitric oxide and cyclic GMP formation upon electrical field stimulation cause relaxation of corpus cavernosum smooth muscle. *Biochem Biophys Res Commun* 1990; 170:843–850.
40. Veldhuis JD, King JC, Urban RJ, et al. Operating characteristics of the male hypothalamo-pituitary-gonadal axis: pulsatile release of testosterone and follicle-stimulating hormone and their temporal coupling with luteinizing hormone. *J Clin Endocrinol Metab* 1987; 65:929–941.
41. MacDonald PC, Madden JD, Brenner PF, et al. Origin of estrogen in normal men and women with testicular feminization. *J Clin Endocrinol Metab* 1979; 49:905–916.
42. Gooren L. Androgens and estrogens in their negative feedback action in the hypothalamo-pituitary-testis axis: site of action and evidence of their interaction. *J Steroid Biochem* 1989; 33:757–761.
43. Sandow J. Clinical applications of LHRH and its analogues. *Clin Endocrinol* 1987; 18:571–592.
44. Vogelzang NJ, Chodak GW, Soloway MS, et al. Goserelin versus orchiectomy in the treatment of advanced prostate cancer: final results of a randomized study. Zoladex Prostate Study Group. *Urology* 1995; 42:220–226.
45. Davis JS. Mechanisms of hormone action: luteinizing hormone receptors and second-messenger pathways. *Curr Opin Obstet Gynecol* 1994; 6:254–261.

# 2
# Office Evaluation of the Infertile Man

R. Dale McClure

Infertility affects approximately 15% of couples who are attempting their first pregnancy. In the United States alone, this amounts to approximately 5 million couples yearly. Few disease entities are of this magnitude. Investigations have found significant pathology related to the male alone in approximately one third of infertile cases, and in 20% abnormalities are found both in the man and in the woman.[1] As the male factor is so prominent, the initial screening evaluation of the male ideally should be performed early in the infertility workup.

Although primary infertility has been defined as the inability to achieve a pregnancy after 1 year of unprotected intercourse, some authorities now suggest couple assessment should commence with their initial presentation, because it has been shown that the longer a couple remains subfertile, the worse their chance for an effective cure. Many couples are generally older at the time of presentation and may be suffering from the detrimental effects of aging on the reproductive process. The increasing awareness of infertility by the lay press has heightened the anxiety and apprehension many couples experience after only a few months of failure to conceive. Couples with long-standing medical diseases, family history of genetic disease, or past history of medical or surgical procedures that would alter their fertility often present earlier than 1 year.

The couple should be considered as a unit and evaluated in a parallel manner until a significant problem is uncovered. Interviewing the couple together during the initial visit allows the physician to gain information about their dynamics as a couple, their individual motivation, and it helps alleviate the stress that the infertility investigation tends to provoke in couples. Cooperation and communication with the woman's physician will allow an efficient and appropriate workup and avoid unnecessary tests and procedures.

At all times during the infertility evaluation, the couple should feel free to question the indications, rationale, and outcomes of various diagnostic procedures. An explanation of the fundamental aspects of male reproductive biology by pamphlets, charts, or diagrams (Fig. 2.1) helps the couple understand the rationale behind various diagnostic tests and therapies. The couple needs also to be reminded that many aspects of both the workup and therapy are subject to controversy. During the evaluation, the physician should take into account both the financial and psychological resources of the couple, for spontaneous cures also can occur with almost every problem in infertility.

The diagnostic evaluation of the man should proceed in a logical, cost-effective sequence to elucidate possible causes of the infertility (Table 2.1).[2] The goals of the treating physicians are to identify both reversible and irreversible causes of infertility and to ascertain the prognosis for the couple.

## History

The cornerstone of the workup of the infertile man is a comprehensive history and physical examination to uncover factors known to be

FIGURE 2.1. Hypothalamic-pituitary-gonadal axis. Testosterone (or its testicular conversion to dihydrotestosterone or estradiol) has an inhibitory effect on the hypothalamic-pituitary axis. Inhibin specifically inhibits serum FSH levels. LH, luteinizing hormone; FSH, follicle-stimulating hormone; GnRH, gonadotropin-releasing hormone. (Reprinted with permission from Singer and Weiner.[64])

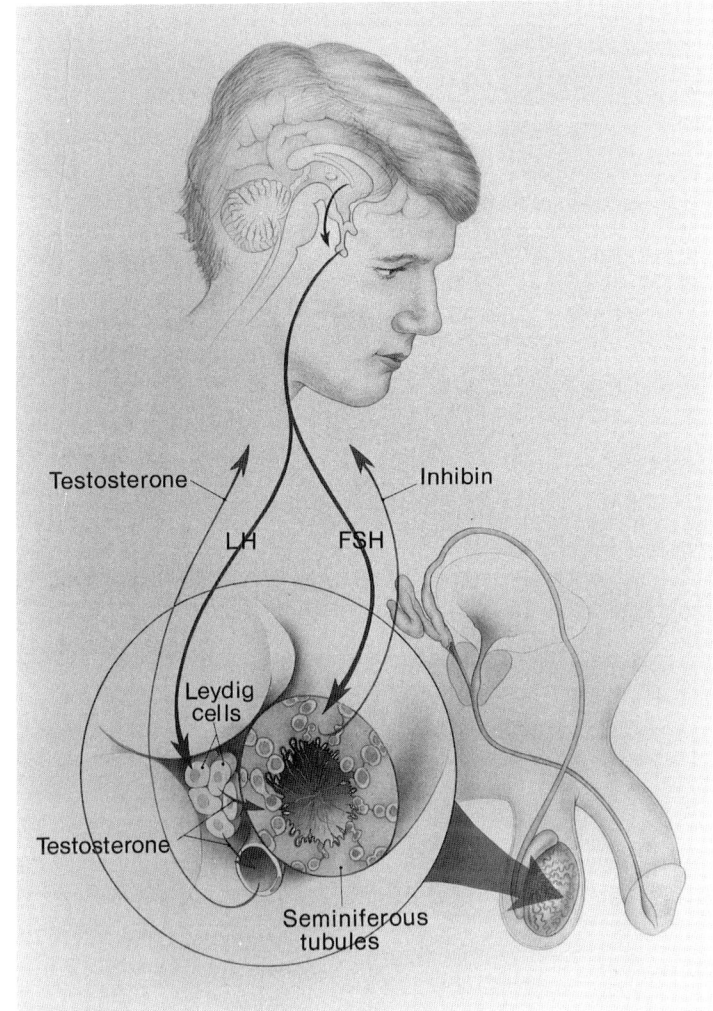

associated with infertility. A workup sheet that addresses most of the pertinent historical points is extremely useful (Table 2.2). Documentation should be made of the duration of unprotected coitus with this or other partners as well as whether the man has fathered children in the past. Notation should be made of the man's previous infertility evaluation, including semen analysis, hormones, and the more sophisticated tests, such as sperm antibody and sperm penetration assays. Determining whether these tests were performed in a physician's office or in a reproductive laboratory may indicate the reliability of the results, for analyses performed in a physician's office or in many general hospital laboratories may fail to match the quality, reliability, and reproducibility of a reproductive laboratory's analyses.

Because the couple should be considered as a unit, it is important that the physician investigating the man be aware of the status of the woman's workup. Details are important in terms of the woman's history: her previous fertility, spontaneous or induced abortions, use of contraceptives, and duration of past exposure to pregnancy. Previous episodes of genital tract infections or acute salpingitis may have led to reproductive tract obstruction. Ovulation should be assessed by a variety of methods, such as menstrual history, basal body tempera-

TABLE 2.1. Differential diagnosis of male infertility.

Potentially treatable causes
  Cryptorchidism
  Varicocele
  Obstruction (acquired, congenital)
  Infection
  Ejaculatory dysfunction
  Hypogonadotropic hypogonadism
  Immunologic problem
  Sexual dysfunction
  Hyperprolactinemia
  Vasal agenesis
  Gonadotoxins (drugs, radiation)
  Idiopathic
Untreatable causes
  Bilateral anorchism
  Germinal cell aplasia
  Primary testicular failure
  Chromosomal anomalies
  Immotile cilia syndrome

ture, urinary luteinizing hormone (LH) kits, as well as serum progesterone. Luteal phase adequacy may be determined by endometrial biopsy or serum progesterone. Tubal patency and assessment of uterine cavity are usually carried out with a hysterosalpingogram. A properly timed postcoital test evaluates the cervical mucus, the delivery of the semen sample, and the survival of sperm within the cervical mucus. Pelvic pathology, including adnexal adhesions, endometriosis, leiomyomata uteri, and tubal pathology, may be identified by laparoscopy.[1]

Documentation of developmental abnormalities in the man is the next step in the investigation. Time of puberty is important, as precocious puberty may indicate the presence of adrenal-genital syndrome, whereas delayed puberty may indicate Klinefelter's syn-

TABLE 2.2. Male infertility history.

| | |
|---|---|
| Male reproductive history | Sexual history |
|   Duration of unprotected coitus |   Potency/libido |
|   Previous marital/extramarital offspring |   Coital technique |
|   Previous infertility evaluation (hormones/semen |   Timing and frequency of intercourse |
|     analysis/sperm antibodies/sperm penetration assay) |   Lubricants |
|   Previous diagnostic conclusions and therapy | |
| | Medications |
| Personal history |   Personal (past/present) |
|   Developmental |   Maternal (diethylstilbestrol) |
|     Onset of puberty (precocious/normal/delayed) |   Recreational drugs (marijuana/cocaine) |
|     Undescended testes | |
|     Gynecomastia | Family history |
|   Surgical |   Hypogonadism/congenital midline defects |
|     Retroperitoneal |   Cystic fibrosis |
|     Pelvic (Y-V plasty bladder neck, transurethral) |   Androgen receptor deficiency (undermasculinization) |
|     Inguinal (herniorrhaphy, orchidopexy) | |
|     Scrotal (trauma/torsion/vasectomy/hydrocele) | Endocrine history |
|   Medical |   Hypothalamic-pituitary |
|     Systemic illnesses and therapy (diabetes mellitus/ |     Headaches/visual changes/polydipsia/impaired ability |
|       ulcerative colitis/respiratory infections/cystic |       to smell |
|       fibrosis) |     Excessive growth of jaw, hands, feet |
|     Mumps orchitis |   Thyroid |
|     History of venereal disease/urethritis/epididymitis/ |     Heat or cold intolerance |
|       orchitis/prostatitis |     Change in bowel movements |
|     Recent (3–6 months) febrile/viral illness |     Increased appetite with weight loss |
|   Gonadotoxins (occupational/environmental) |     Palpitations |
|     Occupation(s) (past/present) |   Adrenal |
|     Thermal exposure (work/saunas/baths/bikini/tights) |     Muscle weakness/anorexia/purpura |
|     Radiation (work/diagnostic/therapeutic) |     Postural hypotension/hyperpigmentation |
|     Chemical exposure (work/insecticides/therapeutic) |   Gonadal |
|     Smoking (amount/duration) |     Retardation of hair growth (facial/body) |
|     Alcohol (amount/duration) |     Breast changes |

drome or idiopathic hypogonadism. Similarly, gynecomastia may indicate an endocrine abnormality. Specific childhood illnesses should be noted, including cryptorchidism,[3,4] postpubertal mumps orchitis,[5] and testicular trauma or pain (torsion).[6] Approximately 50% of men with a history of bilateral cryptorchidism and 30% of men with unilateral cryptorchidism may have sperm counts below normal.[3] Trauma or torsion may result in testicular atrophy, or, if occurring after the time of puberty, may be related to the presence of sperm antibodies.[6,7] Approximately 10% of individuals who develop mumps orchitis bilaterally postpubertally may end up with severe testicular damage.[5]

Previous surgical procedures, such as bladder neck operations (Y-V plasty) or retroperitoneal lymph node dissection for testicular cancer, may cause retrograde ejaculation or absent emission. Similarly, diabetic neuropathy may result in either retrograde ejaculation or impotence. Both the vas deferens and the testicular blood supply can easily be injured during a hernia repair or during scrotal surgery.

Recurrent respiratory infections and infertility may be associated with the immotile cilia syndrome, in which the sperm count is normal but spermatozoa are completely nonmotile due to ultrastructural defects.[8] Kartagener's syndrome, a variant of immotile cilia syndrome, consists of chronic bronchiectasis, sinusitis, situs inversus, and immotile spermatozoa. In Young's syndrome, also associated with pulmonary disease, the cilia ultrastructure is normal, but the epididymis is obstructed due to inspissated material, and these patients present with azoospermia (absence of spermatozoa).[9] Many males with cystic fibrosis have congenital absence of the vas deferens and seminal vesicles.[10] These individuals present with low semen volume, failure of the semen to coagulate, and azoospermia.

Inflammatory processes that involve either the lower urinary tract or the reproductive tract may result in scarring and obstruction of the reproductive ducts or damage to the secondary sex organs. A generalized febrile illness can impair spermatogenesis.[11,12] The ejaculate, however, may not be affected for 3 months after the event, as spermatogenesis takes about 74 days

from initiation to the appearance of mature spermatozoa, and there is also a varied transport time in the ducts.[13] Therefore, events that have occurred in the previous 3 to 6 months are extremely important.

A variety of gonadotoxins—occupational, environmental, or therapeutic—may have detrimental effects on fertility.[14] Cancer chemotherapy has a dose-dependent, potentially devastating effect on the testicular germinal epithelium and may also compromise Leydig cell function.[15] The alkylating agents cyclophosphamide, mustargen, and chlorambucil are particularly damaging. Exposure to x-rays, neutrons, and radioactive materials may also affect spermatogenesis. Radiation effects depend on the total dose received and the developmental stage of the germ cell during exposure.[15] Permanent sterility generally occurs after a single field dose of radiation of 600 to 800 rad. Semen cryopreservation is recommended for men prior to either chemo- or radiotherapy. Although numerous chemicals are known to affect the male reproductive tract, few have been extensively studied. Dibromochloropropane (DBCP), a nematocide used widely in agriculture, appears to be a testicular toxin.[14,16] Lead, known to be a reproductive toxin since the Roman Empire, affects the hypothalamic-pituitary-testicular axis and results in suppression of serum testosterone.[17]

Both cigarette smoking and marijuana have been associated with infertility.[18,19] Although some studies have shown an impairment of sperm density, motility, and morphology among male smokers, other authors have found no statistically significant effect of smoking.[1,19] Individual susceptibility may be responsible for this difference. Human studies have shown that with marijuana usage there is a lowering of serum testosterone and a temporary decrease in sperm counts and motility.[18,20] Among abusers of alcohol, there is a reduction in sperm density, motility, and the number of normal-appearing sperm.[21] Independent of its effect on the liver, alcohol reduces testosterone levels both acutely and chronically. The liver disease concomitant with chronic alcoholism also leads to changes in androgen metabolism and may result in sexual dysfunction.[22] Opiate abuse also inhibits gonadotropin secretion, lowering serum testosterone.[23]

Some authorities suggest that boxer shorts, as compared with briefs, should be worn by individuals with suboptimal semen quality, and studies in the 1960s did show that excessive heat could, with time, alter sperm density.[24] However, the higher-than-normal scrotal temperature in men with cryptorchidism and varicocele may explain abnormal spermatogenesis. It is therefore recommended that use of saunas, hot tubs, or tight nylon bikinis should be discontinued because elevated temperature may impair sperm production.

The type of ejaculation (antegrade/retrograde), sexual habits, including frequency of intercourse and use of coital lubricants, and the patient's understanding of the ovulatory cycle should be discussed. Decreased coital frequency may be related to decreased libido, marital difficulties, or work-related absences from the home as well as religious practices, such as the Mikveh among Orthodox Jews.[25] Caution must be used with lubricants, for substances such as K-Y jelly, Lubrifax, Keri lotion, and saliva have been shown to cause a deterioration of sperm motility when tested in vitro. On the other hand, raw egg white, peanut oil, vegetable oil, and petroleum jelly do not appear to impair in vitro motility.[17]

The optimal timing of intercourse is still not understood by many couples. Recent data have shown that the fertile period for conception lasts about 6 days and ends on the day of ovulation. The drop in conception probability after ovulation may be related to short survival time for ova or perhaps the detrimental effects of the cervical mucus on sperm entry.[26] Historically, it was felt that frequent ejaculations could theoretically reduce the potency of subsequent ejaculates. However, unless the male has severe oligospermia, the present recommendation for couples seeking pregnancy is not to limit the frequency of sexual intercourse during the optimal period.

Medications that disrupt either ejaculation or emission can cause male infertility. Alpha blockers used to control hypertension (e.g., prazosin, terazosin, phentolamine, and phenoxybenzamine), along with ganglion blockers (e.g., methyldopa, guanethidine, and reserpine) can cause retrograde ejaculation or failure of emission. Preventable causes of male infertility can sometimes be found in the careful review of the patient's medications.

A variety of other therapeutic medications may also affect reproductive capability. Prenatal exposure to diethylstilbestrol (DES) may cause an increased incidence of epididymal cysts, slightly increased frequency of cryptorchidism, and may in some individuals affect semen quality.[27] Sulfasalazine, commonly used in treatment of ulcerative colitis, has been associated with a drop in sperm motility and density, which may be reversed upon stopping therapy.[28] Drugs known to inhibit androgen production include spironolactone, cyproterone, ketoconazole (antifungal agent), and cimetidine.[29] These all may significantly affect fertility. During short-term therapy, tetracycline lowers serum testosterone about 20%.[29] Nitrofurantoin depresses spermatogenesis and therefore should be avoided. Other antimicrobial agents (e.g., erythromycin and gentamicin) may also impair spermatozoal function and spermatogenesis.[30] Low-dose androgens, given by some physicians for male infertility, may also affect sperm production by inhibiting gonadotropin secretion. The anabolic steroids used by many professional and amateur athletes also depress gonadotropin secretion, acting as a "male contraceptive."[31] This effect on spermatogenesis appears to be temporary and should be reversible after discontinuing steroids.

Symptoms of other endocrine gland abnormalities (pituitary, thyroid, and adrenal) should be elucidated (Table 2.2). Unless testicular damage is severe or sufficient time has elapsed to regression of male secondary sex characteristics, Leydig cell failure occurring after puberty is difficult to diagnose clinically. Complaints of decreasing libido and poor erections associated with the decreased testicular function may precede changes in shaving pattern, loss of pubic and axillary hair, and the development of gynecomastia. Hot flashes may occasionally be seen in men with declining testicular function. A rapid loss of beard and body hair (over 6 to 12 months) suggests concomitant adrenal insufficiency.[29]

# Physical Examination

A careful physical examination on the initial visit may delineate abnormalities indicating a male factor in infertility (Table 2.3). Particular attention should be given to discerning any features of hypogonadism: poorly developed secondary sexual characteristics; eunuchoidal skeletal proportion (arm span 2 inches greater than height); ratio of upper body segment (crown to pubis) to lower body segment (pubis to floor) less than 1; lack of normal male hair distribution (sparse axillary, pubic, facial, and body hair), and lack of temporal hair recession (Table 2.4).[29,32–34] Excessive wrinkling is often noted with hypogonadism.

Abnormal skin pigmentation may be related to adrenal disease. Headache, visual field defects, galactorrhea, and signs of other tropic hormone deficiencies may point to a secondary (hypothalamic-pituitary) cause.[35] A man with congenital hypogonadism may have associated midline defects, such as anosmia, color blindness, cerebellar ataxia, harelip, and cleft palate.[36]

Gynecomastia is a consistent finding of a feminizing state. Its presence may be a clue to

TABLE 2.4. Features of eunuchoidism.

*Eunuchoid skeletal proportions*
  Upper body to lower body ratio below 1
  Arm span more than 2 inches greater than height
*Lack of male hair distribution*
  Sparse axillary, pubic, and body hair
  Lack of temporal hair recession
*Infantile genitalia*
  Small penis, testes, and prostate
*Diminished muscular development and mass*

testicular dysfunction, whether the failure is primary testicular or secondary to disease in the hypothalamic-pituitary axis. Because palpation by the flat of the hand with the patient supine may fail to detect minimal breast enlargement, gynecomastia may be more easily found by examining the patient sitting, using the fingers to grasp the glandular tissue.

Particular emphasis should be placed on the male's genitalia. Testicular size correlates well with semen quality and fertility. Seminiferous tubules account for approximately 95% of testicular volume. The normal adult testis averages 4.6 cm in length (range, 3.6 to 5.5 cm) and 2.6 cm in width (2.1 to 3.2 cm) with a mean volume of 18.6 ± 4.8 (SD) ml[32,37] (Fig. 2.2). The lower limit of normal length and width for a mature testis is approximately 4 × 2.5 cm, equivalent to a testicular volume of 15 ml. A ruler, caliper, or Prader orchidometer may be used to measure testicular size (Fig. 2.3). When the seminiferous tubules are damaged before puberty, the testes are small and firm; with postpubertal damage, they are usually soft and small. Small testicular volumes, features of eunuchoidism, and the presence of gynecomastia on physical examination are all highly suggestive of endocrine disease. The finding of a unilateral smaller testis may indicate the presence of a varicocele or a previous inflammatory or vascular injury to that testis.

Irregularities in the epididymis or vas may suggest a previous infection and possible obstruction. Examination may reveal a small prostate in men with androgen deficiency or slight tenderness (bogginess) in those with prostatic infection. The penis, which should be at least 5 cm in length when stretched, should be examined for abnormality (hypospadias, abnormal

TABLE 2.3. Infertility physical examination.

Height
Weight
Arm span
Hair
  Pubic
  Axillary
  Chest
Skin (wrinkles/pigmentation)
Virilization (poor/normal)
Visual fields
Sense of smell
Breasts (gynecomastia/galactorrhea)
Abdomen (hepatomegaly/previous surgical scars)
Penis (length/meatus/deformities)
Prostate (size/consistency/tenderness)

| Testes | Right | Left |
| --- | --- | --- |
| Size (length × width or volume by Prader) | | |
| Consistency | | |
| Vas deferens | | |
| Epididymis | | |
| Varicocele (grade I–III) | | |

NORMAL RANGES FOR TESTICULAR VOLUME (Mean)

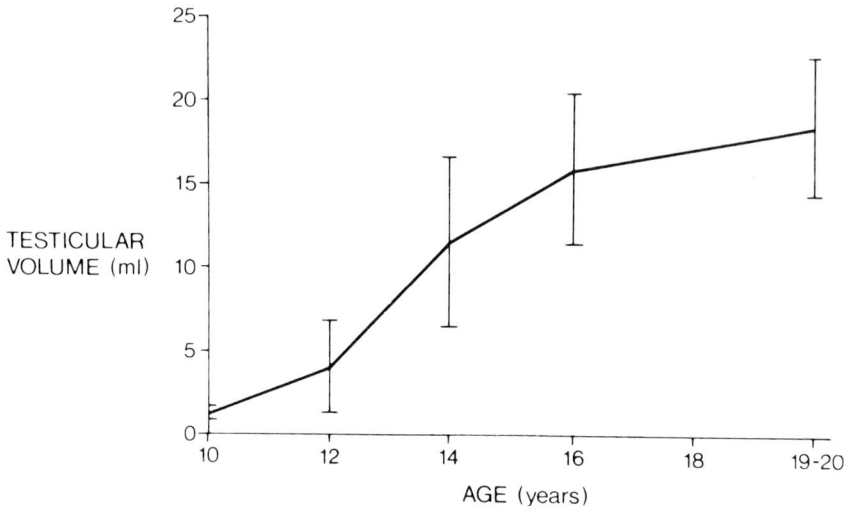

FIGURE 2.2. Normal values for testicular volume in relation to age. (Modified from Zachmann et al.[37]; reprinted from McClure[34] by permission of W.B. Saunders Co.)

curvature, phimosis), because such a problem may interfere with the deposition of the ejaculate in the vagina. Both vasa should be palpated, as 2% of infertile men have congenital absence of the vasa and seminal vesicles.

There should be a careful search for a varicocele, a frequent finding in the infertile male.[38] The patient should be examined in a warm environment, both in the supine and the standing position, with and without the Valsalva maneuver. Spermatic cord structures from both sides should be palpated and compared. With the patient performing the Valsalva maneuver, the examiner secures the cord between index finger and thumb. During this maneuver, an increase in the thickness of the cord or a discrete pulse wave indicative of a venous reflex indicates the presence of a

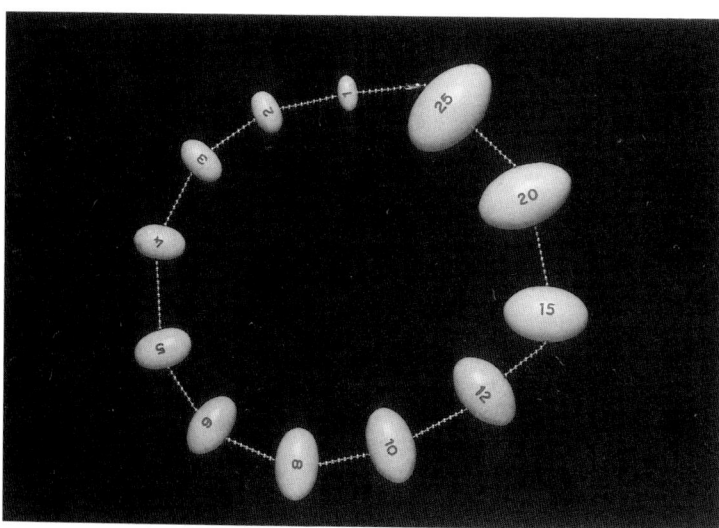

FIGURE 2.3. A Prader orchidometer for measuring testicular volume.

varicocele. On occasion, the cremasteric muscle will contract, foreshortening the cord and leading to an erroneous positive diagnosis. A smaller left testis and a boggy feeling in the surrounding scrotal tissue (bag of worms) even in the supine position will suggest that a varicocele is present.

The examination is not complete without a thorough physical examination to rule out chronic or unsuspected systemic disease that may contribute to the infertility. Proper neck examination will rule out thyromegaly, a bruit, or nodularity associated with thyroid disease. Liver disease may represent undiagnosed cirrhosis, and lymphadenopathy may be the early sign of Hodgkin's disease. Although previously undiagnosed systemic disease is usually very unlikely in the workup of an infertile man, correction of this illness may improve the man's overall health and improve his semen quality.

## Laboratory Investigation and Interpretation

Although completeness of history and thoroughness of physical examination are extremely important, the laboratory testing should be more selective.

### Semen Analysis

A carefully performed semen analysis provides important information concerning the male reproductive hormonal cycle, spermatogenesis, and the patency of the reproductive tract.[39] A past history of paternity or an adequate postcoital test does not eliminate the need for semen analysis that may reveal subtle, but important, abnormalities. However, interpretation of semen analysis must take into consideration the variations in an individual's samples. The minimum number of specimens to define good or poor quality of semen is three samples over a 2-month period with a consistent period of prior abstinence (48 to 72 hours). In a longitudinal analysis of semen from both fertile and infertile men, Sherins et al[40] found that 97% of men with initial good sperm concentration would continue to show good density after as many as

three to six specimens. Those rated poor at the first specimen also remained poor at the third and sixth specimens. For those rated equivocal, the first specimen was of little value and at least three specimens were needed to obtain stability. Conventional semen analysis is an indirect assessment of fertility potential, but pregnancy is the only irrefutable proof of sperm capability to fertilize.

Despite its limitation, semen analysis is a simple, inexpensive screening test. If the first analysis is normal, repeat the analysis for confirmation. If, however, the first one is abnormal, obtain at least three analyses to document abnormalities.

## Normal Values

Semen specimens should be regarded as abnormal if the following values and characteristics persist: volume, less than 1.5 ml or more than 5 ml; sperm concentration, less than $20 \times 10^6$ per ml; total sperm number of fewer than 50 million; sperm motility of less than 50% of cells with forward progression and quality graded below 2 (scale 0 to 4); and sperm morphology of less than 30% oval forms (Table 2.5).[39,41] The terms *oligospermia, asthenospermia*, and *teratospermia* refer to individual semen samples with abnormalities in sperm numbers, motility, and morphology, respectively.

## Categories of Male Infertility

Upon completion of a history and physical examination and evaluation of semen parameters, the patient's infertility can usually be classified into one of nine categories: azoospermia, ejaculatory dysfunction, varicocele, gonadotoxins,

TABLE 2.5. Semen analysis: normal values.

| Ejaculate volume | ≥1.5 ml |
|---|---|
| Sperm concentration | ≥20 million/ml |
| Total sperm count | ≥40 million |
| Motility | ≥50% with forward progression |
| Rapid progression | ≥25% |
| Morphology | >30% normal form |

Data from World Health Organization.[39]

antisperm antibodies, infection, endocrinopathy, idiopathic infertility, or miscellaneous.

## Azoospermia

Azoospermia, a complete absence of sperm within a centrifuged semen specimen, is a relatively infrequent but absolute cause of male factor infertility. Semen samples with less than 1 million sperm per milliliter should be evaluated in the same manner. Investigation should be carried out to differentiate between pretesticular (hormonal deficiency), testicular (sperm production abnormality), and posttesticular (delivery problem) causes. Ejaculatory volume, serum hormones, and testicular size are useful factors in determining the diagnosis (Fig. 2.4).

Low ejaculatory volume (<1.5 ml) is consistent with either ejaculatory dysfunction (failure of emission or retrograde ejaculation), ejacula-

tory duct obstruction, congenital abnormalities of the Wolffian duct structures (absence of the vas), or hypogonadism. Physical examination can easily identify patients with bilateral congenital absence of the vas. A postejaculatory urinalysis revealing sperm within the bladder is consistent with retrograde ejaculation. Although the standard fructose test has been used to evaluate the presence or absence of the seminal vesicles, this test is qualitative rather than quantitative and the results are often misleading in cases of incomplete obstruction or hypoplasia. Transrectal ultrasonography (TRUS) of the prostate, seminal vesicles, and ejaculatory ducts may reveal an obstructive etiology of the azoospermia. Individuals with low volume, severe oligospermia, or severe motility defects should also be evaluated by TRUS.

Hypogonadism can be ruled out on the basis of testes size and hormonal testing. A low

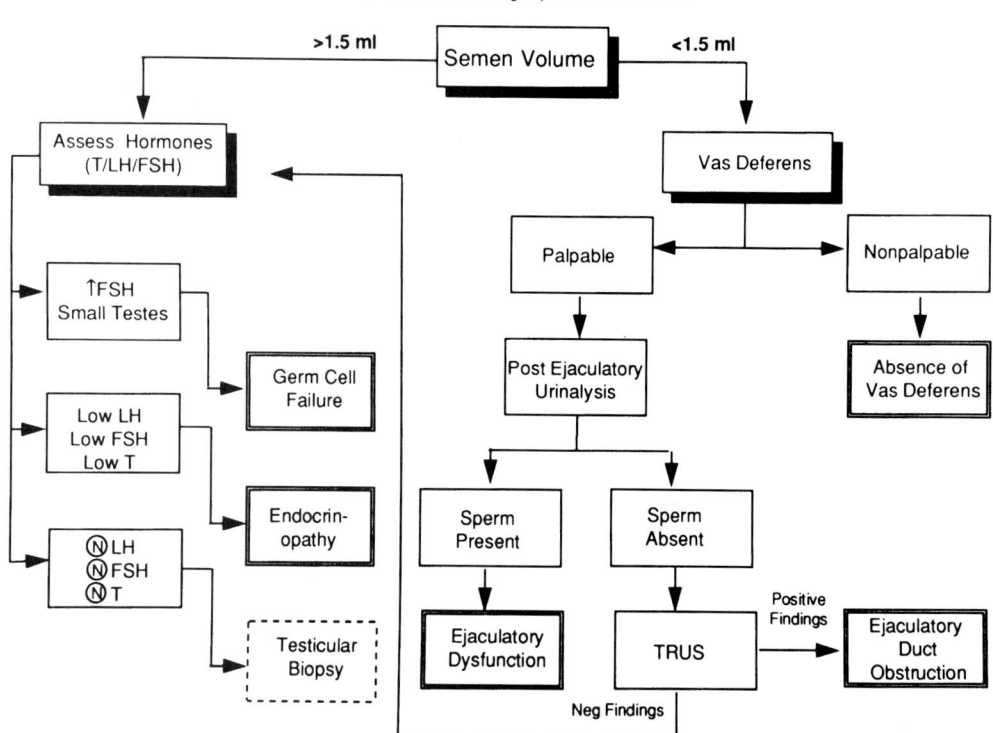

FIGURE 2.4. Azoospermia algorithm.

serum testosterone level is one of the best indicators of hypogonadism. Low LH and follicle-stimulating hormone (FSH) values concurrent with low serum testosterone indicate hypogonadotropic hypogonadism, which may be apparent clinically. Although uncommon, this is a readily treatable form of male infertility.

Elevated serum FSH and LH values help to distinguish primary (hypergonadotropic hypogonadism) from secondary testicular failure (hypogonadotropic hypogonadism). Most patients with primary testicular failure usually have severe, irreversible testicular defects.

In azoospermic and severely oligospermic patients with normal FSH, primary spermatogenic defects cannot be distinguished from obstructive lesions by normal investigation alone; scrotal exploration, testicular biopsy, and vasography should be considered. An elevated serum FSH associated with small atrophic testes, however, implies irreversible infertility secondary to germ cell failure and biopsy may not be warranted.

## Ejaculatory Dysfunction

Ejaculatory dysfunction should be suspected in individuals with cloudy urine after ejaculation or low-volume azoospermic samples, or in individuals presenting with anejaculation. The microscopic examination of the postejaculatory urine for sperm easily reveals a diagnosis of retrograde ejaculation. Therapy for retrograde ejaculation has been highly successful with both medical therapy (sympathomimetic medication) and harvesting the sperm from the bladder. Failure of emission is diagnosed by the absence of sperm in the ejaculate or in the voided urine. In anejaculatory individuals with a typical history of spinal cord injury, retroperitoneal surgery, or a neurologic disorder, vibratory stimulation or electroejaculation is often required to obtain a semen sample.[42]

Injury to the sympathetic nervous system will cause bladder neck incompetence and result in retrograde ejaculation. Retroperitoneal lymph node dissection for nonseminous germ cell tumors performed in the traditional manner often results in sympathetic ganglia damage and either retrograde ejaculation or lack of emission.

Other extensive retroperitoneal surgery, such as colorectal surgery, aneurysmectomy, or aortoiliac bypass, may damage the sympathetic chain. Neurologic conditions affecting the spinal cord, such as multiple sclerosis and transverse myelitis, may also affect ejaculation. In men with diabetes, sympathetic neuropathy is a common occurrence. Many psychotropic and antihypertensive medications are known to affect the ejaculatory process by interfering with the sympathetic nervous system[42] (Table 2.6).

A variety of surgical procedures on the genitourinary tract may either cause sympathetic nerve damage, disturb closure of the bladder neck through disruption of the normal anatomy, or obstruct the ejaculatory duct (Table

TABLE 2.6. Etiology of ejaculatory dysfunction.

| |
|---|
| Bladder neck incompetence |
|   Congenital |
|     Posterior urethral valves/polyps |
|     Exstrophy |
|   Acquired |
|     Bladder neck surgery |
|     Trauma (pelvic fracture) |
|     Postprostatectomy |
| Neurogenic |
|   Spinal cord lesions |
|   Surgical injury |
|     Retroperitoneal lymphadenectomy |
|     Abdominal vascular surgery |
|     Colorectal surgery |
|   Neuropathies |
|     Diabetes mellitus |
|     Multiple sclerosis |
|     Transverse myelitis |
| Pharmacologic |
|   Alpha-adrenergic blockers |
|     Phenoxybenzamine |
|     Bethanidine |
|     Prazosin |
|   Peripheral sympatholytics |
|     Guanethidine |
|   Ganglion blockers |
|     Hexamethonium |
|   Antipsychotics |
|     Chlorpromazine |
|     Haloperidol |
| Mechanical obstruction |
|   Urethral stricture/meatal stenosis |
|   Urethral valves |
|   Ureterocele |
|   Postprostatectomy surgery |
|   Epispadias |

2.6). Some of the newer procedures, including laser prostatectomy and bladder neck incision, may be less harmful to the ejaculatory process. Congenital causes of retrograde ejaculation are uncommon and may include epispadias, exstrophy, or posterior urethral valves. The congenital condition itself or its corrective surgery may interfere with the normal ejaculatory process.

## Varicocele

Numerous clinical studies have demonstrated an association of varicoceles with male infertility and have shown an improvement in semen parameters following surgical repair. A seminal improvement rate of approximately 65% and a pregnancy rate of approximately 35% have been noted.[38,43] Although varicocelectomy is presently the most common surgical therapy for the infertile male, and 15% of the adult male population have a varicocele, its mere presence in an individual undergoing an infertility evaluation is not in itself an indication for surgery. Other less invasive and treatable causes of both male and female infertility should be ruled out before undertaking varicocele correction. Males presenting with a varicocele and normal semen parameters should have a sperm penetration assay (SPA) to evaluate the functional aspects of the sperm. In spite of "normal" conventional semen parameters, 16.3% of males have a functional defect in their sperm.[44] A negative SPA warrants surgical correction of the varicocele.

## Gonadotoxins

Gonadotoxins are drugs, chemicals, or other substances (radiation or heat) that have a suppressive or toxic effect on spermatogenesis. Usually the effect is reversible if the substance is identified and discontinued. Cryopreservation of sperm should be considered in anyone undergoing chemotherapy or radiation, as full recovery of spermatogenesis may not be guaranteed. With the expanded use of in vitro fertilization and in particular with the advent of micromanipulation, successful pregnancies are being obtained even with the severest oligospermic, teratosperinic, or asthenospermic samples.

## Sperm Antibodies

Sperm antibodies have been reported in 3% to 7% of infertile men and may be a relative cause of infertility.[1,7] A history of inflammation of the genitourinary tract, testicular injury or torsion, and a previous vasectomy may lead to the development of sperm antibodies.[7,45] Although the majority of infertile men with sperm immunity have normal findings on semen analysis, the presence of a spontaneous agglutination or poor motility should alert the clinician to the possibility of antibodies. Often sperm agglutination is nonspecific and may be related to the presence of bacteria or cellular debris and may not reflect an immunologic problem. Postcoital testing provides an excellent means to screen for antisperm antibodies. If fewer than five motile sperm per field are seen in a well-estrogenized mucus sample or if the sperm seem to shake or vibrate, sperm antibody testing should be performed.

Sperm antibodies can be found in the circulation, in the seminal plasma, or directly on the sperm surface. Several studies have shown a discordance between results of sperm antibody testing in matched serum and sperm samples. Although humoral antibodies may be detected in blood but not in sperm, locally secreted antisperm antibodies within the genital tract may be detected on sperm with no evidence in the blood. In 166 of 856 matched samples, Bronson[45] found human antibodies in blood but not on the sperm. Conversely, he found antibodies in the genital tract with no evidence in the serum in 14% of cases. The presence of human antibodies directed against sperm is not relevant to fertility unless these circulating antibodies are also present within the reproductive tract. It appears, therefore, that tests capable of detecting immunoglobulins on living motile sperm retrieved from the ejaculate are the most direct way to determine whether significant autoimmunity to sperm exists.

Although found in the circulation of men, antisperm antibodies of the immunoglobulin M (IgM) class are not present within the male genital tract. Therefore, testing for sperm-associated immunoglobulins of the IgM class is unwarranted. On the other hand, IgG found within the male genital tract is either derived from local antibody production or from transudation from the circulation. IgA is assumed to be from local production, because seminal plasma IgA is of the secretory IgA type. Sperm antibody testing should include both IgG and IgA.

There are several useful assays that detect immunoglobulins present on the surface of motile spermatozoa. These include the mixed antiglobulin reaction (MAR), the radiolabeled antiglobulin test (RAT), and the immunobead test (IBT).[7,46] Each of these tests can be used either as a *direct* test for detecting immunoglobulins already bound to a patient's spermatozoa or as an *indirect* test.[17] In the indirect test, passive antibody is transferred to donor sperm (previously tested and found to be negative) from any body fluid (e.g., cervical mucus, seminal plasma, or serum).

The IBT or the immunobead rosette test is one of the most informative and specific of all assays currently available to detect antisperm antibodies bound to the surface of the sperm. This test determines the isotope of immunoglobulin bound, the percentage of sperm bound with antibody, and, in contrast to RAT and MAR assay, it determines the region of sperm to which specific antibodies are bound.

The end point of the immunobead assay is the percentage of motile sperm that bind to immunobeads. Exactly what degree of sperm immunobead binding may indicate a clinically significant level of any sperm antibodies is controversial. From observations of sperm immunobead binding, postcoital test results and pregnancy, Bronson[45] concluded that bead bind of 50% or more of the population is clinically significant. If 50% of the sperm were antibody bound, there was a significant reduction in fertility (21.8%) compared with a similar group with less than 50% bound sperm (45.3%).[45,47] Clark et al,[48] on the other hand, suggested that if 20% or more sperm bind to beads, the antibody level should be considered significant. The information provided by the IBT on location and the class of antibody can be used in conjunction with the couple's clinical history to provide the clinician important information for management of their infertility problem.

## Infection

Symptoms of infection usually include urethral discharge, dysuria, urgency, frequency, testicular/suprapubic or perineal discomfort, as well as hematospermia or pain with ejaculation. The findings of greater than five white blood cells per high power field on the first 10 ml of voided bladder urine 1 ($VB_1$) are considered abnormal and indicative of urethral inflammation. There should be appropriate intervention and treatment of the organism, including therapy for the female partner if sexually transmitted. If the expressed prostatic secretions show more than 10 to 15 white blood cells per high power field, the diagnosis should be prostatitis. Culture of the urine immediately after prostatic massage should identify the infected organism, and treatment can be initiated.[49]

Gram-positive aerobic bacteria, primarily *Staphylococcus epidermidis*, diphtheroids, and streptococcal species, frequently colonize in the male urethra. The ubiquitous nature of the gram-positive bacteria is responsible for urethral contamination of the ejaculate during semen culture and makes routine semen cultures usually useless. On the other hand, the gram-negative enteric bacteria—*Chlamydia trachomatis*, *Neisseria gonorrhoeae*, and *Trachomatis vaginalis*—are rarely isolated from the urethra of normal asymptomatic men and, when isolated, indicate infection.[50]

In asymptomatic infertile men, evaluation for a subclinical infection focuses on the accurate determination of seminal white blood cells. Leukocytospermia or pyospermia has been defined by the World Health Organization (WHO) as the presence of greater than $1 \times 10^6$ white blood cells per milliliter of semen.[39] Increases in seminal leukocytes adversely affect sperm motility and fertilization functions.[51,52] Under routine wet mount light microscopy, both immature germ cells and white blood cells appear as round cells and are difficult to differentiate. Traditional staining techniques, such as Papanicolaou stain and Bryan-Leishman stain, differentiate the cell types based on nuclear morphology. The widely used peroxidase method primarily detects polymorphonuclear leukocytes, which compose 50% to 80% of white blood cells in semen.[53] More recently, labeled monoclonal antibodies directed against leukocyte surface antigen have been used to develop immunohistochemical stains that allow for easy differentiation between white blood cells and immature germ cells.[54] Although leukocytospermia is usually thought to be caused by bacterial pathogens, other factors may also be responsible, including viral infections, recruitment of white blood cells to scavenged defective sperm, and exposure to environmental toxins (alcohol and cigarettes).[53]

The evidence is still inconclusive as to whether asymptomatic genital tract infections are a significant cause of male infertility. Therefore, there appears to be little justification for empiric antibiotic therapy. The commonly sexually transmitted organisms—*Chlamydia*

*trachomatis*, *Mycoplasma hominis*, and *Ureaplasma urealyticum*—have been implicated, but not proven, as a cause of male infertility.[55]

## Endocrine Infertility

Most cases of male infertility are nonendocrine in origin. Routine hormonal evaluation is not warranted unless sperm density is extremely low or there is a clinical suspicion of an endocrinopathy. The incidence of primary endocrine defects in infertile men is less than 3% and is rare in men with sperm concentrations greater than $5 \times 10^6$/ml. Individuals with a history of birth anomalies, delayed or premature sexual maturation, erectile difficulties, or libido loss may need hormonal evaluation. Small testicular volumes, features of eunuchoidism, and the presence of gynecomastia on physical examination are highly suggestive of endocrine disease. Suspect patients should have serum gonadotropins (LH and FSH) and serum testosterone drawn. The algorithm presented in Figure 2.5 demonstrates common patterns

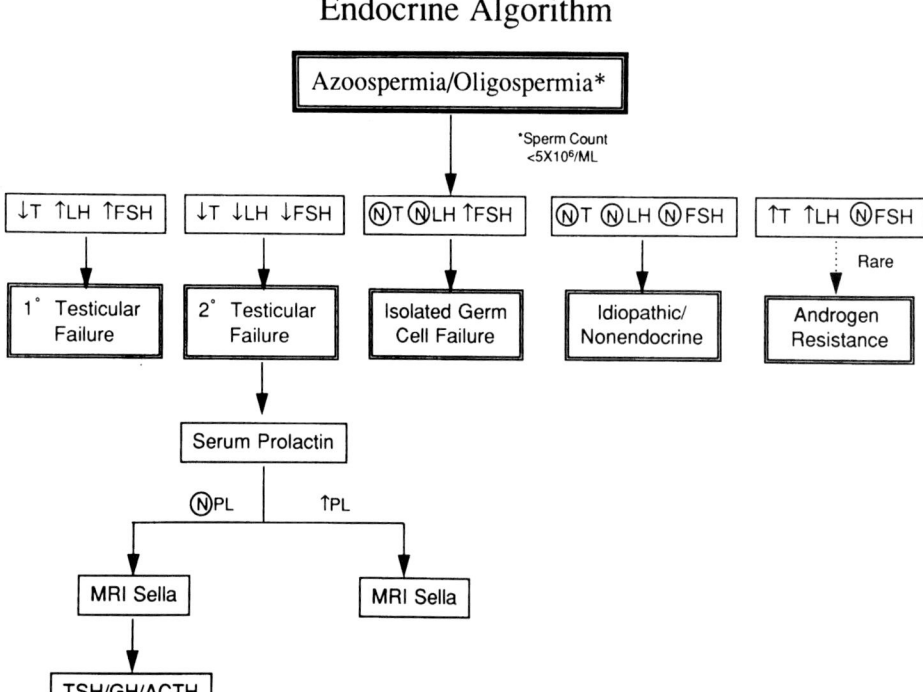

FIGURE 2.5. Endocrine algorithm.

of serum gonadotropins and testosterone by which a diagnosis can be made.

A single LH determination has an accuracy of approximately ±50% because of the episodic nature of LH secretion and its short half-life. Similarly, testosterone secreted episodically in response to LH pulses has a diurnal pattern with early morning peak.[32] To overcome these sampling inaccuracies, three blood samples can be drawn at least 15 to 20 minutes apart, and an equal volume of serum from each can be pooled for a single determination.[56] Serum FSH has a longer half-life and fluctuations are less obvious.

A low serum testosterone level is one of the best indicators of hypogonadism of either hypothalamic or pituitary origin. Mean serum LH and FSH concentrations are significantly lower in hypogonadotropic than in normal men, although in some individuals they can overlap with the lower limits of normal. Low LH and FSH values concurrent with low serum testosterone indicate hypogonadotropic hypergonadism. Individuals presenting with hypogonadotropic hypogonadism should have other pituitary hormones assessed, including thyroid-stimulating hormone (TSH), adrenal corticotropic hormone (ACTH), and growth hormone (GH). Further evaluation should include magnetic resonance imaging (MRI) of the patient's sella.

Elevated serum FSH is a reliable indicator of germinal epithelial damage and is usually associated with azoospermia or severe oligospermia. This elevation is indicative of significant, usually irreversible, germ cell damage.[34]

Elevated serum FSH and LH will help distinguish primary testicular failure (hypergonadotropic hypogonadism) from secondary testicular failure (hypogonadotropic hypogonadism). Patients with primary hypogonadism usually have severe, irreversible testicular defects. Secondary hypogonadism has a hypothalamic or pituitary origin, and in these patients infertility may be medically correctable.

Hyperprolactinemia has been reported to cause oligospermia, but the diagnostic evaluation of routine prolactin measurements is extremely low in men with semen abnormalities, unless associated with decreased libido, impotence, or evidence of hypogonadism.[35,57] Prolactin measurements are warranted in patients with low serum testosterone without an associated increase in serum LH. In individuals with hyperprolactinemia and testosterone deficiency, serum LH levels are inappropriately low, indicating that the hypothalamic-pituitary axis fails to respond to the reduced testosterone level.[35] MRI of the pituitary is required to rule out a pituitary adenoma.

Individuals with gynecomastia or suspected androgen resistance (elevated serum testosterone and LH levels with undermasculinization) should have a serum estradiol determination. The diagnosis can be confirmed by measuring androgen receptor levels in cultured skin fibroblasts.[33]

Individuals with a rapid loss of secondary sexual characteristics, implying both testicular and adrenal failure (adrenal androgen), should undergo investigation of adrenal function. In men with a history of precocious puberty, congenital adrenal hyperplasia should be considered.[58] In the common variant (21–hydroxy deficiency), serum levels of 17–hydroxyprogesterone are elevated, as is urinary pregnanetriol.

## Idiopathic Infertility

In approximately 40% of infertile men, the impairment of sperm count, motility, and morphologic features can be defined, but the cause remains unknown. In the absence of definitive pathogenesis, logical treatment is difficult. Many drugs have been used empirically with varying claims of success, but the few placebo-controlled studies have failed to show any efficacy. Fortunately, the remarkable advances in reproductive biology are now being applied to male infertility. A variety of assisted reproductive techniques (ART) attempt to overcome the problems of reduced sperm motility and number. These procedures circumvent specific stages in the fertilization process without correcting the actual basis of the disorder. These techniques include intrauterine insemination (IUI), in vitro fertilization and embryo transfer (IVF-ET), and gamete intrafallopian tube transfer (GIFT). Recently, micromanipulation techniques have been developed that allow by-passing of further steps of fertilization by mechanically facilitating contact between sperm and oocyte. Intracytoplasmic sperm injection (ICSI), one form of micromanipulation, has been very successful in treating men with severe quantitative and qualitative disorders of spermatogenesis.[59,60] Successes are now being obtained in the ICSI technique both with epididymal and testicular-retrieved sperm.[61] In another advance, investigators have used immature sperm precursors (spermatids) for oocyte insemination.[62] Pregnancies also have been reported with this round spermatid nuclear injection (ROSNI) technique.[62,63]

## Miscellaneous

### Immotile Cilia Syndrome

In this condition, the sperm count is normal, but spermatozoa are completely nonmotile because of ultrastructural defects. The estimated prevalence of this condition is approximately 1 in 20,000. Kartagener's syndrome is a variant of immotile cilia syndrome and has a prevalence of 1 in 40,000. Electron microscopic examination of flagellar or ciliary axonemal structure is diagnostic of this syndrome.[8]

### Increased Semen Viscosity

This appears to be unrelated to the coagulation-liquefaction phenomenon and may signify accessory gland dysfunction. It often interferes with accurate assessment of sperm density and motility. It only becomes clinically relevant when there are but a few sperm in the postcoital test (PCT).

## Conclusion

Reproductive difficulties encountered by couples are receiving increased attention both in the news media and in medical literature. Several factors are responsible for this increasing awareness of infertility. The baby boom generation, born 1946 through 1964, has been delaying childbearing into the ages when their reproductive potential has decreased. Widespread availability and improved methods of contraception as well as increased numbers of abortions have decreased the number of babies available for adoption. Major advances in reproductive techniques are giving new avenues of hope for couples with diagnoses previously thought to be untreatable.

## References

1. Jaffe SB, Jewelewicz R. The basic infertility investigation. *Fertil Steril* 1991; 56:599–613.
2. McClure RD. Male Infertility. In: Tanagho E, McAninch J, eds. *Smith's General Urology*. 14th ed. New York: Appleton & Lange; 1995.
3. Kogan SJ. Cryptorchidism. In: Kelalis PP, King LR, Belman AB, eds. *Clinical Pediatric Urology*. Philadelphia: W.B. Saunders; 1985: 864–887.
4. Yavetz H, Harash B, Paz G, et al. Cryptorchidism: incidence and sperm quality in infertile men. *Andrologia* 1992; 24:293–297.
5. Werner CA. Mumps orchitis and testicular atrophy. *Ann Intern Med* 1950; 32:1066.
6. Nagler HM, Deitch AD, de Vere White R. Testicular torsion: temporal considerations. *Fertil Steril* 1984; 42:257–262.
7. Bronson R, Cooper G, Rosenfeld D. Sperm antibodies: their role in infertility. *Fertil Steril* 1984; 42:171–183.
8. Zamboni L. The ultrastructural pathology of the spermatozoon as a cause of infertility: the role of electron microscopy in the evaluation of semen quality. *Fertil Steril* 1987; 48:711–734.
9. Handelsman DJ, Conway AJ, Boylan LM, et al. Young's syndrome: obstructive azoospermia and chronic sinopulmonary infections. *N Engl J Med* 1984; 310:3–9.
10. Kaplan E, Shwachman H, Perlmutter AD, et al. Reproductive failure in mates with cystic fibrosis. *N Engl J Med* 1968; 279:65–69.
11. MacLeod J, Hotchkiss RS. The effects of hyperpyrexia on spermatozoa counts in men. *Endocrinology* 1941; 28:780.
12. Buch JP, Havlovec SK. Variation in sperm penetration assay related to viral illness. *Fertil Steril* 1991; 55:844–846.
13. Heller CG, Clermont Y. Kinetics of the germinal epithelium in man. *Recent Prog Horm Res* 1964; 20:545.

14. Whorton MD. Male occupational reproductive hazards. *West J Med* 1982; 137:521–524.
15. Oates RD, Lipshultz LI. Fertility and testicular function in patients after chemotherapy and radiotherapy. In: Lytton B, ed. *Advances in Urology*. Chicago: Yearbook Medical Publishers, 1989; 2:55–84.
16. Lipshultz LI, Ross CE, Whorton D, et al. Dibromochloropropane and its effect on testicular function in man. *J Urol* 1980; 124:464–468.
17. Sigman M, Lipshultz LI, Howards SS. Evaluation of the subfertile male. In: Lipshultz L, Howards SS, eds. *Infertility in the Male*. St. Louis: Mosby-Year Book; 1991:179–210.
18. Kolodny RC, Masters WH, Kolodner RM, et al. Depression of plasma testosterone levels after chronic intensive marijuana use. *N Engl J Med* 1974; 290:872–874.
19. Stillman RJ, Rosenberg MJ, Sachs BP. Smoking and reproduction. *Fertil Steril* 1986; 46:545–546.
20. Mendelson JH, Kuehnle J, Ellingbone J, et al. Plasma testosterone levels before, during, and after chronic marijuana smoking. *N Engl J Med* 1974; 291:1051–1055.
21. Smith CG, Asch RH. Drug abuse and reproduction. *Fertil Steril* 1987; 48:355–373.
22. Van Thiel DH, Lester R, Sherins RJ. Hypogonadism in alcoholic liver disease: evidence for a double defect. *Gastroenterology* 1974; 67:1188–1199.
23. Berul CI, Harclerode JE. Effects of cocaine hydrochloride on the male reproductive system. *Life Sci* 1989; 45:91–95.
24. Rock J, Robinson D. Effect of induced intrascrotal hyperthermia on testicular function in man. *Am J Obstet Gynecol*, 1965; 91:793.
25. Feldman P. Sexuality, birth control and childbirth in orthodox Jewish tradition. *Can Med Assoc J* 1992; 146:29–33.
26. Wilcox AJ, Weinberg CR, Baird DD. Timing of sexual intercourse in relation to ovulation: effects on the probability of conception, survival of pregnancy, and sex of the baby. *N Engl J Med* 1995; 333:1517–1521.
27. Whitehead ED, Leiter E. Genital abnormalities and abnormal semen analyses in male patients exposed to diethylstilbestrol in utero. *J Urol* 1981; 125:47–50.
28. Toth A. Reversible toxic effect of salicylazosulfapyridine on semen quality. *Fertil Steril* 1979; 31:538–540.

29. Griffin JE, Wilson JD. Disorders of the testes and male reproductive tract. In: Wilson JD, Foster DW, eds. *Textbook of Endocrinology*. 8th ed. Philadelphia: W.B. Saunders; 1991: 259–311.
30. Schlegel PN, Chang TSK, Marshall FF. Antibiotics: potential hazards to male fertility. *Fertil Steril* 1991; 55:235–242.
31. Swerdloff RS, Palacios A, McClure RD, et al. Male contraception: clinical assessment of chronic administration of testosterone enanthate. In: *Endocrine Approach to Male Contraception*. Copenhagen: Scriptor, 1978: 731–747.
32. Bardin CW, Paulsen CA. The testes. In: Wilson JD, Foster DW, eds. *Textbook of Endocrinology*. 6th ed. Philadelphia: W.B. Saunders; 1981: 293–354.
33. Griffin JE, Wilson ID. The syndromes of androgen resistance. *N Engl J Med* 1980; 302:198–209.
34. McClure RD. Endocrine investigation and therapy. *Urol Clin North Am* 1987; 14:471–488.
35. Carter JN, Tyson JE, Tolis G, et al. Prolactin-secreting tumors and hypogonadism in 22 men. *N Engl J Med* 1978; 299:847–852.
36. Lieblich JM, Rogol AD, White BJ, et al. Syndrome of anosmia with hypogonadotropic hypogonadism (Kallmann syndrome): clinical and laboratory studies in 23 cases. *Am J Med* 1982; 73:506–519.
37. Zachmann M, Prader A, Kind HP, et al. Testicular volume during adolescence. Cross-sectional and longitudinal studies. *Helv Paediatr Acta* 1974; 29:61–72.
38. Howards SS. Varicocele. *Infertil Reprod Med Clin North Am* 1992; 3:429–441.
39. World Health Organization. *Laboratory Manual for the Examination of Human Semen and Semen-Cervical Mucus Interaction*. Cambridge: Cambridge University Press; 1992.
40. Sherins RJ, Brightwell D, Sternthal PM. Longitudinal analysis of semen of fertile and infertile men. In: Troen P, Nankin HR, eds. *The Testis in Normal and Infertile Men*. New York: Raven Press; 1977: 473–488.
41. MacLeod J, Gold RZ. The male factor in fertility and infertility. *J Urol* 1951; 66:436.
42. Lipshultz LI, Witt MA, Grantmyre JE. Electroejaculation. *Infertil Reprod Med Clin North Am* 1992; 3:455–468.
43. Schlesinger MH, Wilets IF, Nagler HM. Treatment outcomes after varicocelectomy: a critical analysis. In: Lipshultz LI, ed. *Urologic Clinics of North America. Male Infertilty*. Philadelphia: W.B. Saunders, 1994; 21:517–529.

44. Rogers BJ. The sperm penetration assay: its usefulness reevaluated. *Fertil Steril* 1985; 43:821–940.

45. Bronson RA. Current concepts on the relation of antisperm antibodies and infertility. *Semin Reprod Endocrinol* 1988; 6:364.

46. Haas GG Jr. How should sperm antibody tests be used clinically? *Am J Reprod Immunol Microbiol* 1987; 15:106–111.

47. Ayvaliotis B, Bronson R, Rosenfeld D, et al. Conception rates in couples where autoimmunity to sperm is detected. *Fertil Steril* 1985; 43:739–742.

48. Clarke GN, Stofanoff A, Cauchi MN, et al. The immunoglobulin class of antispermatozoal antibodies in serum. *Am J Reprod Immunol Microbiol* 1985; 7:143–147.

49. Hellstrom WJG, Neal DE. Diagnosis and therapy of male genital tract infections. *Infertil Reprod Med Clin North Am* 1992; 3:399–411.

50. Bar-Chama N, Goluboff E, Fisch H. Infection and pyospermia in male infertility. Is it really a problem? *Urol Clin North Am* 1994; 21:469–475.

51. Wolf H, Poltich JA, Martinez A, et al. Leukocytospermia is associated with poor semen quality. *Fertil Steril* 1990; 53:528–534.

52. Berger RE, Smith WD, Critchlow CW, et al. Improvement in the sperm penetration (hamster ova) assay (SPA) results after doxycycline treatment of infertile men. *J Androl* 1983; 4:126–130.

53. Anderson DJ. Should male infertility patients be tested for leukocytospermia? *Fertil Steril* 1995; 63:246–248.

54. Politch JA, Wolff H, Hill JA, et al. Comparison of methods to enumerate white blood cells in semen. *Fertil Steril* 1993; 60:372–375.

55. Hellstrom WJ, Schachter J, Sweet RL, et al. Is there a role for *Chlamydia trachomatis* and genital *Mycoplasma* in male infertility? *Fertil Steril* 1987; 48:337–339.

56. Goldzieher JW, Dozier TS, Smith KD, et al. Improving the diagnostic reliability of rapidly fluctuating plasma hormone levels by optimized multiple-sampling techniques. *J Clin Endocrinol Metab* 1976; 43:824–830.

57. Segal S, Polishuk WZ, Ben-David M. Hyperprolactinemic male infertility. *Fertil Steril* 1976; 27:1425–1427.

58. Urban MD, Lee PA, Migeon CJ. Adult height and fertility in men with congenital virilizing adrenal hyperplasia. *N Engl J Med* 1978; 299:1392–1396.

59. Van Steirteghem AC, Liu J, Joris H, et al. Higher success rate by intracytoplasmic sperm injection than subzonal insemination. Report of a second series of 300 consecutive treatment cycles. *Hum Reprod* 1993; 8:1055–1060.

60. Tucker MJ, Wright G, Morton PC, et al. Practical evolution and application of direct intracytoplasmic sperm injection for male factor and idiopathic fertilization failure infertilities. *Fertil Steril* 1995; 63:820–827.

61. Nagy Z, Liu J, Cecile J, et al. Using ejaculated, fresh, and frozen-thawed epididymal and testicular spermatozoa gives rise to comparable results after intracytoplasmic sperm injection. *Fertil Steril* 1995; 63:808–815.

62. Sofikitis N, Miyagawa I, Sharlip I, et al. Human pregnancies achieved by intraooplasmic injections of round spermatid (RS) nuclei isolated from testicular tissue of azoospermic men. *J Urol* 1995; 153:320A (abstract; part 2).

63. Tesarik J, Mendoza C, Testart J. Viable embryos from injection of round spermatids into oocytes. *N Engl J Med* 1995; 333:525–526.

64. Singer C, Weiner WS. *Sexual Dysfunction: A Neuromedical Approach.* Armonk, NY: Futura; 1994.

# 3
# Semen Analysis and Other Tests for Male Infertility

James W. Overstreet

Semen analysis includes the basic laboratory tests for initial assessment of the male partner of an infertile couple. The basic semen evaluation provides the clinician not only with information on testicular function but also with evidence for patency of the reproductive tract and of the man's ability to ejaculate. Despite the basic importance of these tests, neither the methods for semen evaluation nor the criteria for interpretation of results have been fully standardized. These problems are well illustrated by the current controversy over the suggested decline in sperm counts worldwide during the past 50 years.[1–3] Scientific criticism has been based not only on the statistical methodology used in the original analysis but also on the realization that the methods for collection and analysis of semen have varied widely in the past five decades.[3] Although much progress has been made recently in the standardization of semen evaluation procedures, the results of previous studies must be evaluated carefully. Nevertheless, when infertility is suspected, a semen evaluation should be obtained at the initiation of the clinical workup.

## Standard Semen Evaluation, Specimen Collection, and Initial Assessment of Semen Properties

There may be significant variability in ejaculate quality from day to day.[4] Transient semen abnormalities may be caused by systemic infection, genitourinary infection, or any febrile illness. Therefore, one abnormal semen evaluation cannot be accepted as evidence of male subfertility. The number of semen evaluations required for assessment of male fertility potential depends on both the characteristics of the semen and the variability in semen parameters for a given individual. It is important to standardize the period of sexual abstinence prior to semen evaluation, because sexual activity also affects semen quality.[5] The period of abstinence before semen evaluation conventionally is set at 48 to 72 hours. However, it is important to recognize that frequent ejaculations may have different effects on men with abnormal semen as compared with those who have normal semen. For normospermic men, an ejaculation frequency of 24 hours or less can result in a decrease in semen volume, sperm concentration, and sperm motility.[6,7] In contrast, men with abnormal semen may experience either little change in semen quality[8] or an improvement in semen parameters with frequent ejaculation.[8,9] In some cases, it may be appropriate to evaluate the semen at the same interval that the couple has sexual intercourse.

The semen specimen may be collected by masturbation or with a semen collection condom.[10] Contraceptive condoms should not be used because most are spermicidal. Coitus interruptus also is not recommended for semen collection.[11] The laboratory should supply the container for semen collection, and quality control procedures should be followed to ensure that these containers are free of spermicidal activity. The laboratory should provide a private room for semen collection to avoid artifacts that may arise because of changes in the semen that may occur during transport from the home.

The semen evaluation may be as simple as a sperm count or may include a variety of sophisticated measurements. The parameters that are reported in most clinical evaluations include semen volume, number of sperm in the semen, and measurements of sperm motility and sperm morphology. In modern andrology laboratory practice, most semen parameters are measured objectively. Objective measurements can be made manually (e.g., with a counting chamber) or with computer-aided sperm analysis (CASA) systems. Even with automated CASA systems, rigorous technician training and quality control procedures are required to achieve precision in measurements of semen parameters.[12]

Following ejaculation, semen normally coagulates and remains clot-like for 15 to 30 minutes. Semen that does not liquefy within 1 hour should be considered abnormal.[13] As liquefaction takes place, the semen becomes more homogeneous, and in the final stages of liquefaction the semen is fluid with only small areas of coagulation remaining. Semen coagulation is different from semen viscosity, which is measured after the completion of liquefaction. In general, the semen viscosity should be considered abnormal if the semen is insufficiently fluid to flow into a counting chamber. Semen viscosity can be measured on a subjective scale of 0 (water-like) to 4 (gel-like), or more objective methods can be used.[14] If the semen is abnormally viscous, it may be necessary to reduce the viscosity by repeated aspiration through a 15-gauge blunt needle before further analysis can take place.

The semen should be evaluated as soon as possible after ejaculation and always within 1 hour of collection. Semen volume is measured to the nearest 0.1 ml using a 1-, 5-, or 10-ml serologic pipette. The specimen as a whole is examined for color and odor. It is normally opaque and gray-white in color; yellow, pink, or red coloration is abnormal. Abnormal odors, such as urine or putrefaction, should be noted.

Semen pH, measured with an instrument or with pH paper, is typically 7.2 to 7.8.[14]

## Microscopic Evaluation of Semen

### Sperm Motility

After the macroscopic characteristics of the semen are recorded, the specimen is evaluated microscopically. The semen is evaluated with phase-contrast microscopy at 37°C. Sperm motility is scored visually to determine the percentage of motile sperm and the characteristics of sperm progression. Percent motility is determined by evaluation of at least two different slide preparations. Sperm motility can be assessed in a commercially available counting chamber (see below), or a standardized slide preparation with a specified volume and coverslip can be used. Sperm are classified as motile if they have a moving flagellum, regardless of whether the sperm is progressive. One hundred sperm are scored on each slide to determine percentage of motility, and at least five microscopic fields per slide should be sampled. An ocular grid is a useful aid for standardizing the sample of sperm counted in each field. When the values for percentage of motility are compared for the two separate slides, the percentage of difference between the two values should be ≤10%. If the difference is greater than 10%, then a third slide should be prepared and counted. When two slides are counted, the mean value of the two percentages is reported; when three slides are counted, the median value is used. This procedure for counting multiple slides and comparing results between slides is an important internal quality control procedure in the visual evaluation of sperm motility.

Sperm progression also can be assessed visually. When the sperm population is given an overall rating, the precision of assessment cannot be as good as for percentage of motility. A common practice is to use a scale of 1 to 4: 1, no sperm progression; 2, sluggish-to-fair progression; 3, good progression; and 4, very vigorous forward progression. This evaluation also should be based on observations of at least five different fields in two preparations. In other protocols, better precision can be obtained by counting the percentage of progressive sperm in addition to the overall percent motility.[15] Some laboratories calculate a "sperm drive" based on sperm velocity as a measure of sperm progression.[16]

## Sperm Concentration

Sperm concentration is determined following dilution of the semen with a spermicidal solution. The number of sperm in the diluted semen is then estimated with a counting chamber, such as a hemocytometer,[17] a Makler chamber,[18] or a Microcell chamber.[19] Errors can occur during semen dilution, during chamber filling, or during sperm counting. Suspensions of latex beads of known concentration can be used for quality control of counting procedures.[20] In a recent comparative study, the Microcell chamber was found to be the most accurate and precise of the counting chambers for determining sperm concentrations.[21] Quality control of the dilution and counting procedures can be attained by routinely preparing and counting two separate dilutions of the specimen. When the difference in the sperm concentration as determined in the two dilutions is ≤10%, the mean value is reported. If the percentage of difference is greater than 10%, a third dilution is prepared and counted, and the median of the three values is reported.

CASA instruments also can be used to measure sperm concentration, and the Microcell chamber has been reported to be the most appropriate for this application.[21] It is important to recognize the limitations of CASA instruments for counting sperm. These instruments are particularly prone to error when the sperm concentration is very high or very low, or when there is sperm agglutination or seminal debris.[22] In such situations, a manual sperm count should always be performed.

## Sperm Agglutination

Sperm agglutination can be assessed using the same slide preparation as for motility assessment, and at least five microscopic fields (20× objective) should be scanned for this determination. Any motile sperm that is stuck to another sperm by the sperm head, midpiece, or tail is considered agglutinated. Immotile sperm clumps or motile sperm stuck to other cells or debris are not classified as agglutinated. The degree of agglutination can be scored on a scale of 0 to 3: 0, no agglutination; 1, one or fewer agglutination clumps per three or more microscopic fields; 2, one clump per one to two fields; and 3, one or more clumps in every field. Other scoring methods for agglutination may also be used.[23]

## Other Microscopic Observations

During microscopic observation of the semen, other unusual constituents should be noted, including epithelial cells, protozoa, bacteria, and round cells. Round cells are not necessarily leukocytes and many are prematurely exfoliated immature germ cells. The identity of round cells cannot be determined with phase contrast microscopy, but most round cells can be classified on a stained seminal smear (see below).

## Sperm Morphology

Sperm morphology is assessed subjectively on stained seminal smears. This semen parameter generally is measured with poor precision.[24] Reasons for high variability in results between laboratories include differences in slide preparation and staining, differences in technician proficiency, and differences in the interpretation and implementation of protocols.[24] Sperm morphology is commonly assessed on Papanicolaou-stained slides with bright-field oil-immersion optics. The percentage of "normal" spermatozoa on the slide is reported.

There is no widely accepted definition of the characteristics of a morphologically normal sperm. The classic descriptions of normal versus abnormal sperm were based on the visual perception of an oval-shaped head with regular contours, and a slender, straight midpiece and flagellum.[25,26] More recently, metric standards for sperm-head length and width have been proposed, but even these standards are controversial. Most clinical laboratories use some version of the World Health Organization (WHO) criteria.[15,27] More strict morphologic criteria can be used to define a normal sperm, with the result that more sperm are excluded from the normal category because of subtle abnormalities in head shape and staining properties.[28] Thus, semen from fertile men may have as few as 14% normal sperm by strict criteria,[28] in comparison with a 50% cutoff when the WHO criteria of 1987[27] are used. The situation has been further confused by the 1992 revisions of the WHO criteria that include new metric standards and stricter requirements for a normal classification; the recommended cutoff for normal sperm morphology with this new protocol is 30%.[15] These arbitrary cutoff points have not been established with comparative studies of semen from fertile and subfertile men. The value of any cutoff point is further reduced by the low precision of the morphology assessment. It was recently pointed out that given a coefficient of variation for repeated measures of 20% (rarely achieved for assessments of percent normal sperm), when the measured value is 50%, the true value for the measure will be between 30% and 70%.[29] Such uncertainty makes any sperm morphology cutoff point suspect.

Many morphology protocols also assign abnormal sperm to separate categories on the basis of structural abnormalities, but there is also no consensus on the definitions of abnormal sperm types. Electron microscopy has been used to enumerate the morphologic abnormalities of sperm,[30] but this approach is not widely used. There are only a few specific situations in which a knowledge of the types of abnormal sperm has proven useful in the clinical assessment of subfertile males. Sperm with a "round-head defect" have agenesis of the acrosome and are nonfunctional. This condition appears to be congenital, and when present in all sperm, the abnormality leads to complete sterility.[31] Tapered sperm are found more frequently in the semen of infertile men if they have a varicocele.[32] Epididymal dysfunction may be suspected when there is coiling of the sperm tail or other flagellar abnormalities.[33] Although concern is often expressed regarding the relationship of abnormal sperm morphology to abnormalities of pregnancy, there is no correlation between sperm morphology and sperm chromosomal complement,[34] nor is there any association between abnormal sperm morphology and recurrent spontaneous abortion.[35]

## Evaluation of Round Cells in Semen

The stained seminal smear also can be used to evaluate round cells. Most of these cells are likely to be either leukocytes or immature germinal cells, but definite identification of the cell type is not possible without special staining procedures, such as those that use monoclonal antibodies to leukocyte antigens.[36] For a less definitive assessment, seminal granulocytes can be counted in a hemocytometer following peroxidase staining.[15] Polymorphonuclear leukocytes can be recognized on a Papanicolaou-stained smear on the basis of nuclear morphology, and their concentration in semen can be estimated from the ratio of leukocytes to sperm cells on the seminal smear.[19]

## Automated Semen Analysis

CASA instruments are used routinely in many andrology laboratories. These instruments can be used to make precise measurements of sperm concentration, percent motility, and sperm movement characteristics.[37] Standardization of procedures and strict quality control are essential for obtaining reproducible results. Semen specimens with low sperm concentrations may not be accurately assessed by CASA because of misclassification of seminal debris as sperm cells. Similarly, semen with high sperm concentrations may prove difficult for CASA because sperm collisions that result in overlap of sperm trajectories are erroneously interpreted by the instrument. Therefore, it is recommended that semen specimens be diluted before CASA analysis when the sperm concentrations are greater than $50 \times 10^6$/ml.[22] More recently, a number of instruments have become available for automated sperm morphology assessment.[38] Such instruments are particularly attractive because of the poor precision that is generally attained when sperm morphology is assessed visually.[24] The major problem with current instruments is that they are not capable of assessing most midpiece and tail abnormalities.[38] Also, the time required to measure 100 sperm cells can be as long as 100 minutes.[38]

## Interpretation of Semen Parameters

Clinical criteria for distinguishing men with normal semen from men with subfertile semen are based on older studies that compared semen parameters in populations of fertile men and infertility patients.[39–41] Unfortunately, these studies did not use modern methods of semen analysis or strict quality control. Some prospective studies, in which semen parameters were used to predict fertility, have found that sperm numbers, sperm motility, and normal sperm morphology are correlated with the chance for conception.[42–44] These studies suggest that the results of semen evaluation have the potential to diagnose male subfertility. Nevertheless, until large-scale studies are carried out with contemporary laboratory methodology, the clinical application of semen analysis will remain limited to a more general categorization of patients.

The semen parameters can be used to classify sperm into the general categories of normal, marginal, or abnormal (Table 3.1). Because both large and small semen volumes have been associated with male infertility,[45] the range of normal semen volume (2.0 to 5.0 ml) has a lower and upper boundary. Interpretation of abnormal semen volume is often improved when the result of the postcoital test is known.[46] Large semen volumes may result in reduction

of the sperm density as a consequence of dilution. Small semen volumes may not have adequate buffering capacity in the acidic vagina. Either of these circumstances (low sperm density or inadequate buffer) would result in an abnormal postcoital test. Therefore, when the postcoital test is normal, semen volume can usually be discounted as a direct cause of male subfertility. Low semen volume still may be indicative of other clinical conditions, such as retrograde ejaculation or obstruction in the male reproductive tract.

The number of sperm in semen is often considered the most reliable parameter of semen quality. There is a biologic basis for this assumption because this is the most direct measurement of sperm production by the testis. This parameter is measured with greater precision in the manual semen evaluation than either sperm motility or morphology. Sperm concentration or sperm count is usually considered to be abnormal when the value is less than $20 \times 10^6$/ml,[47] although there is evidence that the more accurate cutoff point may be as low as $5 \times 10^6$/ml.[48] Sperm production by the testis is most accurately described by the total number of sperm in the ejaculate, calculated by multiplying the sperm concentration by the semen volume. The normal value for total sperm numbers is widely agreed to be $40 \times 10^6$ sperm per ejaculate.[15] Prospective studies have shown that this parameter is correlated with conception.[49] The likelihood that low sperm numbers are compatible with male fertility is suggested by reports of treatment failures with male contraceptive agents,[50] and by the well-known clinical condition of hypogonadal males being successfully treated with exogenous gonadotropins.[51] In both examples, fertile men may have very low numbers of sperm in their semen. Logic leads to the conclusion that men with low sperm counts may have additional defects in sperm function as the actual cause of their infertility (see below).

Several large prospective studies have shown that subjective measurements of sperm motility are correlated with fertility,[44,52,53] and recent studies have indicated that sperm motility data obtained by CASA also may be predictive of fertility.[49] However, reliable data with which to

TABLE 3.1. Classification of semen from the results of a standard semen evaluation.

| Semen parameter | Normal semen | Marginal semen | Abnormal semen |
|---|---|---|---|
| Semen volume (ml) | 2–5* | 1–2 | <1 |
| Sperm concentration ($\times 10^6$/ml) | 20–250* | 10–20 | <10 |
| Sperm motility (% motile) | >50 | 40–50 | <40 |
| Straight-line velocity (μm/s) | >25 | 20–25 | <20 |
| Sperm morphology (% normal) | >50 | 40–50 | <40 |

*Values that exceed the upper range of normal may result in classification of the semen as marginal or abnormal.

establish cutoff points for normal and abnormal sperm motility are lacking. The widely accepted value for the lower limit of percent motile sperm is 40% to 50% motile (Table 3.1). However, the data on sperm motility from older clinical studies[40,41,54] were obtained by subjective methods and may not be applicable for interpretation of contemporary motility parameters. CASA instruments can measure many parameters of sperm velocity,[55] and there are data to suggest that these measures of sperm progression may be correlated with fertility.[49,56] Ultimately, it may be possible by use of CASA data to calculate the probability of conception over a given time.[49] Until more definitive information is available, the cutoff point for normal sperm progression is a straight-line velocity of 25 $\mu$m/s.[57]

As previously discussed, the results obtained for sperm morphology assessment depend on the definition of a normal sperm, and there is still no consensus on this definition. Applying the original WHO criteria for normal sperm morphology,[27] the recommended cutoff point of 50% normal sperm is an indicator of normal semen quality (Table 3.1). Subjective assessment of sperm morphology is likely to result in considerable variation of results, both within and between technicians and laboratories.[58,59] The use of CASA instruments for sperm morphometry[38] will reduce this variability, but large, well-controlled clinical studies are still needed to determine a normal range of sperm-head sizes and shapes.

Sperm numbers, motility, and morphology must all be taken into account in assessing male fertility, but multiplication of individual parameters (e.g., semen volume $\times$ sperm concentration $\times$ percent motility) is no more predictive than single parameters alone.[48] The semen parameters can be used to assign patients to clinical categories,[19,60] but these categories are useful primarily for planning the future clinical workup. They cannot be considered reliable for predicting fertility, except in extreme cases. The following categories may be used: 1, semen quality within normal limits, no evidence for infertility; 2, marginal semen quality, infertility is possible; and 3, abnormal semen quality, in-

fertility is likely (Table 3.1). Assignment of patients to clinical categories is subjective because of the many unresolved issues regarding the methodology and interpretation of semen data as well as the normal variability in semen properties. When one or more semen parameters are abnormal or in the marginal range of values (for example, marginal sperm motility), the patient is usually assigned to the corresponding clinical category (in this case, marginal semen quality). Patients usually are assigned to the clinical category that reflects the poorest of the semen parameters recorded.

Because of normal variability, several semen evaluations may be required to correctly classify a patient. Normal semen quality should be confirmed by repeat evaluation, and three or more evaluations may be needed to classify some individuals. As previously discussed, the basic semen evaluation is an initial step in the fertility evaluation, and it indicates the appropriate direction of subsequent clinical workups for the infertile couple. A finding of marginal or abnormal semen quality should lead to a complete clinical evaluation of the male. When the semen quality is normal or even marginal, complete evaluation of the female is also warranted because there is a significant possibility that female factors are contributing to the couple's infertility.

## Specialized Laboratory Tests on Sperm

Semen evaluations often are followed by other specialized tests carried out to gain additional information on the functional capabilities of sperm. These tests may be indicated because of abnormal results on the standard semen evaluation or when there is normal semen but unexplained infertility. Although most of these tests have a strong foundation in basic science, their clinical application is hampered by many of the same problems that affect the routine semen evaluation, particularly a lack of standardization and the absence of rigorous assessment in controlled studies.

# Tests of Sperm Structures or Organelles

## Plasma Membrane Integrity

The sperm plasma membrane must be intact for sperm to reach the oocyte and complete the complex functions required for fertilization. The approaches for assessing the integrity of the sperm plasma membrane generally rely on the detection of a cytologic stain that is too large to enter the sperm unless the plasma membrane is disrupted. Sperm that exclude these vital stains are often called "viable" sperm, but sperm viability should not be confused with sperm motility. Abnormal semen may contain many cells that are viable yet immotile. Sperm with abnormalities of the flagellar structure[61] might be viable even though they lack the capability for flagellar movement. Conventional stains, such as eosin or trypan blue,[15] can be used for testing sperm viability. Fluorescent nuclear stains, such as the Hoechst dye 258 (H258), also have been used to assess sperm viability, often in combination with other cytologic probes.[62] Sperm viability is considered normal if more than 75% of the sperm exclude the vital dye.[15] Flow cytometry can be used for automated and objective assessment of sperm membrane integrity, and dual fluorescent staining technology has been applied for simultaneous assessment of both the plasma membrane and mitochondrial membrane integrity.[63]

The hypoosmotic swelling (HOS) test measures sperm viability without the use of vital dyes.[64] In this test, sperm are challenged with a hypoosmotic medium, and sperm membrane integrity is assessed by evaluation of osmotic function. Therefore, in addition to sperm viability, the HOS test is sensitive to other functions of the sperm membrane involved in transport of water. The normal value for this test is reached when more than 60% of the sperm tails swell in hypoosmotic medium; the test is abnormal if less than 50% swell.[64] A number of clinical studies have reported this to be a useful test in assessing male fertility.[64]

## Acrosomal Integrity and Function

The acrosome is a complex organelle of the sperm head that functions at the time of fertilization to enable sperm penetration of the oocyte cumulus and zona pellucida. The acrosome reaction must take place for sperm to fuse with the oolemma.[65] In rare fertility disorders, the acrosome may be completely missing from spermatozoa.[31] More commonly, the acrosome is present but is either nonfunctional or dysfunctional.[66]

The presence or absence of the acrosome can be evaluated most thoroughly with electron microscopy,[31] but cytologic techniques also can be used to visualize the acrosome with the light microscope. Conventional staining techniques have been used,[67] as well as fluoresceinated lectins[62] and monoclonal antibodies[68] that bind to acrosomal constituents. All of these techniques can be used to score the percentage of acrosome-reacted sperm. Because acrosomal loss may be a normal consequence of sperm death, most cytologic approaches employ a second supravital stain to identify viable, acrosome-reacted sperm.[62,67] A recently developed clinical diagnostic test uses monoclonal antibodies that are coated on immunobeads and can bind to acrosome-reacted sperm.[69] Aggregates of beads and motile, acrosome-reacted sperm can be identified microscopically.

Acrosomal function is evaluated with bioassays, such as tests of sperm–zona pellucida interaction or sperm penetration assays (SPA), using zona-free hamster oocytes (see below). Another approach is to treat sperm with chemical or biologic agonists of the acrosome reaction, and then observe the presence or absence of acrosome reactions using one of the tests discussed above. These agonists include the calcium ionophore A23187,[70] progesterone,[71] human follicular fluid,[72] human cumulus oophorus,[73] or human zona pellucida.[74] No cutoff points for male infertility have been established with these acrosomal function tests, although many have been used to screen for normal fertilizing capacity prior to assisted reproduction technology (ART) procedures.

## Hyperactivated Motility

Prior to fertilization, spermatozoa must undergo a physiologic change termed *capacitation*, which involves alterations of the sperm surface and other changes in the subcellular compartments of the cell.[65] Capacitation is a prerequisite for the acrosome reaction and also for a specialized type of movement called hyperactivated motility.[75] Hyperactivation is a marker for capacitation and may be required specifically for sperm transport through the fallopian tube and for penetration of the oocyte investments.[75] Hyperactivated motility of human sperm is characterized by an increase in flagellar amplitude and a decrease in the linearity of the sperm swimming trajectory. Hyperactivation can be measured manually[76] or with CASA instruments.[77] There is some evidence that hyperactivated motility may be abnormal in sperm of subfertile men,[78] but there are no data to establish normal values for this sperm function.

## Bioassays of Sperm Function

These laboratory tests use reproductive tract cells or secretions from humans or animals or both to assess functions of the sperm cell required for fertility. The sperm functions being evaluated are complex, and some are not well understood at the basic cell biology level. Therefore, interpretation of the test results is often empirical. As with any bioassay, the tests are not well standardized; therefore, quality control has proven difficult. However, these tests have been shown to be useful diagnostic tools for assessing sperm function. It is likely that in the future many of the bioassays will be replaced with specific tests, such as the tests of acrosomal function described previously.

### Sperm–Cervical Mucus Interaction

The most basic test of sperm–cervical mucus interaction is the postcoital test (PCT). This test assesses the capability of sperm to enter the cervix and to survive in cervical mucus for a number of hours.[46] The PCT measures interaction between the sperm and the female tract, so abnormal female reproductive function may result in abnormal findings. There are many versions of this test, and there is no consensus on the method for the PCT or the interpretation of results.[46] However, prospective studies have suggested that the results of the PCT are closely related to the probability of a couple's conceiving.[43,44,79]

Laboratory tests of sperm–cervical mucus interaction are usually performed in follow-up to an abnormal PCT. These tests address the cause of sperm–cervical mucus incompatibility[46] and involve observations of sperm interaction with cervical mucus in vitro. The methodology for these tests varies widely. Sperm–mucus interaction can be observed on a microscope slide[80] or in capillary tubes.[81,82] The tests require use of normal, midcycle cervical mucus, so that female factors will not confound the assay results. Many of the sperm functions that are assessed in these tests involve sperm motility, which is required both for entry into mucus and for progression through mucus.[83] In addition, normal interaction between the sperm surface and the cervical mucus macromolecules is necessary for a normal test result.[84] The presence of antisperm antibodies on the sperm surface is usually revealed in tests of sperm–cervical mucus interaction,[85] although specific tests for antisperm antibodies are required to make the diagnosis. There are no widely accepted values for normal sperm–cervical mucus interaction tests although standard protocols have been published.[15]

### Sperm Penetration Assay (SPA) with Zona-Free Hamster Oocytes

The SPA is possible because the zona pellucida of the golden hamster oocyte is the primary block to interspecies fertilization.[86] When the zona is removed from hamster oocytes in the laboratory, human sperm can fuse with the plasma membrane of the oocyte and decondense in the ooplasm.[86] This event, in itself, is required for fertilization, but sperm-oocyte fusion also requires a number of other functions of the sperm cell, including capacitation and the acrosome reaction.[65] It seems logical, therefore, that a single bioassay that measures so many fertilization-related sperm functions would have clinical value in identifying subfertile males. Nevertheless, the SPA has been a controversial test since its inception in 1976,[86] and there is still no consensus either on the best methodology for a clinical assay or on the interpretation of the SPA results.[87]

It is now generally recognized that many subfertile men can have normal SPA results (so-called false-positive results), because a number of important sperm functions including sperm transport to the oocyte and sperm penetration of the oocyte investments are not measured by the assay.[88] A negative result with the assay (no oocytes penetrated) should be diagnostic of male subfertility, yet a high incidence of false-negative results has been reported in some studies.[89] The occurrence of false-negative SPA results has been attributed to biologic variation in the in vitro capacitation requirements of sperm from different men.[87] This problem has been obviated by use of calcium ionophore to induce acrosome reactions, thereby eliminating differences between men in the occurrence of capacitation-mediated, spontaneous acrosome reactions. The results obtained with this version of the SPA correlate with fertility.[90]

An important methodologic problem that must be addressed in all bioassays is the requirement for appropriate laboratory quality control. In the case of the SPA, frozen human semen from fertile donors has been used for quality control. A high degree of precision and low interassay variability have both been reported for the SPA when this approach was used.[91]

The SPA also has been widely used as a screening tool for in vitro fertilization (IVF) programs. The same methodologic problems must be addressed when the SPA is used in this context, and in some studies the test has proven valuable in predicting the results of IVF.[92,93] Results of the SPA also can be used to devise modifications of sperm preparations and IVF conditions for subfertile semen.[94]

### Sperm–Zona Pellucida Interaction

Tests of sperm–zona pellucida interaction are used less frequently than the SPA because they require zonae pellucidae of human oocytes, which are much less plentiful than hamster oocytes. These assays, like the SPA, provide information on sperm functions required for fertilization. Zona pellucida assays can be used to assess sperm capacitation and the acrosome reaction as well as specific functions, such as sperm binding to the zona and sperm penetration through the zona. The specific functions measured are complementary to those measured in the SPA, and in some experimental studies the assays have been used together as a mixed gamete assay.[66]

These assays are used primarily to predict IVF success, and the hemizona assay (HZA) is the most widely used test of this type. This bioassay uses bisected zonae pellucidae to compare the sperm–zona binding capability of a patient's sperm (which are incubated with one hemizona) with sperm from a fertile control sample (which are incubated with the other hemizona).[95] For each hemizona pair, a hemizona index (HZI) is calculated from the ratio of the number of patient sperm bound and the number of control sperm bound. Receiver operating characteristics (ROC) analysis has been used to determine diagnostic cutoff points for the HZA.[96] Other sperm–zona binding assays used clinically measure sperm binding to whole zonae.[97] False-positive results with these assays can be expected because only a limited number of sperm functions are measured.

## Biochemical Tests of Sperm Functions

The seminal plasma is a highly complex biologic fluid, and there are numerous biochemical tests that have been employed to characterize its properties.[98] Relatively little is known of the biologic functions of the seminal fluid, and this lack of information has limited the clinical value of these tests. Nevertheless, the WHO laboratory manual[15] lists measurements of α-glucosidase, zinc, citric acid, acid phosphatase, and fructose as optional tests, and the manual provides normal values for each of these measurements.

There are also components of the sperm cell that can be measured biochemically and that may have clinical relevance. Acrosin is an intraacrosomal, trypsin-like enzyme that may have functions in sperm–zona binding and in sperm penetration of the zona pellucida.[65] There is also some evidence that this enzyme may be involved in sperm–oolemma interaction.[99] Clinical studies have demonstrated that acrosin activity is lower in sperm samples from infertile men as compared with those of fertile men.[100–102] Similar differences from normal sperm have been noted in sperm samples that failed to fertilize oocytes during IVF.[103,104] Adenosine triphosphate (ATP) also has been investigated as a marker for sperm fertility, but its clinical value is controversial.[105]

One of the most promising biochemical tests under current investigation is the measurement of sperm creatine kinase (CK). Clinical studies have demonstrated an inverse correlation between per-sperm CK activity and sperm concentrations, as well as a lower CK activity in sperm selected by swim-up as compared with unselected sperm in the total ejaculate.[106,107] In men with oligospermia who were fertile, the per-sperm CK activities were significantly different from those of men with oligospermia who did not produce a pregnancy.[108] Immunohistochemical studies showed that high CK-staining intensity was found in sperm with abnormal structure, and it was concluded that CK is a marker for a defect in spermatogenesis that is characterized by incomplete cytoplasmic extrusion from sperm.[109] Investigation of the isoforms of CK in sperm led to the conclusion that the percentage of M (muscle) type of CK increases and the percentage of B (brain) type of CK decreases as cytoplasmic extrusion becomes more complete.[110] The ratio of the CK isoforms has been shown to be predictive of IVF success.[111]

Another contemporary approach for prediction of the fertilizing capacity of semen samples focuses on measurements of the biochemical properties of individual sperm cells. Studies of sperm membrane components involved in zona pellucida recognition have focused on the capability of sperm to bind mannose, a saccharide believed to be critical for human sperm–zona interaction.[112] Using a fluoresceinated, mannosylated, neoglycoprotein probe, Benoff et al[113] demonstrated mannose-specific receptors

on the surface of capacitated human sperm and a reduced expression of these receptors on sperm that failed to fertilize oocytes in vitro. This laboratory approach for assessing sperm function also may be useful in identifying subfertile men with fertilization failure in vivo.[114]

## Conclusion

For many years, clinicians and laboratory scientists have worked to develop methods for assessing male fertility by evaluations of semen. In spite of this substantial effort, the goal of accurate male fertility prediction has not been reached. The biologic and technical problems that have limited progress in this area have been discussed in detail by Amann and Hammerstedt.[115] They point to the heterogeneous nature of the ejaculate, which contains sperm in different stages of maturity and probably with different functional capabilities. The mean values of any semen parameters, therefore, are unlikely to describe the sperm that reach and fertilize the oocyte.

The spermatozoon undergoes a continuous process of change that begins during spermatogenesis and continues in the female reproductive tract. Reasonable hope exists that abnormalities of the sperm that occur in the male tract will be detected with appropriate tests on semen. There is less likelihood that abnormalities expressed or induced in the female tract will be detected by tests on seminal sperm. The fact that so many cases of male subfertility can be successfully treated with ART suggests that such postejaculatory sperm dysfunctions are important causes of human reproductive failure.

Jeyendran and Zaneveld[116] have argued that it is important to develop the widest possible array of sperm function tests, providing different tests to measure activities of different sperm organelles. The true measure of the sperm's fertilizing capability is the "combined effective amount" of functional attributes associated with these organelles.[115] Neither the number of sperm attributes required for fertility nor the level of their expression has been determined. Therefore, any battery of contemporary test results on sperm that are "normal" will have limited clinical value because other, unrecognized attributes of the sperm cells may still be defective.[115,116] Only true abnormal tests can be considered definitive proof of male infertility.[115,116] The definition of an abnormal test is critical for this classification, and for every test a cutoff point must be selected, below which fertility rarely occurs. When the outcome to be predicted is fertilization of oocytes in vitro, then IVF data are appropriate for these analyses. However, when prediction of male infertility with natural coitus is the goal, data from populations of untreated couples with normal female partners must be studied. In many cases, these fertility data are available only in animal models, and extrapolation of results between species must be carried out.[115] A major challenge for clinical investigators is to develop comparable databases for human populations.

# References

1. Carlson E, Giwercman A, Keiding N, et al. Evidence for decreasing quality of semen during past 50 years. *Br Med J* 1992; 305:609–613.
2. Stone R. Environmental estrogens stir debate. *Science* 1994; 265:308–310.
3. Olsen GW, Bodner KM, Ramlow JM, et al. Have sperm counts been reduced 50 percent in 50 years? A statistical model revisited. *Fertil Steril* 1995; 63:887–893.
4. Overstreet JW. Assessment of disorders of spermatogenesis. In: Lockey JW, Lemasters GK, Keye WR, eds. *Reproduction: The New Frontier in Occupational and Environmental Health Research*. New York: Alan Liss; 1984: 275–292.
5. Swartz D, Laplanche A, Jouannet P, et al. Within subject variabilities of human semen in regard to sperm count, volume, total number of spermatozoa and length of abstinence. *J Reprod Fertil* 1979; 57:391–395.
6. Oldereid NB, Gordeladze JO, Kirkhus B, et al. Human sperm characteristics during frequent ejaculation. *J Reprod Fertil* 1984; 71:135–140.
7. Levin RM, Latimore J, Wein AJ, et al. Correlation of sperm count with frequency of ejaculation. *Fertil Steril* 1990; 54:906–909.
8. Baker HWG, Burger HG, de Kretser DM, et al. Factors affecting the variability of semen analysis results in infertile men. *Int J Androl* 1981; 4:609–622.
9. Tur-Kaspa I, Maor Y, Levran D, et al. How often should infertile men have intercourse to achieve conception? *Fertil Steril* 1994; 62:370–375.
10. Zavos PM. Seminal parameters of ejaculates collected from oligospermic and normospermic patients via masturbation and at intercourse with the use of a Silastic seminal fluid collection device. *Fertil Steril* 1985; 44:517–520.
11. Zavos PM, Kofinas GD, Sofikitis NV, et al. Differences in seminal parameters in specimens collected via intercourse and incomplete intercourse (coitus interruptus). *Fertil Steril* 1988; 61:1174–1176.
12. Holt W, Watson P, Curry M, et al. Reproducibility of computer-aided semen analysis: comparison of five different systems used in a practical workshop. *Fertil Steril* 1994; 62:1277–1282.
13. Overstreet JW. Semen liquefaction and viscosity problems. In: Tanagho EA, Lue TF, McClure RD, eds. *Contemporary Management of Impotence and Infertility*. Baltimore: Williams & Wilkins; 1988: 311–312.
14. Eliasson R. Analysis of semen. In: Behrman SJ, Kistner RW, eds. *Progress in Infertility*. 2nd ed. Boston: Little, Brown; 1975: 691–713.
15. World Health Organization. *WHO Laboratory Manual for the Examination of Human Semen and Sperm-Cervical Mucus Interaction*. 3rd ed. Cambridge, England: Press Syndicate of the University of Cambridge; 1992.
16. Zanaveld LJD, Jeyendran RS. Modern assessment of semen for diagnostic purposes. *Sem Reprod Endocrinol* 1988; 6:324–337.
17. Freund M, Carol B. Factors affecting hemocytometer counts of sperm concentration in human semen. *J Reprod Fertil* 1964; 8:149–155.
18. Makler A. The improved ten-micrometer chamber for rapid sperm count and motility evaluation. *Fertil Steril* 1980; 33:337–338.
19. Overstreet JW, Davis RO, Katz DF. Semen evaluation. *Infertil Reprod Med Clin North Am* 1992; 3:329–340.
20. Peters AJ, Zaneveld LJD, Jeyendran RS. Quality assurance for sperm concentration using latex beads. *Fertil Steril* 1993; 60:702–705.
21. Johnson JE, Boone WR, Blackhurst DW. Manual versus computer-automated semen

analyses. Part 1. Comparison of counting chambers. *Fertil Steril* 1996; 65:150–155.
22. Davis RO, Katz DF. Operational standards for CASA instruments. *J Androl* 1993; 14:385–394.
23. Mortimer D. The male factor in infertility: semen analysis. *Curr Probl Obstet Gynecol* 1985; 8:4–87.
24. Davis RO, Gravance CG. Consistency of sperm morphology classification methods. *J Androl* 1994; 15:83–89.
25. Freund M. Standards for the rating of human sperm morphology: a cooperative study. *Int J Fertil* 1966; 11:97–118.
26. Eliasson R. Standards for investigation of human semen. *Andrologia* 1971; 3:49–52.
27. World Health Organization. *WHO Manual for the Examination of Human Semen and Semen-Cervical Mucus Interaction*. 2nd ed. Cambridge, England: Press Syndicate of the University of Cambridge; 1987.
28. Menkveld R, Stander FSH, Lotze TJ, et al. The evaluation of morphological characteristics of human spermatozoa according to stricter criteria. *Hum Reprod* 1990; 5:586–592.
29. Davis RO, Gravance CG, Overstreet JW. A standardized test for visual analysis of human sperm morphology. *Fertil Steril* 1995; 63:1058–1063.
30. Baccetti B, Bernieri G, Burrini AG, et al. Notulae Seminologicae. 5. Mathematical evaluation of interdependent submicroscopic sperm alterations. *J Androl* 1995; 16:356–367.
31. Zamboni L. Sperm ultrastructural pathology as a cause of infertility. In: Asch RH, Balmaceda JP, Johnston I, eds. *Gamete Physiology*. Norwell, MA: Serono Symposia, USA; 1990: 119–126.
32. Naftulin BN, Samuels SJ, Hellstrom WJG, et al. Semen quality in varicocele patients is characterized by tapered sperm cells. *Fertil Steril* 1991; 56:149–151.
33. Pelfrey RJ, Overstreet JW, Lewis EL. Abnormalities of sperm morphology in cases of persistent infertility after vasectomy reversal. *Fertil Steril* 1982; 28:112–114.
34. Rosenbusch B, Strehler E, Sterzik K. Cytogenetics of human spermatozoa: correlations with sperm morphology and age of fertile men. *Fertil Steril* 1992; 58:1071–1072.
35. Hill JA, Abbott AF, Politch JA. Sperm morphology and recurrent abortion. *Fertil Steril* 1994; 61:776–778.
36. Wolff H, Anderson DJ. Immunohistologic characterization and quantitation of leukocyte

subpopulations in human semen. *Fertil Steril* 1988; 49:497–504.
37. Davis RO, Katz DF. Standardization and comparability of CASA instruments. *J Androl* 1992; 13:81–86.
38. Garrett C, Baker HWG. A new fully automated system for the morphometric analysis of human sperm heads. *Fertil Steril* 1995; 63:1306–1317.
39. MacLeod J, Gold RZ. Semen quality in 1000 men of known fertility and 800 cases of infertile marriage. *Fertil Steril* 1951; 2:115–139.
40. Rehan NE, Sobrero AJ, Fertig JW. The semen of fertile men: statistical analysis of 1300 men. *Fertil Steril* 1975; 26:492–502.
41. Zuckerman Z, Rodriguez-Rigau LJ, Smith KD, et al. Frequency distribution of sperm counts in fertile and infertile males. *Fertil Steril* 1977; 28:1310–1313.
42. Dunphy BC, Neal LM, Cooke ID. The clinical value of conventional semen analysis. *Fertil Steril* 1989; 51:324–329.
43. Glazener CMA, Kelly NJ, Weir MJA, et al. The diagnosis of male infertility. A prospective time-specific study of conception rates related to seminal analysis and postcoital sperm-mucus penetration and survival in otherwise unexplained infertility. *Hum Reprod* 1987; 2:665–671.
44. Eimers JM, te Velde ER, Gerritse R, et al. The prediction of the chance to conceive in subfertile couples. *Fertil Steril* 1994; 61:44–52.
45. Dubin L, Amelar RD. Etiologic factors in 1294 consecutive cases of male infertility. *Fertil Steril* 1971; 22:169.
46. Boyers S. Evaluation and treatment of disorders of the cervix. In: Keye WR, Chang RJ, Rebar RW, Soules MR, eds. *Infertility Evaluation and Treatment*. Philadelphia: W.B. Saunders; 1995: 195–229.
47. MacLeod J, Wang Y. Male fertility potential in terms of semen quality: a review of the past, a study of the present. *Fertil Steril* 1979; 21:103–116.
48. Peng H-Q, Collins JA, Wilson EH, et al. Receiver-operating characteristics curves for semen analysis variables: methods for evaluation of diagnostic tests of male gamete function. *Gamete Res* 1987; 17:229–236.
49. Barratt CLR, Tomlinson MJ, Cooke ID. Prognostic significance of computerized motility analysis for in vivo fertility. *Fertil Steril* 1993; 60:520–525.

50. Wallace EM, Aitken RJ, Wu FCW. Residual sperm function in oligozoospermia induced by testosterone enanthate administered as a potential steroid male contraceptive. *Int J Androl* 1992; 15:416–424.

51. Burris AS, Clark RV, Vantman DJ, et al. A low sperm concentration does not preclude fertility in men with isolated hypogonadotropic hypogonadism after gonadotropin therapy. *Fertil Steril* 1988; 50:343–347.

52. Bostofte E, Bagger P, Michael A, et al. Fertility prognosis for infertile men: results of follow-up study of semen analysis in infertile men from two different populations evaluated by the Cox regression model. *Fertil Steril* 1990; 54:1100–1106.

53. Barratt CLR, Macleod ID, Dunphy BC, et al. Prognostic significance of two putative sperm function tests: hypoosmotic swelling and bovine sperm mucus penetration test (Penetrak). *Hum Reprod* 1992; 7:1240–1244.

54. MacLeod J, Gold RZ. The male factor in fertility and infertility. III. An analysis of motile activity in the spermatozoa of 1000 fertile men and 1000 men in infertile marriage. *Fertil Steril* 1951; 2:187–204.

55. Boyers SP, Davis RO, Katz DF. Automated semen analysis. *Curr Probl Obstet Gynecol Fertil* 1989; 12:165–200.

56. Marshburn PB, McIntire D, Carr BR, et al. Spermatozoal characteristics from fresh and frozen donor semen and their correlation with fertility outcome after intrauterine insemination. *Fertil Steril* 1992; 58: 179–186.

57. Davis RO. The promise and pitfalls of computer-aided sperm analysis. *Infertil Reprod Med Clin North Am* 1992; 3:341–352.

58. Baker HWG, Clarke GN. Sperm morphology: consistency of assessment of the same sperm by different observers. *Clin Reprod Fertil* 1987; 5:37–43.

59. Dunphy BC, Kay R, Barratt CLR, et al. Quality control during the conventional analysis of semen, an essential exercise. *J Androl* 1986; 10:378–385.

60. Clark RV, Sherins RJ. Use of semen analysis in the evaluation of the infertile couple. In: Santen RJ, Swerdloff RS, eds. *Male Reproductive Dysfunction.* New York: Marcel Dekker; 1986: 253–266.

61. Baccetti B, Burrini AG, Pallini V. Spermatozoa and cilia lacking axoneme in an infertile man. *Andrologia* 1980; 12:525–532.

62. Cross NL, Morales P, Overstreet JW, et al. Two simple methods for detecting acrosome-reacted human sperm. *Gamete Res* 1986; 15:213–226.

63. Evenson DP, Darzynkiewicz Z, Melamed MR. Simultaneous measurement by flow cytometry of sperm cell viability and mitochondrial membrane potential related to cell motility. *J Histochem Cytochem* 1982; 30:279–280.

64. Zanaveld LJD, Jeyendran RS. Sperm function tests. *Infertil Repro Med Clin North Am* 1992; 3:353–371.

65. Yanagimachi R. Mammalian fertilization. In: Knobil E, Neill J, eds. *The Physiology of Reproduction.* 2nd ed. New York: Raven Press; 1994: 189–317.

66. Overstreet JW, Yanagimachi R, Katz DF, et al. Penetration of human spermatozoa into the human zona pellucida and zona-free hamster egg—a study of fertile donors and infertile patients. *Fertil Steril* 1980; 33:534–542.

67. Talbot P, Chacon RS. A new procedure for rapidly scoring acrosome reaction of human sperm. *Gamete Res* 1980; 3:211–216.

68. Wolf DP, Boldt J, Byrd W, et al. Acrosomal status evaluation in human ejaculated sperm with monoclonal antibodies. *Biol Reprod* 1985; 32:1157–1162.

69. Ohashi K, Saji F, Kato M, et al. Acrobeads test: a new diagnostic test for assessment of the fertilizing capacity of human spermatozoa. *Fertil Steril* 1995; 63:625–630.

70. Cummins JM, Pember SM, Jequier AM, et al. A test of the human sperm acrosome parameters. *J Androl* 1991; 12:98–103.

71. Falsetti C, Baldi E, Krausz C, et al. Decreased responsiveness to progesterone of spermatozoa in oligozoospermic patients. *J Androl* 1993; 14:17–22.

72. Calvo L, Vantman D, Banks SM, et al. Follicular fluid-induced acrosome reaction distinguishes a subgroup of men with unexplained infertility not identified by semen analysis. *Fertil Steril* 1989; 52:1048–1054.

73. Tesarik J. Comparison of acrosome reaction-inducing activities of human cumulus oophorus, follicular fluid and ionophore A23187 in human sperm populations of proven fertilizing ability in vitro. *J Reprod Fertil* 1985; 74:383–388.

74. Cross NL, Morales P, Overstreet JW, et al. Induction of acrosome reactions by the human zona pellucida. *Biol Reprod* 1988; 38:235–244.

75. Katz DF, Davis RO, Drobnis EZ, et al. Sperm motility measurement and hyperactivation. *Semin Reprod Endocrinol* 1993; 11:27–39.

76. Burkman LJ. Discrimination between non-hyperactivated and classical hyperactivated motility patterns in human spermatozoa using computerized analysis. *Fertil Steril* 1991; 55:363–371.

77. Hurrowitz EH, Leung A, Wang C. Evaluation of the CellTrak computer-assisted sperm analysis system in comparison to the Cellsoft system to measure human sperm hyperactivation. *Fertil Steril* 1995; 64:427–432.

78. Wang C, Leung A, Tsoi WL, et al. Evaluation of human sperm hyperactivated motility and its relationship with the zona-free hamster oocyte sperm penetration assay. *J Androl* 1991; 12:253–257.

79. Hull MGR, Savage PE, Bromhan DR. Prognostic value of the post-coital test: prospective study based on time-specific conception rates. *Br J Obstet Gynecol* 1982; 89:299–305.

80. Moghissi KS. Cyclic changes of cervical mucus in normal and progestin-treated women. *Fertil Steril* 1966; 17:663–675.

81. Katz DF, Overstreet JW, Hanson FW. A new quantitative test for sperm penetration into cervical mucus. *Fertil Steril* 1980; 33:179–186.

82. Pandya IJ, Mortiner D, Sawers RS. A standardized approach for evaluating the penetration of human spermatozoa into cervical mucus in vitro. *Fertil Steril* 1986; 45:357–360.

83. Feneux D, Serres C, Jouannet P. Sliding spermatozoa: a dyskinesia responsible for human infertility? *Fertil Steril* 1985; 44:508–511.

84. Overstreet JW, Katz DF, Yudin AI. Cervical mucus and sperm transport in reproduction. *Semin Perinatol* 1991; 15:149–155.

85. Kremer J, Jager J. The sperm-cervical mucus contact test: a preliminary report. *Fertil Steril* 1976; 27:335–340.

86. Yanagimachi R, Yanagimachi H, Rogers BJ. The use of zona-free animal ova as a system for the assessment of the fertilizing capacity of human spermatozoa. *Biol Reprod* 1976; 15:471–476.

87. Aitken J. On the future of the hamster oocyte penetration assay. *Fertil Steril* 1994; 62:17–19.

88. Gould JE, Overstreet JW, Yanagimachi H, et al. What functions of the sperm cell are measured by in vitro fertilization of zona-free hamster eggs? *Fertil Steril* 1983; 40:344–352.

89. O'Shea DL, Odem RR, Cholewa C, et al. Long-term follow-up of couples after hamster egg penetration testing. *Fertil Steril* 1993; 60:1040–1045.

90. Aitken RJ, Irvine DS, Wu FC. Prospective analysis of sperm-oocyte fusion and reactive oxygen species generation as criteria for the diagnosis of infertility. *Am J Obstet Gynecol* 1991; 164:542–551.

91. Johnson A, Bassham B, Lipshultz LI, et al. A quality control system for the optimized sperm penetration assay. *Fertil Steril* 1995; 64:832–837.

92. Aitken RJ, Thatcher S, Glasier AF, et al. Relative ability of modified versions of the hamster oocyte penetration test, incorporating hyperosmotic medium or the ionophore A23187, to predict IVF outcome. *Hum Reprod* 1987; 2:227–231.

93. Inoue M. Assessment of male fertility potential by zona-free hamster egg sperm penetration test. *J Assist Reprod Genet* 1993; 10:27.

94. Muller CH. The andrology laboratory in an assisted reproductive technologies program. *J Androl* 1992; 13:349–360.

95. Burkman LJ, Coddington CC, Franken DR, et al. The hemizona assay (HZA): development of a diagnostic test for the binding of human spermatozoa to the human hemizona pellucida to predict fertilization potential. *Fertil Steril* 1988; 49:688–697.

96. Coddington CC, Oehninger SC, Olive DL, et al. Hemizona index (HZI) demonstrates excellent predictability when evaluating sperm fertilizing capacity in in vitro fertilization patients. *J Androl* 1994; 15:250–254.

97. Liu DY, Lopata A, Leung A, et al. A human sperm–zona pellucida binding test using oocytes that failed to fertilize in vitro. *Fertil Steril* 1988; 50:782–788.

98. Glezerman MG, Bartoov B. Semen analysis. In: Insler V, Lunenfeld B, eds. *Infertility*. New York: Churchill Livingstone; 1986: 243–271.

99. Francavilla F, Romano R, Gabriele AR, et al. Impaired hamster egg penetration by human sperm from ejaculates with low acrosin activity but otherwise normal. *Fertil Steril* 1994; 61:735–740.

100. Goodpasture JC, Zavos PM, Cohen MR, et al. Relationship of human sperm acrosin and proacrosin to semen parameters. I. Comparison between symptomatic men of infertile couples and asymptomatic men, and between different split ejaculates. *J Androl* 1982; 3:151–156.

101. Mohsenian M, Syner FN, Moghissi KS. A study of sperm acrosin in patients with unexplained infertility. *Fertil Steril* 1982; 37:223–229.

102. Koukoulis G, Vantman D, Banks SM, et al. Low acrosin activity in a subgroup of men with idiopathic infertility does not correlate with sperm density, percent motility, curvilinear velocity, or linearity. *Fertil Steril* 1989; 52:120–127.

103. Kennedy WP, Kaminski JM, Van der Ven HH, et al. A simple, clinical assay to evaluate the acrosin activity of human spermatozoa. *J Androl* 1989; 10:221–231.

104. Tummon IS, Yuzpe AA, Daniel SAJ, et al. Total acrosin activity correlates with fertility potential after fertilization in vitro. *Fertil Steril* 1991; 56:933–938.

105. Irvine DS, Aitkin RJ. The value of adenosine triphosphate (ATP) measurements in assessing the fertilizing ability of human spermatozoa. *Fertil Steril* 1985; 44:806–813.

106. Huszar G, Corrales M, Vigue L. Correlation between sperm creatine phosphokinase activity and sperm concentrations in normospermic and oligospermic men. *Gamete Res* 1988; 19:67–75.

107. Huszar G, Vigue L, Corrales M. Sperm creatine phosphokinase activity as a measure of sperm quality in normospermic, variable spermic and oligospermic men. *Biol Reprod* 1988; 38:1061–1066.

108. Huszar G, Vigue L, Corrales M. Sperm creatine kinase activity in fertile and infertile oligospermic men. *J Androl* 1990; 11:40–46.

109. Huszar G, Vigue L. Incomplete development of human spermatozoa is associated with increased creatine phosphokinase and abnormal morphology. *Mol Reprod Dev* 1993; 34:292–298.

110. Huszar G, Vigue L. Spermatogenesis-related change in the synthesis of the creatine kinase B-type and M-type isoforms in human spermatozoa. *Mol Reprod Dev* 1990; 25:258–262.

111. Huszar G, Vigue L. Sperm creatine phosphokinase M-isoform ratios and fertilizing potential of men: a blinded study of 84 couples treated with in vitro fertilization. *Fertil Steril* 1992; 57:882–888.

112. Mori K, Daitoh T, Irahara M, et al. Significance of D-mannose as a sperm receptor site on the zona pellucida in human fertilization. *Am J Obstet Gynecol* 1989; 161:207–211.

113. Benoff S, Cooper GW, Hurley I, et al. Human sperm fertilizing potential in vitro is correlated with differential expression of a head-specific mannose-ligand receptor. *Fertil Steril* 1993; 59:854–862.

114. Benoff S, Cooper GW, Hurley IR, et al. Calcium-ion channel blockers and sperm fertilization. *Assist Reprod Rev* 1995; 5:2–13.

115. Amann RP, Hammerstedt RH. In vitro evaluation of sperm quality: an opinion. *J Androl* 1993; 14:397–406.

116. Jeyendran RS, Zaneveld LJD. Controversies in the development and validation of new sperm assays. *Fertil Steril* 1993; 59:726–728.

# 4
# Treating the Sperm: Selection, Stimulation, and Cryopreservation Techniques

Erma Z. Drobnis

In evaluation of an infertile couple, clinicians tend to overlook the male partner or delay his workup. This tendency could become more pronounced if immediate application of intracytoplasmic sperm injection (ICSI) becomes the standard treatment for male-factor infertility. Compelling reasons exist for giving the male partner a thorough evaluation before suggesting appropriate treatment for his infertility.[1] In some cases, a man can be treated directly after the minimal expense of a careful history, physical examination, and semen evaluation.[2] Other men will benefit from having their sperm treated for use in assisted reproductive technology (ART) procedures. Of the ART methods available, less invasive and less costly procedures, such as intrauterine insemination (IUI), may be the most appropriate therapy.[3,4] For patients who have a high likelihood of success with IUI, it is unwarranted to proceed directly to more expensive and risky micromanipulation procedures. To improve the methods of "treating the sperm," meaningful assays of sperm function are required for appropriate evaluation and comparison of various sperm treatments.

## Factors Critical for Collection of Quality Semen Samples

Factors, such as preparation of the patient, semen collection, and sperm-processing methods, can affect the quality and survival of processed sperm. To prepare the best possible sperm sample for a patient, it is important to (1) obtain the highest quality semen possible, (2) minimize iatrogenic damage to the sperm cells during treatment, and (3) improve the functional capacity of the sperm. Sperm treatments used in preparation for IUI, in vitro fertilization (IVF), and other ART procedures include washing to remove seminal plasma, selection of a population of motile sperm, and stimulation of sperm with various bioactive substances.[5-7] For some patients, treatment may involve cryopreservation of sperm prior to use in ART procedures.[6,8,9]

When devising improved sperm treatments and measuring their success in vitro, it is important to consider the complex physiology of normal sperm function in vivo. Diagnostic techniques for analyzing sperm have improved considerably over the past decade and are beginning to provide useful prognostic information for the various ART procedures. Even when optimal techniques are used, however, cryopreservation may result in the death of a significant proportion of sperm and may reduce the functional capacity of those surviving.

Protection of sperm from cellular insult during collection and processing is a primary concern. Human sperm are often considered quite resistant to noxious treatment because they remain motile under a variety of conditions, but sublethal changes difficult to detect can disrupt sperm function, particularly in vivo. Because the sperm chromatin is highly condensed and the DNA is unavailable for transcription, cellular repair mechanisms in sperm are quite limited. Mature sperm incapable of making new proteins or replacing other damaged or lost molecules are unusually susceptible to iatrogenic damage during collection, processing, and cryopreservation. This susceptibility and the sperm cell's minimal cytoplasmic stores may result in a brief life span ex vivo. Selection of the most appropriate methodology for sperm treatment involves use of optimal techniques to maintain or improve the sperm's functional capacity.

## Donor and Patient Factors

Many factors can affect the reproductive status of an individual and consequently influence sperm quality. The age of the man, his general health, his sexual activity, environmental factors, and toxicologic exposure can all influence sperm quality and cellular resistance to suboptimal conditions. Because in vitro treatments and cryopreservation impose significant stresses on these cells, minor defects that are virtually undetectable can have profound effects on the final quality or functional capacity of sperm. Careful selection of sperm donors and preparation of infertility patients can optimize the quality of the sperm collected. Certain patients, regardless of their reproductive health, may be considered for treatment or to cryopreserve semen; for example, a male infertility patient may become a candidate for ART because he has poor semen quality. In these cases, steps must be taken to maximize the survival and function of suboptimal cells. Whenever possible, these factors should be identified in male-factor infertility patients by a careful history, and the patient should be counseled to minimize adverse exposures.

### Age of Patient or Sperm Donor

Sperm production and semen quality are affected by male age.[10] Young men produce fewer testicular sperm and have smaller reserves of epididymal sperm than mature men. After puberty, a rapid increase in sperm production generally accompanies adolescence and continues, but with a more gradual increase in young adulthood. Although total numbers of sperm are relatively low in young males, the quality of sperm produced is high.

Mature men continue to produce large numbers of sperm; however, reproductive function generally declines with advancing age, although there is considerable variation among individuals. Not only is sperm production reduced, but the quality of sperm may also decline. Humans of advanced age tend to produce sperm having lower motility, poorer structure, and altered rates of fusion in the zona-free hamster oocyte assay.[11-13] Some of these changes in sperm quality are undoubtedly related to lower ejaculation frequency, declining health, and lifelong exposure to damaging agents, rather than to the effect of age alone.

A critical effect of age on sperm quality is the increase in chromatin defects in older men. Risk assessment of congenital abnormalities in offspring and direct cytogenetic analysis of sperm have demonstrated that chromosomal abnormalities increase with age.[14] Because there is no correlation between age-related chromosomal abnormalities and sperm morphology,[12,15,16] this condition cannot be detected by standard semen analysis. Concern about chromosomal abnormalities in older men has led to suggested upper age limits of 35 or 40 years for sperm donation.

### Genetic Factors

Several genetic factors are important in the selection of sperm donors. Ideally, donors should be free from genetic disorders and should have outstanding reproductive efficiency. In humans, selection of donors for physical and mental attributes is minimal for ethical reasons.[17] Justified concerns about the misuse of ART technologies have limited use of genetic screening to selection of generally healthy donors. However, efforts to minimize the transmission of known genetic defects necessitates genetic evaluation for sperm donors. Clearly, individuals having congenital abnormalities in their ancestry should be excluded from donation.

Guidelines for genetic screening of human gamete donors have been published by the American Association of Tissue Banks[18] and the American Fertility Society.[19] Potential gamete donors should be interviewed by a medical geneticist and should be excluded from donation if their progeny are more at risk for a disease or abnormality than the general population. All abnormalities reported in the progeny of a donor must be investigated retroactively to determine the chances that a genetically transmitted disorder was transmitted by the donor, and the preserved tissues from the donor must be destroyed if such evidence is obtained.[20] Because approximately 4% of humans are carriers for cystic fibrosis, testing of donors for this disorder has recently been recommended.[21–23]

In addition to screening for inherited diseases, donors should be screened for their potential to produce high-quality gametes that survive cryopreservation. Inheritance is an important factor determining reproductive efficiency. In the most extreme cases, congenital abnormalities cause sterility.[24–26] For the purposes of sperm cryopreservation, more subtle effects must also be considered. Many human sperm banks simply reject potential donors with poor sperm cryosurvival.

## General Health and Nutrition

Reproductive efficiency is highest for individuals with good nutritional status and health. The effects of health and nutrition on reproductive efficiency have been studied for many years in agricultural species, suggestive of strong economic incentives to maximize productivity. To maintain sperm production, a lower plane of nutrition is required in adulthood compared with adolescence, but general health and a minimal plane of nutrition must be maintained.[27] Specific deficiencies of vitamins and minerals are known to decrease male fertility; in particular, low dietary vitamin C levels have been associated with DNA oxidation and damage in the sperm of young, otherwise healthy, humans.

Over the years, there has been some interest in specific nutritional strategies to improve sperm quality and cryosurvival. Because the lipid composition of membranes underlies some differences in sperm cryosurvival,[28,29] several researchers have attempted to improve cryosurvival by dietary alterations, but these attempts have been disappointing. Poor health can have a negative effect on reproduction in both males and females, such as temporary reduction in semen quality following a high fever. Another well-documented example is the poor semen quality, and the accompanying poor sperm cryosurvival, seen in cancer patients. Men often elect to have sperm cryopreserved prior to treatment for leukemia, testicular cancer, or renal failure, treatments that can result in both genetic damage and permanent damage to the spermatogenic epithelium. A sizable proportion of these patients have existing marginal or poor semen quality, low resistance of their sperm to cryodamage, or both.[30–37] Disease conditions apparently contribute to impaired testicular function. Stress can also impair sperm production and quality.[37]

## Infectious Diseases

The potential for transmission of infectious disease by ART has been recognized since the early use of artificial insemination (AI) in domestic species.[38] Although genitally transmitted diseases can be spread by AI, insemination with cryopreserved sperm can actually be used to reduce the danger of such infection by allowing for quarantine and testing of frozen semen. The importance of screening human sperm donors for infectious diseases has been recognized.[18,19,39] The relatively recent change from the widespread use of fresh semen for donor insemination to the exclusive use of cryopreserved sperm was driven by recognition of the potential for transmitting human immunodeficiency virus (HIV).[40] Currently, individuals judged to be at risk for HIV, hepatitis infection, or both are excluded from semen donation.

Each specimen is cultured for gonorrhea and other pathogenic microorganisms. In addition, donors are tested for chlamydia, *Ureaplasma urealyticum*, cytomegalovirus (CMV), hepatitis B virus surface antigen, hepatitis C virus antibody, HIV type 1 and type 2 antibodies, human T-lymphotropic virus (HTLV) type I, and syphilis. The semen is then cryopreserved and held in quarantine for at least 6 months, after which the donor is retested. Units are released from quarantine for use only after negative results are received. The use of CMV-positive donors remains controversial.[41] Active CMV infection during pregnancy can result in severe birth defects and low birth weight.[42] Because some 40% of prospective donors are CMV positive, exclusion of these individuals from donation makes it difficult to find adequate numbers of qualified donors to satisfy the demand for therapeutic donor insemination. For this reason, some programs do offer cryopreserved semen from CMV-positive donors. If semen from a donor seropositive for CMV is to be used, the recipient should be restricted to a patient who is also CMV positive. Each specimen from CMV-positive donors should be tested for viral shedding and rejected if CMV culture is positive.

## Abstinence Period

The frequency of sexual activity can affect the number of sperm per ejaculate as well as sperm quality. During periods of sexual rest, sperm accumulate in the caudal epididymides. An insufficient abstinence period depletes this sperm reserve and decreases the number of sperm produced per ejaculate. During extended periods of sexual activity, sperm stored in the epididymides begin to age. Semen collected following a long abstinence period tends to have high numbers of sperm but generally with a lower percentage of motile sperm, poorer sperm function in vitro, and reduced sperm cryosurvival.[43,44] In general, semen quality is maximized by regular sexual activity followed by a short period of abstinence prior to collection.

For humans, sperm numbers are increased after 2 to 3 days' abstinence, and both the percentage of motile sperm and sperm quality are higher if no more than 5 days have elapsed since the last ejaculation. Men with normal semen parameters have significantly reduced sperm numbers in semen specimens produced after an abstinence period of 1 day or less.[45–48] Although an abstinence period of 2 to 5 days has been suggested, studies of oligozoospermic men have consistently demonstrated that these patients often produce equivalent sperm numbers for two samples collected within a day.[48,49] Collection of successive ejaculates can be attempted in these patients to allow for pooling of samples prior to sperm cryopreservation.

## Iatrogenic Damage to Sperm In Vitro

### Sperm Aging In Vitro

Cellular aging can decrease the resistance of sperm to the stresses imposed during washing, incubation, and cryopreservation. Aging processes occur in vivo for sperm within both the male and female reproductive tracts and are accelerated under most in vitro conditions. After sperm collection, aging phenomena may be compounded by suboptimal culture conditions and damage resulting from preparative techniques. It is desirable to collect sperm before significant aging has begun in vivo and to begin processing as soon after collection as possible.

The initial manifestations of sperm senescence are subtle, and it may be difficult to detect the sublethal defects in sperm that reduce their functional capacity. As sperm age, membrane integrity and motility are retained longer than is the ability to complete gamete fusion.[50] Sperm lose the ability to penetrate the zona pellucida while still capable of fusion with the oolemma.[51] There is recent evidence that aging sperm also develop chromosomal abnormalities; when mouse sperm were aged in vitro, fertilization rates decreased.[52,53] The same was true of male pronuclei in zona-free hamster oocytes arising from human sperm incubated in protein-free media.[54]

### Seminal Plasma Effects

From the standpoint of in vitro treatments for sperm, the seminal plasma is a nuisance variable. There is considerable variation among males and among ejaculates in seminal plasma constituents, and whole seminal plasma can have both cytotoxic and protective activity. Individual males vary in the toxicity of their seminal fluids.[55–57] In some species, the seminal plasma is quite toxic to sperm cells, so the time between collection and processing must be minimized, or the semen must be diluted or washed soon after collection or both.[58–61] Although phospholipase $A_2$ activity is present in human seminal plasma, the levels are much lower.[62] Nevertheless, the seminal plasma in most species contains some cytotoxic activity, and sperm survive longer if diluted or washed and resuspended in a more appropriate culture medium.[61–68] Human sperm function is irreversibly impaired by relatively brief exposure to seminal plasma.[55,69–72] Cryosurvival is reduced if human semen is held for an hour or more before processing, even though the motility is usually unaffected at this time point. Although it seems surprising that sperm survive poorly in seminal plasma, the sperm do not remain in contact with whole seminal plasma in vivo. After ejaculation, the semen is quickly diluted by secretions of the female reproductive tract, and strongly motile sperm migrate into the cervical mucus and secretions overlying the epithelial surfaces of the female reproductive tract.[73,74]

Cytoplasmic droplets are another potentially toxic constituent of semen. These membrane-bound structures are remnants of the final spermatogenic stages during which sperm lose most of their cytoplasm. Cytoplasmic droplets remain attached to sperm following their release from the residual bodies on the seminal vesicle epithelium.[75–77] Under normal circumstances, the cytoplasmic droplets are shed by sperm as they traverse the epididymis, and in some species they appear in semen in equal numbers to sperm cells.[78] These structures are rich in hydrolytic enzyme activity.[79–82] The cytoplasmic droplet membrane is susceptible to damage by cold shock and freeze-thawing and is rendered more fragile by some media, notably Tris buffer.[83] Rupture of these structures has the potential to release damaging enzyme activity.[75]

Some inhibitory substances present in seminal plasma are probably not a concern with respect to sperm processing and storage. Soon after techniques for IVF were developed, it was discovered that seminal plasma inhibits fertilization.[84] This inhibition has been attributed to protein decapacitation factors in semen that adsorb to the sperm surface at ejaculation. Certain proteins become strongly associated with the sperm surface during epididymal maturation or at ejaculation and are lost during capacitation.[85–89] In addition to seminal proteins, cholesterol, which is present in seminal plasma, can act as a decapacitation factor, inhibiting the acrosome reaction and fertilization.[90–97] Decapacitation factors are eventually lost during capacitation, allowing fertilization to proceed. Because premature capacitation and acrosomal lability are now known to be manifestations of cryoinjury to sperm,[98] decapacitation factors (although inhibitory when present during fertilization) are not damaging if present during cryopreservation.

In addition to various cytotoxic activities, the seminal plasma can also be protective, even cryoprotective.[28,99] For sperm collected from the caudal epididymides, addition of seminal plasma constituents stimulates motility and improves fertility.[57,100,101]

## Microbial Contamination

A major concern is that microorganisms are preserved when conditions are optimized to protect sperm from damage during collection and processing. In fact, these cells are generally less sensitive to adverse conditions than are spermatozoa. When the media and conditions employed are designed for optimal preservation of cellular function, they provide ideal environments for microorganismal growth. Although some investigators speculated that key pathogenic microorganisms would be killed by cryopreservation, the careful methods employed to preserve sperm function are generally sufficient to preserve pathogens as well. Even CMV, which is quite cold labile, survives cryopreservation in human semen.[102] When sperm are being prepared for deposition in the uterus by IUI or for IVF procedures, the sample must be essentially free of contamination with bacteria, fungi, and viruses. For cryopreserved samples, there is the concern that microorganisms may leak from stored samples and contaminate the coolant in freezers and storage tanks, thereby gaining access to other specimens. Several strategies are generally employed to control microbial contamination of tissues: donor screening for disease, aseptic or sterile processing techniques, inclusion of antibiotics in media, and testing of tissue. Some of the semen separation techniques efficiently remove bacterial contaminants during sperm processing. Rigorous and sustained quality control (QC) procedures are critical to ensuring that contamination is minimized on a continuous basis.

Ejaculated semen is not sterile. Even in healthy males, microorganisms are present in the urethra and on the external surfaces of the penis.[103] Ideally, a dedicated room, which can be cleaned and sanitized daily, should be available for semen collection. Each donor or patient should be provided with a sterile towelette and instructed to clean the penis before semen collection. Sterile or aseptic containers and media should be used for all steps in semen collection and processing.

Because blood products are often used as constituents of semen diluents and culture media, they represent a source of potential contamination of sperm. Serum albumin preparations are subject to viral contamination,[104] although the actual risk of infection from the usual fraction V human serum albumin (HSA) used in most laboratories is very low due to the ethanol precipitation step used in its preparation.[6] Donors of human serum and HSA to be used in sperm preparation must be screened for diseases (e.g., hepatitis, HIV) in a similar manner to sperm donors. The importance of this is illustrated by a case in which 79 women, and a significant number of their husbands, contracted hepatitis B after undergoing IVF in which contaminated serum was used to prepare media.[105] Cells used for coculture with sperm are also a potential source of pathogens, particularly if they derive from human cells.

Although not a substitute for aseptic collection and processing conditions, antibiotics are sometimes included in sperm diluents and media. Selection of motile sperm by self-migration or gradient centrifugation efficiently removes bacteria from sperm suspensions, but inclusion of antibiotics in media further reduces microbial contamination.[106] Penicillin and streptomycin are most commonly used in media and diluents for human sperm.[107] These drugs have minimal toxicity to gametes and embryos and

inhibit the growth of a broad spectrum of microorganisms.[38,108]

There are some concerns regarding the use of antimicrobial drugs for ART procedures. These agents may have adverse effects on gamete function, on embryo development, or both.[109] A second concern is the potential for an allergic response in the sperm or embryo recipient. Women allergic to penicillin have developed hypersensitivity reactions following intrauterine insemination (IUI) and embryo transfer.[110]

## Toxicity of Labware and Media

Strict QC of materials used in collection of sperm has not always been used. Although bioassays to evaluate labware and media were introduced into human IVF laboratories in some early programs,[111–113] these methods have been less common in andrology laboratories. Over the past decade, numerous materials used in the collection and preparation of gametes and embryos have proved cytotoxic. Ironically, it was the desire to use more reliable and controlled materials that led to the widespread use of sterile, disposable labware in place of laboratory glassware. The cytotoxic properties of plastics have been known for some time,[113–115] but many research programs had not appreciated the toxicity of disposable syringes to sperm and embryos[116–120] or the toxicity of other disposable labware, such as culture dishes, pipettes, micropore filters, blood-collection tubes, and plastic catheters.[121–126] Most ART programs now realize that any plastic surface is potentially cytotoxic.[127] An in-house program for toxicity testing of materials is an essential component of QC.

Among the most toxic materials used in ART laboratories are disposable plastic examination gloves.[128] Touching a culture dish on the spot later used for the bioassay culture drop can cause developmental arrest of embryos or complete immobility of sperm. All types of examination gloves, whether latex or vinyl, powdered or powder-free, can be toxic. In fact, it is likely to be the more flexible plastics, such as those used in gloves, that are toxic because the plasticizers used to impart flexibility are themselves cytotoxic. As with plasticware, rinsing the gloves can reduce toxicity. However, careful screening to find gloves of low toxicity is important, and new lots should always be tested for cytotoxicity.

Lubricants have also been identified as a source of toxicity to sperm. They are often provided to patients and donors for use during semen collection. Lubricants are also used before inserting vaginal probes and speculums during insemination. Because sperm may become contaminated by these substances, lubricants should be evaluated for cytotoxicity or their use should be avoided. A similar problem exists with the ultrasound transmission gel commonly used in ultrasound-guided oocyte retrievals.[129,130]

Medium contamination by bacterial endotoxins may be present even after ultrapurification. Endotoxins, shed during bacterial growth, are lipopolysaccharide components of the outer cell wall of gram-negative bacteria. Because they remain after bacteria are killed or removed by filtration, sterilization of media does not eliminate these toxic compounds. Serum albumin preparations are a potential source of endotoxins and can damage both sperm and embryos.[131,132] Serum albumin preparations, as well as lots of whole serum, are quite variable[133] and can contain substances detrimental to embryo development.[104,134] Fatty acid-free preparations are less likely to contain toxic contaminants and are, therefore, recommended for use in handling of gametes and embryos.[104] The concentrated HSA solutions that are available commercially and licensed for clinical use are primarily intended for intravenous administration and may contain detergents that stabilize the HSA molecule and prevent flocculation.[6] Clearly these cytotoxic detergents are undesirable for sperm preparation. Density gradients used to prepare sperm suspensions are another source of toxic contamination. Percoll, commonly used to provide density gradients, can also be toxic to embryos.[135] Biologic fluids and cells can also contain cytotoxic activity. Serum, follicular fluid, and oviductal fluid are undefined solutions that can contain inhibitory substances, partially masked by their protective properties.[134,136–142]

## Cold Shock and Ultraviolet Light

Sperm of some species are irreversibly damaged when cooled rapidly to room temperature.[143,144] Although relatively resistant to cold shock,[145,146] human sperm are damaged if cooled rapidly to below 20°C.[147–151] When semen is collected off-site, patients should be instructed to protect their specimen from cooling after collection and during transport to the laboratory.

Sperm cells are also sensitive to ultraviolet light,[108] which catalyzes the formation of reactive oxygen species (ROS) and peroxidation of membrane lipids. Sperm become particularly sensitive to oxidative stress when the antioxidants present in seminal plasma are diluted or removed. Lipid peroxidation increases the permeability of the sperm membrane, decreasing the cell's ability to maintain homeostasis. Because sperm cryopreservation itself results in increased lipid peroxidation, it is particularly important to minimize this damage during prefreeze processing. Facilities used for sperm collection and processing should use incandescent lighting if possible, and measures should be taken to minimize the exposure of sperm to light.

# Semen Separation and Sperm Selection Techniques

Semen contains a variety of cellular and soluble elements other than motile sperm, including dead sperm, epithelial cells, leukocytes, microorganisms, cellular debris, lytic enzymes, and oxidizing molecules. These elements can have cytotoxic effects on sperm, can cause painful cramping if deposited in the uterus during IUI, and can damage the oocyte and early embryo if present during IVF.

## Sperm Dilution and Washing

Initial processing of sperm usually involves dilution in a specially formulated medium. Immediate dilution or washing can be used to minimize sperm exposure to damaging seminal constituents. Dilution or washing of sperm with specially formulated semen extenders, cryo-diluents, or culture medium produces a more favorable and controlled extracellular environment for the sperm during incubation or cryopreservation. In many cases, more sophisticated techniques designed to separate sperm from other seminal constituents are used during processing, including preferential selection of motile sperm.

## Centrifugation and Washing

The term *washing* in cell biology refers to dilution of cells (or other particles) with medium, centrifugation to sediment the cells, removal of the supernatant, and resuspension of the cells in fresh medium. Similarly, washing has traditionally been used to describe this procedure of dilution and centrifugation for sperm. Inclusion of other preparative techniques, such as gradient centrifugation, under the description of washing techniques can be misleading.

After collection and liquefaction of semen, many preparative techniques include washing to remove the soluble components of the semen. The seminal plasma must be removed from human sperm prior to IUI because spasmogens in the whole semen can cause painful cramping of the uterus. Washing alone is one method used clinically to prepare sperm for IUI. Of the methods available for seminal plasma removal, washing by dilution and centrifugation is rapid, simple, and results in recovery of most motile sperm while removing many constituents of the seminal plasma. Most methods for separation of semen include at least one washing step.

Unfortunately, washing is damaging to sperm. In some species, severe damage to sperm results from simple washing.[152,153] For most species, including humans, sperm are more resistant to washing, and damage can be reduced by various methods; however, even when gentle washing techniques are employed, sublethal damage is sustained by motile sperm during dilution and washing,[148,154–160] with consequent reduction in functional capacity and longevity. This damage is not caused by centrifugation alone, because cellular injury is reduced when centrifugation is followed by

resuspension in the original solution instead of fresh medium.[153,161–163] Some of the damage apparently results from removal of the seminal plasma. Nevertheless, the process of centrifugation itself is damaging to sperm.[164]

Washing damage can be minimized by various techniques. Variables involved in washing methodology include temperature, washing medium, dilution, volume, centrifugal force, and centrifugation time. It is generally agreed that forces exceeding $800g$ are damaging to human sperm,[154,155] and forces in the range of 300 to $400g$ are usually recommended.[5] However, lower forces sediment a smaller proportion of the motile sperm. There is a direct negative correlation between the proportion of the motile sperm recovered and the centrifugation force.[165] Although it is often assumed that all of the motile sperm are recovered after a washing procedure, this is inaccurate. In fact only 60% to 80% of the motile sperm are recovered at suggested centrifugal forces of 300 to $600g$. This can be easily verified by examination of the supernatant. Sedimentation can be improved and centrifugal force minimized by decreasing the volume in individual tubes. Because the time required to sediment sperm is a function of the volume, dividing samples into multiple tubes for centrifugation can improve recovery.[5]

## Selection of Motile Sperm

Simple washing can efficiently remove soluble constituents of the seminal plasma; however, it does not remove dead sperm and other cells. Even without sedimentation during washing, the presence of dead sperm cells is detrimental to sperm function[166,167] and cryosurvival.[168] Semen separation methods, which have been devised to select motile sperm and remove potentially harmful elements from semen, fall into three general categories: (1) solid-phase adhesion, (2) self-migration, and (3) gradient centrifugation. An ideal separation method would recover all of the motile sperm and remove all other seminal constituents without damaging motile sperm. In practice, however, each method has advantages and disadvantages.[6,7] The method of choice depends on the importance of these factors for each application. Current methods of sperm selection involve loss of some fraction of the motile sperm present in the original sample. Swim-up and Percoll gradient are the methods most widely used in clinical practice, and each involves loss of the majority of the motile sperm. At present, simple washing remains the most efficacious method of preparing samples with very low sperm numbers for IUI.[169]

## Solid-Phase Adhesion

A rapid method for removing dead sperm from semen is column separation, based on the principle that dead sperm become sticky and adhere to glass and plastics. Semen is placed at the top of a column filled with glass beads,[170–175] glass wool,[175–180] or Sephadex.[181–183] As the semen percolates through the solid material, dead sperm are retained in the column while living sperm continue through and are collected below. These techniques have the advantages of being very rapid, not requiring dilution or sedimentation of sperm, and separating a very high proportion of the motile sperm. However, seminal plasma components and cellular contaminates are not removed. Sperm collected in the filtrate must be washed. It is possible that column filtration may be most useful prior to initial washing in order to reduce the cytotoxic effects of sedimenting motile sperm with dead sperm.

A relatively new strategy[184,185] involves incubation of sperm with the lectin peanut agglutinin agent.[186] This method has potential for isolation of high-quality sperm without centrifugation. Monoclonal antibodies that recognize epitopes on the inner acrosomal membrane or acrosomal contents have been used to isolate acrosome-reacted human sperm.[187–190] This technique could also be adapted to removal of sperm with damaged acrosomes.

## Self-Migration

Column separation alone does not remove soluble components of seminal plasma and nonsperm cellular material, including cytoplasmic droplets and microorganisms. Migration methods rely on sperm motility to isolate motile sperm from semen and are thus capable of reducing these undesirable semen constituents. The most common of these methods are the swim-up or rise techniques, in which sperm migrate from semen[154,191–194] or from the washed pellet[5,167,195–198] into overlying culture medium. With the albumin methods, sperm migrate from semen into an underlying layer of solution containing bovine serum albumin (BSA) or HSA.[199–203] Not only dead sperm are removed during migration methods, but other contaminating cellular elements, including microorganisms,[71,104,204–206] are significantly reduced.

The main disadvantage of self-migration methods is that they recover only a small fraction of the motile sperm. When motile sperm are selected by swim-up, only about 20% are recovered.[154,167] This can be a problem if sperm are being prepared for IUI, in which case large numbers of motile sperm are required. It is also a consideration for oligozoospermic samples in which sperm numbers are low to begin with.[170] In addition, all migration methods involve an incubation period, usually an hour, to achieve separation. This added incubation can be damaging, particularly if sperm with impaired longevity are being treated.

Variables involved in sperm migration methods include the temperature and incubation time,[193] the medium used, and whether the sperm are washed prior to migration. An additional factor is the method used to produce the maximum surface area of the interface between the sperm suspension and the fresh medium, generally achieved by increasing the number of tubes[198–207] and positioning the tubes in a nearly horizontal position.[193] In a migration method, which is unique because it does not require washing before or after separation, the sperm migrate into a viscous, hyaluronate medium, which can then be used directly for IVF or IUI.[197,208–211] Another strategy proposed to improve the recovery is to treat the sperm with substances that stimulate motility during the migration procedure.

## Gradient Centrifugation

Gradient centrifugation methods are more rapid and generally recover a higher proportion of the motile sperm than do migration methods.[194,212,213] Dense solutions of sucrose, Ficol, dextran, and polyvinyl pyrrolidone (PVP) can be used to remove most soluble constituents of seminal plasma plus many cellular elements. Because sperm cells are unusually dense, solutions can be prepared having a density intermediate to the sperm and the other seminal constituents. After loading the semen on top of the gradient solution, centrifugation will sediment the sperm while retaining the seminal plasma and lower density cellular elements above the gradient. This method selects sperm from other semen constituents in a single centrifugation step but does not separate motile from immotile sperm.

The density medium Percoll, a colloidal suspension of PVP-coated silica particles, has the advantage of producing high-density solutions with minimal increase in osmolality and has been used successfully to select motile sperm during gradient separation.[160,194,214–217] The semen specimen is loaded on top of a continuous or discontinuous gradient of increasing density. During centrifugation, sperm are drawn into an underlying, high-density solution, isolating them from seminal plasma.[77,214,218] After sperm are recovered from Percoll gradients, they must be washed in order to return them to solutions of normal density.

It is not known with certainty how Percoll gradient separation selects for motile sperm. The strongest evidence[219] suggests that because the sperm head has higher density than the tail, sperm become oriented in the centrifugal field. Continued migration into the higher density medium isolates the motile sperm from nonmotile material of similar density. Thus, the Percoll method actually does involve selection by self-migration. Other data[220] suggest that the immature, morphologically abnormal sperm in some poor-quality samples actually have lower density and are retained at a lower-density level than more normal sperm. These sperm, characterized by the immature isoform of creatine kinase and incomplete replacement of histones with protamines, may not have completed the final maturational changes that normally produce sperm of high density.

The sperm population that is recovered after Percoll separation can have almost 100% motility, although, as with migration methods, there is a trade-off between recovery of motile sperm and percentage motility.[221] Usually, a high percentage of motile sperm is associated with relatively low recovery rates, comparable to those obtained using swim-up procedures.[198,215,222] On the other hand, efficient recovery of sperm from poor quality semen is usually associated with minimal increase in the percentage of motile sperm. For these poor-quality samples, it may not be possible to select motile sperm by standard Percoll gradient methods, unless very few sperm are required for the ART procedure. One strategy used to improve the recovery of motile sperm from oligoasthenozoospermic samples is the mini-Percoll method. Multiple gradients having very low volume are used, and the sperm are washed and concentrated before applying the pellet to the gradients.[223,224]

Percoll gradient separation is widely used to prepare human sperm for ART procedures and in a number of clinical trials has proved superior to swim-up methods of preparing sperm for IVF.[160,216,225,226] There is some evidence that Percoll separation may result in alteration of sperm function, which has generally been viewed as beneficial.[198,217,227] However, these changes in sperm function resemble those produced during capacitation (e.g., motility changes similar to hyperactivation and early fusion with zona-free hamster oocytes). Although early capacitation could be an advantage for IVF, it is potentially damaging for IUI and sperm cryopreservation. Another concern about the use of Percoll is that it has not been approved for human use. Although many programs use Percoll for clinical procedures regardless of its status, the advisability of this practice is questionable. As a possible alternative to Percoll, Nycodenz is another density medium that has been used to prepare human sperm.[228] This molecule is a constituent of an x-ray contrast medium commonly used for angiography.

# Sperm Stimulation Techniques

## End Points Used to Measure Sperm Stimulation

An important consideration when choosing or developing a method of sperm treatment is the end point to be taken as evidence of improved sperm function. The natural history of sperm in the female reproductive tract is complex, involving significant changes in sperm physiology (Table 4.1). Before choosing which sperm attributes or functions to evaluate, it is important to determine what is expected of the sperm after treatment. The end points used to detect improved sperm function for IUI may be quite different from those used to evaluate improved capacity for IVF. The underlying sperm abnormalities being treated are another important consideration. Current ability to measure these various functional capacities of sperm remains quite limited, as does the ability to determine the underlying lesions in the sperm being treated. An example of this problem is the proportion of sperm that are acrosome-reacted after treatment, typically interpreted as a positive outcome for human sperm; indeed, if sperm are being prepared for IVF, and the sperm of this particular patient do not acrosome-react normally, then this is an appropriate end point. However, if sperm are to be used for IUI, the sperm of this patient have unusually labile acrosomes or both, increased acrosome reactions are actually a negative outcome because

TABLE 4.1. Treating the sperm: selection, stimulation, and cryopreservation techniques.

| | |
|---|---|
| I. Factors critical for collection of quality semen samples<br>  A. *Donor and patient factors*<br>    1. Age of patient or sperm donor<br>    2. Genetic factors<br>    3. General health of patients or sperm donors<br>    4. Environmental effects and toxicologic exposure<br>    5. Infectious diseases<br>    6. Abstinence period<br>  B. *Iatrogenic damage to sperm in vitro*<br>    1. Sperm aging in vitro<br>    2. Seminal plasma effects<br>    3. Microbial contamination<br>    4. Toxicity of labware and media<br>    5. Cold shock and ultraviolet light<br>  C. *Semen collection*<br>    1. Collection of ejaculated semen<br>    2. Semen coagulation and liquefaction<br>    3. Electroejaculation and retrograde ejaculation<br>    4. Collection of testicular and epididymal sperm | II. Semen separation and sperm selection techniques<br>  A. *Sperm dilution and washing*<br>    1. The dilution effect<br>    2. Centrifugation and washing<br>    3. Dialysis<br>  B. *Selection of motile sperm*<br>    1. Solid-phase adhesion<br>    2. Self-migration<br>    3. Gradient centrifugation<br>III. Sperm stimulation techniques<br>  A. *End points used to measure sperm stimulation*<br>  B. *Culture media for sperm*<br>  C. *Substances used to stimulate sperm*<br>    1. Methylxanthines and modulation of intracellular cAMP<br>    2. Metabolites, hormones, lytic enzymes<br>    3. Antioxidants<br>    4. Promoters of capacitation and induction of the acrosome reaction<br>  D. *Coculture*<br>  E. *Treatment of sperm bearing antisperm antibodies*<br>IV. Sperm cryopreservation techniques<br>  A. *End points used to measure sperm cryosurvival*<br>  B. *Fecundability with cryopreserved human sperm* |

Summary of normal sperm function in the female reproductive tract and requirements for membrane, cell surface, and motility. The mammalian sperm displays complex physiology during sperm transport and fertilization in vivo. In the course of these processes, the surface characteristics and motility pattern change dramatically. In choosing end points to assess methods of sperm stimulation, it is important to consider which of these functions will be required of the sperm after treatment, and what the underlying lesions in sperm function are for the patient to be treated. Some end points commonly accepted as indicators of improved sperm function, such as fusion with zona-free hamster oocytes, may not be desirable if sperm are to be deposited in the uterus.

sperm survival after the acrosome reaction is quite brief.[229] Available evidence indicates that the fertilizing sperm remain acrosome-intact until interaction with the oocyte.[230,231] In fact, the acrosome reaction can be viewed as a sign of sperm damage and can be induced by detergents and other membrane-disrupting agents.[232,233] For similar reasons, the ability of sperm to fuse with zona-free hamster oocytes, which can also be enhanced by membrane-disrupting agents,[234] is not necessarily a positive outcome, although it does measure the ability of sperm to survive, capacitate, and acrosome-react in vitro. In general, changes associated with capacitation (e.g., acrosome reaction, hyperactivation) are not beneficial until sperm reach the site of fertilization.[231,235,236]

The remarkable success of ICSI is an indication that most functional lesions in the sperm of male-factor patients involve impaired sperm transport and perfusion before fertilization. Lack of strong motility and inappropriate surface characteristics could reduce the ability of sperm to penetrate cervical mucus, to avoid phagocytosis in the uterine lumen, to cross the uterotubal junction (UTJ), to penetrate the zona pellucida, or all of these. Reduced sperm longevity could result in an inadequate population of surviving oviductal sperm when the oocyte is ready for fertilization. Inappropriate membrane changes could result in failure to capacitate, failure to associate appropriately with the oviductal isthmus, failure to undergo the acrosome reaction, failure to bind to the zona pellucida, failure to fuse with the oolemma, or all of these.

## Substances Used to Stimulate Sperm

Many substances have been evaluated for their ability to enhance human sperm function in vitro,[237] including substances that increase the concentration of cyclic adenosine monophosphate (cAMP) within the sperm (caffeine, pentoxifylline, other methylxanthines, dbcAMP, kallikrein), antioxidants (α-tocopherol, β-hydroxytheophylline [BHT], catalase), biologic fluids and molecules that promote capacitation (serum, serum albumin, follicular fluid, egg yolk, Percoll, urea), meta-

bolically active substances (creatine kinase), membrane-active lipids (cholesterol, phospholipids), hormones, platelet activating factor (PAF), steroids, prostaglandins, relaxin, proteases and other lytic enzymes (trypsin, chymotrypsin, α-amylase, hyaluronidase, plasminogen activators), and sulfhydryl reducing agents (dithiothreitol [DTT]).

### Motility Stimulation by Modulation of Intracellular cAMP

The most extensively studied additives to stimulate sperm function are substances that act to increase intracellular cAMP levels ($[cAMP]_i$) in sperm. Of the methylxanthine derivatives, caffeine and pentoxifylline have received the most attention. Methylxanthines act primarily to inhibit the breakdown of cAMP by cAMP-phosphodiesterase, allowing $[cAMP]_i$ to increase. The adenosine analogue 2-deoxyadenosine and the enzyme kallikrein have also been studied and apparently act by increasing $[cAMP]_i$. Various other methylxanthines and substances that modulate $[cAMP]_i$ have been evaluated for sperm stimulation, but they have not been studied as completely as other additives.[237] It is well known that $[cAMP]_i$ acts as a second messenger system in many cell types, including sperm. The understanding of the role of $[cAMP]_i$ in sperm functional capacity and how this signal interacts with other signal transduction systems is somewhat sketchy. The response of an individual sperm cell depends on other factors, such as (1) the intracellular concentration of free calcium ions ($[Ca^{2+}]_i$), (2) the intracellular pH, and (3) inositol phosphate turnover. These other components of sperm physiology interact with the cAMP system, having profound effects on sperm function.[231,238–240] Some of the diverse and seemingly inconsistent actions these drugs have on sperm undoubtedly derive from the complexity of the interaction between $[cAMP]_i$ and other components of sperm physiology.

Caffeine stimulates sperm motility[241,242] and is more effective in this activity than several other methylxanthines (theophylline, isobutylmethylxanthine) or dbcAMP.[243–245] The percentage of motile sperm is increased by appropriate concentrations of caffeine, as is the velocity of swimming sperm in some studies.[246] Although the results with caffeine have not been completely consistent, most investigators have reported stimulation of sperm motility, particularly an increase in the percentage of motile sperm in cases involving a large proportion of viable sperm (sperm with intact membranes) that are nonmotile.[247] It is often the case that sperm samples with a low percentage of motile sperm actually have a high proportion of viable, nonmotile (VNM) sperm. There are significant numbers of VNM sperm following cryopreservation,[184] and caffeine increases the percentage of motile sperm by more than 15% in cryopreserved human semen.[248–250] Caffeine increases the percentage of motility for sperm from asthenozoospermic semen, which also tends to contain a significant proportion of VNM sperm.[251] Senescent sperm also lose motility in advance of viability, and this loss of motility is delayed by caffeine.[242,245,246]

One explanation for the ability of methylxanthines to increase the percentage of motile sperm is the interaction between $[cAMP]_i$ and $[Ca^{2+}]_i$.[237] Sperm generally become immotile under conditions that are damaging to membranes. Until induction of the acrosome reaction, the $[Ca^{2+}]_i$ of sperm is normally maintained in the nanomolar range by active export of $Ca^{2+}$ from the cytosol.[252–256] In contrast, seminal plasma contains some $100\,\mu M$ free calcium ions, and culture media generally contain 1 to $5\,\mu M$ concentrations. The difference between intracellular and extracellular concentrations of this crucial ion is some 10,000-fold for sperm in medium. Small increases in $[Ca^{2+}]_i$ normally accompany capacitation, causing the increased curvature of flagellar bends and asymmetry of the flagellar wave, which are hallmarks of hyperactivation. This process can be reversible, with motility returning to normal following reduction of $[Ca^{2+}]_i$. Large elevations of sperm $[Ca^{2+}]_i$ (i.e., into the micromolar range) cause complete inactivation of the sperm flagellum.[257,258] This process can also be reversed in some cases. Increased $[Ca^{2+}]_i$ resulting from membrane leakage during cold shock immobilizes a significant proportion of sperm in some species—that is, they become nonmotile. However, motility of many sperm returns as they export the excess calcium. Thus, increasing $[Ca^{2+}]_i$ can both stimulate and inhibit sperm motility. High levels of VNM sperm produced by procedures that damage sperm membranes undoubtedly result from leakage of calcium ions into the sperm. Although the interaction between $[cAMP]_i$ and $[Ca^{2+}]_i$ is quite complex, increased cAMP can stimulate transport of $Ca^{2+}$ from sperm under some conditions,[237,259] a process that may enable the VNM sperm to return $[Ca^{2+}]_i$ levels to those compatible with flagellar motility.

Although caffeine stimulates sperm motility, this enhancement is retained only in the presence of the drug,[250] and only when extracellular $[Ca^{2+}]$ is very low.[260] Therefore, the potential of this drug to treat sperm prior to IUI is limited. In a clinical trial, caffeine treatment of sperm prior to artificial insemination was not beneficial.[259–262] Caffeine treatment also has a negative effect on the function of cryopreserved sperm as assessed by fusion with zona-free hamster oocytes,[250] and scanning electron microscopy of caffeine-treated human sperm revealed damage to the sperm surface over the acrosome, especially in asthenozoospermic samples.[251] However, these alterations may be indicative of suboptimal conditions of caffeine treatment. In principle, caffeine could help stimulate the motility of sperm prepared for IVF, prolonging the maintenance of motility during co-incubation and enhancing their ability to penetrate the zona pellucida. However, the safety of co-incubation of the gametes and the early embryo in the presence of this drug is not known. Results using the zona-free hamster oocyte assay have been mixed,[237] and this may be due in part to disruptive effects at high concentrations of caffeine.

Pentoxifylline (another methylxanthine) and caffeine have very similar effects on sperm in vitro. The percentage of motile sperm and the sperm velocity are increased at an appropriate dose,[263,264] which improves the motility of sperm from electroejaculates[265] and from asthenozoospermic patients.[266–268] Pentoxifylline also increases the percentage of motile sperm and the swimming velocity in cryopreserved sperm[269] and in sperm with poor morphology.[270]

It also increases penetration of zona-free hamster oocytes,[269,271,272] and this activity may be related to its stimulation of capacitation or the acrosome reaction or both.[237,268,273,274] Results with IVF have been promising,[267,268] although some researchers have not obtained improved fertilization results, even when motility was improved.[275] It has been suggested that part of the beneficial effect of pentoxifylline on motility and longevity in vitro is due to its activity as a free radical scavenger, reducing oxidative stress rather than by elevation of $[cAMP]_i$ alone.[6,276]

The adenosine analogue 2-deoxyadenosine has been shown to cause an increase in sperm $[cAMP]_i$.[277] In contrast to the transient motility improvement produced by the methylxanthines, 2-deoxyadenosine stimulates a sustained rise in $[cAMP]_i$ and improves motility for several hours after its removal. This molecule also increases the motility of cryopreserved sperm and improves penetration of zona-free hamster oocytes.

Kallikrein is a pancreatic protease that releases the active molecules kinins. The kinins are peptides that must act via membrane receptors. In sperm, the kallikrein-kinin system, apparently improving uptake of substrate by sperm by elevation of $[cAMP]_i$, increases the motility of cryopreserved and poor quality sperm. This effect may not occur when sperm are held at 37°C rather than at room temperature.[237,269] However, clinical results of treating sperm with kallikrein for IUI and IVF are inadequate to draw conclusions about its efficacy for ART procedures.

The clinical value of these molecules that increase sperm $[cAMP]_i$ is probably limited to procedures that bypass sperm transport. However, their application for IVF and perhaps gamete intrafallopian transfer (GIFT) are promising for asthenospermic samples, cryodamaged sperm, and sperm having impaired longevity.

## Coculture

Coculture with primary cell cultures or cell line monolayers has been primarily applied by reproductive biologists to improve the survival and development of embryos. This strategy has also been applied to sperm, with the goal of improving sperm longevity, functional capacity in vitro, or both. In embryology, coculture has been most advantageous for improving the results with poor-quality embryos and has been proposed as a means of rescuing embryos with original quality judged too poor for transfer or cryopreservation. Similarly, coculture may be useful for the treatment of poor-quality sperm and cryopreserved sperm. Human sperm have been incubated with cumulus cells, oviductal cells, and other cells of human reproductive tract origin. This strategy may sustain sperm having poor longevity until they are able to undergo capacitation in vitro. Because normal sperm will undergo capacitation if they are incubated in culture medium, it is not surprising that capacitation and spontaneous acrosome reactions occur during coculture. The presence of the cultured cells increases the proportion of sperm undergoing capacitation in vitro and improves their performance in assays of sperm function. The cells used for coculture in these experiments are not immortal cell lines; thus, freshly prepared cell cultures must be available at the time of sperm preparation. Currently, only the largest ART programs have a ready supply of these cells for routine application in sperm preparation, but it is possible that these cells could be cryopreserved and banked for this purpose. Cells of nonreproductive tract origin, Vero cells, and human skin fibroblasts have also been used for sperm; however, improved culture techniques and scrupulous attention to the quality of media may obviate the need for these complex techniques.

## Sperm Cryopreservation Techniques

In the current treatment of infertility, artificial insemination (AI) with donor semen is a widely used therapy for selected donors with exceptional semen quality and cryosurvival. Using current methods of donor selection, sperm cryopreservation, and timing of insemination, results with cryopreserved human sperm are acceptable, even approaching those with nonfrozen sperm. It is considerably more difficult to preserve sperm for patients who request sperm banking. Cryosurvival of patient sperm is often low, and continued efforts are required to improve cryopreservation methods for patient sperm by minimizing cryodamage.

## End Points Used to Measure Sperm Cryosurvival

There are a number of detectable and consistent changes in sperm morphology and physiology following cryopreservation, but there is limited understanding of what a given cellular change means in terms of function. Large changes in some parameters may have a minimal impact on the functional capacity of sperm, but small changes in other parameters may have profound effects on fertility. Sublethal cryoinjury to sperm can also be quite difficult to detect. Exposure to even relatively low concentrations of glycerol, even without freezing, can dramatically reduce sperm fertility without measurably affecting motility. Although many sperm attributes altered by cryopreservation have been identified, it is less clear which of these are predictive of post-thaw fertility.

Cell membranes are the major site of injury to cells during freezing.[39,144] Cryoinjury to cell membranes, and consequent disruption of permeability barriers, results in death or diminished function of the cell. During freezing and thawing, even if intracellular ice formation is avoided, many forces stress the membrane, including the increased solute concentration that accompanies intracellular dehydration, mechanical shear, osmotic damage during warming, lipid-phase separation, and disruption of temperature-sensitive molecular relationships. Large increases in membrane permeability will render sperm immotile; however, among the surviving motile cells, sublethal increases in membrane permeability and other membrane damage can have profound and diverse effects on sperm function.

A significant consequence of cryodamage to membranes is reduced longevity of sperm in vitro, and it is widely accepted that the fertile life span of cryopreserved sperm in vivo is significantly shorter than that of nonfrozen sperm. Consistent with this notion, cryopreserved sperm disappear more rapidly from the cervix after AI in comparison with nonfrozen sperm. Because of reduced sperm longevity, the timing of insemination is much more critical for cryopreserved sperm.

Cryopreserved sperm swim with reduced velocity. This diminished sperm vigor may be responsible for the impaired transport of cryopreserved sperm in the female reproductive tract. For cryopreserved human sperm, even when postthaw motility remains high, penetration of cervical mucus is reduced and cryopreserved sperm move more slowly within this biopolymer than do nonfrozen sperm. It is likely that abnormalities of the sperm surface result in increased resistance of the mucus microstructure to penetration by these sperm. Such cryodamage to the sperm surface may also underlie the diminished ability of cryopreserved sperm to remain in the cervix or form appropriate associations with the biopolymers that coat the epithelial surfaces of the female reproductive tract and invest the oocyte. Because cryopreserved sperm have reduced ability to penetrate cervical mucus, best results are obtained with cryopreserved sperm if they are placed in the uterus rather than in the cervix.

The acrosome has long been recognized as a significant site of cryoinjury to sperm. Cryopreservation induces swelling of the acrosome and considerable ultrastructural damage to the acrosomal membranes of sperm. Abnormal acrosomal function is a known consequence of cryodamage to sperm and can facilitate premature acrosome reactions.[98,278] Significantly, cryopreserved human sperm have the ability to fuse with zona-free hamster oocytes immediately after separation from seminal plasma but rapidly lose this ability during subsequent incubation.[279] In contrast, nonfrozen sperm require several hours of preincubation to complete capacitation in vitro and retain the ability to fuse with oocytes for many hours, suggesting that the kinetics of sperm capacitation can be altered by cryopreservation and the longevity reduced. If oocyte fusion rates are compared at an early time point, cryopreserved sperm penetrate oocytes at higher rates than do fresh sperm. Therefore, the emphasis on high rates of oocyte fusion does not always indicate more normal sperm physiology.

Other aspects of fertilization are also affected by cryopreservation of sperm. The results of in vitro fertilization have indicated that cryopreserved sperm have lower fertilizing potential in vitro than fresh sperm. In the hemizona assay, cryopreserved human sperm exhibit decreased binding to the zona pellucida compared with fresh sperm.

One component of cryodamage to sperm membranes involves lipid peroxidation. In cryopreserved human sperm, superoxide dismutase (SOD) activity is reduced, particularly in sperm with low motility after thawing, and membranes undergo changes in lipid composition consistent with peroxidative damage. Antioxidants are not in widespread use in human sperm cryodiluents.

## Fecundability with Cryopreserved Human Sperm

Over the past decade, fecundability with cryopreserved sperm (i.e., probability of conception in the first cycle of insemination) has improved as a consequence of several important factors: (1) improved donor selection procedures, (2) improved cryopreservation and storage methods, (3) IUI for cryopreserved sperm, and (4) improved ovulation detection that allows more accurate timing of insemination. In the absence of female-factor infertility, fecundability using cryopreserved sperm is nearly equivalent to that with nonfrozen sperm.

## Cryopreservative Methodology

During the 40 years that cryopreservation of sperm has been used successfully for AI in humans and domestic species, the methods for cryopreservation of human sperm have changed relatively little, particularly following the application of liquid nitrogen to sperm freezing and storage. Human sperm freeze remarkably well relative to sperm of other mammals. Only in humans are reasonable fertility rates achieved by simply adding glycerol to whole semen, packaging in screw-top, plastic cryovials, and freezing in nitrogen vapor in the neck of a storage Dewar. Attempts to improve methodology have been hampered by a lack of meaningful end points to assess cryodamage and the large variation among men in the response of their sperm to cryopreservative treatments. For many years, human semen was nearly always frozen either without dilution or after dilution with an egg-yolk citrate (EYC) diluent, usually containing glycine. In these early days, EYC diluents were common for cryopreservation of sperm from domestic species as well. When freezing without dilution, glycerol alone was added to the whole semen after liquefaction. Using the EYC diluent, the semen was diluted 1:1 or less with EYC, which contained the glycerol. More recently, two new diluents have been applied: human sperm preservation medium (HSPM), developed from a Tyrode's culture medium containing sucrose and HSA [737]; and TEST-yolk, adopted based on its success in a variety of species. Overall, EYC preserves sperm motility and function somewhat better than seminal plasma alone,[280] but TEST-yolk and HSPM are somewhat superior to these earlier techniques.[102,149,281] At the present time, TEST-yolk diluent is available from a variety of commercial sources and is the most widely used diluent in the United States. Because large foreign proteins such as BSA can induce severe allergic reactions in women undergoing IUI and embryo transfer (ET), it is possible that other large proteins, such as those found in egg yolk, could cause similar reactions if they are not removed from sperm prior to deposition in the uterus.

The dilution factor used when adding cryodiluent depends on the desired volume of the final cryopreserved unit and the number of motile sperm required for insemination. Several studies have considered pregnancy rates achieved with varying numbers of motile sperm inseminated. In general, pregnancy rates are higher when larger numbers of motile sperm are used. A major problem with retrospective studies is that the sperm dose is statistically confounded with postthaw survival and sperm quality, but samples in which initial sperm concentration was high and sperm cryosurvival was superior produced higher doses of motile sperm for insemination. The low-dose samples were those with low initial concentration or poorer cryosurvival or both. Based on these studies and practical experience, most programs in the United States use 10 to 20 million motile sperm (postthaw) per insemination dose. In other countries, where 0.25- or 0.5-ml cryostraws are used to package a semen dose instead of 1.0-ml cryovials, somewhat lower doses of motile sperm are generally used. Pregnancy rates over the first six cycles of insemination were not different for the two doses of sperm, although fecundability for both treatments was low (7%).

The concentration of sperm in human semen is relatively low; thus, it is difficult to provide adequate sperm numbers in a 1-ml cryopreserved unit. Sperm banks in the United States commonly guarantee 20 million motile sperm per unit postthaw. Assuming that approximately 50% of the motile sperm will become immotile during the process of freezing and thawing, the prefreeze sperm concentration must be at least 40 million motile sperm per milliliter. To take advantage of the protective activity of the cryodiluent, it is desirable to dilute the semen at least 1:1. Thus, the concentration of motile sperm before processing must be at least 80 million per milliliter. To attain this standard, donors accepted by sperm banks must have exceptionally concentrated sperm or sperm with exceptional cryosurvival or both.

To maximize the number of cryopreserved units produced from each ejaculate, donor semen should be diluted more than 1:1 if possible, maintaining the appropriate dose of motile sperm per unit postthaw (Table 4.2). The total number of motile sperm in the specimen is first calculated from the semen volume, sperm concentration, and percentage of motile sperm. If the freezability (percentage of motile sperm retaining motility postthaw) is known for each donor, this factor may be included in the calculation to allow more appropriate dilution rates. A running average of freezability values of the last three or four samples for each donor can be calculated for this purpose.

By far the most common packaging method for frozen semen is plastic cryostraws. Even for human semen, cryostraws are the preferred

TABLE 4.2. Dilution of human donor semen.

| Sperm function | Location in vivo | Membrane and surface requirements | Motility requirements |
|---|---|---|---|
| Sperm transport/storage | | | |
| Mucus penetration | Cervix | Negative surface charge (avoid adhesion, phagocytosis) | Strong |
| Cervical storage | | High membrane cholesterol | Some (avoid flushing into lumen) |
| Uterine transport | Uterus | Membrane stability | |
| UTJ penetration | | Low $Ca^{2+}$ permeability | Strong |
| Isthmic storage | Isthmus | Capacitation | Quiescent |
| Isthmic release | | | |
| Cumulus penetration | Ampulla | Neutral surface charge | Hyperactivated |
| | | | |
| Fertilization | | | |
| ZP binding | | Receptors expressed | |
| Acrosome reaction | | Fusigenic membrane | |
| ZP penetration | | Increased $Ca^{2+}$ permeability | |
| Gamete binding | | | |
| Gamete fusion | | | |
| Chromatin decondensation | Ooplasm | | |
| Pronuclear formation | | | |
| ONA replication | | | |
| Sperm aster and syngamy | | | |

Example of how to calculate the appropriate dilution for a sample of human donor semen. By this method, more efficient use is made of donor samples by increasing the number of units produced from specimens with exceptional quality.

method worldwide. The shape and heat transfer properties of cryostraws provide a high surface-area-to-volume ratio, and promote even cooling throughout the sample volume. However, concern about potential contamination of freezers and Dewars resulting from straw breakage or loss of straw seals has limited the use of cryostraws in the United States, where human sperm are generally cryopreserved in screw-top, plastic cryovials with Teflon sealing rings to prevent contamination of other samples. Although not ideal for cryopreservation purposes, these cryovials also hold a larger volume (cryostraws hold 0.25 or 0.5 ml), are easier to label, and are easy to thaw and empty in a clinical setting. These containers are not optimal for sperm cryopreservation, and improved results may be possible for some patients if more appropriate packaging is used. Flexible and essentially unbreakable cryostraws that may prove ideal for sperm storage are now available from the company that invented cryostraws (IMV, L'Aigle, France), and they are actually less likely to cause contamination of freezing and shipping equipment than are cryovials. Pathology laboratories are presently using them to store infectious organisms.

Freezing of human sperm is sometimes carried out rapidly by holding the containers in liquid nitrogen vapor for several minutes, although most sperm banks freeze at a more moderate rate (usually 10°C per min) in an automatic freezer. Semen samples are generally thawed at room temperature, in a thermos containing 37°C water, or stepwise using both temperatures. As is true for other cell types, rapid freezing rates (e.g., in the vapor above liquid nitrogen) must be followed by rapid thawing rates to minimize cryoinjury, and slow freezing must be followed by gradual thawing.[282] Human sperm are unusually resistant to differences in these factors, and it has been difficult to demonstrate a significant and consistent difference among the various freezing and thawing rates.[146,150,269] For the most common cooling rate used during freezing of human sperm (10°C/min), rapid warming rates during thawing best preserve motility, membrane integrity, and mitochondrial function.

After thawing, cryopreserved sperm must be processed for insemination. When these sperm are first exposed to culture media or other solutions (e.g., isotonic Percoll) having physiologic osmolality, significant osmotic shock occurs. For IUI-ready sperm, this process takes place when sperm are deposited in the female reproductive tract. The glycerolized sperm have quite high intracellular osmolality. Rapid dilution results in irreversible damage. As is the case with cryopreserved oocytes and embryos, thawed sperm should be diluted gradually into physiologic media to allow glycerol to leave the cell slowly.

## Conclusion

Over the past two decades, andrologists have made some progress in efforts to treat sperm from male-factor patients. This success has largely resulted from improved methods of detecting sperm dysfunction. Continued improvements will require better understanding of normal sperm function. As knowledge regarding the cellular and molecular mechanisms underlying sperm physiology and pathophysiology increases, it will be possible to devise more effective therapies for poor quality sperm. Development of new methodologies for sperm should focus on (1) obtaining the best sample possible from each patient, (2) minimizing iatrogenic damaging to sperm during treatment, and (3) choosing appropriate functional and cellular end points of treatment success.

## References

1. Cummins JM, Jequier AM. Treating male infertility needs more clinical andrology, not less. *Hum Reprod* 1994; 9:1214–1219.
2. Schill W-B, Haidl G. Medical treatment of male infertility. In: Insler V, Lunenfeld B, eds. *Infertility: Male and Female*. 2nd ed. Edinburgh: Churchill Livingstone; 1990: 575–622.
3. Martinez AR, Bernardus RE, Voorhorst FJ, et al. Intrauterine insemination does and clomiphene citrate does not improve fecundity in couples with infertility due to male or idiopathic factors: a prospective, randomized, controlled study. *Fertil Steril* 1990; 53:847–853.

4. Batzofin JH, Lipshultz LI. Assisted reproductive treatments for oligospermia. In: Seibel MM, ed. *Infertility. A Comprehensive Text.* Norwalk, CN: Appleton & Lange; 1990: 189–197.

5. Fulgham DL, Alexander NJ. Spermatozoa washing and concentration techniques. In: Keel BA, Webster BW, eds. *Handbook of the Laboratory Diagnosis and Treatment of Infertility.* Boca Raton, FL: CRC Press; 1990: 193–211.

6. Mortimer D. *Practical Laboratory Andrology.* New York: Oxford University Press; 1994.

7. Byrd W. Sperm preparation and homologous insemination. In: Keye WR, Chang RJ, Rebar RW, Soules MR, eds. *Infertility Evaluation and Treatment.* Philadelphia: W.B. Saunders; 1995: 696–711.

8. Schoysman R, Schoysman-Doboeck A, Van Roosendaal E, et al. Cryopreservation of sperm and its clinical applications. In: Asch RH, Balmaceda JP, Johnston I, eds. *Gamete Physiology.* Norwell, MA: Serono Symposia, USA; 1990: 197–208.

9. Sherman JK. Cryopreservation of human semen. In: Keel BA, Webster B, eds. *CRC Handbook of the Laboratory Diagnosis and Treatment of Infertility.* Boca Raton, FL: CRC Press; 1990: 229–259.

10. Harman SM, Blackman MR. Is there an andropause, the analog to menopause, and if so what tissues are affected and how? In: Robaire B, Pryor JL, Trasler J, eds. *Handbook of Andrology.* American Society of Andrology; 1995: 72–75.

11. Zenzes MT, Reed TE, Nieschlag E. Non-Poisson distribution of sperm from grandfathers in zona-free hamster ova. *J Androl* 1991; 12:71–75.

12. Rosenbusch B, Strehler E, Sterzik K. Cytogenetics of human spermatozoa: correlations with sperm morphology and age of fertile men. *Fertil Steril* 1992; 58:1071–1072.

13. Mladenovic I, Micic S, Papic N, et al. Sperm morphology and motility in different age populations. *Arch Androl* 1994; 32:197–205.

14. Bordson BL, Leonardo VS. The appropriate upper age limit for semen donors: a review of the genetic effects of paternal age. *Fertil Steril* 1991; 56:397–401.

15. Martin RH, Rademaker AW. The effect of age on the frequency of sperm chromosomal abnormalities in normal men. *Am J Hum Genet* 1987; 41:484–492.

16. Martin RH, Rademaker A. The relationship between sperm chromosomal abnormalities and sperm morphology in humans. *Mutat Res* 1988; 207:159–164.

17. American Fertility Society. Ethical considerations of assisted reproductive technologies. *Fertil Steril* 1994; 62(suppl 1):1S–125S.

18. American Association of Tissue Banks. Reproductive cells and tissues. In: *Technical Manual for Tissue Banking.* 2nd ed. McLean, VA: American Association of Tissue Banks; 1992.

19. American Fertility Society. Guidelines for therapeutic donor insemination: sperm. *Fertil Steril* 1993; 59(suppl 1):1S–4S.

20. Schroeder-Jenkins M, Rothmann SA. Causes of donor rejection in a sperm banking program. *Fertil Steril* 1989; 51:903–906.

21. Fugger EF, Maddalena A, Schulman JD. Results of retroactive testing of human semen donors for cystic fibrosis and human immunodeficiency virus by polymerase chain reaction. *Hum Reprod* 1993; 8:1435–1437.

22. Traystman MD, Schulte NA, MacDonald M, et al. Mutation analysis for cystic fibrosis to determine carrier status in 167 sperm donors from the Nebraska genetic semen bank. *Hum Mutat* 1994; 271:275.

23. Findlay I, Cuckle H, Lilford RJ, et al. Screening sperm donors for cystic fibrosis. *Br Med J* 1995; 310:1533.

24. Olds D. Inherited, anatomical, and pathological causes of lowered reproductive efficiency. In: Salisbury GW, VanDemark NL, Lodge JR, eds. *Physiology of Reproduction and Artificial Insemination of Cattle.* 2nd ed. San Francisco: W.H. Freeman; 1978: 611–646.

25. Jainudeen MR, Hafez ESE. Genetics and reproductive failure. In: Hafez ESE, ed. *Reproduction in Farm Animals.* 5th ed. Philadelphia: Lea & Febiger; 1987: 423–435.

26. Vogt PH. Genetic aspects of artificial insemination. *Hum Reprod* 1995; 10(suppl 1): 128–137.

27. Leatham JH. Nutritional influences on testicular composition and function in mammals. *Handbook Physiol* 1975; 5(section 7):397–428.

28. Watson PF. The effects of cold shock on sperm cell membranes. In: Morris GJ, Clark A, eds. *Effects of Low Temperatures on Biological Membranes.* London: Academic Press; 1981: 189–218.

29. Parks JE, Graham JK. Effects of cryopreservation procedures on sperm membranes. *Theriogenology* 1992; 38:209–222.

30. Sanger WG, Armitage JO, Schmidt MA. Feasibility of semen cryopreservation in patients with malignant disease. *JAMA* 1980; 244:789.

31. Sanger WG, Olson JH, Sherman JK. Semen cryobanking for men with cancer—criteria change. *Fertil Steril* 1992; 58:1024–1027.

32. Chapman RM, Sutcliffe SB, Malpas JS. Male gonadal dysfunction in Hodgkin's disease: a prospective study. *JAMA* 1981; 245:1323–1328.

33. Berthelsen JG, Skakkebaek NE. Gonadal function in men with testis cancer. *Fertil Steril* 1983; 39:68–75.

34. Hendry WFF, Stedronska J, Jones CR, et al. Semen analysis in testicular cancer and Hodgkin's disease: pre-freeze and post-treatment findings and implications for cryopreservation. *Br Urol J* 1983; 55:769–773.

35. Agarwal A, Tolentino MV, Sidhu RK, et al. Effect of cryopreservation on semen quality in patients with testicular cancer. *Urology* 1995; 382:389.

36. Shekarriz M, Tolentino MV Jr, Ayzman I, et al. Cryopreservation and semen quality in patients with Hodgkin's disease. *Cancer* 1995; 75:2732–2736.

37. Applegarth LD. The psychological aspects of infertility. In: Keye WR, Chang RJ, Rebar RW, Soules MR, eds. *Infertility Evaluation and Treatment.* Philadelphia: W.B. Saunders; 1995: 25–41.

38. Foote RH. Extenders and extension of unfrozen semen. In: Salisbury GW, VanDemark NL, Lodge JR, eds. *Physiology of Reproduction and Artificial Insemination of Cattle.* 2nd ed. San Francisco: W.H. Freeman; 1978: 442–493.

39. Quigley MM, Collins RL, Schover LR. Establishment of an oocyte donor program. *Ann NY Acad Sci* 1991; 626:445–451.

40. American Fertility Society. New guidelines for the use of semen donor insemination: 1990. *Fertil Steril* 1990; 53(suppl 1):1S–13S.

41. Chauhan M, Barratt CLR, Cooke S, et al. Screening for cytomegalovirus antibody in a donor insemination program: difficulties in implementing the American Fertility Society guidelines. *Fertil Steril* 1989; 51:901–902.

42. McGowan MP, Hayes K, Kovacs GT, et al. Prevalence of cytomegalovirus and Herpes simplex virus in human semen. *Int J Androl* 1983; 6:331.

43. O'Dell WT, Almquist JO, Amann RP. Freezing bovine semen. V. Practicability of collecting and freezing large numbers of successive ejaculates. *J Dairy Sci* 1959; 42:1209–1215.

44. Seidel GE, Foote RH. Influence of semen collection interval and tactile stimuli on semen quality and sperm output in bulls. *J Dairy Sci* 1969; 52:1074–1079.

45. Lampe EH, Masters WH. Problems of male fertility. *Fertil Steril* 1956; 7:123–127.

46. Freund M. Effects of frequency of emission on semen output and an estimate of daily sperm production in man. *J Reprod Fertil* 1963; 6:269.

47. Blackwell JM, Zaneveld LJD. Effect of abstinence on sperm acrosin, hypoosmotic swelling, and other semen variables. *Fertil Steril* 1992; 58:798–802.

48. Tur-Kaspa I, Maor Y, Levran D, et al. How often should infertile men have intercourse to achieve conception. *Fertil Steril* 1994; 62:370–375.

49. Barash A, Lurie S, Weissman A, et al. Comparison of sperm parameters, in vitro fertilization results, and subsequent pregnancy rates using sequential ejaculates, collected two hours apart, from oligoasthenozoospermic men. *Fertil Steril* 1995; 64:1008–1011.

50. Barros C, Jedlicki A, Bize I, et al. Relationship between the length of sperm preincubation and zona penetration in the golden hamster. *Gamete Res* 1984; 9:31–43.

51. Gould JE, Overstreet JW, Hanson FW. Interaction of human spermatozoa with the human zona pellucida and zona-free hamster oocyte following capacitation by exposure to human cervical mucus. *Gamete Res* 1985; 12:47–54.

52. Munné S, Estop A. The effect of in-vitro ageing on mouse sperm chromosomes. *Hum Reprod* 1991; 6:703–708.

53. Estop AM, Munné S, Jost LK, et al. Studies on sperm chromatin structure alterations and cytogenetic damage of mouse sperm following in vitro incubation. Studies on in vitro-incubated mouse sperm. *J Androl* 1993; 14:282–288.

54. Munné S, Estop AM. Chromosome analysis of human spermatozoa stored in vitro. *Hum Reprod* 1993; 8:581–586.

55. Rogers BJ, Perreault SD, Bentwood BJ, et al. Variability in the human-hamster, in vitro assay for fertility evaluation. *Fertil Steril* 1983; 39:204.

56. Sofikitis N, Takahashi C, Kadowaki H, et al. The role of the seminal vesicles and coagulating glands in fertilization in the rat. *Int J Androl* 1992; 15:54–61.

57. Henault MA, Killian GJ, Kavanaugh JF, et al. Effect of accessory sex gland fluid from bulls of differing fertilities on the ability of cauda epi-

didymal sperm to penetrate zona-free bovine oocytes. *Biol Reprod* 1995; 52:390–397.

58. Corteel JM. Viabilité des spermatozoïdes de bouc conservés et congelés avec ou sans leur plasma séminal: effet du glucose. *Ann Biol Anim Biochem Biophys* 1974; 14:741–745.

59. Corteel JM. Effets du plasma séminal sur la survie et la fertilité des spermatozoïdes conserves in vitro. *Reprod Nutr Dev* 1979; 20:115–127.

60. Corteel JM, Paquignon M. Preservation of the male gamete (ram, buck, boar). *Proc Int Congr Anim Reprod Artif Insem* 1984; 10(4):II-20–II-27.

61. Mann T. *The Biochemistry of Semen and of the Male Reproductive Tract*. New York: Wiley; 1964: 17–36.

62. Rönkkö S. Immunohistochemical localization of phospholipase $A_2$ in the bovine seminal vesicle and on the surface of the ejaculated spermatozoa. *Int J Biochem* 1992; 24:869–876.

63. Shannon P. Presence of a heat-labile toxic protein in bovine seminal plasma. *J Dairy Sci* 1965; 48:1362–1365.

64. Eliasson R, Treichl L. Supravital staining of human spermatozoa. *Fertil Steril* 1971; 22:134–137.

65. Sexton TJ, Fewlass TA. A new poultry semen extender. *Poultry Sci* 1978; 57:277.

66. Dott HM, Harrison RAP, Foster GCA. The maintenance of motility and the surface properties of epididymal spermatozoa from bull, rabbit and ram in homologous seminal and epididymal plasma. *J Reprod Fertil* 1979; 55:113–124.

67. Baas JW, Molan PC, Shannon P. Factors in seminal plasma of bulls that affect the viability and motility of spermatozoa. *J Reprod Fertil* 1983; 68:275–280.

68. England GCW, Allen WE. Factors affecting the viability of canine spermatozoa. *Theriogenology* 1992; 37:373–381.

69. Rogers BJ. Mammalian sperm capacitation and fertilization in vitro: a critique of methodology. *Gamete Res* 1978; 1:165–223.

70. Rogers BJ. The sperm penetration assay: its usefulness reevaluated. *Fertil Steril* 1985; 43:821–840.

71. Mortimer D. Semen analysis and sperm washing techniques. In: Gagnon C, ed. *Controls of Sperm Motility: Biological and Clinical Aspects*. Boca Raton, FL: CRC Press; 1990: 263–284.

72. Yavetz H, Yogev L, Homonnai Z, et al. Prerequisites for successful human sperm cryobanking: sperm quality and prefreezing holding time. *Fertil Steril* 1991; 55:812–816.

73. Katz DF, Drobnis EZ, Overstreet JW. Factors regulating mammalian sperm migration through the female reproductive tract and oocyte vestments. *Gamete Res* 1989; 22:443–469.

74. Drobnis EZ, Overstreet JW. Natural history of mammalian spermatozoa in the female reproductive tract. *Oxford Rev Reprod Biol* 1992; 14:1–45.

75. Allison AC, Hartree EF. Lysosomal enzymes in the acrosome and their possible role in fertilization. *J Reprod Fertil* 1970; 21:501.

76. Harrison RAP, White IG. Some methods for washing spermatozoa from bull, boar and ram: a comparison using biochemical and other criteria. *J Reprod Fertil* 1972; 29:271.

77. Mayol RF, Longenecker D. Separation of non-sperm components from seminal preparations and their effect on the analysis of sperm proteins (38744). *Proc Soc Exp Biol Med* 1975; 149:64–69.

78. Cortadellas N, Durfort M. Fate and composition of cytoplasmic droplet of hamster epididymal spermatozoa. *J Morphol* 1994; 221:199–210.

79. Garbers DL, Wakabayashi T, Reed PW. Enzyme profile of the cytoplasmic droplet from bovine epididymal spermatozoa. *Biol Reprod* 1970; 3:327.

80. Gottlieb W, Meizel S. Biochemical studies of metalloendoprotease activity in the spermatozoa of three mammalian species. *J Androl* 1987; 8:14–24.

81. Dowing TW, Garner DL, Ericsson SA, et al. Alteration of sperm metabolism by the addition of excess cytoplasmic droplets. *ARTA* 1992; 3:289–293.

82. Oko R, Hermo L, Chan PTK, et al. The cytoplasmic droplet of rat epididymal spermatozoa contains saccular elements with Golgi characteristics. *J Cell Biol* 1993; 123:809–821.

83. Dott HM, Dingle JT. Distribution of lysosomal enzymes in the spermatozoa and cytoplasmic droplets of bull and ram. *Exp Cell Res* 1968; 52:523.

84. Chang MC. A detrimental effect of seminal plasma on the fertilizing capacity of sperm. *Nature* 1957; 179:258–260.

85. Dukelow WR, Chernoff HN, Williams WL. Properties of decapacitation factor and presence in various species. *J Reprod Fertil* 1965; 14:393–399.

86. Yanagimachi R. Mechanisms of fertilization in mammals. In: Mastroianni L, Biggers JD, eds. *Fertilization and Embryonic Development In Vitro.* New York: Plenum Press; 1981: 81–182.

87. O'Rand MG. Modification of the sperm membrane during capacitation. *Ann NY Acad Sci* 1982; 383:392–404.

88. Oliphant G, Reynolds AB, Thomas TS. Sperm surface components involved in the control of the acrosome reaction. *Am J Anat* 1985; 174:269–283.

89. Eddy EM, O'Brien DA. Biology of the gamete: maturation, transport, and fertilization. In: Working PK, ed. *Toxicology of the Male and Female Reproductive Systems.* New York: Hemisphere; 1989: 31–100.

90. Davis BK, Hungund BJ. Effects of modified membrane vesicles from seminal plasma on the fertilizing capacity of rabbit spermatozoa. *Biochem Biophys Res Commun* 1976; 69:1004–1010.

91. Davis BK. Inhibitory effect of synthetic phospholipid vesicles containing cholesterol on the fertilizing capacity of rabbit spermatozoa. *Proc Soc Biol Med* 1976; 152:257–261.

92. Davis BK. Interaction of lipids with the plasma membrane of sperm cells. I. The antifertilization action of cholesterol. *Arch Androl* 1980; 5:249–254.

93. Fleming AD, Yanagimachi R. Effects of various lipids on the acrosome reaction and fertilizing capacity of guinea pig spermatozoa with special reference to the possible involvement of lysophospholipids in the acrosome reaction. *Gamete Res* 1981; 4:253–273.

94. Go KJ, Wolf DP. Albumin-mediated changes in sperm sterol content during capacitation. *Biol Reprod* 1985; 32:145–153.

95. Ehrenwald E, Parks JE, Foote RH. Cholesterol efflux from bovine sperm. *Gamete Res* 1988; 20:145–157.

96. Cross NL. Multiple effects of seminal plasma on the acrosome reaction of human sperm. *Mol Reprod Dev* 1993; 35:316–323.

97. Cross NL. Human seminal plasma prevents sperm from becoming acrosomally responsive to the agonist, progesterone: cholesterol is the major inhibitor. *Biol Reprod* 1996; 54:138–145.

98. Drobnis EZ, Clisham PR, Brazil CK, et al. Detection of altered acrosomal physiology of cryopreserved human spermatozoa after sperm residence in the female reproductive tract. *J Reprod Fertil* 1993; 99:159–165.

99. Graham JK. Effect of seminal plasma on the motility of epididymal and ejaculated spermatozoa of the ram and bull during the cryopreservation process. *Theriogenology* 1994; 41:1151–1162.

100. Inskeep PB, Magargee SF, Hammerstedt RH. Alterations in motility and metabolism associated with sperm interaction with accessory sex gland fluids. *Arch Biochem Biophys* 1985; 1:1–9.

101. Peitz B. Effects of seminal vesicle fluid components on sperm motility in the house mouse. *J Reprod Fertil* 1988; 83:169–176.

102. Hammitt DG, Aschenbrenner DW, Williamson RA. Culture of cytomegalovirus from frozen-thawed semen. *Fertil Steril* 1988; 49:554.

103. Cohen MS, Collen S, Mardh PA. Mucosal defenses. In: Holmes KK, Mardh PA, Sparling PF, Wiesner PJ, eds. *Sexually Transmitted Diseases.* New York: McGraw-Hill; 1984: 173.

104. Bavister BD. Culture of preimplantation embryos: fact and artifacts. *Hum Reprod Update* 1995; 1:91–148.

105. Grosheide PM, Van Osand HC, Schalm SW, et al. Immunoprophylaxis to limit a hepatitis B epidemic among women undergoing in vitro fertilization. *Vaccine* 1991; 9:682–687.

106. Karlström P-O, Hjelm E, Lundkvist Ö. Comparison of the ability of two sperm preparation techniques to remove microbes. *Hum Reprod* 1991; 6:386–389.

107. Wong PC, Balmaceda JP, Blanco JD, et al. Sperm washing and swim-up technique using antibiotics removes microbes from human semen. *Fertil Steril* 1986; 45:97–100.

108. Foote RH. Buffers and extenders. *Tech Conf Artif Insem Reprod* 1982; 9:62–70.

109. Dunn HO, Larson GL, Willett EL. The effects of freezing bovine spermatozoa in extenders containing antibacterial agents. *J Dairy Sci* 1953; 728:732.

110. Smith YR, Hurd WW, Menge A, et al. Allergic reactions to penicillin during in vitro fertilization and intrauterine insemination. *Fertil Steril* 1992; 847:849.

111. Purdy JM. Methods for fertilization and embryo culture in vitro. In: Edwards RG, Purdy JM, eds. *Human Conception In Vitro.* London: Academic Press; 1982.

112. Sokoloski JE, Wolf DP. Laboratory details in an in vitro fertilization and embryo transfer program. In: Wolf DP, Quigley MM, eds. *Human In Vitro Fertilization and Embryo Transfer.* New York: Plenum Press; 1984: 275–296.

113. Ackerman SB, Swanson RJ, Stokes GK, et al. Culture of mouse preimplantation embryos as a quality control assay for human in vitro fertilization. *Gamete Res* 1984; 9:145–152.

114. Inchiosa MA. Water-soluble extractives of disposable syringes. *J Pharm Sci* 1965; 54:1379.

115. Jaeger RJ, Rubin RJ. Plasticizers from plastic devices: extraction, metabolism and accumulation by biological systems. *Science* 1970; 170:460.

116. Driscoll D, Douglas-Hamilton DH. Toxic effects of commonly used syringes on equine semen. *Theriogenology* 1985; 2–7.

117. Takeda T, Hasler JF. Effect of plastic disposable syringes on development of mouse embryos in culture. *Theriogenology* 1986; 25:205.

118. de Ziegler D, Cedars MI, Hamilton F, et al. Factors influencing maintenance of sperm motility during in vitro processing. *Fertil Steril* 1987; 48:816–820.

119. Johnson DE, Hodgen GD. Syringe-associated toxicity of culture media on mouse and monkey preembryos. *J In Vitro Fertilization Embryo Transfer* 1991; 8:198–201.

120. Broussard JR, Goodeaux SD, Goodeaux LL, et al. The effects of different types of syringes on equine spermatozoa. *Theriogenology* 1993; 39:389–399.

121. Quinn P, Warnes GM, Kerin JF, et al. Culture factors in relation to the success of human in vitro fertilization and embryo transfer. *Fertil Steril* 1984; 41:202–209.

122. Bavister BD, Andrews JC. A rapid sperm motility bioassay procedure for quality-control testing of water and culture media. *J In Vitro Fertilization Embryo Transfer* 1988; 5:67–75.

123. Boone WR, Shapiro SS. Quality control in the in vitro fertilization laboratory. *Theriogenology* 1990; 33:23–50.

124. Findley WE, Gibbons WE. Mouse pre-embryo culture as an evaluation for human pre-embryo requirements. In: Keel BA, Webster BW, eds. *CRC Handbook of the Laboratory Diagnosis and Treatment of Infertility*. Boca Raton, FL: CRC Press; 1990: 329–344.

125. Harrison PE, Barratt CLR, Robinson AJ, et al. Detection of white blood cell populations in the ejaculates of fertile men. *J Reprod Immunol* 1991; 19:95–98.

126. Davis NS, Rothmann SA, Tan M, et al. Effect of catheter composition on sperm quality. *J Androl* 1993; 14:66–69.

127. Naz RK, Janousek JT, Moody T, et al. Factors influencing murine embryo bioassay: effects of proteins, aging of medium, and surgical glove coatings. *Fertil Steril* 1986; 46:914.

128. Althouse GC, Ko JCH, Hopkins SM, et al. Effect of latex and vinyl examination gloves on canine spermatozoal motility. *J Am Vet Med Assoc* 1991; 199:227–229.

129. Sheean LA, Goldfarb JJ, Kiwi R, et al. Arrest of embryo development by ultrasound coupling gels. *Fertil Steril* 1986; 45:568.

130. Shimonovitz S, Yagel S, Zacut D, et al. Ultrasound transmission gel in the vagina can impair sperm motility. *Hum Reprod* 1994; 9:482–483.

131. Dumoulin JCM, Menheere PPCA, Evers JLH, et al. The effects of endotoxins on gametes and preimplantation embryos cultured in vitro. *Hum Reprod* 1991; 6:730–734.

132. Randall GW, Gantt PA. Preimplantation murine embryos are more resistant than human embryos to bacterial endotoxins. *J In Vitro Fertilization Embryo Transfer* 1991; 7:280–284.

133. Bronson RA, Rogers BJ. Pitfalls of the zona-free hamster egg penetration test: protein source as a major variable. *Fertil Steril* 1988; 50:851–854.

134. Maurer HR. Towards serum-free, chemically defined media for mammalian cell culture. In: Freshney RI, ed. *Animal Cell Culture: a Practical Approach*. 2nd ed. Oxford: Oxford University Press; 1992: 15–46.

135. Arora M, Carver-Ward JA, Jaroudi KA, et al. Is Percoll safe for in vivo use? *Fertil Steril* 1994; 61:979–981.

136. Kille JW, Hamner CE. The influence of oviductal fluid on the development of one-cell rabbit embryos in vitro. *J Reprod Fertil* 1973; 35:415–423.

137. Richardson LL, Hamner CE, Oliphant G. Some characteristics of and an inhibitor of embryonic development from rabbit oviductal fluid. *Biol Reprod* 1980; 22:553–559.

138. Caro CM, Trounson A. The effect of protein on preimplantation mouse embryo development in vitro. *J In Vitro Fertilization Embryo Transfer* 1984; 1:183.

139. Shirley B, Wortham JWE, Witmyer J, et al. Effects of human serum and plasma on development of mouse embryos in culture media. *Fertil Steril* 1985; 43:129.

140. Shirley B, Wortham JWE, Peoples D, et al. Inhibition of embryo development by some maternal sera. *J In Vitro Fertilization Embryo Transfer* 1987; 4:93.

141. Archibong AE, Petters RM, Johnson BH. Development of porcine embryos from one-cell

and two-cell stages to blastocysts in culture medium supplemented with porcine oviductal fluid. *Biol Reprod* 1989; 41:1076–1083.

142. Bavister BD. Co-culture for embryo development: is it really necessary? *Hum Reprod* 1992; 7:1339–1341.

143. Quinn PJ. A lipid-phase separation model of low-temperature damage to biological membranes. *Cryobiology* 1985; 22:128–146.

144. Hammerstedt RH, Graham JK, Nolan JP. Cryopreservation of mammalian sperm: what we ask them to survive. *J Androl* 1990; 11:73–88.

145. Sherman JK. Temperature shock in human spermatozoa. *Proc Soc Exp Biol Med* 1955; 88:6–7.

146. Sherman JK. Preservation of bull and human spermatozoa by freezing in liquid nitrogen vapour. *Nature* 1962; 194:1291–1292.

147. Sherman JK. Improved methods of preservation of human spermatozoa by freezing and freeze-drying. *Fertil Steril* 1963; 14:49–64.

148. Freund M, Wiederman J. Factors affecting the dilution, freezing and storage of human semen. *J Reprod Fertil* 1966; 11:1–17.

149. Graham EF, Crabo BG. Some methods of freezing and evaluating human spermatozoa. *Proc Natl Acad Sci USA* 1978; 274–303.

150. Mahadevan MM, Trounson AO. Effect of cooling, freezing and thawing rates and storage conditions on preservation of human spermatozoa. *Andrologia* 1984; 16:52–60.

151. Drobnis EZ, Crowe LM, Berger T, et al. Cold shock damage is due to lipid phase transitions in cell membranes: a demonstration using sperm as a model. *J Exp Zool* 1992; (submitted).

152. Quinn PJ, White IG, Cleland KW. Chemical and ultrastructural changes in ram spermatozoa after washing, cold shock and freezing. *J Reprod Fertil* 1969; 18:209–220.

153. Jones RC, Holt WV. The effects of washing on the ultrastructure and cytochemistry of ram spermatozoa. *J Reprod Fertil* 1974; 41:159–167.

154. Lopata A, Patullo MJ, Chang A, et al. A method for collecting motile spermatozoa from human semen. *Fertil Steril* 1976; 27:677–684.

155. Makler A, Jakobi P. Effect of shaking and centrifugation on human sperm motility. *Arch Androl* 1981; 7:21.

156. Padilla AW, Foote RH. Extender and centrifugation effects on the motility patterns of slow-cooled stallion spermatozoa. *J Anim Sci* 1991; 69:3308–3313.

157. Jeulin C, Serres C, Jouannet P. The effects of centrifugation, various synthetic media and temperature on the motility and vitality of human spermatozoa. *Reprod Nutr Dev* 1982; 22:81.

158. Tarlatzis BC, Laufer N, Murillo O, et al. Semen evaluation following preparation for in vitro fertilization of human oocytes. *Arch Androl* 1986; 17:215–222.

159. Tarlatzia BC, Bontis J, Kolibianakis EM, et al. Evaluation of intrauterine insemination with washed spermatozoa from the husband in the treatment of infertility. *Hum Reprod* 1991; 6:1241–1246.

160. Mortimer D. Clinical significance of antisperm antibodies. *J Soc Obstet Gynecol Can* 1991; 13:69.

161. Alvarez JG, Lasso JL, Blasco L, et al. Centrifugation of human spermatozoa induces sublethal damage. *Hum Reprod* 1993; 8:1087–1092.

162. White IG. The effect of washing on the motility and metabolism of ram, bull and rabbit spermatozoa. *J Exp Biol* 1953; 3:200.

163. Dott HM, Walton A. Effects of dilution and washing on ram spermatozoa. *J Reprod Fertil* 1960; 1:350.

164. Brackett BG. Effects of washing the gametes on fertilization in vitro. *Fertil Steril* 1969; 20:127.

165. Salamon S. Deep freezing of boar semen. *Aust J Biol Sci* 1973; 26:231–237.

166. Iwasaki A, Gagnon C. Formation of reactive oxygen species in spermatozoa of infertile patients. *Fertil Steril* 1992; 57:409–416.

167. Russell LD, Rogers BJ. Improvement in the quality and fertilization potential of a human sperm population using the rise technique. *J Androl* 1987; 8:25–33.

168. Rana N, Jeyendran RS, Holmgren WJ, et al. Glass wool-filtered spermatozoa and their oocyte penetrating capacity. *J In Vitro Fertilization Embryo Transfer* 1989; 6:280–284.

169. Pérez-Sánchez F, Cooper TG, Yeung CH, et al. Improvement in quality of cryopreserved human spermatozoa by swim-up before freezing. *Int J Androl* 1994; 17:115–120.

170. Kerin J, Quinn P. Washed intrauterine insemination in the treatment of oligospermic infertility. *Sem Reprod Endocrinol* 1987; 5:23–33.

171. Bangham AK, Hancock JL. A new method for counting live and dead bull spermatozoa. *Nature* 1955; 176:656.

172. McGrath J, Hillman N, Nadijcka M. Separation of dead and live mouse spermatozoa. *Dev Biol* 1977; 61:114–117.

173. Liu DY, Clarke GN, Baker HWG. Inhibition of human sperm–zona pellucida and sperm-oolemma binding by antisperm antibodies. *Fertil Steril* 1991; 55:440–442.

174. Daya S, Gwatkin RBL, Bissessar H. Separation of motile human spermatozoa by means of a glass bead column. *Gamete Res* 1987; 17:375–380.

175. Casey PJ, Robertson KR, Liu IKM, et al. Column separation of motile spermatozoa from stallion semen. *J Androl* 1993; 14:142–148.

176. Paulson JD, Polakoski KL. A glass wool column procedure for removing extraneous material from the human ejaculate. *Fertil Steril* 1977; 28:178–181.

177. Paulson JD, Polakoski KL, Salvatore L. Further characterization of glass wool column filtration of human semen. *Fertil Steril* 1979; 32:125–126.

178. Sherman JK, Paulson JD, Liu KC. Effect of glass wool filtration on ultrastructure of human spermatozoa. *Fertil Steril* 1981; 36:643–647.

179. Jeyendran RS, Van der Ven HH, Perez-Pelaez M, et al. Separation of viable spermatozoa by standardized glass wool column. In: Ratnam SS, Teoh E-S, Ng S-C, eds. *In Vitro Fertilization*. Carnforth: Parthenon; 1987: 49–53.

180. Rhemrev J, Jeyendran RS, Vermeiden JPW, et al. Human sperm selection by glass wool filtration and two-layer, discontinuous Percoll gradient centrifugation. *Fertil Steril* 1989; 51:685–690.

181. Katayama KP, Stehlik E, Roesler M, et al. Treatment of human spermatozoa with an egg yolk medium can enhance the outcome of in vitro fertilization. *Fertil Steril* 1989; 52:1077–1079.

182. Graham EF, Vasquez IA, Schmehl MKL, et al. An assay of semen quality by use of Sephadex filtration. *Proc Int Congr Anim Reprod Artif Insem* 1976; 8:896–899.

183. Weeda AJ, Cohen J. Effects of purification or split ejaculation of semen and stimulation of spermatozoa by caffeine on their motility and fertilizing ability with the use of zona-free hamster ova. *Fertil Steril* 1982; 37:817–822.

184. Drobnis EZ, Zhong CQ, Overstreet JW. Separation of cryopreserved human semen using Sephadex columns, washing, or Percoll gradients. *J Androl* 1991; 12:201–208.

185. Singer R, Sagiv M, Allalouf D, et al. Separation of normozoospermic human spermatozoa into subpopulations by selective agglutination with peanut agglutinin. *Andrologia* 1986; 18:17–24.

186. Ravid A, Sagiv M, Bartoov B, et al. Separation of sub-populations of sperm with higher fertility potential from normal and pathological semen by peanut agglutinin. *Andrologia* 1990; 22:225–230.

187. Okabe M, Matzno S, Nagira M, et al. Collection of acrosome-reacted human sperm using monoclonal antibody-coated paramagnetic beads. *Mol Reprod Dev* 1992; 32:389–393.

188. Ying X, Okabe M, Mimura T. Selection of acrosome-reacted human spermatozoa and their fusing ability by micro-injection into the perivitelline space of hamster eggs. *Hum Reprod* 1993; 8:1074–1078.

189. Parinaud J, Vieitez G, Labal B, et al. Selection and micro-injection of acrosome-reacted human spermatozoa. *Hum Reprod* 1994; 9:128–129.

190. Ohashi K, Saji F, Wakimoto A, et al. Selection of acrosome-reacted sperm with MH61-immunobeads. *J Androl* 1994; 15:78–82.

191. Overstreet JW, Yanagimachi R, Katz DF, et al. Penetration of human spermatozoa into the human zona pellucida and the zona-free hamster egg: a study of fertile donors and infertile patients. *Fertil Steril* 1980; 33:534–542.

192. Wolf DP, Sokoloski JE. Characterization of the sperm penetration bioassay. *J Androl* 1982; 3:445–451.

193. Makler A, Murillo O, Huszar G, et al. Improved techniques for collecting motile spermatozoa from human semen. *Int J Androl* 1984; 7:61–70.

194. Berger T, Marrs RP, Moyer DL. Comparison of techniques for selection of motile spermatozoa. *Fertil Steril* 1985; 43:268–273.

195. Drevius LO. The "sperm-rise" test. *J Reprod Fertil* 1971; 24:427–429.

196. Cruz RI, Kemmann E, Brandeis VT, et al. A prospective study of intrauterine insemination of processed sperm from men with oligoasthenospermia in superovulated women. *Fertil Steril* 1986; 46:673–677.

197. Wikland M, Wik O, Steen Y, et al. A self-migration method for preparation of sperm for in-vitro fertilization. *Hum Reprod* 1987; 2:191–195.

198. Tanphaichitr N, Millette CF, Agulnick A, et al. Egg-penetration ability and structural proper-

ties of human sperm prepared by Percoll-gradient centrifugation. *Gamete Res* 1988; 20:67.

199. Ericsson RJ, Langevin CN, Nishino M. Isolation of fraction rich in human Y sperm. *Nature* 1973; 246:421–424.

200. Broer KH, Dauber U. A filtering method for cleaning up spermatozoa in cases of asthenospermia. *Int J Fertil* 1978; 23:234–237.

201. Koper A, Evans PR, Witherow RON, et al. A technique for selecting and concentrating the motile sperm from semen in oligozoospermia. *Br J Urol* 1979; 51:587–590.

202. Dmowski WP, Gaynor L, Lawrence M, et al. Artificial insemination homologous with oligospermic semen or albumin columns. *Fertil Steril* 1979; 31:58–62.

203. Perrone D, Testart J. Use of bovine serum albumin column to improve sperm selection for human in vitro fertilization. *Fertil Steril* 1985; 44:839–841.

204. Wolf DP, Byrd W, Dandekar P, et al. Sperm concentration and the fertilization of human eggs in vitro. *Biol Reprod* 1984; 31:837–848.

205. Sun L-S, Gastaldi C, Peterson EM, et al. Comparison of techniques for the selection of bacteria-free sperm preparations. *Fertil Steril* 1987; 48:659–663.

206. Kuzan FB, Hillier SL, Zarutskie PW. Comparison of three wash techniques for the removal of microorganisms from semen. *Obstet Gynecol* 1987; 70:836.

207. Harris SJ, Milligan MP, Masson GM, et al. Improved separation of motile sperm in asthenospermia and its application to artificial insemination homologous (AIH). *Fertil Steril* 1981; 36:219–221.

208. Huszar G, Willetts M, Corrales M. Hyaluronic acid (Sperm Select) improves retention of sperm motility and velocity in normospermic and oligospermic specimens. *Fertil Steril* 1990; 54:1127–1134.

209. Zavos PM, Centola GM. Qualitative and quantitative improvements in human spermatozoa recovered via the swim-up and a new semen filtration method. *Infertility* 1990; 13:25–34.

210. Centola GM, Zavos PM. Qualitative/quantitative improvements in post-thaw human semen using Spermprep. *ARTA* 1991; 11:335–339.

211. Zimmerman ER, Robertson KR, Kim H, et al. Semen preparation with the Sperm Select system versus a washing technique. *Fertil Steril* 1994; 61:269–275.

212. Lessley BA, Garner DL. Isolation of motile spermatozoa by density gradient centrifugation in Percoll. *Gamete Res* 1983; 7:49–61.

213. Dravland JE, Mortimer D. A simple discontinuous Percoll gradient procedure for washing human spermatozoa. *IRCS Med Sci* 1985; 13:375–380.

214. Forster MS, Smith WD, Lee WI, et al. Selection of human spermatozoa according to their relate motility and their interaction with zona-free hamster eggs. *Fertil Steril* 1983; 40:655–660.

215. Bolton VN, Braude PR. Preparation of human spermatozoa for in vitro fertilization by isopycnic centrifugation on self-generating density gradients. *Arch Androl* 1984; 13:167–176.

216. Hyne RV, Stojanoff A, Clarke GN, et al. Pregnancy from in vitro fertilization of human eggs after separation of motile spermatozoa by density gradient centrifugation. *Fertil Steril* 1986; 45:93–96.

217. Leventhal A, Margalioth EJ, Schenker JG. Testing the fertilizing ability of motile spermatozoa separated by Percoll in patients with abnormal sperm analysis or sperm penetration. *Int J Androl* 1987; 32:302–305.

218. Bolton VN, Warren RE, Braude PR. Removal of bacterial contaminants from semen for in vitro fertilization or artificial insemination by the use of buoyant density centrifugation. *Fertil Steril* 1986; 46:1128–1132.

219. Gorus FK, Pipeleers DG. A rapid method for the fractionation of human spermatozoa according to their progressive motility. *Fertil Steril* 1981; 35:662–665.

220. Aitken J, Krausz C, Buckingham D. Relationships between biochemical markers for residual sperm cytoplasm, reactive oxygen species generation, and the presence of leukocytes and precursor germ cells in human sperm suspensions. *Mol Reprod Dev* 1994; 39:268–279.

221. Kaneko S, Sato H, Kobanawa K, et al. Continuous-step density gradient centrifugation for the selective concentration of progressively motile sperm for insemination with husband's semen. *Arch Androl* 1987; 19:75–84.

222. McClure RD, Nunes L, Tom R. Semen manipulation: improved sperm recovery and function with a two-layer Percoll gradient. *Fertil Steril* 1989; 51:874–877.

223. Ord T, Patrizio P, Marello E, et al. Mini-Percoll: a new method of semen preparation for IVF in severe male factor infertility. *Hum Reprod* 1990; 5(suppl 8):987.

224. Ng FLH, Liu DY, Gordon Baker HW. Comparison of Percoll, mini-Percoll and swim-up methods for sperm preparation from abnormal semen samples. *Hum Reprod* 1992; 7:261–266.

225. Guérin JF, Mathieu C, Lornage J, et al. Improvement of survival and fertilizing capacity of human spermatozoa in an IVF programme by selection on discontinuous Percoll gradients. *Hum Reprod* 1989; 4:798–804.

226. Junca AM, Chabi N, Plachot M, et al. Amélioration in vitro et fécondance des spermes déficients. *Contracept Fertil Sexual* 1989; 17:730–731.

227. Arcidiacono A, Walt H, Campana A, et al. The use of Percoll gradients for the preparation of subpopulations of human spermatozoa. *Int J Androl* 1983; 6:433–445.

228. Gellert-Mortimer ST, Clarke GN, Baker HWG, et al. Evaluation of Nycodenz and Percoll density gradients for the selection of motile human spermatozoa. *Fertil Steril* 1988; 49:335.

229. Fleming AD, Yanagimachi R. Fertile life of acrosome-reacted guinea pig spermatozoa. *J Exp Zool* 1982; 220:109–116.

230. Tesarik J. Appropriate timing of the acrosome reaction is a major requirement for the fertilizing spermatozoon. *Hum Reprod* 1989; 4:957–961.

231. Yanagimachi R. Mammalian Fertilization. In: Knobil E, Neill JD, eds. *The Physiology of Reproduction.* 2nd ed. New York: Raven Press; 1994: 189–317.

232. Yanagimachi R. Acceleration of the acrosome reaction and activation of guinea pig spermatozoa by detergents and other reagents. *Biol Reprod* 1975; 13:519–526.

233. Meizel S, Turner KO. Stimulation of an exocytotic event, the hamster sperm acrosome reaction by cis-unsaturated fatty acids. *FEBS Lett* 1983; 161:315–318.

234. Fleming AD, Kosower NS, Yanagimachi R. Promotion of capacitation of guinea pig spermatozoa by the membrane motility agent, $A_2C$ and inhibition by the disulfide-reducing agent DTT. *Gamete Res* 1982; 5:19–33.

235. Olds-Clarke P. Genetic analysis of sperm function in fertilization. *Gamete Res* 1988; 20:241–264.

236. Shalgi R, Smith TT, Yanagimachi R. A quantitative comparison of the passage of capacitated and uncapacitated hamster spermatozoa through the uterotubal junction. *Biol Reprod* 1992; 46:419–424.

237. Lanzafame F, Chapman MG, Guglielmino A, et al. Pharmacological stimulation of sperm motility. *Hum Reprod* 1994; 9:192–199.

238. Tash JS. Role of cAMP, calcium, and protein phosphorylation in sperm motility. In: Gagnon C, ed. *Controls of Sperm Motility: Biological and Clinical Aspects.* Boca Raton, FL: CRC Press; 1990: 229–250.

239. Fraser LR, Monks NJ. Cyclic nucleotides and mammalian sperm capacitation. *J Reprod Fertil* 1990; 42(suppl):9–21.

240. Kopf GS, Gerton GL. The mammalian sperm acrosome and the acrosome reaction. In: Wassarman PM, ed. *Elements of Mammalian Fertilization.* Boca Raton, FL: CRC Press; 1991: 153–203.

241. Garbers DL, Lust WD, First NL, et al. Effects of phosphodiesterase inhibitors and cyclic nucleotides on sperm respiration and motility. *Biochemistry* 1971; 10:1825–1831.

242. Garbers DL, First NL, Sullivan JJ, et al. Stimulation and maintenance of ejaculated bovine spermatozoan respiration and motility by caffeine. *Biol Reprod* 1971; 5:336–339.

243. Haesugcharern A, Chulavatnatol M. Stimulation of human spermatozoal motility by caffeine. *Fertil Steril* 1973; 24:662–665.

244. Homonnai ZT, Gedalia P, Sofer A, et al. Effect of caffeine on the motility, viability, oxygen consumption and glycolytic rate of ejaculated human normokinetic and hypokinetic spermatozoa. *Int J Androl* 1976; 21:163–170.

245. Read MD, Schnieden H. Effect of two methylxanthine derivatives and four prostaglandins on the motility of spermatozoa from volunteers and oligozoospermic patients. *Int J Androl* 1978; 1:220–224.

246. Ruzich JV, Harcharan G, Wein AJ, et al. Objective assessment of the effect of caffeine on sperm motility and velocity. *Fertil Steril* 1987; 48:891–893.

247. Schoenfeld CY, Amelar RD, Dubin L. Stimulation of ejaculated human spermatozoa by caffeine. *Fertil Steril* 1975; 26:158–161.

248. Barkay J, Zuckerman H, Sklan D, et al. Effect of caffeine on increasing the motility of frozen human sperm. *Fertil Steril* 1977; 28:175–176.

249. Schill W-B, Pritsch W, Preissler G. Effect of caffeine and kallikrein on cryopreserved human spermatozoa. *Int J Fertil* 1979; 24:27–32.

250. Aitken RJ, Best F, Richardson DW, et al. Influence of caffeine on movement characteristics, fertilizing capacity and ability to pen-

etrate cervical mucus of human spermatozoa. *J Reprod Fertil* 1983; 67:19–27.

251. Harrison RF, Sheppard BL, Kaliszer M. Observations on the motility, ultrastructure and elemental composition of human spermatozoa incubated with caffeine. *Andrologia* 1980; 12:34–42.

252. Irvine DS, Aitken RJ. Measurement of intracellular calcium in human spermatozoa. *Gamete Res* 1982; 15:57–71.

253. Brokaw CJ. Regulation of sperm flagellar motility by calcium and cAMP-dependent phosphorylation. *J Cell Biochem* 1987; 35:175–264.

254. Babcock DF, Pfeiffer DR. Independent elevation of cytosolic $[Ca^{2+}]$ and pH of mammalian sperm by voltage-dependent and pH-sensitive mechanisms. *J Biol Chem* 1987; 262:15041–15047.

255. Thomas P, Meizel S. An influx of extracellular calcium is required for initiation of the human sperm acrosome reaction induced by human follicular fluid. *Gamete Res* 1988; 20:397–412.

256. Fraser LR, Abeydeera LR, Niwa K. $Ca^{2+}$-regulating mechanisms that modulate bull sperm capacitation and acrosomal exocytosis as determined by chlortetracycline analysis. *Mol Reprod Dev* 1995; 40:233–241.

257. Gibbons BH, Gibbons IR. Calcium-induced quiescence in reactivated sea urchin sperm. *J Cell Biochem* 1980; 84:13–27.

258. Mohri H, Yanagimachi R. Characteristics of motor apparatus in testicular, epididymal and ejaculated spermatozoa. *Exp Cell Res* 1980; 127:191–196.

259. Peterson RN, Seyler D, Bundman D, et al. The effect of theophylline and dibutyryl cyclic AMP on the uptake of radioactive calcium and phosphate ions by boar and human spermatozoa. *J Reprod Fertil* 1979; 55:385–390.

260. Lanzafame F, Chapman MG, Guglielmino A, et al. Pharmacological stimulation of sperm motility. *Hum Reprod* 1994; 9:192–199.

261. Harrison RF. Insemination of husband's semen with and without the addition of caffeine. *Fertil Steril* 1978; 29:532–534.

262. Barkay J, Bartoov B, Ben-Ezra S, et al. The influence of in vitro caffeine treatment on human sperm morphology and fertilizing capacity. *Fertil Steril* 1984; 14:913–918.

263. Shen MR, Chiang PH, Yang RC, et al. Pentoxifylline stimulates human sperm motility both in vitro and after oral therapy. *Br J Clin Pharmacol* 1991; 31:711–714.

264. Moohan JM, Winston RML, Lindsay KS. Variability of human sperm response to immediate and prolonged exposure to pentoxifylline. *Hum Reprod* 1993; 8:1696–1700.

265. Sikka SC, Hellstrom WJG. The application of pentoxifylline in the stimulation of sperm motion in men undergoing electroejaculation. *J Androl* 1991; 12:165–170.

266. Maramma P, Baraghini GF, Carani C, et al. Further studies on the effects of pentoxifylline on sperm count and sperm motility in patients with idiopathic oligoasthenozoospermia. *Andrologia* 1985; 17:612–616.

267. Yovich JM, Edirisinghe WR, Cummins JM, et al. Influence of pentoxifylline in severe male factor infertility. *Fertil Steril* 1990; 53:715–722.

268. Tesarik J, Thébault A, Testart J. Effect of pentoxifylline on sperm movement characteristics in normozoospermic and asthenozoospermic specimens. *Hum Reprod* 1992; 7:1257–1263.

269. Hammitt DG, Martin PA, Callanan T. Correlations between heterospermic fertility and assays of porcine semen quality before and after cryopreservation. *Theriogenology* 1989; 32:385–399.

270. Kaskar K, Franken DR, Van der Horst G, et al. The effect of pentoxifylline on sperm movement characteristics and zona pellucida binding potential of teratozoospermic men. *Hum Reprod* 1994; 9:477–481.

271. Chiang PH, Tsai EM, Shen MR, et al. Effect of pentoxifylline in the hamster zona-free oocyte, spermatozoa penetration assay and on spermatozoa transmembrane migration motility. *Eur Urol* 1992; 21:151–154.

272. Lambert H, Serpa N, Steinleitner A, et al. Enhanced gamete interaction in the sperm penetration assay after coincubation with pentoxifylline and human follicular fluid. *Fertil Steril* 1992; 58:1205–1208.

273. Carver-Ward JA, Jaroudi KA, Einspenner M, et al. Pentoxifylline potentiates ionophore (A23187) mediated acrosome reaction in human sperm: flow cytometric analysis using CD46 antibody. *Hum Reprod* 1994; 9:71–76.

274. Gearon CM, Mortimer D, Chapman MG, et al. Artificial induction of the acrosome reaction in human spermatozoa. *Hum Reprod* 1994; 9:77–82.

275. Dimitriadou F, Rizos D, Mantzavinos T, et al. The effect of pentoxifylline on sperm motility, oocyte fertilization, embryo quality, and preg-

nancy outcome in an in vitro fertilization program. *Fertil Steril* 1995; 63:880–886.

276. Gavella M, Lipovac V, Marotti T. Effect of pentoxifylline on superoxide anion production by human sperm. *Int J Androl* 1991; 14:320–327.

277. Aitken RJ. Andrology and semen preparation for IVF. In: Fishel S, Symonds EM, eds. *In Vitro Fertilisation: Past, Present, Future.* Oxford: IRL Press; 1986: 89–106.

278. Centola GN, Mattox JH, Burde S, et al. Assessment of the viability and acrosome status of fresh and frozen-thawed human spermatozoa using single-wavelength fluorescence microscopy. *Mol Reprod Dev* 1990; 27:130–135.

279. Critser JK, Arneson BW, Aaker DV, et al. Cryopreservation of human spermatozoa. II. Postthaw chronology of motility and of zona-free hamster ova penetration. *Fertil Steril* 1987; 47:980–984.

280. Cohen J, Felten P, Zeilmaker GH. In vitro cryopreserved human spermatozoa: a comparative study of freezing and thawing procedures. *Fertil Steril* 1981; 36:356–362.

281. Keel BA, Webster BW, Roberts DK. Effects of cryopreservation on the motility characteristics of human spermatozoa. *J Reprod Fertil* 1987; 81:213–220.

282. Mazur P. Freezing of living cells: mechanisms and implications. *Am J Physiol* 1984; 247:C125–C142.

# 5
# What Every Andrologist Should Know About Female Reproduction

Gloria Richard-Davis and P. Ronald Clisham

The reproductive cycle in the female is a coordinated interaction between the hypothalamus and pituitary in concert with the ovary, uterus, endometrium, and fallopian tubes. Any derangement in the function of the reproductive system may result in infertility or subfertility.

## Anatomy

### Hypothalamic-Pituitary Axis

#### Hypothalamus and Pituitary

The hypothalamus lies at the base of the brain superior to the optic chiasm. The pituitary gland lies below the hypothalamus within a bony cavity called the sella tursica. The diaphragm sella, a condensation of dura mater, separates the pituitary from the cranial cavity.

The pituitary gland is divided into two parts: a neurohypophysis and an adenohypophysis. The neurohypophysis comprises the pars nervosa (posterior lobe) and the neural stalk (infundibulum). It is derived from neural tissue and is in direct contact with the hypothalamus and central nervous system. The adenohypophysis consists of a pars distalis (anterior lobe), pars intermedia (intermediate lobe), and a pars tuberalis that surround the neural stalk. The adenohypophysis results from an invagination of ectoderm (Rathke's pouch) and has no direct contact with the hypothalamus or central nervous system.

Within the hypothalamus, there are three nuclei that have primary significance to the neuro- and adenohypophysis. The supraoptic and paraventricular nuclei contain cell bodies of neurons that are responsible for the production of oxytocin and vasopressin (antidiuretic hormone). The axons of these neurons terminate in the neurohypophysis where secretion of these hormones occurs and gains access to the circulatory system. The arcuate nucleus contains tuberoinfundibular neurons that are responsible for the production of the gonadotropin-releasing hormone (GnRH). The axons of these neurons terminate on fenestrated blood vessels of the hypophysial portal system located in the median eminence of the neural stalk. The hypophysial portal system is the arterial blood supply to the neural stalk and serves as the major avenue of transport for hypothalamic secretions to the adenohypophysis.

Within the adenohypophysis, five different cell types produce six different peptide hormones: (1) the gonadotroph—follicle-stimulating hormone (FSH) and leutinizing hormone (LH); (2) the thyrotroph—thyroid-stimulating hormone (TSH); (3) the corticotroph—adrenocorticotrophic hormone (ACTH); (4) the lactotroph—prolactin (PRL); and (5) the somatotroph—growth hormone (GH).[1,2]

GnRH is produced in the axonal terminals of the tuberoinfundibular neurons and released into fenestrated capillaries of the hypophysial portal system located in the median eminence. The GnRH is then delivered to the anterior pituitary where it binds to receptors on the gonadotrophs and initiates gonadotropin release (FSH, LH). Gonadotropins circulate systemically and perfuse the ovary to initiate follicular development.

The FSH and LH released from the anterior pituitary are mediated by changes in the pulse frequency of GnRH release. Modulation of the pulse frequency of GnRH may occur by several methods. Feedback inhibition is mediated by neighboring opiodergic neurons with steroid receptors whose axons terminate on neurons in the arcuate nucleus. The degree of GnRH inhibition is dependent on ovarian steroid hormone production. GnRH pulse frequency is inhibited most during the luteal phase when the ovary is producing large amounts of estrogen and progesterone from the corpus luteum. This inhibition is relieved following the disruption of the corpus luteum and the subsequent decrease in steroid hormone production. The increase in GnRH pulse frequency increases the release of FSH and LH and results in a cycle of follicular development. At midcycle, higher levels of estradiol enhance hypothalamic release of GnRH and help to induce the midcycle LH surge, either by increasing the release of GnRH or by increasing the sensitivity of the pituitary to the GnRH decapeptide. Gonadotropins may have an inhibitory effect on GnRH release. Catecholamines also appear to have regulatory effects on GnRH release: dopamine and serotonin have inhibitory effects, whereas norepinephrine is stimulatory.[3]

## Female Pelvic Anatomy

The vagina, uterus, fallopian tubes, and ovaries are the main components of the female reproductive tract. Functionally, these components provide a means for gamete production, collection and transport, fertilization, implantation, incubation, and parturition.

### Ovary

The ovaries are flattened, compressed, oval structures responsible for the periodic release of gametes and the production of the steroid hormones.[4,5] Each ovary consists of three regions: the outer cortex, the central medulla, and the rete ovarii (the hilum). The outer cortex is composed of a superficial layer of cuboidal cells (the germinal epithelium), the tunica albu-

ginea, and an inner cortex. Within the inner cortex are numerous follicles that contain oocytes surrounded by a supporting stroma. The stroma comprises connective tissue and interstitial cells (theca cells) that are responsive to gonadotropins (LH, human chorionic gonadotropin [HCG]) in the production of androgens. Central to the cortex is the medullary layer of the ovary, which is composed of cells that are derived from the mesonephros. The hilum provides a more central point of attachment for the ovary to the ovarian and infundibulopelvic ligaments, through which the major blood supply courses. In addition to blood vessels, nerves and hilus cells are present in this area. Hilus cells, similar in function to Leydig cells, can secrete steroids and have been known to produce androgen-secreting tumors, primarily in elderly women.

### Vagina

The vagina is a flattened tube extending from the hymenal ring at the introitus up to the fornices that surround the cervix. Its epithelium is formed from stratified squamous epithelium and it is nonkeratinized. The vaginal mucosa is devoid of mucous glands and hair follicles. The vagina has a very acid environment (pH 4.3), maintained by the presence of lactobacillus in the vaginal secretions.

### Uterus

The uterus functions as the incubation site for developing gestation and is mechanically responsible for the expulsion and delivery of the conception at parturition. The uterus consists of the cervix and the uterine corpus, which join at the isthmus.

### Cervix

The uterine cervix projects into the vagina and serves as the point of entry for the spermatozoa. The cervix is about 2 to 3 cm in length and is covered with a nonkeratinizing squamous epithelium. The endocervical canal is a tubular structure composed primarily of connective tissue lined by many deep crypts. These crypts are lined with a secretory, ciliated and nonciliated columnar epithelium covered with microvilli. The microvilli present on the epithelium in the endocervix direct mucus outward from the cervix into the vagina. The quality and quantity of cervical mucus can change, depending on the phase of the menstrual cycle. In the follicular phase under estrogenic influence, the cervical mucus is watery and abundant and can serve as a medium for sperm access to the upper reproductive tract. In the secretory phase, under progestational influence, the cervical mucus thickens and forms a plug over the endocervical canal. This mucous barrier may serve to prevent the upward ascent of bacteria, thus preventing reproductive tract infections.

### Uterine Corpus

The uterine corpus is pear-shaped, composed of interlacing smooth muscle fibers. Within the uterine corpus lies the endometrium, the site of implantation for developing gestations. The external surface of the uterine corpus is covered with visceral peritoneum.

### Fallopian Tubes

The fallopian tubes are muscular tubes between 8 and 10 cm in length that are contiguous with the uterus. These structures have a lumen that connects with the endometrial cavity, providing access between the peritoneal cavity and the uterus. The tubes have internal rugae and are lined by a ciliated columnar epithelium. This type of epithelium may be crucial in the fallopian tube because of its function in the transport of the egg/embryo to the uterus. In rabbits, the reversal of a segment of the ampullar portion of the tube, reversing the direction of the ciliary beat, interferes with pregnancy without inhibiting fertilization.[6] However, the cilia do not beat in women with Kartagener's syndrome (the congenital absence of dynein arms in the cilia). Pregnancies have been reported in these women, which suggests that cilia play a less important role in the human.[7]

The secretory characteristics of the fallopian tube epithelium also vary, depending on the phase of the menstrual cycle. During the late follicular phase when estradiol levels are the highest, the secretions in the region of the isthmus become more abundant and viscous. This mucous column is analogous to the mucous column observed in the endocervix and may play an important role in the transport of sperm through the isthmus toward the isthmic-ampullar junction where fertilization occurs. During the luteal phase, when progesterone is present, this mucous secretion is suppressed.

## The Menstrual Cycle

The menstrual cycle can be divided into four phases based on ovarian and endometrial histology: follicular, ovulatory, luteal, and menstrual.

## Follicular Phase

The follicular phase coincides in the ovary with the development of the graafian follicle. During the preceding cycle, as the corpus luteum begins to fail, levels of steroid hormones and inhibin begin to fall, allowing for a rise in FSH secretion. The rising FSH rescues a cohort of developing primary oocytes from atresia (days 27 to 28). Follicular recruitment proceeds for several days. From this cohort of follicles a dominant follicle is selected (days 5 to 7), matures (days 8 to 12), and ovulates (days 13 to 14). The remaining follicles undergo atresia. The follicular phase lasts on average about 13 days, the time required for a follicle to become mature and ovulate.

## Ovulatory Phase

As the dominant follicle develops, estradiol levels increase. With the rising levels of estradiol, the granulosa cells of the follicle acquire the LH receptor and the ability to secrete progesterone (leutinization). About 12 hours later, a rise in LH and FSH occurs, signaling the beginning of the ovulatory phase. This is associated with a peak in estradiol in the serum that occurs about 24 to 36 hours prior to ovulation.[8] The LH surge occurs and results in three events: the final maturation of the oocyte, the initiation of an inflammatory process that will eventually result in ovulation, and further leutinization of the follicle to establish the corpus luteum.

## Luteal Phase

The luteal phase is characterized by progesterone dominance as compared with the estrogen dominance of the follicular phase. The corpus luteum is responsible for progesterone secretion, produced in the luteal cells. Maximal production of progesterone occurs during the midluteal phase. During this time, the endometrium becomes secretory in response to progesterone and is most receptive for implantation of an embryo. If pregnancy is initiated, the syncytiotrophoblast of the fetal placenta secretes HCG, which signals the corpus luteum to continue hormonal support. If pregnancy fails to occur, luteolysis ensues, leading to a decline in progesterone, estradiol, and inhibin.

## Menstrual Phase

The failure of the corpus luteum and loss of hormone production initiates a sequence of events within the endometrium and results in the onset of menses. With the regression of the corpus luteum, basal levels of FSH increase and begin the recruitment of a subsequent cohort of follicles for development in the ensuing cycle.

# Sperm Transport Through the Female Reproductive Tract

With respect to the entry of male gametes into the female reproductive system, the vagina serves as the repository for the male ejaculate following intercourse. The environment in the vagina is extremely acidic and hostile to sperm (pH < 5.0) because of resident lactobacilli. Seminal plasma has an alkaline pH that supports sperm motility and buffers the effect of the acid vaginal pH. However, even with the deposition of this alkaline buffer into the vagina, the acid environment returns within 3 to 4 minutes.[9] Sperm that do not find their way into the cervical mucus or cervical crypts within this time period after ejaculation usually die.

During intercourse, intromission and ejaculation may cause negative changes in vaginal pressure. Female orgasm may cause a positive vaginal pressure followed by a rapid drop after relaxation.[9] Both phenomena may lead to the drawing of sperm into the endocervical canal.

Prostaglandins have been postulated as having a role in promoting uterine contractility (PGE and $PGF_{2\alpha}$)[10–12] and sperm transport; however, the types of prostaglandins primarily present in the seminal fluid (19-hydroxylated) are known to be less biologically active.[13,14] PGE has been found in the seminal plasma of fertile men.[15] $PGF_{2\alpha}$, added to a sperm suspension, has been noted to increase the penetration of sperm through cervical mucus in vitro.[16] However, there are very low quantities of prostaglandin present in seminal plasma, and the relationship between fertility and prostaglandins remains largely unknown. Relaxin, another compound found in seminal plasma[17] has been shown to increase sperm motility and to enhance the movement of sperm through bovine cervical mucus.[18]

In the cervix, the endocervical glands are responsible for the secretion of a cervical mucus that provides sperm with a medium through which they may gain access to the lower uterine cavity. Cervical mucus is penetrable by sperm as early as the ninth day of the menstrual cycle. The rate of sperm penetration increases until the peak penetration is observed around the periovulatory period. During the periovulatory period, the mucus serves to protect sperm from the hostile vaginal environment, prevent entry of seminal plasma into the uterus, exclude morphologically abnormal sperm, and serves as a reservoir for sperm for later migration to the upper tract. One to two days after ovulation, sperm penetration is inhibited because of mucus thickening secondary to progesterone secretion.

Rapid delivery of sperm from the endocervix to the uterotubal junction is probably due to contraction of the uterine musculature. Sperm motility may only serve to maintain the cells in suspension within the uterine fluid.[19] Uterine activity may be stimulated by a number of different mediators, including catecholamines,[20] prostaglandins,[21] and platelet activating factor;[22] all of which propel sperm to the vicinity of the fallopian tubes.

Within the uterus, the endometrium provides an environment that supports the transport of sperm through the uterus and to the fallopian tube. At the time of ovulation, the human endometrium secretes a fluid that is rich in amino acids and proteins. An amino acid found in substantial quantities is taurine, which serves to sustain motility by protecting sperm from high potassium concentrations.[23]

Intimate contact of sperm with the endometrium has been noted to cause changes in the swimming characteristics of sperm. Sperm incubated with monolayers of uterine or tubal epithelium exhibit a higher degree of hyperactivation when compared with sperm incubated with cells from a kidney cell line.[24] Hyperactivated swimming movements may give sperm the ability to penetrate the viscous fluid of the oviduct and the cumulus mass.[25] Polypeptides from uterine fluid may also play a role in capacitation following passive absorption to the sperm surface.[26] In addition to the cervix, the tubal isthmus may serve as an additional storage site for sperm.

## Capacitation

After transit through the male reproductive tract, spermatozoa are active but do not have the ability to fertilize the female gamete. The acquisition of this capability is termed capacitation. It is achieved by the sperm's residence in the female reproductive tract. In the human, capacitation most likely begins as the sperm pass through the cervical mucus.[27]

In the human, capacitation is not an organ-specific phenomenon. Pregnancies have resulted from sperm that have been deposited in the peritoneal cavity following direct intraperitoneal insemination (DIPI)[28-30] as well as in the fallopian tube via the gamete intrafallopian transfer (GIFT) procedure.[31-33] Transit through the cervix and uterus is not required. Capacitation is not species-specific, for sperm capacitation may be facilitated by co-incubation with cells from the reproductive tracts of other species.[34] Capacitation may also occur in vitro with the use of various biologic fluids and chemically

defined capacitation media.[35] The acrosome reaction has been used as an indicator of the completion of the capacitation process. Sperm will not undergo acrosome reaction, either by contact with egg vestments or spontaneously, unless they have been capacitated.[36-44]

## Fertilization

Because the eggs of mammals are covered with a protective glycoprotein coat (zona pellucida), the sperm must possess a means to either enzymatically or mechanically disrupt this protective barrier to gain access to the plasma membrane of the egg. Covering the sperm head is a caplike structure or acrosome that contains enzymes capable of dissolving the vestments of the egg. During the acrosome reaction, the overlying plasma membrane and outer acrosomal membrane undergo multiple sites of fusion, which allows the acrosomal contents to escape. Numerous enzymes have been identified in the acrosomal contents. The two most extensively studied are hyaluronidase and acrosin. It is thought that hyaluronidase dissolves the cumulus matrix and acrosin aids in the passage of the sperm through the zona pellucida.[45-50]

After traversing the zona pellucida, the postacrosomal region of the sperm head fuses with the oocyte membrane and triggers the cortical granule reaction, activation of the oocyte, and the completion of meiosis. The second polar body is then released, leaving the egg with a haploid complement of chromosomes. The sperm nucleus is then incorporated into the ooplasma of the oocyte. The cortical reaction results in changes to the oocyte membrane and zona pellucida that prevent the penetration of another sperm into the oocyte.[51] This forms a block to polyspermy. Following penetration of the oocyte, the sperm nucleus decondenses to form the male pronucleus, which eventually fuses with the female pronucleus at syngamy to form the zygote.[47]

## Implantation

Implantation is a process of attachment between the embryo and endometrium and establishment of a vascular connection to the mother. The process begins with the initial transport of the embryo from the fallopian tube to the uterus. The embryo arrives in the uterus about 3 to 4 days after ovulation. After 2 to 3 days in the uterus, the blastocyst begins to lose its zona pellucida (hatches) due to lytic factors within the uterine fluid. Attachment begins as microvilli on the surface of the embryo interdigitate with those on the luminal surface of the endometrium. Junctional complexes form between the embryo and endometrial epithelium. Three types of interactions between the embryo and the endometrial epithelium have been described: an interdigitation of trophoblast cells between endometrial cells, an undermining of the trophoblast between the endometrial cell and the basement membrane,[52] and fusion of the trophoblast with the endometrial cell.[53]

The trophoblast produces plasminogen activator, an enzyme activity that is important in the early establishment of the trophoblast in the endometrium.[54,55] Plasminogen is converted to plasmin by urokinase produced by the trophoblast. The amount of conversion is regulated by HCG, which is also produced by the trophoblast and inhibits the activity of the urokinase.[56]

At later stages, the embryo can digest the normal intracellular matrix with a number of proteolytic enzymes.[57,58] The space made by this process allows spreading of the trophoblast, gaining further access to the endometrium.[59,60]

# Infertility and Disturbances in Female Reproduction

Disturbances in the normal function of the reproductive cycle generally result in infertility or subfertility. Infertility is defined differently by epidemiologists, public health planners, and clinicians. Its incidence, prevalence, and demographics vary in the population, depending on which definition is used. In the United States, the currently accepted medical definition of infertility is 1 year of unprotected intercourse without conception. Based on this definition, 10% to 20% of married couples in the United States in which the wives were 15 to 44 years

old were infertile in 1982.[61] Without contraception, about 25% of couples will conceive in the first month, 60% within 6 months, and 80% within 1 year.[62] Of the remaining 20% of couples, a significant number will conceive within an additional year. Therefore, the World Health Organization Scientific Group has proposed 2 years of unprotected intercourse without conception as a more conservative definition of infertility.[63] It has been estimated that 3% to 5% of couples worldwide have never conceived despite 2 years of exposure.[63] These couples represent a core population with nearly irreducible infertility.

# Causes of Infertility

The incidence of any individual factor as a cause of infertility can only be estimated and varies with the study population. Among women seeking treatment for infertility, the proportion of reported causes has been similar in several studies.[62] The causes reported include ovulatory dysfunction in 20% to 30%, tubal disease in 15% to 30%, endometriosis in 4% to 6%, cervical and uterine factors in 10%, sperm defects in 30%, and unexplained infertility in 15% of the couples.[62] Furthermore, infertility in many couples has multiple causes (Table 5.1). The prognosis is best for women with failure of ovulation secondary to amenorrhea or oligomenorrhea, with 2-year conception rates of 96% and 78%, respectively. Only 20% to 25% of reported patients with tubal damage conceived despite surgery.[63] Couples with sperm defects have a poor chance of pregnancy

TABLE 5.1. Etiology of infertility.

| Cause | Percentage of infertile couples |
|---|---|
| Female factors | |
|   Ovulatory dysfunction | 20–30 |
|   Uterine/tubal factor | 15–30 |
|   Cervical factor | 5 |
|   Endometriosis | 5–10 |
|   Immunological | <3 |
|   Unexplained | 10–15 |
| Male factor | 30–40 |

Data taken from Speroff et al.[62]

without donor insemination or assisted reproductive technology (ART).

## Epidemiology

Several epidemiologic factors contribute to infertility. Many couples are delaying childbearing, which makes age a major factor. In the female, reproductive ability is maximal between age 21 and 24 years and gradually declines thereafter.[64] The male is most fertile around 24 to 25 years of age.[64] In addition to the inherent effects of age on the reproductive organs, advancing age increases the risk for exposure to diseases with potentially damaging effects on fertility, such as endometriosis, sexually transmitted diseases, and pelvic inflammatory disease (PID). The fertility rate is also related to frequency of intercourse and such factors as cigarette smoking and illicit drug use. Excessive coital activity may result in a decline in sperm density, whereas infrequent coital activity reduces the chance of sperm and egg encounter. Nicotine and other components of smoke adversely affect cervical mucus, tubal motility, spermatogenesis, and oocyte viability. Illicit drugs, such as marijuana or narcotics, affect hypothalamic-pituitary secretion of hormones.[65]

Environmental and occupational exposures to ionizing radiation, textile dyes, and numerous chemicals may have an adverse effect on female or male fertility.

## Infertility Evaluation

### History

Every effort should be made to initiate the fertility survey by a joint interview with both partners. The couple should be encouraged to appear at the initial consultation together. At this visit, a comprehensive medical and surgical history of both partners should be obtained. The female partner should be questioned regarding menstrual cycle, previous pregnancies, contraceptive use, and sexual history. Details relating to coital frequency and timing, sexual dysfunction, and possible use of lubricants should be obtained. The male partner's history should also have a comprehensive evaluation. A social history and prior exposure to environmental and occupational toxins should be elicited from both partners. Finally, the history must include information generated by any prior workup or treatment for infertility. Every effort should be made to obtain the pertinent records.

### Physical Examination

The gynecologist is generally the woman's primary-care physician. The general examination should be a complete one. Special attention should be directed to height, weight, presence of galactorrhea, acne, breast size, and hair distribution. The pelvic examination should screen for any anatomic or pathologic abnormalities, such as masses, infection, and signs of endometriosis.

## Infertility Factors in Female Patients

The factors that affect fertility in couples may be either singular or multifactorial. A systematic and methodical approach to evaluate the individual partners must be comprehensive.

### Ovulation Dysfunction

All infertile women should have an evaluation of their ovulatory status as to whether they have regular menstrual cycles or evidence of menstrual dysfunction. Ovulation disorders account for approximately 20% to 30% of all infertility. If only female factors are considered, ovulatory dysfunction accounts for at least 40% of infertility.[62] Ovulation, the key event in the ovarian cycle, usually occurs in most women who are menstruating normally and regularly, i.e., uterine bleeding occurring at 21- to 36-day intervals. However, even in women who exhibit cyclic bleeding, occasional anovulatory cycles may occur. Abnormal menstrual function can be a symptom reflecting both an ovulation problem and an underlying medical condition. Ovulatory disturbance may result from thyroid, pituitary, or adrenal disease; eating disorders; drugs; or chronic illnesses.

## Polycystic Ovarian Syndrome

Most commonly, polycystic ovarian syndrome (PCOS) accounts for the majority of ovulatory dysfunction. The characteristic polycystic ovary emerges when a state of anovulation persists for any unusual length of time. The precise initiating event in this complex process is yet unknown, but it involves the hypothalamus, pituitary, ovaries, adrenal, and peripheral adipose tissues, all contributing to an endocrine imbalance usually associated with oligo-ovulation, hirsutism, and infertility. In contrast to the characteristic fluctuating hormonal pattern in PCOS, there is a "steady state" of gonadotropins and sex steroids associated with chronic anovulation. The daily production of estrogen and androgens is both increased by and dependent on LH stimulation,[66] which is reflected in higher circulating levels of testosterone, androstenedione, dehydroepiandrosterone (DHA), dehydroepiandrosterone sulfate (DHAS), 17-hydroxyprogesterone (17-OHP), and estrone.[67] Insulin resistance and a hyperinsulinemia resulting from an insulin receptor defect have been associated with PCOS. An increase in insulin results in increased thecal androgen production in response to LH. Insulin binding to insulin-like growth factor-I (IGF-I) receptors augments the LH response.[68] After appropriate evaluation and diagnosis, treatment for fertility patients generally involves ovulation induction using clomiphene citrate or gonadotropins. In rare cases, it may be necessary to institute surgical treatment, such as ovarian wedge resection or ovarian drilling. The goal of medical or surgical treatment is to overcome the excess androgen production and thereby to interrupt the chronic anovulatory cycles.

## Hyperprolactinemia

Elevation in prolactin level (normal range 0 to 25 ng/ml) may also cause ovulatory disturbances. Increasing levels of prolactin can cause a woman to progress through a spectrum beginning with an inadequate luteal phase to anovulation to the amenorrhea associated with complete GnRH suppression. Elevated prolactin inhibits the pulsatile release of GnRH necessary for follicular development, which culminates in ovulation. Prolactin may be elevated as a result of pregnancy, pituitary adenoma, hypothyroidism, stress, amino acid-rich foods, sleep, and multiple drug intake (particularly drugs affecting the central nervous system [CNS] and drugs containing estrogen). A detailed drug history, exclusion of thyroid disease, and the imaging studies of the pituitary (computed tomography [CT] or magnetic resonance imaging [MRI]) are generally necessary in the evaluation process. Once a life-threatening CNS tumor is excluded by imaging studies, the patient with hyperprolactinemia will respond readily to dopamine agonist therapy. The treatment of choice is bromocriptine mesylate (Parlodel, Sandoz Pharmaceuticals). Additional choices of medications include pergolide mesylate and nonergoline dopamine agonist CV205-502.

## Hypothyroidism

Thyroid hormone is needed for the normal function of most organs, and the clinical presentation of hypothyroidism varies according to the magnitude and duration of thyroid hormone deficiency. Thyroid dysfunction, by contribution to anovulation, luteal-phase defect, or hyperprolactinemia, may be associated with infertility. Thyroid hormone profiles are recommended in women presenting with infertility. Generally, treatment is simply the replacement of the deficient thyroid hormone after the etiology has been determined. Replacement of thyroxine ($T_4$) is the method of choice and is usually administered lifelong. Other thyroid hormone preparations available for replacement therapy besides $T_4$ include triiodothyronine ($T_3$), the combination of $T_3$ and $T_4$, desiccated thyroid, and thyroglobulin. The dose for healthy patients will almost always restore TSH to normal values.

## Luteal Phase Defect

Luteal phase defect (LPD) is a disturbance of the ovulatory process associated with inadequate secretion of progesterone to support the luteal or secretory phase of the menstrual cycle. In general terms, this means a malfunction of the corpus luteum. The standard diagnosis is made by endometrial biopsy performed in the late secretory phase. Diagnosis and treatment of LPD remain controversial. It is generally accepted that the diagnosis of LPD requires two endometrial biopsies to be 2 or more days out of phase. The luteal phase is inadequate in up to 30% of cycles in normal females. The incidence of recurrent LPD in the infertile population ranges from 3% to 14%.[65] Serum progesterone levels have been used as a noninvasive method of diagnosing LPD. If the levels are below 10pg/ml when serum progesterone is drawn at the midluteal phase (cycle day 21), LPD is suspected. Additionally, on a basal body temperature (BBT) chart, if the patient's temperature does not remain elevated ($>0.4°C$ above baseline) for 10 days or greater, LPD should be suspected. The treatment for LPD may include the use of ovulation-induction drugs to improve corpus luteum function or to produce more than one corpus luteum or progesterone supplementation in the luteal phase.

### Tubal, Uterine, and Peritoneal Factors

Tubal factors are responsible for approximately 15% to 30% of infertility, and uterine abnormalities are a factor in less than 10%.[69] Tubal dysfunction is one of the most common causes of infertility, its incidence increased primarily due to rising rates of sexually transmitted infection and resultant PID. Other etiologic factors in tubal disease include scarring from endometriosis, previous abdominal surgery, intrauterine device usage, or diethylstilbestrol (DES) exposure. Uterine abnormalities are most commonly congenital or DES related. The most common congenital uterine abnormalities include uterine septum, bicornuate or unicornuate uterus, or uterine didelphis. Congenital uterine anomalies are most commonly associated with recurrent pregnancy losses, rather than with impaired conception.

The most common procedure for initial evaluation of uterine and tubal factors is the hysterosalpingogram (HSG). Further diagnostic evaluation may include laparoscopy, hysteroscopy, or hysterosonography.

## Endometriosis

### Definition, Incidence, and Pathogenesis

Endometriosis is a disease, commonly associated with infertility, which occurs in women of reproductive age. The mean age of diagnosis has been reported to be 25 to 29 years.[70,71] Endometriosis occurs in approximately 10% of women in reproductive age and in up to 50% of women with a history of infertility.[72,73] It is defined as the presence of endometrial tissue in an ectopic location (any place outside of the uterine cavity). Endometrial implants are commonly located in the posterior cul de sac, and on the ovaries, fallopian tubes, bladder, sigmoid, and other pelvic structures. The American Society for Reproductive Medicine (formerly the American Fertility Society) in 1978 organized an expert panel to develop a consensus for a classification system of the staging of endometriosis (Fig. 5.1). This system, revised in 1985, is based on scores assigned according to the size of endometrial implants and adhesions and allows for more accurate comparisons of the effect of treatment modalities on pain and fertility.

The pathogenesis of endometriosis includes histogenesis, etiology, and factors critical for growth and maintenance. The existence of endometriosis may be by coelomic metaplasia of cells lining the pelvic peritoneum or by transplantation and dissemination of shed uterine endometrium to ectopic locations by a number of routes (lymphatic dissemination, vascular spread, iatrogenic transplantation, retrograde menstruation, of all of these). Olive and Hammond[74] have suggested that retrograde menstruation and deficient cellular immunity are both important etiologic factors. A familial tendency for endometriosis has been documented by a number of investigators, and recent reports suggest that genetic transmission is highly likely, with the most probable mode of inheritance being polygenic and multifactorial.[75,76]

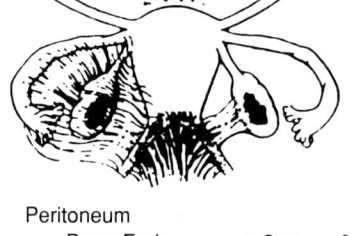

**Stage I (Minimal)**

| Peritoneum | | |
|---|---|---|
| Superficial Endo | 1–3 | 2 |
| R. Ovary | | |
| Superficial Endo | <1 cm | 1 |
| Filmy Adhesions | <1/3 | 1 |
| **Total Points** | | **4** |

**Stage II (Mild)**

| Peritoneum | | |
|---|---|---|
| Deep Endo | >3 cm | 6 |
| R. Ovary | | |
| Superficial Endo | <1 cm | 1 |
| Filmy Adhesions | <1/3 | 1 |
| L. Ovary | | |
| Superficial Endo | <1 cm | 1 |
| **Total Points** | | **9** |

**Stage III (Moderate)**

| Peritoneum | | |
|---|---|---|
| Deep Endo | >3 cm | 6 |
| Cul-de-Sac | | |
| Partial Obliteration | | 4 |
| L. Ovary | | |
| Deep Endo | 1–3 cm | 16 |
| **Total Points** | | **25** |

**Stage III (Moderate)**

| Peritoneum | | |
|---|---|---|
| Superficial Endo | >3 cm | 4 |
| R. Tube | | |
| Filmy Adhesions | <1/3 | 1 |
| R. Ovary | | |
| Filmy Adhesions | <1/3 | 1 |
| L. Tube | | |
| Dense Adhesions | <1/3 | 16* |
| L. Ovary | | |
| Deep Endo | <1 cm | 4 |
| Dense Adhesions | <1/3 | 4 |
| **Total Points** | | **30** |

**Stage IV (Severe)**

| Peritoneum | | |
|---|---|---|
| Superficial Endo | >3 cm | 4 |
| L. Ovary | | |
| Deep Endo | 1–3 cm | 32** |
| Dense Adhesions | <1/3 | 8** |
| L. Tube | | |
| Dense Adhesions | <1/3 | 8** |
| **Total Points** | | **52** |

*Point assignment changed to 16
**Point assignment doubled

**Stage IV (Severe)**

| Peritoneum | | |
|---|---|---|
| Deep Endo | >3 cm | 6 |
| Cul-de-Sac | | |
| Complete Obliteration | | 40 |
| R. Ovary | | |
| Deep Endo | 1–3 cm | 16 |
| Dense Adhesions | <1/3 | 4 |
| L. Tube | | |
| Dense Adhesions | >2/3 | 16 |
| L. Ovary | | |
| Deep Endo | 1–3 cm | 6 |
| Dense Adhesions | >2/3 | 16 |
| **Total Points** | | **114** |

FIGURE 5.1. Stages of endometriosis. Endo, endometrial involvement. (Reproduced from American Fertility Society[87] with permission.)

## Symptoms

Although many patients with the disease are entirely asymptomatic, endometriosis is associated with a wide variety of symptoms, such as infertility, noncyclic pelvic pain, dysmenorrhea, dyspareunia, backache, and dysfunctional uterine bleeding.[77] The cause of dysmenorrhea in patients with endometriosis remains speculative, although prostaglandins appear to be a plausible factor. Recent investigations have revealed that the depth of endometrial implants correlates with both pelvic pain experienced and hormonal responsiveness of the implants.[78] Infertility associated with endometriosis may be related to adhesions impairing normal tubal function. In the absence of pelvic distortion, endometriosis can still affect conception rates; however, the exact mechanism by which endometriosis affects fertility is controversial. In general, it is accepted that women with moderate-to-severe disease experience decreased fecundity rates. The hypothesized mechanisms for the decrease include ovulatory disturbances, luteinized unruptured follicles, and immunologic factors affecting fertilization and implantation.[72]

### Treatment

Treatment directed against endometriosis may be medical or surgical. Medications currently available are designed to create a pseudopregnancy, postmenopausal state, or chronic anovulatory pattern. Medical options include danazol, continuous oral contraceptives, high-dose progestins, and GnRH analog therapy. Medical therapy directed at endometriosis appears to be of value in diminishing the anatomic extent of disease or reduction of pain, but the role of medical therapy in the promotion of fertility is less evident.

Surgery is the most commonly used treatment for endometriosis. Conservative surgery can be efficacious in the reduction of disease and relief of pain and has been used extensively to enhance fertility; however, it is not a panacea. Although a variety of surgical instruments and techniques, such as sharp dissection, cauterization, endocoagulation, and laser vaporization, have been used, there has been no clear advantage of any one approach, and the surgeon should use instruments of personal choice and experience.[79,80]

### Cervical Factor

A cervical factor accounts for approximately 10% of infertility.[81] Although the postcoital test (PCT), also known as the Sims-Huhner test, is an accepted integral part of the infertility workup, its interpretation is controversial. Gross and microscopic examination of the cervical mucus should be performed at, or immedi-

ately before, the time of ovulation. The motility of spermatozoa and the cervical mucus grade observed in this test have been classified by Moghissi.[81] Grossly, the quantity (ranging from 0 to 3cc), viscosity (viscous to watery), and stretchability or spinnbarkeit (0 to 8cm) are assessed and assigned a score of 0 to 3. Microscopically, fern pattern (ranging from simple to tertiary branching), cellularity (many cells to <5/high-power field [HPF]), and motile sperm/HPF (immotile to vigorous forward motility) are observed and scored 0 to 3. Under ideal conditions, more than 10 sperm/HPF ($\times$400) with grade 3+ motility constitutes a normal result. The optimal time to obtain PCT after intercourse is debatable. Recommendations vary from 2 to 24 hours after intercourse. Complement-dependent reactions that immobilize sperm require 8 to 10 hours.[82] Therefore, to optimize information obtained from a PCT, an 8- to 12-hour time interval may be best. Abnormal PCT may result from inappropriate timing, inadequate estrogen levels, vaginal or cervical infection, inadequate cervical mucus production, or the presence of sperm antibodies. Treatment for abnormal PCT is generally intrauterine insemination, which bypasses the hostile cervical mucus.

### Other Factors

Studies have reported a greater prevalence of genital mycoplasma in cervical mucus and semen of infertile couples than in fertile couples.[62,83–85] Two types of organisms recovered from the genital tract of infertile women are *Mycoplasma hominis* and *Ureaplasma urealyticum*. Although correlation of genital mycoplasma and infertility remains debatable, cultures should be obtained and infertile patients treated with doxycycline, if positive. Antisperm antibodies to cervical mucus, sperm, and blood should be obtained if the PCT is abnormal or if there is presence of sperm agglutination on semen analysis or in cases of unexplained infertility.

## Diagnostic Evaluation

Preliminary laboratory tests should include urinalysis, complete blood count, rubella titer, serologic test for syphilis for both partners, and screening for sexually transmitted diseases (STD). Additional laboratory tests for the female partner may include thyroid function tests (for suspected thyroid disease), serum prolactin, FSH and LH (for gonadal disorders), testosterone, dehydroepiandrosterone sulfate (DHEAS), and 17-hydroxyprogesterone (for hirsutism or adrenal disorders), and chromosomal studies (for genetic disorders) when indicated.

Each couple's infertility evaluation should include evaluation for the potential of all possible factors, including ovulatory dysfunction,

tubal factor, male factor, and cervical factor. If indicated or if the basic evaluation is within the normal range, specific testing should be instituted for immunologic factors, endometriosis, and fertilization problems. In the female patient, the timing of the diagnostic tests should be based on her menstrual cycle (Fig. 5.2).

### Ovulation Assessment

Ovulation is evaluated indirectly. The investigator usually relies on presumptive evidence of ovulation, generally determined by basal body

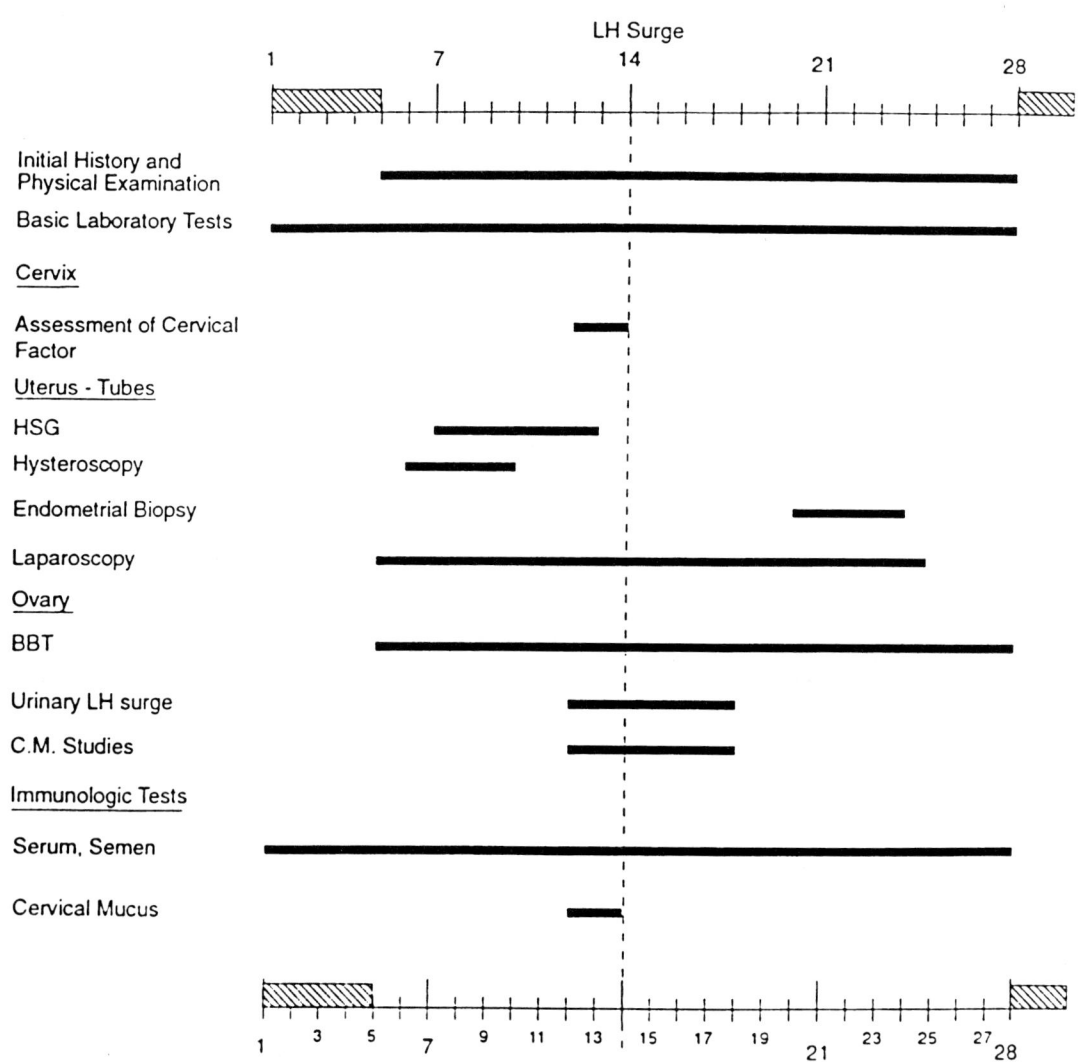

FIGURE 5.2. Optimal time for various infertility investigations (in days).

temperature (BBT), steroid or gonadotropin hormone assays, ultrasonography (US), cervical mucus changes, endometrial biopsy or all of these.[65] Ovulation should be evaluated during several menstrual cycles.

BBT is the oldest, most widely used method of ovulation detection. A sharp rise of 0.4° to 0.6° F within 2 consecutive days is indicative of ovulation. Ovulation has been reported to occur in 3% to 20% of monophasic BBT and may be absent in a small percent of biphasic BBT.[65] The midcycle serum LH surge is the most reliable predictor of ovulation, but this test is expensive and requires frequent blood sampling. Urinary LH kits are now available commercially and offer a reasonable alternative. The evening radioimmunoassay (RIA) urine LH kit was found to detect the day of surge correctly in 98% of the women studied. Endometrial biopsy confirms ovulation as well as evaluating the adequacy of the luteal phase. Diagnosis and treatment of LPD remains controversial, but it is generally accepted that the diagnosis of LPD requires that two endometrial biopsies be 2 or more days out of phase. The luteal phase has been found to be inadequate in up to 30% of isolated cycles in normal females. However, the incidence of recurrent LPD in the infertile population ranges from 3% to 14%.[65]

## Uterine and Tubal Assessment

Although hysteroscopy and laparoscopy can be used effectively, the most common procedure for initial evaluation of uterine and tubal factors is the hysterosalpingogram (HSG). The current techniques of HSG have about a 75% correlation with laparoscopy or hysteroscopy for accuracy.[62] The procedure should be done in the early follicular phase after menses has stopped, but it should be postponed if there is evidence of infection or a pelvic mass. The risk of infection is <1% in a low-risk population and 3% with a high-risk population, e.g., history of pelvic PID, septic abortion, intrauterine device (IUD) usage, ruptured appendix, pelvic or tubal surgery, or history of ectopic pregnancy. The therapeutic effects of an HSG remain controversial. If the HSG is normal, a 6-month interval should elapse to allow time for possible therapeutic benefits before proceeding with operative procedures. Hysterosonography is the most recent nonradiologic method of evaluating the endometrial cavity and fallopian tubes. In an office setting, a small catheter is placed in the endometrial cavity and a balloon is inflated to form a closed system. Sterile saline is instilled under ultrasound visualization, allowing visualization of the endometrial cavity and the flow through the fallopian tubes.[86]

Hysteroscopy should be done preferably after menses and before ovulation, and it should be performed by an experienced gynecologist capable of performing an operative procedure if indicated. Laser or operative laparoscopy, when used as a diagnostic procedure, has a high incidence of detecting endometriosis, pelvic adhesions, or other pathologies and should be available for a trained specialist. In the event that the fallopian tubes are irreparably damaged, assisted reproductive technologies are recommended for treatment.

## Treatment

Treatment options vary widely depending on the etiologic factors involved. Ovulation induction drugs, such as clomiphene citrate, human menopausal gonadotrophin (hMG), human follicle-stimulating hormone (hFSH), and gonadotropin-releasing hormone agonist, are most commonly used to correct ovulatory dysfunction. Newer, purified, or recombinant forms of gonadotropins will soon be available for clinical use. Male or cervical factor may be treated with intrauterine inseminations. However, severe male factor may require ART. Tubal or uterine factors are generally corrected surgically when possible. If these factors are not amenable to surgical corrections, then ART is a viable option. ART includes in vitro fertilization (IVF), GIFT, and micromanipulation of gametes (Table 5.2). Micromanipulation is the most recent and advanced technique in ART, primarily used for the treatment of severe male factor infertility. A couple may undergo a single treatment or combination of the treatment regimens, depending on the factors involved.

TABLE 5.2. Treatment options for infertility.

| Condition | Treatment |
|---|---|
| Ovulatory dysfunction | Ovulation induction |
| | Clomiphene citrate |
| | Human menopausal gonadotrophins (hMG) |
| | Follicle-stimulating hormone (FSH) |
| | Pulsatile gonadotropin-releasing hormone |
| | High-purified FSH* (HPFSH) |
| | Recombinant FSH* (rFSH) |
| Hyperprolactinemia | Dopamine agonist |
| | Bromocriptine |
| | Pergolide |
| Hypothyroidism | Thyroxine (T₄) |
| Tubal disease | Surgical treatment |
| | Tuboplasty, neosalpingostomy |
| | In vitro fertilization (IVF) |
| Endometriosis | Surgical treatment |
| | Laser, cautery |
| | Medical treatment |
| | GnRH agonist |
| | Danazol |
| | Oral contraceptive pill |
| | Progestins |
| Male factor | Intrauterine insemination |
| | Husband or donor |
| | Assisted reproductive technologies |
| | IVF, GIFT, micromanipulation |

## Conclusion

The female reproductive system and the reproductive process involve a very complex well-orchestrated interaction between the hypothalmus, pituitary gland, ovaries, uterus, fallopian tubes, adrenals, and thyroid. Minor dysfunction in any one of these organ systems may render the entire reproductive process nonfunctional and result in infertility. Some patients with infertility may suffer from physical disability, but their mental anguish may severely undermine their physical well-being, marital fulfillment, and family life. A well-informed and sympathetic physician who is capable of establishing good rapport and initiating an orderly, meticulous, and comprehensive program of investigation and management may provide them with an immense measure of physical and mental comfort. With careful study and search, the etiology of infertility may be identified in almost 85% to 90% of couples, and pregnancies will occur in 40% to 50% of adequately evaluated and treated infertile couples. Sophisticated and innovative therapeutic modalities, such as induction of ovulation, microsurgery, and assisted reproductive technologies, provide the promise of ever-improving results.

## References

1. Everett JW. Pituitary and hypothalamus: perspective and overview. In: Knobil E et al, eds. *The Physiology of Reproduction*. 2nd ed. New York: Raven Press; 1994: 1509–1619.
2. Yen SSC. The hypothalamic control of pituitary hormone secretion. In: Yen SSC, Jaffe R, eds. *Reproductive Endocrinology*. 3rd ed. Philadelphia: W.B. Saunders; 1991: 65–104.
3. Yen SSC. The human menstrual cycle: neuroendocrine regulation. In: Yen SSC, Jaffe R, eds. *Reproductive Endocrinology*. 3rd ed. Philadelphia: W.B. Saunders; 1991: 273–308.
4. Gore-Langton RE, Armstrong DT. Follicular steroidogenesis and its control. In: Knobil E. et al, eds. *The Physiology of Reproduction*. 2nd ed. New York: Raven Press; 1994: 571–627.
5. Adashi EY. The ovarian life cycle. In: Yen SSC, Jaffe R, eds. *Reproductive Endocrinology*. 3rd ed. Philadelphia: W.B. Saunders; 1991: 181–237.
6. Eddy CA, Flores JJ, Archer DR, et al. The role of cilia in infertility: an evaluation by selective microsurgical modification of the rabbit oviduct. *Am J Obstet Gynecol* 1978; 132:814–821.
7. Jean Y, Langlais J, Roberts KD, et al. Fertility of a woman with nonfunctional ciliated cells in the fallopian tubes. *Fertil Steril* 1979; 31:349–350.
8. Pauerstein CJ, Eddy CA, Croxatto HD, et al. Temporal relationships of estrogen, progesterone, and luteinizing hormone levels to ovulation in women and infra human primates. *Am J Obstet Gynecol* 1978; 130:876–886.
9. Fox CA, Meldrum SJ, Watson BW. Continuous measurement by radiotelemetry of vaginal pH during human coitus. *J Reprod Fertil* 1973; 33:69–75.
10. Bygdeman M, Eliasson R. The effect of prostaglandin from human seminal fluid on the motility of the non-pregnant human uterus in vitro. *Acta Physiol Scand* 1963; 59:43–51.

11. Bygdeman M, Hamberg M, Samuelsson B. The content of different prostaglandin in human seminal fluid and their threshold dose on the human myometrium. *Mem Soc Endocrinol* 1976; 14:49–63.

12. Karim SMM, Sharma SD. Therapeutic abortion and induction of labour by the intravaginal administration of prostaglandin E2 or F2a. *J Obstet Gynaecol Br Commonw* 1971; 78:294–300.

13. Bygdeman M, Samuelsson B. Analysis of prostaglandin in human semen. Prostaglandin and related factors. *Clin Chim Acta* 1966; 13:465–474.

14. Bygdeman M, Fredericsson B, Svanborg K, et al. The relation between fertility and prostaglandin content of seminal fluid in man. *Fertil Steril* 1970; 21:622–629.

15. Templeton AA, Cooper I, Kelly RW. Prostaglandin concentrations in the semen of fertile men. *J Reprod Fertil* 1978; 52:147–150.

16. Eskin BA, Azarbal S, Sepic R, et al. In vitro responses of the spermatozoa-cervical mucus system treated with prostaglandin F2a. *Obstet Gynecol* 1973; 41:436–439.

17. Colon JM, Gagliardi C, Schoenfeld C, et al. Human relaxin stimulates human sperm penetration of bovine cervical mucus. *Fertil Steril* 1989; 52:340–342.

18. Weiss G, Goldsmith LT, Schoenfeld C, et al. Partial purification of relaxin from human seminal plasma. *Am J Obstet Gynecol* 1986; 154:749–755.

19. White IG, Kar A. Aspects of the physiology of sperm in the female genital tract. *Contraception* 1973; 3:183–194.

20. Levi L. The urinary output of adrenalin and noradrenalin during pleasant and unpleasant emotional states. A preliminary report. *Psychosom Med* 1965; 27:80–85.

21. Gottlieb C, Andersson E, Fried G. The effect of 19-hydroxyprostaglandins on the human myometrium in-vitro. *Prostaglandin* 1991; 41:607–613.

22. Braquet P, Touqui L, Shen TY, et al. Perspectives in platelet-activating research. *Pharmacol Rev* 1987; 39:97–145.

23. Casslen B. Free amino acids in human uterine fluid. Possible role of high taurine concentration. *J Reprod Med* 1987; 32:181–184.

24. Guerin JF, Ouhibi N, Regnier-Vigouroux G, et al. Movement characteristics and hyperactivation of human sperm on different epithelial cell monolayers. *Int J Androl* 1991; 14:412–422.

25. Suarez SS, Katz DF, Owen DH, et al. Evidence for the function of hyperactivated motility in sperm. *Biol Reprod* 1991; 44:375–381.

26. Voglmayr JK, Sawyer RF Jr. Surface transformation of ram spermatozoa in uterine, oviduct and cauda epididymal fluids in vitro. *J Reprod Fertil* 1986; 78:315–325.

27. Lambert H, Overstreet JW, Morales P, et al. Sperm capacitation in the human female reproductive tract. *Fertil Steril* 1985; 43:325–327.

28. Forrler A, Dellenbach P, Nisand I, et al. Direct intraperitoneal insemination in unexplained and cervical infertility. *Lancet* 1986; 1:916–917.

29. Lesec G, Manhes H, Hardy RI, et al. In-vivo transperitoneal fertilization. *Hum Reprod* 1989; 4:521–526.

30. Rowland IW. Insemination of the guinea-pig by intraperitoneal injection. *J Endocrinol* 1957; 16:98–106.

31. Borrero C, Ord T, Balmaceda JP, et al. The GIFT experiences: an evaluation of the outcome of 115 cases. *Hum Reprod* 1988; 3:227–230.

32. Leeton J, Healy D, Rogers P, et al. A controlled study between the use of gamete intrafallopian tube transfer (GIFT) and in-vitro fertilization and embryo transfer in the management of idiopathic and male infertility. *Fertil Steril* 1987; 48:605–607.

33. McGaughey RW, Nemiro JS. Correlation of estrogen levels with oocytes aspirated and with pregnancy in a program of clinical tubal transfer. *Fertil Steril* 1987; 48:98–106.

34. Saling PM, Bedford JM. Absence of species-specificity for mammalian sperm capacitation in vivo. *J Reprod Fertil* 1981; 63:119–123.

35. Toyodo Y, Yokoyama M, Hoshi T. Studies on the fertilization of mouse eggs in vitro. *Jpn J Anim Reprod* 1971; 16:147–157.

36. Storey BT, Kopt GS. Fertilization in the mouse, II. Spermatozoa. In: Dunbar SB, O'Rand MG, eds. *A Comparative Overview of Mammalian Fertilization.* New York: Plenum Press; 1991: 167–216.

37. Storey BT. Sperm capacitation and the acrosome reaction. *Ann NY Acad Sci* 1991; 637:457–473.

38. Sidhu KS, Guraya SS. Cellular and molecular biology of capacitation and acrosome reaction in mammalian spermatozoa. *Int Rev Cytol* 1989; 118:321–328.

39. Saling PM. Mammalian sperm interaction with extracellular matrices of the egg. In: Milligan SR, ed. *Oxford Review of Reproductive Biology.* Oxford: Oxford University Press; 1989; 2:339–388.

40. Fraser LR. Requirements for successful mammalian sperm capacitation and fertilization. *Arch Pathol Lab Med* 1992; 116:345–350.

41. Fraser LR, Ahuja KK. Metabolic and surface events in fertilization. *Gamete Res* 1988; 20:491–519.

42. Fraser LR. Sperm capacitation and its modulation. In: Bavister BD et al, eds. *Mammalian Fertilization*. Norwell, MA: Serono Symposia USA; 1990: 141–153.

43. Cummins JM, Woodall PE. On mammalian sperm dimensions. *J Reprod Fertil* 1985; 5:153–175.

44. Bedford JM, Hoskins DD. The mammalian spermatozoa: morphology, biochemistry and physiology, In: Lamming GE, ed. *Marshall's Physiology of Reproduction*. Edinburgh: Churchill Livingstone; 1990: 379–568.

45. Zaneveld LJD, De Jonge CJ, Anderson RA, et al. Human sperm capacitation and the acrosome reaction. *Hum Reprod* 1991; 6:1265–1274.

46. Zaneveld LJD, DeJonge CJ. Mammalian sperm acrosmal enzymes and the acrosome reaction. In: Dunbar BS, O'Rand JG, eds. *A Comparative Overview of Mammalian Fertilization*. New York: Plenum Press; 1991: 63–79.

47. Yanagimachi R. Mammalian fertilization. In: Knobil E et al, eds. *The Physiology of Reproduction*. 2nd ed. New York: Raven Press; 1994; 1:189–317.

48. Sidhu KS, Guraya SS. Cellular and molecular biology of capacitation and acrosome reaction in mammalian spermatozoa. *In Rev Cytol* 1989; 118:231–280.

49. Saling PM. How the egg regulates sperm function during gamete interaction: facts and fantasies. *Biol Reprod* 1991; 44:246–251.

50. Saling PM. Mammalian sperm interaction with extracellular matrices of the egg. In: Milligan SR, ed. *Oxford Review of Reproductive Biology*. Oxford: Oxford University Press; 1989; 2:339–388.

51. Barros C, Yanagimachi R. Induction of zona reaction in golden hamster eggs by cortical granule material. *Nature* 1971; 233:268–269.

52. Schlafke S, Enders AC. Cellular basis of interaction between trophoblast and uterus at implantation. *Biol Reprod* 1975; 12:41–65.

53. Larsen JF. Electron microscopy of the implantation site in the rabbit. *Am J Anat* 1961; 109:319–325.

54. Queenan JT, Kao LC, Arboleda CE, et al. Regulation of urokinase-type plasminogen activator production by cultured human cytotrophoblasts. *J Biol Chem* 1987; 262:10903–10906.

55. Strickland S, Reich E, Sherman MI. Plasminogen activator in early embryogenesis: enzyme production by trophoblast and parietal endoderm. *Cell* 1976; 9:231–240.

56. Milwidsky A, Finci-Yehesel Z, Yagel S, et al. Gonadotropin-mediated inhibition of proteolytic enzymes produced by human trophoblast in culture. *J Clin Endocrinol Metab* 1993; 76:1101–1105.

57. Glass RH, Aggeler J, Spindle A, et al. Degradation of extracellular matrix by mouse trophoblast outgrowths: a model for implantation. *J Cell Biol* 1983; 96:1108–1116.

58. Moll UM, Lane BL. Proeolytic activity of first trimester human placenta: localization of interstitial collagenase in villous and extravillous trophoblast. *Histochemistry* 1990; 94:555–560.

59. Boving BG. Implantation. *Ann NY Acad Sci* 1959; 75:700–725.

60. Weitlauf HM. Biology of Implantation. In: Knobil E et al, eds. *The Physiology of Reproduction*. 2nd ed. New York: Raven Press; 1994; 1:391–440.

61. Pratt WF, Mosher WD, Bachrach C, et al. *Infertility—United States, 1982. MMWR* 1985; 34:197–205.

62. Speroff L, Glass RH, Kase NG. *Clinical Gynecologic Endocrinology and Infertility*. 5th ed. Baltimore: Williams & Wilkins; 1994.

63. Barad D. *Workup of the Infertile Couple. Infertility and Reproductive Medicine Clinics of North America*. Philadelphia: W.B. Saunders; 1991: 255–267.

64. Richard-Davis G, Moghissi K. Basic work-up and evaluation of infertile couples. *Female Patient* 1993; 18:71–78.

65. Jaffe S, Jewelewicz R. The basic infertility investigation. *Fertil Steril* 1991; 56:599–613.

66. Chang RJ. Ovarian steroid secretion in polycystic ovarian disease. *Semin Reprod Endocrinol* 1984; 2:244–251.

67. Laatikainen TJ, Apter DL, Paavonen JA, et al. Steroids in ovarian and peripheral venous blood in polycystic ovarian disease. *Clin Endocrinol* 1980; 13:125–134.

68. Bergh C, Carlsson B, Olsson J-H, et al. Regulation of androgen production in cultured human thecal cells by insulin-like growth factor I and insulin. *Fertil Steril* 1993; 59:323–331.

69. Hammond MG, Talbert LM. *Infertility: a Practical Guide for the Physician*. 2nd ed. Oradell, NJ: Medical Economics Books; 1985.

70. Norwood GE. Sterility and fertility in women with pelvic endometriosis. *Clin Obstet Gynecol* 1960; 3:456–462.

71. Olive DL, Haney AF. Endometriosis. In: DeCherney AH, ed. *Reproductive Failure*. New York: Churchill Livingstone; 1986: 153–201.

72. Burns WN, Schken RS. Pathophysiology. In: Schenken RS, ed. *Endometrioisis: Contemporary Concepts in Clinical Management*. Philadelphia: J.B. Lippincott; 1989: 83–126.

73. Wheeler JM. Epidemiology of endometriosis-associated infertility. *J Reprod Med* 1989; 34:41–46.

74. Olive DL, Hammond CB. Endometriosis: pathogenesis and mechanisms of infertility. *Postgrad Obstet Gynecol* 1985; 5:1–12.

75. Simpson JL, Elias S, Malinak LR, et al. Heritable aspects of endometriosis. I. Genetic studies. *Am J Obstet Gynecol* 1980; 137:327–331.

76. Malinak LR, Buttram VC Jr, Elias S. Heritable aspects of endometriosis. *Am J Obstet Gynecol* 1980; 137:332–337.

77. Ranney B. Endometriosis. III. Complete operations. Reasons, sequelae, treatment. *Am J Obstet Gynecol* 1971; 109:1137–1144.

78. Cornillie FJ, Oosterlynck D, Lauwerns JM, et al. Deeply infiltrating pelvic endometriosis: histology and clinical significance. *Fertil Steril* 1990; 53:978–983.

79. Guzick DS, Rock JA. A comparison of danazol and conservative surgery for the treatment of infertility due to mild or moderate endometriosis. *Fertil Steril* 1983; 40:580–584.

80. Olive DL, Lee KL. Analysis of sequential treatment protocols for endometriosis-associated infertility. *Am J Obstet Gynecol* 1986; 154:613–619.

81. Moghissi K. The cervix in infertility. *Clin Obstet Gynecol* 1979; 22:27–42.

82. Bronson RA, Cooper GW, Rosenfeld DL. Autoimmunity to spermatozoa effect in sperm penetration of cervical mucus as reflected by postcoital testing. *Fertil Steril* 1984; 41:609–614.

83. Friberg J. Mycoplasmas and ureaplasmas in infertility and abortion. *Fertil Steril* 1980; 33:351–359.

84. Fowlkes DM, MacLeod J, O'Leary WM. T-mycoplasmas and human infertility: correlation of infection with alterations in seminal parameters. *Fertil Steril* 1975; 26:1212–1218.

85. Cassel GH, Younger JB, Brown MB, et al. Microbiologic study of infertile women at the time of diagnostic laparoscopy-association of *Ureaplasma Urealyticum* with a defined subpopulation. *N Engl J Med* 1983; 308:502–505.

86. Dubinsky TJ, Parvey HR, Gormaz G, et al. Transvaginal hysterosonography in the evaluation of small endoluminal masses. *J Ultrasound Med* 1995; 14:1–6.

87. American Fertility Society. Revised American Fertilty Society Classification of Endometriosis: 1985. *Fertil Steril* 1985; 43:351–352.

# 6
# Leukocytospermia, Oxidative Stress, and Sperm Function

R. John Aitken

Defective sperm function is not only the most prevalent, defined cause of human infertility, but it is one that, until recently, was extremely difficult to treat.[1] Part of this difficulty is derived from incomplete understanding of the factors contributing to male infertility. Environmental conditions have been implicated, notably in the proposed role of estrogens in precipitating the decline in sperm counts observed in men in several European countries during the past half century.[2,3] Genetic factors have also been implicated, particularly in cases of severe oligospermia or nonobstructive azoospermia where microdeletions in the Y chromosome or sex chromosome abnormalities such as XXY have been observed.[4,5] Even in cases of obstructive azoospermia, genetic factors may be involved, as evidenced by the association between congenital absence of the vas deferens and mutations in the cystic fibrosis gene.[6]

Resolving the relative importance of environmental and genetic factors in the etiology of male infertility is of relevance to the development of methods to both prevent and treat this condition. Thus, although techniques, such as intracytoplasmic sperm injection, offer considerable promise to patients who had hitherto been considered untreatable,[7] there are dangers in the indiscriminate use of such treatments while the cause of male infertility is still so poorly understood. Such action might lead to the inadvertent transmission of defective genes that will either perpetuate the infertility or give rise to other pathologies with a related genetic

background. To keep the risk of such complications to a minimum, it will be necessary to identify conditions affecting male fertility where genetic factors are not involved. Leukocytospermia (the presence of leukocyte concentrations in semen exceeding $1 \times 10^6$/ml) is one of the few conditions where this requirement is satisfied, and, moreover, it is a condition that might be amenable to treatment.

## Leukocytes in Semen

### Leukocyte Composition

Given the potential importance of seminal leukocytes in the etiology of male infertility and the transmission of human immunodeficiency virus (HIV), it is surprising how few studies have attempted to define the composition of this cell population in the ejaculates of normal men. Furthermore, the way in which the leukocyte population becomes altered in cases of autoimmunity against sperm surface antigens or genital tract infection has received scant attention. The few studies that have been conducted using monoclonal antibodies to identify the leukocyte subpopulations are in general agreement that the major leukocyte species in the human ejaculate is the granulocyte.[8–10] Lower concentrations of macrophages, B cells, and both CD4$^+$ and CD8$^+$ T cells are also present in many human ejaculates (Table 6.1), and occasional specimens are found in which one or other of these cell types predominates.

TABLE 6.1. Analysis of the leukocyte subpopulations in human semen.

| Leukocyte phenotype ($10^4$/ml) | Aitken et al[8] | Wolff and Anderson[9]* | Tomlinson et al[10†] |
|---|---|---|---|
| Pan leukocyte | 39.19 ± 9.05 (120) | 205.68 ± 560.37 (51) | 13.28 ± 2.69 (512) |
| Neutrophils/granulocytes | 39.69 ± 7.643 (91) | 154.49 ± 468.22 (51) | 6.70 ± 1.46 (512) |
| Monocytes/macrophages | 3.83 ± 2.01 (91) | 27.96 ± 51.10 (51) | 2.39 ± 0.32 (512) |
| CD4+ T cells | 6.06 ± 1.58 (91)** | 4.44 ± 15.87 (51) | 0.09 ± 0.01 (512) |
| CD8+ T cells | | 2.46 ± 6.03 (51) | 0.12 ± 0.02 (512) |
| B cells | 3.77 ± 0.98 (91) | 2.53 ± 11.86 (51) | 0.16 ± 0.05 (512) |

*Original data presented as leukocytes/ejaculate; to aid comparison, these data have been recalculated as leukocytes/ml, assuming a mean semen volume of 3.5 ml.[9] Numbers in parentheses are the number of samples analyzed.
† Pan T-cell marker.

Thus, in a recent analysis of 120 patients attending an infertility clinic, 97% were found to possess detectable numbers of leukocytes, and in 82.5% of these samples the predominant leukocyte species was the granulocyte.[8] Within the same population of patients, macrophages, B cells, and T cells dominated in 3.3%, 4.4%, and 6.6% of specimens, respectively.

Although this general picture of human semen as a medium dominated by granulocytes is common to all recent investigations of this subject, there are some interesting differences between studies in the absolute number of leukocytes identified within each subpopulation (Table 6.1). In particular, Wolff and Anderson[9] observed much higher concentrations of monocytes/macrophages and granulocytes in their patient population than did investigators in the other studies.[8–11] This is in keeping with a significantly higher level of general leukocyte contamination in their patient population compared with the data sets presented by Aitken et al[8] and Tomlinson et al.[10] Moreover, these differences are also reflected in the higher incidence of leukocytospermia recorded by these authors (23%) when compared with other studies where immunocytochemical detection systems have been applied to cohorts containing more than 100

TABLE 6.2. Prevalence of leukocytospermia.

| Study | No. of subjects (prevalence) |
|---|---|
| Aitken et al[8] | 9/120 (7.5%) |
| Wolff and Anderson[9] | 41/179 (22.9%) |
| Tomlinson et al[10] | 14/512 (2.8%) |
| Wang et al[11] | 8/101 (7.9%) |

subjects (2.7% to 7.9%) (Table 6.2). Such disparities indicate the existence of considerable differences between patient groups in the size of the seminal leukocyte population.

## Origin of Leukocytic Infiltration

The site and cause of leukocytic infiltration into the male reproductive tract is very poorly understood. A reasonable assumption would be that leukocytospermia involves inflammatory changes in the male reproductive tract secondary to infection in the urethra or secondary sexual glands. Leukocytospermia is recognized as one of the criteria by which male genital tract infection can be diagnosed, and the incidence of this condition is certainly higher in samples containing pathogenic bacteria, or even nonpathogenic bacteria if present in sufficiently high concentrations.[12] Nevertheless, in general, the relationship between leukocytospermia and seminal microbiology is surprisingly weak.[13]

In those rare cases in which a high level of lymphocytic infiltration into the ejaculate is observed,[8] low-grade orchitis might be involved. Independent studies of testicular biopsies taken from male infertility patients have revealed evidence of lymphocytic infiltration in the testes of 5% to 8% of such specimens.[14,15] The sites of lymphocytic infiltration were associated with local degeneration of the seminiferous epithelium and bore a strong resemblance to the testicular lesions observed in experimental autoimmune orchitis. Such histopathologic findings might therefore suggest a role for cell-mediated immunity in the etiology of male infertility.

Other factors that might contribute to the degree of leukocytic infiltration observed in human semen include viral infections, sensitization to sperm surface antigens, and low-grade toxicants, such as cigarette smoke, marijuana, or alcohol.[12,16] It is also possible that leukocytic infiltration is induced by the spermatozoa themselves. It is known in many species, including the human,[17] that insemination results in a sudden infiltration of leukocytes into the female reproductive tract. Moreover, it has been demonstrated that both spermatozoa and sperm-free seminal plasma can provide the chemotactic signals responsible for eliciting this leukocytic response to insemination.[18,19] However, the nature of these chemotactic signals is still poorly understood.

One possible mechanism by which spermatozoa might attract neutrophils would be through the activation of complement. Thus, if spermatozoa are incubated with complement-fixing antisperm antibodies, they are readily recognized and phagocytosed in vitro by polymorphs. Intriguingly, this phagocytic response is "silent" in the sense that it does not result in an oxidative burst.[20] Under these circumstances, the free radical–generating machinery of the leukocytes appears to be fully functional in that it can still be activated by soluble (phorbol esters) or particulate (opsonized zymosan) stimuli.[20] In addition, cytochemical techniques have confirmed the localized generation of reactive oxygen species at the sites of sperm-leukocyte contact. However, this oxidative response appears to be locally restricted and does not develop into a full-blown oxidative burst.[20]

The biologic significance of such a "silent" phagocytic mechanism is clear in the context of both the epididymis and the female reproductive tract. In both situations, there is a need to remove the defective, senescent, or moribund cells without damaging the large numbers of normal spermatozoa in the immediate vicinity. Given the highly reactive and penetrating nature of the toxic oxygen metabolites generated by activated leukocytes, and the susceptibility of spermatozoa to oxidative stress,[21] the evolution of mechanisms to prevent the development of an oxidative burst in sites such as the cervix and epididymis might be anticipated. Whether

complement can be fixed by defective spermatozoa in the absence of antibodies and whether complement fixation is the only mechanism whereby spermatozoa express chemoattractant activity have not been investigated. It is also unclear as to whether defects in the spermatozoa mediated by complement fixation or some other mechanism are ever responsible for pathologic levels of leukocytic infiltration into the male reproductive tract. The observation that vasectomy significantly reduces the size of the leukocyte population in human semen[12] strongly suggests that the chemoattractant activity of spermatozoa is a significant factor in the etiology of leukocytic infiltration into the male reproductive tract. However, the fact that a recent study revealed a significant correlation between the size of the seminal leukocyte population and the spontaneous generation of reactive oxygen species by the human ejaculate[22] suggests that leukocytes enter the semen in an activated state (Fig. 6.1). Moreover, the ejaculates of nine patients recruited into this study with leukocytospermia exhibited a significantly higher rate of reactive oxygen species generation than did the rest of the population ($n = 115$), giving median luminol-dependent chemiluminescent counts of 34,400 and 477 counts/10 s, respectively.[22] Given that sperm-induced phagocytosis is thought to be a silent process, it would seem unlikely that the leukocytic infiltration observed in such cases is due to the generation of chemoattractants by the spermatozoa. More plausible would be the attraction of leukocytes into the seminal compartment under conditions, such as bacterial infection, where they become activated. Alternatively, sperm-derived chemoattractants might be responsible for bringing the leukocytes into the male reproductive tract where they become activated by alternative mechanisms.

Whatever the causal factors of leukocytospermia, the existing data suggest that the leukocytes arrive in the ejaculate in an activated state and, as a consequence, are actively generating reactive oxygen species. Because spermatozoa are exquisitely sensitive to oxidative stress, leukocytospermia involving free radical–generating phagocytes might be expected to have a profound effect on fertility.

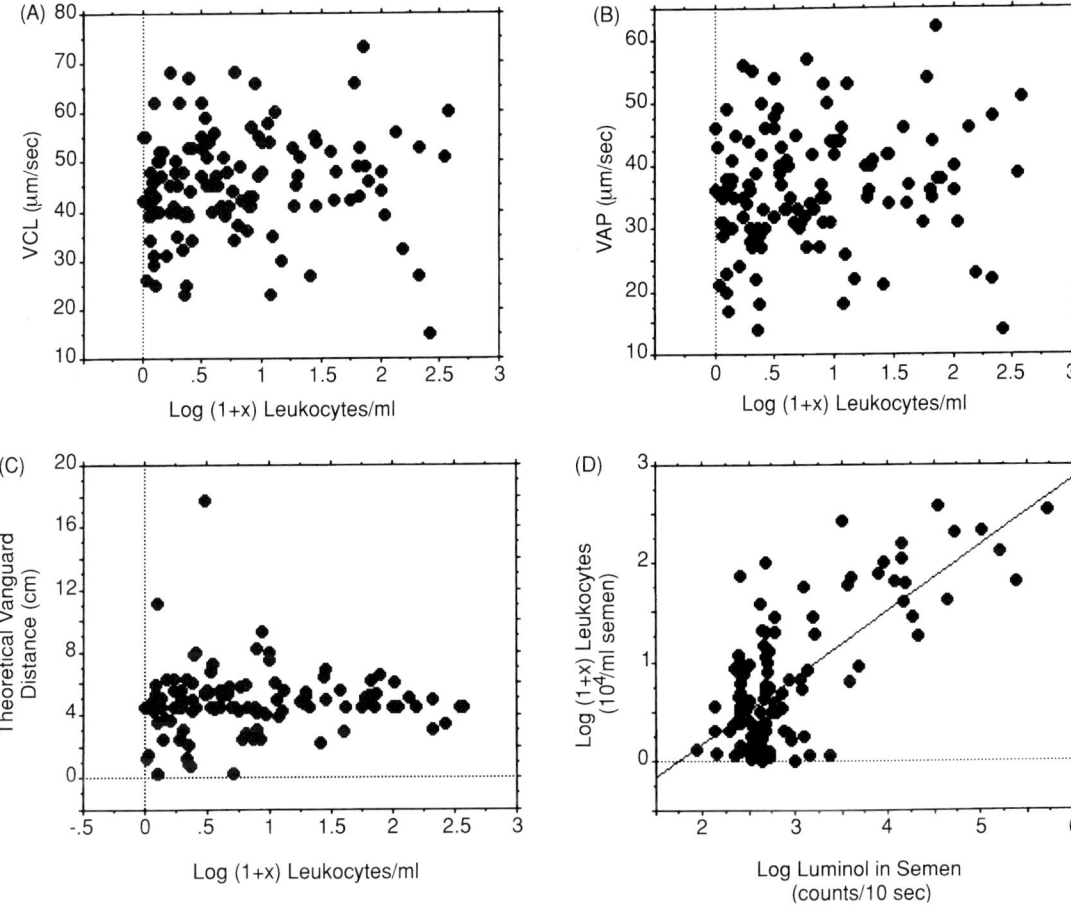

FIGURE 6.1. Lack of a relationship between the level of leukocyte contamination in human semen samples and sperm motility despite the active generation of toxic oxygen metabolites by the phagocyte subpopulation. Graphs show the concentration of leukocytes plotted against (A) the curvilinear velocity (VCL) of the spermatozoa, (B) the velocity of the average path (VAP) of the spermatozoa, and (C) the ability of the spermatozoa to penetrate a hyaluronic acid polymer.[43] (D) The positive correlation between the leukocyte concentration and the spontaneous generation of reactive oxygen species by human semen samples.[22]

## Leukocytosis and Fertility

The impact of leukocytospermia on semen quality and sperm function is extremely controversial. Some authors have observed that leukocytospermia is associated with significant changes in the semen profile, as reflected by reductions in sperm number, percentage of motility, velocity, motility index, and total motile sperm count.[23] Others[8,10] have found no correla-

tion between the concentration of leukocytes in human semen and any component of the semen profile. Moreover Tomlinson et al[10] found that the size of the seminal leukocyte population in a prospective trial bore no relationship with the conception rates subsequently observed on follow-up. These researchers concluded that the analysis of seminal leukocytes was of little prognostic value and could be ignored as a component of the routine diagnostic workup of the infertile male. For several reasons, however, such a conclusion may be premature.

The analysis of Tomlinson et al[10] assumed that the severity of leukocytic infiltration is a phenomenon that will remain constant over time, so that the levels of leukocytic infiltration observed at the beginning of the study could be meaningfully correlated with the incidence of pregnancy recorded at its conclusion.[10] However, the limited studies that have been performed in this area indicate that leukocytic infiltration into the human ejaculate is a relatively labile phenomenon with the result that leukocytospermia exhibits a high rate of spontaneous resolution.[24] Furthermore, the severity of the leukocytospermia may well have a bearing on the consequences of this condition. Tomlinson et al found that leukocytospermia occurred in only 2.7% of the subjects analyzed, and the median leukocyte count in the entire patient population was only $1.5 \times 10^4$/ml. In contrast, the analysis of Wolff et al,[23] in which an impact of leukocytospermia on semen quality was observed, exhibited an incidence of leukocytospermia of 23%, with median leukocyte counts some 10- to 100-fold higher than the patient population analyzed by Tomlinson et al. Clearly, the incidence of clinically significant, leukocytic infiltration observed in the patients analyzed by Tomlinson et al is too small to allow conclusions to be drawn about the impact of this condition on semen quality. It should also be emphasized that even where poor semen quality is observed in association with leukocytospermia, the relationship is not necessarily directly causative. In one recent study, leukocytospermia was found to induce a change in semen quality only if the leukocytic infiltration was accompanied by the impairment of seminal vesicle function.[25] The disruption of vesicular function was associated with significant declines in sperm motility and vitality and a higher incidence of antisperm antibodies.

Such results emphasize the difficulty of drawing clinical conclusions on the basis of leukocytospermia alone. The impact of this condition will depend on the composition of the leukocyte population, their site of origin, the nature of the stimulus that induced their infiltration, the extent of collateral damage to the male reproductive tract, and the concomitant presence of antisperm antibodies. In the case of phagocytes, much will depend on the state of activation of these cells, where they became activated, and for how long they have been activated. When activated leukocytes originate from the secondary sexual glands, the first time the spermatozoa will come in contact with these cells will be at the moment of ejaculation. Under these circumstances, the amount of damage that the spermatozoa sustain as a consequence of oxidative stress will depend on the antioxidant status of seminal plasma.

## Leukocytes and Seminal Plasma

One of the major functions of seminal plasma is to provide the spermatozoa with protection against free radical attack. Spermatozoa are extremely susceptible to this form of damage because they possess high concentrations of unsaturated fatty acids, particularly 22:6. Although these unsaturated lipids help create the membrane fluidity needed to achieve fertilization, they are also extremely vulnerable to peroxidation.[26] In addition, spermatozoa possess a relative paucity of antioxidant enzymes with which to protect their store of unsaturated fatty acids, because of the lack of cytoplasmic space. What residual cytoplasm is present in human spermatozoa is concentrated in the midpiece of the cell. It is clear that antioxidant enzymes restricted to this location[27] are in no position to protect the vulnerable membranes overlying the flagellar or acrosomal domains of this cell. As a consequence of these factors, spermatozoa rely very heavily on the provision of extracellular antioxidant protection during most of their life history. For example, the ejaculated spermatozoon is covered with an extracellular coat of lactoferrin that serves to limit the penetration of free iron to the sperm plasma membrane where it might initiate a lipid peroxidation cascade.[28,29] Human seminal plasma also contains high concentrations of superoxide dismutase- and catalase-like activities[30,31] as well as nonenzymatic antioxidants, such as ergothionine, vitamin C, and urate—all of which will protect the spermatozoa from oxidative stress.

Given the wealth of antioxidants present in human seminal plasma, it is not surprising that human spermatozoa are quite resistant to the oxidative stress created by infiltrating leukocytes. The concentration of leukocytes in human semen exhibits no discernible relationship with either the movement characteristics of the spermatozoa or their performance in a hyaluronate penetration assay (Fig. 6.1), despite the production of reactive oxygen species.[22] These results underline the important physiologic function of seminal plasma as an antioxidant protective medium[26] and explain why low-to-moderate levels of leukocytic infiltration are not detrimental to semen quality or the semen profile.[10,22] However, this protective system has finite limits to its effectiveness and in patient populations exhibiting extremely high levels of leukocytic infiltration, the spermatozoa can be damaged by the resultant oxidative stress and fertility compromised.[12,23,32]

## Leukocytes and Sperm Function In Vitro

Although seminal plasma may protect human spermatozoa from moderate levels of oxidative stress in the fresh ejaculate, quite a different situation arises during the preparation of spermatozoa for fertilization in vitro. In contrast to the complex mixture of antioxidants present in seminal plasma, most assisted conception protocols involve the use of simple defined culture media in which the only extracellular antioxidant protection afforded to the spermatozoa comes in the form of albumin or serum. Some culture media, such as Ham's F-10, are even supplemented with milligram quantities of pro-oxidant transition metals, such as iron and copper, which can initiate a lipid peroxidation cascade in the spermatozoa and seriously impair sperm function.[33] In addition to the removal of extracellular antioxidants, some sperm preparation protocols call for the centrifugation of the unfractionated, washed ejaculate prior to the isolation of the spermatozoa using a "swim-up" procedure. Such treatment results in the compaction of free radical–generating defective spermatozoa and leukocytes together with functional spermatozoa in the absence of significant extracellular protection. The act of centrifuging the mixture of leukocytes and defective spermatozoa triggers the additional release of reactive oxygen species.[34] As a consequence, sperm-preparation protocols involving centrifugation of the unfractionated, washed ejaculate have the potential to inflict serious damage on the spermatozoa and to impair their capacity for fertilization.[34] The severity of such damage depends on the extent to which the original semen sample was contaminated with leukocytes and defective spermatozoa.[35] However, this may frequently be the case in patients exhibiting male-factor infertility. It is damage that can be avoided simply by isolating the functional spermatozoa directly from semen, prior to the introduction of any centrifugation procedures. These conditions are satisfied by "swim-up from semen" protocols or the discontinuous Percoll gradient centrifugation technique.

Although the latter is an efficient procedure, it should also be recognized that it is not completely effective in removing leukocytes from human sperm suspensions. Sperm suspensions prepared from high-density Percoll fractions will frequently give a chemiluminescent response to agonists, such as formyl methionyl leucyl phenylalanine (FMLP) or opsonized zymosan, indicating the existence of low-level leukocyte contamination.[36,37] Such contamination, although slight, may have a profound effect on the outcome of in vitro fertilization therapy. In two independent assisted conception programs, the presence of low-level leukocyte contamination has been shown to be one of the major factors determining fertilization rate.[38,39] In one of these studies,[39] a stepwise multiple regression analysis was performed that gave an $\gamma$ value of 0.78 with fertilization rate on the basis of six parameters of semen quality. The earliest incorporated and most important of these criteria were (1) sperm morphology and (2) a chemiluminescence test of leukocyte contamination (Fig. 6.2). In the second study,[38] significant leukocyte contamination was observed in 28.5% of the sperm suspensions prepared by discontinuous Percoll gradient

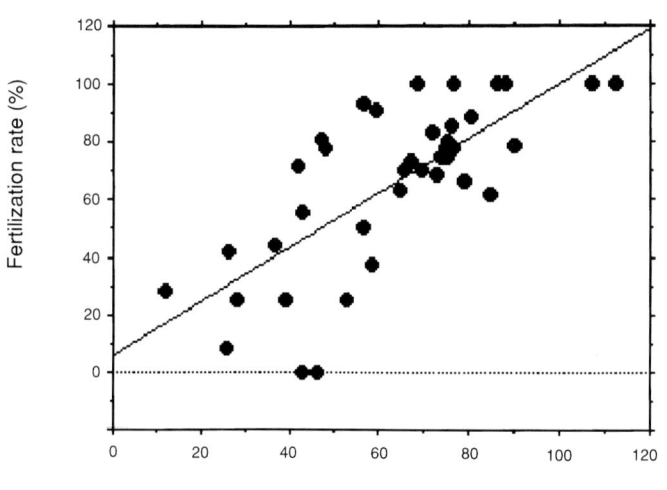

FIGURE 6.2. Correlations observed between the in vitro fertilization rates observed in a clinical IVF program and fertilization rates predicted on the basis of a multiple regression equation incorporating various criteria of sperm function. The regression equation was based on six criteria of which the most important was an FMLP provocation test for leukocyte contamination and percentage normal morphology.[39]

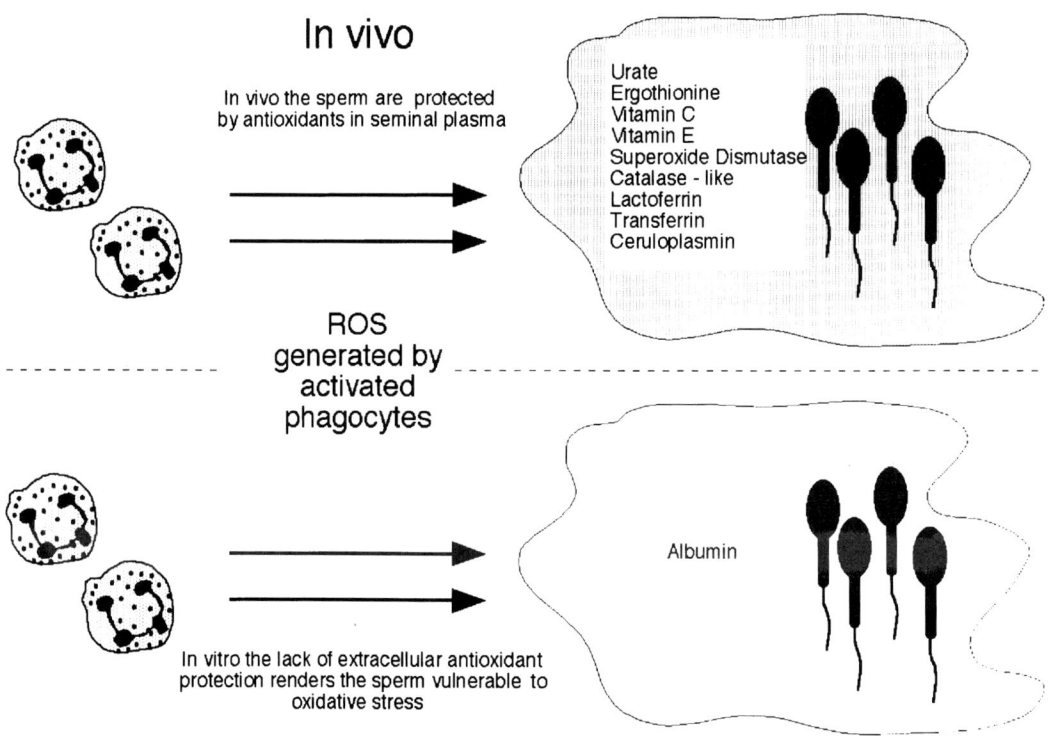

FIGURE 6.3. Seminal leukocytes, particularly polymorphs, generate reactive oxygen species (ROS), but in vivo the spermatozoa are protected by the antioxidants present in seminal plasma. In washed sperm preparations, the free radicals generated by contaminating leukocytes are able to attack the spermatozoa, and the only extracellular antioxidant protection afforded to the latter is, frequently, just albumin.

centrifugation. These leukocyte-contaminated samples were associated with enhanced reactive oxygen species generation, decreased motility, and a decreased capacity for fertilization in vitro.

These results emphasize that leukocyte contamination of human sperm suspensions significantly impairs the fertilizing capacity of the spermatozoa in vitro. A rational solution to this problem would be to incorporate antioxidants into the incubation medium to intercept the toxic oxygen metabolites generated by the leukocytes before they have an opportunity to damage the spermatozoa. A recent comparative study of the ability of antioxidants to protect human spermatozoa from the oxygen radicals generated by phorbol ester-activated granulocytes demonstrated the particular potential of N-acetylcysteine, glutathione, and hypotaurine in this context.[40] These studies were limited to the ability of these antioxidants to preserve sperm motility in the face of oxidative stress. As a prelude to clinical trials, further studies are now needed to determine whether these antioxidants can support other aspects of sperm function, including the acrosome reaction and sperm-oocyte fusion.

## Conclusion

Leukocytospermia is a relatively rare condition affecting 5% to 10% of the patient population in the United Kingdom and China, but the incidence can rise to >20% in certain patient groups. Granulocytes are the most abundant leukocyte species in human semen, although the existence of occasional cases where macrophages or lymphocytes predominate is proof that leukocytospermia is a condition with multiple underlying causes. The phagocytes present in human semen spontaneously generate reactive oxygen species, and yet sperm function does not appear, in most cases, to be significantly altered. Although this situation seems paradoxical, the preservation of sperm function in the presence of free radical–generating leukocytes is simply a reflection of the powerful antioxidant properties exhibited by seminal plasma. However, when spermatozoa

are washed free of seminal plasma, they are extremely susceptible to oxidative stress. In the context of assisted conception therapy, even low levels of leukocyte contamination appear to have a detrimental effect on the fertilizing potential of the spermatozoa (Fig. 6.3). A rational solution to this problem would be to incorporate antioxidants into the culture media used for in vitro fertilization. Because arrested embryonic development also appears to involve oxidative stress,[41,42] the development of media containing antioxidants might also promote the postfertilization development of the zygote. Systematic efforts are now being made to engineer such media and bring them into clinical practice.

## References

1. Hull MGR, Glazener CMA, Kelly NJ, et al. Population study of causes, treatment and outcome of infertility. *Br Med J* 1985; 291:1693–1697.
2. Carlsen E, Giwercman A, Keiding N, et al. Evidence for decreasing quality of semen during the past 50 years. *Br Med J* 1992; 305:609–613.
3. Sharpe RM, Skakkebaek NE. Are oestrogens involved in falling sperm counts and disorders of the male reproductive tract? *Lancet* 1993; 341:1392–1395.
4. Ma K, Inglis JD, Sharkey A, et al. A Y chromosome gene family with RNA-binding protein homology: candidates for the azoospermia factor AZF controlling human spermatogenesis. *Cell* 1993; 75:1287–1295.
5. Vogt P, Chandley AC, Hargreave TB, et al. Microdeletions in interval 6 of the Y chromosome of males with idiopathic sterility point to disruption of AZF, a human spermatogenesis gene. *Hum Genet* 1992; 89:491–496.
6. Patrizio P, Asch RH, Handelin B, et al. Aetiology of congenital absence of vas deferens. *Hum Reprod* 1993; 8:215–220.
7. Palermo G, Joris H, Derde M-P, et al. Sperm characteristics and outcome of human assisted fertilization by subzonal insemination and intracytoplasmic sperm injection. *Fertil Steril* 1993; 59:826–835.
8. Aitken RJ, West K, Buckingham D. Leukocyte infiltration into the human ejaculate and its association with semen quality, oxidative stress and sperm function. *J Androl* 1994; 15:343–352.

9. Wolff H, Anderson DJ. Immunohistologic characterization and quantification of leukocyte subpopulations in human semen. *Fertil Steril* 1988; 49:497–504.

10. Tomlinson MJ, Barratt CLR, Cooke ID. Prospective study of leukocytes and leukocyte subpopulations in semen suggests that they are not a cause of male infertility. *Fertil Steril* 1993; 60:1069–1075.

11. Wang AW, Politch J, Anderson D. Leukocytospermia in male infertility patients in China. *Andrologia* 1994; 26:167–172.

12. Comhaire F, Verschraegen G, Vermeulen L. Diagnosis of accessory gland infection and its possible role in male infertility. *Int J Androl* 1980; 3:32–45.

13. Wolff H. The biological significance of white blood cells in semen. *Fertil Steril* 1995; 63:1143–1157.

14. Suominen J, Söderström K-O. Lymphocyte infiltration in human testicular biopsies. *Int J Androl* 1982; 5:461–466.

15. Hofmann N, Kuwert E. Chronic orchitis of unknown cause. [Die chronische, nicht-Erreger-bedingte Orchitis.] [German] *Z Hautkr* 1979; 54:173–180.

16. Close CE, Roberts PL, Berger RE. Cigarettes, alcohol and marijuana are related to pyospermia in infertile men. *J Urol* 1990; 144:900–903.

17. Pandya IJ, Cohen J. The leukocytic reaction of the human uterine cervix to spermatozoa. *Fertil Steril* 1985; 43:417–421.

18. Yanagimachi R, Chang MC. Infiltration of leukocytes into the uterine lumen of the golden hamster during the oestrus cycle and following mating. *J Reprod Fertil* 1963; 5:389–396.

19. Maroni ES, Symon DNK, Wilkinson PC. Chemotaxis of neutrophil leukocytes towards spermatozoa and seminal fluid. *J Reprod Fertil* 1972; 28:359–368.

20. D'Cruz OJ, Wang B-L, Haas GG. Phagocytosis of immunoglobulin G and C3–bound human sperm by human polymorphonuclear leukocytes is not associated with the release of oxidative radicals. *Biol Reprod* 1992; 46:721–732.

21. Aitken RJ. Pathophysiology of human spermatozoa. *Curr Opin Obstet Gynaecol* 1994; 6:128–135.

22. Aitken RJ, Buckingham D, Brindle J, et al. Analysis of sperm movement in relation to the oxidative stress created by leukocytes in washed sperm preparations and seminal plasma. *Hum Reprod* 1995; 10:2061–2071.

23. Wolff H, Politch JA, Martinez A, et al. Leukocytospermia is associated with poor semen quality. *Fertil Steril* 1990; 53:528–536.

24. Yanushpolski EH, Politch JA, Hill JA, et al. Antibiotic therapy and leukocytospermia: a prospective, randomized, controlled study. *Fertil Steril* 1995; 63:142–147.

25. Gonzales GF, Kortebani G, Mazzolli AB. Leukocytospermia and function of the seminal vesicles on semen quality. *Fertil Steril* 1992; 57:1058–1065.

26. Jones R, Mann T, Sherins R. Peroxidative breakdown of phospholipids in human spermatozoa, spermicidal properties of fatty acid peroxides, and protective action of seminal plasma. *Fertil Steril* 1979; 31:531–537.

27. Aitken RJ, Buckingham DW, Carreras A, et al. Superoxide dismutase in human sperm suspensions: relationships with cellular composition, oxidative stress and sperm function. *Free Rad Biol Med* 1996; 4:495–504.

28. Aitken RJ, Harkiss D, Buckingham D. Relationship between iron-catalysed lipid peroxidation potential and human sperm function. *J Reprod Fertil* 1993; 98:257–265.

29. Aitken RJ, Harkiss D, Buckingham DW. Analysis of lipid peroxidation mechanisms in human spermatozoa. *Mol Reprod Dev* 1993; 35:302–315.

30. Jeulin C, Soufir JC, Weber P, et al. Catalase activity in human spermatozoa and seminal plasma. *Gamete Res* 1989; 24:185–196.

31. Zini A, de Lamirande E, Gagnon C. Reactive oxygen species in semen of infertile patients: levels of superoxide dismutase- and catalase-like activities in seminal plasma and spermatozoa. *Int J Androl* 1993; 16:183–188.

32. Aitken RJ, Baker G. Seminal leukocytes: passengers, terrorists or good Samaritans? *Hum Reprod* 1995; 10:1736–1739.

33. Gomez E, Aitken RJ. Impact of IVF-ET culture media on peroxidative damage to human spermatozoa. *Fertil Steril* 1994; 45:880–882.

34. Aitken RJ, Clarkson JS. Significance of reactive oxygen species and antioxidants in defining the efficacy of sperm preparation techniques. *J Androl* 1988; 9:367–376.

35. Aitken RJ. A free radical theory of male infertility. *Reprod Fert Dev* 1994; 6:19–24.

36. Aitken RJ, West K. Relationship between reactive oxygen species generation and leukocyte infiltration in fractions isolated from the human ejaculate on Percoll gradients. *Int J Androl* 1990; 13:433–451.

37. Krausz C, West K, Buckingham D, et al. Analysis of the interaction between N-formylmethionyl-leucyl phenylalanine and human sperm suspensions: development of a

technique for monitoring the contamination of human semen samples with leukocytes. *Fertil Steril* 1992; 57:1317–1325.

38. Krausz C, Mills C, Rogers S, et al. Stimulation of oxidant generation by human sperm suspensions using phorbol esters and formyl peptides: relationships with motility and fertilization in vitro. *Fertil Steril* 1994; 62:599–605.

39. Sukcharoen N, Keith J, Irvine DS, et al. Predicting the fertilizing potential of human sperm suspensions in vitro: importance of sperm morphology and leukocyte contamination. *Fertil Steril* 1995; 63:1293–1300.

40. Baker HWG, Brindle J, Irvine DS, et al. Protective effect of antioxidants on the impairment of sperm motility by activated polymorphonuclear leukocytes. *Fertil Steril* 1994; 45:411–419.

41. Nasr-Esfahani M, Aitken RJ, Johnson MH. The measurement of $H_2O_2$ levels in preimplantation embryos from blocking and nonblocking strains of mice. *Development* 1990; 109:501–507.

42. Nasr-Esfahani M, Johnson M, Aitken RJ. The effect of iron and iron chelators on the in vitro block to development of the mouse preimplantation embryo: BTT6 a new medium for improved culture of mouse embryo in vitro. *Hum Reprod* 1990; 5:743–747.

# 7
# Imaging the Reproductive Tract

Brett C. Mellinger

Imaging the reproductive tract is indicated in numerous clinical situations, most commonly during an infertility evaluation. Several imaging modalities are available for the clinician to assess the reproductive tract, each with distinct advantages and disadvantages. Because plain radiography is currently of limited value for imaging the reproductive tract, the more common modalities used are ultrasonography, magnetic resonance imaging (MRI), and computed tomography (CT).

Ultrasound is the modality of choice when evaluating the prostate, seminal vesicles, ejaculatory apparatus, and the scrotal compartment. It is relatively inexpensive, readily available, and used and interpreted by many non-radiologist physicians. Ultrasound offers the advantage of avoiding ionizing radiation, and the high-frequency probes currently available provide excellent spatial resolution.

Nuclear magnetic resonance (NMR) refers to the physical property of atomic nuclei when submitted to an external magnetic field. MRI represents the intensity of the radiofrequency signal generated by the atomic nuclei of the tissues under study. MRI is the best imaging technique for evaluating the pituitary gland and the prostate when transrectal ultrasonography (TRUS) is inconclusive. The principal advantage of MRI is its superior contrast resolution as compared with either plain radiographic or CT imaging. Another advantage of MRI is its ability to obtain direct transverse, sagittal, oblique, and coronal plane images. MRI images are obtained directly from the NMR signals and not from stacked transverse images as in CT imaging. Another advantage of MRI is the possibility to perform in vivo spectroscopy. Areas of interest can be evaluated for the NMR spectrum, which reveals the molecular nature of the abnormality.[1]

## Imaging the Pituitary Gland

Since its development as an application for medical imaging, MRI has been most useful for examination of the central nervous system. Inflammatory disease, neoplasms, ischemic changes, degenerative disease of the white matter, hemorrhage, and other conditions are more easily identified with MRI than any other imaging technique.[1] Because of the advantages afforded by MRI, CT imaging of the brain is used less frequently.

## Indications

In reproductive medicine, the most common indication for obtaining an MRI of the brain is for imaging of the pituitary gland for hypogonadism associated with gonadotropin insufficiency, which is most often due to hyperprolactinemia from a prolactin-secreting pituitary adenoma. Routine testing of prolactin for men presenting for an infertility or impotence evaluation is not cost-effective, and endocrine screening with testosterone and follicle-stimulating hormone (FSH) will detect significant endocrinopathies. Other causes of elevated prolactin should be evaluated before an MRI of the pituitary gland is ordered.

## Technical Considerations

The principal advantages of MRI as compared with CT imaging are its multiplanar capability and exquisite contrast resolution. CT imaging of the pituitary gland offers less contrast resolution because of bone around the sella tursica. Additionally, positioning patients for coronal scanning—the best plane for imaging—is difficult if not impossible with CT imaging.

Many MRI experts recommend the use of contrast agents for imaging the pituitary gland, although this is not universally accepted. Several contrast agents are available, but the most frequently used agents are metal ion chelates, such as gadolinium chelated to a carrier compound. These agents alter the MRI signal indirectly by shortening relaxation times.[1] During coronal scanning, pituitary lesions are best detected with thin slices and rapid scanning after administration of a contrast agent.

## Images of the Pituitary Gland

### Pituitary Gland Adenoma

Prolactin-secreting tumors of the pituitary gland are classified as microadenomas (diameter ≥10mm) or macroadenomas (diameter ≥10mm). With MRI, a pituitary tumor often appears as a hypointense lesion on the T1-weighted image (Figs 7.1 and 7.2). CT imaging may demonstrate a nonenhancing lesion after administration of contrast (Fig. 7.3).

## Imaging the Scrotum

Ultrasonography is the imaging modality of choice for examination of the scrotal compartment. High-frequency ultrasound examination provides superior resolution to distinguish solid lesions from fluid collections. Ultrasound examination can be performed quickly and safely with no ionizing radiation. Gray-scale imaging is improved with spectral waveform analysis (duplex Doppler ultrasonography) and color Doppler ultrasonography for determination of blood flow. A limitation of scrotal sonography is that benign lesions mimic tumors, but MRI imaging can differentiate tumors from benign lesions.[2]

## Indications

The indications for ultrasound imaging of the scrotum include any palpable abnormalities of the scrotal compartment, e.g., varicocele, testicular mass, epididymal abnormalities, scrotal swelling and fluid collections. To rule out intratesticular masses, patients presenting with testicular pain should be evaluated with ultrasound even when palpation is normal.[3] Ultrasound examination following scrotal trauma can distinguish between simple hematoma versus rupture of the tunica albuginea of the testis, which may require immediate surgical exploration and repair. Color duplex Doppler ultrasonography can distinguish between testicular torsion and epididymoorchitis in patients presenting with acute testicular pain.[4]

## Technical Considerations

A careful detailed history and focused physical examination is necessary prior to scrotal imaging. Palpable findings and direction by the patient to areas of concern are helpful for the sonographer in correlating physical examination with ultrasound examination. With the patient in the supine position in a warm examination room, the penis is draped over the abdomen and the scrotum supported with a rolled towel or the sonographer's gloved hand. Imaging frequencies of 7.5 to 13MHz provide the best resolution, and most modern ultrasound instrumentation comes equipped with 10- or 13-MHz probes. A generous amount of ultrasound gel is applied to the scrotum and minimal pressure is applied, which is especially important for the painful scrotum. The overall gain is adjusted to provide optimum gray-scale information. Each testis and epididymis is examined with both transverse and longitudinal views. Transverse imaging of both testes in the same image allows for direct comparison of the ultrasound images.

Duplex sonography of the testis and spermatic cord should be performed for suspected testicular torsion and to facilitate the diagnosis of varicocele. In cases of suspected torsion, the patient should be examined while in the supine position. With ultrasound Doppler examination, the measured blood flow velocity is dependent on the speed of red blood cells in the vessel and the angle of the incident sound beam. Therefore, it is important to keep the angle of the beam between 30° and 70°. Color Doppler sonography should indicate the presence of intratesticular arterial flow in nontorsional testes.

Patients evaluated for varicocele should be examined both supine and standing, with and without Valsalva's maneuver. Standing for a

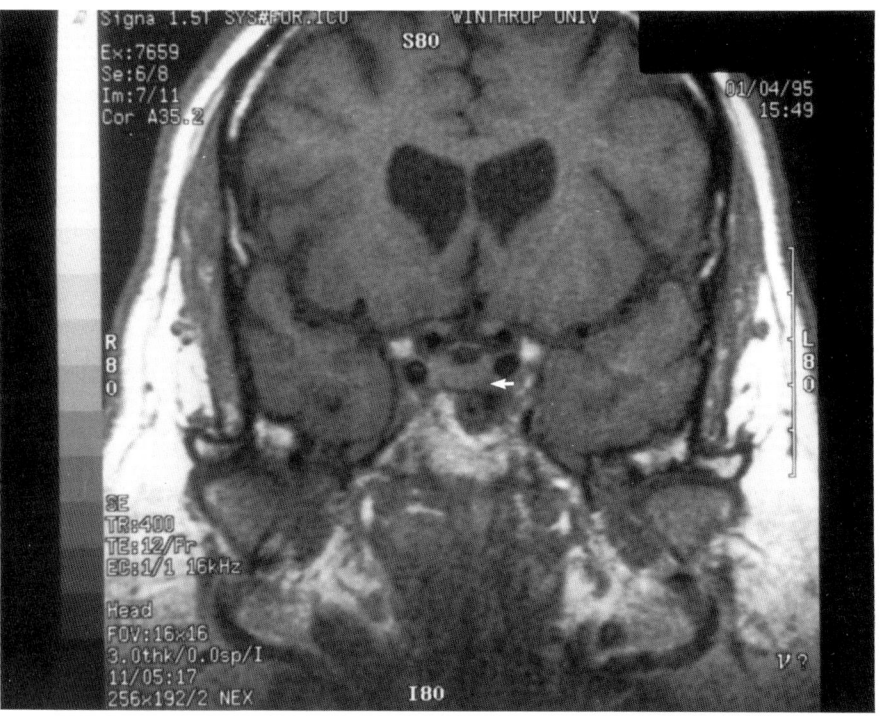

FIGURE 7.1. MRI of 60-year-old man presenting with complaints of impotence and found to have low serum testosterone levels associated with hyper- prolactinemia. A lesion is suspected before administration of contrast.

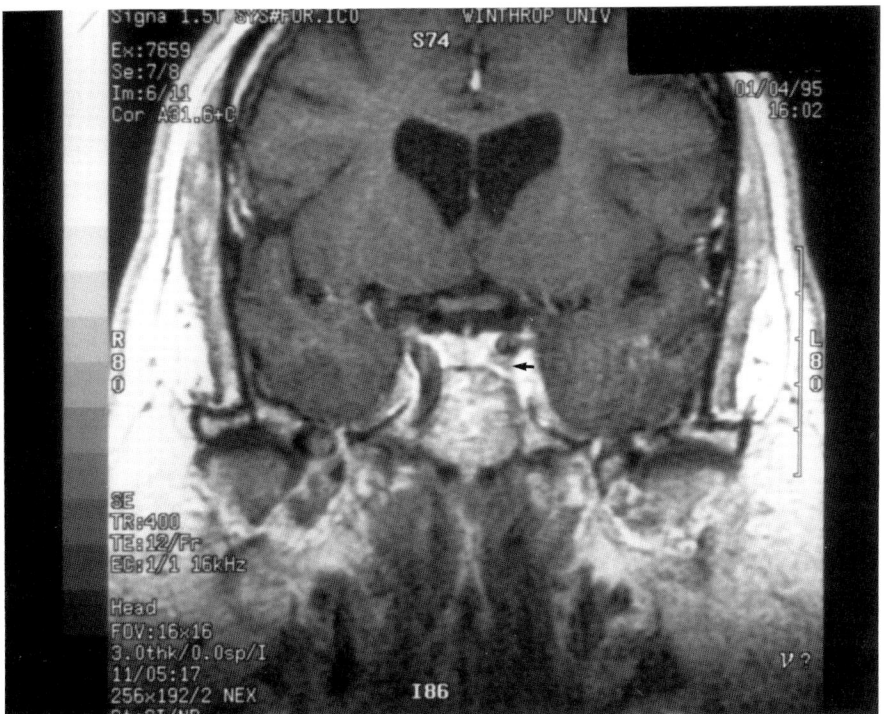

FIGURE 7.2. MRI of same patient as in Figure 7.1 after contrast revealing a hypointense pituitary lesion (arrow).

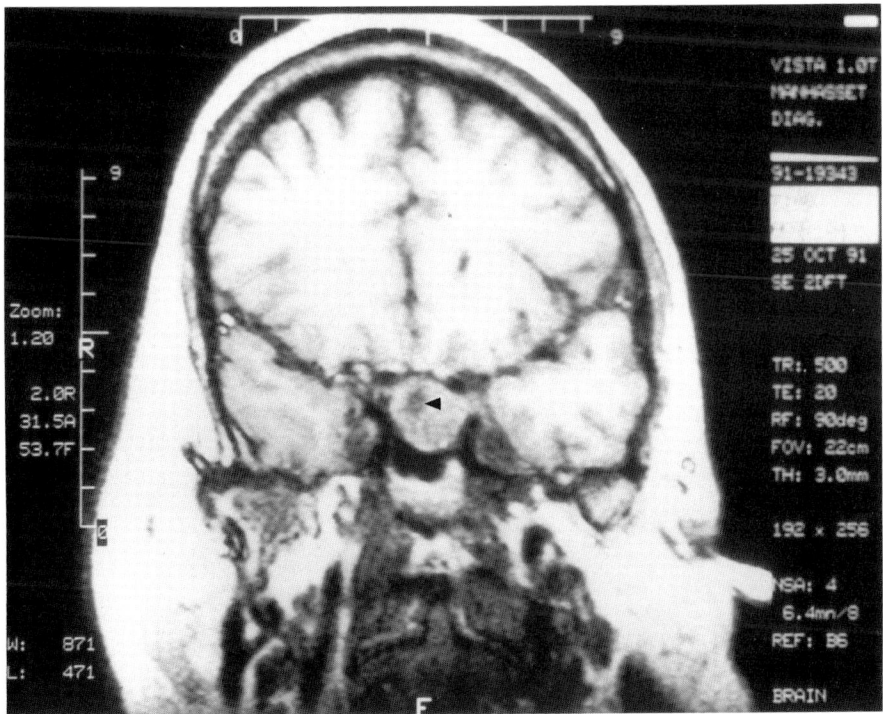

FIGURE 7.3. CT of pituitary revealing a macro-adenoma with an area of probable necrosis (arrow-head). The patient presented for an infertility evaluation and was found to have marked elevation of the serum prolactin level.

short period allows for hydrostatic pressure filling of the pampiniform plexus, which permits easier identification and measurement of dilated veins. Measurement of the greatest vein diameter should be performed during Valsalva's maneuver. Doppler sonography should also be performed on the most prominent veins during a Valsalva maneuver to detect reversal of blood flow consistent with varicocele.

## Scrotal Ultrasound Images

### Normal Testis

The normal testis demonstrates medium homogeneous echogenicity, is ovoid-shaped, and measures 3 to 5 cm in length along the vertical axis and 2 to 3 cm in width. Both testes should be equal in size and echogenicity. On ultrasound, the mediastinum testis is identified as a bright echogenic band that extends into the testicular parenchyma (Fig. 7.4). The appendix testis is readily seen when a hydrocele is

present and appears as a small round appendage between the caput epididymis and upper pole of the testis. The epididymis usually displays similar or slightly increased echogenicity as compared to the testis.

### Inflammation

In a patient with acute epididymitis, gray-scale sonography demonstrates enlargement of the epididymis, mixed hypoechogenicity, hydrocele, and scrotal skin thickening (Fig. 7.5). These ultrasound findings are not restricted to acute epididymitis. Doppler sonography of the normal epididymis detects few blood vessels; however, with inflammation, the number and size of vessels identified increases.[5]

Infection may spread from the epididymis to the testis with development of epididymoorchitis. With orchitis, there may be testicular enlargement and decreased echogenicity. With focal involvement, gray-scale sonography

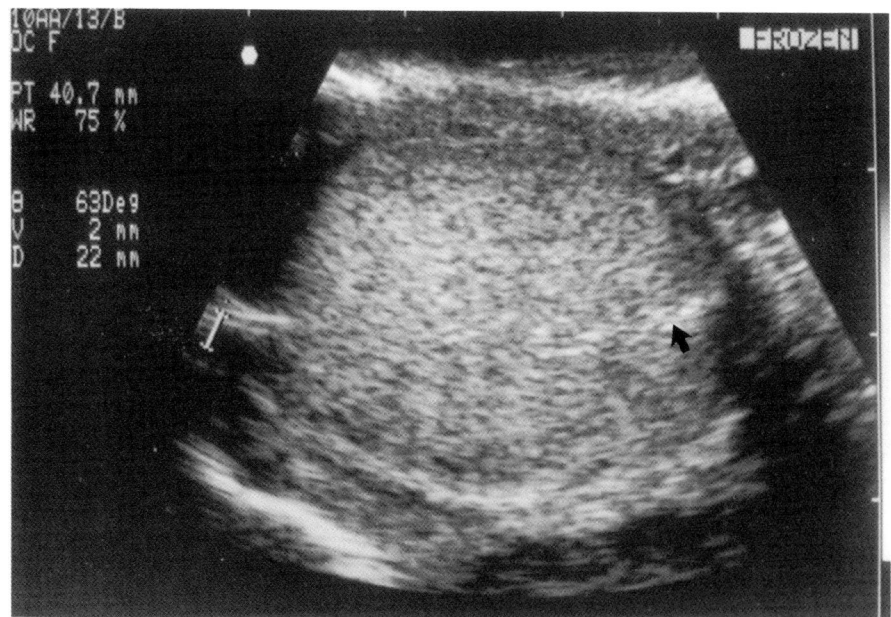

FIGURE 7.4. Normal testicular ultrasound demonstrating a linear echogenic band (arrow) of the mediastinum testis.

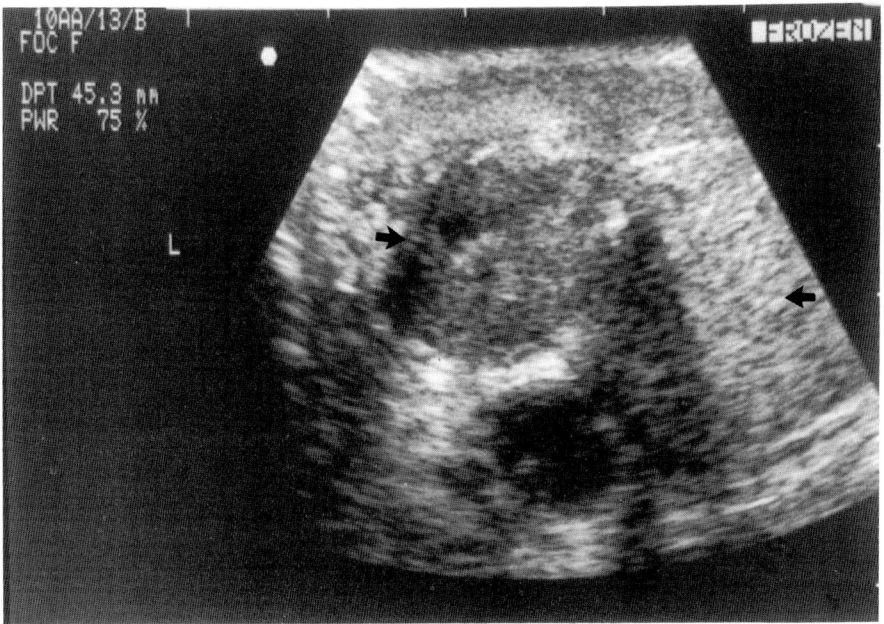

FIGURE 7.5. Acute epididymitis revealing enlargement and mixed echogenicity of the caput epididymis (arrow) adjacent to the testis.

of the testis may reveal a hypoechoic, crescent-shaped intratesticular lesion adjacent to an enlarged epididymis. Doppler sonography will reveal increased blood flow in these hypoechoic lesions.[5]

## Testicular Torsion

Gray scale ultrasound may reveal diffuse, decreased echogenicity, but this is nonspecific. Color duplex Doppler ultrasonography has been shown to be sensitive in the diagnosis of complete testicular torsion.[6,7] Intermittent torsion and blood flow in prepubertal testes may present false positives and false negatives.[8,9]

## Varicocele

A clinically significant varicocele is usually detected with a thorough physical examination with the patient in both the supine and upright positions, with and without a Valsalva maneuver, although ultrasound and Doppler examinations often facilitate the diagnosis. Several clinical investigations have attempted to establish ultrasound criteria for the diagnosis of varicocele; however, these are not universally accepted and some controversy remains. Vein-diameter cutoff points for clinical varicocele have been suggested at 2mm,[10] 3mm,[11] and 3.6mm[12] (Fig. 7.6). Doppler sonographic demonstration of reversal of blood flow during a Valsalva maneuver is generally accepted as evidence of a varicocele (Fig. 7.7). Subclinical varicocele remains controversial, as do the ultrasound criteria for establishing the diagnosis.

## Testicular Masses

Until proven otherwise, an intratesticular mass must be considered malignant. Testicular masses are usually palpable; however, nonpalpable masses are encountered more frequently due to the liberal use of scrotal sonography for evaluation of testicular pain or detection of varicocele in an infertility evaluation. Ultrasound characteristics may be useful in differentiating seminoma from other germ-cell tumors. Sonographic findings consistent with seminoma include a hypoechoic mass, homogeneous echogenecity, round- or

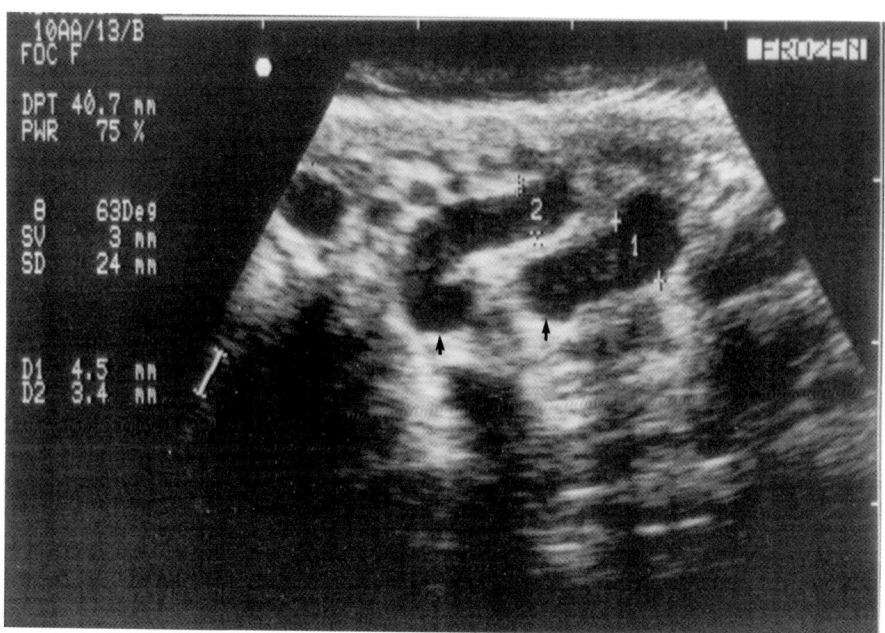

FIGURE 7.6. Varicocele (arrows) imaged with a 13-MHz probe. Vein measurements are obtained during Valsalva's maneuver revealing dilatation that meets the sonographic criteria for a varicocele.

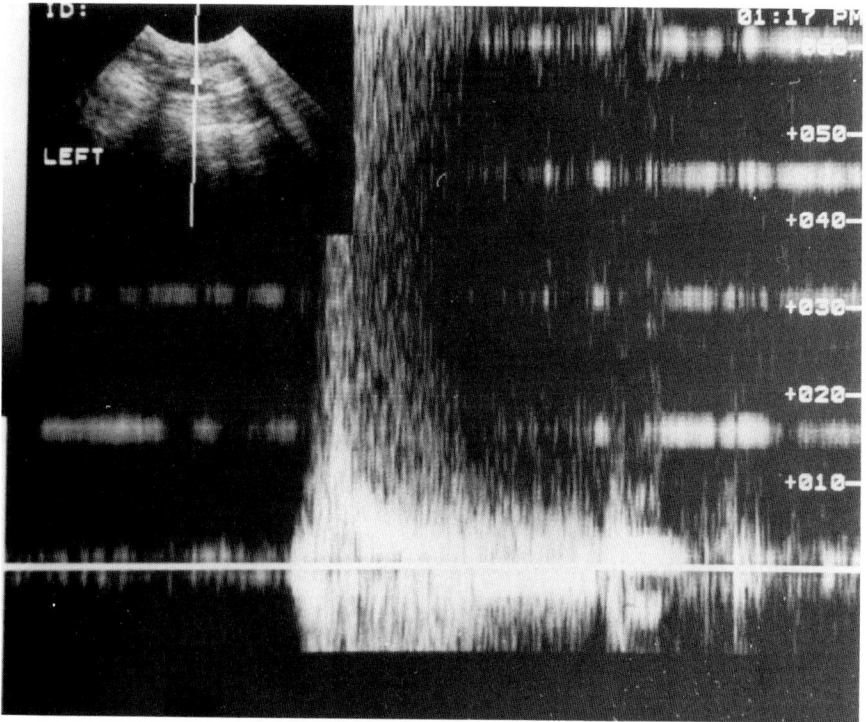

FIGURE 7.7. Black and white duplex Doppler in a patient with a palpable varicocele. The Doppler tracing reveals a typical pattern seen with venous reflux.

oval-shaped lesion with sharp demarcation from normal testicular parenchyma, and possible multifocal lesions.[5] Embryonal carcinoma is usually associated with other germ-cell tumors. Sonographically, it may appear as a heterogeneous mass with cystic components or calcification. Teratoma appears as a heterogeneous mass with multiple cystic areas, echogenic foci, and possible acoustic shadowing.[5] Epidermoid cyst is a rare benign tumor, which may appear as an echogenic central lesion with a surrounding hypoechoic rim.[13] Non–germ-cell tumors are usually benign and do not demonstrate any specific sonographic pattern (Fig. 7.8).

*Cysts*

Detection of testicular or epididymal cysts has improved with high-resolution ultrasonography. Cysts of the tunica albuginea are detected outside the testicular parenchyma, and benign intratesticular cysts are usually identified near the mediastinum testis. When these lesions are benign, they meet sonographic criteria for simple cysts and can be managed conservatively.[14]

Epididymal cysts are commonly reported in adult males. They frequently occur on the caput epididymis and may cause obstruction of the epididymal tubule (Fig. 7.9). Spermatoceles are also commonly found on the caput epididymis but demonstrate internal echoes on imaging. Differentiating between a simple cyst and a spermatocele can be difficult if they demonstrate similar echo patterns.

*Fluid Collections*

The potential space between the parietal and visceral layers of the tunica vaginalis often fills with fluid to create a hydrocele. This can be congenital or associated with inflammation or tumors. It is, therefore, important to assess the testis for an intratesticular lesion when a hydrocele is detected. Occasionally, diffuse swirling echoes may be seen during sonography. This ultrasound appearance is similar to hematocele (Fig. 7.10) or pyocele, but may also be due to protein aggregates in the hydrocele.[15]

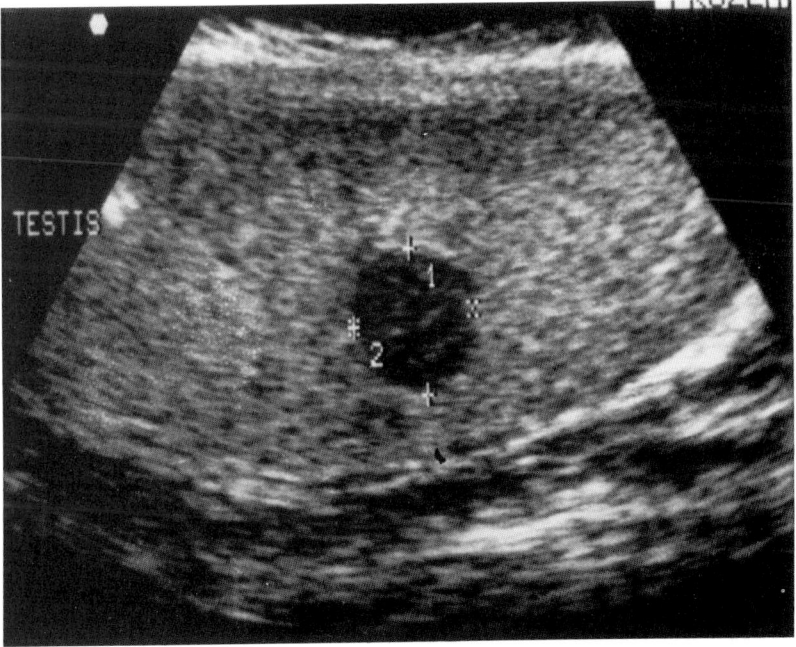

FIGURE 7.8. Nonpalpable intratesticular mass measuring 7.8 × 6.7 mm detected during sonography for evaluation of varicocele. The lesion was found to be a Leydig cell tumor at surgery.

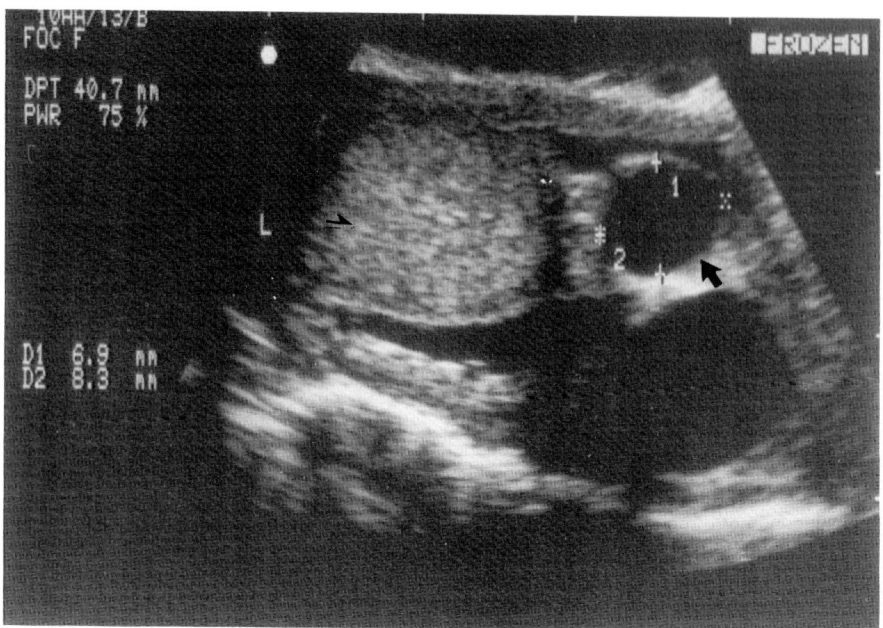

FIGURE 7.9. Epididymal cyst (arrowhead) of the caput that was detected by palpation. The testis (arrow) appears normal, and there is a small fluid collection around the testis consistent with a hydrocele.

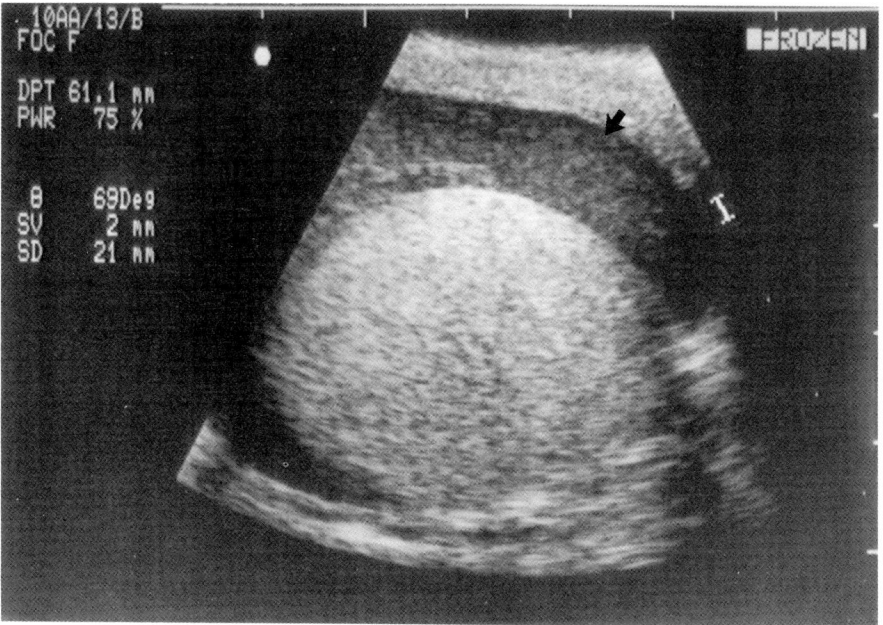

FIGURE 7.10. Acute hematocele (arrow) following needle biopsy of the testis. Immediate drainage resulted in minimal residual swelling.

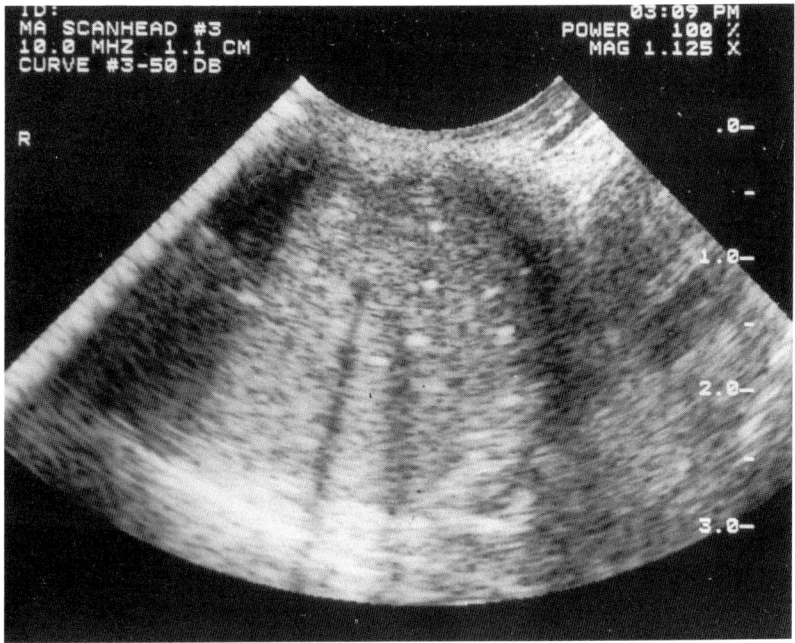

FIGURE 7.11. Testicular microlithiasis detected during sonography for evaluation of small palpable varicocele. This image demonstrates acoustic shadowing that is not normally seen in this condition.

## Microlithiasis

Testicular microlithiasis is a rare condition associated with various entities, including neoplasm and infertility. It is characterized by the presence of diffuse hyperechoic nonshadowing foci throughout the testis[16] (Fig. 7.11). Although associated with infertility and conditions that lead to infertility, its presence does not necessarily imply a poor prognosis for achieving pregnancy, as the condition is also found in otherwise normal patients.[17] Because of the frequent association of microlithiasis with testicular tumors, it has been suggested that patients have follow-up scans at frequent intervals and monitoring of serum tumor markers.[18]

## Imaging the Prostate and Ejaculatory Apparatus

The development of high-resolution ultrasonography for the detection of prostate cancer has led to the application of transrectal ultrasound (TRUS) for the evaluation and treatment of ejaculatory disorders. MRI with endorectal coil provides exquisite detail of the anatomy of the prostate, seminal vesicles, and ejaculatory apparatus. MRI is especially useful in cases where TRUS fails to provide a definitive diagnosis. CT imaging is used much less frequently and offers no advantage as compared with TRUS or MRI with endorectal coil.

## Indications

TRUS is the initial imaging modality of choice for evaluation of ejaculatory disorders because of its ease of performance and relative low cost. MRI with endorectal coil is indicated when TRUS fails to provide a definitive diagnosis despite strong clinical suspicions. It can be particularly useful for evaluation of chronic hematospermia in older patients when TRUS fails to reveal any pathology.

Ejaculatory dysfunction is any disorder of the seminal vesicles and ejaculatory apparatus that may cause symptoms of or lead to infertility. Ejaculatory disorders associated with infertility diagnosed with TRUS include complete or partial obstruction of the ejaculatory ducts and bilateral congenital absence of the vas deferens. Hematospermia is often benign and self-limiting in young men, but in older patients may be due to a urologic malignancy.

The indications for performing imaging of the prostate, seminal vesicles, and ejaculatory apparatus during an infertility evaluation include azoospermia, low semen volume, low sperm motility not explained by other findings (e.g., varicocele), and low sperm viability. Lower genital tract imaging is also indicated for all men presenting with ejaculatory pain and chronic hematospermia and hematospermia in men greater than 40 years of age because of the increased incidence of prostatic malignancy.

## Technical Considerations

### Transrectal Ultrasound (TRUS)

Ultrasound imaging of the ejaculatory apparatus is best performed with imaging frequencies of 7 to 10 MHz. Biplanar probes are preferable, to allow for easy switching from sagittal to transverse images. End-fire probes are of value for reaching the superior aspect of the seminal vesicles for transverse images.

The patient is positioned in the left lateral decubitus position. Digital rectal examination is performed prior to inserting the ultrasound probe. Sagittal imaging better demonstrates the anatomical relationship between the seminal vesicles, prostate, and ejaculatory ducts. The bladder is best left somewhat full to allow for easier orientation. Just lateral to the midline, the seminal vesicles are easily identified posterior to the bladder. The ultrasound appearance at the junction of the seminal vesicles and prostate should be carefully noted, as the ejaculatory ducts are seen at this level.

### MRI

MRI's exceptional soft tissue contrast and multiplanar capability permit evaluation of the lower genital tract when TRUS is indeterminate. Conventional body coil techniques fail to provide detailed anatomy of the prostate and ejaculatory apparatus. The experience with endorectal surface coils to stage prostate malig-

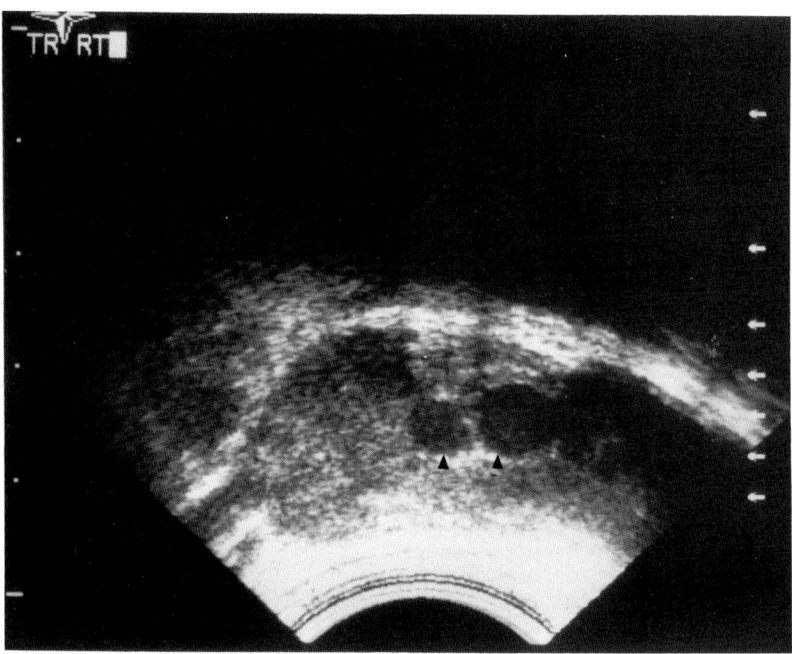

FIGURE 7.12. Transverse image of the prostate revealing dilated ejaculatory ducts (arrowheads). The patient presented with low volume azoospermia and acid pH.

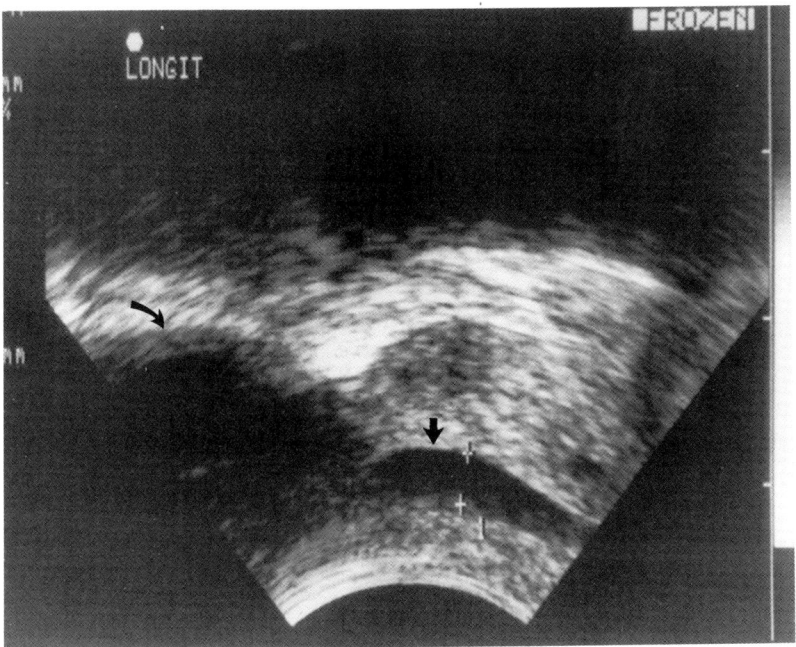

FIGURE 7.13. Longitudinal image of the junction of the seminal vesicle (curved arrow) and prostate revealing dilated ejaculatory duct (arrow) that measured 3.6 mm. This patient presented with normal volume, absent sperm motility, and low sperm viability.

nancy has demonstrated the superiority of this technique in providing detailed anatomic information. MRI imaging with endorectal surface coil is the study of choice if TRUS is indeterminate.[19] In preparation for performance of MRI with endorectal coil, intramuscular glucagon is administered to induce bowel hypotonia. T1 and T2-weighted images complement each other, but contrast resolution is better with T2-weighted images.[20]

## Images of the Prostate, Seminal Vesicles, and Ejaculatory Apparatus

### Partial and Complete Ejaculatory Obstruction

With complete obstruction of the ejaculatory ducts, semen analysis demonstrates low volume, azoospermia, absent or low quantitative seminal fructose, and usually acid pH. These seminal findings are also consistent with bilateral congenital absence of vas deferens (BCAVD). In BCAVD, vasa deferentia are not palpated, and TRUS usually demonstrates absent or hypoplastic seminal vesicles. With partial ejaculatory duct obstruction, semen analysis demonstrates normal or low volume, normal or low sperm count, impaired motility, and low sperm viability due to delay in transit through the ductal system. In complete or partial ejaculatory duct obstruction, TRUS or MRI may demonstrate markedly dilated ejaculatory ducts and dilated seminal vesicles (Figs. 7.12 and 7.13). The seminal vesicles are usually 15 mm or less when measured in the anterior-posterior diameter,[21] and values greater than this suggest obstruction (Fig. 7.14). Partial obstruction may be due to müllerian duct cyst, which can splay the ejaculatory ducts laterally and lead to compression and partial obstruction (Fig. 7.15). Midline cysts usually appear as bright white cystic structures on MRI if only clear fluid is present. The relationship of the cyst to the seminal vesicles is best appreciated with sagittal images (Figs. 7.16 and 7.17). Ejacu-

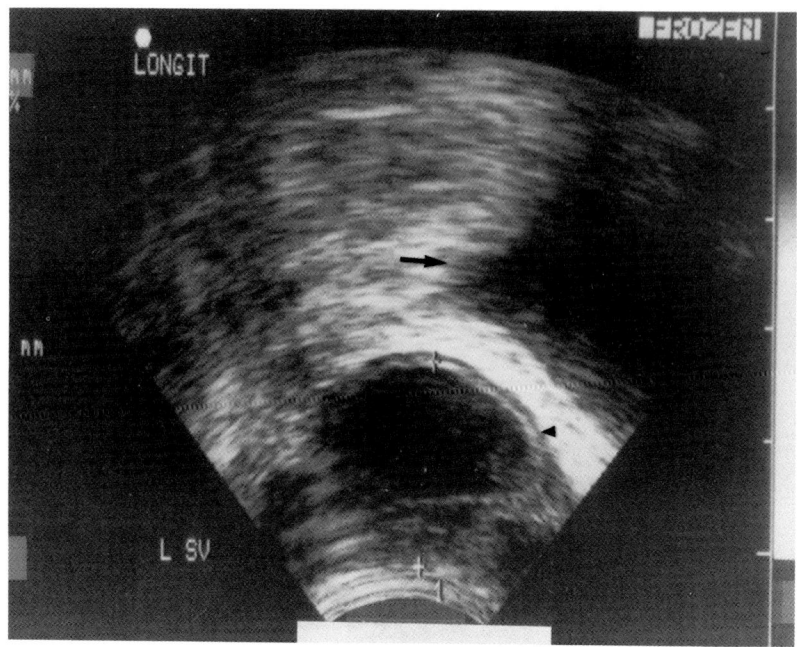

FIGURE 7.14. Same patient as in Figure 7.13, the seminal vesicle (arrowhead) measured 18.5 mm at the anterior-posterior diameter. Keeping the bladder (arrow) full permits easier orientation.

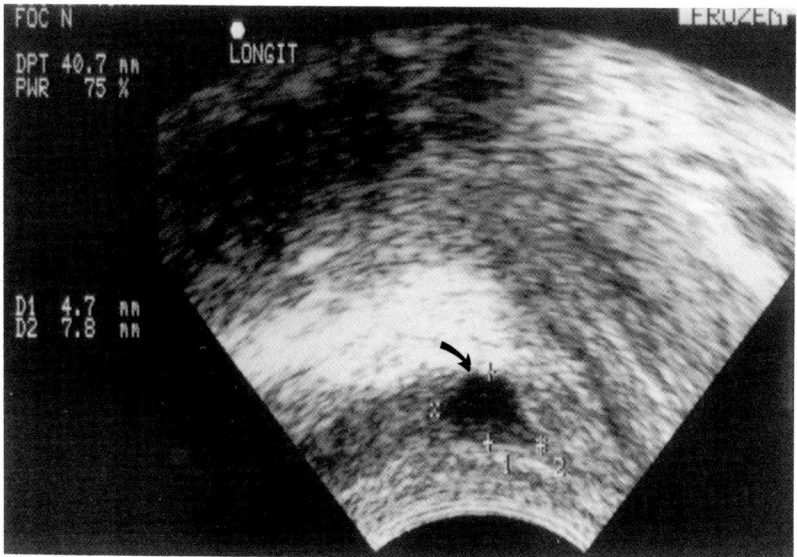

FIGURE 7.15. Longitudinal image demonstrating a müllerian-duct cyst (curved arrowhead). This patient presented with consistently impaired sperm motility, normal semen volume, and a normal physical examination.

11. Meacham RB, Townsend RR, Rademacher D, et al. The incidence of varicoceles in the general population when evaluated by physical examination, gray scale sonography and color doppler sonography. *J Urol* 1994; 151:1535–1538.

12. Eskew LA, Watson NE, Wolfman N, et al. Ultrasonographic diagnosis of varicoceles. *Fertil Steril* 1993; 60:693–697.

13. Maxwell AJ, Mamtora H. Sonographic appearance of epidermoid cyst of the testis. *J Clin Ultrasound* 1990; 18:188–190.

14. Hamm B, Fobbe F, Loy V. Testicular cysts: differentiation with US and clinical findings. *Radiology* 1988; 168:19–23.

15. Collings C, Cronan JJ, Grusmark J. Diffuse echoes within a simple hydrocele: an imaging caveat. *J Ultrasound Med* 1994; 13:439–442.

16. Janzen DL, Mathieson JR, Marsh JI, et al. Testicular microlithiasis: sonographic and clinical features. *AJR* 1992; 158:1057–1060.

17. Kessaris DN, Mellinger BC. Incidence and implication of testicular microlithiasis detected by scrotal duplex sonography in a select group of infertile men. *J Urol* 1994; 152:1560–1561.

18. Backus ML, Mack LA, Middleton WD, et al. Testicular microlithiasis: imaging appearances and pathologic correlation. *Radiology* 1994; 192:781–785.

19. Schnall MD, Pollack HM, Van Arsdalen K, et al. The seminal tract in patients with ejaculatory dysfunction: MR imaging with an endorectal surface coil. *AJR* 1992; 159:337–341.

20. Weintraub MP, De Mouy E, Hellstrom WJG. Newer modalities in the diagnosis and treatment of ejaculatory duct obstruction. *J Urol* 1993; 150:1150–1154.

21. Carter SS, Shinohara K, Lipshultz LI. Transrectal ultrasonography in disorders of the seminal vesicles and ejaculatory ducts. *Urol Clin North Am* 1989; 16:773–790.

# 8
# Immunologic Infertility

John E. Gould

Among the multitude of factors that impair human fertility is a biologic system whose purpose is to protect us from a hostile environment. The immune system is a complex network of cells and cell products that is called upon every day to defend against microorganisms and deleterious foreign material. But the immune system can also turn on its host with catastrophic consequences: lupus erythematosis, rheumatoid arthritis, Hashimoto's thyroiditis, Graves' disease, pernicious anemia, hemolytic anemia, and polyarteritis nodosa. The impairment of fertility by the immune system has characteristics that may be unique. In a sense, the recognition of sperm antigens by men and women represents a proper functioning of immune surveillance. With respect to human reproductive function, we ask the immune system to make an exception. Usually, foreign reproductive antigens are tolerated.

It has been stated that immunity to sperm is a relative, not absolute, cause of infertility.[1] It therefore follows that it is difficult to precisely identify how many couples are afflicted with immunologic infertility. The incidence of antisperm antibodies in infertile couples is thought to range between 10% and 30%,[2,3] with background rates in fertile couples <2% in serum, semen, and cervical mucus.[4] The presence of immune reactivity to sperm in an infertile couple will reveal little about their fertility. More detailed information will allow more accurate fertility prognoses: the concentration of antibodies present, the percent of sperm cells bound, isotype (e.g., immunoglobulins

IgG, IgA), locations of antibody binding on sperm cells, body fluid containing the antibodies (serum, semen), the type of assay used to detect the antibodies, and complement titers in the female tract[5-8] (Table 8.1). In this context, it becomes easier to understand why immunologic infertility is not an "all-or-none" phenomenon.

## Sperm Autoimmunity

Sperm production in males begins at puberty, long after the immune system has matured. The process of spermatogenesis results in the expression of new sperm-surface antigens.[9] It is therefore entirely appropriate that if the immune system and the sperm antigens come in contact, immune recognition occurs. Under normal circumstances, the new antigens are isolated from the immune system by the blood-testis barrier. The anatomical definition of this barrier is a series of tight junctions between neighboring Sertoli cells, which separate the adluminal spaces of the seminiferous tubules from the basal area.[10] The new antigens on sperm cells do not normally appear until the developing sperm cells enter the adluminal compartment (late pachytene). The antigens are not present on spermatogonia. These observations have therefore suggested that the function of the blood-testis barrier is to prevent new sperm antigens from contacting elements of the immune system. It is generally believed that the sequestration of the sperm antigens from

TABLE 8.1. Factors to consider in antisperm antibody literature.

Which antibodies (isotype)?
How are they detected?
Concentration, % bound?
In what fluid (semen, serum, etc.)?
Which sperm surface domain (head, tail)?
Are there controls?

the immune system continues along the epididymis, vas deferens, and urethra, but the exact nature of this isolation barrier is not well understood. Nevertheless, the sequestration appears to be quite efficient: fluid from the seminiferous tubules is low in immunoreactive elements, such as immunoglobulins and leukocytes.[11]

The appearance and modification of sperm surface antigens begin in the seminiferous tubules; further modifications are likely to occur with the addition of seminal vesicle and prostate fluid and through the cellular events of capacitation and the acrosome reaction. The functions and characteristics of sperm-surface antigens are not well understood. Efforts to characterize antigens are increasing, because not all antigens are necessarily functionally relevant and not all necessarily impair fertility.[12,13] It is known that the ability of sperm to undergo capacitation usually requires sperm transit through the epididymis.[14] It might soon be possible to characterize surface antigens involved in sperm capacitation, verify their appearance after epididymal transport, and demonstrate that antibodies to these antigens account for capacitation failure and infertility. Perhaps epididymal proteins involved in the acquisition of sperm motility might also be characterized in this fashion. Such studies will greatly enhance our ability to precisely define the mechanisms of immunologic infertility.

Potential sites for sperm contact with the immune system include the rete testis and efferent ducts. It has been observed that the tight junctions between cells lining these areas are weak.[9] It has also been observed that T-suppressor cells are abundant in between the epithelial cells in the rete testis, epididymis, vas deferens, seminal vesicles, and prostatic acini.[15] The ratio of T-suppressor to T-helper cells in

these environments and the magnitude of antigenic leak may be important factors in immune infertility. Further evidence for rete testis involvement in antigenic leakage comes from the experimental allergic orchitis model in which passive transfer of leukocytes activated by testicular antigens produces an orchitis in the recipient animal.[16] Furthermore, immune complexes can be observed outside the efferent ducts following vasectomy in rhesus monkeys.[9]

On the basis of these data, one might postulate a number of mechanisms that influence the development of antisperm antibodies in men. Four of these mechanisms were summarized by Witkin:[17]

1. A breakdown in the blood-testis barrier or other sequestration barriers, allowing sperm and immune elements to come into contact with each other.
2. A decrease in T-suppressor cell numbers or activity in areas where sperm antigens might leak out of their sequestered environment.
3. A deficiency in genital-tract fluid soluble factors that modulate suppressor cell activity (e.g., interferons, prostaglandins).
4. A deficiency in the ability of sperm cells themselves to suppress immune responses. (There is evidence that spermatozoa and developing sperm cells are capable of suppressing immune responses.[18,19])

The female reproductive tract must provide protection against invading organisms, but it must be tolerant of foreign antigens on sperm cells and the developing fetus. This subject has been recently reviewed by Naz and Menge[20] and provides another important mechanism of immunoinfertility. A detailed review of female immunoinfertility is beyond the scope of this chapter. However, a few important points should be made on this subject.

Most women do not develop antisperm antibodies despite coital inoculation with huge numbers of foreign cells. Immunosuppressive factors are thought to play an important role in this phenomenon. The majority of intraepithelial lymphocytes in the female genital tract seem to be T-suppressor cells.[21] Seminal plasma itself contains numerous immunosuppressive factors,[9] although these factors are probably only important in the lower female tract. When antibodies to sperm do form despite these immunosuppressive factors, some failure of these mechanisms must occur. An erosion of vaginal mucosa from trauma or infection is one presumed mechanism of sperm antigen presentation.

## Etiology

It is widely believed that conditions that disrupt the sequestration of sperm antigens from the immune system have the potential to result in antisperm antibody formation. However, it is also true that men who have no identifiable risk factor for immunologic infertility may develop antisperm antibodies. Furthermore, it is also true that there is no clinical event that uniformly leads to antisperm antibody formation in all men. An association between antisperm antibodies and human leukocyte antigen (HLA) has been observed,[22] suggesting that genetic factors may modulate immunologic responses in men.

Gonadal trauma has been associated with antisperm antibody formation.[23] Iatrogenic trauma in the form of testicular biopsy might also predispose to antisperm antibody formation. This possibility has been refuted[24] and supported.[25] Testicular torsion may impair fertility, in part by immunologic mechanisms.[26,27] Prepubertal torsion has no immunologic consequence, because sperm antigens are not yet present.[28]

Other postulated mechanisms of antisperm antibody formation include obstruction,[29] cryptorchidism,[30] varicocele,[31] and genital tract infection.[32]

Previous vasectomy is recognized as a leading cause of clinical immunologic infertility.[33] Antisperm antibodies develop in the serum of approximately two thirds of men who have undergone vasectomy.[34,35] Sperm autoimmunity is often seen in the first few months after a vasectomy,[36] but may decrease to lower levels in the ensuing years.[37] The advisability of testing for circulating antisperm antibodies prior to a vasovasostomy is controversial. Although serum IgG has been shown to be a good predictor

of sperm surface antibodies,[5] the predictive value of serum antisperm antibodies to eventual fertility is controversial. Alexander[38] showed diminished fertility in vasectomized men with sperm agglutinating antibodies in serum, whereas Silber[39] found no such correlation. No clear relationship has been shown between the formation of sperm granulomas and antisperm antibodies,[40] although granulomas may have good prognostic value, presumably through testicular decompression.[41]

Finally, laboratory risk factors for antisperm antibodies include sperm agglutination on semen evaluation, an abnormal postcoital test in the presence of good-quality mucus, a normal semen evaluation, and fertilization failure (as in negative sperm-penetration assay or failed in vitro fertilization). An abnormal postcoital test may also indicate the presence of antisperm antibodies in the cervical mucus. The postcoital test may show no sperm and good-quality mucus or sperm stuck in mucus with a "shaking" type of motion.[42]

## Antisperm Antibody Detection

There are now numerous tools to detect antisperm antibodies on sperm, in seminal plasma, in serum, in cervical mucus, and in any reproductive secretions (Table 8.2). Correlation between circulating and sperm surface antibodies may be poor.[5,43] It is assumed that sperm surface antibodies are biologically more relevant than antibodies in seminal plasma or serum. Circulating immunoglobulins include IgG, IgM, and monomeric IgA. Male genital tract immunoglobulins comprise the IgG and secretory IgA isotypes. Much has been written comparing assay results,[44,45] and a basic understanding of these tools is needed (Table 8.2).

The *immunobead test* is widely used to detect sperm surface antibodies.[46,47] In this test, polyacrylamide beads are linked to isotype-specific rabbit antihuman antibodies. Immunobeads bind to the sperm surface where antibodies are found and, under light microscopy, the regional specificity is determined. Immunobeads therefore may be used to indicate the immunoglobulin class and its location on the sperm surface.

TABLE 8.2. Assays for antisperm antibodies (ASAB).

| Name | Description | Application |
|------|-------------|-------------|
| Immunobead test (IBT) | Polyacrylamide beads with isotype-specific antihuman antibodies bind to ASAB | Determines isotype and location of ASAB on live sperm; good sensitivity and specificity |
| Sperm agglutination tests | Multivalent antibodies cross-link sperm | Determines IgM or IgA; poor specificity due to possible agglutination by bacteria nonimmunoglobulin proteins |
| Mixed agglutination reaction (MAR) | Sperm and red blood cells with surface IgG agglutinate in presence of anti-IgG | Nonquantitative way to screen for sperm-surface IgG |
| Sperm immobilization test | Sperm cells with ASAB are exposed to complement and lose motility | Detects IgG and IgM, not IgA |
| Indirect immunofluorescence | ASABs bind to fluorescent-labeled antibodies | Determines surface location for ASAB but specificity is poor |
| Enzyme-linked immunosorbent assay (ELISA) | Enzyme-antiglobulin complex binds to ASAB; color change when substrate added | Allows for quantitative determination of ASABs but sensitivity is poor |

The beads are used both as a direct test of sperm-surface antibodies and as an indirect test of serum antibodies after passive transfer to donor sperm cells. Passive transfer of antibodies to donor sperm is also possible using follicular fluid, cervical mucus, and seminal plasma. False-positive results are low with this test, but false-negative results may occur in that only motile cells are tested. The immunobead test has become one of the most clinically useful antisperm antibody tests.[48]

*Sperm agglutination tests* are based on the principle that large, multivalent isotypes, such as IgM or secretory IgA, may be able to cross-link large numbers of sperm. In its simplest form, the agglutination test is composed of a mixing of test serum with sperm cells and performing a microscopic evaluation of sperm clumping after 1- to 2-hour incubation at 37°C. The agglutination tests are known by several different names, including the tray-slide agglutination test (Franklin and Dukes[49]), the tray agglutination test (Friberg[50]), and the gelatin agglutination test (Kibrick et al[51]). False-positive results are possible with all of these agglutination techniques because bacteria and nonimmunoglobulin proteins in semen and serum may cause significant sperm agglutination. A variation of these tests is the mixed agglutination reaction,[52] which was designed to detect antibodies directly on the sperm cells (no serum

added). In this test, a mixture of human red blood cells with IgG on their surface and test sperm cells is combined with a rabbit anti-IgG. A mixed agglutination of blood cells and sperm cells is indicative of sperm surface IgG. The ensuing agglutination is macroscopic and does not allow for a determination of the proportion of sperm with antibodies or the sperm surface regional specificity.

The *sperm immobilization test* (Isojima et al[53]) is based on the principle that sperm cells with surface antibodies, in the presence of complement, lose their ability to move. This test may recapitulate a mechanism of immunologic infertility because complement is present in the female reproductive tract and may interfere with the progression of antibody-coated sperm. False-positive results are rare, and this test therefore has high specificity. A disadvantage to the sperm immobilization test is a lack of sensitivity. IgA, which does not fix complement, is not detected. Head-directed antibodies may also go undetected, because even in the presence of complement such antibodies may not impair motility.

*Indirect immunofluorescence*[54,55] is another method to detect antibody-bound sperm. A fluorescent label is attached to an antihuman antibody. When this antibody recognizes sperm surface antibodies, fluorescence is observed under fluorescence microscopy. This test is sensitive, as false-negative results are uncommon. The location of the antibody on the sperm surface can also be determined. False-positive results are encountered because the method allows internal sperm antigens to be released. Internal sperm antigens are not thought to be related to immunologic infertility. A variation on this idea is the *radiolabeled antiglobulin assay*.[56] Here the antihuman immunoglobulin is labeled to a radioisotope, and the washed sperm suspension is counted for residual radioactivity. False-positive results are possible here, again owing to internal antigens released from dead cells. When this test is applied to motile cells, such as in a swim-up preparation, it is highly specific and sensitive. It does not give information on the regional specificity of binding or on the proportion of sperm that are antibody bound.

The *enzyme-linked immunosorbent assay*[57,58] is a calorimetric assay for antisperm antibodies. An enzyme is linked to an antiglobulin that recognizes sperm surface antibodies. When the enzyme is placed in the presence of its substrate, a color change develops that is measured photometrically. The methods involved in this assay may expose internal antigens or damage surface antigens; therefore, false-positive and false-negative results may occur.

# Mechanisms of Immunologic Infertility

The rapid advances in assisted reproductive technology (ART) have provided the tools to investigate the effects of antisperm antibodies on fertile functions. One might hypothesize that antisperm antibodies could inhibit fertilization in three broad areas. First, sperm function that occurs prior to fertilization could be affected. This might include sperm maturation in the epididymis, sperm transport through the cervix and uterus, and entry into the oviduct. Second, events around the time of fertilization, such as penetration of the cumulus oophorus and zona pellucida, as well as fusion with the vitellus, might be affected. Finally, the events of embryogenesis and embryo implantation after

fertilization might be influenced by sperm surface antibodies. To further complicate the matter, the polyclonal response to sperm in men and women would suggest that different sperm surface antibodies have different effects on this spectrum of fertilization events.

There is considerable evidence that sperm surface antibodies hinder the ability of sperm to enter and survive in cervical mucus.[59,60] Mathur et al[61] showed that 64% of 66 couples without significant sperm surface antibodies had adequate sperm motility in cervical mucus and improved fertility compared with 26% of 122 couples with sperm surface antibodies. The impairment of cervical mucus penetration appears to be directly proportional to the proportion of sperm with antibodies, and IgA is a much more potent inhibitor of mucus penetration than IgG.[6] It appears that the Fc portion of the antibody molecule is responsible for the impairment of sperm entry into mucus. Bronson et al[60] have shown that when the Fc portion of the antibody is removed proteolytically, the sperm so treated have an improved ability to penetrate cervical mucus. Furthermore, Jaeger et al[62] have shown that the Fab portion of antisperm IgG does not impair sperm entry into cervical mucus.

Sperm survival and its migration through the female reproductive tract may be impaired by sperm surface antibodies for other reasons, possibly by macrophage phagocytosis and complement-mediated cytotoxicity.[63,64] Complement proteins have been identified in cervical mucus and follicular fluid.[65] Further problems may occur with capacitation and the acrosome reaction. Major antigenic differences exist between capacitated and noncapacitated sperm, but the effect of these surface antibodies on the capacitation process itself is unknown.[66] Ultrastructural studies of antibody-bound human sperm do not show significant alteration in acrosomal morphology, suggesting that this is not an important mechanism of infertility.[67] However, Bandoh et al[68] showed that sperm-immobilizing antibodies in vitro inhibit the acrosome reaction. Benoff et al[69] showed that antisperm antibodies to sperm surface progesterone receptors may impair acrosome reactions. There are some data that even suggest a facilitation of the acrosome reaction by antisperm antibodies.[70]

It is widely accepted that sperm surface antibodies have the potential to significantly impair sperm/egg interactions. The precise mechanism of this impairment is unclear. Presumably, the surface antibodies may cover or alter important sperm surface proteins. Penetration of the zona pellucida, for example, requires tight binding of the sperm to the zona surface.[71] This binding is thought to involve specific receptors between the zona surface and specialized regions on the sperm head. Blockage of these specialized regions could produce fertilization failure.[72–74] Further support for this idea comes from in vitro fertilization (IVF) cycles. Zouari et al[75] showed that in patients with sperm head-directed antibodies there were higher IVF fertilizations observed when oocytes showed good sperm binding, and lower fertilization rates when oocytes showed poor sperm–zona binding. Shibahara et al[76] demonstrated that sperm immobilizing antibodies may significantly block sperm–zona tight binding as measured by the hemizona assay (HZA). Sperm surface antibodies may also interfere with fusion of sperm and hamster vitelli.[77,78] It is reasonable to hypothesize that human sperm and human vitelli may have impaired fusion events when antisperm antibodies are present. There is recent evidence from Wolf et al[79] that showed that IgG inhibits fusion between sperm and vitellus in a dose-dependent fashion. IgA antibodies did not appear to inhibit the fusion to the same extent. The authors used patients undergoing subzonal insemination (SUZI) to make these observations.

The degree to which antisperm antibody isotypes impair in vitro fertilization seems to be significantly influenced by the amount of antibody binding and the isotype. Yeh et al[80] reviewed retrospectively 80 IVF cycles with sperm surface antibodies by immunobead test. IgA binding levels of >68%, particularly when head-associated, as well as IgM binding of >40% were particularly deleterious to IVF. Lower levels of IgA and any level of IgG did not significantly impair fertilization. Clarke and coworkers[81] showed that high levels of sperm surface IgA significantly impaired fertilization

rates in IVF cycles. When the male patient had 80% or more of his motile sperm covered with IgG and IgA (i.e., both isotypes strongly present), overall fertilization rates were only 27%. In nine male patients with sperm surface antibodies but in whom <80% were coated with IgA antibodies, the fertilization rate was 78%. High fertilization rates were observed in patients even when IgG surface binding alone was quite high. No problems with subsequent implantation and pregnancy were observed. Other workers have shown reduced fertilization rates in IVF cycles only when both IgA and IgG are present together, but no reduction in fertilization when only one of the two isotypes was present.[82] The geography of sperm surface antibodies may be another important variable. Mandelbaum et al[83] studied 40 couples in IVF cycles in whom antisperm antibodies were present in serum, semen, or follicular fluid. Antibodies to the sperm tail tip did not adversely affect fertilization rates, and head-directed antisperm antibodies were similarly unimportant when observed in semen or male serum. However, head-directed antibodies detected in female serum reduced fertilization rates. A similar effect was seen when head-directed antibodies were detected in female follicular fluid. Witkin et al[84] found that tail-directed antibodies reduced fertilization rates. Finally, the impairment of IVF success by antibodies may be additive to other poor prognostic indicators, such as abnormal morphology.[85]

A detrimental effect of female circulating antisperm antibodies on in vitro fertilization has been shown,[86–88] but has also been challenged.[89,90] Some groups have advocated substitution of antibody-negative serum for antibody-positive serum in IVF cycles.[86] Furthermore, it is not universally accepted that sperm surface antibodies formed in the male are always deleterious. Pagidas et al[89] showed no impairment of IVF using sperm with surface antibodies even when antibody levels were high. Human epididymal sperm with surface antibodies do not appear to impair IVF.[91] The polyclonal immunologic response to sperm may well account for some of these inconsistencies between studies.

Little is known about the potential for antisperm antibodies to impair embryogenesis. Observations of lower rates of pregnancies and embryonic quality in IVF cycles exposed to antisperm antibodies suggest that early embryonic development may be adversely affected.[88]

Given that polyclonal responses confound our precise understanding of immunologic infertility, it follows that monoclonal antibodies will provide important tools to identify mechanisms of subfertility. Mouse myeloma cells have been fused with lymphocytes from an infertile female patient to produce an IgM monoclonal antibody.[92] This antibody has been successfully used to identify an internal lactosaminoglycan that is a specific site for sperm immobilizing antibody binding. This internal protein may offer clues to the molecular basis for infertility in women who possess this antibody. Antibodies and antigens that result in sperm agglutination and immobilization[93] as well as those that follow vasectomy[94] have been characterized using monoclonal antibodies. Riedel et al[95] have examined the effect of specific monoclonal antisperm antibodies on penetration rates of hamster ova. A monoclonal antibody to fertilization antigen-1 inhibits sperm capacitation and the acrosome reaction.[96] These types of studies will continue to offer important clues as to the mechanisms of immunologic infertility.

## Treatment

An approach to the treatment of couples with immunologic infertility is summarized in Table 8.3. Broadly speaking, treatment may be aimed at eliminating or disabling antisperm antibodies by treating patients or treating the ejaculate. Alternatively, assisted reproductive technologies may be applied to appropriate couples to circumvent the detrimental effects of sperm surface antibodies. Many studies in the area of immunologic infertility treatment suffer from a lack of controls. Controls are critically important because antisperm antibodies impair fertility but don't absolutely prevent it.

The use of condoms to prevent female sensitization to sperm antigens has been advocated,[49,97] but the effectiveness of this therapy has been questioned.[98] Couples use condoms for several months and then stop condom use for ovulatory coitus. No controlled studies have shown benefit to this therapy.

Systemic steroids have been advocated in men and women to diminish or eliminate antisperm antibodies.[99] There are several questions to consider in reviewing the literature on steroid use for immunologic infertility: (1) Which antibody isotypes was the study detecting, using what assay? (2) Were the antibodies in serum, seminal plasma, cervical mucus, or sperm surface? (3) What steroid regimen was used? (4) What were the outcome parameters used (e.g., pregnancy, antisperm antibody (ASAB) levels, semen analysis)? A comprehensive review of corticosteroid literature between 1970 and 1988 is provided by Haas[100] in table form. The majority of studies to date have been uncontrolled. A discussion of some of the controlled studies is warranted here (Table 8.4).

In 1985 De Almeida et al[101] published a randomized double-blind study using 10 subjects with serum and seminal plasma antisperm antibodies detected by agglutination and "sperm toxicity" assays. The small group of subjects was randomized to placebo versus prednisolone, 1 mg/kg/day for 9 days; a total of three cycles was completed. The authors did not observe any effect on fertility and no effect was seen on serum or semen antisperm antibodies. They did observe a slight decrease in seminal plasma antibodies in the steroid-treated group.

TABLE 8.3. Treatment of immunologic infertility.

A. Eliminate ASAB
   1. Treat patient
      a. Barrier methods
      b. Steroid
   2. Treat ejaculate
      a. Proteolytic enzymes
      b. Immunoabsorption
      c. Magnetic isolation
      d. Dextram column
      e. Percoll gradient
      f. Immunobead processing
B. Circumvent ASAB (ART)
   1. IUI
   2. IVF
   3. ICSI

TABLE 8.4. Fecundity rate per cycle and per couple with immunologic male infertility treated with oral corticosteroids.

| First author/ Year | Number of pregnancies | Number of cycles | Fecundity per cycle | Number of couples | Fecundity per couple |
|---|---|---|---|---|---|
| Hendry/79 | | | | | |
|     Treated | 14 | 222 | 0.06 | 47 | 0.30 |
| Shulman/82 | | | | | |
|     Treated | 31 | 641 | 0.05 | 71 | 0.31 |
| Alexander/83 | | | | | |
|     Treated | 7 | 76 | 0.09 | 19 | 0.37 |
|     Control | 3 | 100 | 0.03 | 25 | 0.12 |
| Haas/87 | | | | | |
|     Treated | 3 | 66 | 0.045 | 24.125 | |
|     Control | 1 | 50 | 0.02 | 19 | 0.05 |
| Hendry/90 | | | | | |
|     Treated | 9 | 261 | 0.03 | 29 | 0.31 |
|     Control | 2 | 189 | 0.01 | 21 | 0.09 |

Two years later Haas and Manganiello[102] studied 43 subjects whose sperm were positive for IgG or IgA by direct radiolabeled antiglobulin assay. The design was double-blind, controlled, and prospective over a 3-month study period. Female workup was performed to rule out concurrent female problems. Thirty-five subjects completed the study and were randomized to placebo versus methylprednisolone. The authors treated the men during their partners' luteal phase, using methylprednisolone 96 mg/day × 7 days, 32 mg on day 8, and 16 mg on day 9. The subjects were given three courses on three consecutive cycles. The authors did not observe any improvement in the semen evaluation parameters, fertility, or antisperm antibodies except that sperm surface IgG was lowered in subjects receiving methylprednisolone.

The strongest data to date advocating steroid use in antisperm antibodies resulted from Hendry et al.[103] This study had a double-blind prospective design with crossover. Forty-three couples with clinical infertility of at least 1 year's duration were entered into the trial. To be included, the male subjects had to have positive mixed agglutination reaction (sperm surface antibodies) and positive triglutination tests (serum, seminal plasma antibodies, or both). Female inclusion criteria included one patent oviduct, normal ovulation, and abnormal postcoital test. Twenty-seven subjects completed the 18-month study. Subjects were randomized to prednisolone or placebo for 9 months and then crossover occurred. The prednisolone dose was 20 mg twice daily on days 1 to 10 of the female partner's menstrual cycle, followed by 5 mg on days 11 and 12. The authors observed nine pregnancies in the steroid group and two pregnancies in the placebo group. Antisperm antibody levels were assayed in seminal plasma and were diminished by steroid treatment. No effect on antisperm antibody levels was seen in serum. The semen analysis was minimally affected by this regimen. The authors also point out that there was no difference in the two groups until after 6 months of treatment. Sixty percent of subjects experienced mild steroid side effects compared with 19% taking placebo.

The background fecundity of couples with antisperm antibodies is unknown. Table 8.4 shows fecundity per cycle and fecundity per couple data from several representative studies in which pregnancies occurred. Small numbers of pregnancies in treated and untreated couples produce a wide scatter of fecundity data. The use of corticosteroids remains controversial, and long-term, prospective, multi-institutional trials would assist in evaluation of this treatment modality. Although rare, the devastating complications of steroid use, such as aseptic necrosis of the hip,[104] require cautious use of steroids in infertile couples.

In summary, there is no consensus on the therapeutic benefits of steroids in immunologic infertility, but data do exist that would justify steroid use in an informed patient willing to endure potential side effects, some of which carry significant morbidity.

Elder et al[105] provided data that suggest an improved fertilization and conception rate when antibody-positive semen was collected into a small volume of medium containing 50% serum. The study was retrospective and not controlled. It is presumed that the serum inhibited the binding of antibodies to the sperm surface.

The next type of treatment option would be the removal or alteration of sperm surface antibodies by means of treating the sperm directly. Proteolytic enzymes such as subtilisin, chymotrypsin, trypsin, and papain have been investigated for this use.[106] Some of these agents may be shown to have a beneficial effect on sperm disagglutination, but a concomitant impairment of sperm/mucus interaction or zona-free hamster egg penetration may also result.[107] Trypsin seems to improve penetration of zona-free hamster eggs but does not improve sperm/mucus interaction. An IgA protease can be used to improve in vitro sperm cervical mucus penetrating ability.[60] Immunoabsorption techniques have also been investigated. Bronson et al[108] had subjects collect semen in a suspension of freeze/thawed sonicated human sperm and observed improved penetration of cervical mucus by the sperm so treated. Kiser et al[109] added immunobeads to sperm and allowed the sperm to swim up out of the bead suspension. The authors did not observe an improvement in motility or motile density and had poor recovery of sperm with this technique.

Magnetic isolation of sperm has been investigated. Magnetic spheres can be linked to immunobead complexes mixed with semen, and the suspension can be placed in a magnetic field.[109] However, separation is suboptimal and the motility of treated sperm deteriorates rapidly. Magnetic separation has been observed to reduce the number of sperm with surface antisperm antibodies,[110] but the method has not been used in any large clinical trials. Diluted ejaculates have been passed through a column of dextran beads with improved motility and hamster egg penetration in sperm undergoing

this treatment.[109] Percoll gradients have also been used to select antibody-free sperm,[111] but no testing of the fertility potential of such sperm has yet been undertaken.

The same immunobeads that are used to detect sperm surface antibodies can be used to lower the proportion of sperm bound with antisperm antibodies.[112] Co-incubation of immunobeads with sperm results in a decrease in the number of sperm bound to immunobeads. The decreased binding results in a transference, at least in part, of the antisperm antibody from the sperm to the immunobead.[113] This technique has not been applied clinically.

No current technique for in vitro antisperm antibody processing has been shown to improve fecundity in a clinical setting.

Various forms of assisted reproductive technology (ART) are used to circumvent antibodies. These techniques can be used in conjunction with the other treatment modalities discussed so far. One might consider intrauterine insemination (IUI) as the simplest form of ART. IUI has been used to treat sperm surface antibodies. Applied without controls to women with serum antisperm antibodies, there was a suggestion of an improved pregnancy rate,[114] similarly for sperm surface antibodies in men.[115] A controlled study of IUI with high levels of sperm surface antibodies showed no therapeutic benefit to IUI.[116] There are no controlled data to support IUI as a treatment for immunologic infertility. Also, IUI does not appear to cause female serum or cervical mucus antisperm antibodies.[117]

IVF is a tool to define the pathophysiology of immunologic infertility, particularly as it relates to failure of sperm/egg interaction. A separate but related question is whether IVF is a reasonable treatment for immunologic infertility. Again, a few fundamental questions must be kept in mind when reviewing the literature on IVF as a treatment option. What assay was used to detect the antibodies and which domain (serum, semen, cervical mucus) was tested? What antisperm antibody level was considered significant?

There are considerable data to suggest that IVF is a reasonably good treatment option for antisperm antibodies. Janssen et al[118] reviewed

1074 antibody-negative IVF cycles, 61 IVF cycles with sperm surface antibodies ($\geq$ 10% IBT), and 67 IVF cycles with female serum antisperm antibody (TAT). The authors found no difference in fertilization rates with female serum antibodies and lower fertilization rates only when the sperm surface antibody levels were >50%. There was no difference in ongoing pregnancy rates between the antibody-negative and -positive groups when semen quality was similar. The authors concluded that, in general, IVF provides a similar chance of conception in couples with or without antibodies unless the levels were quite high. These results were confirmed by Lähteenmäki.[119] Daitoh et al[120] confirmed a lower fertilization rate in IVF cycles involving women with sperm immobilizing antibodies. However, this group showed that subsequent implantation and pregnancy rates were higher in the women with sperm immobilizing antibodies and concluded that IVF is a reasonable treatment option. Other studies have shown decreased embryo quality and decreased pregnancy rates in the presence of female serum antibodies, using tubal factor as a control.[88]

Even if IVF pregnancy rates for antisperm antibody-positive couples approach control levels, both cost and inconvenience of this technology are considerable. Simpler and less costly in vitro procedures would be useful. Intracytoplasmic sperm injection (ICSI) may offer yet another alternative with high pregnancy rates. Nagy et al[121] achieved high fertilization rates with ICSI in 55 cycles using sperm with surface antibody (MAR test); compared with ICSI cycles using antibody negative sperm, the antibody positive sperm seemed to improve fertilization rates and yield the same pregnancy rates but to decrease the proportion of good quality embryos.

## Summary

The development of antisperm antibodies is an appropriate but unwelcome immune phenomenon. The polyclonal response to sperm surface antigens has a variable effect on fertile functions and is not necessarily detrimental. However, the most common result of immunoreactivity to sperm is a relative impairment in fertility. This impairment may affect the spectrum of sperm functions all the way from entry into the female tract to embryogenesis. Therapy is currently suboptimal, with highest success rates associated with highest monetary costs. It is hoped lower cost sperm processing techniques will become available to help infertile couples with antisperm antibodies. Moreover, the complex molecular events that comprise the expression and recognition of sperm surface proteins may help unlock the mysteries of human fertility.

*Acknowledgment.* The author gratefully acknowledges the assistance of Ms. Cynthia Kolp in the preparation of this chapter.

## References

1. Bronson R, Cooper G, Rosenfeld D. Sperm antibodies: their role in infertility. *Fertil Steril* 1984; 42:171–183.
2. Bronson RA, Tung KSK. Human spermatozoa antibodies: detection and clinical significance. In: Rose NR, de Macario ER, eds. *Manual of Clinical Laboratory Immunology.* 4th ed. Washington, DC: American Society for Microbiology; 1992: 775–780.
3. Clarke GN, Elliott PJ, Smaila C. Detection of sperm antibodies in semen using the immunobead test: a survey of 813 consecutive patients. *Am J Reprod Immunol Microbiol* 1985; 7:118–123.
4. Kutteh WH, McAlister D, Byrd W, et al. Antisperm antibodies: current knowledge and new horizons. *Mol Androl* 1992; 4:183–193.
5. Hellstrom WJG, Overstreet JW, Samuels SJ, et al. The relationship of circulating antisperm antibodies to sperm surface antibodies in infertile men. *J Urol* 1988; 140:1039–1044.
6. Clarke GN. Immunoglobulin class and regional specificity of antispermatozoal autoantibodies blocking cervical mucus penetration by human spermatozoa. *Am J Reprod Immunol Microbiol* 1988; 16:135–138.
7. Menge AC, Beitner O. Interrelationships among semen characteristics, antisperm antibodies, and cervical mucus penetration assays in infertility human couples. *Fertil Steril* 1989; 51:4886–4892.

8. Eggert-Kruse W, Christmann M, Gerhard I, et al. Circulating antisperm antibodies and fertility prognosis: a prospective study. *Hum Reprod* 1989; 4:513–520.

9. Alexander NJ, Anderson DJ. Immunology of semen. *Fertil Steril* 1989; 47:192–205.

10. Gilula NB, Fawcett DW, Aoki A. The Sertoli cell occluding junction and gap junctions in mature and developing mammalian testis. *Dev Biol* 1976; 50:142–168.

11. Haas GG Jr. Antibody-mediated causes of male infertility. *Urol Clin North Am* 1987; 14:539–550.

12. Snow H, Ball GD. Characterization of human sperm antigens and antisperm antibodies in infertile patients. *Fertil Steril* 1992; 58:1011–1019.

13. Kurpisz M, Alexander NJ. Carbohydrate moieties on sperm surface: physiological relevance. *Fertil Steril* 1995; 63:158–165.

14. Overstreet JW. Human sperm function: acquisition in the male and expression in the female. In: Santen RJ, Swerdloff RW, eds. *Male Reproductive Function*. New York: Marcel Dekker; 1986: 29–47.

15. El-Demiry NIM, Hargreave TB, Busuttil A, et al. Lymphocyte subpopulations in the male genital tract. *Br J Urol* 1985; 57:769–774.

16. Tung KSK, Yule TD, Mahi-Brown CA, et al. Distribution of histopathology and Iga positive cells in actively induced and passively transferred experimental autoimmune orchitis. *J Immunol* 1987; 138:752–759.

17. Witkin SS. Mechanisms of active suppression of the immune response to spermatozoa. *Am J Reprod Immunol Microbiol* 1988; 17:61–64.

18. Hurtenback U, Shearer GM. Germ cell-induced immune suppression in mice. Effect of inoculation of syngeneic spermatozoa on cell-mediated immune responses. *J Exp Med* 1982; 155:1719–1729.

19. Hurtenback U, Morgensern F, Bennett D. Induction of tolerance in vitro by autologous murine testicular cells. *J Exp Med* 1980; 151:827–838.

20. Naz RK, Menge AC. Antisperm antibodies: origin, regulation, and sperm reactivity in human infertility. *Fertil Steril* 1994; 61:1001–1013.

21. Boehme M, Donat H. Identification of lymphocyte subsets in the human fallopian tube. *Am J Reprod Immunol* 1992; 28:81–84.

22. Law HY, Bodmer WF, Mathews JD, et al. The immune response to vasectomy and its relation to the HLA system. *Tissue Antigens* 1979; 14:115–139.

23. Rapaport FT, Sampath A, Kano K, et al. Immunological sequelae of experimental thermal injury to the testis. *Surg Forum* 1969; 20:503–505.

24. Ansbacher R, Gangai MP. Testicular biopsy: sperm antibodies. *Fertil Steril* 1975; 26:1239–1242.

25. Hjort T, Husted S, Linnet-Jepsen P. The effect of testis biopsy on autosensitization against spermatozoal antigens. *Clin Exp Immunol* 1974; 18:201–212.

26. Harrison RG, Lewis-Jones DI, Moreno de Marvel MJ, et al. Mechanism of damage to the contralateral testis in rats with an ischaemic testis. *Lancet* 1981; 2:723–725.

27. Nagler HM, deVere White R. The effect of testicular torsion on the contralateral testis. *J Urol* 1982; 128:1343–1348.

28. Henderson JA IV, Smey P, Cohen MS, et al. The effect of unilateral testicular torsion on the contralateral testicle in prepubertal Chinese hamsters. *J Pediatr Surg* 1985; 20:592–597.

29. Hendry WF, Parslow JM, Stedronska J, et al. The diagnosis of unilateral testicular obstruction in subfertile males. *Br J Urol* 1982; 54:774–779.

30. Koskimies AL, Hovatta O. Hypothalamopituitary-gonadal axis and sperm-agglutinating antibodies in infertile men treated for cryptorchidism. *Arch Androl* 1982; 8:181–183.

31. Golomb J, Vardinon N, Hommonnai ZT, et al. Demonstration of antispermatozoal antibodies in varicocele-related infertility with an enzyme-linked immunosorbent assay (ELISA). *Fertil Steril* 1986; 45:397–403.

32. Witkin SS, Toth A. Relationship between genital tract infections, sperm antibiodies in seminal fluid, and infertility. *Fertil Steril* 1983; 40:805–808.

33. Alexander NJ, Anderson DJ. Vasectomy: consequences of autoimmunity to sperm antigens. *Fertil Steril* 1979; 32:253–260.

34. Shulman S, Zappi E, Ahmed U, et al. Immunologic consequences of vasectomy. *Contraception* 1972; 5:269–278.

35. Fuchs EF, Alexander NJ. Immunologic considerations before and after vasovasostomy. *Fertil Steril* 1983; 40:497–506.

36. Witkin SS, Zelikovsky G, Bongiovanni AM, et al. Sperm-related antigens, antibodies, and circulating immune complexes in sera of recently vasectomized men. *J Clin Invest* 1982; 70:33–40.

37. Phadke AM, Padukone K. Presence and significance of autoantibodies against spermatozoa in

the blood of men with obstructed vas deferens. *J Reprod Fertil* 1964; 7:162–170.

38. Alexander NJ. Antibody levels and immunologic infertility. In: Isojima S, Billington WE, eds. *Reproductive Immunology 1983*. Amsterdam: Elsevier Science; 1983: 207–212.

39. Silber SJ. The relationship of abnormal semen parameters to pregnancy outcome. In: Seibel MM, ed. *Infertility: A Comprehensive Text*. Norwalk: Appleton & Lange; 1990: 149–155.

40. Alexander NJ, Schmidt SS. Incidence of antisperm antibody levels and granulomas in men. *Fertil Steril* 1977; 28:655–657.

41. Belker AM, Thomas AJ, Fuchs EF, et al. Results of 1469 microsurgical vasectomy reversals by the vasovasostomy study group. *J Urol* 1991; 145:505–511.

42. Haas GG. Immunologic male infertility. *Infert Reprod Med Clin North Am* 1992; 3:413.

43. Haas GG Jr, Schrieber AD, Blasco L. The incidence of sperm-associated immunoglobulins and C3, the third component of complement, in infertile men. *Fertil Steril* 1983; 39:542–547.

44. Peters AJ, Ivanovic M, Jeyendran RS. Variation in antisperm antibody results using different assays. *Am J Reprod Immunol* 1995; 33:140–143.

45. Andreou E, Mahmoud A, Vermeulen L, et al. Comparison of different methods for the investigation of antisperm antibodies on spermatozoa, in seminal plasma and in serum. *Hum Reprod* 1995; 10:125–131.

46. Bronson RA, Cooper GW, Rosenfeld DL. Correlation between regional specificity of antisperm antibodies to the spermatozoan surface and complement-mediated sperm immobilization. *Am J Reprod Immunol* 1982; 2:222–224.

47. Bronson R, Cooper G, Rosenfeld DL. Membrane-bound sperm-specific antibodies: their role in infertility. In: Jangiello G, Vogel H, eds. *Bioregulators of Reproduction*. New York: Academic Press; 1981: 521–527.

48. Rajah SV, Parslow JM, Howell RJS, et al. Comparison of mixed antiglobulin reaction and direct immunobead test for detection of sperm-bound antibodies in subfertile males. *Fertil Steril* 1992; 57:1300–1303.

49. Franklin RR, Dukes DC. Antispermatozoal antibody and unexplained infertility. *Am J Obstet Gynecol* 1964; 89:6–9.

50. Friberg J. A simple and sensitive micro-method for demonstration of sperm-agglutinating activity in serum from infertile men and women. *Acta Obstet Gynecol Scand* 1974; 36:21–29.

51. Kibrick S, Belding DL, Merrill B. Methods for the detection of antibodies against mammalian spermatozoa. II. A gelatin agglutination test. *Fertil Steril* 1952; 3:430.

52. Jager S, Kremer J, van Slochteren-Draaisma T. A simple method of screening for antisperm antibodies in the human male: detection of spermatozoal surface IgG with the direct mixed antiglobulin reaction carried out on untreated fresh human semen. *Int J Fertil* 1978; 23:12–21.

53. Isojima S, Tsuchiya K, Koyama K, et al. Further studies on sperm-immobilizing antibody found in sera of unexplained cases of sterility in women. *Am J Obstet Gynecol* 1972; 112:199–207.

54. Hjort T, Hansen KB. Immunofluorescent studies on human spermatozoa. 1. The detection of different spermatozoal antibodies and their occurrence in normal and infertile women. *Clin Exp Immunol* 1971; 8:9–23.

55. Tung KSK, Cooke WD Jr, McCarty TA, et al. Human sperm antigens and antisperm antibodies. II. Age-related incidence of antisperm antibodies. *Clin Exp Immunol* 1976; 25:73–79.

56. Haas GG Jr, Cines DB, Schreiber AD. Immunologic infertility: identification of patients with antisperm antibody. *N Engl J Med* 1980; 303:722–727.

57. Alexander NJ, Bearwood D. An immunosorption assay for antibodies to spermatozoa: comparison with agglutination and immobilization tests. *Fertil Steril* 1984; 41:270–276.

58. Paul S, Baukloh V, Mettler L. Enzyme-linked immunosorbent assays for sperm antibody detection and antigenic analysis. *J Immunol Methods* 1983; 56:193–199.

59. Bronson RA, Cooper GW, Rosenfeld DL. Auto-immunity to spermatozoa: effects on sperm penetration of cervical mucus as reflected by post coital testing. *Fertil Steril* 1984; 41:609–614.

60. Bronson RA, Cooper GW, Rosenfeld DL. The effect of IgA1 protease on immunoglobulins bound to the sperm surface and sperm cervical mucus penetrating ability. *Fertil Steril* 1987; 47:985–991.

61. Mathur S, Williamson HO, Baker ME, et al. Sperm motility on postcoital testing correlates with male autoimmunity to sperm. *Fertil Steril* 1984; 41:81–87.

62. Jaeger S, Kremer J, Kuiken J, et al. The significance of the Fc part of antispermatozoal anti-

bodies for the shaking phenomenon in the sperm-cervical mucus contact test. *Fertil Steril* 1984; 36:792–797.

63. Schumacher GFB. Immunology of spermatozoa and cervical mucus. *Hum Reprod* 1988; 3:289–300.

64. Cohen J, Werrett DJ. Antibodies and sperm survival in the female tract of the mouse and rabbit. *J Reprod Fertil* 1975; 42:301–310.

65. Price RJ, Boettcher B. The presence of complement in human cervical mucus and its possible relevance to infertility in women with complement-dependent sperm-immobilizing antibodies. *Fertil Steril* 1979; 32:61–66.

66. Margalloth EH, Cooper GW, Taney FH, et al. Capacitated sperm cells react with different types of antisperm antibodies than fresh ejaculated sperm. *Fertil Steril* 1992; 57:393–398.

67. Bronson RA, Cooper GW, Phillips DM. Effects of anti-sperm antibodies on human sperm ultrastructure and function. *Hum Reprod* 1989; 4:653–657.

68. Bandoh R, Yamano S, Kamada M, et al. Effect of sperm-immobilizing antibodies on the acrosome reaction of human spermatozoa. *Fertil Steril* 1992; 57:387–392.

69. Benoff S, Rushbrook JI, Hurley IR, et al. Coexpression of mannose-ligand and non-nuclear progesterone receptors on motile human sperm identifies an acrosome-reaction inducible subpopulation. *Am J Reprod Immunol* 1995; 34:100–115.

70. Saragüeta P, Lanuza G, Miranda PV, et al. Immunoglobulins from human follicular fluid induce the acrosome reaction in human sperm. *Mol Reprod Dev* 1994; 39:280–288.

71. Bleil JD, Wasserman PM. Sperm-egg interactions in the mouse: sequence of events and induction of the acrosome reaction by a zona pellucida glycoprotein. *Dev Biol* 1983; 95:317–324.

72. Bronson RA, Cooper GW, Rosenfeld, DL. Sperm-specific isoantibodies and autoantibodies inhibit the binding of human sperm to the human zona pellucida. *Fertil Steril* 1982; 38:724–729.

73. Tsukui S, Noda Y, Yano J, et al. Inhibition of sperm penetration through human zona pellucida by antisperm antibodies. *Fertil Steril* 1986; 46:92–96.

74. Naz RK, Brazil C, Overstreet JW. Effects of antibodies to sperm surface fertilization antigen-1 on human sperm-zona pellucida interaction. *Fertil Steril* 1992; 57:1304–1310.

75. Zouari R, De Almeida M, Rodrigues D, et al. Localization of antibodies on spermatozoa and sperm movement characteristics are good predictors of in vitro fertilization success in case of male autoimmune infertility. *Fertil Steril* 1993; 59:606–612.

76. Shibahara H, Burkman LJ, Isojima S, et al. Effects of sperm-immobilizing antibodies on sperm-zona pellucida tight binding. *Fertil Steril* 1993; 60:533–539.

77. Dor J, Rudak E, Aitken RJ. Antisperm antibodies: their effect on the process of fertilization studies in vitro. *Fertil Steril* 1981; 35:535–541.

78. Haas GG, Sokoloski JE, Wolf DP. The interfering effect of human IgG antisperm antibodies on human sperm penetration of zona-free hamster eggs. *Am J Reprod Immunol* 1980; 1:40–43.

79. Wolf JP, De Almeida M, Ducot B, et al. High levels of sperm-associated antibodies impair human sperm-oolemma interaction after subzonal insemination. *Fertil Steril* 1995; 63:584–590.

80. Yeh W-R, Acosta AA, Seltman HJ, et al. Impact of immunoglobulin isotype and sperm surface location of antisperm antibodies on fertilization in vitro in the human. *Fertil Steril* 1995; 63:1287–1292.

81. Clarke GN, Lopata A, McBain JC, et al. Effect of sperm antibodies in males on human in vitro fertilization (IVF). *Am J Reprod Immunol Microbiol* 1985; 8:62–66.

82. Junk SM, Matson PL, Yovich JM, et al. The fertilization of human oocytes by spermatozoa from men with antispermatozoal antibodies in semen. *J In Vitro Fert Embryo Transfer* 1986; 3:350–352.

83. Mandelbaum SL, Diamond MP, DeCherney AH. Relationship of antisperm antibodies to oocyte fertilization in in vitro fertilization-embryo transfer. *Fertil Steril* 1987; 47:644–651.

84. Witkin SS, Viti D, David SS, et al. Relation between antisperm antibodies and the rate of fertilization of human oocytes in vitro. *J Assist Reprod Gen* 1992; 9:9–13.

85. Acosta AA, van der Merwe JP, Doncel G, et al. Fertilization efficiency of morphologically abnormal spermatozoa in assisted reproduction is further impaired by antisperm antibodies on the male partner's sperm. *Fertil Steril* 1994; 62:826–833.

86. Clarke GN, Lopata A, Johnston WIH. Effect of sperm antibodies in females on human in vitro fertilization. *Fertil Steril* 1986; 46:435–441.

87. Mandelbaum SL, Diamond MP, DeCherney AH. Relationship of antibodies to sperm head to etiology of infertility in patients undergoing in vitro fertilization/embryo transfer. *Am J Reprod Immunol* 1989; 19:3–5.

88. Vazquez-Levin M, Kaplan P, Guzman I, et al. The effect of female antisperm antibodies on in vitro fertilization, early embryonic development, and pregnancy outcome. *Fertil Steril* 1991; 56:84–88.

89. Pagidas K, Hemmings R, Falcone T, et al. The effect of antisperm autoantibodies in male or female partners undergoing in vitro fertilization-embryo transfer. *Fertil Steril* 1994; 62:363–369.

90. Hershlag A, Napolitano B, Cangemi C, et al. The value of routine screening of female serum for antisperm antibodies in assisted reproductive technology cycles. *Fertil Steril* 1994; 61:867–871.

91. Patrizio P, Silber SH, Ord T, et al. Relationship of epididymal sperm antibodies to their in vitro fertilization capacity in men with congenital absence of the vas deferens. *Fertil Steril* 1992; 58:1006–1010.

92. Gill TJ. Human antisperm antibodies. *Immunol Today* 1989; 10:91.

93. Batova I, Kameda K, Hasegawa A, et al. Monoclonal antibody recognizing an apparent peptide epitope of human seminal plasma glycoprotein and exhibiting sperm immobilizing activity. *J Reprod Immunol* 1990; 17:1–16.

94. Ben KL, Hamilton MS, Alexander NJ. Vasectomy-induced autoimmunity: monoclonal antibodies affect sperm function and in vitro fertilization. *J Reprod Immunol* 1988; 13:73–84.

95. Riedel HH, Wellnitz K, Lehmann-Willenbrock E. Effect of monoclonal antisperm antibodies on the penetration rates of human spermatozoa in zona pellucida-free hamster oocytes. *J Reprod Med* 1990; 35:128–132.

96. Kaplan P, Naz RK. The fertilization antigen-1 does not have proteolytic/acrosin activity, but its monoclonal antibody inhibits sperm capacitation and acrosome reaction. *Fertil Steril* 1992; 58:396–402.

97. Haas GG. Immunologic infertility. *Obstet Gynecol Clin North Am* 1987; 14:1069–1085.

98. Isojima S, Li TS, Ashitaka Y. Immunologic analysis of sperm immobilizing factor found in sera of women with unexplained infertility. *Am J Obstet Gynecol* 1969; 101:677–683.

99. Sharma KK, Barratt CLR, Pearson MJ, et al. Oral steroid therapy for subfertile males with antisperm antibodies in the semen: prediction of the responders. *Hum Reprod* 1995; 10:103–109.

100. Haas GG. Male infertility and immunity. In: Lipshultz LI, Howards SS, eds. *Infertility in the Male*. St Louis: Mosby-Year Book; 1991: 287–290.

101. De Almeida M, Feneaux D, Rigand C, et al. Steroid therapy for male infertility associated with antisperm antibodies. Results of a small randomized clinical trial. *Int J Androl* 1985; 8:111–117.

102. Haas GG Jr, Manganiello P. A double-blind, placebo-controlled study of the use of methylprednisolone in infertile men with sperm-associated immunoglobulins. *Fertil Steril* 1987; 47:295–301.

103. Hendry WF, Hughes I, Scammel G, et al. Comparison of prednisolone and placebo in subfertile men with antibodies to spermatozoa. *Lancet* 1990; 335:85–88.

104. Hendry WF. Bilateral aseptic necrosis of the femoral heads following intermittent high dose steroid therapy. *Fertil Steril* 1982; 38:120.

105. Elder KT, Wick KL, Edwards RG. Seminal plasma anti-sperm antibodies and IVF: the effect of semen sample collection into 50% serum. *Hum Reprod* 1990; 5:179–184.

106. Pattinson HA, Mortimer D, Curtis EF, et al. Treatment of sperm agglutination with proteolytic enzymes. I. Sperm motility, vitality, longevity and successful disagglutination. *Hum Reprod* 1990; 5:167–173.

107. Pattinson HA, Mortiner D, Taylor PJ. Treatment of sperm agglutination with proteolytic enzymes. II. Sperm function after enzymatic disagglutination. *Hum Reprod* 1990; 5:174–178.

108. Bronson RA, Cooper GW, Rosenfeld D. Use of freeze-thawed sonicated human sperm as an in vitro immunoabsorbent. *Am J Reprod Immunol* 1982; 2:162.

109. Kiser GC, Alexander NJ, Fuchs EF, et al. In vitro immune absorption of antisperm antibodies with immunobead-rise, immunomagnetic, and immunocolumn separation techniques. *Fertil Steril* 1987; 47:466–474.

110. Foresta C, Varotto A, Caretto A. Immunomagnetic method to select human sperm without sperm surface-found autoantibodies in male autoimmune infertility. *Arch Androl* 1990; 242:221–225.

111. Grundy CE, Robinson J, Grodon AG, et al. Selection of an antibody-free population of

spermatozoa from semen samples of men suffering from immunological infertility. *Hum Reprod* 1991; 6:593–596.

112. Gould JE, Brazil CK, Overstreet JW. Sperm-immunobead binding decreases with in-vitro incubation. *Fertil Steril* 1994; 62:167–171.

113. Gould JE, Ordorica RC. Removal of sperm surface antibodies using immunobeads. Abstract presented at the American Fertility Society 48th Annual Meeting, New Orleans, November 4, 1992.

114. Margalloth EJ, Sauter E, Bronson RA, et al. Intrauterine insemination as treatment for antisperm antibodies in the female. *Fertil Steril* 1988; 50:441–446.

115. Check JH, Bollendorf A. Effect of antisperm antibodies on postcoital results and effect of intrauterine insemination of pregnancy outcome. *Arch Androl* 1992; 28:25–31.

116. Francavilla F, Romano R, Santucci R, et al. Failure of intrauterine insemination in male immunological infertility in cases in which all spermatozoa are antibody-coated. *Fertil Steril* 1992; 58:587–592.

117. Goldberg JM, Haering PL, Friedman CI, et al. Antisperm antibodies in women undergoing intrauterine insemination. *Am J Obstet Gynecol* 1990; 163:65–68.

118. Janssen HJG, Bastiaans BA, Goverde HJM, et al. Antisperm antibodies and in vitro fertilization. *J Assist Reprod Gen* 1992; 9:345–349.

119. Läteenmäki A. In-vitro fertilization in the presence of antisperm antibodies detected by the mixed antiglobulin reaction (MAR) and the tray agglutination test (TAT). *Hum Reprod* 1993; 8:84–88.

120. Daitoh T, Kamada M, Yamano S, et al. High implantation rate and consequently high pregnancy rate by in vitro fertilization-embryo transfer in infertile women with antisperm antibody. *Fertil Steril* 95; 63:87–91.

121. Nagy ZP, Verheyen G, Liu J, et al. Results of 55 intracytoplasmic sperm injection cycles in the treatment of male-immunological infertility. *Hum Reprod* 1995; 10:1775–1780.

# 9
# Genetics for the Clinician

Robert D. Oates

Male reproductive medicine and surgery have seen notable advances in the past several years. We now possess a greater understanding of the basic processes that underlie development of the ductal system and the external genitalia. We are beginning to solve the mystery of spermatogenesis and its regulation. We are even starting to comprehend the enormous complexity of the human spermatozoan. However, our most magnificent achievements have involved strategies to compensate for inherent deficiencies in the system, such as anatomical/structural disease that prevents natural conception or inadequate spermatogenesis that essentially precludes paternity through intercourse alone. Intracytoplasmic sperm injection can overcome almost all potential male factors, even allowing for the use of sperm retrieved from the testicular tissue of a man with such a low level of spermatogenesis that fully formed sperm cannot be isolated from the ejaculate but can only be found after an exhaustive search of the testicular parenchyma. However, with these types of therapies, both the physician and the couple need to completely understand the genetic basis of the disorder being treated. Without this knowledge, genetic disease may be propagated unwittingly.

## Basic Human Genetic Concepts

The normal human cell contains a diploid complement of 46 chromosomes—22 pairs of autosomes and 1 pair of sex chromosomes. The long and short arms of a chromosome are designated q and p, respectively. In the male, the sex chromosomes consist of a Y and an X, and in the female two Xs are present. A male karyotype is abbreviated 46,XY and that of a female 46,XX. During spermatogenesis, not only is a motile cell formed that can deliver its genetic package to the oocyte, but the diploid state is reduced to a haploid one containing only one half the original number of chromosomes and either the X or the Y. When syngamy occurs, the diploid state is reconstituted from the combination of the haploid sperm and the haploid oocyte. The sex of the embryo depends on whether the fertilizing sperm carries an X or a Y.

## Embryonic Reproductive Development

The testicle develops from the primitive, bipotential gonad during weeks 5 to 7 of gestation.[1] A gene on Yp named SRY is known to be one of the most important genes in the testis determination cascade.[2] If present and functionally normal, and if all of the downstream genes are also adequate, the gonad is directed to become a testis. SRY is located adjacent to the "pseudoautosomal boundary" within Yp and is the "testis determining factor" (TDF).[3] The product of SRY binds DNA and probably regulates transcription of an autosomal or X-linked gene. In some cases, but not all, of pure gonadal dysgenesis, SRY has been found to be defective.[4] This implies that other genes are required for proper testicular differentiation.[5] Arn et al[6] have mapped a sex-reversal locus (SRVX) to Xp2l.2-p22.11. Cases of gonadal dysgenesis are also found in association with Wilms' tumor, aniridia, genitourinary abnormalities, and mental retardation (WAGR) syndrome (vide infra), and campomelic dwarfism, implicating participating autosomal loci.[7,8] Ogata and Matsuo[9] hypothesize that SRY acts via suppression of SRVX, which in turn represses the function of an autosomal testis-determining gene. If SRY is normal and able to inhibit SRVX, repression of the autosomal locus is prevented, and active differentiation of the primitive gonad into a testis takes place.

In both internal and external genital development, there may be a role for the Wilms' tumor 1 (WT 1) gene, as patients with the WAGR complex are born with aniridia, genitourinary malformations (cryptorchidism and hypospadias), and various levels of cognitive disability, and develop Wilms' tumor early in life.[8] The chromosomal locus underlying this syndrome is located at 11p13. The aniridia gene (AN 2) lies in close molecular proximity to WT 1, and in cases involving a deletional defect AN 2 is simply lost along with WT 1, thereby explaining the association of aniridia with Wilms' tumor (1:100 patients). There may be sequences within exon 1 of WT 1 that are prone to deletion.[10] Clarkson et al[11] have shown that WT 1 is expressed in embryonic renal and gonadal tissues, fortifying the hypothesis of van Heyningen et al[8] that WT 1 may also play a role in genital development. An aberration in WT 1 may be found in cases where reproductive anomalies exist in association with either Wilms' tumor or early-onset nephropathy but is unlikely to be present if the genital abnormalities are solitary clinical findings.[11] WT 1 may be a transcription repressor and has 10 exons. Denys-Drash syndrome presents in the newborn period with ambiguous genitalia, but Wilms' tumor and renal failure due to mesangial sclerosis evolve clinically in childhood.[12] Denys-Drash syndrome is also due to mutations in WT 1.[13] In this syndrome, the gonads are typically dysgenic or an admixture of testicular and ovarian tissue.

Gonadal development itself is not testosterone dependent. During week 8 of gestation, Leydig cells located between the evolving sex cords/seminiferous tubules begin to secrete testosterone. Proper morphogenesis of each mesonephric duct is critically dependent on ipsilateral testicular testosterone production. However, the precursors of the external genitalia require the conversion of circulating testosterone into intracellular dihydrotestosterone by the enzyme 5α-reductase. Both testosterone and dihydrotestosterone have their action mediated by the androgen receptor that transports either hormone to the nucleus and helps regulate transcription of androgen responsive genes. Syndromes affecting the elaboration of testosterone, its conversion into dihydrotestosterone, or the action of either hormone result in a spectrum of internal ductal and external genital virilization deficiency. As a default mode, if no active virilization of the external genitalia occurs, these genitalia will develop along female lines.

Antimüllerian hormone (AMH) (müllerian inhibiting factor or substance [MIF, MIS]) is secreted by the Sertoli cell of the developing gonad. Its role is to actively cause regression of the paramesonephric (müllerian) duct—the precursor of the uterus, fallopian tubes, and upper vagina. In the normal circumstance, AMH will prevent any of these structures from developing while the adjacent mesonephric duct, under the influence of testosterone, differentiates into the male internal genitalia.

The AMH gene has been localized to 19p13.3 and contains 5 exons.[14,15] Exonic mutations have been detected in patients with the persistent müllerian duct syndrome (vide infra). AMH is a l40-kd glycoprotein and a member of the transforming growth factor-β (TGF-β) family. Its expression may be regulated negatively by androgen, as AMH secretion ceases at puberty, but Leydig cell testosterone production increases.[16] AMH is posttranslationally processed, and it appears that carboxy terminus dimers are the biologically active moieties. AMH also plays a role in limiting embryonic Leydig cell proliferation as well as being in-

changes. Hypothalamic anatomy and function are severely abnormal with resultant complete lack of GnRH secretion. The pituitary (intrinsically normal) is, therefore, not stimulated to elaborate either FSH or LH. The testes do not produce testosterone and pubertal virilization is absent. Spermatogenesis is not initiated and the size of the testes remains small. Kallmann's is one of the forms of primary hypogonadotropic hypogonadism. Prader-Willi syndrome (PWS) also has hypogonadotropic hypogonadism as one of its principal features, along with obesity, infantile hypotonia, cognitive disability, and cryptorchidism. PWS is caused by a microdeletion or mutation in paternal 15q11q13 or maternal uniparental disomy for chromosome 15 in which both chromosomes are inherited from the mother.[56]

Kallmann's occurs in 1:10,000 to 1:60,000 births. Inheritance is mostly X-linked, but other patterns have been documented.[57] The genetic pathophysiology that underlies the X-linked form of Kallmann's has been defined. The gene itself, known as Kalig-1 (Kallmann's syndrome interval gene 1) maps to Xp22.3.[57] The product of Kalig-1 is a neural cell adhesion molecule that assists in the directional growth and spatial orientation of the axons that will eventually help form the GnRH secreting portion of the hypothalamus.[58] Deletions have been found in Kalig-1 and point mutations will most likely be discovered soon.[57] Associated features of Kallmann's include other midline defects, such as anosmia and cleft palate. Distant anomalies also occur, including cryptorchidism, micropenis, deafness, craniofacial asymmetry, spastic paraplegia, and renal defects.[59] Virilization can be induced with human chorionic gonadotropin (hCG) (initiates testosterone production by the Leydig cells) or by parenteral administration of testosterone. Spermatogenesis requires both intratesticular testosterone secretion and Sertoli cell stimulation by circulating FSH. FSH may be given exogenously in the form of injection. Finally, to accomplish both purposes, pulsatile replacement GnRH may be used to activate pituitary secretion of endogenous FSH and LH.

# Bioinactive FSH, LH, and Their Receptors

As do all hormones, LH and FSH have specific receptors that help mediate their eventual effect. All must be functionally sound for that effect to be optimal. FSH and LH are heterodimers, composed of a common α subunit and a unique β subunit. The α subunit has been localized to chromosome 6. The LH β gene has been mapped to 19q13.2, and the FSH β gene resides at 11pter-p11.2.[60,61] The FSH β gene lies in close proximity to WT 1 (vide supra).[62] The LH receptor gene has been assigned to 2p21.[63] Biologically inactive LH may present as a phenotype reflective of inefficient virilization ranging from ambiguous genitalia to only infertility.[64,65] The serum LH value (an immunoreactive measurement) should be elevated while the value for testosterone is markedly reduced due to deficient stimulation of the Leydig cells.

Isolated FSH deficiency is mentioned as one of the rare causes of spermatogenic failure. FSH cannot be detected in serum while LH levels are normal. Certainly this could result from a specific lack of pituitary FSH secretion but more likely reflects a defect in the FSH molecule itself, perhaps due to a mutation in the FSH β gene. Matthews et al[66] described a female with a truncated FSH β subunit transcript due to homozygosity for a frame shift deletion in exon 3, and the resultant FSH was functionally inadequate. Conclusions from these data include the possibility that men who are azoospermic or severely oligospermic may have high levels of immunoreactive, biologically inactive LH or FSH and replacement therapy may be warranted. As the β-subunit genes become refined and assays for them routine, perhaps this will be found true in a certain percentage of men with azoospermia.

LH receptor gene mutations have been detected in two siblings with the condition of Leydig cell agenesis.[67] LH receptor inadequacy has also been found in males with pseudohermaphroditism.[68] FSH receptor anomalies may soon be discovered as well.

## Errors in Androgen Biosynthesis

The pathway that leads from cholesterol to testosterone is a long and complex one, requiring five separate enzymes.[43] Any enzymatic defect will lead not only to failure of testosterone synthesis but also to formation of all postenzymatic products. Figure 9.3 outlines this cascade and the syndromes associated with deficiency of that particular enzyme. Adrenal steroidogenesis is also impaired when one of the first three steps in the process is imperfect, eventuating in one of the congenital adrenal hyperplasia syndromes. Affected genetic and gonadal males may present with incomplete masculinization. Most inheritance patterns are either autosomal recessive or X-linked.

## Androgen Insensitivity Syndrome

If androgen production is normal but tissue response is not, syndromes reflecting deficient androgen action will result.[69,70] Collectively, these are known as androgen insensitivity syndromes (AIS) and comprise a spectrum of conditions from complete lack of androgen effect

(CAIS) to partial androgen effect (PAIS).[71,72] All are manifestations of abnormalities (point mutations, deletions, etc.) in the androgen receptor (AR) gene that lead to qualitative or quantitative defects or both in the AR protein itself.

The AR gene has eight distinct exons and intervening introns, and it measures 90 kb in length[73] (Fig. 9.4). The AR gene maps to Xq 11-12. The AR protein has three regions, each with a different, although interrelated, function. The entire protein consists of roughly 910 amino acids (the AR gene exons totaling 2730 base pairs).[74] Exon 1 ($\approx$ 1586 bp) codes entirely for the AR's N-terminal transactivation domain, which is responsible for the regulation of transcription of the targeted, hormonally responsive nuclear gene with both activating and repressing functions.[71] It also assists in gene recognition. Within exon 1 lies an expandable (CAG)n trinucleotide repeat, which, when abnormally large, may result in the AR dysfunction that underlies Kennedy's disease (vide infra). Exons 2 (152 bp) and 3 (117 bp) encode for the DNA-binding domain of the AR, which is critical in the recognition of and binding to

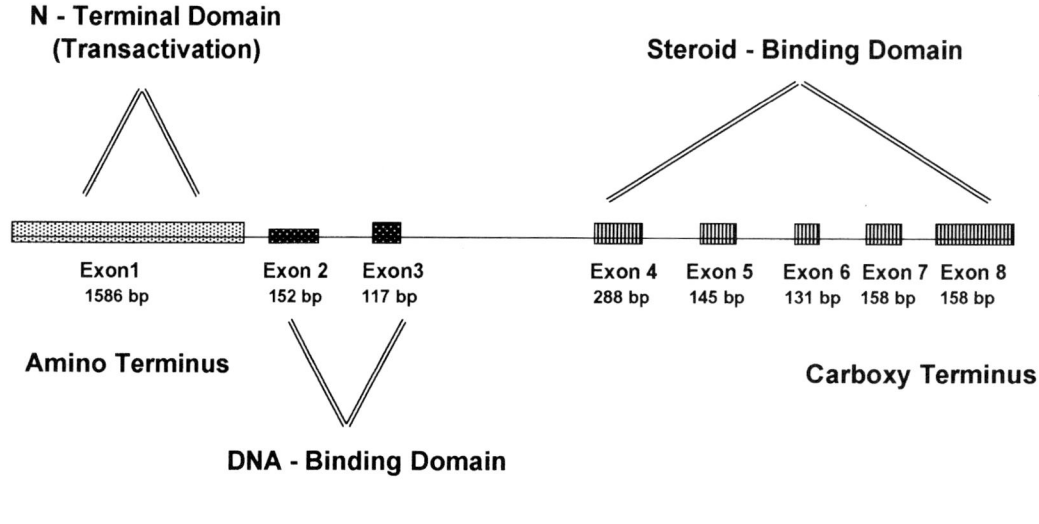

FIGURE 9.3. The androgen receptor gene with its eight exons and the three protein domains that they code for.

specific hormonally responsive nuclear DNA sequences termed androgen response elements (AREs). This domain has an N-terminal zinc finger (a single zinc atom bound to four cysteine residues) important for DNA recognition and a C-terminal zinc finger that assists in AR dimerization. The third AR domain is responsible for coupling the AR to androgen, which, once accomplished, induces a conformational change in the AR/androgen complex that results in disassociation of the AR from several bound proteins, allowing for migration of the new complex across the nuclear membrane. A portion of exon 4 is also required for nuclear translocation.[75] This steroid-binding domain is encoded for by exon 4 (288 bp), exon 5 (145 bp), exon 6 (131 bp), exon 7 (158 bp), and exon 8 (153 bp). AIS may be the phenotypic or clinical result or both of a defect in any one of the three AR domains.[74]

The severity of the phenotypic aberration depends on how a mutation affects AR action—the more profound the quantitative or qualitative resultant AR deficiency, the more abnormal the consequent anatomical aberrations are. CAIS is commonly known as "testicular feminization." Under the influence of SRY, the primitive gonads differentiate into testes, the Leydig cells secrete testosterone, and the Sertoli cells produce müllerian-inhibiting factor (MIF). Due to a total paucity of androgen effect, male internal ductal development is absent and the external genitalia develop along female lines. The paramesonephric duct degenerates under the influence of MIF so that both fallopian tubes, the uterus, and the upper one third of the vagina are also missing. Patients typically present at puberty for the evaluation of primary amenorrhea. Breast development, which is unopposed by androgen, occurs in response to the estrogen secreted by the Leydig cells. After the full development of female secondary sex characteristics, the gonads should be removed, for fear of subsequent malignant tumor development. In PAIS, internal and external virilization may be less than normal, ranging from completely ambiguous genitalia to hypospadias alone. The most subtle form of impaired androgen action may be inefficient spermatogenesis or undervirilization. It is unclear what percentage of men who are azoospermic/severely oligospermic have AR abnormalities.[76–78]

Many gene aberrations have been detected in patients with CAIS and PAIS. Exonic deletions are rare, but point mutations causing a change in the ultimate amino acid sequence are most common.[73,79–87] An exon 6 base pair mutation was detected in a patient who only presented with a mild degree of undervirilization.[88] Exons 5 and 7 seem to contain a high proportion of the total number of identified base pair alterations.[74] Intronic anomalies leading to messenger RNA (mRNA) splicing inefficiency have been noted as well.[89] As McPhaul et al[90] have shown, the same mutation may present in one individual as PAIS and in another as CAIS, indicating that there is no strict genotype/phenotype relationship. Infants with a CAIS or PAIS phenotype should be evaluated for mutations in the Wilms' tumor gene that predisposes to Wilms' tumor or renal failure (Denys-Drash syndrome) (vide supra).[11] Because the AR gene is located on the X chromosome, no direct transmission of the trait for PAIS, CAIS, or Kennedy's disease will occur if biological paternity is realized either through natural intercourse or the use of ejaculated or testicular sperm in conjunction with the advanced reproductive technologies.[91] However, a daughter of the affected individual may pass the inherited abnormal AR gene on to a son (the grandson of the original affected individual). This male may express either PAIS or CAIS. Therefore, patients with recognized AR defects must be counseled that it may not be that they will pass on only their infertility or a minor genital anomaly to a grandson but potentially they may pass on a more severe phenotypic manifestation.

## Spinal and Bulbar Muscular Atrophy (Kennedy's Disease)

Kennedy's disease or X-linked spinal and bulbar muscular atrophy (SBMA) is an adult-onset α motor neuron disease characterized by progressive bulbar and spinal muscle weakness. The sensory nervous system, the pyramidal tracts, and the cerebellum remain unaffected. Symptoms first appear in the fourth or fifth decade but may arrive as early as the teen years or as late as the sixth decade. A majority of males with SBMA have significantly reduced spermatogenesis but normal male internal and external genital differentiation.[92]

The molecular basis of SBMA is dysfunctional androgen receptor due to $(CAG)_n$ trinucleotide expansion within the transcriptional domain (exon 1) of the AR gene.[93-95] These CAG repeats code for multiple glutamine residues in the amino terminal portion of the mature AR protein. Patients with SBMA typically have 40 to 55 more repeat sequences than normal controls, potentially affecting transactivation function.[96-99] The affected AR also demonstrates decreased high affinity binding, implying that an altered amino terminal domain may functionally affect the action of the ligand binding domain.[94,98,99] MacLean et al[94] showed a correlation between binding affinity and the degree of testicular atrophy. However, they found no correlation between repeat size and severity of neurologic/muscular symptoms. Therefore, these authors hypothesize that there may be two independent effects of CAG expansion of the AR. The first would be an androgen-dependent effect leading to progressive testicular atrophy and gynecomastia. The second would be an androgen-independent effect in which the expanded AR negatively interacts with other cellular components, impairing or inhibiting them in some nonspecific way, most of this indirect effect manifested in spinal and bulbar neurons. However, the mechanism underlying neuronal degeneration is speculative at this time.

## 5α-Reductase Deficiency

Testosterone is converted intracellularly to dihydrotestosterone (DHT) by a 3-oxo-5α-steroid:Δ4-oxidoreductase termed 5α-reductase. DHT is required for proper external genital differentiation from bipotential precursors. If 5α-reductase is unable to perform this conversion adequately, masculinization of the external genitalia is not complete. Because internal ductal morphogenesis is only dependent on testosterone, the epididymis, vas deferens, seminal vesicles, and ejaculatory ducts are fully formed. There are two 5α-reductase isoenzyme genes known as SRD5A1 and SRD5A2. The active form is SRD5A2 and has 5 exons and 4 introns, and it maps to 2p23.[100] This gene codes for the 254 amino acid reductase enzyme. A variety of mutations in SRD5A2 have been detected in patients with the 5α-reductase deficiency syndrome.[101] The syndrome has an autosomal recessive pattern of inheritance. The external genitalia are incompletely masculinized, with varying degrees of hypospadias.[102] DHT levels are markedly depressed. Spermatogenesis may still be adequate, but the ejaculatory dysfunction created by the anatomical abnormalities is most responsible for the reduction in fertility these patients experience. Patients raised as females often change their gender role at puberty secondary to the increased levels of effective testosterone.

# Syndromes That Affect the Morphogenesis of the Internal Ductal System

The internal male reproductive ductal system comprises the seminiferous tubules, rete testis, efferent ductules, epididymal tubule proper, the vas deferens, the seminal vesicle, and the ejaculatory duct. Three separate embryologic precursors must not only form normally but also must join and establish patency so that the flow of sperm is uninterrupted from the testis to the prostatic urethra. Syndromes that affect ductal development may have a genetic basis and often result in azoospermia. With treatment options, such as direct microsurgical sperm aspiration in conjunction with intracytoplasmic sperm injection, it is important to understand the genetic bases for these various conditions prior to proceeding with therapy in order that the afflicted couple can be educated about the chances of transmission. Vasal aplasia is found in three clinical disorders: cystic fibrosis (CF), congenital bilateral absence of the vas deferens (CBAVD), and congenital unilateral absence of the vas deferens (CUAVD). CBAVD and CF both present with bilateral absence of the vasa deferentia, although there is some overlap with unilateral absence.

## Congenital Bilateral Absence of the Vas Deferens

Clinical CF is the most common lethal disease with autosomal recessive inheritance present in Caucasians of Northern European descent with an incidence approaching 1 in 2500 along with a carrier frequency of 1 in 25.[103] Obstructive debilitating pulmonary disease and exocrine pancreatic dysfunction are the two most prominent features of CF and are not present in patients with CBAVD. As Anguiano et al[104] initially pointed out, CF and most cases of CBAVD are two ends of a genotypic/phenotypic spectrum resulting from mutations in the CFTR gene.

The CF gene encodes for a protein known as the CF transmembrane conductance regulator (CFTR). It is located at 7q3l, is 250 kb in length, and comprises 27 exons, intervening introns, and various other regulatory elements.[105] Greater than 500 CF gene mutations have been identified (CF Genetic Analysis Consortium). ΔF508 is a three-base pair deletion in exon 10, which accounts for approximately 70% of CFTR mutations worldwide[106,107] and is categorized as a "severe" mutation. Patients homozygous for ΔF508 have serious respiratory and gastrointestinal dysfunction. If a "mild" mutation occurs in conjunction with a "severe" mutation in the opposite CF gene (compound heterozygote), the "mild" mutation is dominant in determining phenotypic expression. By implication, if a patient has CF diagnosed due to either pulmonary or pancreatic disease, the combination of mutations must be relatively "severe" in terms of overall CFTR dysfunction. Nearly all males with CF lack vasa bilaterally.[108] CFTR is responsible for the regulation of chloride ion efflux/influx across epithelial cell membranes. When CFTR is dysfunctional, thick and viscous luminal fluids occlude the respiratory and pancreatic ductal systems. Hypothetically, a proper electrolyte and fluid milieu, as occurs when a certain critical threshold of normal CFTR quantity is superseded, must be present for vasal morphogenesis to be optimal; otherwise, vasal agenesis may result.[109]

CBAVD occurs in 1.4% of males with azoospermia. The seminal vesicles (also derivatives of the mesonephric ducts) are atrophic, absent, or hypoplastic and nonfunctional. The caput epididymis, however, is uniformly present, as it derives from a different embryologic precursor than the remainder of the epididymis. The diagnosis of CBAVD is secure when the semen volume is low, the pH is acidic, the vasa are nonpalpable on physical examination, and the epididymal remnants are firm and obstructed. In those patients with detectable CF mutations (vide infra), no renal anomalies are usually discovered, although up to 40% of patients with no CF mutations upon analysis will demonstrate unilateral renal agenesis. Scrotal exploration is not required to diagnose CBAVD. If CFTR function is compromised to a lesser degree than that seen in patients with CF, CBAVD may be the only manifestation of that dysfunction as approximately 60% to 80% of patients with CBAVD will have at least one CF mutation identified (15% compound heterozygotes, 65% simple heterozygotes, and 20% with no detectable mutation).[110] In patients in whom only one mutation has been identified, the opposite gene may possess a cryptic exonic mutation or a mutation/polymorphism in a "regulatory" region, such as a promoter or one of the many introns leading to quantitatively reduced amounts of potentially normal CFTR protein. Chillon et al[111] have shown that the most common genotype present in their CBAVD population was a combination of a recognized mutation in one CF copy, and the other copy possessed the 5T allele variant in intron 8 that quantitatively reduces the amount of normal CFTR ultimately derived from that particular gene. These data dramatically increase the percentage of CBAVD patients that are found to have "abnormalities" in both CF genes and strengthen the argument that CFTR dysfunction is implicated in a high proportion of CBAVD cases. If the level of properly functioning CFTR drops below 10%, phenotypic signs begin to occur. It appears that vasal maldevelopment may be the most sensitive expression of CFTR dysfunction. Therefore, a great percentage of patients with CBAVD will have an autosomal recessive pattern of inheritance.

Of the 20% or so of CBAVD patients with no presently detectable alterations in the CF gene, there are two potential explanations. Some patients may harbor two undefined CF gene alterations, but others may possess another etiology altogether for their vasal aplasia that is unrelated to CF gene status, as suggested by Augarten et al[112] as well as by Mulhall and Oates,[113] and may be related to improper morphogenesis of the early mesonephric duct. If the mesonephric duct is developmentally affected prior to week 7 of gestation, both ureteral and reproductive ductal derivatives may be deficient and lead to vasal and renal agenesis. Because so few patients with CBAVD with CF mutations have renal anomalies of position or of number, it is likely that CFTR abnormalities do not compromise the morphogenesis of the mesonephric duct proper prior to the critical time of separation of the two portions. Therefore, CBAVD may have two distinct etiologies, distinguishable both genetically (the presence or absence of CFTR gene aberrations) and phenotypically (the presence or absence of renal agenesis or ectopy). If improper mesonephric ductal morphogenesis is genetically determined, transmission may be possible in either an autosomal recessive or dominant mode.

If a second genetic mechanism does exist that affects the development of the mesonephric ducts prior to week 7 of gestation, the most severe manifestation comparable with life would be bilateral vasal aplasia and unilateral renal agenesis. Any patient with this anatomical combination and no CFTR mutations detectable should have counseling prior to attempts at conception and have prenatal ultrasonography to detect renal anomalies in the offspring, including the potential for bilateral renal agenesis.

## Congenital Unilateral Absence of the Vas Deferens

CUAVD is defined when only one scrotal vas deferens is palpable. If the palpable vas deferens is patent from its origin to its termination at the confluence with the duct of the seminal vesicle to form the ejaculatory duct, it is unlikely that a CF mutation will be detected. However, if the palpable vas abruptly terminates in either the inguinal or pelvic region, CF mutation analysis will reveal a mutation in over 90% of patients. Therefore, if the anatomical patency of the vasa is disrupted bilaterally (CF, CBAVD, CUAVD with pelvic or inguinal occlusion of the existant vas, or both), most patients will harbor mutations in their CF genes.[114]

For patients with CF, CBAVD, or CUAVD, prior to microsurgical sperm aspiration to retrieve sperm for intracytoplasmic sperm injection each patient and his partner should have CF mutation analysis to define and provide an estimate of their risks of transmitting CF/CBAVD to any offspring.[115] If both are positive for mutations, then amniocentesis or chorionic villous sampling are options to elucidate the genetic status of the fetus. Preimplantation genetic diagnosis of each embryo has been reported with uterine transfer of only those embryos that are not at risk for CF or CBAVD.[116]

## Young's Syndrome

Young's syndrome is often confused with either immotile cilia syndrome or cystic fibrosis. It is a condition that combines bronchiectasis and sinusitis with obstructive azoospermia secondary to inspissated epididymal secretions. Most commonly, this occlusion occurs at the junction of the corpus and caput. The obstructive process may not become clinically manifest until after pregnancy has been achieved, distinct from CBAVD in which the anatomical defect is present at birth.[117] Spermatozoa are motile and capable of fertilization and the vasa are anatomically and structurally normal, distinguishing Young's from immotile cilia syndrome and CF, respectively.[118] Wilton et al,[119] however, debate this point and claim that axonemal substructure may show subtle defects. Therefore, whether Young's is caused by a primary ciliary or by mucus abnormality is still unclear. No specific pattern of inheritance has been defined. Two conflicting reports exist as to whether Young's is actually a mild form of CF. Hirsch et al[120] found ΔF508 in 2/7 patients with Young's syndrome, but Le Lannou et al,[121] in a more extensive study, did not find any CF mutations upon analysis of 12 Young's syndrome patients.

Hendry et al[122] have proposed a completely different potential etiology related to childhood mercury exposure. Treatment options include vasoepididymostomy or microsurgical epididymal sperm aspiration or both.

## Persistent Müllerian Duct Syndrome

Persistent müllerian duct syndrome (PMDS) is a rare condition in which müllerian duct–derived structures remain in an otherwise phenotypically normal male. External genital and internal ductal development occur along male lines so that testes, epididymides, vasa deferential, seminal vesicles, prostate, scrotum, and penis are all present. However, the testicles are often cryptorchid, tethered by a uterus and fallopian tubes that are mature derivatives of the embryonic müllerian (paramesonephric) ducts. The condition is first detected when these anomalous structures are discovered at the time of hernia repair or orchidopexy or both.[123] Transverse testicular ectopia, in which both testes reside in the same hemiscrotum, may occasionally occur.[124–126] Surgery is aimed at bringing the testes into the scrotum, but the müllerian duct remnants need not be detached from the vasa, as this may compromise vasal integrity or vasal blood supply.[126] Spermatogenesis is usually normal so that iatrogenic vasal injury may preclude natural conception.

Patients with PMDS have a normal 46,XY chromosomal constitution. PMDS is the phenotypic consequence of abnormalities in AMH, the AMH receptor, or the timing of AMH release during gonadal and reproductive ductal morphogenesis.[127] Mutations in the AMH gene have been detected in patients with PMDS.[128-131] Transmission of PMDS is thought to be autosomal dominant with sex-limited expression, but the exact genetic pattern may depend on the molecular etiology (AMH or AMH receptor defect).

## Syndromes That Negatively Affect Sperm Function

Spermatozoa must do many things properly to be considered functionally competent. Motility must be directional and sufficiently rapid. Penetration of the outer investments of the oocyte must occur. Deposition of the nucleus and centrosome into the egg cytoplasm is required for proper early embryo development. Any defect in the structural components or the intrinsic biochemical actions of the sperm may result in failure of any or all of these sequential steps. Considered below are disorders of motility that severely limit biologic paternity in the man so affected.

## Syndromes of Primary Ciliary Dyskinesia

The primary ciliary dyskinesias (PCD) (also known as the immotile cilia syndromes) are a diverse group of clinical syndromes resulting from abnormalities in the axoneme (motor apparatus) of ciliated cells. PCD occurs in approximately 1:16,000 live births.[132] Kartagener's syndrome is a specific PCD characterized by chronic sinusitis, bronchiectasis, situs inversus, and immotile spermatozoa. Secondary to the consequent respiratory pathology, PCD is typically diagnosed in childhood but may be first considered in the young adult.[133] Any organ with active, beating cilia or a framework supported by a nonfunctional axonemal substructure may be affected, including the fallopian tube (result: reduced fertility), middle ear (result: deafness; vide infra), cerebral ventricle, retina (result: retinitis pigmentosa), and spermatozoa (result: immotile sperm).[134] Ineffective or absent sperm motility results in male factor infertility, although the sperm counts are normal and the viability is adequate. Morphology may be quite bizarre if the axonemal substructure is unstable or missing altogether. The sperm nucleus is unaffected and intracytoplasmic injection of sperm may be the most appropriate treatment option. Subzonal sperm insemination has been shown to result in embryo development, but no pregnancy.[135]

Inheritance of the PCD syndromes is predominantly autosomal recessive, although a case illustrating autosomal dominant or X-linked transmission has been described.[136] Because there are at least 200 to 300 separate proteins required for proper assembly and function of the sperm tail, defects in axonemal ultrastructure are potentially numerous. The sperm tail is divided into three portions.[137] The middle piece originates from the neck or connecting piece and terminates in the annulus. The axoneme (vide infra) is surrounded by nine distinct outer dense fibers (ODF), each of which is intimately related to one of the outer doublet microtubule pairs. Surrounding the ODFs is a circumferential band of helically oriented mitochondria. The principal piece continues on from the annulus, and the mitochondria are replaced by a fibrous sheath that now encloses the ODFs and the axoneme. The fibrous sheath consists of two longitudinal bands that run the length of the principal piece and are supported by bridging ribs. These columns replace ODFs 3 and 8. The fibrous sheath is thought to allow movement only in the plane perpendicular to its longitudinal axis. The sperm tail terminates in the end piece. The axoneme is the adenosine triphosphate (ATP)-driven motor of the sperm cell. Its structure is highly conserved across vertebrate and invertebrate species. Nine outer doublet pairs encircle two central single tubules. Each doublet pair consists of an A tubule and a B tubule.[138] The A tubule is made up of 13 protofilaments that themselves are formed from alternating α and β tubulin subunits. The β tubule has 10 or 11 protofilaments and rides on the back of the A tubule. Inner and outer dynein arms extend out from the A tubule, reaching for the posterior aspect of the B tubule of the next doublet pair. Dynein is actually a group of proteins that, in aggregate, possess adenosine triphosphatase (ATPase) activity and provide the energy for microtubule sliding that is the mechanism of movement generation. In *Chlamydomonas*, each dynein arm has at least 10 subunits with none being common to both arms.[139] The outer arm consists of three heavy chains, two intermediate chains, and several light ones.[139] The inner arm is also complex and probably most responsible for movement, especially the beat frequency.[140] As Kamiya[139] points out, different dynein heavy chains possess "different properties as mechanicochemical transducers." Radial spokes also originate from the base of the A tubule to make connection with the inner central twin tubules.[141] They consist of a head and a stalk, which contain, in total, several protein

species. Nexin also links the A and B tubules in a direct fashion.

Described aberrations of the axoneme in men with PCD include absence of the inner or outer dynein arms or both, structural defects of the outer doublet, disarrangement or absence of the radial spokes, and missing central tubules.[134] Short or stump tail syndrome may be a manifestation of a severe axonemal defect, either in directed growth or in stability. Polycystic kidney disease has been noted in a patient with immotile cilia syndrome.[142] No specific mutations in the human have as yet been recognized to account for cases of PCD or morphologic tail abnormalities. Narayan et al[136] found no gross abnormalities of chromosomes 12, 14, or X chromosome in a PCD patient and her affected male child by cytogenetic and fluorescent in situ hybridigation (FISH) analysis. Autosomes 12 and 14 are syntenic with mouse chromosomes 6 and 12, on which mutations have been found that result in a PCD phenotype. Kaplan et al[143] believe that there may exist a gene at 14q32 that is required for normal ciliary function. Phillips et al[144] describe a case that appears to show defective somatic cilia (absence of the dynein arms) but normal spermatozoal axonemes, perhaps due to differential gene expression in the different organ systems. During early development, ciliated cells help direct the orientation of asymmetric structures, such as the heart and abdominal organs. The normal ciliary beat causes the embryo to twist in a right helical fashion, shifting the heart to the left side. If this ciliary action is deficient, chance alone determines left-right orientation.[145]

Retinitis pigmentosa (RP) is a genetically and phenotypically heterogeneous disease characterized by progressive loss of night and peripheral field vision. Autosomal dominant, autosomal recessive, and X-linked forms have been described.[146] The autosomal dominant form may be caused by mutations in any one of seven different genes. X-linked RP has had at least two responsible loci identified. Many forms of autosomal dominant RP are associated with defects in rhodopsin and peripherin/ RDS;[147] at least one form of X-linked disease may be associated with defects in axonemal substructure,[148] and males with RP3 have been described having immotile cilia.[149] Usher's syndrome (US) is an autosomal recessive disorder characterized by hearing loss and RP as well as by vestibular dysfunction; it is a subtype of RP and has multiple subforms.

US accounts for 3% to 6% of deaf children and is present in 4.4/100,000 people in the United States. Three broad subdivisions of US exist.[150] Type 1 (USH1) is the most severe, with congenital deafness, early onset RP, and vestibular dysfunction. Three subsets are distinguished genetically with linkage to USH1A—14q32;[151] USH1B—11q13.5;[152] USH1C—11p15.1.[153] Type 2 (USH2) is milder in its severity, with moderate deafness and a late onset of RP. USH2A maps to 1q41[154] but the approximate gene locus of USH2B is undetermined. Type 3 (USH3) has progressive hearing loss, pubertal onset of RP, and vestibular hypoactivity, and maps to 3q2lq25.[155]

It is known that auditory, vestibular, and photoreceptor cells develop from ciliated precursors.[156] Mature photoreceptor and vestibular cells contain nonmotile ciliary structures but spermatozoa contain functionally motile axonemes. Therefore, it would not be unusual if a global ciliary abnormality would be found to underlie the defect responsible for the diverse system pathogenesis found in Usher's syndrome. Because the axoneme comprises over 200 different proteins, there are numerous possible genetic aberrations that could lead to phenotypic axonemal/ciliary dysfunction and consequent disease in any or all of these systems. Hunter et al[157] studied the sperm tail axoneme in 10 patients with USH2 (nine men) and USH1 (one man) and concluded that the sperm motility and velocity were decreased in the patient group as compared with the control group; light microscopic morphologic sperm tail abnormalities were seen in increased numbers versus controls; transmission electron microscopy imaged an increase in defective tail axonemes in the sperm of their study population as well as in the photoreceptor cilia of a patient with US. Their study suggests that the recognized pathology arises from an inherently unstable axoneme that eventually collapses upon itself. Hunter et al[148] also found a similar sperm and photoreceptor defect in patients with X-linked RP. Photoreceptors are nonrenewing cells and would, theoretically, accumulate progressive damage to their substructure over time, which may be the reason for the later onset of RP in these patients. USH1B appears to be related to a defect in a type VII myosin involved in the axonemal motor apparatus as a cytoskeletal protein.[158]

The fact that the phenotypic manifestations of an axonemal defect may be so different (immotile spermatozoa and respiratory disease but no retinal/auditory dysfunction or normal respiratory status in a patient with Usher's syndrome) implies that the specific defect (? mutation) that affects a single component of the axonemal substructure may affect the cilia in such diverse ways that each ciliary-dependent system responds in a unique fashion. For example, auditory and retinal photoreceptor cells are nonmotile, but those lining the respiratory tree and spermatozoa are motile. Hypothetically, if an axonemal aberration affects only those aspects concerned with motility and not with structural integrity, perhaps only sperm and respiratory cilia will be affected, whereas auditory and photoreceptor cells will be spared.

# Nonspecific Syndromes with Variable Effects on the Reproductive Axis

## Noonan Syndrome

Noonan syndrome (NS) is characterized by phenotypic features similar to those found in Ullrich-Turner syndrome and include pulmonary stenosis, hypertrophic cardiomyopathy, short stature, webbing of the neck, low set ears, hypertelorism, cubitus valgus, bleeding diatheses, sternal deformities, and learning and behavioral difficulties.[159,160] NS is occasionally referred to as male Turner syndrome, although the inheritance pattern is autosomal dominant with both normal male (46,XY) and female (46,XX) karyotypes found in affected persons. In up to 50% of cases, some clinical aspects of NS will be apparent in one of the parents. No increased parental age effect has been noticed.[161] No specific chromosomal locus has been rigidly defined, although Jamieson et al[162] and Robin et al[163] suggest that one may be located on 12q. Cryptorchidism occurs in up to 77% of males with NS and predicts poor spermatogenic potential with appropriately elevated serum FSH values.[161,164,165] Erectile function and libido are normal. In males without cryptorchidism, biologic paternity is likely. Pubertal onset may be delayed in a small percentage of males.[165]

## Myotonic Dystrophy

Myotonic dystrophy (DM) is a common form of inherited adult muscular dystrophy with a prevalence of 1:1800.[166] Muscle weakness, myotonia, cataracts, arrhythmias, and hypogonadism are prominent manifestations of this disease. Mental retardation occurs in congenital forms.

DM is caused by the expansion of an unstable CTG trinucleotide repeat sequence located in the 3′ UTR of the DM protein kinase gene on chromosome 19. Anticipation occurs in which the disease severity increases, and the age of onset decreases with each passing generation as the size of the CTG repeat grows larger (up to 2000 copies).[167] Other trinucleotide repeat disorders include Kennedy's disease (vide supra), Huntington's chorea, and fragile X syndrome. Transmission is typically maternal, although paternal passage has been documented.[168] The reason for this apparent discrepancy can be found in the reduced fertility in males with DM, severely reducing their ability to pass the disorder along. Spermatogenesis is significantly reduced in males with DM, and it appears that the size of the CTG repeat indirectly correlates with the level of spermatogenic failure.[169] Vasquez et al[170] examined 70 men with DM and found that 66% had testicular atrophy. Oligospermia and azoospermia were reported in 12 and 8 patients, respectively, out of 27 who provided semen samples. Testicular biopsy in 45 patients showed severe spermatogenic deficiency in 71%. The greater the size of the expansion, the worse the level of sperm production. FSH values elevated proportionally, implicating a primary testicular cause as the etiology of the reduced spermatogenesis.[171] Sertoli cell function as it relates to inhibin production appears intact, but the inhibin/FSH axis may be slightly disrupted.[172]

Although expansion occurs in both somatic and germ line tissues as the patient ages, early embryonic cell division in a conceived offspring also drives expansion so that the child may be more severely affected than the parent. Male germ-line contraction of the repeat may actually transpire as well.[173] Jansen et al[174] found that there was a wide expansion range in the sperm of males with small or intermediate expansions in the blood, but similarly sized or smaller increases were detected in the sperm of males with large somatic expansions (>700 repeats). Therefore, DM patients are gonosomal mosaics in which the genetic constitution of the germ-line is different from that of somatic cells. These authors also reported that the offspring's CTG repeat length was significantly different from the expansion size found in the father's sperm, implying that early embryonic somatic and germ-line CTG length increases.[174]

# Conclusion

It may not be wise or appropriate for patients with heritable disorders of phenotype to conceive, especially if the manifestations in the offspring are potentially worse than in the parent. By defining the condition and its responsible genetics, clinicians can provide valuable information to the couple, allowing them to make an informed reproductive choice. For some men, the knowledge that their situation is one of an autosomal recessive pattern and that their partner is not a carrier will eliminate the uncertainty of passage to an offspring and can alleviate some of the fears of paternity.

## References

1. Moore KL. *Clinically Oriented Embryology.* Philadelphia: W.B. Saunders; Co., 1982.
2. Blythe B. The genetic blueprint for maleness. *Contemp Urol* 1995; 7:37–44.

3. Mittwoch U. Sex determination and sex reversal: genotype, phenotype, dogma and semantics. *Hum Genet* 1992; 89:467–479.

4. Hawkins JR, Taylor A, Goodfellow PN, et al. Evidence for increased prevalence of SRY mutations in XY females with complete rather than partial gonadal dysgenesis. *Am J Hum Genet* 1992; 51:979–984.

5. Moore CC, Grumbach MM. Sex determination and gonadogenesis: a transcription cascade of sex chromosome and autosomal genes. *Semin Perinatol* 1992; 16:266–278.

6. Arn P, Chen H, Tuck-Muller CM, et al. SRVX, a sex reversing locus in Xp21.2–p22.11. *Hum Genet* 1994; 93:389–393.

7. Hall BD, Spranger JW. Campomelic dysplasia: further elucidation of a distinct entity. *Am J Dis Child* 1980; 134:285–289.

8. van Heyningen V, Bickmore WA, Seawright A, et al. Role for the Wilms' tumor gene in genital development? *Proc Natl Acad Sci USA* 1990; 87:5383–5386.

9. Ogata T, Matsuo N. Testis determining gene(s) on the X chromosome short arm: chromosomal localization and possible role in testis determination (letter). *J Med Genet* 1994; 31:349–350.

10. Huff V, Jaffe N, Saunders GF, et al. WT 1 exon 1 deletion/insertion mutations in Wilms' tumor patients, associated with di- and trinucleotide repeats and deletion hotspot consensus sequences. *Am J Hum Genet* 1995; 56:84–90.

11. Clarkson PA, Davies HR, Williams DM, et al. Mutational screening in the Wilms' tumor gene, WT 1, in males with genital abnormalities. *J Med Genet* 1993; 30:767–772.

12. Mueller RF. The Denys-Drash syndrome. *J Med Genet* 1994: 471–476.

13. Coppes MJ, Huff V, Pelletier J. Denys-Drash syndrome: relating a clinical disorder to genetic alterations in the tumor-suppressor gene WT 1. *J Pediatr* 1993; 123:673–678.

14. Cohen-Haguenauer O, Picard J Y, Mattei M-G, et al. Mapping of the gene for anti-müllerian hormone to the short arm of human chromosome 19. *Cytogenet Cell Genet* 1987; 44:2–6.

15. Cate RL, Mattaliano RJ, Hession C, et al. Isolation of the bovine and human genes for müllerian inhibiting substance and expression of the human gene in animal cells. *Cell* 1986; 45:685–698.

16. Rey R, Lordereau-Richard I, Carel JC, et al. Anti-müllerian hormone and testosterone serum levels are inversely proportional during normal and precocious pubertal development. *J Clin Endocrin Metab* 1993; 77:1220–1226.

17. Behringer RR, Finegold MJ, Cate RL. Müllerian-inhibiting substance function during mammalian development. *Cell* 1994; 79:415–425.

18. Behringer RR. The in vivo roles of müllerian inhibiting substance. *Curr Topics Dev Biol* 1994; 29:171-187.

19. Grootegoed JA, Baarends WM, Themmen AP. Welcome to the family: the anti-müllerian hormone receptor. *Mol Cell Endocrinol* 1994; 100:29–34.

20. Magro G, Grasso S. Expression of cytokeratins, vimentin and basement membrane components in human fetal male müllerian duct and perimüllerian mesenchyme. *Acta Histochem* 1995; 97:13–18.

21. Shen WHM, Ikeda Y, Parker KL, et al. Nuclear receptor steroidogenic factor 1 regulates the müllerian inhibiting substance gene: a link to the sex determination cascade. *Cell* 1994; 77:651–661.

22. Morton NE. Parameters of the human genome. *Proc Natl Acad Sci USA* 1991; 88:7474–7476.

23. Foote S, Vollrath D, Hilton A, et al. The human Y chromosome: overlapping DNA clones spanning the euchromatic region. *Science* 1992; 258:60–66.

24. Vollrath D, Foote SAH, Hilton A, et al. The human Y chromosome: a 43 interval map based on natural occurring deletions. *Science* 1992; 258:52–59.

25. Tiepolo L, Zuffardi O. Localization of factors controlling spermatogenesis in the nonfluorescent portion of the human Y chromosome long arm. *Hum Genet* 1976; 38:119–124.

26. Reijo R, Lee T-Y, Salo P, et al. Diverse spermatogenic defects in humans caused by Y chromosome deletions encompassing a novel RNA-binding protein gene. *Nature Genet* 1995; 10:383–393.

27. Ismail SR, el-Beheiry AH, Hashishe MM, et al. Cytogenetic study in idiopathic infertile males. *J Egypt Public Health Assoc* 1993; 68:179–204.

28. Vogt P, Chandley AC, Hargreave TB, et al. Microdeletions in interval 6 of the Y chromosome of males with idiopathic sterility point to disruption of AZF, a human spermatogenesis gene. *Hum Genet* 1992; 89:491–496.

29. Nagafuchi S, Namiki M, Nakahori Y, et al. A minute deletion of the Y chromosome in men with azoospermia. *J Urol* 1993; 150:1155–1157.

30. Kobayashi K, Mizuno K, Hida A, et al. PCR analysis of the Y chromosome long arm in azoospermic patients: evidence for a second locus required for spermatogenesis. *Hum Mol Genet* 1994; 3:1965–1967.

31. Nielsen J, Wohlert M. Sex chromosome abnormalities found among 34,910 newborn children: results from a 13-year incidence study in Arhus, Denmark. *BD:OAS* 1990; 26:209–223.

32. Hachimi-Idrissi S, Desmyttere S, Goossens A, et al. Retroperitoneal teratoma as first sign of Klinefelter's syndrome. *Arch Dis Child* 1995; 72:163–164.

33. Derenoncourt AN, Castro-Magana M, Jones KL. Mediastinal teratoma and precocious puberty in a boy with mosaic Klinefelter syndrome. *Am J Med Genet* 1995; 55:38–42.

34. Kiffer JD, Sandeman TF. Primary malignant mediastinal germ cell tumors: a study of eleven cases and a review of the literature. *Int J Radiat Oncol Biol Phys* 1989; 17:835–841.

35. Dexeus F, Logothetis C, Chong C, et al. Genetic abnormalities in men with germ cell tumors. *J Urol* 1988; 140:80–83.

36. Hasle H, Mellemgaard A, Nielsen J, et al. Cancer incidence in men with Klinefelter syndrome. *Br J Cancer* 1995; 71:416–420.

37. Therman E, Susman M. *Human Chromosomes: Structure, Behavior, and Effects.* New York: Springer-Verlag; 1993.

38. Lorda-Sanchez I, Binkert F, Maechler M, et al. Reduced recombination and paternal age effect in Klinefelter syndrome. *Hum Genet* 1992; 89:524–530.

39. Gordon DL, Krmpotic E, Thomas W, et al. Pathologic testicular findings in Klinefelter's syndrome. *Arch Intern Med* 1972; 130:726–730.

40. Terzoli G, Lalatta F, Lobbiani A, et al. Fertility in a 47, XXY patient: assessment of biological paternity by deoxyribonucleic acid fingerprinting. *Fertil Steril* 1992; 58:821–822.

41. Harari O, Bourne H, Baker G, et al. High fertilization rate with intracytoplasmic sperm injection in mosaic Klinefelter's syndrome. *Fertil Steril* 1995; 63:182–184.

42. Cozzi J, Chevret E, Rousseaux S, et al. Achievement of meiosis in XXY germ cells: study of 543 sperm karyotypes from an XY/XXY mosaic patient. *Hum Genet* 1994; 93:32–34.

43. Griffin JE, Wilson JD. Disorders of sexual differentiation. In: Walsh PC, Retik AB, Stamey TA, Vaughn ED, Jr, eds. *Campbell's Urology.* Philadelphia: W.B. Saunders; 1992; 2:1496–1542.

44. Bauder F, Ramond S, Delmer A, et al. Acute myelomonocytic leukemia in a XYY man. *Cancer Genet Cytogenet* 1993; 69:156–157.

45. Thapar A, Gottesman II, Owen MJ, et al. The genetics of mental retardation. *Br J Psychiatry* 1994; 164:747–758.

46. Han TH, Ford JH, Flaherty SP, et al. A fluorescent in situ hybridization analysis of the chromosome constitution of ejaculated sperm in a 47,XYY male. *Clin Genet* 1994; 45:67–70.

47. Speed RM, Faed MJW, Batstone PJ, et al. Persistence of two Y chromosomes through meiotic prophase and metaphase 1 in an XYY man. *Hum Genet* 1991; 87:416–420.

48. Schweikert HU, Weissbach L, Leyendecker G, et al. Clinical, endocrinological, and cytological characterization of two 46, XX males. *J Clin Endocrinol Metab* 1982; 54:745–752.

49. Weil D, Wang I, Dietrich A, et al. Highly homologous loci on the X and Y chromosomes are hot-spots for ectopic recombinations leading to XX maleness. *Nature Genet* 1994; 7:414–419.

50. Page DC, de la Chapelle A, Weissenbach J. Chromosome Y specific DNA in related human XX males. *Nature* 1985; 315:224–226.

51. Page DC, Brown LG, de la Chapelle A. Exchange of terminal portions of X and Y chromosomal short arms in human XX males. *Nature* 1987; 328:437–439.

52. Fechner PY, Marcantonio SM, Jaswaney V, et al. The role of the sex determining region Y gene in the etiology of 46, XX maleness. *J Clin Endocrinol Metab* 1993; 76:690–695.

53. Andersson M, Page DC, Pettay D, et al. Y, Autosome translocations and mosaicisms in the aetiology of 45, X maleness: assignment of fertility factor to distal Yqll. *Hum Genet* 1988; 79:2–7.

54. Sugarman ID, Crolla JA, Malone PS. Mixed gonal dysgenesis and cell line differentiation: Case presentation and literature review. *Clin Genet* 1994; 46:313–315.

55. Wegner HEH, Ferst A, Wegner RD, et al. Primary infertility due to mixed gonadal dysgenesis—report of two cases and review of the literature. *Urologe* 1994; 33:342–346.

56. Smeets DFCM, Hamel BCJ, Nelen MR, et al. Prader-Willi syndrome and Angelman syndrome in cousins from a family with a translocation between chromosome 6 and 15. *N Engl J Med* 1992; 326:807–810.

57. Bick D, Franco B, Sherins RJ, et al. Original articles: brief report: intragenic deletion of the Kalig-1 gene in Kallmann's syndrome. *N Engl J Med* 1992; 326:1752–1755.

58. Swanzel-Fukada M, Bick D, Pfaff DW. Luteinizing hormone releasing hormone (LHRH) expressing cells do not migrate normally in an inherited hypogonadal (Kallmann) syndrome. *Brain Res Mol Brain Res* 1989; 6:311–326.

59. Sigman M, Howards SS. Male Infertility. In: Walsh PC, Retik AB, Stamey TA, Vaughn DE Jr, eds. *Campbell's Urology*. Philadelphia: W.B. Saunders; 1992; 1:661–705.

60. Watkins PC, Eddy R, Beck AK, et al. DNA sequence and regional assignment of the human follicle-stimulating hormone beta-subunit gene to the short arm of chromosome 11. *DNA* 1987; 6:205–212.

61. Mohrenweiser HW, Tynan KM, Branscomb EW, et al. Development of an integrated genetic, functional and physical map of human chromosome 19 (Abstract). *Cytogenet Cell Genet* 1991; 58:20–21.

62. Glaser T, Lewis WH, Bruns GAP, et al. The beta-subunit of follicle-stimulating hormone is deleted in patients with aniridia and Wilms' tumor, allowing a further definition of the WAGR locus. *Nature* 1986; 321:882–887.

63. Rousseau-Merck MF, Misrahi M, Atger M, et al. Localization of the human luteinizing hormone choriogonadotropin receptor gene (LHCGR) to chromosome 2p2l. *Cytogenet Cell Genet* 1990; 54:77–79.

64. Park IJ, Burnett LS, Jones HW, et al. A case of male pseudohermaphroditism associated with elevated LH, normal FSH, and low testosterone possible due to the secretion of an abnormal LH molecule. *Acta Endocrinol* 1976; 83:173–181.

65. Axelrod L, Neer RM, Kliman B. Hypogonadism in a male with immunologically active, biologically inactive leuteinizing hormone: an exception to a venerable rule. *J Clin Endocrinol Metab* 1979; 48:279–287.

66. Matthews CH, Borgato S, Beck-Peccoz P, et al. Primary amenorrhea and infertility due to a mutation in the beta-subunit of follicle-stimulating hormone. *Nature Genet* 1993; 5:83–86.

67. Kremer H, Kraaij R, Toledo SPA, et al. Male pseudohermaphroditism due to a homozygous missense mutation of the luteinizing hormone receptor gene. *Nature Genet* 1995; 9:160–164.

68. Perez-Palacios G, Scaglia HE, Kofman-Alfaro S, et al. Inherited male pseudohermaphrodi- tism due to gonadotrophin unresponsiveness. *Acta Endocrinol* 1981; 98:148–155.

69. Griffin JE, Wilson JD, McPhaul MJ. The spectrum of molecular defects in androgen resistance syndromes. XIIth North American Testis Workshop: function of somatic cells in the testis. Tampa, Florida, April 13–16, 1993, Serono Symposia, USA.

70. Griffin JE. Androgen resistance: the clinical and molecular spectrum. *N Engl J Med* 1992; 326:611–618.

71. Brown TR. Human androgen insensitivity syndrome. *J Androl* 1995; 16:299–303.

72. Malchoff CD. Syndromes of androgen resistance. *Infert Reprod Clin North Am* 1992; 3:267–283.

73. Sultan S, Lumbroso S, Poujol N, et al. Mutations of androgen receptor gene in androgen insensitivity syndromes. *J Steroid Biochem Mol Biol* 1993; 46:519–530.

74. Brinkman AO, Jenster G, Ris-Stalpers C, et al. Androgen receptor mutations. *J Steroid Biochem Mol Biol* 1995; 53:443–448.

75. Zhou Z-X, Sar M, Simental JA, et al. A ligand-dependent bipartite nuclear targeting signal in the human androgen receptor. *J Biol Chem* 1994; 269:13115–13123.

76. Aiman J, Griffin JE, Gazak JM, et al. Androgen insensitivity as a cause of infertility in otherwise normal men. *N Engl J Med* 1979; 300:223–227.

77. Puscheck EE, Behzadian MA, McDonough PG. The first analysis of exon 1 (the transactivation domain) of the androgen receptor in infertile men with oligospermia or azoospermia. *Fertil Steril* 1994; 62:1035–1038.

78. Schulster A, Ross L, Scommegna A. Frequency in androgen insensitivity in infertile phenotypically normal men. *J Urol* 1983; 130:699–671.

79. Beitel LK, Kazemi-Esfarjani P, Kaufman M, et al. Substitution of arginine-839 by cysteine or histidine in the androgen receptor causes different receptor phenotypes in cultured cells and coordinate degrees of clinical androgen resistance. *J Clin Invest* 1994; 94:546–554.

80. Imasaki K, Hasegawa T, Okabe T, et al. Single amino acid substitution (840 Arg to His) in the hormone-binding domain of the androgen receptor leads to incomplete androgen insensitivity syndrome associated with a thermolabile androgen receptor. *Eur J Endocrinol* 1994; 130:569–574.

81. Jakubiczka S, Werder EA, Wieacker P. Point mutation in the steroid-binding domain of the

androgen receptor gene in a family with complete androgen insensitivity syndrome (CAIS). *Hum Genet* 1992; 90:311–312.

82. Quigley CA, Evans BAJ, Simental JA, et al. Complete androgen insensitivity due to deletion of exon C of the androgen receptor gene highlights the functional importance of the second zinc finger of the androgen receptor in vivo. *Mol Endocrinol* 1992; 6:1103–1112.

83. DeBellis A, Quigley CA, Cariello NF, et al. Single base mutations in the human androgen receptor gene causing complete androgen insensitivity: rapid detection by a modified denaturing gradient gel electrophoresis technique. *Mol Endocrinol* 1992; 6:1909–1920.

84. Kasumi H, Komori S, Yamasaki N, et al. Single nucleotide substitution of the androgen receptor gene in a case with receptor-positive androgen insensitivity syndrome (complete form). *Acta Endocrinol* 1993; 128:355–360.

85. Kazemi-Esfarjani P, Beitel LK, Trifiro M, et al. Substitution of valine-865 by methionine or leucine in the human androgen receptor causes complete or partial androgen insensitivity, respectively with distinct androgen receptor phenotypes. *Mol Endocrinol* 1993; 7:37–46.

86. Saunders PTK, Padayachi T, Tincello DG, et al. Point mutations detected in the androgen receptor gene of three men with partial androgen insensitivity syndrome. *Clin Endocrinol* 1992; 37:214–220.

87. Zopi S, Wilson CN, Harbison MD, et al. Complete testicular feminization caused by an amino-terminal truncation of the androgen receptor with downstream initiation. *J Clin Invest* 1993; 91:1105–1112.

88. Tsukada T, Inoue M, Tachibana S, et al. An androgen receptor mutation causing androgen resistance in undervirilized male syndrome. *J Clin Endocrinol Metab* 1994; 79:1202–1207.

89. Ris-Stalpers C, Verleun-Mooijman MCT, de Blaeij TJP, et al. Differential splicing of human androgen receptor pre-mRNA in X-linked Reifenstein's syndrome, because of a deletion involving a putative branch site. *Am J Hum Genet* 1994; 54:609–617.

90. McPhaul MJ, Marcelli M, Zoppi S, et al. Mutations in the ligand-binding domain of the androgen receptor gene cluster in two regions of the gene. *J Clin Invest* 1992; 90:2097–2101.

91. Yong EL, Ng SC, Roy AC, Yun G, et al. Pregnancy after hormonal correction of severe spermatogenic defect due to mutation in androgen receptor gene (letter to the editor). *Lancet* 1994; 344:826–827.

92. Stefanis C, Papetropoulos T, Scarpelazos S, et al. X-linked spinal and bulbar muscular atrophy of late onset. *J Neurol Sci* 1975; 24:493–503.

93. LaSpada AR, Wilson EM, Lubahn DB, et al. Androgen receptor gene mutations in X-linked spinal and bulbar muscular atrophy. *Nature* 1991; 352:77–79.

94. MacLean HE, Choi W-T, Rekaris G, et al. Abnormal androgen receptor binding affinity in subjects with Kennedy's disease (spinal and bulbar muscular atrophy). *J Clin Endocrinol Metab* 1995; 80:508–516.

95. Yamamoto Y, Kawai H, Nakahara K, et al. A novel primer extension method to detect the number of CAG repeats in the androgen receptor gene in families with X-linked spinal and bulbar muscular atrophy. *Biochem Biophys Res Commun* 1992; 182:507–513.

96. Ferlini A, Patrosso MC, Guidetti D, et al. Androgen receptor gene (CAG)n repeat analysis in the differential diagnosis between Kennedy disease and other motoneuron disorders. *Am J Med Genet* 1995; 55:105–111.

97. Chamberlain NL, Driver ED, Miesfeld RL. The length and location of CAG trinucleotide repeats in the androgen receptor N-terminal domain affect transactivation function. *Nucleic Acids Res* 1994; 22:3181–3186.

98. Matsura T, Demura T, Aimoto Y, et al. Androgen receptor abnormality in X-linked spinal and bulbar muscular atrophy. *Neurology* 1992; 42:1724–1726.

99. Warner CL, Griffin JE, Wilson JD, et al. X-linked spinomuscular atrophy: a kindred with associated abnormal androgen receptor binding. *Neurology* 1992; 42:2181–2184.

100. Davis DL, Russell DW. Unusual length polymorphism in human steroid 5 alpha-reductase type 2 gene (SRD5A2). *Hum Mol Genet* 1993; 2:820.

101. Wigley WC, Prihoda JS, Mowszowicz BB, et al. Natural mutagenesis study of the human steroid 5 alpha reductase 2 isoenzyme. *Biochemistry* 1994; 33:1265–1270.

102. Carpenter TO, Imperato-McGinley J, Boulware SD, et al. Variable expression of 5 alpha-reductase deficiency: presentation with male phenotype in a child of Greek origin. *J Clin Endocrinol Metab* 1990; 71:318–322.

103. McCrae WM, Williamson R. Cystic fibrosis. In: Emery AEH, Rimoin DL, eds. *Principles and Practices of Medical Genetics*. Edinburgh: Churchill Livingstone; 1990: 1165–1178.

104. Anguiano A, Oates RD, Amos JA, et al. Congenital bilateral absence of the vas deferens: a

primarily genital form of cystic fibrosis. *JAMA* 1992; 267:1794–1797.

105. Rommens JM, Iannuzzi MC, Kerem B, et al. Identification of the cystic fibrosis gene: chromosome walking and jumping. *Science* 1989; 245:1059–1065.

106. Consortium TCFGA. Worldwide survey of the ΔF508 mutation Report from the Cystic Fibrosis Genetic Analysis Consortium. *Am J Hum Genet* 1990; 47:354–359.

107. Kerem B, Rommens JM, Buchanan JA, et al. Identification of the cystic fibrosis gene: genetic analysis. *Science* 1989; 245:1073–1780.

108. Kaplan E, Shwachman H, Perlmutter AD, et al. Reproductive failure in males with cystic fibrosis. *N Engl J Med* 1968; 279:65–69.

109. Oates RD, Amos JA. Congenital bilateral absence of the vas deferens and cystic fibrosis: a genetic commonality. *World J Urol* 1993; 11:82–88.

110. Mickle JE, Collin A, Wu HQ, et al. Cystic fibrosis and congenital absence of the vas deferens: genetic analysis of 100 men suggests locus heterogeneity. In press, 1995.

111. Chillon M, Casals T, Mercier B, et al. Mutations in the cystic fibrosis gene in patients with congenital absence of the vas deferens. *N Engl J Med* 1995; 332:1475–1480.

112. Augarten A, Yahav Y, Kerem BS, et al. Congenital bilateral absence of the vas deferens in the absence of cystic fibrosis (letter). *Lancet* 1994; 344:1473–1474.

113. Mulhall J, Oates RD. Vasal aplasia and cystic fibrosis. *Curr Opinion Urol* 1995; 5:316–319.

114. Mickle JE, Milunsky A, Amos JA, et al. Congenital unilateral absence of the vas deferens (CUAVD): a heterogeneous disorder with two distinct subpopulations based upon etiology and mutational status of the cystic fibrosis gene. *Hum Reprod* 1995; 10:1728–1735.

115. Oates RD, Amos JA. The genetic basis of congenital bilateral absence of the vas deferens and cystic fibrosis. *J Androl* 1994; 15:1–8.

116. Liu J, Silber Sj, Devroey P, et al. Birth after the preimplantation diagnosis of the cystic fibrosis ΔF508 mutation by polymerase chain reaction in human embryos resulting from intracytoplasmic sperm injection with epididymal sperm. *JAMA* 1994; 272:1858–1860.

117. Handelsman DJ, Conway AJ, Boylan LM, et al. Young's syndrome: obstructive azoospermia in chronic sinopulmonary infections. *N Engl J Med* 1984; 310:3–9.

118. de Iongh R, Ing A, Rutland J. Mucociliary function, ciliary ultrastructure, and ciliary orienta-

tion in Young's syndrome. *Thorax* 1992; 47: 184–187.

119. Wilton LJ, Teichtal H, Temple-Smith PD, et al. Young's syndrome (obstructive azoospermia and chronic sinobronchial infection): a quantitative study of axonemal ultrastructure and function. *Fertil Steril* 1991; 55:144–151.

120. Hirsch A, Williams C, Williamson B. Young's syndrome and cystic fibrosis mutation delF508 (letter). *Lancet* 1993; 342:118.

121. Le Lannou D, Jezequel P, Blayou M, et al. Obstuctive azoospermia with agenesis of the vas deferens or with bronchiectasia (Young's syndrome): a genetic approach. *Hum Reprod* 1995; 10:338–341.

122. Hendry WE, A'Hern RP, Cole PJ. Was Young's syndrome caused by mercury exposure in childhood? *Br Med J* 1993; 307:1579–1582.

123. Beheshti M, Churchill BM, Hardy BE, et al. Familial persistent müllerian duct syndrome. *J Urol* 1984; 131:968–969.

124. Martin EL, Bennett AH, Cromie WJ. Persistent müllerian duct syndrome with transverse testicular ectopia and spermatogenesis. *J Urol* 1992; 147:1615–1617.

125. Mouli K, McCarthy P, Ray P, et al. Persistent müllerian duct syndrome in a man with transverse testicular ectopia. *J Urol* 1988; 139:373–375.

126. Thompson ST, Grillis MA, Wolkoff MH, et al. Transverse testicular ectopia in a man with persistent müllerian duct syndrome. *Arch Pathol Lab Med* 1994; 118:752–755.

127. Loeff DS, Imbeaud S, Reyes HM, et al. Surgical and genetic aspects of persistent müllerian duct syndrome. *J Pediatr Surg* 1994; 29:61–65.

128. Carre-Eusebe D, Imbeaud S, Harbison M, et al. Variants of the anti-müllerian hormone gene in a compound heterozygote with the persistent müllerian duct syndrome and his family. *Hum Genet* 1992; 90:389–394.

129. Guerrier D, Tran D, Vanderwinden JM, et al. The persistent müllerian duct syndrome: a molecular approach. *J Clin Endocrinol Metab* 1989; 68:46–52.

130. Guerrier D, Boussin L, Mader S, et al. Expression of the gene for anti-müllerian hormone. *J Reprod Fertil* 1990; 88:695–706.

131. Knebelmann B, Boussin L, Guerrier D, et al. Anti-müllerian hormone Bruxelles: a nonsense mutation associated with the persistent müllerian duct syndrome. *Proc Natl Acad Sci USA* 1991; 88:3767–3771.

132. Schidlow DV. Primary ciliary dyskinesia (the immotile cilia syndrome). *Ann Allergy* 1994; 73:457–468.
133. Perraudeau M, Scott J, Walport M, Oakley C, Bloom S, Brooks D. Late presentation of Kartagener's syndrome. *Br Med J* 1994; 308:519–521.
134. Yokota T, Ohno N, Tamura K, et al. Ultrastructure and function of cilia and spermatozoa flagella in a patient with Kartagener's syndrome. *Int Med* 1993; 32:593–597.
135. Bongso TA, Sathananthan AH, Wong PC, et al. Human fertilization by micro-injection of immotile spermatozoa. *Hum Reprod* 1989; 4:175–179.
136. Narayan D, Krishnan SN, Upender M, et al. Unusual inheritance of primary ciliary dyskinesia (Kartagener's syndrome). *J Med Genet* 1994; 31:493–496.
137. Oko R, Clermont Y. Mammalian spermatozoa: structure and assembly of the tail. In: Gagnon C, ed. *Controls of Sperm Motility: Biological and Clinical Aspects.* Boca Raton, FL: CRC Press; 1990: 3–28.
138. Song Y-H, Mandelkow E. The anatomy of flagellar microtubules: polarity, seam, junctions, and lattice. *J Cell Biol* 1995; 128:81–94.
139. Kamiya R. Exploring the function of inner and outer dynein arms with *Chlamydomonas* mutants. *Cell Motil Cytoskeleton* 1995; 32:98–102.
140. Hamasaki T, Barkalow K, Satir P. Regulation of ciliary beat frequency by a dynein light chain. *Cell Motil Cytoskeleton* 1995; 32:121–124.
141. Piperno C. Regulation of dynein activity within *Chlamydomonas* flagella. *Cell Motil Cytoskeleton* 1995; 32:103–105.
142. Saeki H, Kondo S, Morita T, et al. Immotile cilia syndrome associated with polycystic kidney. *J Urol* 1984; 132:1165–1166.
143. Kaplan J, Gerber S, Bonneau D, et al. A gene for Usher syndrome type 1 (USH1A) maps to chromosome 14q. *Genomics* 1992; 14:979–987.
144. Phillips DM, Jow WW, Goldstein M. Testis factors that may regulate gene expression: evidence from a patient with Kartagener's syndrome. *Andrology* 1995; 16:158–162.
145. Pansera F. Development of left/right symmetry and asymmetry, Kartagener's syndrome, and cerebral laterality. *Med Hypotheses* 1994; 42:283–284.
146. Dryja TP, Berson EL. Retinitis pigmentosa and allied diseases. *Invest Ophthalmol Vis Sci* 1995; 36:1197–2000.

147. Shastry BS. Retinitis pigmentosa and related disorders: phenotypes of rhodopsin and peripherin/RDS mutations. *Am J Med Genet* 1994; 52:467–474.
148. Hunter DG, Fishman GA, Kretzer FL. Abnormal axonemes in X-linked retinitis pigmentosa. *Arch Ophthamol* 1988; 106:362–368.
149. van Dorp DB, Wright AF, Carothers AD, et al. A family with RP3 type of X-linked retinitis pigmentosa: an association with ciliary abnormalities. *Hum Genet* 1992; 88:331–334.
150. Smith RJH, Lee EC, Kimberling WJ, et al. Localization of two genes for Usher syndrome type I to chromosome 11. *Genomics* 1992; 14:995–1002.
151. Larget-Piet D, Gerber S, Bonneau D, et al. Genetic heterogeneity of Usher syndrome type 1 in French families. *Genomics* 1994; 21:138–143.
152. Kimberling WJ, Möller CG, Davenport S, et al. Linkage of Usher syndrome type 1 gene (USH 1B) to the long arm of chromosome 11. *Genomics* 1992; 14:988–994.
153. Keats BJB, Nouri N, Pelias MZ, et al. Tightly linked flanking microsatellite markers for the Usher syndrome type 1 locus on the short arm of chromosome 11. *Am J Hum Genet* 1994; 54:681–686.
154. Kimberling WJ, Weston MD, Möller C, et al. Gene mapping of Usher syndrome type IIa: localization of the gene to a 2.1-cM segment on chromosome 1q4l. *Am J Hum Genet* 1995; 56:216–223.
155. Sankila E-M, Pakarinen L, Kaariainen H, et al. Assignment of an Usher syndrome type III (USH 3) gene to chromosome 3q. *Hum Mol Genet* 1995; 4:93–98.
156. Shinkawa H, Nadol JB. Histopathology of the inner ear in Usher's syndrome as observed by light and electron microscopy. *Ann Otol Rhinol Laryngol* 1986; 95:313–318.
157. Hunter DG, Fishman GA, Mehta RS, et al. Abnormal sperm and photoreceptor axonemes in Usher's syndrome. *Arch Ophthalmol* 1986; 104:385–389.
158. Weil D, Blanchard S, Kaplan J, et al. Defective myosin VIIA gene responsible for Usher syndrome type 1B. *Nature* 1995; 374:60–61.
159. Sharland M, Patton MA, Burch M, et al. A clinical study of Noonan syndrome. *Arch Dis Child* 1992; 67:178–183.
160. Wood A, Massarano A, Super M, et al. Behavioral aspects and psychiatric findings in

Noonan's syndrome. *Arch Dis Child* 1995; 72:153–155.

161. Sharland M, Morgan M, Smith G, et al. Genetic counselling in Noonan syndrome. *Am J Med Genet* 1993; 45:437–440.

162. Jamieson CR, van der Burgt I, Brady AF, et al. Mapping a gene for Noonan syndrome to the long arm of chromosome 12. *Nature Genet* 1994; 8:357–360.

163. Robin NH, Sellinger B, McDonald-McGinn D, et al. Classical Noonan syndrome is not associated with deletions of 22q11. *Am J Med Genet* 1995; 56:94–96.

164. Sasagawa I, Nakada T, Kubota Y, et al. Gonadal function and testicular histology in Noonan's syndrome with bilateral cryptorchidism. *Arch Androl* 1994; 32:135–140.

165. Elsawi MM, Pryor JP, Klufio G, et al. Genital tract function in men with Noonan syndrome. *J Med Genet* 1994; 31:468–470.

166. Wong L-JC, Ashizawa T, Monckton DG, et al. Somatic heterogeneity of the CTG repeat in myotonic dystrophy is age and size dependent. *Am J Hum Genet* 1995; 56:114–122.

167. Harley HG, Rundle SA, MacMillan JC, et al. Size of the unstable CTG repeat sequence in relation to phenotype and parental transmission in myotonic dystrophy. *Am J Hum Genet* 1993; 52:1164–1174.

168. Nakagawa M, Yamada H, Higuchi I, et al. A case of paternally inherited myotonic dystrophy. *J Med Genet* 1994; 31:397–400.

169. Jaspert A, Fahsold R, Grehl H, et al. Myotonic dystrophy: correlation of clinical symptoms with the size of the CTG trinucleotide repeat. *J Neurol* 1995; 242:99–104.

170. Vasquez JA, Pinies JA, Martul P, et al. Hypothalamic-pituitary-testicular function in 70 patients with myotonic dystrophy. *J Endocrinol Invest* 1990; 13:375–379.

171. Mastrogiacomo I, Pagani E, Novelli GA, et al. Male hypogonadism in myotonic dystrophy is related to (CTG)n triplet mutation. *J Endocrinol Invest* 1994; 17:381–383.

172. Lou XY, Nishi Y, Haji M, et al. Reserved Sertoli cell function in the hypogonadic male patients with myotonic dystrophy. *Fukuoka Igaku Zasshi Fukuoka Acta Medica* 1994; 85:168–174.

173. Monckton DG, Wong LJ, Ashizawa T, et al. Somatic mosaicism, germline expansions, germline reversions, and intergenerational reductions in myotonic dystrophy males: small pool PVR analyses. *Hum Mol Genet* 1995; 4:1–8.

174. Jansen G, Willems P, Coerwinkel M, et al. Gonadosoma mosaicism in myotonic dystrophy patients: involvement of mitotic events in (CTG)n repeat variation and selection against extreme expansion in sperm. *Am J Hum Genet* 1994; 54:575–585.

# 10
# Medical and Endocrine Therapy of the Infertile Male

Rebecca Z. Sokol

The differential diagnosis of male factor infertility can be subdivided into four major diagnostic categories: (1) irreversible germ cell failure, (2) hypogonadotropic hypogonadism, (3) anatomic defects, and (4) idiopathic infertility. Therapies for germ cell failure and hypogonadotropic hypogonadism are clearly delineated. Anatomic defects are surgically corrected. A specific therapy for idiopathic infertility has yet to be defined, but a number of medical therapies have been proposed for its treatment. Because of the heterogeneity of the disorders that fall into this category, specific etiologic factors for each are not yet defined, which prevents identification of specific therapies. No single empiric medical therapy proposed has proven efficacious when studied in a controlled, prospective fashion. Placebo-controlled trials are necessary because the treatment-independent pregnancy rate is 30% in 1 year.[1] A 30% improvement in pregnancy rate in a noncontrolled study is therefore meaningless.

## Treatment Options

The selection of a treatment regimen for the infertile man depends on the history, the underlying endocrine abnormality that may be contributing to the infertility, and the patient's semen analysis (Tables 10.1 and 10.2).

## Irreversible Germ Cell Failure

Men with irreversible infertility can be subdivided into two major groups: (1) men with spermatogenic failure who present with elevated serum follicle-stimulating hormone (FSH) levels, normal luteinizing hormone (LH) and testosterone levels, and small testes; and (2) men who present with classic hypergonadotropic hypogonadism identified by elevated gonadotropins, low testosterone, and azoospermia. Klinefelter's syndrome (47,XXY), occurring in approximately 0.2% of adults, is the most common cause of hypergonadotropic hypogonadism. At present, there is no therapy available for the treatment of infertility in these two groups of men. Artificial insemination with donor (AID) semen or adoption are the recommended options.[2] The combination of intratesticular sperm aspiration along with intracytoplasmic sperm injection or round spermatid nuclear injection (ROSNI) may revolutionize the treatment of the male with testicular failure.[3]

Men with hypergonadotropic hypogonadism should be treated with androgens to maintain their secondary sexual characteristics.[4] The traditional replacement dose is testosterone enanthate 200 mg intramuscularly every 10 to 14 days (Fig. 10.1). An alternative dosing method now available is a transdermal therapeutic system consisting of a polymeric membrane containing 5 to 10 mg of testosterone that

TABLE 10.1. Hormone therapy.

Hypergonadotropic hypogonadism (androgen
   replacement)
   Intramuscular testosterone ester, 200 mg q 10 to 14
    days
   Transdermal patch 5–10 mg q 24 hrs
Hypogonadotropic hypogonadism (spermatogenesis
   stimulation)
   hCG, 1500–2000 IU 2–3×/week for up to 24 weeks
   If poor return of spermatogenesis add
    hMG, 75 IU 2–3×/week for up to 24 weeks
  or
    GnRH 5–20 μg/pulse every 90–120 minutes via
     portable pump

TABLE 10.2. Empiric medical treatments for idiopathic oligospermic.

| Testosterone | Corticosteroids |
|---|---|
| Low dose | Others |
| Rebound therapy | Vitamins |
| Gonadotropins | Minerals |
| LH | Antioxidants |
| FSH | Kallikrein |
| GnRH | Pentoxyfylline |
| Antiestrogens | Thyroid hormone |
| Clomiphene citrate | Bromocriptine |
| Tamoxifen | |
| Testolactone | |

is applied to the scrotal skin every 24 hours.[5,6]
The advantage of this method is that physiologic levels of serum testosterone are maintained (Fig. 10.2).[6]

## Hypogonadotropic Hypogonadism

A small number of infertility patients carry the
diagnosis of hypogonadotropic hypogonadism.
Men with hypogonadotropic hypogonadism are

deficient in LH and FSH secretion. As a result,
these men are also deficient in testosterone and
spermatogenesis. The congenital form of this
disorder, Kallmann's syndrome or idiopathic
hypogonadotropic hypogonadism, is an abnormality of the secretion of gonadotropin-
releasing hormone (GnRH). Acquired causes
include tumor, infection, infiltrative diseases,
and autoimmune hypophysitis. The exclusion
of coincident pituitary deficiencies and appro-

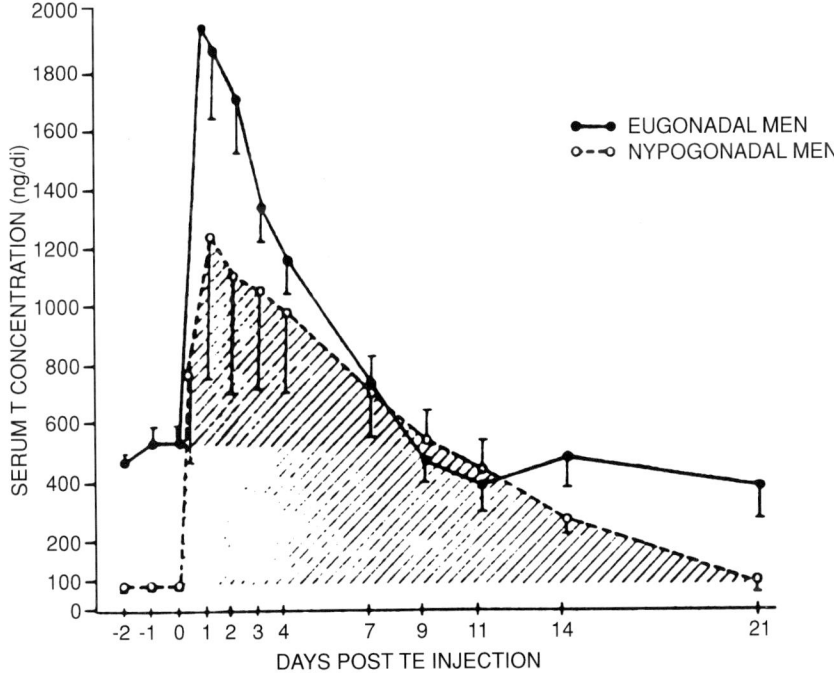

FIGURE 10.1. Mean and standard error of testosterone levels in eugonadal and hypogonadal men before and
at various time intervals after an intramuscular injection of 200 mg of testosterone enathate. (From
Cunningham GR, Cordero E, Thornby JI. "Testosterone Replacement with Transdermal Therapeutic Systems." *JAMA* 1989: 2526.)

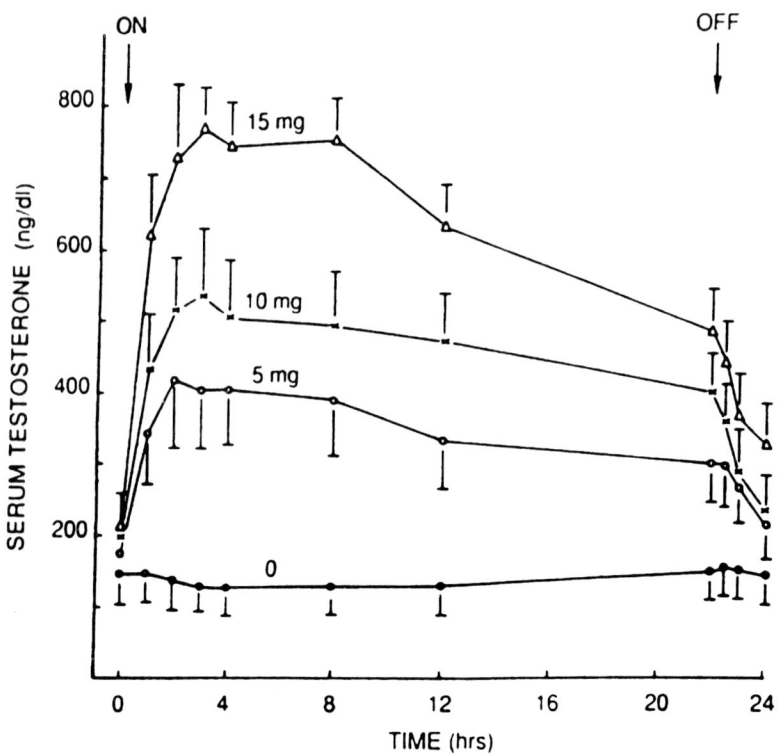

FIGURE 10.2. The time course of the mean ($\pm$ SE) serum testosterone concentrations in six hypogonadal men in the 22 hours following the application to the scrotum of thin flexible membranes containing 0, 5, 10, or 15 mg testosterone and in the 2 hours after their removal. The arrows indicate when the membranes were applied (ON) and removed (OFF). (From Sokol RZ, Palacios A, Campfield LA, Saul C, Swerdloff RS. "Comparison of the kinetics of injectible testosterone in eugonadal and hypogonadal men." Fertil Steril 1982; 37:425–430. Reproduced with permission of the publisher, the American Society of Reproductive Medicine [The American Fertility Society].)

priate radiologic investigation is required prior to initiation of therapy for fertility. Prolactin-secreting tumors may require surgery, treatment with dopamine agonists, or both.[7]

Spermatogenesis can be initiated and pregnancies achieved in many of these hypogonadotropic hypogonadal men when they are treated with exogenous gonadotropins or GnRH. Selection of the type of hormonal therapy as well as its ultimate success depends on the severity of the defect. The most frequently prescribed preparations are human chorionic gonadotropin (hCG) and human menopausal gonadotropin (hMG).

The usual first-line drug for the treatment of nonhyperprolactinemic hypogonadotropic hypogonadism directed toward the restoration of spermatogenesis is a course of hCG. Human chorionic gonadotropin is comparable to LH in that it stimulates Leydig cell secretion of testosterone and estradiol. Treatment with hCG alone in patients with partial gonadotropin deficiency may increase sperm counts and result in pregnancies.[8] The degree of re-

sponse correlates with the size of the testis prior to treatment. Human chorionic gonadotropin is administered at a dosage of 1500 to 2000 IU two to three times per week for 18 to 24 weeks. This dose will result in normal serum testosterone levels. When there is no further increase in testicular growth or improvement in sperm production, hMG (a compound that contains both LH and FSH) is added to the regimen to further stimulate spermatogenesis. Human menopausal gonadotropin is administered at a dose of 75 IU two to three times weekly until the patient produces ejaculates containing 5 million or more sperm per milliliter, or until pregnancy is achieved. The hMG then can be withdrawn and spermatogenesis usually maintained by continued administration of hCG.[9]

Patients not interested in maintenance of spermatogenesis for fertility should be treated with testosterone replacement as previously outlined. Prior chronic treatment of hypogonadotropic hypogonadal men with testosterone does not affect the subsequent success of gonadotropin therapy.[9,10] A few side effects during hCG/hMG treatment have been reported: headaches, gynecomastia, breast tenderness, further suppression of spermatogenesis, and the development of anti-hCG antibodies.[11]

A more specific treatment for men with idiopathic hypogonadotropic hypogonadism (IHH) is replacement therapy with GnRH. By definition, GnRH therapy is effective only in cases in which the pituitary gland is intact. GnRH is administered at 90- to 120-minute intervals via a portable automatic-infusion pump at doses ranging between 5 and 20 µg/per pulse.[12–14]

Because insulin and insulin-like growth factor-I (IGF-I) may be involved in modulating gonadal steroidogenesis, growth hormone (GH) treatment has been proposed as an adjuvant to gonadotropin therapy for men with hypogonadotropia who fail conventional treatment. In a preliminary study, cotreatment with GH improved spermatogenesis in two of four men.[15] Definitive conclusions regarding the efficacy of this GH regimen await the results of a larger clinical trial.

## Idiopathic Infertility

Patients with idiopathic oligospermia present with normal gonadotropins and a normal serum testosterone in the face of low sperm counts. This is a heterogeneous group of patients. Their oligospermia is the result of a variety of abnormalities, each causing a reduction in sperm concentration. Thus, treating all patients with the same drug will not uniformly result in improvement of fertility. A number of empiric therapies have been proposed (Table 10.2). However, few placebo-controlled studies are published that evaluate the efficacy of these drugs in the treatment of male infertility.

### Androgen Therapy

Therapies with both low-dose testosterone and high-dose testosterone regimens have been suggested. In the low-dose testosterone regimen, androgens are given in oral doses of either 10 to 50 mg/day of methyltestosterone, 50 to 70 mg/day of mesterolone, or 5 to 20 mg/day of fluoxymesterone for a least 3 months in an effort to supplement allegedly inadequate endogenous production of testosterone and thus stimulate spermatogenesis. These regimens have been shown to be ineffective.[16,17]

Rebound therapy involves the administration of higher doses of testosterone preparations, most frequently testosterone enanthate, 200 to 500 mg intramuscularly every 2 weeks. These doses suppress LH and spermatogenesis. Following the cessation of therapy, sperm production usually resumes, and in some patients sperm concentrations may rebound to a higher level than at the initiation of therapy. Two recent studies verify that the treatment does not improve fertility. Fifty-two patients with idiopathic oligoesthenospermia or teratospermia or both were treated with either 150 mg per day of mesterolone or placebo for 12 months.[18] Similar semen improvement was noted in both the treated and control patients. The pregnancy rate in the mesterolone-treated cases was 26%. The pregnancy rate in the placebo control cases was 48%.

In a similar controlled study, 25 men with idiopathic oligospermia, asthenospermia, or teratozospermia were treated with either 240 mg per day of testosterone undecanoate or placebo for 3 to 6 months.[19] Changes in sperm concentration, motility, and morphology were similar in both groups. Two pregnancies occurred, one during the first month of placebo intake and the other during the second month of testosterone undecanoate treatment.

### Gonadotropins

Investigators have administered gonadotropin therapy to patients with idiopathic oligospermia in a manner similar to that for patients with hypogonadotropic hypogonadism without improvement in fertility.[20,21]

Therapy with purified human FSH may play a role in the treatment of men with severe oligospermia whose partners are enrolled in an in vitro fertilization (IVF) program.[22] Fifty men with a history of infertility and abnormal semen analyses were treated with intramuscular injections of purified FSH three times per week for at least 3 months. Although no significant changes were observed in serum LH, testosterone levels, or semen parameters, the fertilization rates of preovulatory oocytes were significantly improved. Unfortunately, no control arm was included in the study, and the number of men in some of the groups was too low to reach definite conclusions regarding significance.

In a related study, the potential of short-term systemic administration of FSH to improve sperm quality was assessed, including ultrastructure in patients with teratozoospermia with normal endocrine profiles. A significant improvement in agenesis of the acrosome and in the amorphous heads was observed. No significant changes were observed in basic semen analysis parameters. The relationship between these induced morphologic changes and pregnancy rates was not reported.[23] The efficacy of FSH treatment of infertile men as adjunctive treatment during IVF remains to be proven. Additionally, the advent of intracytoplasmic sperm injection (ICSI) may render this adjuvant therapy obsolete.

## GnRH Therapy

Pulsatile GnRH therapy as a treatment for idiopathic oligoasthenospermia does not improve sperm parameters or pregnancy rates. Investigators in Switzerland treated 28 infertile men with either GnRH or placebo for 3 months in a crossover study. They theorized that men with low bioactive FSH, possibly because of inadequate GnRH pulsatility, would benefit from GnRH therapy. They concluded from their data that low bioactive FSH was not the cause of idiopathic oligospermia and was not predictive of response to GnRH.[24]

## Antiestrogens

A number of antiestrogens have been proposed as male fertility drugs. These include clomiphene, tamoxifen, and testolactone. Clomiphene and tamoxifen act as competitive inhibitors of estrogen action by occupying estrogen receptors. Testolactone, an aromatase inhibitor, prevents the conversion of testosterone to estradiol.[2] These drugs exert their effects in at least two ways. Androgens and estrogens modulate hypothalamic and pituitary functions to regulate gonadotropin production.

Antiestrogens displace estrogens from their receptors and interfere with the normal feedback of signals of circulating or locally produced estrogens. As a result, secretion of GnRH stimulates increased gonadotropin secretion, which, in turn, increases testosterone production and, theoretically, induces germ cell maturation. Antiestrogens may also have a direct effect on the testis by blocking the inhibitory action of estradiol on Leydig cell function.[25]

Of this group of drugs, the estrogen competitive inhibitor clomiphene is the most commonly prescribed drug in the treatment of male infertility. Until recently, studies reporting on the efficacy of clomiphene were not well controlled. Results stemming from these studies have been variable. Some indicated improvement of sperm motility and fertility on clomiphene regimens, whereas others reported no improvement in fertility. In the few studies that did include controls, the investigators concluded that clomiphene could not be considered an effective agent. In general, placebo-controlled studies indicate that clomiphene citrate may improve sperm concentration without improving pregnancy rates.[26–32]

In one controlled study, pregnancy rates were marginally increased in the partners of men with initial sperm concentrations greater than 10 million sperm per milliliter. The authors concluded that the prognosis for fertility with treatment was more favorable for patients with higher initial sperm concentrations.[29] However, two similar studies did not find any differences in pregnancy rates between partners of placebo- and clomiphene-treated men.[30,31] Negative results were also reported by the World Health Organization multicenter double-blind study.[32]

Investigators evaluating testolactone and tamoxifen citrate as antiestrogen therapies for men with idiopathic oligospermia have similarly reported variable results.[33–38] Tamoxifen citrate is an antiestrogen with weaker intrinsic estrogenic activity than clomiphene. Tamoxifen increases serum concentrations of LH, FSH, testosterone, and estradiol. Similar to the clomiphene studies, nonplacebo-controlled trials of tamoxifen suggested improvement in sperm concentration and pregnancy rates. However, in a placebo-controlled trial no differences in pregnancy rates between tamoxifen-treated men were found. These data indicate that tamoxifen does not improve fertility.

Similar negative results have been reported with testolactone. A preliminary uncontrolled study suggested an improvement in pregnancy rates.[39] However, in a controlled crossover trial, no differences between placebo and testolactone treatment groups were found, leading to the conclusion that testolactone does not improve fertility.[40]

A variety of other pharmacologic agents have been empirically administered to men with idiopathic infertility. These include tri-iodothyronine, vitamins A, C, and E, zinc, and bromocriptine. None of these has proven successful in the treatment of idiopathic male infertility.

## Corticosteroids

Corticosteroid immunosuppression as a therapy for antisperm antibodies is controversial. In the majority of clinical trials supporting their efficacy, men were selected for corticosteroid therapy because of the presence of circulating antibodies, not sperm-directed antibodies.[41] A double blind, placebo-controlled study of the use of 3 months of high-dose methylprednisolone in men with antisperm antibodies on their sperm surface failed to demonstrate a significant effect of such therapy on pregnancy rates, seminal, or plasma immunoglobulin G (IgG) antisperm activity, or sperm-associated IgG antisperm antibody activity. However, a significant decrease of serum associated IgG antibody was reported.[42] In a similar study, a longer treatment period improved pregnancy rates.[43] However, the risks of corticosteroid therapy increase with prolonged duration of therapy. Even with short-term therapy, cases of aseptic necrosis of the hip have occurred.[44]

# Summary

A small percentage of men with fertility problems will present with a clearly definable disorder that has a specific treatment approach, but the majority of men will not have a clearly defined cause of their infertility. Nonetheless, each man is entitled to a careful evaluation by a physician committed to the care of the male partner of an infertile couple. Empiric therapies should not be offered unless the results from controlled clinical trials indicate that they are efficacious.

# References

1. Glazner CMA, Kelly NJ, Weir MJA, et al. The diagnosis of male infertility: Prospective time-specific study of conception rates related to seminal analysis and post coital sperm-mucus, penetration and survival in otherwise unexplained infertility. *Hum Reprod* 1987; 8:665–671.

2. Sokol RZ. Medical endocrine therapy of male factor infertility. In: Overstreet JW, ed. *Infertility Reproductive Medicine Clinics of North America*. Philadelphia: W.B. Saunders, Harcourt, Brace, Jovanovich; 1992; 3:389–397.

3. Nagy Z, Liu J, Cecile J, et al. Using ejaculated, fresh, and frozen-thawed epididymal and testicular spermatozoa gives rise to comparable results after intracytoplasmic sperm injection. *Fertil Steril* 1995; 63:808–815.

4. Sokol RZ, Palacios A, Campfield LA, et al. Comparison of the kinetics of injectable testosterone in eugonadal and hypogonadal men. *Fertil Steril* 1982; 37:425–430.

5. Findlay JAC, Place VA, Snyder PJ. Transdermal delivery of testosterone. *J Clin Endocrinol Metab* 1987; 64:266–268.

6. Cunningham GR, Cordero E, Thornby JI. Testosterone replacement with transdermal therapeutic systems. *JAMA* 1989; 261:2525–2530.

7. Molitch ME, Etton RL, Blackwell RE, et al. Bromocriptine as primary therapy for prolactin secreting macroadenomas: results of a prospective multicenter study. *J Clin Endocrinol Metab* 1985; 60:698–705.

8. Sherins RJ, Howards SS II. Male infertility. In: Walsh PC, Retik AB, Stamey TA, Vaughan ED, eds. *Campbell's Urology*. Philadelphia: W.B. Saunders; 1986: 640–697.

9. Ley SB, Leonard JM. Male hypogonadotropic hypogonadism: factors influencing response to human chorionic gonadotropic and human menopausal gonadotropin, including prior endogenous androgens. *J Clin Endocrinol Metab* 1985; 61:746–752.

10. Hamman M, Berg AA. Long-term androgen replacement therapy does not preclude gonadotropin-induced improvement of spermatogenesis *Scand J Urol Nephrol* 1990; 24:17–19.

11. Sokol RZ, McClure RD, Peterson M, et al. Gonaodotropin therapy failure secondary to hCG induced antibodies. *J Clin Endocrinol Metab* 1981; 52:929–933.

12. Hoffman AR, Crowley WF. Induction of puberty in men by long-term pulsatile administration of low-dose gonadotropin-releasing hormone. *N Engl J Med* 1982; 307:1237–1241.

13. Skarin G, Nillius SJ, Wibell I. Chronic pulsatile low dose GnRH therapy for induction of testosterone production and spermatogenesis in a man with secondary hypogonadotropic hypogonadism. *J Clin Endocrinol Metab* 1982; 55:723–726.

14. Donald RA, Wheeler M, Sonksen PH, et al. Hypogonadotropic hypogonadism resistant to hCG and responsive to GnRH: report of a case. *Clin Endocrinol* 1983; 18:385–389.

15. Shoham Z, Conway CS, Ostergaard H, et al. Co-treatment with growth hormone for induction of spermatogenesis in patients with hypogonadotropic hypogonadism. *Fertil Steril* 1992; 57:1044–1051.

16. Steinberger A. Clinical assessment of treatment results in male infertility. In: Santen RJ, Swerdloff RS, eds. *Male Reproductive Dysfunction.* New York: Marcel Dekker; 1986: 373–386.

17. Keough EJ, Burger HG, DeKretser DM, et al. Non-surgical management of male infertility. In: Hafez ESP, ed. *Human Semen and Fertility Regulation in Men.* St. Louis: C.V. Mosby; 1976: 452–463.

18. Gerris J, Comhaire F, Hellemans P, et al. Placebo-controlled trial of high-dose mesterolone treatment of idiopathic male infertility. *Fertil Steril* 1991; 55:603–607.

19. Comhaire FH. Treatment of idiopathic testicular failure with high-dose testosterone undecanoate: a double-blind pilot study. *Fertil Steril* 1990; 54:689–693.

20. Rosenberg E. Medical treatment of male infertility. *Andrologia* 1976; 8(suppl 1):95–107.

21. Lunenfeld B, Mor A, Mani M. Treatment of male infertility I. Human gonadotropins. *Fertil Steril* 1967; 18:581–592.

22. Acosta AA, Khalifa E, Oehninger S. Pure human follicle stimulating hormone has a role in the treatment of severe male infertility by assisted reproduction: Norfolk's total experience. *Hum Reprod* 1992; 7:1067–1072.

23. Bartov Z, Eltes F, Lunenfeld E, et al. Sperm quality of subfertile males before and after treatment with follicle stimulating hormone. *Fertil Steril* 1994; 61:727–734.

24. Crottaz B, Senn RF, Germond M, et al. Stimulating hormone bioactivity in idiopathic normogonadotropic oligoasthenozoospermia: double-blind trial with GnRH. *Fertil Steril* 1992; 57:1034–1043.

25. Adashi EY. Clomiphene citrate. Mechanism(s) and site(s) of action: a hypothesis revisited. *Fertil Steril* 1985; 42:331–344.

26. Weiland RG, Anasar AH, Klein DE, et al. Idiopathic oligospermia: control observations and response to cis-clomiphene. *Fertility Steril* 1972; 23:471–474.

27. Mascala A, Delitala G, Alagna S, et al. Effect of clomiphene citrate on plasma levels of immunoreactive luteinizing hormone-releasing hormone, gonadotropin, and testosterone in normal subjects and in patients with idiopathic oligospermia. *Fertil Steril* 1978; 29:424–427.

28. Foss GL, Tindal VR, Birkett JP. The treatment of subfertile men with clomiphene citrate. *J Reprod Fertil* 1973; 37:167–170.

29. Wang C, Chan CW, Wong KK, et al. Comparison of the effectiveness of placebo, clomiphene citrate, mesterolone, pentoxifylline, and testosterone rebound therapy for the treatment of idiopathic oligospermia. *Fertil Steril* 1983; 40:358–365.

30. Micic S, Dotlic M. Evaluation of sperm parameters in clinical trial with clomiphene citrate of oligospermic men. *J Urol* 1985; 133:221–222.

31. Sokol RZ, Steiner BS, Bustillo M, et al. A controlled comparison of the efficacy of clomiphene citrate in male infertility. *Fertil Steril* 1988; 49:865–870.

32. World Health Organization. *Special Programme of Research, Development and Research Training in Human Reproduction Annual Technical Report 1990.* Geneva: WHO; 1991: 146–147.

33. AinMelk Y, Belisle S, Caimel M, et al. Tamoxifen citrate therapy in male infertility. *Fertil Steril* 1987; 48:113–117.

34. Buvat J, Ardaens K, Lemaire A, et al. Increased sperm count in 25 cases of idiopathic normogonadotropic oligospermia following treatment with tamoxifen. *Fertil Steril* 1983; 39:700–703.

35. Comhaire FH. Treatment of oligospermia with tamoxifen. *Int J Fertil* 1976; 21:232–238.

36. Comhaire FH. Tamoxifen. In: Bain J, Schill WB, Schwarzstein L, eds. *Treatment of Male Infertility.* New York: Springer-Verlag; 1982: 45.

37. Vermeulen A, Comhaire F. Hormonal effects of an antiestrogen, tamoxifen, in normal and oligospermic men. *Fertil Steril* 1978; 29:320–327.

38. Willis KJ, London DR, Bevis MA, et al. Hormonal effects of tamoxifen in oligospermic men. *J Endocrinol* 1977; 73:171–178.

39. Vigersky RA, Glass AR. Effects of delta-1-testolactone on the pituitary-testicular axis in oligospermic men. *J Clin Endocrinol Metab* 1981; 52:897–902.

40. Clark RV, Sherins RJ. Clinical trail of testolactone for treatment of idiopathic male infertility. *J Androl* 1989; 10:240–247.

41. Haas GG. Evaluation of sperm antibodies in autoimmunity in the infertile male. In: Santen RJ, Swerdloff RS, eds. *Male Reproductive Dysfunction.* New York: Marcel Dekker; 1986: 439–456.

42. Haas GG Jr, Manganiello P. A double-blind, placebo-controlled study of the use of methyl-prednisolone in infertile men with sperm-associated immunoglubulins. *Fertil Steril* 1987; 47:295–301.

43. Hendry WF, Hughes L, Scammell G, et al. Comparison of prednisolone and placebo in subfertile men with antibodies to spermatozoa. *Lancet* 1990; 335:85–88.

44. Hendry WF. Bilateral aseptic necrosis of femoral heads following intermittent high-dose steroid therapy (letter). *Fertil Steril* 1982; 38:120.

# 11
# Testicular Biopsy and Vasography

Ira D. Sharlip and Seck L. Chan

## Testis Biopsy

Testis biopsy is performed to identify the quality of spermatogenesis in patients who may have obstructive male infertility or to identify the presence of testicular sperm cells, which may be aspirated and used for intracytoplasmic sperm injection (ICSI). Testis biopsy may also be used to identify the presence of round spermatids, which may be aspirated and used for round spermatid nuclear injection (ROSNI).

## Indications

The primary indication for testis biopsy is to aid in the diagnosis of obstruction of the male reproductive system. In the azoospermic patient, the findings of normal volume and consistency of the testes with normal serum follicle-stimulating hormone (FSH) should create suspicion that obstruction is present. A testicular biopsy is needed in these patients to identify whether spermatogenesis is normal or subnormal. If normal, obstruction must be present at some level. Testis biopsy to rule out obstruction is indicated not only in men who are azoospermic but also in men who are oligozoospermic and have normal volume and consistency of the testes with normal FSH. The severity of oligozoospermia, which is compatible with obstruction, is a matter of controversy. There is general agreement that testicular biopsy should be performed on men whose sperm counts are consistently less than 5 million/ml and on men with sperm counts in the range of 5

to 10 million/ml if sperm motility also is markedly reduced. Testicular biopsy is not helpful, and therefore is not indicated, in men whose sperm counts are consistently greater than 10 million/ml, except in some specific cases in which there is a particularly high degree of suspicion of obstructive infertility. Such cases include men with partial ejaculatory duct obstruction, previous vasectomy reversal, or previous bilateral hernia or scrotal surgery. In the clinical setting in which there is a particularly high degree of suspicion of obstruction, testicular biopsy may be useful even if sperm counts are as high as 20 million/ml as long as there is also marked reduction of motility.

Transrectal ultrasonography of the prostate, seminal vesicles, and ejaculatory ducts should be a routine part of the evaluation of the patient with azoospermia or marked oligoasthenozoospermia. This simple noninvasive procedure may show evidence of ejaculatory duct obstruction, further increasing the suspicion of an obstructive cause for infertility.

A recently developed indication for testicular biopsy is azoospermia, or very severe oligoasthenospermia of nonobstructive origin, in which no clinical treatment is available to improve spermatogenesis and insufficient numbers of sperm are present in the ejaculate for use in ICSI. Men with nonobstructive infertility may be candidates for sperm aspiration by either open or percutaneous needle biopsy of the testicle if at least a minimal amount of spermatogenesis is present. Sperm may be isolated from testicular biopsy specimens and then used

Color Plate I

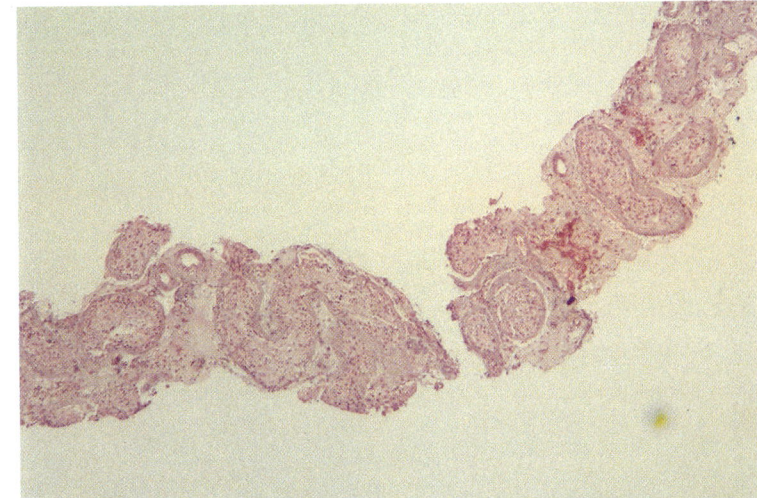

FIGURE 11.1. Human testis biopsy obtained by Biopty gun percutaneously and preserved in Bouin's solution (low-power view).

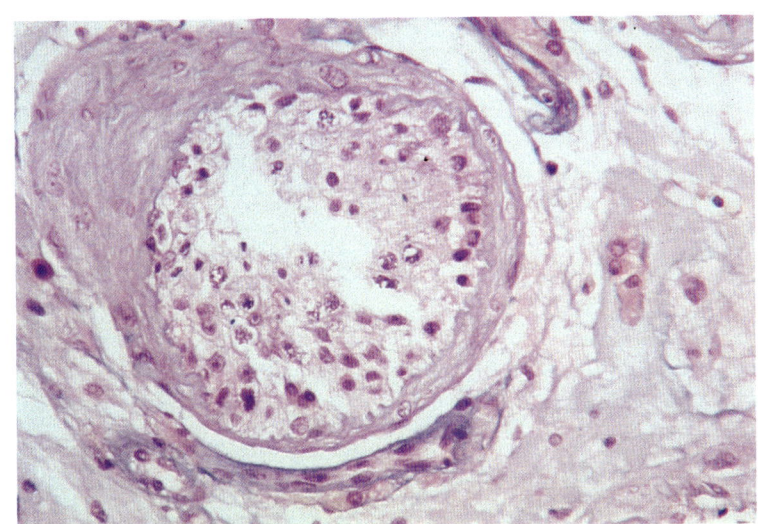

FIGURE 11.2. High-power view of human testis biopsy obtained by Biopty gun percutaneously. The germinal epithelium architecture and cellular relationships are well preserved.

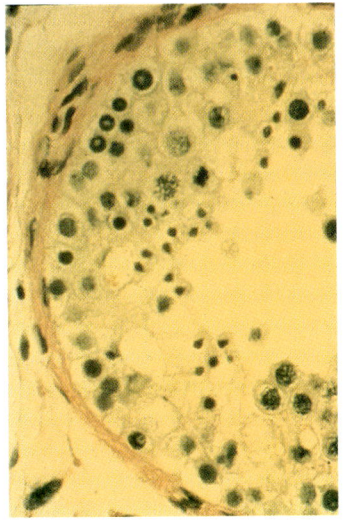

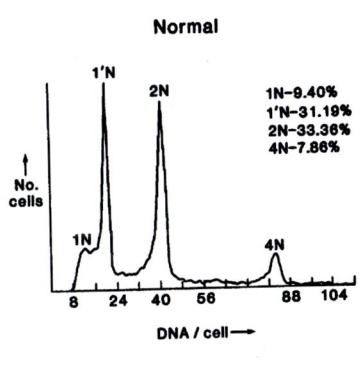

FIGURE 11.4. Normal spermatogenesis—histology and DNA histogram. The proportion of the various cellular elements characterizes the composition of the germinal epithelium.

Color Plate II

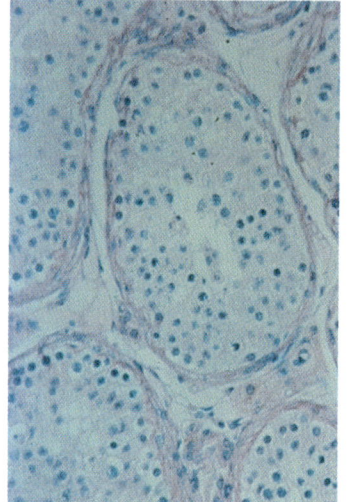

FIGURE 11.6. Maturation arrest at the primary spermatocyte stage—histology and DNA histogram.

**Maturation Arrest**

1N-<1%
1'N-10.68%
2N-69.86%
4N-14.31%

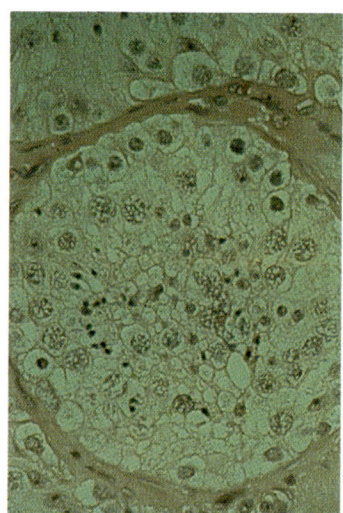

FIGURE 11.7. Hypospermatogenesis—histology and DNA histogram.

**Hypospermatogenesis**

1N-13.96%
1'N-45.45%
2N-22.14%
4N-12.16%

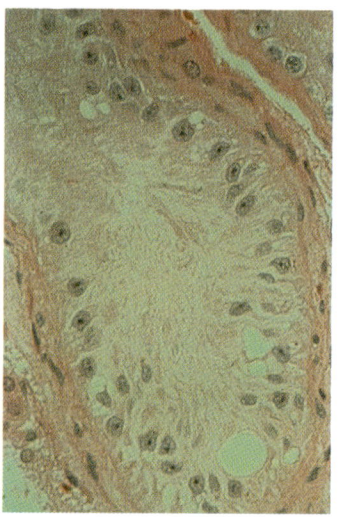

FIGURE 11.8. Germinal Aplasia (Sertoli-cell–only syndrome)—histology and DNA histogram.

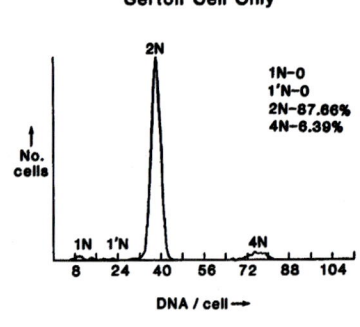

**Sertoli Cell Only**

1N-0
1'N-0
2N-87.66%
4N-6.39%

for ICSI into the human oocyte. Even if spermatogenic arrest has prevented the formation of mature spermatozoa, the finding of round spermatids in testicular tissue is significant. Intracytoplasmic injection of round spermatids or round spermatid nuclei, which have a haploid set of chromosomes, has produced pregnancy and live births in a small number of cases, both animal and human.

In most instances, it is preferable to perform a testicular biopsy as a separate diagnostic procedure. Analysis of permanent sections from a testicular biopsy is much more accurate in identifying normal spermatogenesis than using the fresh-frozen technique or touch-imprint technique. Because testicular biopsy can be performed as a simple, in-office procedure with local anesthesia and minimal postoperative discomfort, it is logical to perform this biopsy prior to planning a therapeutic procedure. Only in unusual cases with a high degree of expectation that obstruction is present should testicular biopsy be performed simultaneously with therapeutic procedures like vasoepididymostomy or ejaculatory duct incision.

## Technique

Open surgical biopsy of the testicle is the standard method for obtaining testicular tissue for diagnostic and therapeutic use. Testicular tissue may also be obtained by percutaneous needle biopsy of the testis.

*Open testicular biopsy* can be performed without an assistant as a 15-minute in-office procedure using local anesthesia. The patient is placed in the supine position, and the skin of the scrotum on the side to be biopsied is shaved and scrubbed with antiseptic solution. The spermatic cord is blocked with 0.25% bupivacaine using a 27-gauge needle, and the skin of the anticipated biopsy site is infiltrated with bupivacaine or 1% lidocaine. After the block is established, it is usually possible to palpate the epididymis. The surgeon uses one hand to immobilize the testicle in the scrotum and to stretch the skin of the anterior scrotal wall over the anterior surface of the testis, making sure to keep the epididymis on the posterior side of the scrotum. With the other hand, a $\frac{1}{2}$- to

$\frac{3}{4}$-cm horizontal incision is made in the anterior scrotal skin. Continuing with the scalpel, the scrotal tunics are incised and the parietal layer of tunica vaginalis is identified and incised. A 5-mm incision is made into the tunica albuginea. By producing counterpressure on the posterior surface of the testicle, testicular tissue may be evaginated into the incision in the tunica albuginea. Tenotomy scissors are used to excise a small piece of testicular tissue. For both diagnostic purposes and for therapeutic isolation of mature spermatozoa from testicular tissue, the amount of testicular tissue needed is approximately 2 to 4 mm in each of the three dimensions. For ROSNI, the goal is to obtain approximately 50 mg of testicular tissue. This is equivalent to a spherical piece of testicular tissue measuring about 4 mm in each of the three dimensions. After the proper amount of tissue has been removed, it is transferred to a special solution (not formalin), with specific care taken not to squeeze or distort the biopsy material. For diagnostic biopsy, Bouin's or Zenker's solution should be used. For therapeutic biopsy, Biggers, Whitten, and Whittingham (BWW) solution, human tubal fluid, or Ham's F-10 solution may be used, or the tissue may be transferred directly to the sperm laboratory in a sterile container with no solution, provided the laboratory is prepared to accept and process the tissue immediately.

The incision in the tunica albuginea is then closed with one or two interrupted sutures of 4-0 polyglycolic acid. The anterior layer of tunica vaginalis is closed with the same material, as is the skin. A mildly compressive gauze dressing and scrotal supporter are applied and worn for 24 hours.

For *needle biopsy of the testis*, the patient should lie supine in a warm environment. The scrotal skin is prepared with alcohol, which is preferable to iodine-based solution because traces of iodine may contaminate the needle and reduce the viability of sperm cells. Cord block is achieved with 0.25% bupivacaine, using a 27-gauge needle to avoid accidental injury to the spermatic vessels. The scrotal skin at the anticipated biopsy site is infiltrated with local anesthetic. With the scrotal skin stretched over the testicle and immobilized with one hand, the

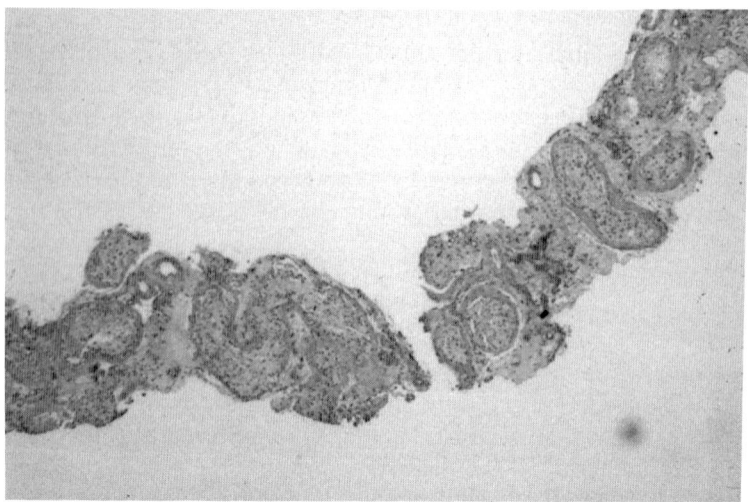

FIGURE 11.1. Human testis biopsy obtained by Biopty gun percutaneously and preserved in Bouin's solution (low-power view). See color plate.

other hand is used to make a 1- to 2-mm skin incision on the inferior aspect of the scrotum. The epididymis is fixed posterolaterally by the opposing hand to avoid accidental puncture.

Several different types of needles have been suggested for use in obtaining the biopsy, such as a Biopty gun armed with a 10-cm, 20-gauge needle that produces tissue specimens sufficient for either diagnostic or therapeutic uses (Figs. 11.1 and 11.2, see color insert). The needle is placed at the puncture site in the lower scrotum and directed away from the epididymis. If the testicle is small, care must be taken not only to avoid puncturing the tunica albuginea on the

opposite side of the scrotum but also to avoid injuring the hand that is immobilizing the testicle. Using a needle with a 22-mm core length will help avoid such a complication. The same skin incision may be used for several passes of the biopsy needle. For diagnostic biopsy, one or two passes are sufficient. Three to four samples usually yield sufficient tissue for selecting spermatozoa to be used for ICSI if there is normal spermatogenesis. Patients with poor sperm production probably require more samples. Once an adequate amount of tissue has been obtained, digital pressure is applied to the puncture site for a few minutes to minimize

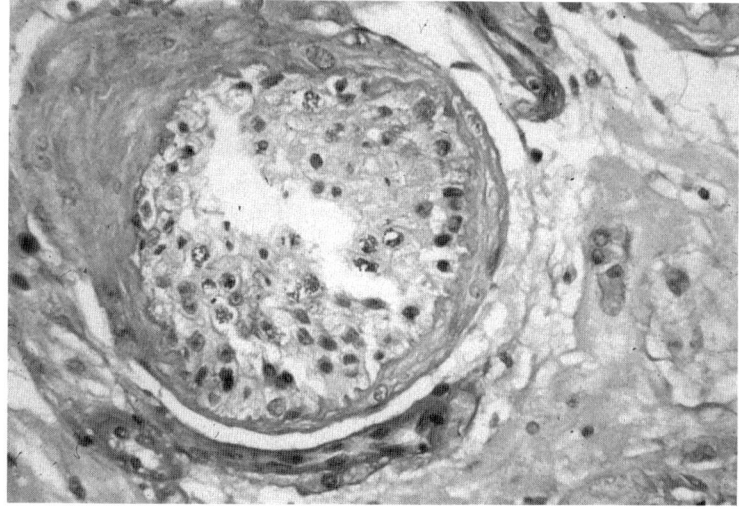

FIGURE 11.2. High-power view of human testis biopsy obtained by Biopty gun percutaneously. The germinal epithelium architecture and cellular relationships are well preserved. See color plate.

hematocele formation. A pressure dressing is not required. The patient is advised to avoid rigorous physical activity and platelet-inhibiting medication for 24 hours. Postoperative pain is managed with acetaminophen, ibuprofen, or Vicodin.

With either open or needle biopsy of the testicle, some surgeons routinely perform diagnostic testicular biopsy bilaterally rather than unilaterally. The argument in favor of bilateral biopsy is that there may be significant discrepancy of spermatogenesis between the two sides. However, unilateral biopsy may be performed when both testicles are equal in volume and consistency. If the testes are not symmetric in volume and consistency, the larger, firmer testis should be biopsied because it is more likely to show good spermatogenesis and therefore more likely to support a diagnosis of obstruction. It is sufficient to perform therapeutic testicular biopsy unilaterally only, unless not enough sperm cells are obtained otherwise. There may be variations in testicular histology within one testis or even within one biopsy specimen. This suggests that it may be advisable to perform more extensive unilateral or even bilateral therapeutic testicular biopsy than has been the practice in the past.

## Interpretation

Standard evaluation of testicular biopsy uses light microscopy. Interpretation of testicular biopsy is purely descriptive and is often subjective.[1] Testicular biopsy does not provide information about the underlying pathophysiology. Electron microscopy of the germinal epithelium has also been studied as a means of identifying additional pathologic features.[2–4] However, electron microscopy has not proven to be specific and, like light microscopy, fails to characterize the pathophysiology and etiology of abnormal spermatogenesis.

Numerous attempts have been made to quantify spermatogenesis on testicular biopsy but none has been well accepted for clinical use.[5–7] One method is based on counting the number of mature spermatids in seminiferous tubules that have been transected transversely.[8] Correlation was noted between the average number of spermatids per seminiferous tubule and sperm concentration in the ejaculate. For example, the finding of greater than 20 spermatids per seminiferous tubule is associated with a sperm count of greater than 10 million/ml. This technique may be used to predict what the sperm count might be if obstruction were not present. If the actual sperm concentration is less than predicted by the biopsy material, evidence of obstruction is thought to be present. This technique, however, is time-consuming, and it cannot be used in instances of maturation-arrest at the spermatid stage. When the amount of tissue biopsied is small, sampling error may be encountered due to the heterogeneous nature of the germinal epithelium. The original study[8] was based on a relatively small number of patients, and the validity of this work has not been verified by other independent authors. As of 1997, testicular biopsy continues to be useful only as a qualitative, rather than as a quantitative, study.

In the search for a reliable and reproducible modality to quantify spermatogenesis, a number of investigators have evaluated DNA flow cytometry.[9–13] Very minute amounts of seminiferous tubules obtained by needle biopsy of the testicle may be used and processed rapidly. The basic principle of pulsatile flow cytometry involves the passage of cells or subcellular components in aqueous solution through a sensing region at speeds of 1000 cells/s. Optical signals indicative of specific biologic properties are generated.[14] In the case of testicular tissue, the heterogeneous cellular population may be characterized by its DNA content as haploid, diploid, or tetraploid. Staining with a DNA-specific fluorochrome is used. Excitation by an illuminating source, such as a laser or mercury arc lamp, will elicit fluorescent emission. This signal is sensed through a collecting lens with a photomultiplier tube, thus generating an electrical impulse proportional to the fluorescent intensity. These impulses are further processed and recorded as a pulse-height distribution or DNA histogram (Fig. 11.3). Each of the peaks represents a cellular subpopulation with specific DNA content or ploidy. The area under these peaks may be integrated by computer analysis to yield quantitative information on

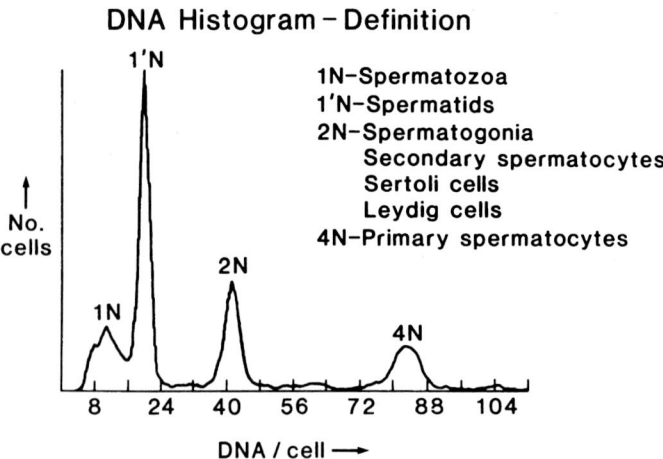

## DNA Histogram – Definition

1N–Spermatozoa
1′N–Spermatids
2N–Spermatogonia
    Secondary spermatocytes
    Sertoli cells
    Leydig cells
4N–Primary spermatocytes

FIGURE 11.3. DNA histogram of human testis by flow cytometry.

the relative proportion of each cell type with respect to the total cell population.

## Histologic Classification

Infertile men exhibit a spectrum of testicular pathology that can be grouped into one of various patterns.

### Normal

Normal testicular tissue is composed predominantly of seminiferous tubules with blood vessels and Leydig cells in the interstitial areas. The seminiferous tubules consist of the progressively maturing germ cells and the nutritive Sertoli cells surrounding them. The germ cells go through an orderly progression from the most immature stages, or spermatogonia, to primary spermatocytes, secondary spermatocytes, spermatids, and mature spermatozoa. The seminiferous tubules are lined by a basement membrane and myoid cells. Spermatogenesis begins in the periphery of the tubule and progresses toward the lumen in specific cellular associations called stages[15] (Fig. 11.4, see color insert). Type A spermatogonia have a diploid set of chromosomes (2n). They undergo mitotic divisions to replenish the stock of type A stem cells and to create type B spermatogonia (2n). The latter differentiate into preleptotene primary spermatocytes that undergo DNA synthe-

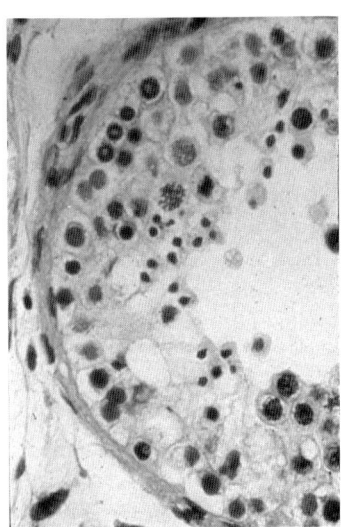

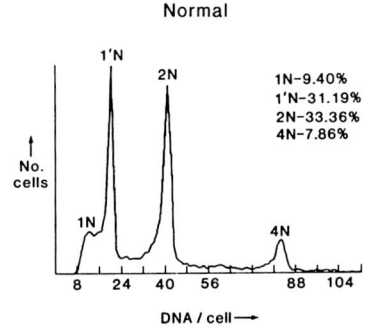

Normal

1N–9.40%
1′N–31.19%
2N–33.36%
4N–7.86%

FIGURE 11.4. Normal spermatogenesis—histology and DNA histogram. The proportion of the various cellular elements characterizes the composition of the germinal epithelium. See color plate.

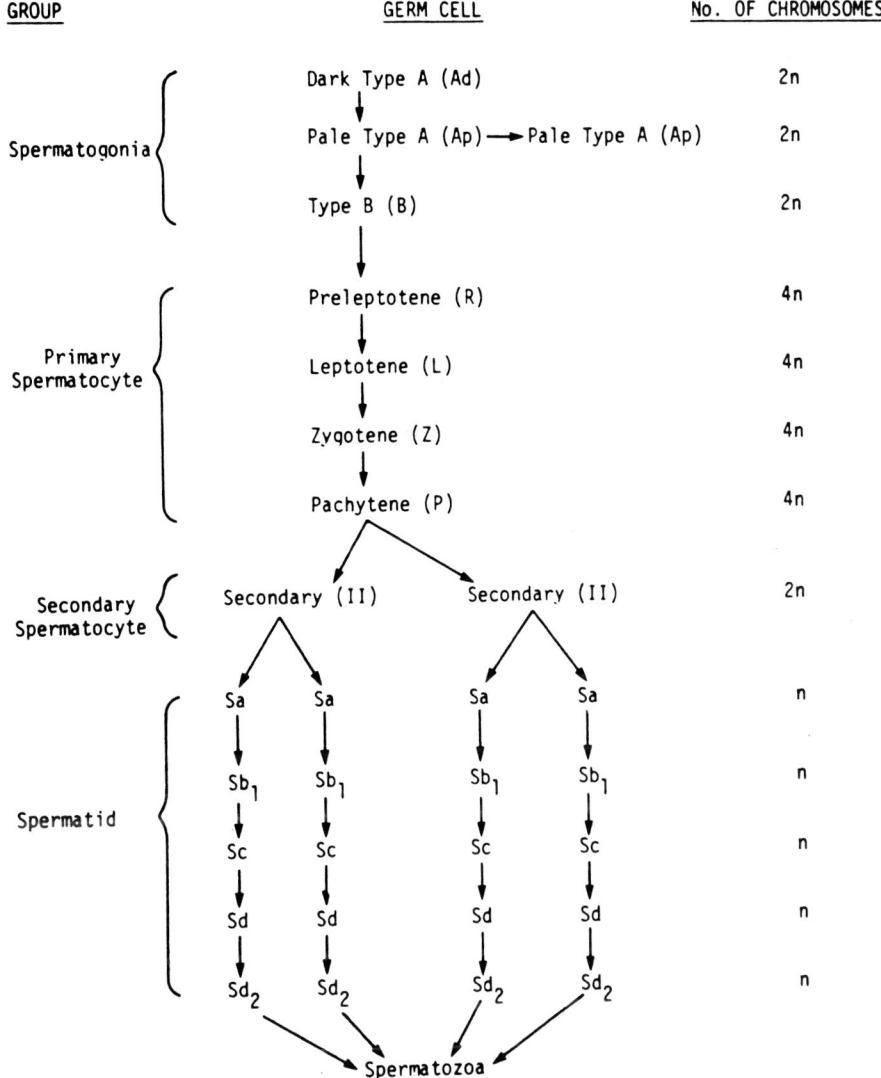

FIGURE 11.5. Spermatogenesis and spermiogenesis in the human testis. (From Chan et al.[27])

sis, which results in a tetraploid number of chromosomes (4n) (Fig. 11.5). Further transformation occurs within the adluminal compartment of the seminiferous tubules as the blood-testis barrier is traversed. The pachytene primary spermatocytes (4n) then undergo meiotic reduction division, resulting in secondary spermatocytes (2n). A second reduction division gives rise to the spermatids that have a haploid number of chromosomes (n). Further differentiation leads to the production of round spermatids, elongated spermatids, and finally mature spermatozoa. The process is completed in about 72 days.

DNA histograms obtained by flow cytometry characterize this heterogeneous population according to its DNA content or ploidy. More than one third of the total cellular population consists of haploid mature spermatozoa (n) and spermatids (1'n). These two peaks are thought to be separate because the chromatin in mature spermatozoa is more compact and less susceptible to fluorochrome staining. The diploid (2n) group constitutes 40% of the cellular elements and is made up of Sertoli cells, Leydig cells, and secondary spermatocytes. Only 12% of the cells are tetraploid primary spermatocytes in various stages of development.

In cases of azoospermia, testis biopsy showing normal spermatogenesis by light microscopy is believed to be pathognomonic of obstruction in the ductal system.[16-18] Hypospermatogenesis, maturation arrest, or both have also been described in the presence of obstruction.[19-21] However, it is not clear whether these abnormalities are actually due to the obstruction or are independent coexisting findings. Camatini et al[2] described subtle changes at the completion of meiosis in patients with congenital absence of the vas. Some histologic abnormalities, such as degeneration of the germinal epithelium, thickening of the basement membrane, and minimal interstitial fibrosis, may be only transient phenomena. In the presence of azoospermia due to obstruction, electron microscopy commonly demonstrates atypical acrosome complexes and deformed headcaps. There is some evidence that spermiation may be affected. Sertoli cells show increased numbers of lysosomes, and their spatial relationships with spermatozoa are altered. No consistent changes in Leydig cells due to obstruction have been noted.

Intraoperative assessment of spermatogenesis is sometimes necessary in cases of suspected ductal obstruction in order to facilitate immediate exploration and microsurgical repair. A frozen section of testicular biopsy material is often inaccurate because of distortion artifacts. A touch imprint technique may be used, which predicts obstruction if mature spermatozoa are found. However, this technique fails to identify motility because the fixation and staining process inactivates sperm cells.[22] Jow and coworkers[23] have described a "wet prep" technique to permit intraoperative assessment of motility. A small piece of testicular tissue mixed with Ringer's lactated solution is compressed between a glass slide and cover slip. The finding of motile sperm around the periphery of the compressed tissue correlates well with ductal obstruction. Motile sperm are a potential source of sperm that may be obtained by needle or open biopsy and used for intracytoplasmic injection into human oocytes, provided microsurgical reconstruction of the ductal obstruction is not feasible.[24]

## Maturation Arrest

In maturation arrest, there is a block of sperm maturation at a specific stage of spermatogenesis with normal numbers of germ cells at stages

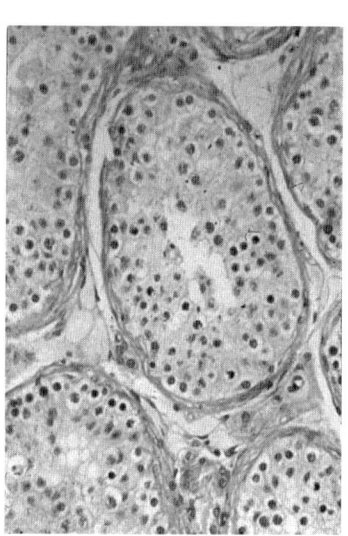
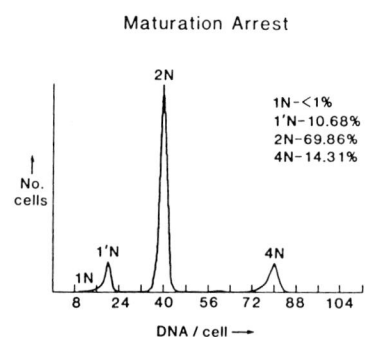

Figure 11.6. Maturation arrest at the primary spermatocyte stage—histology and DNA histogram. See color plate.

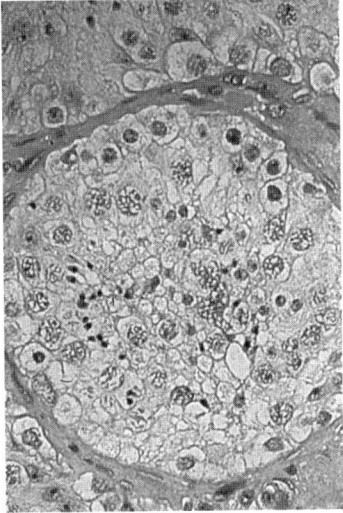

FIGURE 11.7. Hypospermato-genesis—histology and DNA histogram. See color plate.

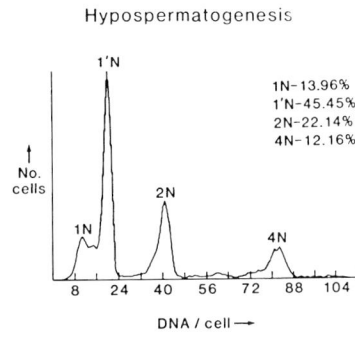

preceding the arrest (Fig. 11.6, see color insert). This point is constant for the individual patient, but varies from one patient to another. The two most common points of spermatogenic arrest are primary spermatocytes or late spermatids. No abnormalities are present in the Leydig cells, Sertoli cells, or in the general architecture of the seminiferous tubules. The DNA histogram in Figure 11.6 shows arrest at the primary spermatocyte stage, with the majority of cells in the diploid and tetraploid state at the expense of the haploid cells. Clinically, patients with maturation arrest have severe oligozoospermia or azoospermia.

## Hypospermatogenesis

In hypospermatogenesis, there is a generalized decrease in the absolute number of all germ cells and a resultant thinning of the germinal epithelium (Fig. 11.7, see color insert). All cell types are present in approximately normal proportion. Narbaitz et al[4] described normal cellular relationships and normal nongerminal elements by electron microscopy. Thick banded collagen fibers are observed in the tunica propria. The presence of these collagen fibers seems to be dependent on the degree of depletion of the germinal epithelium. DNA flow cytometry reveals a relative predominance of tetraploid (4n) and haploid cells (1'n) with a decrease in mature spermatozoa (1n) and

diploid cells (2n). Patients generally have oligospermia of varying degrees.

## Combination

In some biopsies, there is a mixed picture of maturation arrest and hypospermatogenesis with patchy areas containing tubules lined only by Sertoli cells. Peritubular fibrosis is common, and hyalinization of tubules is observed in more severe states. Leydig cells usually appear normal.

## Germinal Aplasia (Sertoli-Cell–Only Syndrome)

Testicular biopsies in patients with germinal aplasia typically show small seminiferous tubules and complete absence of germ cells (Fig. 11.8, see color insert). The basement membrane is normal and only Sertoli cells are present. Their cytoplasm contains large numbers of fat vacuoles. There may be an occasional tubule showing some degree of spermatogenesis. Although some investigators have described normal ultrastructural features, Carpino et al[25] noted several changes in the nuclei and organelles: nuclei were round or oval with no peripheral invagination, and they frequently lacked nucleoli; Golgi's apparatuses appeared well developed to support secretory functions, and there were very few thin filaments and residual bodies. Flow cytometry histograms char-

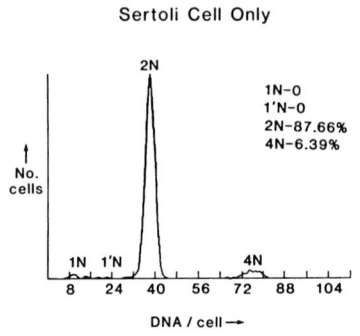

acteristically show only a major diploid (2n) peak, which represents Sertoli and Leydig cells.

### Tubular and Peritubular Sclerosis

This is an untreatable condition with absence of both germ cells and Sertoli cells in the tubules and a paucity of Leydig cells in the interstitium. The tunica propria is thickened with fibrosis. In contrast, men with Klinefelter's syndrome usually show hyperplastic nodules of Leydig cells.

## Vasography

The distal male reproductive system includes the vas deferens, ampulla of the vas, seminal vesicle, ejaculatory duct, prostate, and urethra. The proximal male reproductive system includes the testicle and epididymis.

Vasography is the definitive method of identifying the location of obstruction in the distal male reproductive system. Because vasography is done infrequently, it is best performed by a surgeon with experience in surgical andrology. The inexperienced surgeon runs the risk of injuring the vas at the injection site, causing a secondary obstruction at this location. In addition, accurate interpretation of vasography requires expertise in male reproductive abnormalities.

### Indication

When obstructive male infertility is present, the site of obstruction may be in the epididymis or in the distal male reproductive system. Other than vasal obstruction due to vasectomy, the epididymis is by far the most common location of obstruction of the male reproductive system. Ejaculatory duct obstruction and obstruction due to previous hernia or scrotal surgery are much less common. Obstruction in the retroperitoneal vas or ampulla of the vas is very rare. Unilateral obstruction may be quite common but is rarely diagnosed because patients with unilateral obstruction are usually fertile.

When obstruction occurs, semen analysis reveals either azoospermia when the obstruction is complete or severe oligoasthenozoospermia when the obstruction is incomplete. Men with a history of prior bilateral hernia surgery or scrotal surgery should be considered at risk for bilateral obstruction of the reproductive system. Obstruction should be considered in the differential diagnosis of male infertility if two or more semen analyses show azoospermia or severe oligoasthenozoospermia.

Transrectal ultrasonography of the prostate, ejaculatory duct, and seminal vesicles should be a routine part of the evaluation of the male with azoospermia or severe oligoasthenospermia. This topic is further reviewed in Chapter 12.

All patients being evaluated for male infertility should have at least one serum FSH measurement. The finding of a normal serum FSH is compatible with both obstructive and nonobstructive azoospermia or severe oligozoospermia. However, an FSH that is elevated to more than three times normal is usually pathognomonic of hypospermatogenesis or germinal aplasia. In these instances, testicular biopsy simply confirms the presence of hypo- or aspermatogenesis, and vasography is not necessary. If the serum FSH is not greater than three times normal, obstruction may be present and testicular biopsy should be performed before proceeding to vasography in order to accurately assess the quality of sperm production. If testicular biopsy shows reduced or absent sperm production, vasography is not indicated. If testicular biopsy shows normal spermatogenesis, vasography is necessary to rule out obstruction of the distal male reproductive system. Even if obstruction is present in the epididymis, vasography is still needed to rule out obstruction in the distal reproductive system, a possible cause of secondary epididymal obstruction.

Testicular biopsy with frozen sections, touch preparation, or "wet prep" technique may be performed occasionally at the time of vasography and simultaneous microsurgery and sperm aspiration, rather than prior to these procedures. Deferring testicular biopsy to the time of surgery is appropriate only when there is a very high degree of suspicion that obstruction is present. Such a high degree of suspicion of obstruction exists in the presence of azoospermia or severe oligoasthenozoospermia, normal FSH, normal testicular size and consistency, and a history of bilateral hernia or scrotal surgery, or evidence of ejaculatory duct obstruction by transrectal ultrasonography. In most cases, testicular biopsy should be performed as a separate procedure prior to vasography. Vasography is indicated by the finding of normal or nearly normal testicular histology in the patient with azoospermia or severe oligoasthenozoospermia.

## Technique

Vasography may be performed with local, regional, or general anesthesia. In some instances, the presence of ejaculatory duct obstruction will have been suggested by prevasography transrectal ultrasonography of the prostate and seminal vesicle. In instances where a microsurgical reconstructive procedure or transurethral incision of ejaculatory duct may be expected, it is best to do vasography with general anesthesia so that the therapeutic surgical procedure may be accomplished immediately following vasography.

The preoperative preparation and shave for vasography should include only the scrotum. A small upper vertical scrotal incision should be made in the anterior scrotum. The parietal layer of tunica vaginalis should be opened and the testicle and epididymis inspected. Where chronic obstruction of the distal reproductive tract exists, secondary epididymal obstruction due to sperm extravasation may have occurred on one or both sides. The visceral layer of tunica vaginalis should be opened directly over the proximal portion of the vas in a position where the vas is minimally convoluted or straight. The vas should be isolated from the surrounding tissue for about 1 cm, and a $\frac{1}{4}$-inch Penrose drain should be placed behind it. Using a #11 scalpel blade, vasotomy incision should be made through the vas muscularis and mucosa. This incision should be made through no more than 90° of the circumference of the vasal wall. To make a small vasotomy incision possible, optical magnification is necessary. This may be accomplished with loupes, but it is preferable to use an operating microscope that allows magnification of 10× to 16× normal size.

After incising the mucosa, a 22-gauge Medicut catheter should be placed into the proximal lumen, leading toward the testicle, to obtain intravasal fluid for microscopic examination. A clear plastic catheter with a blunt tip must be used, because a nontransparent catheter prevents the surgeon from knowing whether fluid has been picked up from the vas lumen. The intravasal fluid should be examined microscopically in the operating room, using magnification of 400× normal size. If the vas fluid contains sperm, significant epididymal obstruction is ruled out. However, if the vas fluid does not contain sperm, more proximal obstruction is present and vasoepididymostomy is necessary in addition to surgical correction of any obstruction in the male reproductive system.

Following examination of the vas fluid, a 23-gauge blunt-tipped needle should be placed into the vas lumen leading in the distal direction. Five to 10 ml of saline should be injected distally. In most cases of distal obstruction, less than 1 ml of fluid may be injected distally. However, there are occasional cases of distal obstruction in which there is cystic dilatation of the ejaculatory duct or a dilated müllerian duct remnant proximal to the obstruction. In these cases, it is possible to inject more than 1 ml of saline, although increased hand pressure may be needed to accomplish the injection. Five to 10 ml of 50% radiographic contrast should be injected toward the urethra. A distal vasogram may be obtained either with standard x-rays or fluoroscopy. Either of these techniques will identify the exact position and often the cause of obstruction.

When the volume and pH of the semen are normal and ejaculatory duct obstruction is not suspected, obstruction of the distal male reproductive system may be ruled out by use of saline and dye injection into the distal vas, without x-ray exposure. After the surgical vasotomy incision is made, only a trace of intravasal fluid will be found if distal obstruction is absent. Then 10 ml of sterile saline may be injected into the distal vas with a blunt-tipped 23-gauge needle. Only a small amount of pressure will be necessary to inject all of the saline when distal obstruction is not present. The absence of distal obstruction may be confirmed by the injection of 5 to 10 ml of a dilute methylene blue solution, or 1 ml of methylene blue in 10 ml of saline. After injection of this dilute methylene blue solution, blue urine may be obtained from the bladder by catheterization. In the contralateral vas, 5 to 10 ml of dilute fluorescein solution may be injected distally, or 1 ml of injectable fluorescein

with 25 ml of sterile saline. After injection of this dilute fluorescein solution, yellow, green, or orange urine may be recovered by catheterization of the bladder, proving patency of the other side.

When transrectal ultrasonography of the ejaculatory duct is normal and when the semen volume and pH are normal, saline and dye injection of the vas should replace radiographic vasography, except when intravasal injection of 10 ml of saline fails to proceed easily and completely.

Following the vasogram, the vasotomy incision should be repaired with interrupted sutures of 9-0 nylon, using a microsurgical technique. Three to five sutures should be placed through the full thickness of the vas wall, picking up a small amount of the mucosal edge. Intervening muscular sutures should be used to seal and secure the anastomosis. When a vasotomy incision has been made through just 90° of the vasal circumference and then repaired microsurgically, minimal narrowing of the vasotomy site has been found, and the vas has been noted to be clearly patent at the time of subsequent vasal surgery.

The visceral tunica vaginalis overlying the vas should be closed with 4-0 absorbable suture, and the parietal tunica vaginalis should be closed over the testicle and epididymis with the same material to provide easy access to these tissues if subsequent vasoepididymostomy is necessary. The skin and dartos should be closed in the manner of the surgeon's preference.

## Ejaculatory Duct Obstruction

Ejaculatory duct obstruction is a special category of obstructive infertility.[26] The identifying characteristics for ejaculatory duct obstruction are azoospermia or severe oligoasthenozoospermia, a decrease in the semen volume to 1.0 ml or less, and a decrease in the semen pH to 7.0 or less. In addition, the ejaculate consists of thin, watery fluid that lacks coagulation and the characteristic odor of semen. When these characteristics are present, testing of semen fructose is not necessary. If it is measured, fructose will be found to be low or absent. If the volume and pH of the semen are normal, it is almost certain that the patient does not have ejaculatory duct obstruction. However, if the volume and pH of the semen are abnormally low, there is a likelihood of ejaculatory duct obstruction. In these cases, radiographic vasography is necessary to diagnose and image the obstruction and to plan surgical treatment. When ejaculatory duct obstruction is suspected, transrectal ultrasonography of the prostate, ejaculatory ducts, and seminal vesicles may identify the location of the obstruction. Partial ejaculatory duct obstruction may be associated with azoospermia or severe oligozoospermia and low sperm motility but with normal semen volume and pH. Consequently, transrectal ultrasonography of the prostate, seminal vesicles, and ejaculatory ducts is especially important in all infertile men.

Radiographic vasography may be necessary to identify the exact location of ejaculatory duct obstruction and to plan for treatment. However, when the semen characteristics typical of ejaculatory duct obstruction are not present, ejaculatory duct obstruction may be effectively ruled out using saline and dye injection into the distal vas, rather than using radiographic vasography.

## Discussion

Some surgeons are tempted to inject contrast in the proximal direction toward the epididymis in the hope of identifying proximal obstruction. Strong injection pressure is needed to push the contrast fluid back into the epididymis. However, the wall of the epididymis is so delicate that injection in the proximal direction usually causes extravasation of contrast in the cauda epididymis, inducing a secondary obstruction where none was present previously. For that reason, proximal injection toward the epididymis during vasography is contraindicated.

Some surgeons attempt to perform vasography by percutaneous needle cannulation of the vas lumen or by transmural injection of the vas wall with a needle after exposure of the vas. Although it is possible to accomplish vasography by this method, there is a risk of injury to the vas wall or extravasation of the contrast fluid into the perivasal or intramural tissue. Consequently, needle injection of the vas, either percutaneously or transmurally, may cause vasal obstruction.

Vasography is equally effective whether standard radiographic technique or fluoroscopy is used. An advantage of the standard radiologic technique is that the surgeon may leave the room during the radiographic exposure, eliminating the surgeon's exposure to radiation, because real-time fluoroscopy requires the surgeon's hands to be in the field of fluoroscopic exposure.

The normal unobstructed vas lumen has a diameter 0.3 to 0.5 mm. In cases of significant obstruction of the distal vas or ejaculatory duct, the vas lumen is dilated to 0.6 to 1.0 mm. This increase in vas luminal diameter is a subtle, but consistent, vasographic finding in the presence of distal obstruction.

The orientation of the distal portion of the unobstructed ejaculatory duct is straight and parasagittal to the urethral midline in the anteroposterior (AP) projection. The two ejaculatory ducts run parallel to one another and are separated by only a few millimeters. When fluoroscopy is used during vasography, the injected contrast material may be seen to enter the urethra and bladder within 1 to 5 seconds after injection into the vas lumen.

One of the rare causes of ejaculatory duct obstruction is a midline retroprostatic cyst. In such cases, both vasa may empty into the midline cystic structure. Consequently, injection of contrast into one vas may opacify the ipsilateral distal vas, the midline retroprostatic cyst, or even the distal portion of the contralateral vas. In addition, the retroprostatic cyst may have a small communication with the urethra, and, if such a communication exists, a small amount of the contrast may enter the prostatic urethra and bladder.

Figures 11.9 to 11.14 illustrate normal and abnormal vasograms.

## Complications

The major risk of vasography is the occurrence of partial or complete stenosis at the site of the vasotomy incision. Injury to the intramural

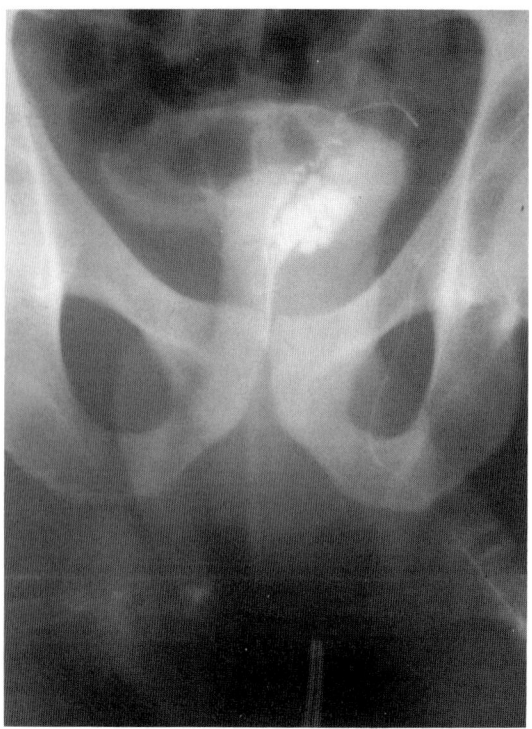

FIGURE 11.9. Normal left vasogram. Note the delicate anatomy of the distal reproductive system.

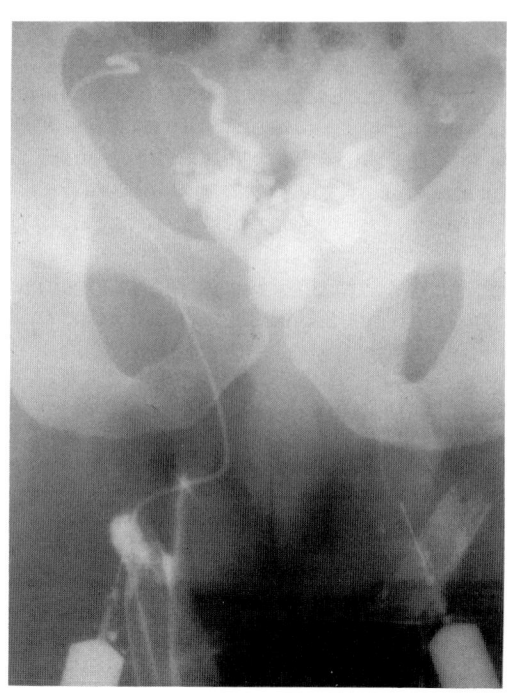

FIGURE 11.11. Midline retroprostatic cyst overlying symphysis pubis. In this position, the cyst is accessible by transurethral incision in the midline of the floor of the prostate.

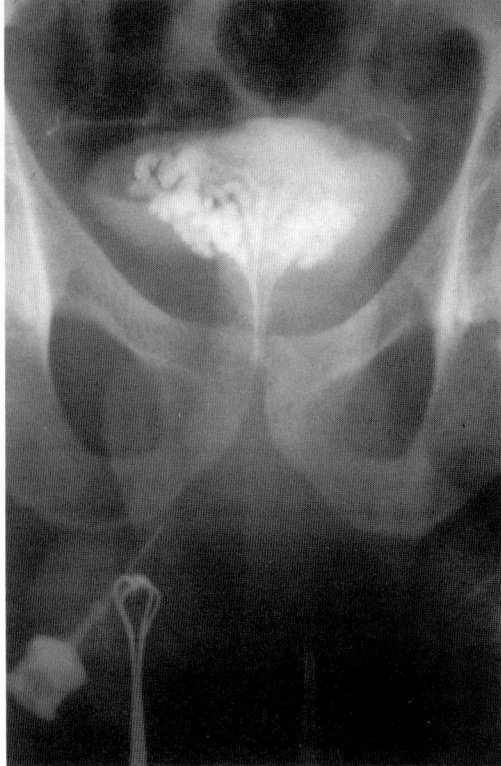

FIGURE 11.10. Normal bilateral vasograms. The ejaculatory ducts are straight and parallel to one another.

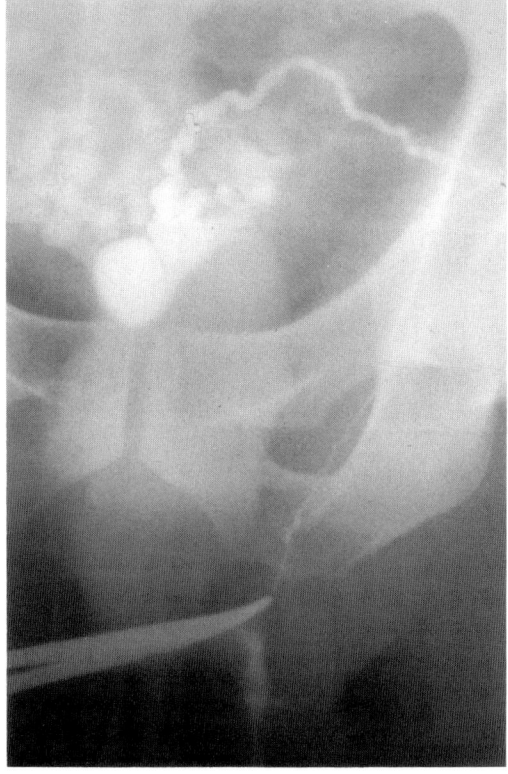

FIGURE 11.12. Midline retrovesical cyst lying superior to the symphysis pubis. This cyst was too cephalad to be accessible through transurethral incision of the prostate.

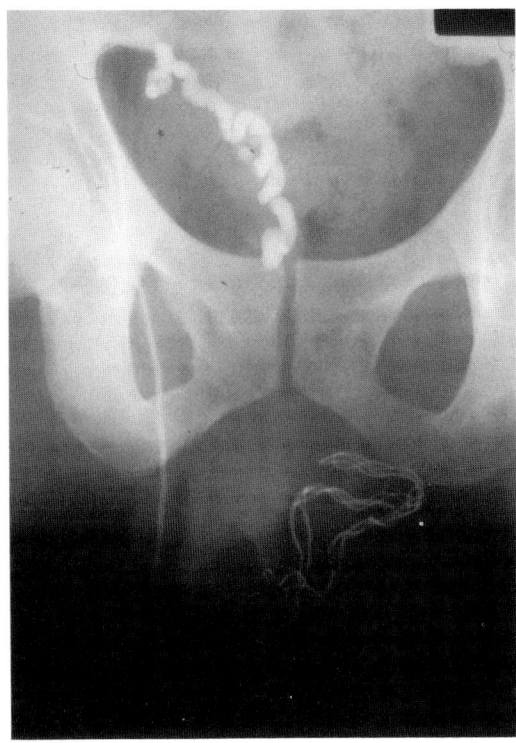

FIGURE 11.13. Obstruction of the ampulla of the right vas deferens due to pull-through anoplasty for imperforate anus.

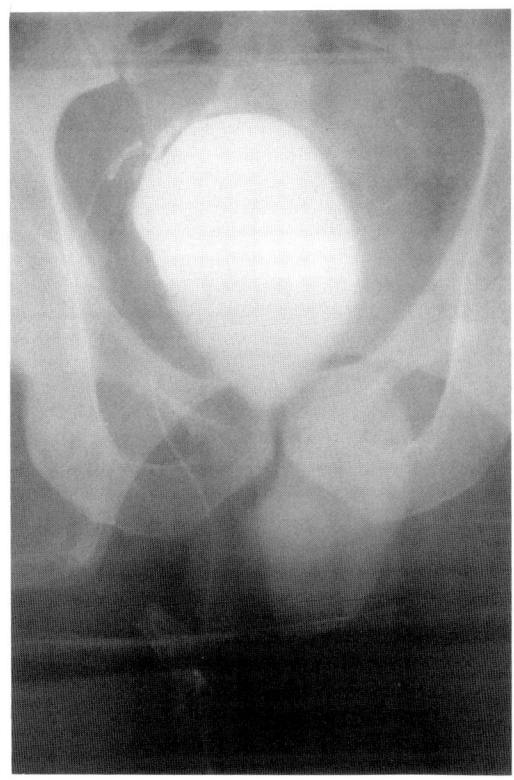

FIGURE 11.14. Huge retrovesical midline cyst simulating the bladder. Contrast was instilled from the vas and filled the large cyst. No contrast was placed into the bladder.

blood supply of the vas may occur, resulting in fibrosis of the vas wall. This may, in turn, result in the absence of muscular contraction during ejaculation, creating a functional obstruction at this site. Perivasal fibrosis, hematoma, and sperm granuloma may also occur.

## Conclusion

The recent development of intracytoplasmic sperm injection has created a new indication for testis biopsy, i.e., "therapeutic" testis biopsy. In the future, it is likely that more needle and open testicular biopsies will be performed. Andrologic surgeons and gamete technicians may be expected to gain increasing familiarity with testis biopsy and histology as this trend develops.

## References

1. Wong TW, Straus FH, Warner NE. Testicular biopsy in the study of male infertility. I. Testicular causes of infertility. *Arch Pathol* 1973; 95:151–159.
2. Camatini M, Franchi E, Faleri M. Ultrastructure of spermiogenesis in men with congenital absence of the vasa deferentia. *Arch Androl* 1979; 3:93–99.
3. Re M, Carpino F, Familiari G, et al. Ultrastructural characteristics of idiopathic spermatidic arrest. *Arch Androl* 1979; 2:283–289.
4. Narbaitz R, Tolnai G, Jolly E, et al. Ultrastructural studies on testicular biopsies from eighteen cases of hypospermatogenesis. *Fertil Steril* 1978; 30:679–686.
5. Clermont Y. The cycle of seminiferous epithelium in man. *Am J Anat* 1963; 112:35–44.

6. Steinberger E, Tjioe DY. A method for quantitative analysis of human seminiferous epithelium. *Fertil Steril* 1968; 19:959–961.

7. Zukerman Z, Rodriguez-Rigau LJ, Weiss D, et al. Quantitative analysis of the seminiferous epithelium in human testicular biopsies, and the relation of spermatogenesis to sperm density. *Fertil Steril* 1978; 30:448–455.

8. Silber SJ, Rodriguez-Rigau LJ. Quantitative analysis of testicle biopsy: determination of partial obstruction and prediction of sperm count after surgery for obstruction. *Fertil Steril* 1981; 36:480–485.

9. Clausen OPF, Purvis K, Hansson V. Quantitation of spermatogenesis by flow cytometric DNA measurements. *Int J Androl* 1978; 1(suppl 2):513–522.

10. Abyholm T, Clausen OP. Clinical evaluation of DNA flow cytometry of fine-needle aspirates from testes of infertile man. *Int J Androl* 1981; 4:505–514.

11. Chan SL, Lipshultz LI, Schwartzendruber D. Deoxyribonucleic acid (DNA) flow cytometry: a new modality for quantitative analysis of testicular biopsies. *Fertil Steril* 1984; 41:485–487.

12. Kaufman DG, Nagler HM. Aspiration flow cytometry of the testes in the evaluation of spermatogenesis in the infertile male. *Fertil Steril* 1987; 48:287–291.

13. Hellstrom WJG, Telsuk H, Deitch AD, et al. Comparison of flow cytometry to routine testis biopsy in male infertility. *Urology* 1990; 35:321–326.

14. Pinkel D, Dean P, Lake D, et al. Flow cytometry of mammalian sperm—progress in DNA and morphology measurement. *J Histochem Cytochem* 1979; 27:353–358.

15. Heller CG, Clermont Y. Kinetics of the germinal epithelium in man. *Recent Prog Horm Res* 1964; 20:545–553.

16. Wong TW, Straus FH, Jones TM, et al. Pathological aspects of the infertile testis. *Urol Clin North Am* 1978; 5:503–530.

17. Hagedoorn JP, David TE. Fine structure of the seminiferous tubules after vasectomy in man. *Physiologist* 1974; 17:236.

18. Gupta I, Dhawan S, Goel GD. Low fertility in vasovasostomy males and its possible immunologic mechanism. *Int Fertil* 1975; 20:183–191.

19. Joshi KY, Ramedo ZN, Sachder K. Effects of vasectomy in testis. *Int Surg* 1972; 57:711–713.

20. Oswin Perera BMA. Changes in the structure and function of the testis and epididymides in vasectomized rams. *Fertil Steril* 1978; 29:354–359.

21. Kubota R. Electron microscopic studies on the testis after vasectomy in rats and men. *Jpn J Urol* 1969; 60:373–397.

22. Coburn M, Wheeler TM, Lipshultz LI. Testicular biopsy: its use and limitations. *Urol Clin North Am* 1987; 14:551–561.

23. Jow WW, Steckel J, Schlegel PN, et al. Motile sperm in human testis biopsy specimens. *J Androl* 1993; 14:194–198.

24. Barnes FL, Zouves C, Rodriguez H, et al. Sperm retrieval from testes biopsy with fertilization and pregnancy following ICSI. Abstract, Pacific Coast Fertil Society Meeting, April 19, 1996, Indian Wells, California.

25. Carpino F, Re M, Familiari G, et al. Ultrastructural study on the Sertoli cell in germinal aplasia. (Sertoli-cell-only syndrome). *Int. J Nephrol Urol Androl* 1980; 1:89–92.

26. Goluboff ET, Stifelman MD, Fisch H. Ejaculatory duct obstruction in the infertile male. *Urology* 1995; 45:925–931.

27. Chan SL, Cunningham GR, Lipshultz LI. Testicular and post-testiculaar causes of male infertility. In: deVere White R, ed. *Aspects of Male Infertility*. Baltimore: Williams and Wilkins; 1982: 116–152.

# 12
# Evaluation and Treatment of Ejaculatory Duct Obstruction in the Infertile Male

Randall B. Meacham and Julia A. Drose

In approximately 50% of infertile couples, a male factor is operative. Male infertility is often difficult to correct because infertile men frequently suffer from intrinsic testicular failure.[1] This condition is composed of hypospermatogenesis, maturation arrest, a combination of these histologic patterns, or Sertoli-cell–only syndrome. Although testicular failure is currently an area of significant research, thus far no reliable treatment options are available for patients with testicular failure. Similarly, some genetic causes, such as Klinefelter's syndrome, are not currently treatable.

On the other hand, subfertile men suffering from an obstructive process are potential candidates for surgical therapy. Such obstruction may occur along any portion of the excurrent ductal system from the epididymis to the ejaculatory ducts. The frequency of azoospermia in the general population has been estimated at approximately 2%.[2] The incidence of azoospermia among patients evaluated at infertilty clinics, however, has been reported to be as high as 10% to 20%. In a review published by Jarow and associates,[2] 37% of patients with azoospermia evaluated in a male fertility clinic were found to have an obstructive process as the cause. Patients found to have an obstruction at the level of the epididymis or vas deferens may be candidates for microsurgical reconstruction.[3]

Within the past decade, clinicians in the field of male reproductive medicine and surgery have gained a greater appreciation for the role of ejaculatory duct obstruction in male infertil-ity. The primary reason for the increased awareness of this lesion is the advent of the widespread use of transrectal ultrasonography in the evaluation of a variety of urologic disorders. Most often used in the evaluation of patients suspected of suffering from prostate malignancy, high-resolution transrectal ultrasound also provides excellent visualization of the excurrent ductal system in the prostatic and periprostatic regions. Prior to the use of transrectal ultrasound, the diagnosis of ejaculatory duct obstruction was most frequently made through the use of vasography. That modality, however, is relatively invasive and poses the risk of scarring and obstruction of the vas deferens at the vasography site.

The use of transrectal ultrasonography in the evaluation of the excurrent ductal system was described by Tanahashi and coworkers[4] in 1975. Other early investigators reporting the use of transrectal ultrasonography in evaluating ductal obstruction include Littrup and coworkers,[5] who in 1988 described the use of this modality in the assessment of patients suffering from conditions such as hematospermia, dysuria, and perineal pain. In 1989 Carter and associates[6] discussed the use of transrectal ultrasonography to investigate prostatic and seminal vesicle cysts. In that same year, Shabsigh and coworkers[7] provided details of the use of transrectal ultrasonography in the diagnosis and management of prostatic and seminal vesicle cysts.

Within the past 5 years, the use of transrectal ultrasonography has become a standard part of the armamentarium for the evaluation and management of male inferility. Ejaculatory duct obstruction can be corrected via transurethral resection of the obstructed ducts or decompression of obstructing müllerian duct cysts. Although it is now recognized that transurethral correction of ejaculatory duct obstruction is not without potential complications, in properly selected patients this treatment can yield excellent results.

## Pathophysiology

The ejaculatory ducts are approximately 1 to 2 cm in length and enter the prostate in an oblique fashion, traveling medially and anteriorly through the substance of the gland and entering the prostatic urethra at the level of the verumontanum. The prostatic utricle is located in the region of the verumontanum between the ejaculatory ducts. The utricle is a remnant of the müllerian duct, is of endodermal origin, and is not believed to communicate with any other structures. Anatomical studies have indicated that under normal circumstances there is no communication between the ejaculatory ducts and the lumen of the utricle.[8]

Obstruction of the ejaculatory ducts may arise from a variety of causes. Congenital atresia or stenosis of the ejaculatory ducts is one proposed mechanism of obstruction. Inflammatory disorders of the prostate or surgical procedures in the prostate region are other proposed causes of this condition. Another possible etiologic factor in ejaculatory duct obstruction is the presence of müllerian duct cysts. Although cysts of müllerian origin should not communicate with the wolffian duct system, extrinsic compression by such cysts may lead to blockage of the ejaculatory ducts.[9,10] Additionally, it appears that cystic dilatation of the distal wolffian system may create a midline prostatic cyst into which the ejaculatory ducts enter directly. In many cases, differentiation between müllerian and wolffian cysts is very difficult when using transrectal ultrasonography. In either case, however, transurethral unroofing of the cystic structure may yield good clinical results.

## Clinical Presentation

Patients suffering from ejaculatory duct obstruction may have an antecedent history that includes prostatitis, urethral catheterization, or transurethral surgical procedures. Frequently, however, the patient's history is negative for such causal factors. Physical examination is most often unremarkable. Because spermatogenesis is commonly intact, the testicles are usually of normal size and consistency. The vasa differentia should be palpably intact bilaterally. In some instances, long-standing obstruction may contribute to epididymal induration. This, however, is a variable finding. Rectal examination is most often unremarkable. Occasionally, a midline cyst may be palpated in the region of the prostate. In circumstances where the seminal vesicles are markedly dilated, they may be palpably enlarged on rectal examination.

As in other types of ductal obstruction, evaluation of serum testosterone and gonadotropins will generally yield normal results. In those cases where testis biopsy is performed, histologic results should show intact sperm production and maturation. It should be borne in mind, however, that patients may potentially suffer from intrinsic testicular failure as well as from ejaculatory duct obstruction. For this reason, semen quality may not return to normal in spite of correction of the obstructing lesion.

Unlike men with pure epididymal or vasal obstruction, those suffering from ejaculatory duct obstruction will generally present with decreased ejaculate volume. A large portion of the seminal fluid generated during ejaculation is derived from the seminal vesicles. In the presence of complete ejaculatory duct obstruction, only the prostatic fraction of the ejaculate emerges. Additionally, patients with ejaculatory duct obstruction will generally be found to have decreased sperm concentration or azoospermia. Individuals with partial ejaculatory duct obstruction may have varying concentrations of sperm in the ejaculate.[11] Such patients, however, will usually be found to have significantly decreased sperm motility. Evaluation of semen fructose content has historically played a role in the evaluation of men suspected of having ejaculatory duct obstruction. Although a negative semen fructose test suggests a diagnosis of complete ejaculatory duct obstruction, it may be positive in the case of partial obstruction. For this reason, a positive semen fructose evaluation does not rule out the possibility of ejaculatory duct obstruction. As in all evaluations of male fertility, two separate semen analyses should be performed on men suspected of suffering from ejaculatory duct obstruction. It is critical to ascertain whether or not a complete semen specimen was collected for each analysis.

Another potential cause of decreased ejaculate volume is retrograde ejaculation. Although retrograde ejaculation is often associated with a history of bladder neck surgery or a neurologic lesion, such as spinal cord injury or diabetes, it may be seen in men with no contributory history. Men presenting with abnormal semen quality and decreased ejaculate volume should undergo assessment for the presence of this condition. The easiest and most effective way to evaluate a patient for the presence of retrograde ejaculation is by examination of a postejaculatory urine specimen. The patient is asked to collect a semen specimen through masturbation and then void into a separate container. This evaluation can be facilitated by asking the patient to void most of his bladder content prior to masturbation. The residual urine that remains in the bladder will be more

manageable for laboratory personnel than would the contents of a full bladder. The voided specimen is centrifuged and the pellet resuspended in an appropriate medium. Detailed analysis of the antegrade and retrograde specimens is performed, and the specimens are compared for sperm content and motility. Laboratory and physical examination findings characteristic of ejaculatory duct obstruction are presented in Table 12.1.

## Ultrasound Evaluation

Ultrasound evaluation of patients suspected of suffering from ejaculatory duct obstruction is performed in much the same way as in men being evaluated for possible prostate neoplasms. Ultrasonography is most appropriately performed using a 5- to 7-MHz endocavitary probe. Scanning should be performed in both the transverse and longitudinal planes. A variety of ultrasound findings may suggest ejaculatory duct obstruction.[12] Ultrasound is generally considered positive if a posterior midline cyst is identified deep to the verumontanum or if dilatation of the seminal vesicles or vasal ampullae is identified (Fig. 12.1). There is no firm consensus regarding what constitutes seminal vesicle dilatation on ultrasonograpy. Carter and associates[6] have defined a dilated seminal vesicle as one that is greater than 15 mm in transverse dimension. Vazquez-Levin et al[13] have described dilated seminal vesicles as those in which the maximum width is greater than 12 mm at any point along their course. Hall and Oates[14] described normal seminal vesicle dimensions as $3 \pm 0.5$ cm in the transverse plane, $1.5 \pm 0.4$ cm in the sagittal plane, and a volume of $13.7 \pm 3.7$ ml.

Normal ejaculatory ducts can be visualized sonographically as small hypoechoic paired structures located centrally within the substance of the prostate (Fig. 12.2). When viewed in the sagittal plane, they appear as linear structures coursing from the seminal vesicles to the prostatic urethra (Fig. 12.3). In patients not suffering from ejaculatory duct obstruction, the ejaculatory ducts may not be visible. Vazquez-Levin and associates[13] defined dilated

TABLE 12.1. Laboratory values and physical findings characteristic of ejaculatory duct obstruction.

Laboratory
  Decreased ejaculate volume (<2.0)
  Decreased sperm concentration (may have complete
    azoospermia)
  Decreased sperm motility
  Negative postejaculatory urine evaluation
  Semen fructose positive or negative
  Normal serum testosterone and gonadotropins
Physical findings
  Normal testicular volume and consistency
  May have:
    Epididymal induration
    Midline prostatic cyst
    Dilated seminal vesicles

From Meacham and Lipshultz,[18] with permission.

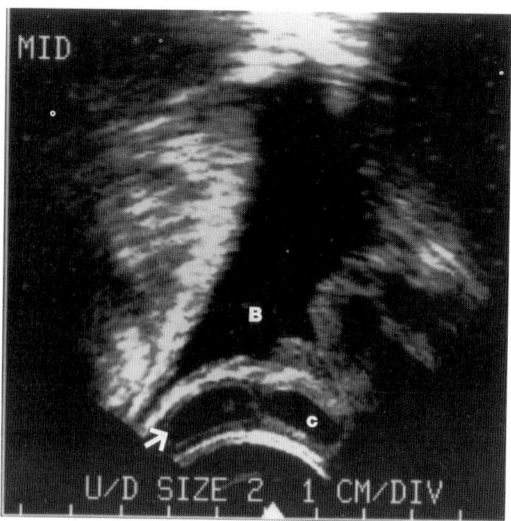

FIGURE 12.1. Sagittal image of the prostate showing a midline cyst (c) in conjunction with a dilated seminal vesicle (arrow). B, bladder.

ejaculatory ducts as those wherein the lumen of the ducts could be readily visualized between the two walls.

A variety of cystic structures may be observed within the prostate. Prostatic retention cysts are thought to occur as a result of benign prostatic hyperplasia. Believed to be cystic dilatations of the prostatic acini, such cysts are usually small and often are scattered within the central zone of the prostate or at the junction between the central and peripheral zones (Fig. 12.4).[15]

A diagnosis of ejaculatory obstruction is suggested by the presence of a cyst posterior to the prostatic urethra. Cysts located in this area may be of several types, including müllerian duct cysts, utricular cysts, and ejaculatory duct cysts. Such cysts may be differentiated based on whether or not they contain sperm.[16] Midline cysts that do not contain sperm are believed to be of müllerian duct origin and may be referred to as müllerian duct cysts or utricular cysts. Such lesions may cause obstruction of the ejaculatory ducts by external compression. Differentiation between müllerian duct cysts and utricular cysts may be problematic. It has been stated that these two types of cysts arise from different embryologic origins, utricular cysts being of endodermal origin and müllerian duct cysts being of mesodermal origin.[8] Müllerian duct cysts may extend well above the prostate and manifest as large pelvic masses. Although utricular cysts are variable in size, they are generally somewhat smaller in size than müllerian duct cysts.[17] Figure 12.5 presents the transverse and longitudinal sonographic images of the prostate in a 29-year-old man. A midline cyst is identified that was thought to be of either müllerian or utricular origin. The patient's semen quality was normal. Fluid aspirated from the cyst was not found to contain spermatozoa.

Midline prostatic cysts that contain sperm are considered to be of wolffian origin.[16] Cysts such as this likely represent dilated ejaculatory ducts. Calcifications in the area of the ejaculatory ducts provide supportive evidence of

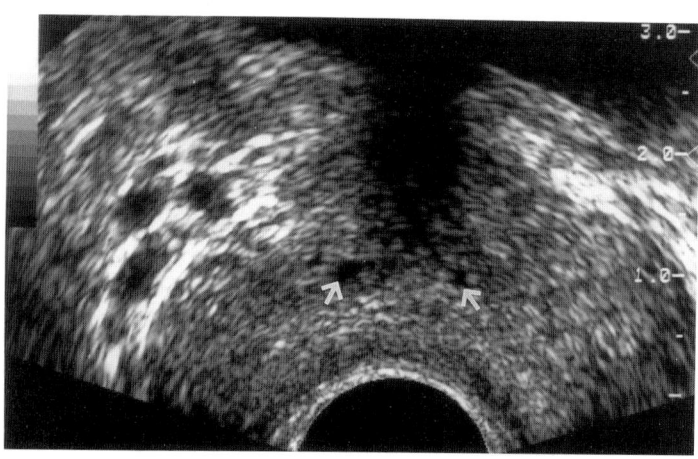

FIGURE 12.2. Transverse image of normal ejaculatory ducts (arrows) within the prostate.

FIGURE 12.3. Sagittal image of a normal ejaculatory duct (arrows) within the prostate.

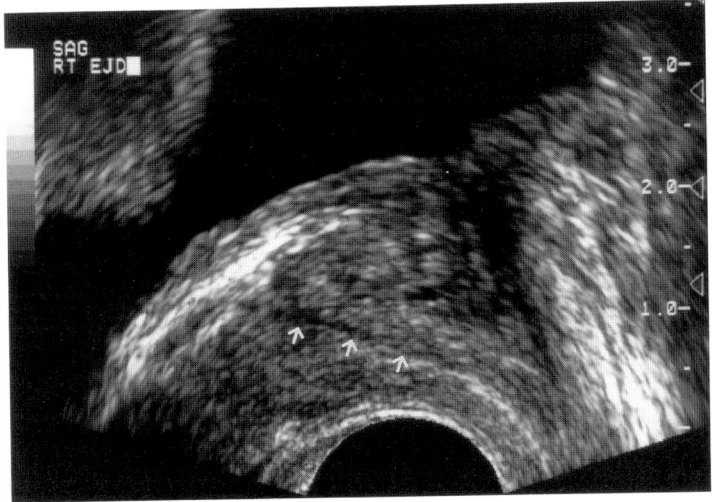

ejaculatory duct obstruction. Although this finding is probably less reliable than the above-described cystic dilatations, it may be significant under appropriate clinical circumstances (Fig. 12.6). Figure 12.7 represents a transverse sonographic image of a midline prostatic cyst. Aspirated fluid contained sperm, indicating that this was an ejaculatory duct cyst. Figure 12.8 shows another transverse sonogram revealing a midline prostatic cyst that was confirmed to be an ejaculatory duct cyst by the presence of sperm in fluid obtained during cyst aspiration.

Table 12.2 represents ultrasound findings in 20 men diagnosed with ejaculatory duct obstruction reported by Meacham and Lipshultz.[18]

Additional techniques have been described for confirming the diagnosis of ejaculatory duct obstruction. Katz and associates[19] reported the use of ultrasound-guided transrectal seminal vesiculography to confirm ejaculatory duct obstruction. Ruiz Rubio et al[20] described the use of ultrasound guided transperineal cyst puncture and instillation of contrast into the cyst and seminal vesicles. Jarow[21] has recently described

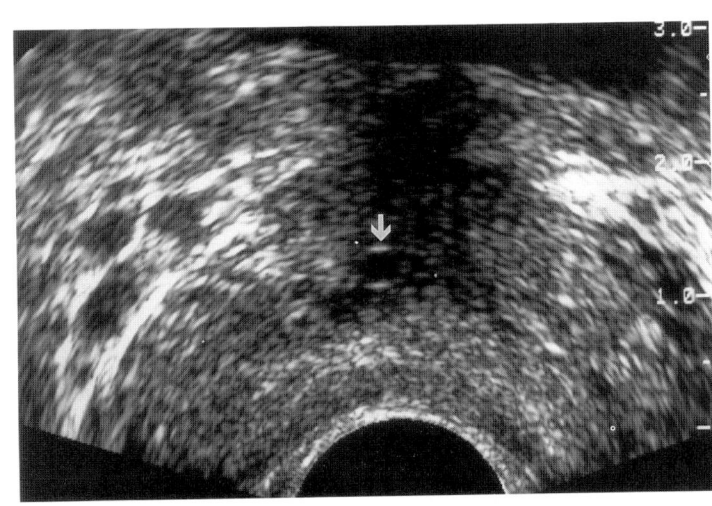

FIGURE 12.4. Transverse image of a prostatic retention cyst (arrow) located within the central portion of the prostate.

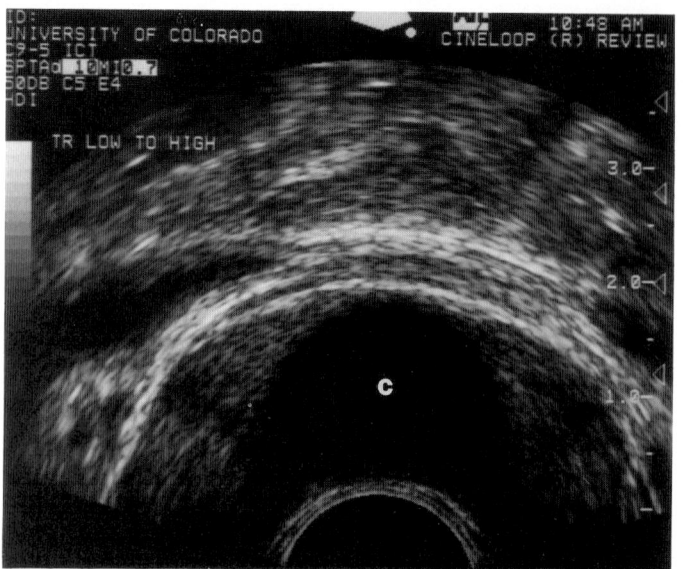

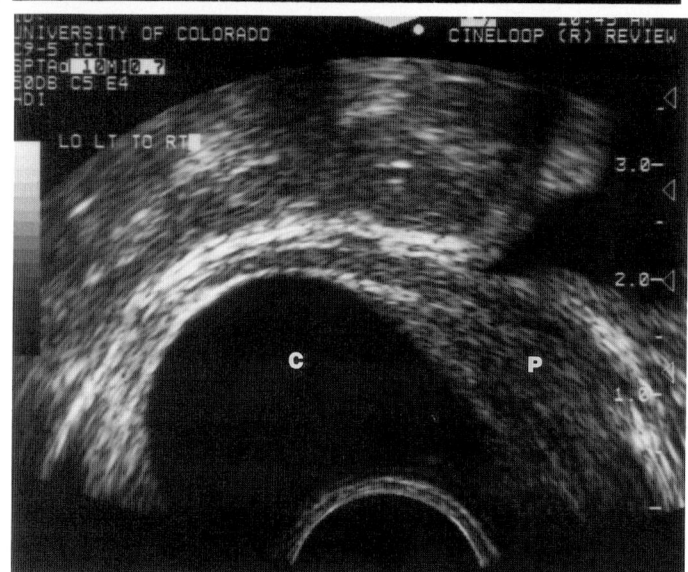

FIGURE 12.5. (A) Transverse image of a midline cyst (c) within the prostate that was thought to be utricular or müllerian in origin. (From Meacham et al,[25] with permission.) (B) Sagittal image of the same patient showing the same midline cyst (c) extending above the prostate (p).

FIGURE 12.6. Sagittal image of calcifications coursing along the ejaculatory duct (arrows).

FIGURE 12.7. Transverse image of an ejaculatory duct cyst (c) within the prostate. B, bladder. (From Meacham et al,[25] with permission.)

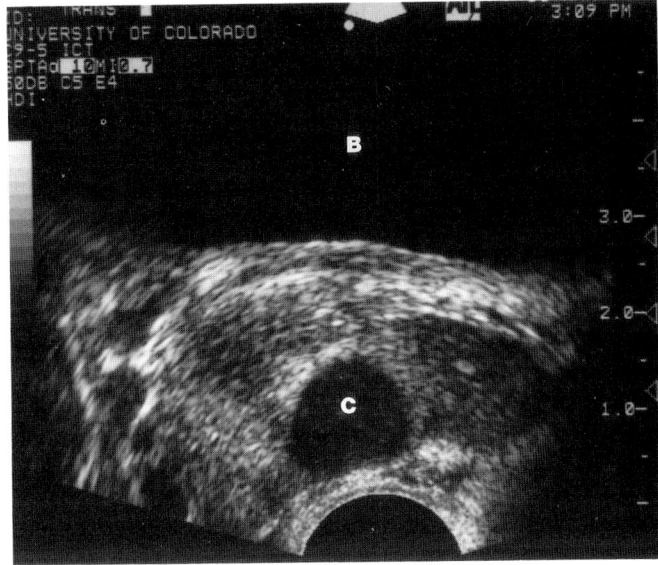

the use of transrectal ultrasound-guided seminal vesicle aspiration in the confirmation of ejaculatory duct obstruction. Results of his investigation indicate that sperm are not usually present within the seminal vesicles and that ejaculatory duct obstruction should be suspected in any patient in whom numerous sperm are identified within fluid aspirated from the seminal vesicles.

# Treatment of Ejaculatory Duct Obstruction

Treatment of ejaculatory duct obstruction is generally accomplished via transurethral unroofing of the obstructed ducts. A variety of approaches to this procedure have been described.[18] Because the ejaculatory ducts enter the prostatic urethra in the region of the

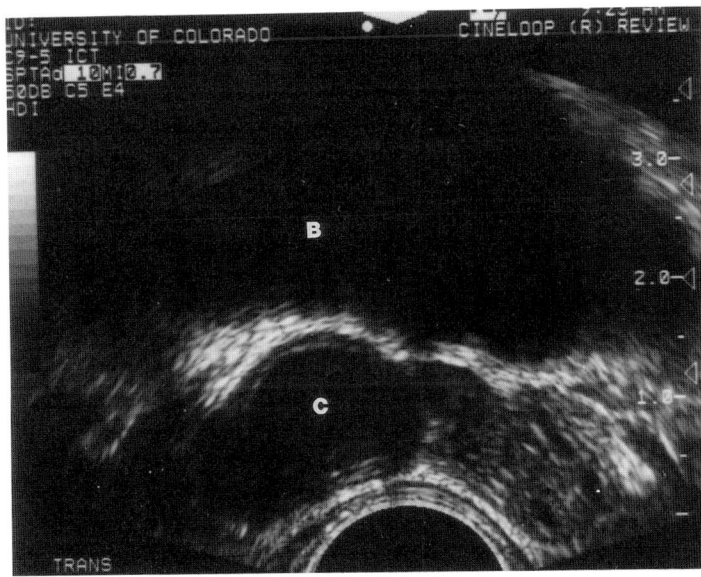

FIGURE 12.8. Transverse image of an ejaculatory duct cyst (c) within the prostate. B, bladder. (From Meacham et al,[25] with permission.)

TABLE 12.2. Results of transrectal ultrasonography.

| Finding | Group 1 | Group 2 | Group 3 |
|---|---|---|---|
| Ejaculatory duct cyst | 4 | 3 | 1 |
| Dilated seminal vesicles | 4 | 2 | 1 |
| Dilated vasal ampullae or ejaculatory ducts | 3 | 0 | 0 |
| Calcification of ejaculatory ducts | 1 | 1 | 0 |

Ultrasound findings in 20 patients diagnosed as having ejaculatory duct obstruction via transrectal sonography. (From Meacham and Lipshultz,[18] with permission.)

verumontanum, the most direct route to surgical unroofing is transurethral resection of the veru itself.[12] Figure 12.9 illustrates the technique used for transurethral unroofing of the ejaculatory ducts. If an ejaculatory duct cyst is present, it will usually be entered less than 1 cm deep to the resected verumontanum. Caution must be exercised to avoid damage to the rectum, bladder neck, or external sphincter during resection. It may prove useful to insert a gloved finger into the rectum during the procedure in order to guard against resecting too deeply.

Intraoperative transrectal sonography may be useful in surgical correction of ejaculatory duct obstruction. Ultrasonography will indicate the exact location of an ejaculatory duct cyst and will allow measurement of the distance between the cyst and prostatic urethra. Figure 12.10 shows a sagittal ultrasound image revealing an ejaculatory duct cyst and its relationship to the bladder neck. During this particular procedure, it was possible to place a flexible guidewire into the ejaculatory duct cyst to provide a guide for further incision. Figure 12.11 shows a sonographic image of the guidewire within the ejaculatory duct cyst. Figure 12.12 is a sonographic image of the ejaculatory duct cyst after it had been incised.

Adequate unroofing of the ejaculatory ducts can be confirmed by placing a gloved finger in the rectum and digitally compressing the seminal vesicles. When the ducts have been adequately resected, seminal fluid should be seen flowing into the prostatic urethra during this maneuver. Care should be taken to minimize coagulation in the area of the resected ducts in order to avoid scarring. A 24-French urinary catheter is usually left in place for 24 to 48

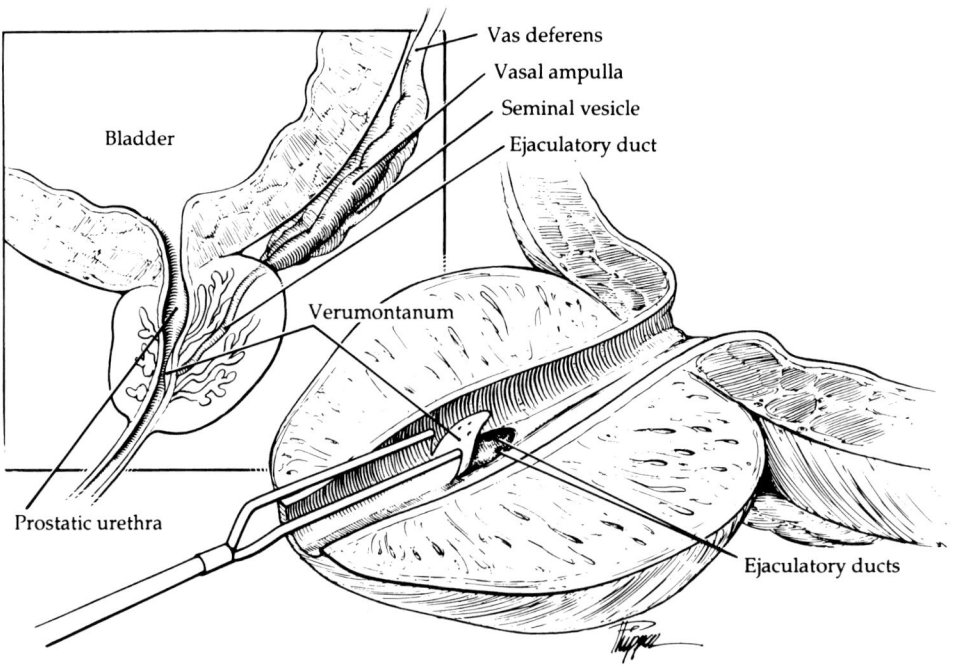

FIGURE 12.9. Technique for resection of the ejaculatory ducts. (From Meacham et al,[12] with permission.)

FIGURE 12.10. Sagittal image showing an ejaculatory duct cyst (c)
within the prostate and its relationship to the bladder neck (arrow).
(From Meacham et al,[25] with permission.)

FIGURE 12.10. Sagittal image showing an ejaculatory duct cyst (c)
within the prostate and its relationship to the bladder neck (arrow).
(From Meacham et al,[25] with permission.)

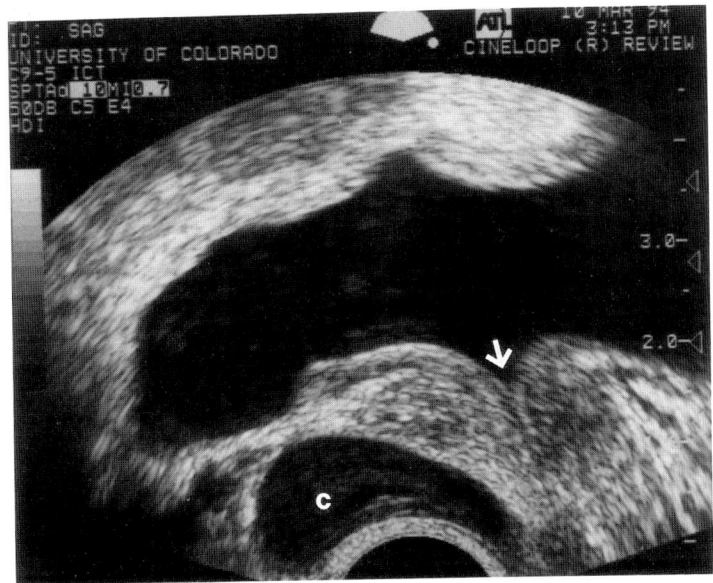

hours to facilitate management of postoperative hematuria.

Ideally, following transurethral unroofing of
the ejaculatory ducts, patients should experience an improvement in ejaculate volume as
well as in sperm quality. Patients with partial
ejaculatory duct obstruction who have an increase in ejaculate volume following transurethral resection but no improvement in sperm
concentration or motility may suffer from intrinsic testicular failure in addition to ejaculatory duct obstruction. Additionally, patients
with complete obstruction of the ejaculatory
ducts who achieve an increase in ejaculate volume postoperatively but do not experience return of sperm to the semen have a second
obstructing lesion at the level of the epididymis.
It is well recognized that patients who have
long-standing obstruction of the vas deferens
secondary to vasectomy may develop epididymal obstruction secondary to pressure within
the ductal system. It is likely that patients with

FIGURE 12.11. Sagittal image of a
guidewire (arrows) being advanced
into an ejaculatory duct cyst (c)
prior to surgical resection. B, bladder. (From Meacham et al,[25] with
permission.)

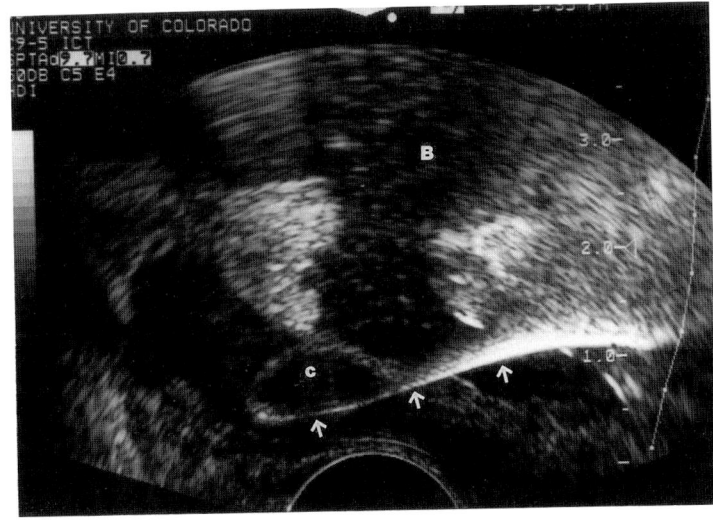

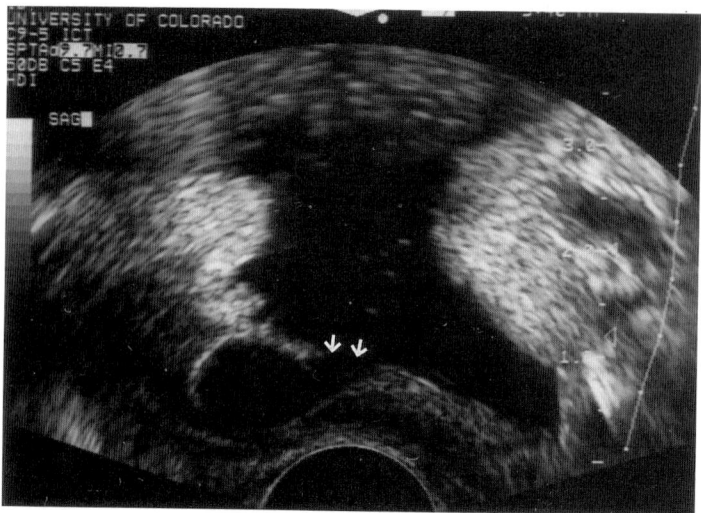

FIGURE 12.12. Sagittal image immediately postresection of an ejaculatory duct cyst (arrows). (From Meacham et al,[25] with permission.)

ejaculatory duct obstruction can suffer a similar epididymal lesion. Patients suffering from a secondary epididymal obstruction may require subsequent scrotal exploration and vasoepididymal reconstruction.[9,22]

In 1993 Meacham and associates[12] reported the results of 26 transurethral resections of the ejaculatory ducts performed in 24 patients (Table 12.3). Twelve patients achieved an improvement in sperm concentration or motility or both. Eight patients were found to have increased ejaculate volume with no improvement in sperm quality, and six patients failed to respond to therapy. Seven patients' wives became pregnant postoperatively. Weintraub et al[23] also reported encouraging results following transurethral resection of the ejaculatory ducts in eight patients. Among the five patients treated primarily for infertility, four achieved improvement in ejaculatory volume or sperm quality or both and fathered children. Among 85 patients who underwent transurethral resection of the ejaculatory ducts in a collected series reported by Vazquez-Levin et al,[13] 55% of the patients obtained an improvement in semen parameters postoperatively, and 33% of the patients' wives achieved a pregnancy.

It should be recognized that transurethral resection of the ejaculatory ducts is not without potential complications. Meacham and associates[12] reported two patients who suffered significant postoperative hematuria. In addition,

Vazquez-Levin and associates[13] reported eight patients in whom assessment of preoperative and postoperative semen creatinine was performed to detect contamination by urine. Seven of eight patients were found to have increased creatinine levels postoperatively within the semen. Although it is not entirely clear what the impact of such urinary contamination of the ejaculate may be, it is possible that this will decrease subsequent fertility.[13] Additionally, Goluboff et al[24] reported a patient who developed significant postvoid dribbling following transurethral resection of the ejaculatory ducts. In this case, it was demonstrated that urine refluxed through the resected ejaculatory ducts into one of the patient's seminal vesicles, leading to postvoid dribbling as the seminal vesicle

TABLE 12.3. Overall response to treatment.

|  | Number of patients | Number of pregnancies |
| --- | --- | --- |
| Group 1* | 12 | 6 (50%) |
| Group 2† | 8 | 1 (12.5%) |
| Group 3‡ | 6 | 0 |
| Total | 26 | 7 (27%) |

*Postoperative improvement in sperm density, motility, or both.
†Improvement in ejaculate volume only.
‡No postoperative improvement in semen parameters.
Results of transurethral resection of the ejaculatory ducts in 24 patients (two patients underwent two procedures). (From Meacham et al,[12] with permission.)

subsequently emptied.[8] Transurethral resection of the ejaculatory ducts may also lead to epididymitis. The etiology of this is most likely retrograde flow of urine into the vas deferens.

When considering transurethral resection of the ejaculatory ducts in a patient with partial obstruction, it should be noted that surgical therapy may result in further stenosis of the ducts. Patients who undergo transurethral resection of the ejaculatory ducts may develop scarring in the region of the prostatic urethra, converting a partial ejaculatory duct obstruction into a complete obstruction. Recent advances in the use of in vitro fertilization technologies have allowed the generation of pregnancies even in the face of significantly impaired semen quality. The patient who presents with decreased semen quality may, therefore, successfully achieve a pregnancy through the use of these technologies. If such a patient is rendered azoospermic through transurethral unroofing of the ejaculatory ducts, his chances for fathering a child will be impaired.

## Conclusion

Over the past 5 years, ejaculatory duct obstruction has become a well-recognized cause of male infertility. The use of transrectal ultrasonography has greatly facilitated identification of this lesion. Used judiciously, transurethral unroofing of the ejaculatory ducts can yield gratifying results in this challenging patient population.

## References

1. Wong T, Jones M. Evaluation of testicular biopsy in male infertility studies. In: Lipshultz LI, Howards SS, eds. *Infertility in the Male*. New York: Churchill Livingstone; 1983: 217–248.
2. Jarow JP, Espeland MA, Lipshultz LI. Evaluation of the azoospermic patient. *J Urol* 1989; 142:62–65.
3. Thomas AJ, Howards SS. Microsurgical treatment of male infertility. In: Lipshultz LI, Howards SS, eds. *Infertility in the Male*. 2nd ed. Chicago: Mosby-Year Book; 1991: 357–369.
4. Tanahashi Y, Wantanabe H, Irari D, et al. Volume estimation of the seminal vesicles by means of transrectal ultrasonotomography: a preliminary report. *Br J Urol* 1975; 47:695–702.
5. Littrup PJ, Lee F, McLeary RD, et al. Transrectal ultrasound of the seminal vesicles and ejaculatory ducts: clinical correlation. *Radiology* 1988; 168:625–628.
6. Carter SSC, Shinohara K, Lipshultz LI. Transrectal ultrasonography in disorders of the seminal vesicles and ejaculatory ducts. *Urol Clin North Am* 1989; 16:773–790.
7. Shabsigh R, Lerner S, Fishman IJ, et al. The role of transrectal ultrasonography in the diagnosis and management of prostatic and seminal vesicle cysts. *J Urol* 1989; 141:1206–1209.
8. Goluboff ET, Stifelman MD, Fisch H. Ejaculatory duct obstruction in the infertile male. *Urology* 1995; 45:925–931.
9. Worischeck JH, Parra RO. Transrectal ultrasound in the evaluation of men with low volume azoospermia. *J Urol* 1993; 149:1341–1344.
10. Elder JS, Mostwin JL. Cyst of the ejaculatory duct/urogenital sinus. *J Urol* 1984; 132:768–770.
11. Hellerstein DK, Meacham RB, Lipshultz LI. Transrectal ultrasound and partial ejaculatory duct obstruction in male infertility. *Urology* 1992; 39:449–452.
12. Meacham RB, Hellerstein DK, Lipshultz LI. Evaluation and treatment of ejaculatory duct obstruction in the infertile male. *Fertil Steril* 1993; 59:393–397.
13. Vazquez-Levin MH, Dressler KP, Nagler HM. Urine contamination of seminal fluid after transurethral resection of the ejaculatory ducts. *J Urol* 1994; 152:2049–2052.
14. Hall S, Oates RD. Unilateral absence of the scrotal vas deferens associated with contralateral mesonephric duct anomalies resulting in infertility: laboratory, physical and radiographic findings, and therapeutic alternatives. *J Urol* 1993; 150:1161–1164.
15. Queralt JA, Gersovich EO, Gould JE, et al. Intraoperative transrectal ultrasonography in the management of ejaculatory duct obstruction caused by midline prostatic cyst. *J Clin Ultrasound* 1993; 21:293–298.
16. Jarow JP. Transrectal ultrasonography of infertile men. *Fertil Steril* 1993; 60:1035–1039.
17. Nghiem HT, Kellman GM, Sandberg SA, et al. Cystic lesions of the prostate. *Radiographics* 1990; 10:635–650.
18. Meacham RB, Lipshultz LI. Transrectal ultrasonography in the evaluation of the infertile male. *Adv Urol* 1992; 5:195–207.

19. Katz D, Mieza M, Nagler HM. Ultrasound guided transrectal seminal vesiculography: a new approach to the diagnosis of male reprodutive tract abnormalities. *J Urol* 1994; 151:310A.

20. Ruiz Rubio JL, Fernandez Gonzalez I, Quijano Barrosso P, et al. The value of transrectal ultrasonography in the diagnosis and treatment of partial obstruction of the seminal duct system. *J Urol* 1995; 153:435–436.

21. Jarow JP. Seminal vesicle aspiration in the management of patients with ejaculatory duct obstruction. *J Urol* 1994; 152:899–901.

22. Worischeck JH, Parra RO. Transrectal ultra-sound in the evaluation of men with low volume azoospermia. *J Urol* 1993; 149:1341–1344.

23. Weintraub MP, DeMouy E, Hellstrom WJG. Newer modalities in the diagnosis and treatment of ejaculatory duct obstruction. *J Urol* 1993; 150:1150–1154.

24. Goluboff ET, Kaplan SA, Fisch H. Seminal vesicle urinary reflux as a complication of trans-urethral resection of ejaculatory ducts. *J Urol* 1995; 153:1234–1235.

25. Meacham RB, Townsend RR, Drose JA. Ejacu-latory duct obstruction: diagnosis and treatment. *AJR* 1995; 165:1463–1466.

# 13
# Varicocele

Armand Zini, Sarah K. Girardi, and Marc Goldstein

A varicocele is dilated testicular veins in the scrotum. Although it is generally agreed that a varicocele represents the most common identifiable pathology in infertile men and that correction of this lesion usually results in improved fertility, the influence of varicoceles and varicocelectomy on fertility remains the subject of ongoing controversy.

## Incidence

The incidence of varicoceles in the general male population is about 15%.[1-4] The incidence in men presenting for infertility is about 35%, and in that subset of men with secondary infertility it is 70% to 80%.[5-7] Although varicoceles are almost always larger and more common on the left side,[5,8] the incidence of bilateral varicoceles is in the range of 15% to 50%. The rare, isolated right-sided varicocele generally suggests that the right internal spermatic vein enters the right renal vein, but this finding may be associated with situs inversus or retroperitoneal tumors.[9] Oster[10] observed that no varicoceles were detected in 188 boys 6 to 9 years of age, but were detected with increasing incidence in boys 10 to 14 years of age, which suggests that varicoceles develop at puberty. Occasionally, varicoceles may be acquired secondary to underlying benign or malignant retroperitoneal pathology.

The significantly higher incidence of varicoceles in men with secondary infertility and the observation that varicoceles generally develop at the time of puberty suggest that the presence of a varicocele can cause a progressive decline in fertility and imply that men with a varicocele and prior fertility are not immune from potential ongoing varicocele-mediated testicular injury.[6,7] Although the high incidence of varicoceles in the general male population suggests that many or even most men with varicoceles are fertile (at least when they are younger), a study by the World Health Organization has shown that semen quality declines in men with untreated varicoceles.[11] In an earlier study, Johnson et al[3] showed that in a cohort of asymptomatic military recruits, nearly 70% of men with a palpable varicocele had an abnormality on semen analysis.

## Etiology

Among the most widely accepted of the proposed theories on the causes of varicoceles are (1) that there are anatomic differences between the left and right internal spermatic vein, (2) that there is an absence or incompetence of venous valves resulting in reflux of venous blood, and (3) that there is increased hydrostatic pressure in the scrotal veins.

The reflux of venous blood into the pampiniform plexus is believed to arise largely as a result of the absence or incompetence of internal spermatic venous valves. The report by Braedel et al[12] on the venographic pattern of 659 consecutive men with varicoceles revealed that the majority of these men (484/659) had absent venous valves. Compression of the left renal vein and narrowing of the left internal spermatic vein were seen in 103 and 3 men, respectively.

The anatomy of the left internal spermatic vein is different from the right. The left vein is about 8 to 10 cm longer, and this is believed to result in an increase in hydrostatic pressure.[13] This pressure is transmitted to the internal spermatic vein at the level of the pampiniform plexus, causing dilatation and tortuosity of the veins.

Compression of the left renal vein between the aorta and the superior mesenteric artery ("nutcracker effect") may also contribute to the increased internal spermatic venous pressure. Radiologic studies have documented a relative distention of the proximal left renal vein, suggesting partial distal obstruction.[14,15]

It is likely that the etiology of varicocele is multifactorial.

# Mechanisms

## Animal Studies

The virtual lack of naturally occurring varicoceles in animals has led numerous researchers to create experimental models of varicoceles in the hope of understanding the mechanisms responsible for testicular dysfunction and infertility associated with varicoceles in humans. Most of these investigators have induced varicoceles by partial ligation of the left renal vein medial to the entrance of the left testicular vein and have assessed one or more of a number of end points, including semen quality, testicular histology, testicular blood flow, testicular temperature, and the bilateral nature of this experimental pathology. In general, a surgically induced varicocele reproduces many of the pathophysiologic manifestations of naturally occurring varicoceles in humans. However, it is important to realize that the validity of extrapolating results obtained from experimental varicoceles and applying them to human pathology has not been confirmed.

Semen quality uniformly declines in animals with induced varicoceles.[16-20] As is observed in infertile men with varicoceles, testicular histology in varicocelized animals reveals abnormalities in the seminiferous epithelium, characterized by abnormal Sertoli cells and germ-cell sloughing. An increase in testicular temperature is reported in most studies. Testicular blood flow has been shown to increase in experimental models of varicoceles;[16,17] however, in one study, a decrease in testicular blood flow was observed, and was attributed to the use of a different animal model.[21] Recently, Turner et al[22] demonstrated that an experimental left varicocele results in increased testicular intravascular volume, bilaterally. They suggested that the increased testicular blood flow in their model could be explained only in part by this increase in intravascular volume together with the focal testicular capillary growth they observed. The inhibition of testosterone synthesis in rats with surgically induced varicoceles was shown to be due principally to a reduction in the activity of the enzyme 17,20-desmolase.[23]

## Human Studies

A number of theories have been proposed to explain the observed pathophysiology of varicoceles. Zorgniotti and MacLeod[24] reported that men with varicoceles have higher intrascrotal temperatures than the controls. They also noted a bimodal intrascrotal temperature distribution in infertile men without varicoceles, demonstrating the nonspecificity of an isolated elevated intrascrotal temperature reading. Goldstein and Eid[25] directly measured intratesticular temperatures and found them elevated in men with varicoceles as did Saypol et al[16] in an animal model of varicoceles. A number of reports have documented the sensitivity of spermatogenesis to temperature elevations.[16,24,26-28] Recently, testicular hyperthermia (generated by inguinal placement of the testes) has been advocated as an effective contraceptive, capable of rendering men azoospermic or severely oligospermic.[29,30] The reduction in scrotal temperature following varicocele ligation supports a causative role of increased temperature on the infertility produced by the varicocele.[17,31,32]

The theory of adrenal and renal metabolite reflux stems from early anatomic radiographic studies documenting reflux of blood from the renal vein into the internal spermatic vein. Despite the reports demonstrating correlations between increased concentrations of these metabolites in the internal spermatic vein and the presence of a varicocele, few of these metabolites have clearly been shown to be gonadotoxic.

Comhaire and Vermeulen[33] measured spermatic vein catecholamine (adrenal metabolite) concentrations in infertile patients with and without varicoceles and found that although internal spermatic vein levels of catecholamines were higher than peripheral levels in both groups, the ratio of spermatic vein to peripheral vein catecholamine was higher in men with varicoceles than in control subjects. Cohen et al[34] performed a small study demonstrating that a subset of patients with both varicoceles and high internal spermatic vein catecholamine levels achieved higher pregnancy rates after varicocelectomy than those men with lower catecholamine levels. However, there are no convincing data showing that catecholamines are gonadotoxic.

Ito et al[35] examined the concentration of prostaglandins and other presumably renal-derived metabolites and found their concentration to be high in the internal spermatic veins of men with varicoceles. Although this study was not controlled, these findings may be relevant in light of the animal work demonstrating that prostaglandins have a gonadotoxic effect.[36,37] It has been shown that prostaglandins depress serum luteinizing hormone (LH) and testosterone levels.[38]

Increased hydrostatic pressure in the internal spermatic vein from renal vein reflux has been proposed by Shafik and Bedeir[13] as a possible mechanism for varicocele-induced pathology. It was postulated that the venous stasis in the internal spermatic vein could lead to inefficient blood transport and result in a decrease in the oxygen tension and subsequent failure of spermatogenesis. Although intuitively logical, this theory is weakened by the reports of Donohue et al[39] and Netto et al[40] showing no significant difference in pH or oxygen tension in the inter-

nal spermatic vein blood of men with varicoceles as compared with controls.

# Pathophysiology

Numerous aspects of testicular function and varicocele-associated pathology have been investigated in the hope of gaining a better understanding of the pathophysiology of varicoceles.

## Testis Atrophy

Testicular atrophy has been documented in men with varicoceles as early as 100 A.D.[41–43] More recently, Lipshultz and Corriere[44] objectively demonstrated, with the use of calipers, that left testicular size in men with a left varicocele was significantly decreased when compared with a control group of men. The World Health Organization (WHO) presented similar data in a multicenter study that evaluated the physical findings and semen characteristics of men presenting for infertility.[11] The WHO study reported that varicoceles (most of which were on the left side) were associated with relative left testicular atrophy as compared with the contralateral testis. In contrast, right and left testicular size was not significantly different in men without a varicocele. This study also demonstrated that combined testicular volume (right plus left sides) decreased with increasing size of the varicocele.

## Testis Histology and Biochemical Function

Some studies have attempted to characterize the changes in testicular histology associated with the development of the varicocele.[41,45–50] Most of these studies have documented the bilateral nature of these changes. The histologic findings have varied from normal to Sertoli-cell–only pattern, with most studies reporting varying degrees of hypospermatogenesis. Additionally, premature sloughing of germ cells into the seminiferous tubule lumen is a histologic feature identified in a number of the studies. Although some investigators have also noted

Leydig cell hyperplasia, this has not been confirmed by all reports.[48]

Evaluation of bilateral testicular histology by use of electron microscopy has revealed changes predominantly in Sertoli and endothelial cells.[50] The Sertoli cells exhibited varying degrees of endoplasmic reticulum dilatation, with vacuolization in extreme cases. These changes were believed to cause breaks in the Sertoli cell plasma membrane and premature release of immature germ cells. Endothelial cells were noted to contain many small pinocytic vesicles and the arterioles appeared contracted.

Using a testicular biopsy score count, before and after varicocelectomy, Johnsen and Agger[47] evaluated the testicular biopsies of 22 men with varicoceles. They reported that varicocelectomy significantly improved the biopsy scores in all men. The magnitude of improvement was independent of the duration or size of the varicocele itself. These results strengthen the concept that varicocelectomy improves testicular function.

The activity of enzymes involved in DNA synthesis (many of which are key in the process of germ cell multiplication) has been shown to decrease in the testes of men with varicoceles as compared with normal controls.[51,52] It is unclear, however, whether a reduction in the activity of these enzymes results in the hypospermatogenesis observed in testis with a varicocele or is secondary to the germ cell depletion seen in this pathology. Other studies have shown that the lipid concentration is increased in the testes of men with varicocele.[53–55] It is speculated that the specific increase in cholesterol may be due to deficient or aberrant androgen biosynthesis in Leydig cells. To date, these studies have not confirmed the specificity of these biochemical changes to varicoceles, as these changes are likely found in idiopathic oligospermia as well.

## Leydig Cell Function

Leydig cell dysfunction has been documented in men with varicoceles. A WHO multicenter study on the influence of varicocele on fertility parameters demonstrated that the mean testosterone concentration of men older than 30 years of age with varicoceles was significantly lower than that of younger patients with varicoceles, whereas this trend was not observed in men without varicoceles.[11] These findings suggest a detrimental time-dependent effect of varicocele on Leydig cell function. Comhaire and Vermeulen[56] evaluated 10 patients with decreased testosterone, impotence, and varicoceles, and observed that after varicocelectomy, the serum testosterone increased in all cases. Recently, Su et al[57] also observed a significant increase in mean testosterone levels after varicocelectomy in a group of 53 infertile men with varicoceles.

Although these studies suggest that a varicocele may impair testicular steroidogenic function, substantial evidence has come from studies that use human chorionic gonadotropin (hCG) stimulation of testosterone release and gonadotropin-releasing hormone (GnRH) stimulation of gonadotropin release. These tests are more sensitive indicators of Leydig cell function than peripheral testosterone concentration. In the normal male, peripheral levels of testosterone show a biphasic response to hCG with an initial peak at 1 to 4 hours and a second peak at 36 to 96 hours. Scholler et al[58] demonstrated that the early peak of testosterone and dihydrotestosterone (DHT) may be blunted in men with varicocele. They suggested that this may be due to a block at the level of the steroidogenic enzyme 17,20-lyase, based on the observed increase in the levels of $17\alpha$-hydroxyprogesterone.

Subsequent studies have employed the gonadotropin response to bolus injection or continuous infusion of GnRH, as it is a more sensitive test of Leydig cell function than hCG stimulation. Hudson and McKay[59] demonstrated that men with varicoceles have an excessive response [LH and follicle-stimulating hormone (FSH) release] to a 4-hour infusion of GnRH. The magnitude of the response was also greater in severely oligospermic men than in those with sperm concentrations between 11 and 30 million/ml. More importantly, Hudson[60] found that the men with exaggerated gonadotropin response to GnRH were most likely to show improvement in semen parameters following varicocelectomy, regardless of the degree of oligospermia. Additionally, the report of Fujisawa et al[61] demonstrated that a normalization of the LH response to GnRH stimulation after varicocelectomy was predictive of improved fertility postoperatively. These findings suggest that men with varicocele and abnormal Leydig cell function are most likely to benefit from varicocelectomy.

## Semen Characteristics/Sperm Function

The abnormalities of semen parameters in infertile men with varicoceles were first objectively described by MacLeod[62] in 1965. In that study, MacLeod observed that the vast majority of semen samples, obtained from 200 infertile men with varicoceles, were found to have an increased number of abnormal forms, decreased motility, and lower mean sperm counts. This "stress pattern," characterized by an increased number of tapered forms and immature cells, was also reported in other studies.[11,63,64] However, some investigators have shown that the characteristic stress pattern is not a sensitive marker for varicocele and believe that it is not diagnostic of this pathology.[65,66]

A large number of studies have evaluated the effects of varicocelectomy on semen parameters.[5,67–71] Most of these studies have demonstrated an improvement in sperm density with or without a concomitant increase in sperm motility and morphology after varicocelectomy, suggesting a cause-and-effect relationship between a varicocele and abnormal semen parameters. However, because the bulk of the reported outcome data on varicocelectomy comes from uncontrolled or poorly designed controlled studies, the value of these results is limited.[72]

The impact of the grade size of varicoceles on the magnitude of improvement in semen quality after varicocelectomy is equivocal. Steckel et al[73] reported that men with larger varicoceles present with lower sperm densities and show greater relative improvement in semen quality than men with smaller varicoceles who present with higher mean sperm densities. Jarow et al[74] reported virtually identical

results and suggested that repair of subclinical varicoceles is of questionable value. At this time, the grade of the varicocele remains of uncertain value in predicting the outcome of varicocelectomy.

## Diagnosis

The diagnosis of a varicocele is generally made on physical examination. A warm examining room promotes relaxation of the scrotal dartos muscle and facilitates accurate evaluation for varicoceles. A number of other modalities have been used to diagnose varicoceles, including venography, Doppler stethoscope, radionuclide angiography, scrotal thermography, and scrotal ultrasonography. Despite some reports demonstrating the potential limitations of venography, when it is performed in experienced hands this modality is generally accepted as the most accurate method of varicocele diagnosis and is thus regarded as the standard against which other tests are to be compared.[75] However, this test is not routinely used because of its invasive nature.

Although it is regarded as the most clinically useful tool in the diagnosis of a varicocele, the limitation of the physical examination has been highlighted by a World Health Organization[76] study comparing this and other diagnostic modalities to venography. The physical examination used had a 23% false-negative and a 24% false-positive rate in the detection of left-sided varicocele in this study. These results in part reflect the limitations of the clinical examination in its ability to detect smaller lesions and may explain the discrepancy between the clinical examination and other more sensitive diagnostic tools, hence the concept of the subclinical varicocele. Despite these limitations, the physical examination remains the primary diagnostic modality in varicocele evaluation.

Doppler stethoscope, radionuclide angiography, and scrotal thermography in the diagnosis of varicocele have been evaluated in a number of studies but these modalities have been largely abandoned in view of their low accuracy.[77–79]

The availability, reproducibility, and non-invasiveness of scrotal ultrasonography have led to its increased use. The ability of scrotal ultrasonography with color flow to accurately measure the testicular vein diameter, and detect reversal of flow with the Valsalva maneuver, often undetectable by physical examination (subclinical varicocele), has prompted investigators to evaluate the potential role of this modality in diagnosing varicoceles and in predicting the outcome of varicocelectomy. McClure and Hricak[80] evaluated 50 infertile men, half with and half without varicoceles, using scrotal ultrasonography. They based their ultrasonographic detection criteria for varicoceles (internal spermatic vein diameter >3mm) on the findings of a control population of 25 normal fertile men without clinically palpable varicoceles. They reported that all palpable varicoceles were detected by ultrasonography and, in addition, a left varicocele was detected in 12 of the 25 patients without palpable (subclinical) varicoceles. Eskew et al[81] critically examined scrotal ultrasonography as a diagnostic tool in the evaluation of varicoceles. They performed physical examination, color duplex scrotal ultrasonography, and internal spermatic vein venography on 64 testicular units in 33 men. They found that the best predictor of a varicocele was the internal spermatic vein diameter with the patient in the supine position. They reported that the optimal criteria for venous diameter in a varicocele was 3.6mm for a clinical and 2.7mm for a subclinical varicocele, but caution that the accuracy in using these optimal criteria (that combine high sensitivity and specificity) is only 63%.

The significance of a subclinical varicocele (one that is not clinically palpable) remains controversial.[82] The lack of standardized criteria for diagnosis and the conflicting treatment outcome reports on subclinical varicoceles raise questions about the existence and significance of this entity.[82–86]

# Varicocelectomy

Varicocelectomy, the most commonly performed operation for the treatment of male infertility, is indicated for the treatment of varicocele-induced infertility, because a varicocele is associated with a progressive and duration-dependent decline in testicular function,[6,7,42,44,87–91] and repair of the varicocele can halt further damage to testicular function and result in improved spermatogenesis.[5,42,70] Varicocelectomy is also indicated in the child or adolescent with decreased ipsilateral testicular volume or an abnormal gonadotropin response to luteinizing hormone–releasing hormone (LHRH) stimulation or both.[92] In adolescents, a good case can also be made for repair of larger varicoceles associated with a softer ipsilateral testis.

Surgical approaches advocated for varicocelectomy include retroperitoneal and conventional inguinal open techniques, microsurgical inguinal and subinguinal approaches, laparoscopic repairs, and radiographic embolization. The importance of using a varicocelectomy technique that minimizes the risk of complications and recurrences cannot be overemphasized. Table 13.1 summarizes these methods of varicocele repair.

The earliest recorded attempts at repair of a varicocele involved external clamping of the scrotal skin, including the enlarged veins. In the early 1900s an open scrotal approach was em-

TABLE 13.1. Techniques of varicocelectomy.

| Technique | Artery preserved | Hydrocele (%) | Failure (%) | Potential for serious morbidity |
|---|---|---|---|---|
| Retroperitoneal | No | 7 | 15–25 | No |
| Conventional inguinal | No | 3–30 | 5–15 | No |
| Laparoscopic | Yes | 12% | ?5–15 | Yes |
| Radiographic embolism | Yes | 0 | 15–25 | Yes |
| Microscopic inguinal | Yes | 0 | 0.5 | No |

ployed, involving the mass ligation and excision of the varicosed plexus of veins. At the level of the scrotum, however, the pampiniform plexus of veins is intimately entwined with the coiled testicular artery. Therefore, scrotal operations are to be avoided because of potential damage to the arterial supply of the testis with subsequent testicular atrophy.

Retroperitoneal repair of varicocele involves incision at the level of the internal inguinal ring, splitting of the external and internal oblique muscles, and exposure of the internal spermatic artery and vein retroperitoneally near the ureter. This approach has the advantage of isolating the internal spermatic veins near the entrance into the left renal vein where only one or two large veins are present and where the testicular artery has not yet branched and is often distinctly separate from the internal spermatic veins. Although this approach is a commonly employed method for the repair of a varicocele, the identification and preservation of the testicular artery and lymphatics via the retroperitoneal approach is difficult, especially in children because these structures are small. Kass and Marcol[93] reported that recurrence of a varicocele can be markedly reduced in children and adolescents by intentional ligation of the testicular artery, because this modification did not result in testicular atrophy in their series of patients. Despite the reassuring results of Kass and Marcol, it should be noted that in adults, bilateral testicular artery ligation has been shown to cause azoospermia and testicular atrophy and in the event that these patients undergo subsequent vasectomy testicular atrophy world likely result.

Laparoscopic repair is essentially a retroperitoneal approach and many of the advantages and disadvantages are similar to those of the open retroperitoneal approach. Using this method, the internal spermatic vessels and vas deferens can be clearly visualized through the laparoscope as they enter the internal inguinal ring. The magnification as provided by the laparoscope allows visualization of the testicular artery and lymphatics and makes their preservation possible.

A number of smaller studies have reported the results of laparoscopic varicocelectomy, but the results cannot be evaluated critically at this time due to the small number of cases and short follow-up.[94–97] In theory, the incidence of varicocele recurrence and complications is expected to be similar to that associated with the open retroperitoneal operations. However, this treatment option is less attractive than open surgery because the potentially shorter postoperative convalescent period is outweighed by the need for general anesthesia, the higher cost of the laparoscopic surgery, and the potential complications associated with it (injury to bowel, vessels, or viscera; air embolism; peritonitis). Nonetheless, in the hands of an experienced laparoscopist, the approach is a reasonable alternative for the repair of bilateral varicoceles.[98]

The inguinal (and subinguinal) varicocelectomy is currently the most popular surgical approach. The advantages of this approach are that it enables the surgeon to easily identify the spermatic cord structures and, if necessary, access the testis, epididymis, and the external spermatic and gubernacular veins.

In the traditional inguinal varicocelectomy, a 5- to 10-cm incision is made over the inguinal canal, the external oblique aponeurosis is opened, and the spermatic cord is encircled and delivered. The internal spermatic veins are ligated and the vas deferens and its vessels are preserved.[5] An attempt is made to identify and preserve the testicular artery and the lymphatics, if possible. In addition, the cord is elevated and external spermatic veins are identified and ligated. The use of magnification enables the surgeon to identify and preserve the testicular artery and lymphatics and thus prevent potential testicular atrophy and hydrocele formation, respectively.[70,99]

The subinguinal approach described by Marmar et al[100] obviates the need for opening any fascial layer and as a result is associated with less postoperative pain and a more rapid recovery. However, at the subinguinal level, significantly more veins are encountered, the artery is more often surrounded by a network of tiny veins that must be ligated, and the testicular artery has often divided into two or three branches, making its identification and preservation more difficult. Subinguinally, the artery is somewhat more difficult to identify because the arterial pulsations are often dampened by compression of the edge of the external ring. A subinguinal operation is recommended in men with a history of prior inguinal surgery; in obese men; in men with high, lax, capacious external rings; and in men with long cords and low-lying testes.

The inguinal approach is recommended in children who have not had prior inguinal surgery. In children, identification of the artery using the subinguinal approach is very difficult because of the very small size of the testicular artery and low systemic blood pressure. An inguinal approach should also be used in men with a solitary testis and in whom preservation of the artery is critical. At this more proximal level, the artery is more easily identified as it has not yet branched and generally has stronger pulsations.

A microsurgical subinguinal approach is recommended for virtually all varicocelectomies. A 2.0- to 3.0-cm incision extending from the external inguinal ring medially is made first (Fig. 13.1). The incision is deepened through Camper's and Scarpa's fascia with the

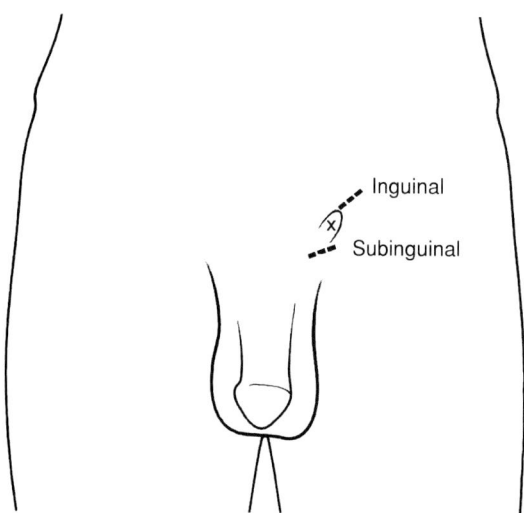

FIGURE 13.1. Schematic representation of inguinal and subinguinal incisions for varicocele repair. A dot is made to mark the external inguinal ring (X). The inguinal incision is then extended laterally in the skin lines, while the subinguinal incision is extended medially.

electrocautery. The spermatic cord is then grasped with a Babcock clamp and delivered. With the cord delivered, the ilioinguinal and genital branches of the genitofemoral nerve are excluded and preserved. The Babcock clamp is replaced with a large Penrose drain and the testicle is delivered. The gubernacular veins and external spermatic perforators are then isolated and divided (Fig. 13.2), because gubernacular veins have been demonstrated radiographically to account for 10% of varicocele recurrences.[101] Once all gubernacular veins have been divided, the testicle is returned to the scrotum and the spermatic cord remains elevated on a large Penrose drain for stabilization in preparation for microscopic examination (Fig. 13.3). The microscope is then brought into the operating field, and the cord is examined under 8 to 15 power magnification.

The internal and external spermatic fascia are incised and the cord is examined. Subtle pulsations will usually reveal the location of the underlying testicular artery. If not, 1% papaverine solution is sprinkled on the cord to facilitate its identification. Once identified, the artery is dissected free of all surrounding veins and encircled with a 0-silk ligature for identification (Fig. 13.4). All remaining internal spermatic veins with the exception of the vasal veins are clipped or ligated and divided (Fig. 13.5). Any additional arteries encountered during inspection of the remainder of the cord are encircled with a 0-silk ligature for identification and preservation. Care must be taken to preserve a majority of lymphatics, as these when divided can contribute to hydrocele formation postoperatively (Fig. 13.6). The vas deferens and its associated vessels should be readily identified posteriorly and outside the internal spermatic fascia. The vas deferens is inspected for any abnormally dilated veins. Veins measuring 3 mm or greater should be divided as these can also lead to postoperative recurrences. There are usually two sets of vessels that accompany the vas deferens in the spermatic cord. At least one of these sets must be preserved to ensure venous return following varicocelectomy.

The entire cord is inspected until no additional internal spermatic veins or abnormally

FIGURE 13.2. (A) A schematic representation of the gubernacular veins and external spermatic perforators. Delivery of the testicle enables the surgeon to identify and ligate these vessels, which are responsible for some varicocele recurrences. (B) An intraoperative photograph of the same.

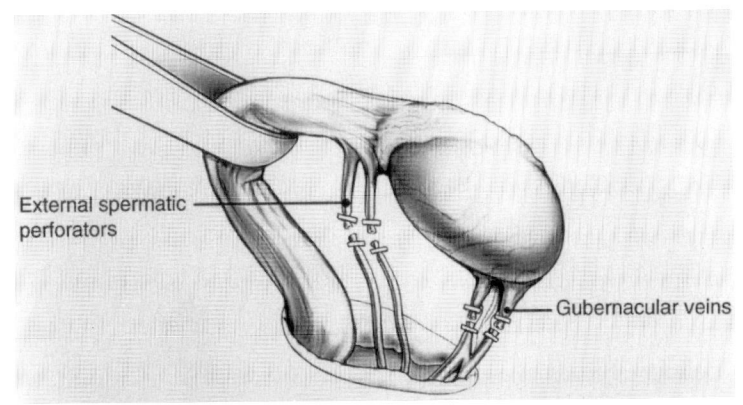

External spermatic perforators

Gubernacular veins

**A**

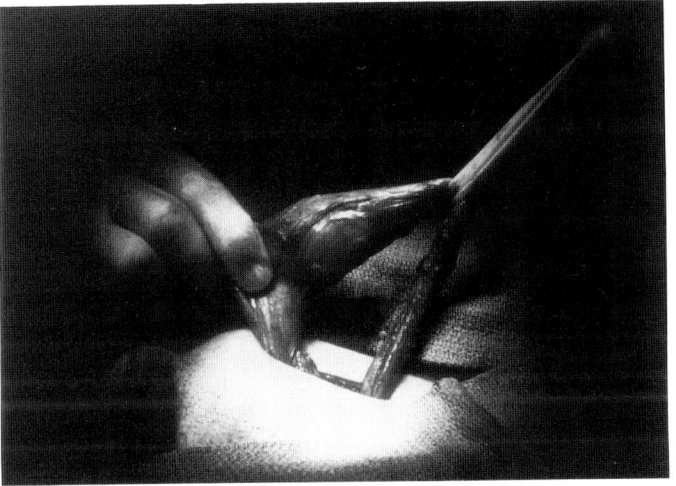

**B**

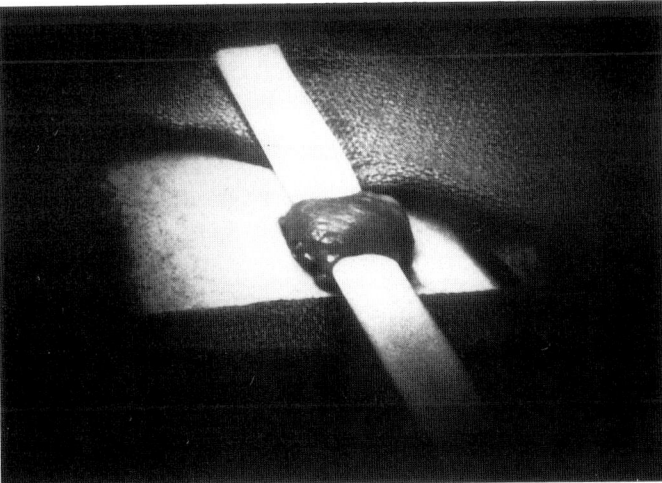

FIGURE 13.3. An intraoperative photograph showing the spermatic cord elevated on a Penrose drain. After the testicle has been returned to the scrotum, the cord is left elevated on a large Penrose drain that serves as a stable stage during microscopic examination of the cord.

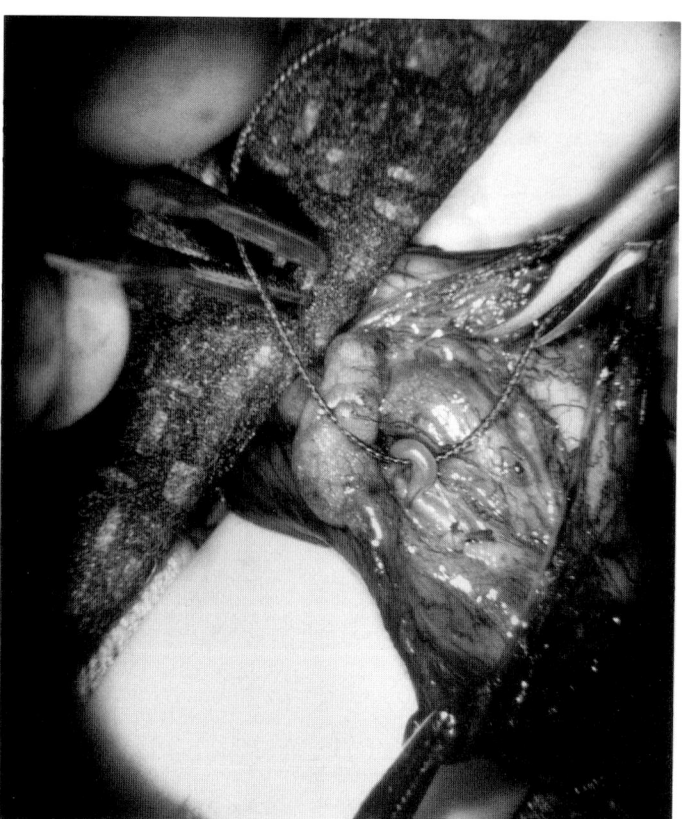

FIGURE 13.4. An intraoperative photograph showing the isolated testicular artery at approximately 10× magnification. Encircle with an 0-silk suture to identify it and preserve it. Any additional arteries encountered are also identified in this way.

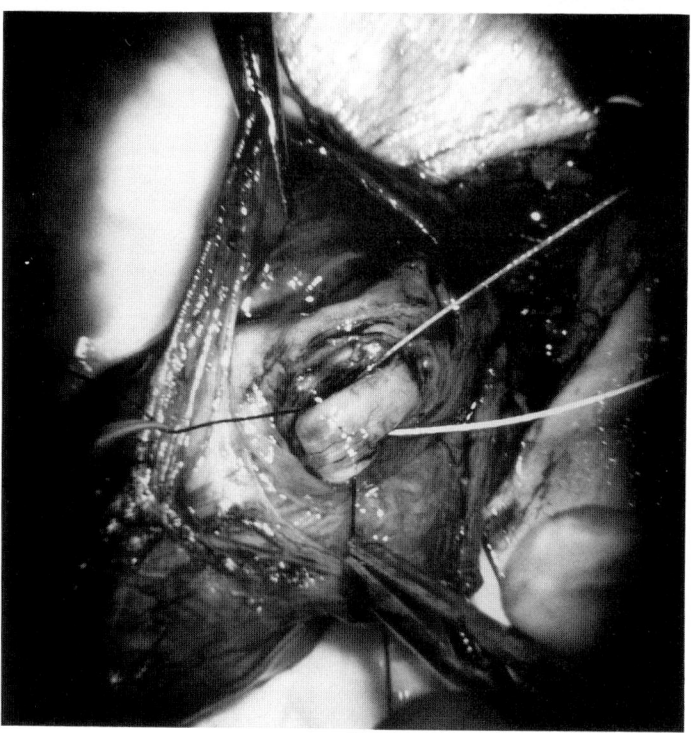

FIGURE 13.5. An intraoperative photograph showing an internal spermatic vein just prior to ligation and division. Two 4-0 silk ties, one black and one white, are used to ligate veins measuring 2mm or less in diameter, while hemoclips are used for veins measuring greater than 2mm.

FIGURE 13.6. An intraoperative photograph of a spermatic cord lymphatic channel at approximately 12× magnification. Lymphatic channels have a characteristic appearance in that they appear as vessels filled with clear fluid.

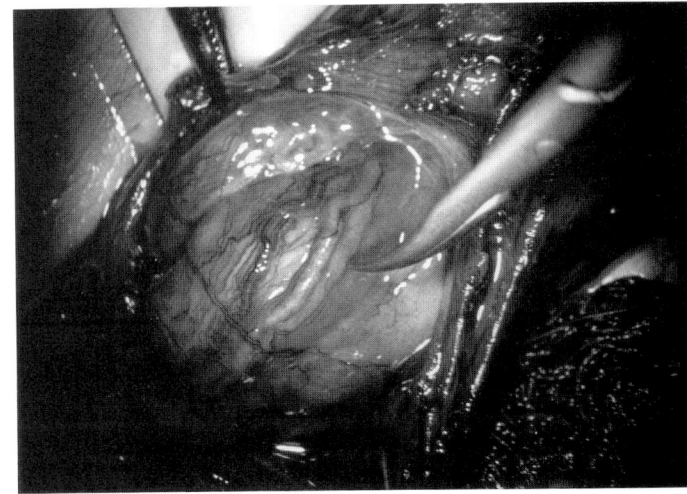

dilated vasal or cremasteric veins are identified on two consecutive inspections of the cord. At the completion of varicocelectomy, the cord should contain only the testicular artery or arteries, vas deferens and associated vessels, cremasteric muscle (with its veins ligated and artery preserved), and spermatic cord lymphatics. A few drops of 1% papaverine solution are then sprinkled on the testicular artery (or arteries) to break any spasm. Once pulsations are seen, the 0-silk ligatures are removed and the spermatic cord is returned to the inguinal canal.

The wound is irrigated with 1% neomycin irrigation, and Scarpa's and Camper's fascia are closed with a single 3-0 monofilament absorbable suture. The incision is infiltrated with 0.025% Marcaine solution with epinephrine, and the skin is closed with a 5-0 Monocryl subcuticular closure reinforced with Steri-Strips (Fig. 13.7). A dry sterile dressing and scrotal fluffs are applied and secured with a well-fitting scrotal support. The patient is sent home on the day of surgery and will return to desk work in 2 to 3 days.

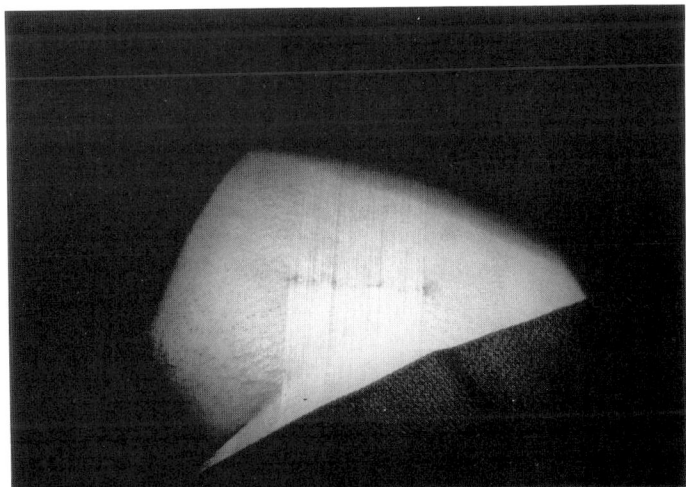

FIGURE 13.7. An intraoperative photograph of the skin incision at the termination of the procedure. After the incision has been infiltrated with Marcaine solution with epinephrine, it is closed with a 5-0 Monocryl subcuticular closure and reinforced with Steri-Strips.

Radiographic balloon or coil occlusion of the internal spermatic veins has been successfully employed for treatment of varicocele.[102–104] These techniques are performed under local anesthesia through a small cut-down incision over the femoral vein. This method is not complicated by hydrocele formation or internal spermatic artery injury. However, the recurrence rate after balloon occlusion varies from 4% to 11%.[105–108] The rate of unsuccessful attempts ranges from 2% to 15%[109–110] and a significant number of men undergoing attempted radiographic occlusion will ultimately require a surgical approach. The radiographic techniques take between 1 and 3 hours to perform, as compared with the 25 to 45 minutes required for surgical repair. Rare, serious complications of radiographic balloon or coil occlusion have included migration of the balloon or coil into the renal vein, resulting in loss of a kidney, pulmonary embolization of the coil or balloon, femoral vein perforation or thrombosis, and anaphylactic reaction to radiographic contrast medium.[108]

Antegrade scrotal sclerotherapy via cannulation of a scrotal vein has been reported in Europe.[111] The recurrence rate is similar to those in balloon or coil techniques, but the generally poor long-term follow-up after percutaneous embolization raises questions about the validity of outcome data.

## Complications of Varicocele Repair

Hydrocele formation is the most common complication reported after nonmicrosurgical varicocelectomy. The incidence of this complication varies from 3% to 33%, with an average incidence of about 7%.[112] The difficulty in identifying and preserving lymphatics using nonmicrosurgical approaches (especially retroperitoneal) results in this complication. Analysis of the hydrocele fluid has indicated that hydrocele formation following varicocelectomy is due to ligation of the lymphatics.[112] At least half of postvaricocelectomy hydroceles grow to a size that produces sufficient discomfort to warrant surgical excision. The effect of hydrocele formation on sperm function and fertility is unknown. It is possible that the development of a large hydrocele may have a negative

impact on testicular function, perhaps by elevating testicular temperature or affecting the diurnal variations in scrotal temperature.[24,27] However, the use of magnification to identify and preserve lymphatics can virtually eliminate the development of a hydrocele after varicocelectomy.[70,99] In addition, radiographic balloon or coil occlusion techniques are not complicated by hydrocele formation.

The incidence of testicular artery ligation during varicocelectomy is unknown, but some studies suggest it is common.[113,114] The identification and preservation of the 0.5- to 1.0 mm testicular artery via the retroperitoneal approach is difficult, especially in children because the artery is small. Injury or ligation of the testicular artery carries with it the risk of testicular atrophy or impaired spermatogenesis or both. Penn et al (Starzl's transplant group)[115] reported a 14% incidence of frank testicular atrophy when the testicular artery was purposefully ligated. Animal studies indicate that the risk of testicular atrophy after testicular artery ligation varies from 20% to 100%.[116,117] In humans, atrophy after artery ligation is probably less likely due to the contribution of the cremasteric and vasal arteries. In children, the potential for neovascularization and compensatory hypertrophy of the vasal and cremasteric vessels is probably greater than in adults, making atrophy after testicular artery ligation even less likely. Use of magnifying loupes, or preferably an operating microscope or a fine-tipped Doppler probe or both, facilitates identification and preservation of the testicular artery and therefore minimizes the risk of testicular injury. Radiographic balloon or coil is not complicated by testicular atrophy.

The incidence of varicocele recurrence following surgical repair varies from 1.0% to 45%. Recurrence is more common after repair of pediatric varicoceles.[118–120] Venographic studies of recurrent varicoceles have identified periarterial, parallel inguinal, midretroperitoneal, or, more rarely, transscrotal collaterals.[106] Retroperitoneal operations are associated with the highest rate of varicocele recurrence. Recurrence rates after retroperitoneal varicocelectomy are in the range of 15%.[121,122] Failure is usually due to preservation of the periarterial plexus of fine veins (venae comitantes). These veins have been shown to communicate with larger internal spermatic veins and if left intact may dilate and cause recurrence. Less commonly, failure is due to the presence of parallel inguinal or retroperitoneal collaterals that may exit the testis, bypass the retroperitoneal area, and join the internal spermatic vein proximal to the site of ligation.[105,123] Cremasteric veins cannot be identified using a retroperitoneal approach and may be a potential site of varicocele recurrence as well.[124] The recurrence rate after balloon occlusion varies from 4% to 11%.[105–108] Nonmagnified inguinal operations have a lower incidence of varicocele recurrence but fail to address the issue of scrotal collaterals or small veins surrounding the testicular artery. The microsurgical approach with delivery of the testis lowers the incidence of varicocele recurrence to less than 1% compared with 9% using conventional inguinal techniques.[70]

## Results

A large number of studies have evaluated the outcome of varicocelectomy on fertility parameters and most of these studies have demonstrated an improvement in semen quality and pregnancy rates.[5,67–71,125] However, because the bulk of the reported outcome data on varicocelectomy comes from uncontrolled or poorly designed controlled studies, the value of these results is limited.[72] In addition, the few reports comparing the various treatment options have not convincingly shown the superiority of one method over another. Overall, varicocelectomy results in significant improvement in semen analysis in 60% to 80% of men, and pregnancy rates after varicocelectomy vary from 20% to 60%.[126] In a series of 1500 microsurgical operations 43% of couples were pregnant at 1 year and a cumulative 69% at 2 years when female-factor couples were excluded.[70] Results were poorer in the 1% of men who had their testicular arteries inadvertently ligated.[127]

Only a small number of properly controlled studies evaluating the outcome of varicocelectomy have been performed. Although the bulk of the literature supports a favorable effect of varicocelectomy on fertility, the effectiveness of varicocelectomy will remain controversial until a larger number of controlled studies are reported. The recent randomized crossover study by Madgar et al[71] demonstrated significantly higher pregnancy rates in the early and delayed varicocelectomy groups compared with the control nonoperated group. Laven et al[69] evaluated the results of varicocelectomy in adolescents with varicoceles in a prospective randomized fashion. They demonstrated improved semen parameters in the surgically treated group but not in the control group. Nieschlag et al[125] recently reported the results of a randomized study of non-microsurgical varicocelectomy in adults. They found no significant difference in pregnancy rates between the control and treatment arms (ligation or embolization), but they did find a significant improvement in semen parameters in the treatment arms.

## Summary

Varicocele is a very common entity. It is present in 15% of the male population, in approximately 35% of men with primary infertility, and in 70% to 80% of men with secondary infertility. A substantial body of evidence suggests that venous dilation results in elevated testicular temperature and blood flow perturbations. There is reasonably good evidence showing that a varicocele causes progressive duration-dependent injury to the testis and that varicocelectomy can restore fertility in some men. Refined methods of varicocele repair have reduced the incidence of complications significantly, thus making prophylactic repair of varicoceles a tenable goal for preventing future infertility and androgen deficiency.

## References

1. Horner JS. The varicocele: a survey among secondary schoolboys. *Med Officer* 1960; 104:377–381.
2. Clarke BG. Incidence of varicocele in normal men and among men of different ages. *JAMA* 1966; 198:1121–1122.
3. Johnson DE, Pohl DR, Rivera-Correa H. Varicocele: an innocuous condition? *South Med J* 1970; 63:34–36.

4. Steeno O, Knops J, Declerk L, et al. Prevention of fertility disorders by detection and treatment of varicocele at school and college age. *Andrologia* 1976; 8:47–53.

5. Dubin L, Amelar R. Varicocelectomy: 986 cases in a 12 year study. *Urology* 1977; 10:446–449.

6. Gorelick J, Goldstein M. Loss of fertility in men with varicocele. *Fertil Steril* 1993; 59:613–616.

7. Witt MA, Lipshultz LI. Varicocele: a progressive or static lesion? *Urology* 1993; 42:541–543.

8. Greenberg SH, Lipschultz LI, Wein AJ. Experience with 425 subfertile male patients. *J Urol* 1978; 119:507–510.

9. Comhaire F, Kunnen M, Hahoum C. Radiological anatomy of the internal spermatic vein in 200 retrograde venograms. *Int J Androl* 1981; 4:379–387.

10. Oster J. Varicoceles in children and adolescents. *Scand J Urol Nephrol* 1971; 5:27–32.

11. World Health Organization (WHO). The influence of varicocele on parameters of fertility in a large group of men presenting to infertility clinics. *Fertil Steril* 1992; 57:1289–1292.

12. Braedel HU, Steffens J, Ziegler M, et al. A possible ontogenic etiology for idiopathic left varicocele. *J Urol* 1994; 151:62–66.

13. Shafik A, Bedeir GA. Venous tension patterns in cord veins. 1. In normal and varicocele individuals. *J Urol* 1980; 123:383–385.

14. Coolsaet BL. The varicocele syndrome: venography determining the optimal level for surgical management. *J Urol* 1980; 124:833–839.

15. Buschi AJ, Harrison RB, Brenbridge AN, et al. Distended left renal vein: CT/sonographic normal variant. *Am J Radiol* 1980; 135:339–342.

16. Saypol DC, Howards SS, Turner TT. Influence of surgically induced varicocele on testicular blood flow, temperature, and histology in adult rats and dogs. *J Clin Invest* 1981; 68:39–45.

17. Hurt GS, Howards SS, Turner TT. Repair of experimental varicoceles in the rat. Long-term effects on testicular blood flow and temperature and cauda epididymal sperm concentration and motility. *J Androl* 1986; 7:271–276.

18. Al-Juburi A, Pranikoff K, Dougherty K, et al. Alterations of semen quality in dogs after creation of varicocele. *Urology* 1979; 13:535–539.

19. Snydle FE, Cameron DF. Surgical induction of varicocele in the rabbit. *J Urol* 1983; 130:1005–1009.

20. Sofikitis N, Miyagawa I. Bilateral effect of varicocele on testicular metabolism in the rat. *Int J Fertil* 1994; 39:239–247.

21. Harrison RM, Lewis RW. Roberts JA. Testicular blood flow and fluid dynamics in monkeys with surgically induced varicoceles. *J Androl* 1983; 4:256–260.

22. Turner TT, Brown KJ, Spann CL. Testicular intravascular volume and microvessel mitotic activity: effect of experimental varicocele. *J Androl* 1993; 14:180–186.

23. Rajfer J, Turner TT, Rivera F, et al. Inhibition of testicular testosterone biosynthesis following experimental varicocele in rats. *Biol Reprod* 1987; 36:933–937.

24. Zorgniotti AW, MacLeod J. Studies in temperature, human semen quality, and varicocele. *Fertil Steril* 1973; 24:854–863.

25. Goldstein M, Eid JF. Elevation of intratesticular and scrotal skin surface temperature in men with varicocele. *J Urol* 1989; 142:743–745.

26. Galil KAA, Setchell BP. Effects of local heating of the testis on testicular blood flow and testosterone secretion in the rat. *Int J Androl* 1987; 11:73–85.

27. Lerchl A, Keck C, Spiteri-Grech J, et al. Diurnal variations in scrotal temperature of normal men and patients with varicocele before and after treatment. *Int J Androl* 1993; 16:195–200.

28. Mieusset R, Bujan L, Mondinat C, et al. Association of scrotal hyperthermia with impaired spermatogenesis in infertile men. *Fertil Steril* 1987; 48:1006–1007.

29. Shafik A. Contraceptive efficacy of a polyester-induced azoospermia in normal men. *Contraception* 1992; 45:439–451.

30. Mieusset R, Bujan L. The potential of mild testicular heating as a safe, effective and reversible contraceptive method for men. *Int J Androl* 1994; 17:186–191.

31. Sofikitis N, Takahashi C, Nakamura I, et al. Surgical repair of secondary right varicocele in rats with primary left varicocele: effects on fertility, testicular temperature, spermatogenesis and sperm maturation. *Arch Androl* 1992; 28:43–52.

32. Wright EJ, Young GP, Goldstein M. Reduction in testicular temperature after varicocelectomy in infertile men. *Urology* 1997; in press.

33. Comhaire F, Vermeulen A. Varicocele sterility: cortisol and catecholamines. *Fertil Steril* 1974; 25:88–95.

34. Cohen MS, Plaine L, Brown JS. The role of internal spermatic vein plasma catecholamine determinations in subfertile men with varicoceles. *Fertil Steril* 1975; 26:1243–1249.

35. Ito H, Fuse H, Kawamura K, et al. Internal spermatic vein prostaglandins in varicocele patients. *Fertil Steril* 1982; 37:218–222.

36. Abbatiello ER, Kaminsky M, Weisbroth S. The effect of prostaglandins and prostaglandin inhibitors on spermatogenesis. *Int J Fertil* 1975; 20:177–182.

37. Tierney WJ, Daly IW, Abbatiello ER. The effect of prostaglandins PGE2 and PGF2A prostaglandin on spermatogenesis in adult male Sprague-Dawley rats. *Int J Fertil* 1979; 24:206–209.

38. Saksena SK, El Sajoury S, Bartke A. Prostaglandin E2 and F2A decrease plasma testosterone levels in male rats. *Prostaglandins* 1973; 4:235.

39. Donohue RE, Brown JS. Blood gases and pH determinations in the internal spermatic veins of subfertile men with varicocele. *Fertil Steril* 1969; 20:365–369.

40. Netto NR, Lemos GS, Goes RM. Varicocele: relation between anoxia and hypospermatogenesis. *Int J Fertil* 1977; 22:174–178.

41. Johnsen SG, Agger P. Quantitative evaluation of testicular biopsies in varicocele. *Fertil Steril* 1978; 29:52–57.

42. Kass EJ, Belman AB. Reversal of testicular growth failure by varicocele ligation. *J Urol* 1987; 137:475–476.

43. Pinto KJ, Kroovand L, Jarow JP. Varicocele related testicular atrophy and its predictive effect upon fertility. *J Urol* 1994; 152:788–790.

44. Lipshultz LI, Corriere JN. Progressive testicular atrophy in the varicocele patient. *J Urol* 1977; 117:175–176.

45. Dubin L, Hotchkiss RS. Testis biopsy in subfertile men with varicocele. *Fertil Steril* 1969; 20:50–57.

46. Ibrahim AA, Awad HA, El-Haggar S, et al. Bilateral testicular biopsy in men with varicocele. *Fertil Steril* 1977; 28:663–667.

47. Johnsen SG, Agger P. Quantitative evaluation of testicular biopsies before and after varicocelectomy. *Fertil Steril* 1978; 29:58–63.

48. Weiss DB, Rodriguez-Rigau LJ, Smith KD, et al. Quantitation of Leydig cells in testicular biopsies of oligospermic men with varicocele. *Fertil Steril* 1978; 30:305–312.

49. Cameron DF, Snydle FE, Ross MH, et al. Ultrastructural alterations in the adluminal testicular compartment in men with varicocele. *Fertil Steril* 1980; 33:526–533.

50. Terquem A, Dadoune JP. Morphological findings in varicocele: an ultrastructural study of 30 bilateral testicular biopsies. *Int J Androl* 1981; 4:515–531.

51. Fujisawa M, Yoshida S, Kojima K, et al. Biochemical changes in testicular varicocele. *Arch Androl* 1989; 22:149–159.

52. Fujisawa M, Yoshida S, Matsumoto O, et al. Decrease of topoisomerase I activity in the testis of infertile men with varicocele. *Arch Androl* 1988; 21:45–50.

53. Rodriguez-Rigau LJ, Weiss DB, Zuckermann Z, et al. A possible mechanism for the detrimental effect of varicocele on testicular function in men. *Fertil Steril* 1978; 30:575–585.

54. Ando S, Giacchetto C, Colpi G, et al. Plasma levels of 17-OH-progesterone and testosterone in patients with varicoceles. *Acta Endocrinol* 1983; 102:463–469.

55. Takayema M, Honjoh M, Kodama M, et al. Testicular steroids in spermatic and peripheral veins after single injection of hCG in patients with varicocele. *Arch Androl* 1990; 24:207–213.

56. Comhaire F, Vermeulen A. Plasma testosterone in patients with varicocele and sexual inadequacy. *J Clin Endocrinol Metab* 1975; 40:824–829.

57. Su LM, Goldstein M, Schlegel PN. The effect of varicocelectomy on serum testosterone levels in infertile men with varicoceles. *J Urol* 1995; 154:1752–1755.

58. Scholler R, Nahoul K, Castanier M, et al. Testicular secretion of conjugated and unconjugated steroids in normal adults and in patients with varicocele. Baseline levels and time course response to hCG administration. *J Steroid Biochem* 1984; 20:203–215.

59. Hudson RW, McKay DE. The gonadotropin response of men with varicoceles to gonadotropin-releasing hormones. *Fertil Steril* 1980; 33:427–432.

60. Hudson RW. The endocrinology of varicoceles. *Fertil Steril* 1986; 49:199–208.

61. Fujisawa M, Hayashi A, Imanishi O, et al. The significance of gonadotropin-releasing hormone test for predicting fertility after varicocelectomy. *Fertil Steril* 1994; 61:779–782.

62. MacLeod J. Seminal cytology in the presence of varicocele. *Fertil Steril* 1965; 16:735–757.

63. Ali JI, Weaver DJ, Weinstein SH, et al. Scrotal temperature and semen quality in men with and

without varicocele. *Arch Androl* 1989; 24:215–219.

64. Naftulin BN, Samuels SJ, Hellstrom WJG, et al. Semen quality in varicocele patients is characterized by tapered sperm cells. *Fertil Steril* 1991; 56:149–151.

65. Rodriguez-Rigau LJ, Smith KD, Steinberger E. Varicocele and the morphology of spermatozoa. *Fertil Steril* 1981; 35:54–57.

66. Ayodeji O, Baker HW. Is there a specific abnormality of sperm morphology in men with varicoceles? *Fertil Steril* 1986; 45:839–842.

67. Nilsson S, Edvinsson A, Nilsson B. Improvement of semen and pregnancy rate after ligation and division of internal spermatic vein: fact or fiction? *Br J Urol* 1979; 51:591–596.

68. Vermeulen A, Vandeghe M. Improved fertility after varicocele correction: fact or fiction? *Fertil Steril* 1984; 42:249–256.

69. Laven JS, Haans LC, Mali WP, et al. Effects of varicocele treatment in adolescents. *Fertil Steril* 1992; 58:756–762.

70. Goldstein M, Gilbert BR, Dicker AP, et al. Microsurgical inguinal varicocelectomy with delivery of the testis: an artery and lymphatic sparing technique. *J Urol* 1992; 148:1808–1811.

71. Madgar I, Weissenberg R, Lunenfeld B, et al. Controlled trial of high spermatic vein ligation for varicocele in infertile men. *Fertil Steril* 1995; 63:120–124.

72. Schlesinger MH, Wilets IF, Nagler HM. Treatment outcome after varicocelectomy: a critical analysis. *Urol Clin North Am* 1994; 21:517–529.

73. Steckel J, Dicker AP, Goldstein M. Influence of varicocele size on response to microsurgical ligation of the spermatic veins. *J Urol* 1993; 149:769–771.

74. Jarow JP, Ogle SR, Eskew LA. Seminal improvement following repair of ultrasound detected subclinical varicoceles. *J Urol* 1996; 155:1287–1290.

75. Comhaire F, Kunnen M. Selective retrograde venography of the internal spermatic vein: a conclusive approach to the diagnosis of varicocele. *Andrologia* 1976; 8:11–24.

76. World Health Organization (WHO). Comparison among different methods for the diagnosis of varicocele. *Fertil Steril* 1985; 43:575–577.

77. Dhabuwala CB, Hamid S, Moghissi KS. Clinical versus subclinical varicocele: improvement in fertility after varicocelectomy. *Fertil Steril* 1992; 57:854–875.

78. Comhaire F, Monteyne R, Kunnen M. The value of scrotal thermography as compared with selective retrograde venography of the internal spermatic vein for the diagnosis of "subclinical" varicocele. *Fertil Steril* 1976; 27:694–698.

79. Comhaire F, Simons M, Kunnen M, et al. Testicular arterial perfusion in varicocele: the role of rapid sequence scintigraphy with technetium in varicocele evaluation. *J Urol* 1983; 130:923–926.

80. McClure RD, Hricak H. Scrotal ultrasound in the infertile man: detection of subclinical unilateral and bilateral varicoceles. *J Urol* 1986; 135:711–715.

81. Eskew LA, Watson NE, Wolfman N, et al. Ultrasonographic diagnosis of varicoceles. *Fertil Steril* 1993; 60:693–697.

82. Howards SS. Subclinical varicocele. *Fertil Steril* 1992; 57:725–726.

83. McClure RD, Khoo D, Jarvi K, et al. Subclinical varicocele: the effectiveness of varicocelectomy. *J Urol* 1991; 145:789–791.

84. Kondoh N, Meguro N, Matsumiya K, et al. Significance of subclinical varicocele detected by scrotal sonography in male infertility: a preliminary report. *J Urol* 1993; 150:1158–1160.

85. Bsat FA, Masabani R. Effectiveness of varicocelectomy in varicoceles diagnosed by physical examination versus Doppler studies. *Fertil Steril* 1988; 50:321–323.

86. Tinga DJ, Jager S, Bruijnen CLAH, et al. Factors related to semen improvement and fertility after varicocele operation. *Fertil Steril* 1984; 41:404–410.

87. Russell JK. Varicocele, age, and fertility. *Lancet* 1957; 2:222.

88. Nagler HM, Li X-Z, Lizza EF, et al. Varicocele: temporal considerations. *J Urol* 1985; 134:411–413.

89. Hadziselimovic F, Herzog B, Liebundgut B, et al. Testicular and vascular changes in children and adults with varicocele. *J Urol* 1989; 142:583–585.

90. Harrison RM, Lewis RW, Roberts JA. Pathophysiology of varicocele in nonhuman primates: long-term seminal and testicular changes. *Fertil Steril* 1986; 46:500–510.

91. Chehval MJ, Purcell MH. Deterioration of semen parameters over time in men with untreated varicocele: evidence of progressive testicular damage. *Fertil Steril* 1992; 57:174–177.

92. Kass EJ, Freitas JE, Bour JB. Adolescent varicocele: objective indications for treatment. *J Urol* 1989; 142:579–582.

93. Kass EJ, Marcol B. Results of varicocele surgery in adolescents: a comparison of techniques. *J Urol* 1992; 148:694–696.

94. Jarow JP, Assimos DJ, Pittaway DE. Effectiveness of laparoscopic varicocelectomy. *Urology* 1993; 42:544–547.

95. Lynch WJ, Badenoch DF, McAnena OJ. Comparison of laparoscopic and open ligation of the testicular vein. *Br J Urol* 1993; 72:796–798.

96. Enquist E, Stein BS, Sigman M. Laparoscopic versus subinguinal varicocelectomy: a comparative study. *Fertil Steril* 1994; 61:1092–1096.

97. Mischinger HJ, Colombo T, Rauchenwald M, et al. Laparoscopic procedure for varicocelectomy. *Br J Urol* 1994; 74:112–116.

98. Donovan JF, Winfield HN. Laparoscopic varix ligation. *J Urol* 1992; 147:77–81.

99. Marmar JL, Kim Y. Subinguinal microsurgical varicocelectomy: a technical critique and statistical analysis of semen and pregnancy data. *J Urol* 1994; 152:1127–1132.

100. Marmar JL, DeBenedictis TJ, Praiss D. The management of varicoceles by microdissection of the spermatic cord at the external inguinal ring. *Fertil Steril* 1985; 43:583–588.

101. Kaufman SL, Kadir S, Barth KH, et al. Mechanisms of recurrent varicocele after balloon occlusion or surgical ligation of the internal spermatic vein. *Radiology* 1983; 147:435.

102. Lima SS, Castro MP, Costa OF. A new method for the treatment of varicocele. *Andrologia* 1978; 10:103–106.

103. Walsh PC, White RI. Balloon occlusion of the internal spermatic vein for the treatment of varicoceles. *JAMA* 1981; 246:1701–1702.

104. Weissbach L, Thelen M, Adolphs H-D. Treatment of idiopathic varicoceles by transfemoral testicular vein occlusion. *J Urol* 1981; 126:354–356.

105. Murray RR, Mitchell SE, Kadir S, et al. Comparison of recurrent varicocele anatomy following surgery and percutaneous balloon occlusion. *J Urol* 1986; 135:286–289.

106. Kaufman SL, Kadir S, Barth KH, et al. Mechanisms of recurrent varicocele after balloon occlusion or surgical ligation of the internal spermatic vein. *Radiology* 1983; 147:435–440.

107. Mitchell SE, White RI, Chang R, et al. Long-term results of outpatient balloon embolotherapy in 300 varicoceles. *Radiology* 1985; 157(suppl):90.

108. Matthews RD, Roberts J, Walker WA, et al. Migration of intravascular balloon after percutaneous embolotherapy of varicocele. *Urology* 1992; 49:373–375.

109. White RI, Kaufman SL, Barth KH, et al. Occlusion of varicoceles with detachable balloons. *Radiology* 1981; 139:327–334.

110. Morag B, Rubinstein ZJ, Goldwasser B, et al. Percutaneous venography and occlusion in the management of spermatic varicoceles. *Am J Roentgen* 1984; 143:635–640.

111. Tauber R, Johnsen N. Antegrade scrotal sclerotherapy for the treatment of varicocele: technique and late results. *J Urol* 1994; 151:386–390.

112. Szabo R, Kessler R. Hydrocele following internal spermatic vein ligation: a retrospective study and review of the literature. *J Urol* 1984; 132:924–925.

113. Silber S. Microsurgical aspects of varicocele. *Fertil Steril* 1979; 31:230–232.

114. Wosnitzer M, Roth JA. Optical magnification and Doppler ultrasound probe for varicocelectomy. *Urology* 1983; 22:24–26.

115. Penn I, Mackie G, Halgrimson CG, et al. Testicular complications following renal transplantation. *Ann Surg* 1972; 176:697–699.

116. Goldstein M, Young GPH, Einer-Jensen N. Testicular artery damage due to infiltration with a fine gauge needle: experimental evidence suggesting that blind cord block should be abandoned. *Surg Forum* 1983; 24:653–656.

117. MacMahon RA, O'Brien B McG, Cussen LJ. The use of microsurgery in the treatment of the undescended testis. *J Pediatr Surg* 1976; 11:521–526.

118. Gorenstein A, Katz S, Schiller M. Varicocele in children: "To treat or not to treat"—venographic and manometric studies. *J Pediatr Surg* 1986; 21:1046–1050.

119. Levitt S, Gill B, Katlowitz N, et al. Routine intraoperative post-ligation venography in the treatment of the pediatric varicocele. *J Urol* 1987; 137:716–718.

120. Reitelman C, Burbige KA, Sawczuk IS, et al. Diagnosis and surgical correction of the pediatric varicocele. *J Urol* 1987; 138:1038–1040.

121. Homonnai ZT, Fainman N, Engelhard Y, et al. Varicocelectomy and male fertility: comparison of semen quality and recurrence of varicocele following varicocelectomy by two techniques. *Int J Androl* 1980; 3:447–456.

122. Rothman LP, Newmark M, Karson R. The recurrent varicocele. A poorly recognized problem. *Fertil Steril* 1981; 35:552–556.

123. Sayfan J, Adam YG, Soffer Y. A natural "venous bypass" causing postoperative recurrence of a varicocele. *J Androl* 1981; 2:108–110.

124. Sayfan J, Adam YG, Soffer Y. A new entity in varicocele subfertility: the "cremasteric reflux." *Fertil Steril* 1980; 33:88–90.

125. Nieschlag E, Hertle L, Fischdick A, et al. Treatment of varicocele: counseling as effective as occlusion of the vena spermatica. *Hum Reprod* 1995; 10:347–353.

126. Pryor JL, Howards SS. Varicocele. *Urol Clin North Am* 1987; 14:499–513.

127. Wright EJ, Goldstein M. Ligation of the testicular artery during microsurgical varicocelectomy: incidence and implications. *J Urol* 1994; 151:141A.

# 14
# Penile Vibratory Stimulation and Electroejaculation

Dana A. Ohl and Jens Sonksen

Ejaculatory dysfunction is an uncommon cause of male infertility. In Dubin and Amelar's[1] classic paper on causes of male sexual dysfunction, only 2% of men presenting for treatment of subfertility were diagnosed with ejaculatory dysfunction as the cause.

There are, however, certain clinical conditions in which infertility is mostly due to ejaculatory dysfunction, such as patients with spinal cord injury (SCI) or who have had a surgical sympathectomy from retroperitoneal lymph node dissection (RPLND). In these individuals, absence of seminal emission represents a formidable therapeutic dilemma for the treating physician.

## Normal Ejaculatory Reflex

The ejaculatory reflex is of very short duration but represents a complex series of events.[2] If these events do not occur in an organized fashion, with all components actively performing their roles, appropriate delivery of sperm will not occur. These events are under the control of several divisions of the nervous system, but the afferent inputs into this reflex are of two major types, cerebral and genital sensory.

The cerebral contribution to the reflex is quite poorly understood, for visual, auditory, and other erotic stimuli are processed and integrated by the brain.[3] In most sexual situations, higher central nervous system (CNS) input alone will not initiate a climax, but helps instead to lower the threshold for climax and ejaculation. However, an ejaculatory reflex may be initiated solely by CNS input, such as in nocturnal emissions.

Sensory information entering the sacral cord must ascend through the spinothalamic tracts to the thoracolumbar ejaculation center, where such input is merged with that coming from cerebral centers in descending tracts. Nerves carrying tactile stimulation information from the penis and genitals enter the sacral cord at levels S2–4, and impulses are carried there via the dorsal nerve of the penis. Integration of information in the cord results in efferent sympathetic signals being generated to effect the peripheral manifestations of the reflex.

Autonomic impulses responsible for seminal emission exit the lateral thoracolumbar cord at levels T10–L2, and these autonomic nerves then enter the sympathetic chains. Postganglionic fibers from each sympathetic chain emerge and course anteriorly at the lateral surface of the aorta. They coalesce on the anterior surface of the aorta just below the inferior mesenteric artery (inferior mesenteric plexus). From there, they again diverge and course somewhat laterally down into the pelvis as the hypogastric outflow. They then travel to the ejaculatory organs where there is a short synapse in or near the walls of these organs.

Activation of these fibers results in contraction of the vas deferens, seminal vesicles, prostate, and bladder neck. Seminal emission into the posterior urethra ensues, and the emitted ejaculate is prevented from going backward into the bladder by the tight contraction of the bladder neck. At the time of seminal emission, there are pleasurable generalized and localized (genital) sensations collectively termed as orgasm.

Shortly after seminal emission, rhythmic contractions of the periurethral muscles cause rhythmic projectile ejaculation of seminal fluid. These involuntary muscle contractions are carried by somatic fibers innervating skeletal muscle. These muscles are normally under full voluntary control, but during the course of the ejaculatory reflex their action becomes completely involuntary.

# Ejaculatory Dysfunction

Neurologic lesions at any of the normal ejaculatory reflex components can lead to ejaculatory dysfunction. The type of neurologic dysfunction dictates the clinical scenario.

## Premature Ejaculation

Premature ejaculation is probably caused by lack of proper cerebral control leading to activation of the ejaculatory reflex prior to the desired time. Most men with premature ejaculation are able to ejaculate intravaginally and to collect semen on command. Fertility, therefore, is not an issue, and ejaculation induction procedures are not necessary.

## Idiopathic Anejaculation

This condition, like premature ejaculation, is thought in most cases to have psychological causes. It is usually diagnosed by history. Men with idiopathic anejaculation suffer total anorgasmia, an inability to climax and ejaculate during sexual activity. Some men with this condition are able to ejaculate with masturbation, but most are unable to reach climax under any circumstances while awake. Typically, intermittent nocturnal emissions are present.[4]

Many of these men awaken during nocturnal emissions and thus have a good idea of what the sensation of orgasm is like. In men who do not have an appreciation for this sensation, a detailed history is necessary to determine whether they are suffering from inability to climax or whether there is totally dry ejaculate at the time of climax.

Men with refractory idiopathic anejaculation are candidates for electroejaculation for the purposes of achieving a pregnancy if more conservative measures fail to result in successful orgasm and ejaculation.[4] A small minority of men with this condition may also respond to penile vibratory stimulation (PVS), but experience with vibration is extremely limited in this patient population.

## Retrograde Ejaculation

Retrograde ejaculation is caused by inability of the bladder neck to close, resulting in ejaculation backward into the bladder. In men with retrograde ejaculation, the other components of the ejaculatory reflex (seminal emission and contraction of the periurethral muscles) are usually intact. Many of the conditions discussed below that cause total absence of seminal emission may also cause retrograde ejaculation.

Because sperm are being emitted into the bladder, ejaculation induction procedures are not necessary, but medical management is indicated to convert retrograde ejaculators to antegrade ejaculators prior to insemination with sperm retrieved from the urine.

## Anejaculation/Absence of Seminal Emission

Anejaculation is the absence of release of seminal fluid due to neurologic causes. Some men with absence of seminal emission, such as those with SCI, will also have anorgasmia, whereas others, such as men with diabetic neuropathy or those who have had a retroperitoneal lymph node dissection, will have orgasm with absence of seminal emission.

### Spinal Cord Injury

Men with SCI may be infertile from a variety of causes, including erectile dysfunction, ejaculatory dysfunction, and poor sperm quality.[5,6] Of the functional deficits, ejaculatory dysfunction is clearly the most important. Only about 5% of men with SCI are able to ejaculate without medical intervention. A detailed history may be helpful in identifying those with preserved ejaculation, but because these men do not usually have the capability to sense whether an orgasm occurs, it is sometimes difficult to fully characterize their level of baseline function. Nevertheless, the physician should inquire about responses to masturbation and sexual activity in order to identify whether characteristic reflexes that are typical during ejaculation are occurring. The appearance of cloudy urine or the presence of clumped material following sexual activity may indicate the presence of occult retrograde ejaculation.

Men with SCI who are anejaculatory may be candidates for either PVS or electroejaculation (EEJ).

## Testicular Cancer/Retroperitoneal Lymph Node Dissection

Retroperitoneal lymph node dissection (RPLND) has an integral role in the treatment of testis cancer. Unfortunately, this operation requires that the surgeon dissect the region where crucial components of the ejaculatory reflex reside.

Classic bilateral radical retroperitoneal lymphadenectomy has resulted in ejaculatory dysfunction in nearly all cases, because the template for such an operation damages all of the sympathetic outflow-controlling ejaculation.[7,8] Although the ejaculatory dysfunction following RPLND has been referred to as retrograde ejaculation, there is evidence that a great deal of ejaculatory dysfunction found in the classic RPLND is, in fact, total absence of seminal emission.[7]

Newer, nerve-sparing operations have been developed to decrease the rate of ejaculatory dysfunction from RPLND. These include modification of the template to narrow the areas of dissection,[9] direct sparing of nerves,[10] or combinations of both techniques.[11] In the template method, it is crucial to preserve the contralateral sympathetic chain, its outflow, and the inferior hypogastric plexus below the inferior mesenteric artery.

With application of modified templates and nerve-sparing techniques, ejaculation rates approaching 100% can be achieved in low-stage disease.[10,11] Men who have residual masses following chemotherapy and those with higher stage disease have a higher rate of ejaculatory dysfunction even when nerve-sparing procedures are attempted, and some of these men with large-volume disease may be better candidates for the classic operation with its inevitable anejaculation.

Men with anejaculation following RPLND are candidates for electroejaculation.[12] Those who have had additional treatment, such as chemotherapy and radiation therapy, may have further compromised sperm quality, despite a successful electroejaculation procedure.[13]

## Peripheral Neuropathy

Autonomic neuropathy involving the sympathetic nerves may occur in a variety of clinical situations. The most common setting is that of advanced diabetic neuropathy where a variety of autonomic functions may be affected, including gastric emptying, cardiac rhythm control, and erectile function. Ejaculatory dysfunction is seen in a minority of diabetic neuropathy patients but, when present, can be an important cause of infertility.

Ejaculatory dysfunction in diabetic patients follows a course typical of other autonomic disruptions. The abnormal function is slowly progressive, beginning with decreased ejaculate volume, followed by retrograde ejaculation, and culminating in the absence of seminal emission. Medical management may result in improvement in such slowly progressive conditions, but continued deterioration is expected.

## Other Neurologic Conditions

The ejaculatory reflex may also be impaired by multiple sclerosis, myelodysplasia, syringomyelia, and different types of retroperitoneal and perirectal surgery. Very rarely, some men with ejaculatory dysfunction will have no definable neurologic explanation for their condition. Men suffering anejaculation from these varied conditions present a greater challenge, because the clinical situation is not as obvious. Evaluation and recommendations for treatment in such individuals must follow a logical progression of steps.

# Evaluation and Initial Therapy of Ejaculatory Dysfunction

The initial history is many times the most useful piece of information leading to a diagnosis of an ejaculatory problem. Some historical points are obvious, such as spinal cord injury and a history of RPLND. Others may be more subtle, such as early diabetic neuropathy or multiple sclerosis, particularly if the diagnosis of the primary condition has not yet been made.

The physician must ask about changes in sexual function and particularly about experiences at the time of ejaculation. Detailing the events surrounding possible orgasm is required in men who have never experienced an orgasm, as such men may have a poor understanding of what is supposed to happen. A precise, step-by-step description of what the patient is experiencing may lead to a diagnosis of anorgasmia. Information as to the amount of seminal fluid and any recent changes in the amount of ejaculate volume is essential. Cloudy urine or clumps in the urine following a sensation of orgasm are important indicators of possible retrograde ejaculation and should be documented if present.

The patient's general medical history and a review of systems may also lead to a diagnosis. Manifestations of systemic neuropathy in a diabetic patient may lead to the suspicion of ejaculatory dysfunction. As with any infertility problem, it is important to survey for other causes of general infertility that may coexist with a possible ejaculatory dysfunction.

The physical examination is used to support the clinical impression made upon taking the patient's history. Other signs of possible infertility, such as sparse body and facial hair (endocrine deficiency) and small testicular volume (spermatogenic defects), may be obvious on examination. The neurologic examination also may uncover clues regarding ejaculatory dysfunction.

As with any male infertility evaluation, the semen analysis is a cornerstone of the treatment of ejaculatory dysfunction. One of the most crucial pieces of information is the semen volume. Men with chronically low volume of semen may have an ejaculatory duct obstruction, diagnosed by transrectal ultrasound of the prostate, but men with low semen volume may also have an abnormal ejaculatory reflex. Those individuals with total absence of seminal emission should be checked for retrograde ejaculation by examination of the postorgasm urine. Men with the absence of any seminal emission, but an excellent history consistent with orgasm, have a high likelihood of neurogenic ejaculatory dysfunction.

Men with psychogenic dysfunction (premature ejaculation and idiopathic anejaculation) are best treated by psychological means, e.g., sex therapy. Premature ejaculation is treated quite readily and with high success rates by a sex therapist, but idiopathic anejaculation can be more problematic. Men with idiopathic anejaculation who are resistant to sex therapy may be considered candidates for EEJ or possibly PVS.[4]

Men with organic absence of seminal emission and those with retrograde ejaculation should be tried initially on sympathomimetic agents in an attempt to induce antegrade ejaculation. Various sympathomimetic agents have been used, including ephedrine, phenylpropanolamine, and tricyclic antidepressants.[14,15] These drugs work poorly in those men who have ejaculatory dysfunction from acute events, such as SCI and RPLND. The best results are seen in individuals who have the recent onset of a slowly progressive condition, such as men with early ejaculatory dysfunction from diabetic neuropathy.

Men with anejaculation who do not respond to medical management can be considered candidates for ejaculation induction procedures.

Men with retrograde ejaculation who do not respond to sympathomimetic agents and do not convert to antegrade ejaculation are candidates for assisted reproductive techniques using sperm retrieved from the bladder. On the day of the partner's ovulation, the man is initially catheterized to empty the bladder and to instill a sperm-friendly medium. He then masturbates to climax, and the sperm are extracted by a second catheterization. Patients are prepped with sodium bicarbonate to balance the pH in the urine, and their fluid intake is restricted prior to sperm retrieval. The fluid restriction is aimed at limiting the urine production between catheterizations, thereby limiting the contact of urine and sperm. By the above-mentioned techniques, the second catheterization yields nearly pure ejaculate with almost no urine. This use of catheterization and fluid restriction versus spontaneous voiding is, however, controversial.[16,17]

Sperm retrieved from the bladder are immediately washed and processed in the laboratory. This yields a clean specimen suitable for artificial insemination, and many pregnancies have been reported by the use of such sperm.[16,18,19]

# Ejaculation Induction Procedures

## Less Commonly Used Procedures

Some ejaculation induction procedures have fallen out of favor. Intrathecal administration of cholinesterase inhibitors is one such procedure.[20] Introduction of neostigmine into the spinal canal of an anejaculatory spinal cord injured man will result in several ejaculations over the ensuing several hours. Unfortunately, many unwanted autonomic adverse effects also occur, such as paroxysmal changes in blood pressure, sweating, and flushing. One death has been reported from malignant hypertension and cerebral hemorrhage following the use of this technique.[20] These autonomic side effects dictate that such a procedure needs to be performed in an intensive care unit. Because of more recent and safer alternatives, intrathecal neostigmine has little place in the modern management of anejaculation.

To decrease the autonomic side effects of intrathecal administration of cholinesterase inhibitors, subcutaneous administration of physostigmine has been suggested by Chapelle and coworkers.[21] Side effects are less severe, but the ejaculation rates are also lower. Furthermore, manual or vibratory stimulation of the penis is also required to optimize ejaculation rates. Be-

cause high ejaculation rates are obtainable with PVS alone, the wisdom of even subcutaneous administration of a cholinesterase inhibitor needs to be questioned.

There have been reports of surgical extraction of sperm from anejaculatory males.[22–24] Although adequate amounts of sperm that can cause pregnancy may be obtained, the potential for scarring of the genital tracts and subsequent obstruction makes this a less appealing option than vibratory simulation or electroejaculation.

## Penile Vibratory Stimulation (PVS)

Vibratory stimulation of the penis can induce ejaculation in the majority of men with SCI. Because this procedure relies on activation of a normal reflex, all components of the lower reflex arc must be present; therefore, men who are anejaculatory from RPLND will not respond to PVS. Further, men with the potential for cerebral inhibition of the ejaculatory reflex, such as those with idiopathic anejaculation, will most likely not respond to the vibrator.

The goal of PVS is to activate a normal ejaculatory reflex. The afferent stimulation used is the genital input from the penis, initiated by application of a vibrating knob against the frenulum of the penis and held there for a period of 3 minutes or until antegrade ejaculation ensues (Fig. 14.1). A series of characteristic responses occur during PVS. Initially, abdominal and leg muscle contractions occur episodically, as well as generalized piloerection and scrotal wall contraction. Penile erection is a common occurrence but is not essential for the ejaculatory response. In the seconds preceding ejaculation, the abdominal and leg muscles become more profoundly and tonically contracted, and the erection rigidity may peak. Men prone to autonomic dysreflexia note severe flushing and may sense that the blood pressure is elevated. Periurethral contractions begin and proceed in a rhythmic fashion, with resultant projectile ejaculation. Almost all patients exhibit antegrade ejaculation exclusively, indicating normal reflex closure of the bladder neck.

At the time that rhythmic periurethral contractions appear, the vibration stimulation should be stopped. By stopping the stimulation

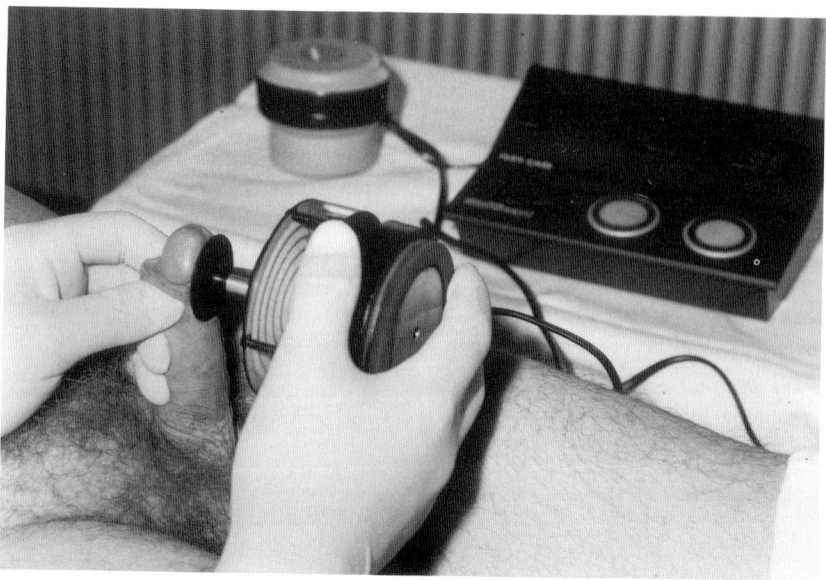

Figure 14.1. Penile vibrator is applied to the frenulum until ejaculation occurs.

at this time, multiple ejaculations over several minutes may be achieved and the risk of autonomic dysreflexia is limited. If no ejaculation ensues for a period of 3 minutes, a rest period of 1 to 2 minutes should be given, followed by a repetition of the stimulation procedure. If no ejaculation occurs in six stimulation cycles, the patient is considered as having a penile vibration failure.

The highest ejaculation rates are seen in individuals who have spastic upper motor neuron lesions (>T9) and intact reflexes below the level of the lesion. Intact hip flexion and bulbocavernosus reflexes predict success from PVS in 77% of cases, whereas absence of these reflexes suggests failure in nearly all cases.[25] The effect of bladder management on ejaculation rates from PVS is controversial.[25,26]

Significant complications from PVS are unusual. Local skin swelling is a common finding but is self-limited and mild. Skin abrasion or frank ulceration is rare. Muscle spasms of the abdomen and lower extremities may be uncomfortable. The most serious potential complication of PVS is autonomic dysreflexia, a condition where autonomic reflexes are expressed in an unchecked fashion, leading to dangerous elevations of the blood pressure.[27]

This response is seen in SCI patients with spinal lesions above T6. In response to noxious stimuli below the level of the injury, activation of sympathetic mechanisms to increase blood pressure is induced and continues unchecked by the brain stem homeostatic mechanisms, because there is no neural communication between the two systems. Application of a penile vibrator may induce these changes with resultant marked increases in blood pressure.

Men with lesions above T6 and/or those with a history of autonomic dysreflexia are at risk for developing this dangerous response during PVS. Blood pressure must be monitored in such individuals to assure it is not reaching dangerous levels. Blood pressure elevation can be limited by avoidance of vibration during ejaculation (as noted above). If the blood pressure rises to unacceptable levels during the procedure, it returns to baseline promptly upon cessation of the stimulation. In men prone to dysreflexia, the blood pressure rise can be blunted by prophylactic administration of nifedipine 10 to 20 mg sublingually 10 minutes prior to PVS.

There are numerous published reports regarding the efficacy of PVS in men with SCI.[28–33] Unfortunately, the ejaculation rates in

TABLE 14.1. Ejaculation rates from selected series of penile vibratory stimulation in SCI males.

| Reference | Ejaculation rate | Number of patients |
|---|---|---|
| Piera, 1973[28] | 27% | 101 |
| Brindley, 1984[29] | 53% | 93 |
| Sarkarati et al, 1987[30] | 24% | 33 |
| Szasz and Carpenter, 1989[31] | 40% | 57 |
| Beretta et al, 1989[32] | 71% | 102 |
| Siösteen et al, 1990[33] | 91% | 32 |

Range: 24–91%.

such reports vary widely, and it is difficult to extract from the older literature optimum vibration parameters (Table 14.1). Recent work by Sonksen et al[26] has shown that the amplitude of the vibration appears to be of utmost importance in achieving success. High ejaculation rates were seen when the peak-to-peak amplitude of a vibrator was 2.5 mm at 100 Hz (96%), in contrast to much lower ejaculation rates (32%) with an amplitude of only 1.0 mm. The efficacy of the high amplitude vibration was verified by Sonksen et al in another group of 41 Danish men with SCI (83% ejaculation rate)[26] and by Ohl et al[25] in an American cohort. In the latter series, 65% of all men with SCI had antegrade ejaculation, but in men with lesions above T10 the ejaculation rate was 81%. Sonksen et al's preliminary work has led to the development of a Food and Drug Administration (FDA)-registered device that reliably delivers the optimum vibration parameters (Fig. 14.2).

Sonksen and Biering-Sorensen[6] reviewed the efficacy of PVS in establishing pregnancies. In 619 men treated with PVS, 102 pregnancies were established. The successes were obtained with a variety of techniques, including home vaginal insemination by the patients and intracervical and intrauterine insemination in the clinic setting. The literature is quite confusing in this field, because of poorly standardized reporting of pregnancies, inaccurate numbers on how many of these men were actively seeking pregnancy, and which types of methods were used to initiate pregnancy. Because of these inconsistencies, it is often difficult to extract accurate pregnancy rates.

## Electroejaculation (EEJ)

In contradistinction to vibratory stimulation, EEJ is suitable for all types of neurogenic and psychogenic anejaculation. This procedure is uniformly successful in inducing seminal

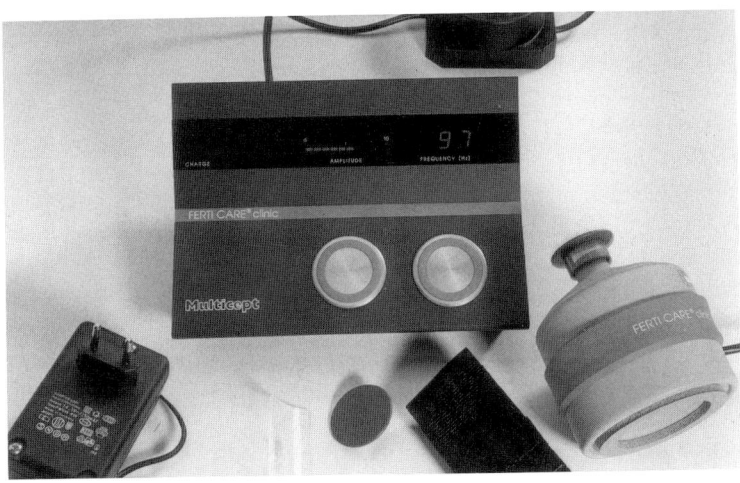

FIGURE 14.2. Commercially available device for penile vibratory stimulation, the FERTI CARE Clinic (Multicept APS, Rungsted, Denmark).

emission in all patients and applies to those SCI men who are PVS failures.

Electroejaculation is carried out via rectal probe. Although the exact mechanism of EEJ is not understood, the procedure does not produce the normal characteristic ejaculatory response seen in PVS. Release of semen may be intermittent following each stimulation, or may be episodic. Another difference is that a significant portion of an electroejaculate is emitted in retrograde direction.

Because of these characteristics of EEJ, it is important to catheterize the patient before a procedure to empty all the urine from the bladder. The urine toxicity is also limited by decreasing acidity with sodium bicarbonate and placing a sperm-friendly medium into the bladder, similar to the recommendations above for men with retrograde ejaculation. An appropriate-sized rectal probe is used to give the stimulation, and then an antegrade ejaculate is collected in a sterile specimen container. The patient is catheterized after the procedure to remove any retrograde ejaculate from the bladder. Both specimens can be processed and used for assisted reproductive techniques. A sigmoidoscopy to 10 cm is performed before and after stimulation to survey for preexisting rectal conditions and injury from the procedure.

Serious complications from EEJ are uncommon. Rectal injury occurs in less than 0.1% of patients, but this complication may require operative repair and diverting colostomy. Autonomic dysreflexia is consistently seen in men with SCI with lesions above T6 and can be quite severe, but extreme blood pressure elevations can be prevented with prophylactic nifedipine. EEJ typically requires more nifedipine than does PVS, with a typical starting dose of 20 mg given sublingually 10 minutes prior to the procedure. If severe hypertension occurs during EEJ, stopping the stimulation and removing the rectal probe allows prompt return to baseline pressures. Abdominal and leg spasms, which may be more uncomfortable than those seen in PVS, are common.

Because PVS is noninvasive, lacks the risk of rectal injury, and entails less discomfort than EEJ, patients universally prefer that PVS be used to procure semen specimens. The current algorithm for patients with SCI is to try PVS first and save EEJ for PVS nonresponders.

Patients with causes of anejaculation other than spinal cord injury and who have normal pelvic and perirectal sensation require an anesthetic before EEJ. This is also true of men with SCI with very low lesions and those with sensory sparing below the lesion. Spinal or general anesthetics have been used in such patients, without altering the universal success in inducing seminal emission.

At the University of Michigan Spinal Cord Fertility Program, EEJ has been in use since 1985. Seminal emission has been routinely obtained, but semen containing sperm in adequate numbers for artificial insemination is seen in only 71% of men with SCI.[34] Of men who were anejaculatory because of RPLND, 87% had adequate sperm numbers. Of the RPLND men who did not have sperm in the EEJ specimen, one had carcinoma in situ of the remaining testis and the others had chemotherapy-induced germ cell failure.[12] One hundred and twenty couples with anejaculatory infertility were treated with EEJ and assisted reproductive technologies. Fifty-three (44%) of the couples achieved 75 pregnancies. Forty-three of these couples achieved their first pregnancy by EEJ in combination with intrauterine insemination, and the remaining ten couples required the gamete intrafallopian transfer (GIFT) procedure.[35]

# Sperm Quality in Ejaculation Induction Procedures

Regardless of the cause of ejaculatory dysfunction, both PVS and EEJ yield semen specimens with poor sperm quality. Specimens typically have normal-to-high counts but poor motility (Table 14.2).[12,25,36,37] The problem of poor basic semen quality is further compounded by the finding of more subtle abnormalities in sperm function.

In a cohort of men undergoing electroejaculation, sperm-function assessments were performed, including viability staining, sperm survival, bovine mucus penetration, hamster

TABLE 14.2. Selected series examining sperm count and motility in specimens obtained by ejaculation induction procedures.

| Series | | Procedure | Total sperm (millions) | Motility |
|---|---|---|---|---|
| Ohl et al, 1989[34] | (Antegrade) | EEJ | 2440 (both fractions) | 18% |
| Denil et al, 1992[36] | (Antegrade) | EEJ | 2752 (both fractions) | 11% |
| Sonksen et al, 1991[37] | (Antegrade) | PVS | 99 (antegrade) | 13% |
| Ohl et al, 1995[25] | (Antegrade) | PVS | 1236 (both fractions) | 26% |

egg sperm penetration assay (SPA), and the direct immunobead test. The sperm had poor viability (which nearly exactly paralleled the motility), poor survival, mildly impaired mucus penetration, and decreased scores on the SPA.[36] Immunologic infertility was not found to be an important cause of poor sperm quality in these patients.[38]

The exact reasons for poor sperm quality are not clear. In men with spinal cord injury, potential etiologies of this poor sperm quality as enumerated in a review article by Linsenmeyer and Perkash[39] include recurrent urinary tract infections, type of bladder management, stasis of prostatic fluid, testicular hyperthermia, abnormal testicular histology, changes in the hypothalamic pituitary testicular axis, sperm antibodies, and long-term use of various medications.

Men with testicular cancer may even suffer spermatogenic defects prior to their retroperitoneal lymphadenectomy, a phenomenon termed "pretreatment subfertility."[40–42] Fertility may be further compromised by ejaculatory dysfunction and by other treatment modalities, such as chemotherapy or radiation therapy.[43,44] Even when these additional treatment modalities have not been used, sperm quality from EEJ is poor in men who are status post retroperitoneal lymphadenectomy.

Because of the poor sperm quality, it is essential that ovulation monitoring and female management be optimized by the gynecology team. The addition of high-level assisted reproductive techniques, such as in vitro fertilization with or without intracytoplasmic injection, may be necessary in extreme cases of poor semen quality or in those couples who do not become pregnant with intrauterine insemination alone.

## Conclusion

Although ejaculatory dysfunction is an uncommon cause of infertility, it may be the sole cause in various clinical situations, such as spinal cord injury and retroperitoneal lymphadenectomy patients. With a stepwise evaluation detailing the exact type of ejaculatory dysfunction and application of ejaculation induction procedures and assisted reproductive technologies, high rates of treatment success may be achieved.

Penile vibratory stimulation should be used first in patients with SCI, and electroejaculation should be used in all other patients with ejaculatory dysfunction and in men with SCI in whom PVS has failed. With these two techniques, a success rate of virtually 100% in inducing ejaculation may be obtained. Even with application of assisted reproductive techniques, fertility rates will probably never approach those of the general population because of poor sperm quality. However, with the continued advances in assisted reproduction techniques, the prospects for procreation for this cohort of infertile couples continue to improve.

Ejaculation induction procedures represent a safe, effective means of achieving pregnancy for couples in which the men have anejaculatory infertility.

## References

1. Dubin L, Amelar RD. Etiologic factors in 1294 consecutive cases of male infertility. *Fertil Steril* 1971; 22:469–474.
2. Thomas AJ. Ejaculatory dysfunction. *Fertil Steril* 1983; 39:445–454.
3. Strasberg PD, Brady SM. Sexual functioning of persons with neurologic disorders. *Semin Neurol* 1988; 8:141–144.

4. Stewart DE, Ohl DA. Idiopathic anejaculation treated by electroejaculation. *Int J Psychiatry Med* 1989; 19:263–268.

5. Biering-Sorensen F, Sonksen J. Penile erection in men with spinal cord or cauda equina lesions. *Semin Neurol* 1992; 12:98–105.

6. Sonksen J, Biering-Sorensen F. Fertility in men with spinal cord or cauda equina lesions. *Semin Neurol* 1992; 12:106–114.

7. Kedia K, Markland C, Fraley E. Sexual function following high retroperitoneal lymphadenectomy. *J Urol* 1975; 114:237–239.

8. Weissback L, Boedefeld EA, Horstmann-Dubral B. Surgical treatment of stage-I non-seminomatous germ cell testis tumor. Final results of a prospective multicenter trial 1982–1987. Testicular Tumor Study Group. *Eur Urol* 1990; 17:97–106.

9. Lange P, Chang W, Fraley E. Fertility issues following therapy for testicular cancer. *Semin Urol* 1984; 2:264–272.

10. Jewett MAS, Kong YS, Goldberg SD, et al. Retroperitoneal lymphadencetomy for testis humor with nerve sparing for ejaculation. *J Urol* 1988; 139:1220–1224.

11. Donohue JP, Foster RS, Rowland RG, et al. Nerve-sparing retroperitoneal lymphadenectomy with preservation of ejaculation. *J Urol* 1990; 144:287–291.

12. Ohl DA, Denil J, Bennett CJ, et al. Electroejaculation following retroperitoneal lymphadenectomy. *J Urol* 1991; 145:980–983.

13. Lange PH, Chang WY, Fraley EE. Fertility issues in the therapy of nonseminomatous testicular tumors. *Urol Clin North Am* 1987; 14:731–747.

14. Stewart BH, Bergant JA. Correction of retrograde ejaculation by sympathomimetic medication: preliminary report. *Fertil Steril* 1974; 25:1073–1074.

15. Brooks ME, Berezin M, Braf Z. Treatment of retrograde ejaculation with imipramine. *Urology* 1980; 15:353–355.

16. Urry RL, Middleton RG, McGavin S. A simple and effective technique for increasing pregnancy rates in couples with retrograde ejaculation. *Fertil Steril* 1986; 46:1124–1127.

17. Shangold GA, Cantor B, Schreiber JR. Treatment of infertility due to retrograde ejaculation: a simple, cost-effective method. *Fertil Steril* 1990; 54:175–177.

18. van der Linden PJ, Nan PM, te Velde ER, et al. Retrograde ejaculation: successful treatment with artificial insemination. *Obstet Gynecol* 1992; 79:126–128.

19. Vernon M, Wilson E, Muse K, et al. Successful pregnancies from men with retrograde ejaculation with the use of washed sperm and gamete intrafallopian tube transfer (GIFT). *Fertil Steril* 1988; 50:822–824.

20. Guttmann L, Walsh JJ. Prostigmine assessment test of fertility in spinal man. *Paraplegia* 1971; 9:39–51.

21. Chapelle PA, Blanquart F, Puech AJ, et al. Treatment of anejaculation in the total paraplegic by subcutaneous injection of physostigmine. *Paraplegia* 1983; 21:30–36.

22. Bustillo M, Rajfer J. Pregnancy following insemination with sperm aspirated directly from vas deferens. *Fertil Steril* 1986; 46:144–146.

23. Berger RE, Muller CH, Smith D, et al. Operative recovery of vasal sperm from anejaculatory men: preliminary report. *J Urol* 1986; 135:948–950.

24. Macourt D, Engel S, Jones RF, et al. Pregnancy by gamete intrafallopian transfer (GIFT) with sperm aspirated from the vasoepididymal junction of spinal injured man: case report. *Paraplegia* 1991; 29:550–553.

25. Ohl DA, Menge AC, Sonksen J. Penile vibratory stimulation in SCI males—does a penile prosthesis impair results? *J Urol* 1995; 153(suppl):260A.

26. Sonksen J, Biering-Sorensen F, Kristensen JK. Ejaculation induced by penile vibratory stimulation in men with spinal cord lesion. The importance of the vibratory amplitude. *Paraplegia* 1994; 32:651–660.

27. Rossier AB, Ziegler WH, Duchose PW, et al. Sexual function and dysreflexia. *Paraplegia* 1971; 9:51–63.

28. Piera JB. The establishment of a prognosis for genito-sexual function in the paraplegic and tetraplegic male. *Paraplegia* 1973; 10:271–278.

29. Brindley GS. The fertility of men with spinal injuries. *Paraplegia* 1984; 22:337–348.

30. Sarkarati M, Rossier AB, Fam BA. Experience in vibratory and electroejaculation techniques in spinal cord injury patients: a preliminary report. *J Urol* 1987; 138:59–62.

31. Szasz G, Carpenter C. Clinical observations in vibratory stimulation of the penis of men with spinal cord injury. *Arch Sex Behav* 1989; 18:461–474.

32. Beretta G, Chelo E, Zanollo A. Reproductive aspects in spinal cord injured males. *Paraplegia* 1989; 27:113–118.

33. Siösteen A, Forssman L, Steen Y, et al. Quality of semen after repeated ejaculation treatment in spinal cord injury men. *Paraplegia* 1990; 28:96–104.

34. Ohl DA, Bennet CJ, McCabe M, et al. Predictors of success in electroejaculation of spinal cord injured men. *J Urol* 1989; 142:1483–1486.

35. Ohl DA, Hurd WW, Wolf LJ, et al. Electroejaculation and assisted reproductive technologies. *Fertil Steril* 1995; 64(suppl):S138.

36. Denil J, Ohl DA, Menge AC, et al. Functional characteristics of sperm obtained by electroejaculation. *J Urol* 1992; 147:69–72.

37. Sonksen JO, Drewes AM, Biering-Sorensen F, et al. Vibration-induced reflex ejaculation in patients with spinal cord injuries [Danish]. *Ugeskr Laeger* 1991; 153:2888–2890.

38. Menge AC, Ohl DA, Denil J, et al. Absence of antisperm antibodies in anejaculatory men. *J Androl* 1990; 11:396–398.

39. Linsenmeyer TA, Perkash I. Infertility in men with spinal cord injury. *Arch Phys Med Rehabil* 1991; 72:747–754.

40. Bouchot O, Plougastel ML, Karam G, et al. Sterility and tumors of the testis. Study of late exocrine and endocrine functions in stage I or IIA

tumors [French]. *J Urol (Paris)* 1989; 95:367–371.

41. Hendry WF, Stedronska J, Jones CR, et al. Semen analysis in testicular cancer and Hodgkin's disease: pre-and post-treatment findings and implications for cyropreservation. *Br J Urol* 1983; 55:769–773.

42. Carroll PR, Whitmore WFJ, Herr HW, et al. Endocrine and exocrine profiles of men with testicular tumors before orchiectomy. *J Urol* 1987; 137:240–223.

43. Fossa SD, Ous S, Abyholm T, et al. Post-treatment fertility in patients with testicular cancer. II. Influence of cis-platin-based combination chemotherapy and of retroperitoneal surgery on hormone and sperm cell production. *Br J Urol* 1985; 57:210–214.

44. Berthelsen JG. Sperm counts and serum follicle-stimulating hormone levels before and after radiotherapy and chemotherapy in men with testicular germ cell cancer. *Fertil Steril* 1984; 41:281–286.

# 15
# Vasovasostomy

Arnold M. Belker

Vasovasostomy is performed exclusively to reverse a vasectomy, whether the vasectomy was a planned scrotal elective sterilization or the consequence of an unfortunate vasal injury, such as might occur during infant inguinal herniorrhaphy. Macrosurgical vasovasostomy is extremely simple and rapid. The results of the more difficult microsurgical anastomosis are sufficiently better now that most surgeons perform microsurgical vasovasostomy.

## Surgical Considerations

### Vasovasostomy or Vasoepididymostomy?

During a planned vasovasostomy, fluid obtained from the testicular end of the vas is examined microscopically to determine if sperm are present. When no sperm are found during the initial examination of vasal fluid, repeated microscopic examination of a series of samples of vasal fluid may reveal that sperm are present. When sperm are not seen, irrigation with Ringer's solution into the vas toward the epididymis in a nonocclusive manner sometimes results in the efflux of fluid containing sperm from the testicular end of the vas. This maneuver must be performed without occluding the vas around the 24-gauge blunt tip needle that is used for irrigation. Such nonocclusive irrigation allows fluid constantly to flow out of the end of the vas around the needle and thereby avoids the danger of rupture of the epididymal tubule that may occur during occlusive irrigation.

If sperm are not present in the testicular end vasal fluid after the previously mentioned procedures have been performed, the cause could be a back-pressure–induced rupture of the epididymal tubule with resulting sperm extravasation and sperm granuloma formation.[1] When the epididymal tubule is thus obstructed, vasoepididymostomy must be performed to restore the patient's fertility. Unfortunately, the surgeon cannot be guided solely by the presence or absence of sperm in the testicular end vasal fluid to determine if vasoepididymostomy is required. The Vasovasostomy Study Group[2] observed that patients who underwent bilateral microsurgical vasovasostomy, instead of vasoepididymostomy when sperm were absent bilaterally from the intraoperative vasal fluid, achieved a postoperative patency rate of 60% (50 of 83 patients), and a pregnancy occurred in the wives of 31% (20 of 65 patients). Therefore, in some instances, factors other than epididymal obstruction appear to play a role in causing the intraoperative absence of sperm from the vasal fluid.

The Vasovasostomy Study Group[2] also studied the relation of the intraoperative absence of sperm from the vasal fluid to the obstructive interval (time from the vasectomy until its reversal). The chance that there would be no sperm in the vasal fluid on either side during a planned vasovasostomy was 9% (5 of 58) if the interval was less than 3 years, 13% (26 of 201) if

cal series. The simplicity of fibrin adhesive used to perform vasovasostomy is very attractive, but the technique's value will not be apparent until more clinical studies are performed.

## Macrosurgical Anastomosis

The inner diameter of the unobstructed lumen of the abdominal end of the vas ranges from 0.3 to 0.5 mm, beyond the resolution of the human eye. Therefore, almost all surgeons who perform what is loosely termed "macrosurgical" vasovasostomy actually use optical loupe magnification to better visualize the anatomic details of the vasal ends during anastomotic suturing. Macrosurgical vasovasostomy has been performed using end-to-end techniques, with or without spatulation, and using side-to-side techniques. Most surgeons who perform macrosurgical vasovasostomy and many who perform microsurgical vasovasostomy use a modified one-layer, end-to-end anastomotic technique popularized by Schmidt.[12] This method involves the placement of four to eight interrupted full-thickness 9-0 nylon sutures through both ends of the vas. After all full-thickness sutures have been placed and tied, 9-0 nylon sutures are placed through the outer muscular wall between adjacent full-thickness sutures. To obtain optimal approximation of opposing mucosal edges, "triangular" placement rather than "square" placement of the full-thickness sutures is preferred (Fig. 15.4). The triangular full-thickness sutures penetrate the adventitial surface of the vas several millimeters from the transected edge of each end of the vas and penetrate the mucosa immediately adjacent to the transected mucosal edge.

## Microsurgical Anastomosis

Microsurgical vasovasostomy may be performed either with the modified one-layer technique described for macrosurgical vasovasostomy or with a two-layer technique.[13–17] Surgeons who perform a microsurgical modified one-layer vasovasostomy generally use six to eight full-thickness sutures of 9-0 or 10-0 nylon and place outer muscular sutures of 9-0 nylon between adjacent full-thickness sutures. The two-layer method may be preferable for two reasons: (1) to help resident surgeons acquire optimal microsurgical skills and (2) to enable the primary surgeon to develop and subsequently maintain the microsurgical skills required to perform the much more difficult microsurgical procedure of vasoepididymostomy.

After the vasal fluid has been examined microscopically and patency of the abdominal end of the vas has been verified, the perivasal tissue at the base of each end of the vas is approximated and the long end of the approximating suture is tagged to the surgical drapes on the surgeon's side of the table (Fig. 15.5). This maneuver assures that the vasal ends will not retract below the edges of the skin during anastomotic suturing.

The use of a hinged folding approximating clamp (Accurate Surgical and Scientific Instruments Corp., Westbury, NY, and Edward Weck & Co., Research Triangle Park, NC) is recommended for the anastomosis.[13] After the clamp is applied, it is folded and the two-layer anastomosis is performed with the clamp in the folded position (Fig. 15.6). A length of umbilical tape is wrapped around the hinge post of the folded approximating clamp and secured to the surgical drapes on the assistant's side (Fig. 15.5). Thus, bilateral stability of the vasal ends is achieved. The approximating clamp always is applied on the assistant's side so the assistant, and not the surgeon, will need to manipulate instruments around the clamp's protruding hinge post. Six to eight interrupted sutures of 10-0 nylon are placed in the inner mucosal layer, and seven to ten interrupted sutures of 9-0 nylon are placed in the outer muscular layer. The mucosal layer sutures must include about one fifth to one fourth of the thickness of the muscular layer; otherwise, the mucosal sutures tend to separate the mucosa from the muscularis. During placement of the outer muscular layer sutures, the underlying inner mucosal sutures should be visualized to prevent the muscular layer sutures from penetrating the lumen. The placement of sutures in both layers is shown in Figure 15.7. After completion of the anastomosis, the approximating clamp is removed, the perivasal fascial approximating su-

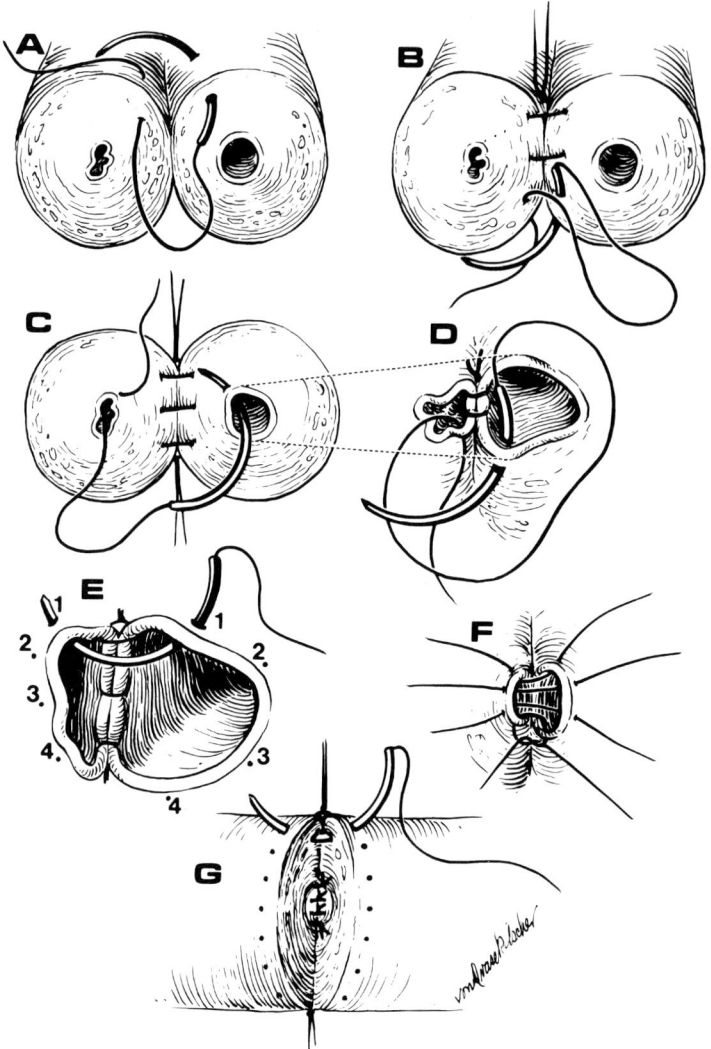

FIGURE 15.6. The author's method of microsurgical two-layer vasovasostomy. Note the discrepancy in luminal diameters. (A and B) Three posterior row muscular layer sutures are placed so that knots are outside. Only 90° of circumference are approximated, leaving full access to mucosa. End sutures are left long. (C and D) Note change in magnification indicated by dotted lines. Two or three posterior row mucosal sutures are placed from assistant's side toward surgeon's side. (E) Four to five anterior row mucosal sutures are placed in order indicated by numbers. (F) Sutures cut long and left untied until all anterior row mucosal sutures are placed. Sutures then are tied in reverse order of placement. (G) Anterior 270° (diagram depicts only 180°) of muscular layer sutures are placed, using traction on the two end posterior muscular layers sutures to aid placement of anterior muscular layer sutures. (From Belker,[13] by permission.)

FIGURE 15.7. Operative photographs. Dilated testicular end lumen on left and smaller abdominal end lumen on right. (A) Two posterior mucosal sutures are placed and tied after posterior muscular sutures have been placed and tied. (B) After an additional mucosal suture was placed and tied on each side, the last three anterior mucosal sutures are all cut long until the last one has been placed. The depth of mucosal suture placement is apparent. The disparity between luminal diameters necessitates wider spacing between sutures on the side of the larger testicular end lumen than on the side of the smaller abdominal end lumen. *(Continued)*

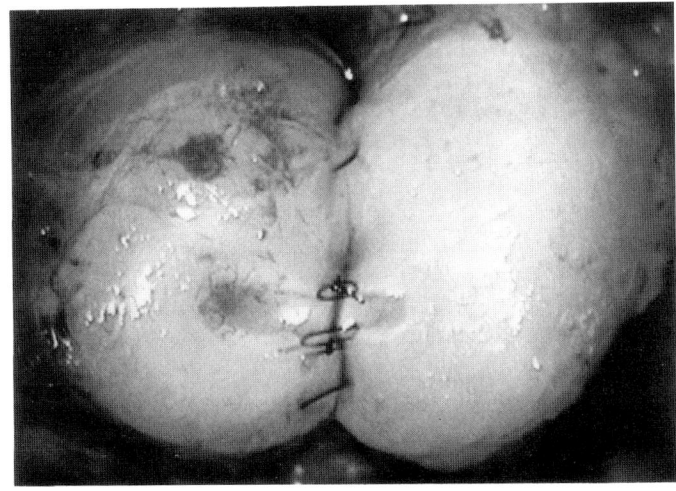

A

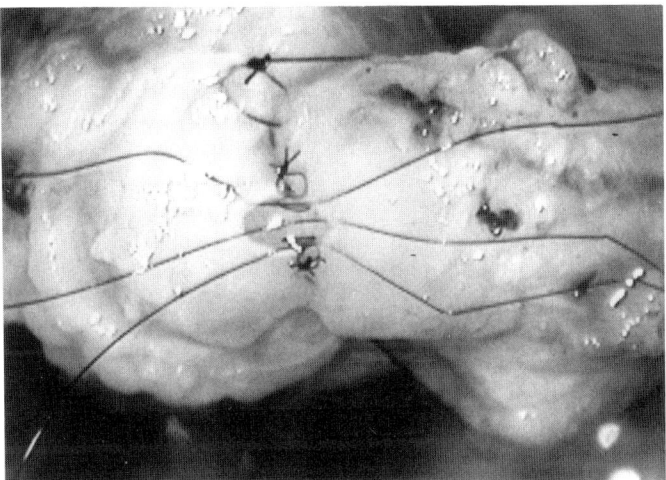

B

ture is cut short, the vas is replaced in its natural position, and routine scrotal wound closure is performed.

## Postoperative Care

Because of the meticulous hemostasis required for microsurgery, drains are not required in most cases, nor are perioperative antibiotics or corticosteroids. Based upon Schmidt's observations of the rate of healing of canine vasovasostomies, patients are requested to avoid ejaculation for 2 weeks postoperatively, remain at home for 1 week, and use a scrotal support and avoid heavy physical activity for 4 weeks postoperatively.[18] Vasectomy reversal patients who are allowed free rein to perform any postoperative activity that does not cause significant discomfort may experience disruption of the anastomosis. This occurred after several of the early reversals, when postoperative activity was not restricted. Semen analyses should be obtained at 2-month intervals starting 2 months postoperatively, until stable semen parameters are maintained, and then at 3- to 6-month intervals until a pregnancy is achieved. Although sperm may not appear in the semen until 4 to 12 months after microsurgical vasoepididymostomy, per-

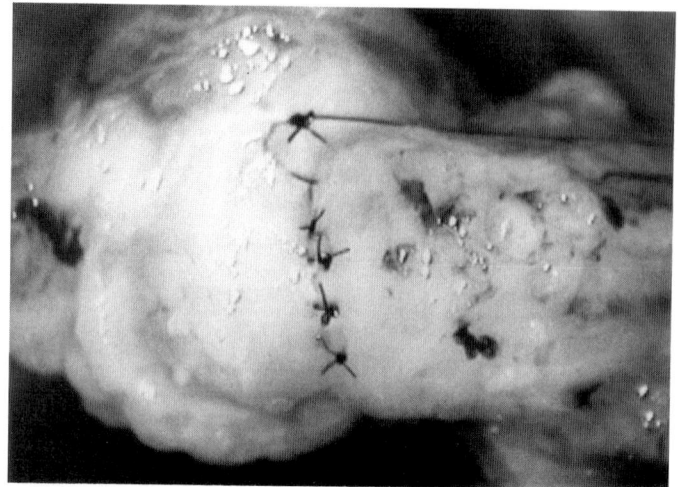

FIGURE 15.7. *Continued* (C) Good mucosal edge approximation after all sutures tied. (D) Anterior muscular suture placement. Note that tension on the last previous muscular suture (top) aids needle placement. Depth of suture placement and ability to visualize underlying mucosal sutures while placing anterior muscular sutures are demonstrated.

C

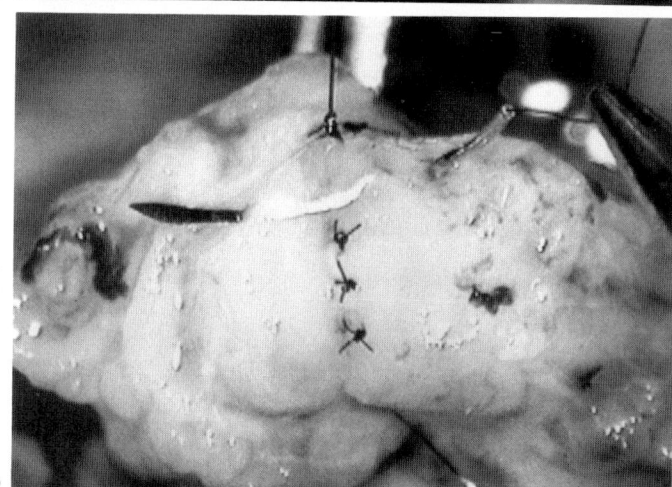

D

sistence of azoospermia beyond 2 to 4 months after vasovasostomy indicates a surgical failure.

## Factors that Influence Results

### Preoperative Factors

#### Obstructive Interval

The obstructive interval, the time from the vasectomy until its reversal, is the single most important preoperative prognostic factor that can be used to predict postoperative results. The Vasovasostomy Study Group[2] defined new obstructive interval guidelines that may be used to advise patients about their chances for fertility after vasectomy reversals (Fig. 15.8). It is apparent from this study that men with shorter obstructive intervals have a much better chance for fertility after vasovasostomy than men with obstructive intervals of 15 years and longer.

#### Sperm Antibodies

Linnet and Hjort[19] suggested that men with high preoperative serum titers of sperm agglutinins were much more likely than men with low preoperative serum titers to have sperm agglu-

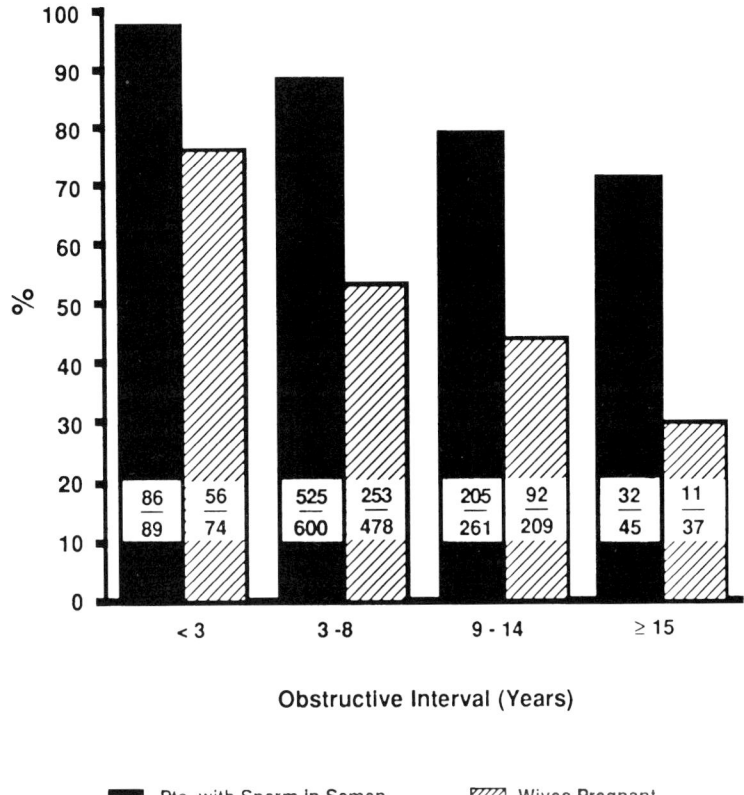

FIGURE 15.8. New obstructive interval guidelines are useful to predict postoperative patency and pregnancy rates. The numerator equals the number of patients achieving patency or pregnancy, and the denominator equals the total number of patients in each group. (From Belker et al,[2] by permission.)

tinins appear in the seminal plasma after vasovasostomy, and that the postoperative appearance of sperm agglutinins in the seminal plasma adversely affected fertility. However, their findings have not been substantiated by others and the sperm agglutinin method no longer is used by most investigators to measure sperm antibody levels. Meinertz et al[20] measured preoperative serum sperm antibodies by the tray agglutination test (TAT) and the gelatin agglutination test (GAT) and measured sperm surface immunoglobulin (Ig) antibodies in the semen of men after vasovasostomy. A preoperative serum GAT titer of $\geq 256$ was associated with significantly reduced fertility after vasovasostomy. When the postoperative sperm surface mixed antiglobulin reaction

(MAR) revealed a pure IgG response, the conception rate was 86%, but only 43% of wives of men with IgA on the sperm surface achieved a pregnancy. When 100% of the sperm were coated with IgA, the conception rate was reduced to 22%, and the combination of IgA on all the sperm and a serum GAT titer of $\geq 256$ was associated with a conception rate of zero.

Men with high percentages of sperm coated with IgA and IgG during direct immunobead tests after vasovasostomy may have poor sperm motility and low rates of conception. Unfortunately, there is no uniformly accepted preoperative test of a patient's sperm antibody status to guide the surgeon in offering a prognosis for fertility after vasovasostomy.

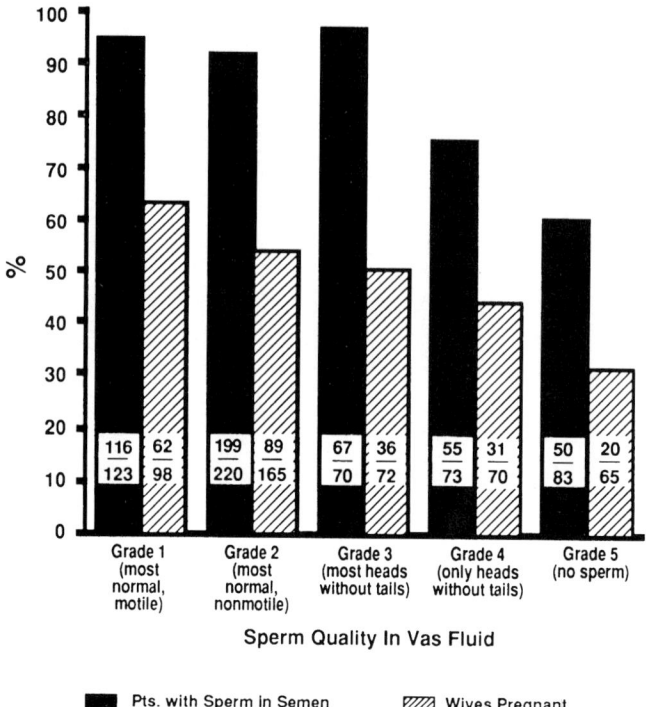

FIGURE 15.9. Patency and pregnancy rates according to the quality of sperm in intraoperative vas fluid when sperm quality is identical bilaterally. The numerator equals the number of patients achieving patency or pregnancy, and the denominator equals the total number of patients in each group. (From Belker et al,[2] by permission.)

## Testicular Effects of Vasectomy

It was believed for many years that there were no testicular abnormalities resulting from vasectomy. However, Jarow et al[21] found that 23% of vasectomized men's testicular biopsies showed focal interstitial fibrosis and such changes were not seen in testicular biopsies of fertile men. The men with focal interstitial fibrosis had significantly lower fertility rates after vasovasostomy than men without such histologic changes. Thus, there is a subset of men predetermined to have poor postoperative fertility rates because of testicular changes caused by the vasectomy. The findings of Jarow et al, however, have not caused urologists to recommend that a testicular biopsy be performed before the procedure in order to make a decision about undergoing vasovasostomy. In a later study, Jarow et al[22] found that the testicular changes seen after vasectomy were not associated with the patient's sperm antibody status; the testicular changes appeared to result from some mechanism other than sperm autoimmunity.

## Age and Fertility Status of Wife

Reproductive gynecologic assessment of the wife should be performed routinely before a man undergoes vasovasostomy. It is pointless for the man to have vasectomy reversal if there is a reason his wife cannot or should not become pregnant. When applicable, couples should be informed of declining female fertility rates after 30 to 35 years of age and particularly of the increased rates of children with congenital abnormalities after a maternal age of 35 years. When semen parameters are normal for 1 year postoperatively and a pregnancy has not occurred, further gynecologic evaluation of the wife should be performed. However, couples should be informed that the average interval until a pregnancy after microsurgical vasovasostomy is 1 year.[2]

# Intraoperative Factors

## Sperm Quality in Vas Fluid

The Vasovasostomy Study Group[2] studied the relationship of the intraoperative sperm quality in the vasal fluid, when the quality was identical bilaterally, to the results of vasovasostomy. Five grades of sperm quality were defined. The patency and pregnancy rates for each grade of sperm quality are shown in Figure 15.9. Results were best and were comparable when grades 1, 2, and 3 sperm quality were present and slightly less good for grade 4. Patency and pregnancy rates were 60% and 31%, respectively, even when no sperm were present (grade 5) in the intraoperative vasal fluid bilaterally. There was no difference in results for various concentrations, excluding zero, of sperm in the intraoperative vasal fluid.[2]

## Sperm Granuloma at Vasectomy Site

A sperm granuloma at the vasectomy site seems to have a beneficial pressure-releasing effect, manifested by less luminal dilation and better vasal fluid sperm quality on the side with a sperm granuloma at the vasectomy site than on the side without one.[23] However, this apparently beneficial effect did not prove to have clinical significance when the results of microsurgical vasovasostomies for patients with and without histologic evidence of bilateral sperm granulomata at the vasectomy site were compared.[2] Patency and pregnancy rates were 96% and 63%, respectively, when a sperm granuloma was present bilaterally, and 85% and 51% when a sperm granuloma was absent bilaterally ($p = 0.05$ for patency and $p > 0.05$ for pregnancy rate comparisons).

# Modified One-Layer Versus Two-Layer Microsurgical Anastomoses

The results of microsurgical modified one-layer and two-layer microsurgical vasovasostomies by the Vasovasostomy Study Group[2] are not statistically different (Fig. 15.10). These findings agree with those reported by Lee.[24]

## Macrosurgery Versus Microsurgery

It is difficult to compare the results of various studies when the results have not been related to obstructive intervals. A review revealed that macrosurgical vasovasostomies achieve patency rates ranging from 35% to 100% and pregnancy rates of 19% to 55%.[25] A survey by Derrick et al[26] of 1,630 macrosurgical procedures performed by 542 urologists revealed a postoperative patency rate of 38% and a postoperative pregnancy rate of 19%. However, Middleton et al[27] reported a patency rate of 81% and a pregnancy rate of 45% after nonmagnified vasovasostomies. The strikingly different results reported in the survey by Derrick et al[26] and the series by Middleton et al[27] suggest that the surgeon's experience with vasovasostomy may be more important than the actual anastomotic technique that is selected.

It is critical that microsurgical techniques and instrumentation be learned in a microsurgical laboratory and practiced *before* clinical application.[28] Failure to do so will produce suboptimal results.

## Repeat Reversals

Overall patency and pregnancy rates, respectively, reported by the Vasovasostomy Study Group[2] were 85% (865 of 1,012) and 52% (421 of 808) for first microsurgical vasovasostomies, and 75% (150 of 199) and 43% (52 of 120) for repeat procedures. It is clear that the results of repeat procedures are not as good as the results of first procedures. It therefore is beneficial for the patient undergoing an initial vasovasostomy to have the procedure performed by an experienced surgeon.

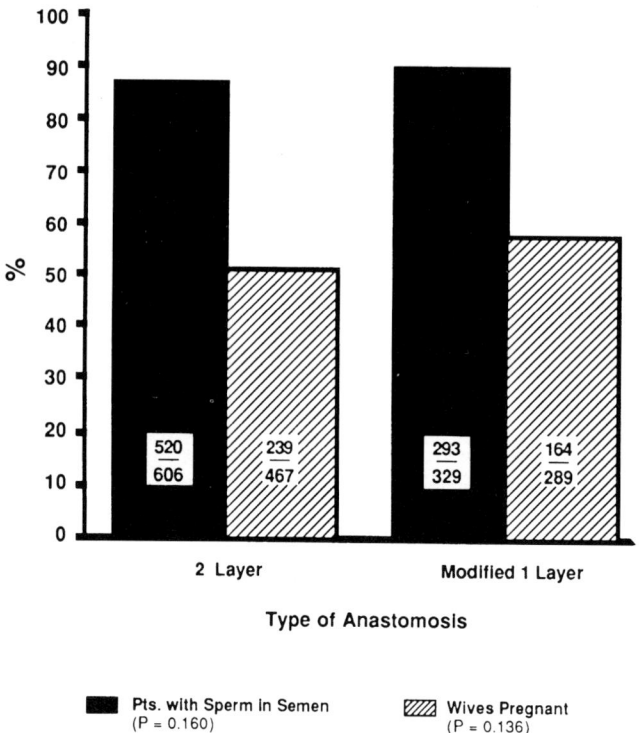

FIGURE 15.10. Patency and pregnancy rates are not significantly different after two-layer and modified one-layer microsurgical vasovasostomy. The numerator equals the number of patients achieving pa-tency or pregnancy, and the denominator equals the total number of patients in each group. (From Belker et al,[2] by permission.)

## Conclusion

Various surgical techniques and factors that influence the results of vasovasostomy should be considered. The obstructive interval appears to be the most important preoperative factor relative to postoperative results. The difficult intraoperative decision regarding the performance of vasovasostomy or of vasoepididymostomy when sperm are absent from the intraoperative vasal fluid is based upon multiple factors. The sperm quality in the vasal fluid and the surgical technique are important intraoperative factors that affect results. When properly performed, microsurgical vasovasostomies are associated with better results than are macrosurgical anastomoses. The importance of the surgeon's experience with vasovasostomy, regardless of the anastomotic technique used, must be considered.

When judging the reported results of vasovasostomies, the reader should be aware of Sharlip's[29] study. Of 95 patients who had normal sperm concentration and normal sperm motility during a consecutive 12-month period after vasectomy reversal, 61% achieved a pregnancy. Allowing for some patients who would have achieved a pregnancy after the follow-up period, Sharlip estimated the maximum pregnancy probability for a vasectomy reversal to be 67%.

There is some difficulty in comparing the results of any one series of vasectomy reversals to the results of other series. Comparisons cannot be made unless comparable data are provided, and surgeons who report their results with any method of vasovasostomy should stratify the results according to established obstructive interval guidelines.[2]

# References

1. Silber SJ. Epididymal extravasation following vasectomy as a cause for failure of vasectomy reversal. *Fertil Steril* 1979; 31:309–315.

2. Belker AM, Thomas AJ, Fuchs EF, et al. Results of 1,469 microsurgical vasectomy reversals by the Vasovasostomy Study Group. *J Urol* 1991; 145:505–511.

3. Belker AM. Infrapubic incision for specific vasectomy reversal situations. *Urology* 1988; 32:413–415.

4. Middleton RG, Henderson D. Vas deferens reanastomosis without splints and without magnification. *J Urol* 1978; 119:763–764.

5. Rowland RG, Nanninga JB, O'Conor VJ Jr. Improved results in vasovasostomies using internal plain catgut stents. *Urology* 1977; 10:260–262.

6. Berger RE, Chapman W, Jessen J. Randomized trial of vasostent-vasovasostomy versus microscopic two-layer vasovasostomy—preliminary results. *J Urol* 1993; 149:389A.

7. Lynne CM, Carter M, Morris J, et al. Laser-assisted vas anastomosis: a preliminary report. *Lasers Surg Med* 1983; 3:261–263.

8. Rosemberg SK. Further clinical experience with $CO_2$ laser in microsurgical vasovasostomy. *Urology* 1988; 32:225–227.

9. Silverstein JI, Mellinger BC. Fibrin glue vasal anastomosis compared to conventional sutured vasovasostomy in the rat. *J Urol* 1991; 145:1288–1291.

10. Niederberger C, Ross LS, Mackenzie B, et al. Vasovasostomy in rabbits using fibrin adhesive prepared from a single human source. *J Urol* 1993; 149:183–185.

11. Holmes SAV, Christmas TJ, Kirby RS, et al. Vasovasostomy using tissue glue: a comparison with microscopic anastomosis. *J Urol* 1993; 149:389A.

12. Schmidt, SS. Vasovasostomy. *Urol Clin North Am* 1978; 5:585–592.

13. Belker AM. Microsurgical two-layer vasovasostomy: simplified technique using hinged, folding-approximating clamp. *Urology* 1980; 16:376–381.

14. Belker AM. Technical aids for vasovasostomy. *Urology* 1982; 20:635–637.

15. Belker AM. Vasovasostomy. In: Resnick MI ed. *Current Trends in Urology*. Baltimore: Williams & Wilkins; 1981; 1:20–41.

16. Belker AM. Microscopic vasovasostomy. In: *Male Infertility*. Urology Today Videotape Series. Norwich: Norwich Eaton Audio-Visual Library; 1985; 4:1.

17. Belker AM. Microsurgical vasectomy reversal. In: Lytton B, Catalona WJ, Lipshultz LI, McGuire EJ eds. *Advances in Urology*. Chicago: Yearbook Medical Publishers; 1988; 1:193–230.

18. Schmidt SS. Anastomosis of the vas deferens: an experimental study. *J Urol* 1956; 75:300–303.

19. Linnet L, Hjort T. Sperm agglutinins in seminal plasma and serum after vasectomy. Correlation between immunological and clinical findings. *Clin Exp Immunol* 1977; 30:413–420.

20. Meinertz H, Linnet L, Fogh-Andersen P, et al. Antisperm antibodies and fertility after vasovasostomy: a follow-up study of 216 men. *Fertil Steril* 1990; 54:315–321.

21. Jarow JP, Budin RE, Dym M, et al. Quantitative pathologic changes in the human testis after vasectomy. *N Engl J Med* 1985; 313:1252–1256.

22. Jarow JP, Goluboff ET, Chang TK, et al. Relationship between antisperm antibodies and testicular histologic changes in humans after vasectomy. *Urology* 1994; 43:521–524.

23. Belker AM, Konnak JW, Sharlip ID, et al. Intraoperative observations during vasovasostomy in 334 patients. *J Urol* 1983; 129:524–527.

24. Lee HY. A 20-year experience with vasovasostomy. *J Urol* 1986; 136:413–415.

25. Belker AM. Urologic microsurgery—current perspectives: I. vasovasostomy. *Urology* 1979; 14:325–329.

26. Derrick FC, Yarbrough W, D'Agostino J. Vasovasostomy: results of questionnaire of members of the American Urological Association. *J Urol* 1973; 110:556–557.

27. Middleton RG, Smith JA, Moore MH, et al. A 15-year follow-up of a nonmicrosurgical technique for vasovasostomy. *J Urol* 1987; 137:886–887.

28. Belker AM. Principles of microsurgery. *Urol Clin North Am* 1994; 21:487–504.

29. Sharlip ID. What is the best pregnancy rate that may be expected from vasectomy reversal? *J Urol* 1993; 149:1469–1471.

30. Belker AM. Repeating the vasectomy reversal. *Contemporary Urology* 1993; 5(9):54–66.

31. Belker AM. Microsurgical vasovasostomy: two-layer technique. In: Goldstein M, ed. *Surgery of Male Infertility*. Philadelphia: W.B. Saunders; 1995: 61–65.

32. Belker AM. Microsurgical repair of obstructive causes of male infertility. *Semin Urol* 1984; 2:91–98.

# 16
# Obstructive Azoospermia and Vasoepididymostomy

Anthony J. Thomas, Jr. and Osvaldo F. Padron

Excurrent duct obstruction is a potentially reversible cause of male infertility. It can occur anywhere along the ductal system from the rete testes (empty epididymis syndrome) to the ejaculatory ducts. The incidence of obstructive azoospermia among infertile men is approximately 7% to 10%. Elective vasectomy is the most common cause of ductal obstruction. Other causes of ductal obstruction include those related to congenital anomalies ranging from total absence of the vasa deferentia, seminal vesicles, and ejaculatory ducts to a minor dysjunction between vasa and epididymides or obstruction secondary to scarring of the tubules as a result of prior infection, inflammation, trauma, or iatrogenic injury to the epididymis or vas deferens. Figure 16.1 is an algorithm suggested for evaluating and treating patients who may have an obstructive or nonobstructive problem causing azoospermia.

## Anatomy and Physiology of the Epididymis

Six to eight efferent ducts derived from the mesonephric tubules coalesce to form the proximal caput epididymis, which unites with the wolffian duct (mesonephric duct) from which is formed the corpus and cauda epididymis as well as the vas deferens. The epididymis lies lateral to the cord structures along the longitudinal axis of the testes and measures approximately $1 \times 1 \times 6$ cm in size. If the epididymal tubule were unfolded, it would be about 4 to 5 m in length. The normal unobstructed epididymal tubule has a luminal diameter of less than 0.2 mm. The wall of the epididymal tubule is thinnest at the caput, becoming thicker and more muscular as it continues to its caudal portion. Here, the muscular mass increases greatly to become the ductus deferens. Sperm transit time through the epididymis varies from 2 to 6 days.

The blood supply of the upper portion of the epididymis is derived from a branch of the testicular artery. It has abundant communications with the artery of the vas deferens. The distal epididymis is supplied by the combined network of cremasteric and vas deferens arteries. The vascular network between the testicular artery and the artery of the vas deferens allows for the mobilization and resection of the distal epididymis without devascularizing the more proximal portion of the epididymis.

The epididymis acts to mature, store, transport, and concentrate sperm. Hydrostatic pressure and peristaltic contractions of the seminiferous tubules move sperm out of the testes to the excurrent ducts. These sperm require a specific microenvironment for maturation to take place. Epididymal sperm are exposed to protein products from the lining cells of the epididymal tubule as they mature. Sperm are concentrated in the epididymis, with the greatest number in the cauda. Certain protein substances and ions secreted in the cauda of the epididymis appear to play an important role in keeping sperm quiescent prior to their expulsion during ejaculation.[1–6]

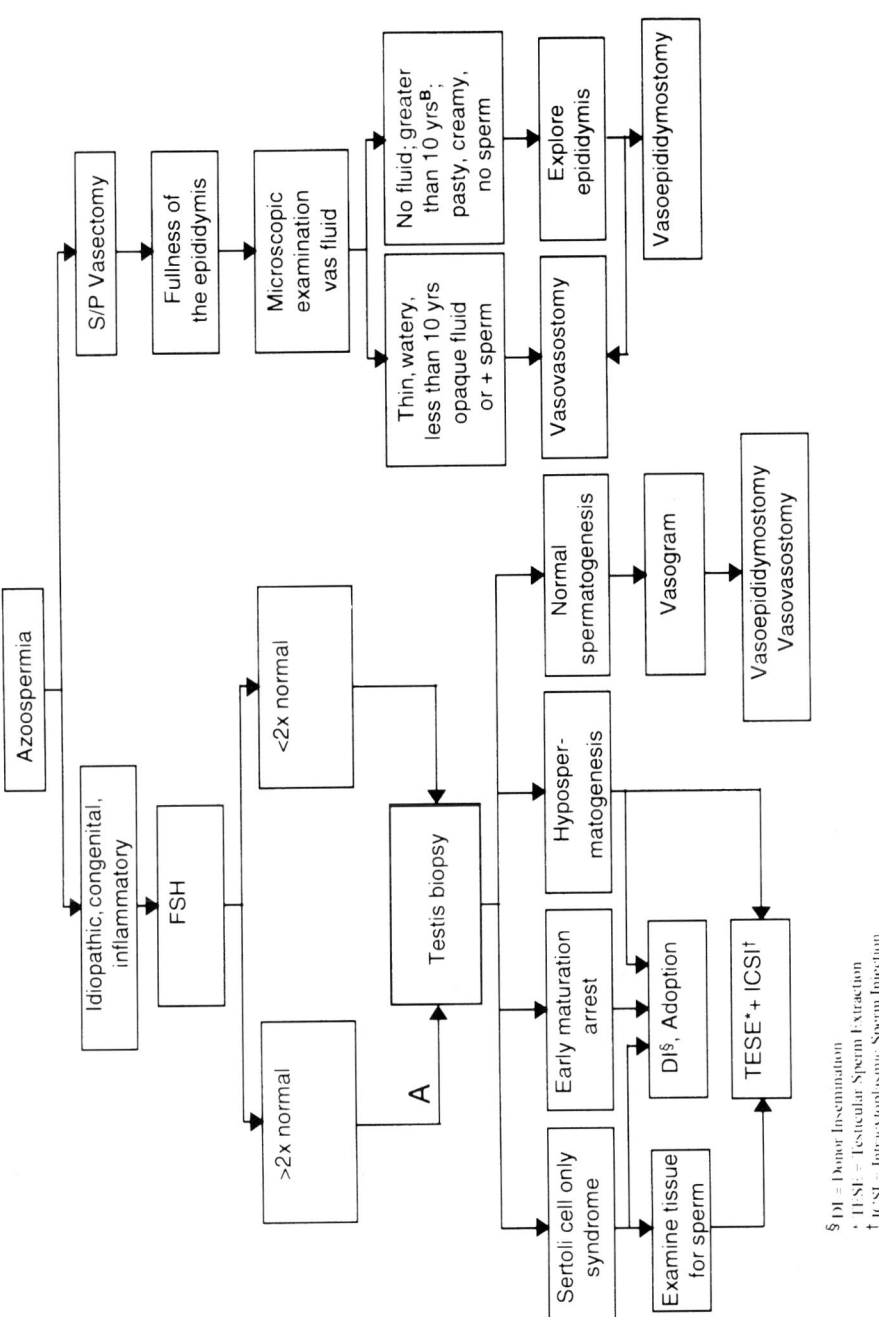

§ DI = Donor Insemination
* TESE = Testicular Sperm Extraction
† ICSI = Intracytoplasmic Sperm Injection

FIGURE 16.1. Algorithm to evaluate and treat obstructive azoospermia. (A) Consider testicular biopsy and examination of testicular tissue for viable sperm if the couple is interested in in vitro fertilization with intracytoplasmic sperm injection. (B) Epididymal blowout can occur at any time after vasectomy but the incidence increases significantly after 8 to 10 years.

# Causes of Epididymal Obstruction

Most males with cystic fibrosis are born with absence of the distal epididymides and the vasa deferentia and often have absent or hypoplastic seminal vesicles. Some apparently healthy men are born with similar genital anomalies. When screened for the more common genetic alterations, approximately two thirds of these males will be found to have at least one gene mutation associated with cystic fibrosis.[7,8] Clinically, these men are azoospermic with a low ejaculate volume ($<1$ ml) that is acidic and watery in appearance, and seminal fructose is either absent or in very low concentrations. No satisfactory corrective surgical treatment is available for this group of men who generally are found to have normal spermatogenesis. Treatment is available, however, by means of epididymal sperm aspiration combined with an assisted reproductive technique, such as in vitro fertilization (IVF) with intracytoplasmic sperm insertion (ICSI).[9–15] Some men with azoospermia will be found to have a unilateral absence of the vas deferens and an otherwise normal vas, although not connected to the epididymis on the contralateral side. Surgical correction is possible in this group. If the ipsilateral testis is atrophic or for other reasons is not making adequate sperm, the vas deferens can be crossed over to the contralateral testis to be anastomosed to the epididymis.[16]

A variety of congenital anomalies of the epididymis and vas deferens have been described by Scorer and Farrington[17] and others.[18] Surgeons involved in treatment of men with congenital causes of obstructive azoospermia should be well acquainted with the variations in anatomy (Fig. 16.2).

Acquired lesions causing excurrent duct obstruction are more common and more easily correctable with surgery than congenital causes of obstructive azoospermia. Epididymitis from a bacterial or viral source may resolve with appropriate treatment but leave sufficient scarring to cause complete obstruction of the epididymis. Clinically evident bilateral acute epididymitis from an infectious source is a rare entity. Therefore, if only one side is affected, the man's fertility may remain intact if the contralateral ductal system is normal. More often than not, when there is bilateral obstruction the patient has no recall of a specific event that afflicted both testicles.

Blunt and penetrating trauma to the scrotal contents may result in disruption of the excurrent ductal pathway. Perhaps the more common trauma is inadvertent injury to the vas deferens or the epididymis during the performance of surgical procedures unrelated to fertility, such as hernia repair or hydrocelectomy. As with the inflammatory causes of obstruction, if only one vas or epididymis is injured and the contralateral side is normal, there will often be no notice taken of the injured side as long as fertility is unaffected. If, however, both sides are injured, the contralateral side is atrophic or hypoplastic, or there is a congenital absence of part or all of the ductal system, the patient with azoospermia or severe oligospermia will usually be referred to the attention of a urologist.

An association has been identified between chronic sinus and pulmonary disease and obstructive azoospermia. Originally described by Young[19] in 1970, other studies have noted chronic sinusitis, bronchitis, or bronchiectasis along with either primary or secondary infertility caused by obstruction within the middle and distal portions of the epididymis, which are found to be filled with thick, yellowish material devoid of sperm. The association with cystic fibrosis has been put forth but not proven.[20] Even when sperm are identified in the more proximal portion of the epididymis, vasoepididymostomy has not proven as successful as in those patients who have postinflammatory causes for their obstruction.

Partial epididymal or vasal obstruction may also occur, but this is more likely to happen following a prior attempt to correct a complete obstruction and is less likely to be found as a primary phenomenon. Patients with obstruction have sperm in their ejaculate in low numbers inconsistent with the higher quality of spermatogenesis demonstrated on testis biopsy, and the sperm in the ejaculate may have little or no motility, with broken tails and dysmorphic-shaped heads.

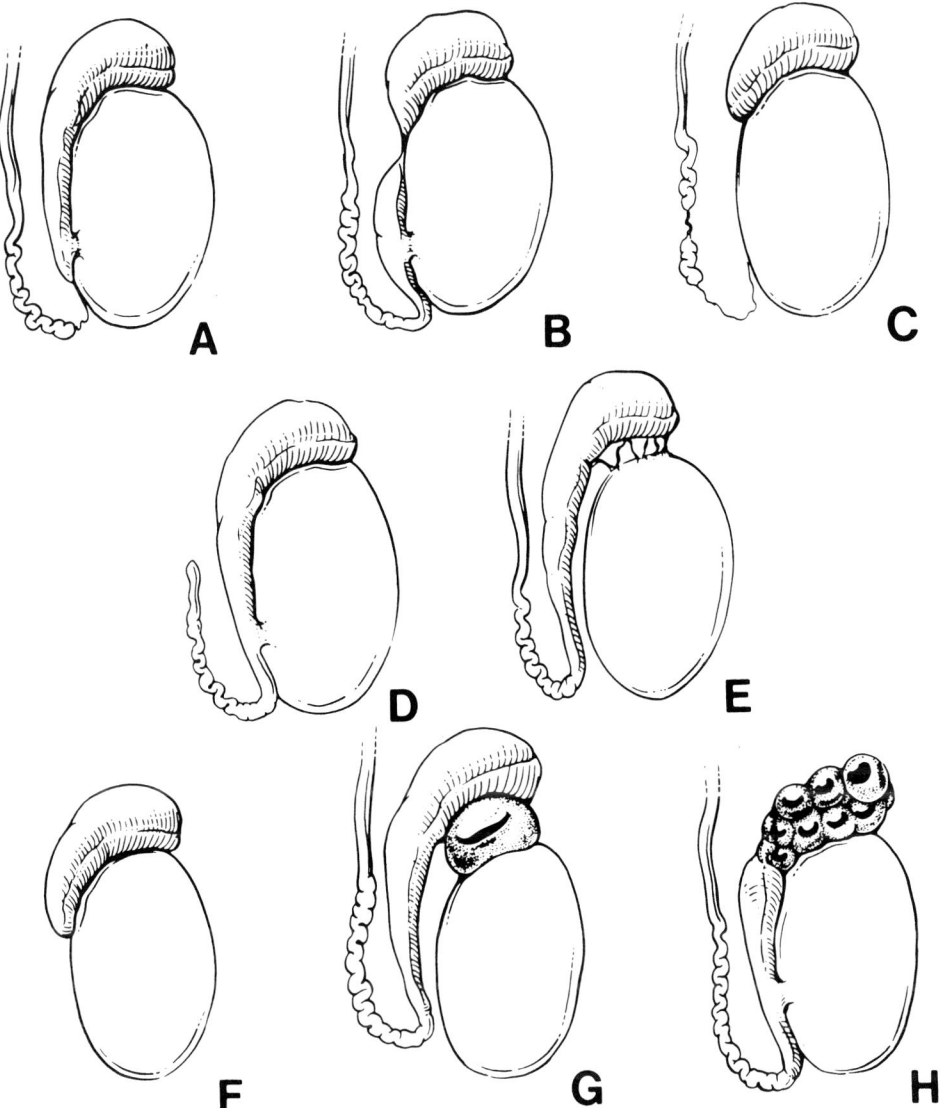

FIGURE 16.2. Congenital abnormalities of the vas deferens and epididymis. (A) Atresia of the distal epididymis. (B) Skip area midepididymis. (C) Absence of the body and tail of the epididymis. (D) Blind-ending vas deferens. (E) No communication between testis and epididymis. (F) Caput present no further excurrent ductal system. (G) Spermatocele between epididymis and testis. (H) Epididymal cysts. (From Thomas,[26] with permission.)

Surgical reconstruction for excurrent duct obstruction following vasectomy is straightforward, except when no sperm are found in the vasal fluid of a patient who has been obstructed for a long interval. Those men who have copious amounts of clear fluid without sperm have been shown to have an excellent prognosis with regard to sperm return after vasovasostomy alone. Examination of the azoospermic vasal fluid in some men will reveal it to be thick, pasty, or altogether absent. These men will have sustained a blowout of the epididymal tubule, probably as a result of increased pressure within the epididymis and vas, although this is speculative. Vasoepididymostomy will be necessary in order to restore sperm to the ejaculate. The incidence of a blowout occurring is related to the number of years postvasectomy, being more common after 10 years. There is at least a 20% chance that there will not be sperm in either vas at an interval of more than 10 years, and the surgeon must be prepared to perform a vasoepididymostomy on one or both sides.[21-23]

# Vasoepididymostomy

## Preoperative Evaluation and Preparation

Most patients with epididymal obstruction have epididymes that are palpably full or even indurated. Their semen volume is normal (>1.5 ml) and has an alkaline pH devoid of sperm. The vasa feel normal and at least one testis is of normal size (>20 ml). Serum gonadotropin levels are normal. Proof of adequate sperm production is needed prior to attempted reconstruction. A testis biopsy can be done as a separate procedure or, in many instances, at the same operative event as the reconstructive surgery. A frozen section, touch preparation, or crushed wet preparation can be easily and quickly examined to verify the presence of active spermatogenesis.

## Surgical Anesthesia and Preparation

Because the time needed for this type of surgery can vary from 2 to 4 or more hours, depending on the degree of scarring encountered and the rapidity with which the surgeon can identify sperm in the epididymal tubule, a general anesthetic or continuous epidural block is preferred. Care in positioning the patient on the operating room table is crucial to both comfort and safety. All pressure points, such as the sacrum, the heels, and the back of the patient's head, should be cushioned with small portions of "egg crate" mattress material. The patient's arms should be tucked at the side of the body or abducted approximately 45°C in order to prevent discomfort and potential nerve injuries that may occur if the arms are hyperextended for a prolonged time.

Anastomosis of the vas deferens to the epididymis can be accomplished by either an end-to-end or end-to-side technique, depending on the surgeon's preference and the level at which the anastomosis is made.[21-26] The end-to-end method is best performed at the caudal level where the loops of the tubule are thicker and fewer in number, which allows for easier identification of the patent portion of the tubule. Mobilization of the distal epididymis may be easier after transection and can provide a few more centimeters in length that might be helpful to bridge a distance between vas and epididymis. The end-to-side method can be done at any level, the primary advantages being no resection necessary of the epididymis, minimal bleeding, and only one opened loop of the epididymal tubule to which the vas lumen is attached.

## Surgical Techniques

Whichever method of anastomosis is preferred, the surgeon must be certain, through testis biopsy, vasography or both, that there is active sperm production and a patent vas deferens before exploring the epididymis. Vasography is useful to identify anatomic abnormalities within the excurrent ductal system or to define and confirm patency.

The vas can be grasped with a towel clip at its straight portion and its blood supply carefully pushed away from the anterior surface. Plastic tubing from a sterile "butterfly" intravenous needle is inexpensive and readily available to be passed beneath the vas and act as a nontraumatic holding device. A 30-gauge lymphangiogram needle (No. 6657, Becton-Dickinson Co., Franklin Lakes, NJ) is used to puncture the vas lumen by sliding the needle in an almost parallel path with the vas lumen (Fig. 16.3). With minimal practice, the surgeon can feel when the needle enters the lumen, as there is an immediate decrease in resistance. Proper position in the lumen is confirmed by injecting 1 to 2 ml of saline. If the saline does not flow easily, the needle should be repositioned. Once proper placement is confirmed, a scout film of the pelvis is obtained, 2 to 4 ml of Renografin 60 (NDC0003-0707-50, Squibb Diagnos-

FIGURE 16.3. Vasography technique. Note the plastic tubing (arrow) used as an atraumatic holder.

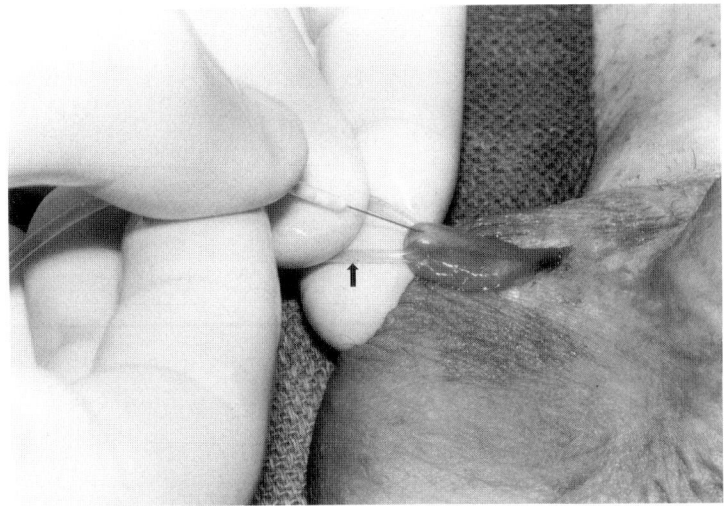

tics, Princeton, NJ) mixed with normal saline in a one-to-one mixture injected, and another radiograph obtained[27] (Fig. 16.4). The same procedure can be repeated on the contralateral side, or 10 ml or more of saline can be flushed through the lumen, and if it flows easily, the lumen is considered patent. If there is a distal (inguinal) obstruction, only a small amount of contrast is needed to fill the vas proximal to the obstruction. If the surgeon places the thumb and forefinger on the vas just distal to the needle, the intermittent dilation of the vas can be felt as the syringe is gently and repeatedly pressed in and released. *It is strongly recommended that vasography be performed at the time of the definitive reconstructive surgery.*

## End-to-End Microsurgical Vasoepididymal Anastomosis

This method of anastomosis was described by Silber[21] in 1978. The testicle is exposed and examined. Even without optical magnification, the point of obstruction in the epididymis may

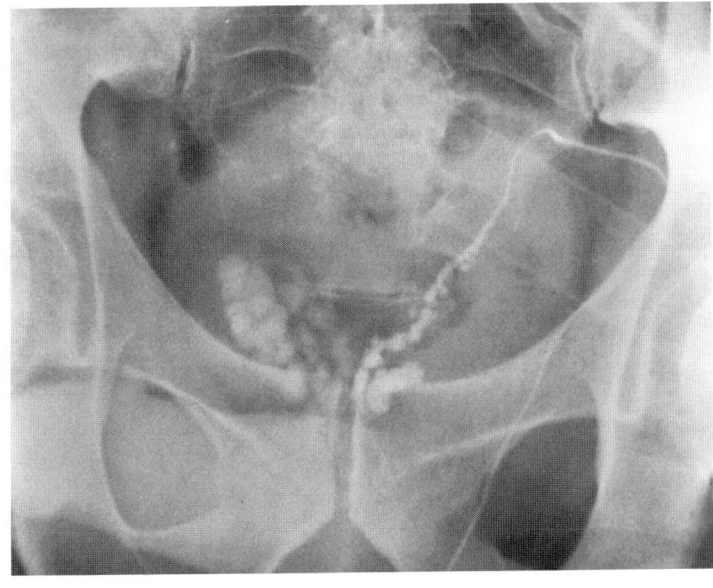

FIGURE 16.4. Normal left vasogram in a patient with epididymal obstruction. Some residual contrast is seen in right seminal vesicle from vasogram done on that side.

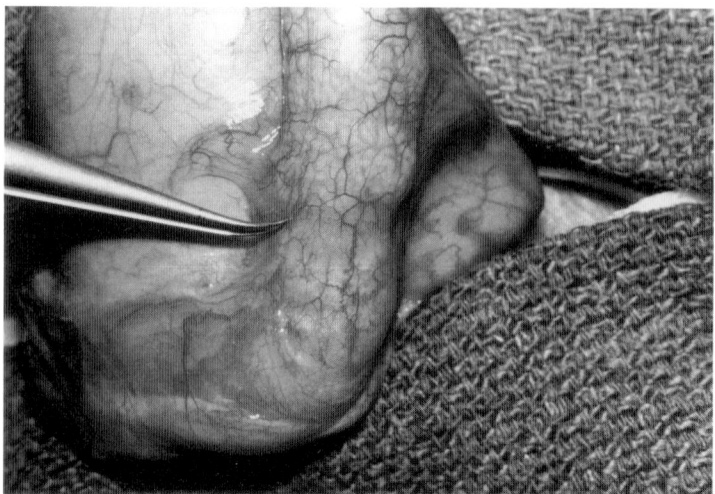

FIGURE 16.5. A distinct point of narrowing within the epididymis (tip of the forceps) indicates the point of obstruction.

be obvious by a distinct narrowing or an area of blue-brown discoloration beneath the epididymal tunic, which may indicate a point of sperm extravasation and cell breakdown (Figs. 16.5 and 16.6). Before the epididymis is cut, it is necessary to separate the proximal end of the vas deferens, along with its blood supply, from the surrounding loose connective tissue. The vas deferens must be sufficiently mobilized to allow the cut abdominal end to be brought from its medial position to lie lateral, in close proximity to the epididymis.

The epididymis is examined under the operating microscope. Beginning at the distal portion of the cauda, the epididymis is transected transversely, and fluid from the cut ends of the epididymal tubule is examined for sperm (Fig. 16.7A). If none are found, the epididymis is transected another half centimeter more proximal and the inspection process repeated until the patent portion of the tubule containing sperm is opened. Defunctionalized tubules will empty quickly, and the patent tubule will be the only cut end that continues to efflux fluid containing long-tailed sperm. It is easier to cut the epididymis if a plane is developed between the epididymis and the testis with a small tongue depressor or knife blade handle against which

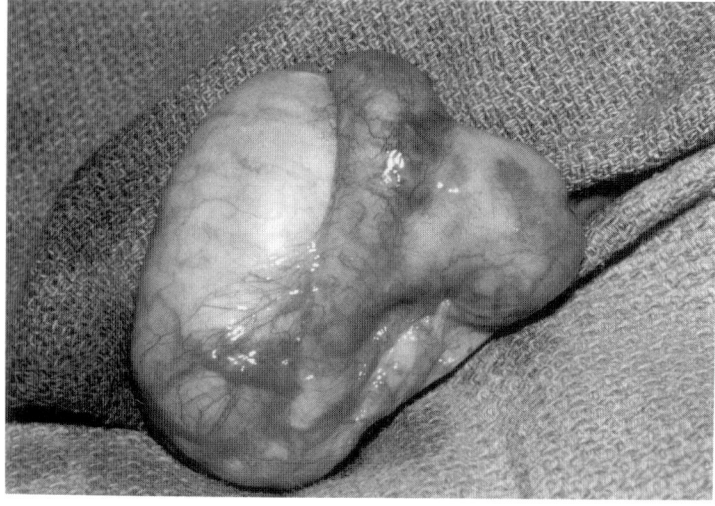

FIGURE 16.6. Blue-brown discoloration is sometimes seen at the site of obstruction of the epididymis.

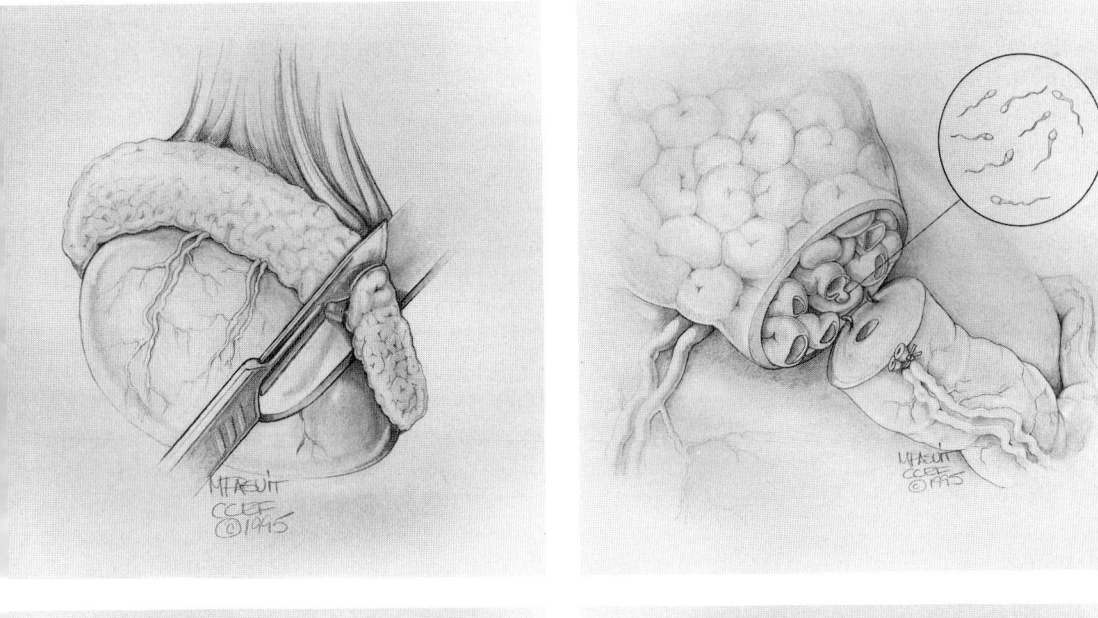

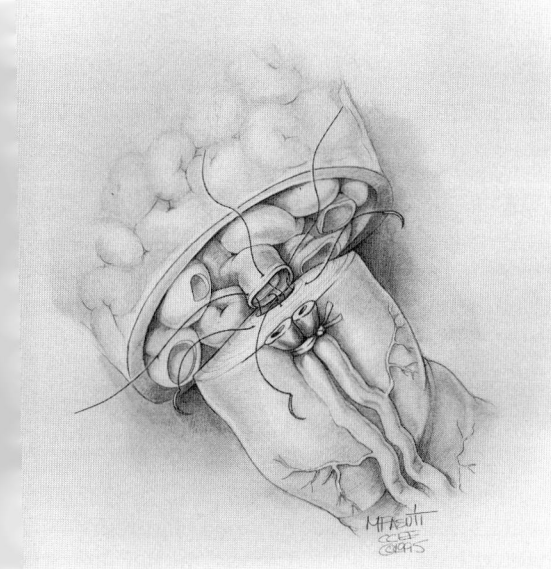

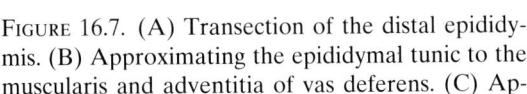

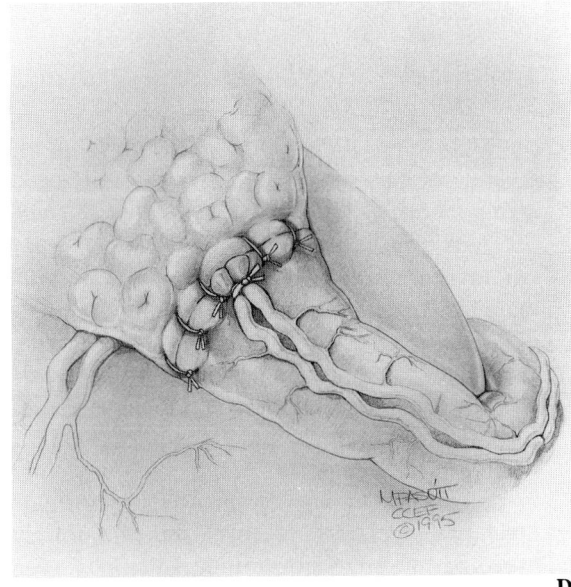

FIGURE 16.7. (A) Transection of the distal epididymis. (B) Approximating the epididymal tunic to the muscularis and adventitia of vas deferens. (C) Approximation of the vasal and epididymal lumina. (D) Completion of end-to-end anastomosis. (Parts A, B, and C from Padron and Thomas,[41] with permission.)

the cut is made beneath the epididymis. This plane between the testis and the epididymis can be developed only along the distal two thirds so as not to interfere with the blood supply of the proximal epididymis and the testis itself. Bipolar cautery is useful to obtain the meticulous hemostasis, which is crucial to this operation in

allowing adequate visualization for the anastomosis to be performed.

The cut abdominal end of the vas is brought to the opened end of the epididymis. The adventitia and muscularis of the vas deferens are approximated to the tunic of the epididymis at the six o'clock position to prevent any undue tension on the mucosal anastomosis (Fig. 16.7B). Four or five equally spaced 10-0 nylon sutures (#1850–38, Davis and Geck, American Cyamed Co., Danbury, CT) are then placed from outside-in on the opened epididymal tubule to inside-out through the edge of lumen of the vas deferens (Fig. 16.7C). The adventitia and muscularis of the vas are then approximated to the epididymal tunic with 9-0 nylon sutures (#2890, Ethicon, Inc., Summerville, NJ) placed in a circumferential pattern (Fig. 16.7D). The testicle is replaced in the scrotum, and the tunica vaginalis is closed with a continuous running absorbable suture. The dartos layer and skin are also closed with absorbable suture. A soft dressing of "fluffs" and some form of support shorts are used to keep the dressing in place. No attempt is made to maintain a compressive-type dressing.

## End-to-Side Microsurgical Vasoepididymostomy

Mobilization of the vas deferens is the same as for the end-to-end technique. It is advantageous to bring the abdominal end of the vas deferens from its medial position lateral to the epididymis, passing it beneath the cord and remaining within the tunica vaginalis. The epididymis is grasped gently between the surgeon's thumb and forefinger to tighten the tunic overlying the dilated convoluted epididymal tubule. Inspection for sperm should begin at the cauda epididymis, moving toward the caput as determined by the finding of long-tailed, normal-appearing sperm. A $\frac{1}{2}$-cm linear incision is made in the epididymal tunic with a Beaver blade (#376400, Becton-Dickinson Co., Franklin Lakes, NJ). A single loop of the tubule is isolated from the others by use of blunt-tipped curved microscissors (#E-3320RX, Karl-Storz, Tuttlingen, Germany). A 1.5-mm microsurgical knife (#AMK8742-K, American Surgical and Scientific Instruments, Inc., Westbury, NY) is used to make a $\frac{1}{2}$- to 1-mm incision in the epididymal tubule (Fig. 16.8A). Fluid obtained from this loop is aspirated with a 24-gauge angiocath (#3828641, Becton-Dickinson Vascular Access, Sandy, UT) attached to a tuberculin syringe, and a drop is placed on a sterile glass

slide diluted with a drop of saline or Ringer's lactate and examined under light microscopy (40×) for the presence of normal-appearing motile or nonmotile sperm. If none are identified, another incision is made in the epididymal tunic $\frac{1}{2}$ to 1 cm more cephalad, and the procedure is repeated until sperm are found. Anastomosis is not carried out unless sperm are identified.

With the tubule open and the presence of sperm confirmed, three 10-0 nylon sutures are placed in the opened edges of the tubule 120° from one another. The vas deferens, having been cut previously and brought to the epididymis, is secured by placing one or two 9-0 nylon sutures from the edge of the cut epididymal tunic through the adventitia and muscularis layers of the vas to hold them in position so that mucosal anastomosis can be performed (Fig. 16.8B). The previously placed 10-0 nylon suture closest to the vas lumen is placed in an inside-out fashion through the edge of the lumen, incorporating a small bit of muscularis. Additional sutures are placed at the 4 and 8 o'clock positions in an outside-in, inside-out pattern from the epididymal tubule to the vas. The two previously placed sutures that were at 120° from the first are now passed in an inside-out pattern through the vas lumen. Before these last two are tied, a final suture is placed at the 12 o'clock position to complete the lumen-to-lumen anastomosis (Fig. 16.8C). Additional 9-0 sutures are then placed from the epididymal tunic to the vas muscularis and adventitia in a circumferential manner until it is completely secured (Fig. 16.8D). Additional sutures of 9-0 nylon are placed along the vas, anchoring it to the parietal portion of the tunica vaginalis.

If the patient has had a prior vasectomy or if the proximal vas has been injured or scarred, the distal (abdominal) vas deferens is sometimes not of sufficient length to reach the epididymis without tension. It is possible to mobilize the distal vas along with its blood supply by placing a holding suture on the end of the vas, passing a finger beneath the vas, and gently pushing away with gentle upward traction the loose surrounding tissues that tether it. If this maneuver is still not sufficient to allow for a tension-free anastomosis, the upper portion of

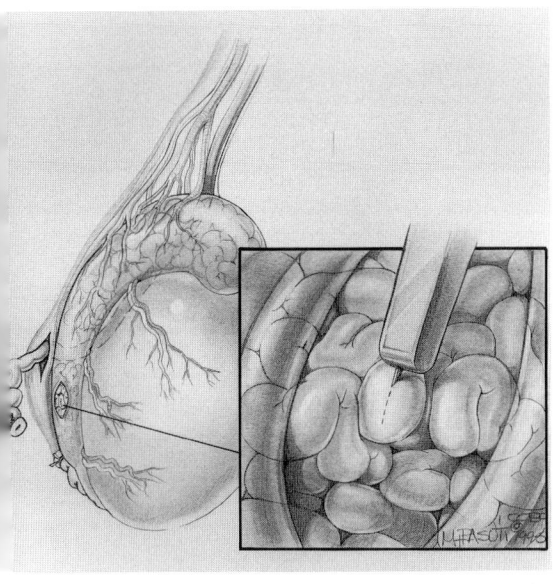
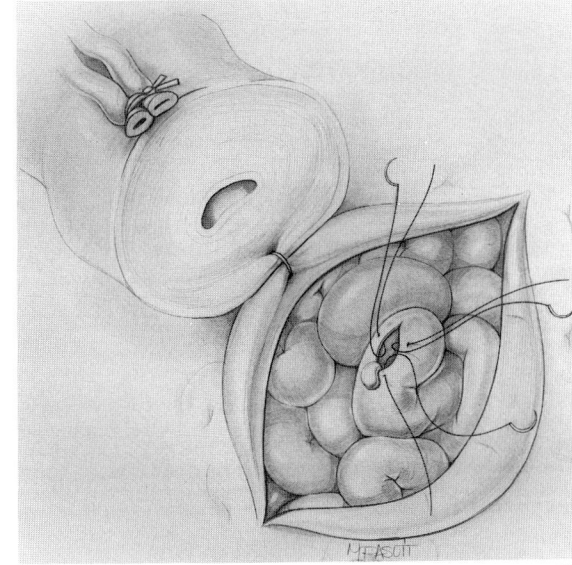

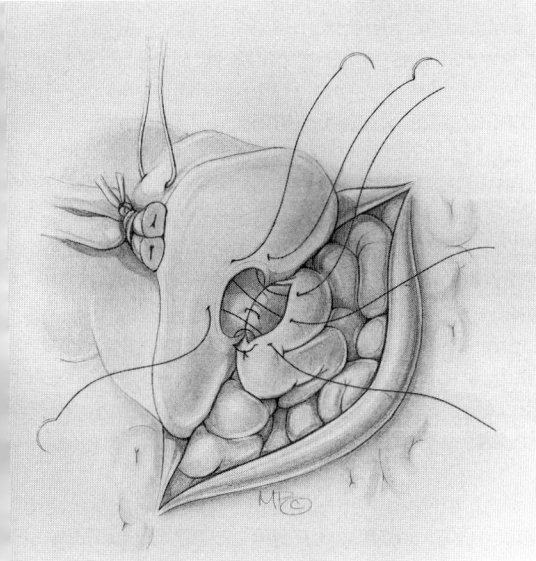
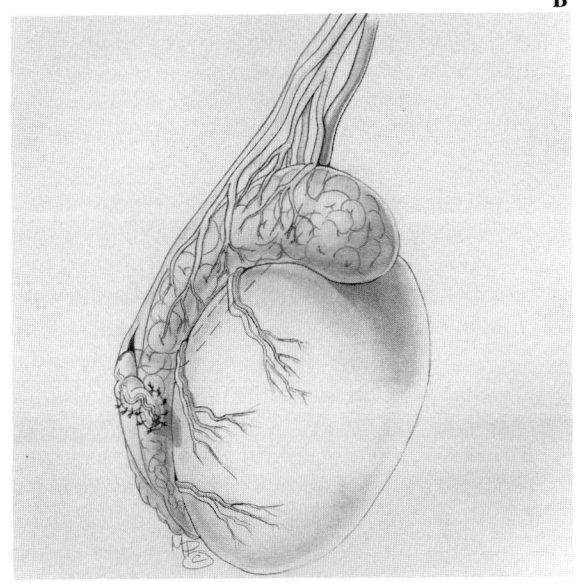

**B**

**D**

FIGURE 16.8. (A) A microknife is used to open a loop of the epididymal tubule. Note that the distal vas deferens has been brought lateral to the epididymis ready for anastomosis. (B) Approximation of the vas muscularis to the epididymal tunic and pre-placement of epididymal sutures. (C) Completion of the anastomosis of the vas and epididymal tubule lumen. (D) Completion of the epididymal anastomosis. (Parts A and B from Padron and Thomas,[41] with permission.)

the incision can be extended to the external ring or beyond and the vas deferens further freed from the cord and brought down to the epididymis. This extensive mobilization, if needed, should be done before the epididymis is inspected or incised.

## Results

The use of the operative microscope has revolutionized surgery for male infertility. Surgeons are able to attain a degree of accuracy in the apposition of two very small lumina that was

TABLE 16.1. Vasoepididymostomy results with the operating microscope.

| Authors | Year | No. of Patients | Patency (%) | Pregnancy (%) |
|---|---|---|---|---|
| Silber[28] | 1989 | 139 | (78) | (56) |
| Fuchs[29] | 1991 | 39 | 23/39 (59) | 8/23 (35) |
| Thomas[30] | 1993 | 153 | 110/145 (76)* | 47/111 (42)* |
| Schlegel and Goldstein[31] | 1993 | 107 | 64/91 (70)* | 25/81 (31)† |

*Patients with follow-up of longer than one year.
†Excludes patients with female factor infertility.

not previously possible. Consequently, the results of their efforts are reflected in the success achieved by their patients (Table 16.1).[28–32]

## Alloplastic Spermatocele

Attempts are being made to develop an artificial reservoir or alloplastic spermatocele from which adequate numbers of motile sperm can be obtained repeatedly through percutaneous puncture. Although some success has been achieved, long-term patency of these devices has been unusual.[31–38] Of note is a more recent variation of the spermatocele reported by Moni and Lalitha,[39] who attempted to create a continuous flow of sperm from an opening made in a single loop of the epididymal tubule to drain sperm into the inner portion of the tunica vaginalis where it could be aspirated under ultrasound guidance. Matthews and associates[40] reported a modification of this procedure using the operating microscope to more carefully open the tubule and secure the edges to the visceral tunic of the epididymis. Volume of fluid and sperm quality have varied from poor to excellent.

## Obstruction of the Vas Deferens Above the Level of the Scrotum

Although the excurrent ductal system can be obstructed anywhere along its path, the most common sites for obstruction, excluding purposeful vasectomy, are either the epididymides or the ejaculatory ducts. Less common are those sites along the course of the vas deferens

that may have sustained injury during the performance of other operative procedures, such as hernia repair, renal transplant, or surgeries within the deep pelvis. Special mention should be made of blockage of the vas deferens in the inguinal canal. Its presence should be suspected in the patient with normal-volume azoospermia who has had prior inguinal surgery and is found to have at least one normal-size testis with a full epididymis and a vas deferens that, on careful palpation, is often tortuous and dilated.

Inguinal obstruction is confirmed by vasography (Fig. 16.9). If the obstruction was inadvertently caused during an infant hernia repair, the abdominal end is usually found below the level of the internal inguinal ring. This is important when planning the incision, taking into account that the surgeon must open the area medial to the ring or incise it in a cephalad direction to get adequate exposure not only to identify the often buried end of the vas but also to have sufficient room to mobilize the two ends in order to anastomose them without tension. The vasovasostomy is performed in a manner similar to that done at the scrotal level. It is important to examine the fluid from the testicular end of the vas deferens. If sperm are found, there is no secondary epididymal obstruction. If sperm are not found, the vasovasostomy is still performed, although the patient should be told that there *may* be a more proximal obstruction that cannot be corrected at the time of the vasovasostomy, as it could jeopardize the blood supply of the vas deferens. It is suggested that an interval of 6 months be allowed, and if the patient still has azoospermia, vasography and vasoepididymostomy may be necessary.

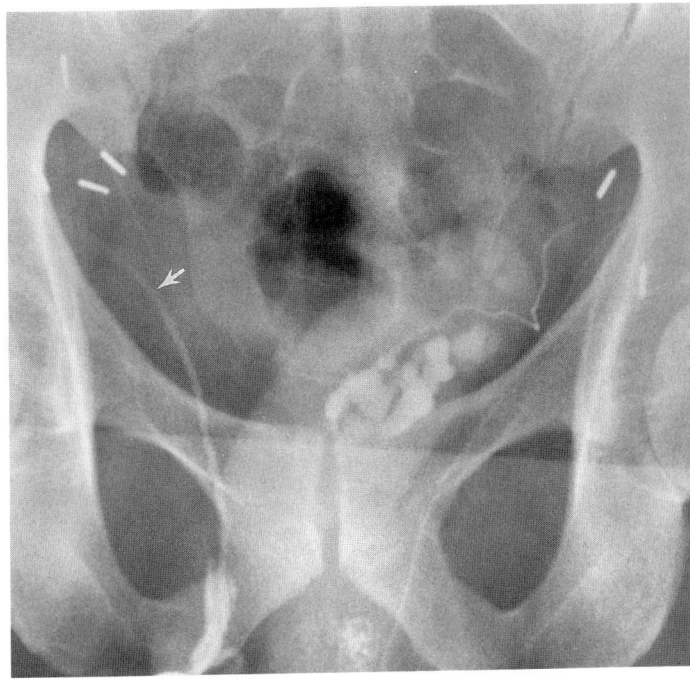

FIGURE 16.9. Bilateral vasogram in a patient with left vas deferens obstruction at the level of the internal inguinal ring (arrow). Note the difference in lumen diameters.

## Sperm Aspiration and Cryopreservation

The ability to offer patients in vitro fertilization with intracytoplasmic sperm injection using few cryopreserved sperm has led to the practice of asking patients undergoing correction of excurrent duct obstruction if they wish to save motile sperm found at the time of reconstructive surgery. It should be clearly explained that the amount and quality of sperm, if any, would almost always require a sophisticated (i.e., expensive) form of assisted reproductive technology. If the couple is not interested or is unable to do this for personal reasons, they simply choose not to cryopreserve. The quality of sperm varies, depending upon where in the ductal system sperm are identified. The best quality is from the vas deferens, then the caput epididymis, followed by the corpus and cauda (Padron OF, Thomas AJ, unpublished data).

Schlegel and Goldstein[31] reviewed their experience with vasoepididymostomy and noted that 16% of men who had sperm in their ejaculate after surgery scarred down the anastomoses and developed azoospermia. This suggests that sperm should be frozen whenever there are live, motile sperm in the ejaculate.[39]

## Summary

Obstructive azoospermia can be caused by a variety of insults. Microsurgical techniques currently employed have dramatically improved patency and pregnancy rates. Simple sperm aspiration combined with intracytoplasmic sperm injection frequently obviates the need for corrective surgery. Current experience indicates that the results of surgery with regard to success and cost outweigh the lesser surgical experience of sperm aspiration for the man and hormonal stimulation of his spouse (Kolettis P, Thomas AJ, unpublished data).

## References

1. Amann RP, Howards SS. Daily spermatozoal production and epididymal spermatozoal reserves of the human male. *J Urol* 1980; 124:211–215.

2. Turner TT, Cesarini DM. The ability of the rat epididymus to concentrate spermatozoa. *J Androl* 1983; 3:197–202.

3. Wong PYD, Au CL, Nagi HK. Electrolyte transport in the rat epididymis: its possible role in sperm maturation. *Int J Androl* 1978; 2 (suppl):608–628.

4. Robaire B, Hermo L. Efferent ducts, epididymis and vas deferens: structure, function and their regulation. In: Knobil E, Neil J, eds. *The Physiology of Reproduction.* New York: Raven Press; 1988: 999–1080.

5. Turner TT. On the epididymis and its role in the development of the fertile ejaculate. *J Androl* 1995; 16:292–298.

6. Bedford JM. The status and state of the human epididymis (review). *Hum Reprod* 1994; 9:2187–2199.

7. Anguiano A, Oates RD, Amos JA, et al. Congenital absence of the vas deferens. A primarily genital form of cystic fibrosis. *JAMA* 1992; 267:1794–1797.

8. Mercier B, Verlingue C, Lissens W, et al. Is congenital bilateral absence of the vas deferens a primary form of cystic fibrosis? Analysis of the CFTR gene in 67 patients. *Am J Hum Genet* 1995; 56:272–277.

9. Silber SJ. Pregnancy with sperm aspiration from the proximal head of the epididymis: a new treatment for congenital absence of the vas deferens. *Fertil Steril* 1988; 50:525–528.

10. Silber S, Ord T, Balmaceda J, et al. Congenital absence of the vas deferens. The fertilizing capacity of human epididymal sperm. *N Engl J Med* 1990; 323:1788–1792.

11. Bourne H, Watkins W, Speirs A, et al. Pregnancies after intracytoplasmic injection of sperm collected by fine needle biopsy of the testis. *Fertil Steril* 1995; 64:433–436.

12. Chen CS, Chu SH, Soong YK, et al. Epididymal sperm aspiration with assisted reproductive techniques: difference between congenital and acquired obstructive azoospermia? *Hum Reprod* 1995; 10:1104–1108.

13. Schlegel PN, Palermo GD, Alikani M, et al. Micropuncture retrieval of epididymal sperm with in vitro fertilization: importance of in vitro micromanipulation techniques. *Urology* 1995; 46:238–241.

14. Tsirigotis M, Craft I. Sperm retrieval methods and ICSI for obstructive azoospermia (review). *Hum Reprod* 1995; 10:758–760.

15. Tucker MJ, Morton PC, Witt MA, et al. Intracytoplasmic injection of testicular and epididymal spermatozoa for treatment of obstructive azoospermia. *Hum Reprod* 1995; 10: 486–489.

16. Sabanegh E, Thomas AJ. Effectiveness of crossover transseptal vasoepididymostomy in treating complex obstructive azoospermia. *Fertil Steril* 1995; 63:392–395.

17. Scorer CG, Farrington GH. *Congenital Deformities of the Testis and Epididymis.* New York: Appleton-Century-Crofts; 1971.

18. Wagenknecht LV. Alloplastic spermatocele. In: Goldstein M, ed. *Surgery of Male Infertility.* Philadelphia: W.B. Saunders; 1995: 142–158.

19. Young D. Surgical treatment of male infertility. *J Reprod Fertil* 1970; 23:541–542.

20. Le Lannou D, Jezequel P, Blayau M, et al. Obstructive azoospermia with agenesis of the vas deferens or with bronchiectasis (Young's syndrome): a genetic approach. *Hum Reprod* 1995; 10:339–341.

21. Silber SJ. Microscopic vasoepididymostomy: specific microanastomosis to the epididymal tubule. *Fertil Steril* 1978; 30:565–571.

22. Silber SJ. Microsurgery for vasectomy reversal and vasoepididymostomy. *Urology* 1984; 23:505–524.

23. Belker AM, Thomas AJ Jr, Fuchs EF, et al. Results of 1469 microsurgical vasectomy reversals by the vasovasostomy study group. *J Urol* 1991; 145:505–511.

24. Goldstein M. Microsurgical vasoepididymostomy: end-to-end anastomosis. In: Goldstein M, ed. *Surgery of Male Infertility.* Philadelphia: W.B. Saunders; 1995: 120–127.

25. Dewire DM, Thomas AJ. Microsurgical end-to-side vasoepididymostomy. In: Goldstein M, ed. *Surgery of Male Infertility.* Philadelphia: W.B. Saunders; 1995: 128–134.

26. Thomas AJ. Vasoepididymostomy. *Urol Clin North Am* 1987; 14:527–538.

27. Thomas AJ, Nagler HM. Testicular biopsy and vasography for evaluation of male infertility. *Urol Clin North Am* 1987; 14:167–176.

28. Silber SJ. Results of microsurgical vasoepididymostomy: role of epididymis in sperm maturation. *Hum Reprod* 1989; 4:298–303.

29. Fuchs EF. Restoring fertility through epididymovasotomy. *Contemp Urol* 1991; 3:27–38.

30. Thomas AJ. Microsurgical end-to-side vasoepididymostomy: analysis and outcome of 161 procedures. Presented at the 88th annual meeting of the American Urological Association, San Antonio TX, May, 1993.

31. Schlegel PN, Goldstein M. Microsurgical vaso-epididymostomy: refinements and results. *J Urol* 1993; 150:1165–1168.

32. Schoysman R. Vasoepididymostomy: a survey of techniques and results with consideration of delay of appearance of spermatozoa after surgery. *Acta Eur Fertil* 1990; 21:239–245.

33. Belker AM, Jimenez-Cruz DJF, Kelami A, et al. Alloplastic spermatocele: poor sperm mobility in intraoperative epididymal contraindicates prosthesis implantation. *J Urol* 1986; 136:408–409.

34. Prins GS, Ross LS. Properties of human epididymal sperm obtained from an alloplastic. Spermatoceles motility assessment and penetration of zona-free hamster oocytes in the presence and absence of caffeine. *Fertil Steril* 1985; 44:401–404.

35. Marmar JL, De Benedictis TJ, Praiss DE. Clinical experience with an artificial spermatocele. *J Androl* 1984; 5:304–311.

36. Wagenknecht LV. Alloplastic spermatocele: 20 years experience and perspectives. *Acta Chir Hung* 1994; 34:207–229.

37. Turner TT. On the development and use of alloplastic spermatoceles. *Fertil Steril* 1988; 49:387–395.

38. Grantmyre JE, Thomas AJ, Falk RM, et al. Development of a new alloplastic spermatocele demonstrating successful sperm retrieval in an animal model. *Fertil Steril* 1995; 64:179–184.

39. Moni VN, Lalitha PA. Moni's window operation: a new surgical technique to create a sperm reservoir in congenital vasal agenesis. *J Urol* 1992; 148:843–844.

40. Matthews GJ, Schlegel PN, Goldstein M. Microsurgical epididymal tubule marsupialization for creation of an autogenous tunica vaginalis sperm reservoir. In: Goldstein M, ed. *Surgery of Male Infertility*. Philadelphia: W.B. Saunders; 1995: 135–141.

41. Padron OF, Thomas AJ. Microsurgical correction of epididymal obstruction: epididymovasostomy. In: Lipshultz LI, ed. The Atlas of Urologic Clinics of North America. Philadelphia: W.B. Saunders; 1996.

# 17
# Micromanipulation of the Male Gamete

Sarah K. Girardi and Peter N. Schlegel

Since the first report in 1983[1] of a live birth resulting from in vitro fertilization, the field of assisted reproduction has virtually exploded. Perhaps the most impressive advances made in the past decade in assisted reproduction have been in the area of male factor infertility. As recently as 10 years ago, couples with infertility due to abnormal semen quality were advised to pursue donor insemination or adoption. Today, those same couples and even men with azoospermia from unreconstructable reproductive tract obstruction are able to contribute to pregnancies through assisted reproductive techniques that facilitate sperm and egg interaction. Such techniques range from the relatively simple intrauterine insemination to the more complicated in vitro fertilization combined with partial zona dissection, subzonal insemination, or intracytoplasmic sperm injection.

## Background

The success of human micromanipulation techniques today is owed to the over 30 years of research into the physiology and manipulation of animal gametes as well as to several serendipitous discoveries. Several landmark results in animal experiments paved the way for successful human trials. Using sea urchin eggs, Hiramoto[2] in 1962 showed that the egg cytoplasm must be activated before injected sperm can successfully decondense in the oocyte cytoplasm. Uehara and Yanagimachi[3] in 1976 were the first to successfully inject isolated hamster sperm nuclei and subsequently frozen/thawed human spermatozoa into hamster eggs with development of two pronuclei. In a series of experiments involving zona free rat oocytes and mouse sperm, Thadani[4] subsequently showed that only the zona free rat oocytes were capable of fertilization by mouse sperm. This finding suggested that the species-specific process of fertilization is mediated by sperm–zona interactions, not by sperm-oocyte plasma membrane events. In further experiments, it was shown that the interaction between oocyte and sperm nuclei is less species-specific than their sperm–zona recognition events. In other words, specific membrane fusion events could be bypassed by microinjection without compromising the initiation of development. In 1983 Markert[5] showed that microinjected sperm heads and grossly defective spermatozoa could induce normal fertilization. Such experiments demonstrated that the events of sperm penetration and fusion with the oocyte are not required for successful fertilization. Direct intracytoplasmic injection of sperm into the oocyte could bypass these events and still result in successful fertilization. All of these experiments naturally set the stage for attempts at micromanipulation of human gametes in the treatment of infertility.

Problems existed, however, with the first applications of micromanipulation in humans. First, although successful fertilizations and cleavage had been achieved in animals, embryos had not yet survived transfer. Also, techniques that had been successful in animal models proved not to be functional for human gametes. Gordon and Talansky[6] reported successful fertilizations in mice after partial zonal digestion using an acidic Tyrode's solution, but the same intervention was deleterious to human oocytes. Experiments in the past several years, therefore, have focused on improving the understanding of the physiology of human gamete interaction and perfecting micromanipulation techniques in humans.

## Barriers to Fertilization

Although great strides had been made in animal gamete micromanipulation, techniques mastered in animals have not always been applicable to humans. The anatomical (if not mechanical) barriers to fertilization that have needed to be fully defined prior to successful fertilization include: (1) the cumulus of the oocyte, (2) the zona pellucida, and (3) the vitelline membrane or oocyte plasma membrane. The cumulus is the first anatomic barrier encountered by the spermatozoon. Although its role is not completely understood, it probably functions less as a barrier than as a facilitator of sperm action. Sperm interaction with cumulus cells normally results in human sperm capacitation including hyperactivation. Capacitated sperm traverse the cumulus without difficulty.[7] Animal studies have shown that cumulus penetration does not require enzyme release,[8] and studies in humans have shown that acrosome-intact spermatids have reached the zona successfully.[9] Data suggest that cumulus cells actually direct the spermatozoa to reach the zona in the proper orientation.[10] Of note, most spermatozoa that attach to the cumulus complex and zona are morphologically normal.

The next anatomic barrier is the zona pellucida. In contrast to the easy passage through the cumulus, penetration of the zona requires enzymatic action and mechanical forces. Binding to the zona is species-specific and receptor mediated. The acrosome intact sperm recognizes a specific region of the zona pellucida sperm receptor molecule. Once recognition has occurred, the spermatozoon binds to the receptor and the acrosome reaction is induced. The acrosome reaction involves fusion of the outer acrosomal membrane and plasma membrane, release of enzymes, and penetration of the zona pellucida.

The sperm then reaches the perivitelline space where it fuses with the oocyte plasma membrane, the final barrier to fertilization. This step requires that the spermatozoon has undergone successful acrosome reaction and capacitation. In addition, the sperm must have a normally shaped head and clearly defined equatorial segment. Spermatozoa with "round head" defects are incapable of oocyte fusion.[11–13] Fusion, in turn, induces a series of changes that result in a block to polyspermia. The fusion of spermatozoon and oocyte plasma membrane causes modifications in the zona pellucida and the zonal sperm receptor molecule. With circumvention of the zona pellucida in human micromanipulation, polyspermia is possible because the zona pellucida receptors can no longer act as sperm receptors or inducers of the acrosome reaction and as a blockade to polyspermia. These observations provide evidence that the prevention of polyspermia is under the control of the zona pellucida and not the oolemma in humans.

Although normal spermatozoa are equipped to penetrate these barriers, impaired sperm—that is, those with abnormal motility, morphology, absent acrosomes, or defective cilia (Kartagener's syndrome)—cannot. Micromanipulation techniques have been designed to overcome these sperm defects and to facilitate the traversal of sperm through these barriers. They are, from least to most invasive, partial zonal dissection (PZD), subzonal insemination (SuZI), and intracytoplasmic sperm injection (ICSI). In general, the more severe the sperm impairment, the more invasive the micromanipulation technique required. However, SuZI and PZD are complementary procedures, with each technique providing fertilization for some couples where the other technique failed. The more invasive the technique, the greater the likelihood of oocyte injury as a result of handling. The consistently superior results achieved with ICSI over the past 2 years have made it the micromanipulation technique of choice for severe impairments in sperm quality and have relegated PZD and SuZI to techniques of historic significance only.

# Candidates for Assisted Reproductive Techniques

Any couple unsuccessful in achieving pregnancy after 1 year of unprotected intercourse warrants an infertility evaluation. The need for assisted reproduction is then determined after both members of the couple have been evaluated and treated. Specific, treatable factors that may affect fertility should be addressed prior to resorting to assisted reproductive procedures. Candidates for assisted reproduction may include couples with identifiable female- or male-factor infertility or both, and couples with idiopathic infertility. Female factors include cervical stenosis, abnormal sperm–cervical mucus interaction, tubal factors, polycystic ovarian disease, endometriosis, and immune-based infertility. Cervical factors can often be successfully treated with intrauterine insemination (IUI). Male factors include anatomical defects, such as severe hypospadias that prevent deposition of sperm in the vagina, congenital and acquired reproductive tract obstruction, neurologic disorders that have resulted in impaired erection or ejaculation, and severely impaired semen quality unresponsive to specific interventions. Male factors with or without female factors often require in vitro fertilization (IVF) with some form of gamete micromanipulation.

# Assisted Reproductive Techniques

Assisted reproductive techniques (ARTs) comprise a large spectrum of interventions ranging from intravaginal deposition of semen to highly specialized micromanipulation techniques that can only be performed during an in vitro fertilization cycle. It is imperative that both members of the infertile couple be examined thoroughly so that the factor responsible for the couple's infertility can be correctly identified. In this way, the couple can be directed to the simplest, most effective and expeditious treatment available.

## Intrauterine Insemination

For couples with male-factor infertility in whom the problem is anatomical (e.g., severe hypospadias preventing successful deposition of semen), physiologic (e.g., retrograde ejaculation, anejaculation, or impotence), or involves impaired semen quality, the least invasive procedures are intravaginal or intracervical insemination. These procedures make use of cervical mucus that acts as a filter, allowing sperm of good quality to progress into the uterus while retaining poor quality sperm, seminal fluid, white blood cells, and debris in the lower reproductive tract. The advantage of this procedure is that unprocessed semen can be used. The disadvantage is that there is a marked reduction in the number of spermatozoa that reach the oocyte, and inferior pregnancy rates have been demonstrated with this technique when compared with intrauterine insemination.

In IUI, processed semen is deposited directly into the uterine fundus via a small catheter. By bypassing the cervical mucus and placing processed semen directly into the uterus, the normal reduction in numbers of sperm that naturally occurs at the level of the cervix is eliminated. In this way, more sperm are able to reach the oocyte. IUI may circumvent one of the positive functions of cervical mucus, however. In addition to serving as a filter, cervical mucus serves as a reservoir allowing a slow release of sperm over 24 to 48 hours, thereby maximizing the delivery of sperm after ovulation. The disadvantage of IUI is that by bypassing the cervical mucus, this reservoir function is also bypassed and insemination has to be timed very precisely to ovulation.

The success of IUI is dependent on semen quality. Ho et al[14] found that the greater the number of sperm defects, the lower the pregnancy rate with IUI. Horvath et al[15] also showed that pregnancy rates were directly related to the total number of motile sperm and the percentage of morphologically normal sperm. Of the three semen parameters (concentration, motility, and morphology), impaired motility has the greatest adverse effect on IUI pregnancy rates. IUI is therefore most successful for couples in whom a known cervical factor exists and good sperm quality has been established. Sigman[16] recommends that IUI be reserved for couples in whom the semen has been evaluated using strict criteria and found to have a normal sperm penetration assay or greater than 4% morphologically normal sperm forms. He further advocates that IUI be used as a first-line therapy in male-factor infertility after treatment of specific factors affecting male fertility but prior to proceeding with other more invasive assisted reproductive techniques. In general, IUI alone for male-factor infertility is of limited benefit. IUI with ovarian stimulation using clomiphene citrate or follicle-stimulating hormone (FSH)/human menopausal gonadotropin (hMG), however, can be beneficial in the treatment of couples with male-factor infertility.

## In Vitro Fertilization

For couples with more severe impairments in sperm quality or defects in sperm fertilizing capacity, in vitro fertilization (IVF) may be beneficial. The term *in vitro* is translated from the Latin for "in glass" and refers to any process that takes place in an artificial environment outside the body. Sperm and egg are retrieved from each partner and fertilization takes place outside the body. The resulting embryo or embryos are then transferred to the female partner's uterus. IVF can be performed with or without manipulation of the egg and sperm. The sperm are processed by washing with centrifugation, swim-up, sedimentation, or Percoll gradient centrifugation to ensure that only the purest, most motile sperm are used for insemination. In couples with male factor infertility, even normal numbers of sperm will not fertilize oocytes as well as sperm from men with normal semen quality. One study showed that insemination with 50,000 to 100,000 motile sperm per oocyte resulted in a 71% fertilization rate

in non–male-factor couples, and only a 23% fertilization rate in male-factor couples.[17] The fertilization rate in male-factor couples was increased to 61% by increasing the sperm concentration to 500,000. For this reason, it is recommended that sperm concentrations of 500,000 to 2 million per oocyte be used for IVF in male-factor couples compared with 50,000 to 100,000 sperm per oocyte in non–male-factor couples.

Sperm morphology has a dramatic effect on fertilization rates. Using very strict criteria for normal sperm shape, where borderline morphologic forms were considered abnormal, Kruger et al[18] reported that abnormal morphology was the single best predictor of fertilization rates during IVF. Using the Kruger criteria, Oehninger et al[19] showed that individuals with >14% normal forms achieved a 94% fertilization rate and 44% per cycle pregnancy rate, those with 4% to 14% normal forms had an 86% fertilization rate and 33% per cycle pregnancy rate, and individuals with <4% normal forms had only a 44% fertilization rate and 8% per cycle pregnancy rate. The same study showed that these poor fertilization rates in couples with <4% normal forms can be partially compensated for by increasing the number of sperm inseminated per oocyte. A fertilization rate of 63% was achieved when the concentration of inseminated sperm was increased to >100,000 sperm per milliliter per oocyte. The pregnancy rate, however, increased to only 9% per cycle. Exclusionary criteria for IVF based on semen parameters have been defined.[20] If a sperm concentration of <2 million and a motility of <5% or normal forms of ≤3% are present, then the chances of oocyte fertilization with standard IVF are so low that micromanipulation should be used to increase fertilization rates.

The low fertilization and pregnancy rates achieved with critically poor sperm quality have paved the way for the study of gamete manipulation. If low fertilization rates in male-factor couples with critically poor semen quality are the result of the spermatozoon's inability to penetrate natural oocyte barriers, then perhaps fertilization rates could be improved by assisting spermatozoa to overcome those barriers. These observations have led to the advent of micromanipulation of human gametes for male-factor infertility.

## Zona Pellucida Drilling and Partial Zonal Dissection

Zona pellucida drilling and partial zonal dissection (PZD) are examples of micromanipulation techniques aimed at breaching the zona pellucida. The technique of zona drilling was first described in mouse oocytes in 1986 by Gordon and Talansky.[6] In this procedure, the zona is digested by chemicals contained within a mi-

cropipette that is used to pierce the zona tangentially. A small amount of zona is thereby removed, leaving a small patch of oolemma exposed for routine insemination. This permitted access to the oocyte plasma membrane by spermatozoa that were otherwise unable to bind and penetrate the zona pellucida. The procedure is of historic significance because, despite its success in mice, zona drilling with acid Tyrode's solution proved detrimental to human oocytes and serves as an example of the difficulty in applying animal models to human gamete micromanipulation.

The principle of zona removal was successfully applied to human oocytes in the develop-

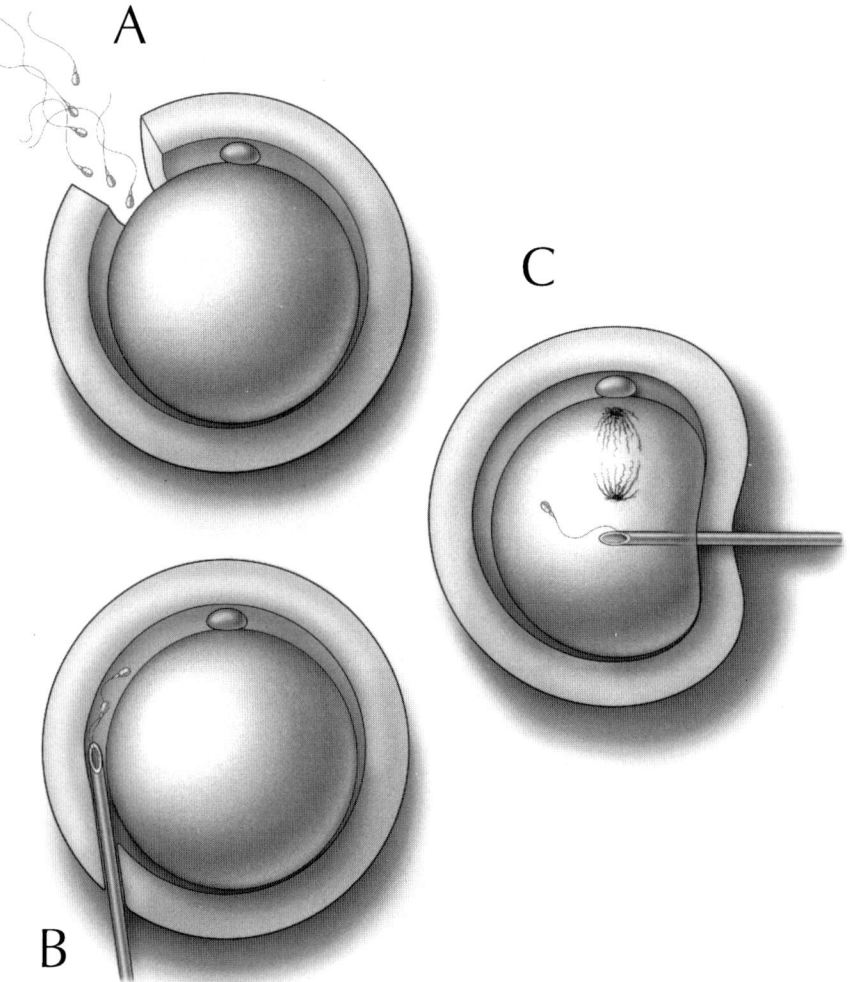

FIGURE 17.1. (A) Partial zonal dissection (PZD). (B) Subzonal insemination (SuZI). (C) Intracytoplasmic sperm injection (ICSI).

ment of PZD. In PZD a hyperosmotic solution is used to treat the oocytes. This results in shrinkage of the ooplasm within the zona pellucida, enlarging the perivitelline space. The oocyte is held with gentle suction on a holding pipette. A microneedle is placed tangentially through the zona pellucida with the insertion point at the 1 o'clock position and the exit point at the 11 o'clock position. The microneedle is then lifted off the zona pellucida, leaving a slit in the zona (Fig. 17.1A). The oocyte is then subjected to routine insemination. Like zona drilling, PZD was aimed at assisting fertilization in couples where the male had a low sperm count or sperm incapable of binding and penetrating the zona or both.

Both of the above techniques have the advantages of avoiding manipulation of the spermatozoa, minimal manipulation of the oocyte, and no disturbance of the oocyte plasma membrane or cytoplasm. The major problem, however, is that by removing the zona pellucida the major block to polyspermy is removed. Therefore, PZD results in an unacceptable rate of oocyte loss due to polyspermy. In addition, oocyte fertilization rates rarely exceed 20% and 36% of couples treated at centers applying PZD and subzonal insemination (SuZI) did not achieve monospermic fertilization of the oocytes.

## Subzonal Insemination

The next step in the process of gamete micromanipulation was to place spermatozoa into the perivitelline space while leaving the zona intact—subzonal insemination.

Subzonal insemination (SuZI) of spermatozoa was first described by Ng et al[21] in 1988. This technique involves gentle deposition of a single or multiple spermatozoa into the perivitelline space with an injecting pipette (Fig. 17.1B). The advantages of this procedure are that it is less damaging to the zona pellucida than zona drilling or PZD, fertilization can be achieved with few spermatozoa, and the oolemma is not disturbed. The disadvantages are that spermatozoa must be capable of undergoing capacitation and the acrosome reaction, and when multiple spermatozoa are inserted,

the procedure still results in high polyspermy rates.

The technique of SuZI demonstrated that fertilizations and pregnancies could be achieved in humans in cases of severe oligospermia, oligoasthenoteratospermia, and azooasthenospermia. Monospermic fertilization rates as high as 37% have been reported with SuZI in cases of moderate-to-severe teratospermia.[22] Cohen[23] reported a fertilization rate of 28% per oocyte and a pregnancy rate per cycle of 27% for couples who underwent SuZI after failed IVF. Although these rates were shown to be better than that achieved with IVF alone in controlled studies, the major limitation of SuZI remains the high rate of polyspermy. This finding and the superior fertilization results achieved with intracytoplasmic sperm injection have led essentially all centers to abandon SuZI in favor of ICSI.

## Intracytoplasmic Sperm Injection

The most invasive, most successful, and most quantitatively efficient of the established micromanipulation techniques for humans is intracytoplasmic sperm injection (ICSI). By direct injection of spermatozoa into the oocyte cytoplasm, all oocyte barriers are effectively bypassed. The procedure involves the deposition of sperm directly into the oocyte cytoplasm with a micropipette (Fig. 17.1C). The success of this procedure in humans depends on several factors: (1) the ability of the human oocyte to withstand piercing of the oocyte plasma membrane, (2) the viability of the spermatozoon, and (3) effective activation of the oocyte. The advantages of this technique are that it bypasses all oocyte barriers so that even severely abnormal spermatozoa can successfully fertilize, and it does not require sperm capacitation or the ability of sperm to undergo an acrosome reaction. The major disadvantages are that it requires manipulation of both gametes, which can result in injury to the gametes, and that injection of spermatozoa is technically demanding and requires extensive experience on the part of the clinician to achieve optimal results.

TABLE 17.1. Fertilization and pregnancy rates from selected series with various techniques of sperm retrieval and IVF/ICSI.

| | Sperm retrieval technique | Fertilization rate per oocyte (%) | Pregnancy rate per cycle (%) |
|---|---|---|---|
| Schlegel et al[25] | MESA | 140/312 (45) | 14/27 (52) |
| Craft et al[26] | PESA | 114/349 (33) | 10/42 (24) |
| Silber et al[27] | Testis biopsy | 56/185 (30) | 5/12 (42) |
| Bourne et al[28] | TESA | 14/22 (64) | 2/2 (100) |

MESA, microsurgical epididymal sperm aspiration; PESA, percutaneous epididymal sperm aspiration; TESA, testicular sperm aspiration.

## Indications for ICSI

Although rigid criteria for any of the assisted reproductive techniques are lacking, most would agree that ICSI is indicated in couples who have failed repeated IVF attempts and in couples with severe male-factor infertility. The latter category includes men with obstructive and nonobstructive azoospermia as well as men with severe oligospermia ($<2 \times 10^6$ sperm per cubic centimeter or $<500,000$ motile sperm per ejaculate). ICSI has been shown to be necessary for optimal results when using sperm retrieved from the testis or epididymis of men who have acquired or congenital reproductive tract obstruction.

## ICSI Technique

### Sperm Retrieval

Spermatozoa for ICSI may be retrieved from the whole ejaculate in nonobstructed men who are neurologically intact, or through electroejaculation in individuals who have failure of emission due to neurologic impairment. In men with obstruction due to bilateral congenital absence of the vas deferens or other reproductive tract obstructions, sperm may be retrieved from the epididymis through open microsurgical techniques[24,25] or percutaneously aspirated from the epididymis with a fine needle.[26] Spermatozoa can also be retrieved from the testis in an open biopsy[27] or percutaneously with fine needle aspiration.[28] Open microsurgical epididymal aspiration with the micropuncture technique[24] is recommended because it yields an adequate number and quality of sperm for immediate use and for cryopreservation, it minimizes contamination by blood cells, and it minimizes the risk of complications, such as hematocele or inadvertent injury to the testis, epididymis, or vascular supply of the testis. Sperm retrieved by all of these techniques can result in successful fertilizations and pregnancies with ICSI (Table 17.1).

### Sperm Processing

Once whole semen is collected or spermatozoa are retrieved, the specimens are washed by centrifugation and then purified on a discontinuous Percoll gradient. Use either a two- or three-layer gradient (47.5% and 95%, or 55%, 70%, and 90%), depending on sperm density and motility.[29] This final sperm preparation is then added to a droplet of polyvinyl pyrrolidone and placed in the middle of a petri dish. A recently motile, immobilized spermatozoon is aspirated from the edge of this droplet and injected into the oocyte.

### Ovarian Stimulation and Oocyte Retrieval

Female partners are downregulated with a gonadotropin-releasing hormone (GnRH) agonist and then stimulated with hMG or FSH or both. Women are followed with daily transvaginal ultrasound to evaluate ovarian follicle development and also with sequential serum estradiol levels. When optimal follicular development is obtained, human chorionic gonadotropin (hCG) is given, and oocytes are retrieved at 35 hours by vaginal ultrasound-guided puncture. Oocytes are examined under an inverted microscope and scored according to degree of maturation. The oocytes are then prepared for micromanipulation.

## Oocyte Processing

Oocytes are prepared by removing the cumulus mass and corona radiata with hyaluronidase. The oocytes are then examined under the inverted microscope to assess the maturation stage by observing the presence of a germinal vesicle, germinal vesicle breakdown, and the extruded first polar body. Metaphase II oocytes are identified by the presence of the extruded first polar body. Intracytoplasmic sperm injection is performed on all metaphase II oocytes. Metaphase II oocytes have their diploid complement of chromosomes delicately arranged on the metaphase plate near the polar body. Mechanical disruption of the metaphase plate can occur by injury from the injection pipette or the presence of a motile sperm in the oocyte cytoplasm.

Each oocyte is placed in a droplet of medium surrounding the central droplet that contains the spermatozoa. The droplets are covered with lightweight paraffin oil, and the petri dish is placed on a heated stage of the microscope. The microscope is equipped with two hydraulic micromanipulators that are fitted to two tool holders for the micropipettes.

During the intracytoplasmic sperm injection procedure, oocytes are stabilized with a holding micropipette, and injected with an injection pipette. Each pipette is hand drawn, forged, and either fire-polished or sharpened. The final outer diameter of the holding pipette is 60 μm, and the inner diameter is 20 μm. The outer diameter of the injection pipette is 5 to 7 μm, and the inner diameter is approximately 4 to 6 μm.

## Oocyte Injury

Results from some of the major centers performing ICSI show rates of oocyte loss after injection of 7% to 14% (Table 17.2). Although the precise reasons for oocyte injury are not known, it is thought to occur as a result of plasma membrane and ultrastructural disturbances associated with injection, damage to the meiotic spindle during injection, or extrusion of the oocyte cytoplasm following injection or both. In addition, other factors, such as changes in temperature, have been reported to cause irreversible changes in the meiotic spindle of the human oocyte.[30]

## Sperm Immobilization

In preparation for injection, spermatozoa are immobilized and then aspirated, tail first, into an injection pipette. Immobilization was initially described as being induced by gentle compression of the sperm tail with the tip of a micropipette.

Two recent studies have investigated the possible beneficial effects of more vigorous immo-

TABLE 17.2. Fertilization and clinical pregnancy rates from IVF/ICSI.

| | No. of couples | No. of cycles | No. of oocytes injected | Oocyte loss (%) | Fertility rate per oocyte (%) | Clin pregnancy rate per cycle (%) | Ongoing or delivered pregnancy rate per cycle (%) |
|---|---|---|---|---|---|---|---|
| Van Steirteghem et al[66]* | — | 1816 | 18,778 | 1997 (11) | 11,629/18,778 (62) | — | 666/1816 (37) |
| Palermo et al[29] | 227 | 227 | 1,923 | 136 (7) | 1142/1923 (59) | 94/227 (41) | 84/227 (37) |
| Tsirigotis et al[67] | 69 | 69 | 789 | 84 (11) | 410/789 (52) | 23/69 (33) | 19/69 (28) |
| Payne et al[68] | 100 | 100 | 1,003 | — | 672/1003 (67) | — | 25/100 (25) |
| Harari et al[69] | 114 | 119 | 1,185 | 112 (9) | 717/1185 (61) | 36/119 (30) | 24/119 (20) |
| Oehninger et al[46] | 92 | 102 | 1,163 | 154 (13) | 708/1163 (61) | 31/102 (30) | 26/102 (25) |
| Sherins et al[47] | 190 | 229 | 1,690 | 237 (14) | 617/1690 (37) | 38/229 (17) | 35/198 (18) |

* Adapted from abstract. Includes results from July 1992 to May 1994 only. Results from April 1990 to June 1992 excluded.

TABLE 17.3. Fertilization and pregnancy rates in ICSI cycles using ejaculated, testicular, and epididymal spermatozoa immobilized by two different methods.

| | Standard immobilization | | Aggressive immobilization | |
|---|---|---|---|---|
| | Fertilization/ oocyte (%) | Clinical pregnancy/ cycle (%) | Fertilization/ oocyte (%) | Clinical pregnancy/ cycle (%) |
| Ejaculated spermatozoa | 3469/4963 | 273/645 | 677/922 | 50/110 |
| | (69.9) | (42.3) | (73.4) | (45.5) |
| Epididymal spermatozoa | 171/354 | 18/35 | 141/172 | 14/17 |
| | (48.3) | (51.4) | (82.0) | (82.4) |
| Frozen/thawed spermatozoa | 58/119 | 3/16 | 48/58 | 6/8 |
| | (48.7) | (18.7) | (82.8) | (75.0) |
| Testicular spermatozoa | 9/22 | 2/3 | 8/12 | 0/2 |
| | (40.9) | (66.7) | (66.7) | (0) |

From Palermo, et al. Human Reprod 11:1023–1029, 1996.

bilization techniques. Gerris et al[31] evaluated the effects of sperm tail breakage on ICSI success by studying the fertilization rates achieved when using sperm with intact tails compared with sperm with damaged tails. Specifically, the tail was cut approximately halfway between the spermatozoal head and the tip of the tail, with the researchers taking care to preserve the spermatozoal midpiece. This technique resulted in a significant increase in the percentage of normally fertilized two-pronuclear oocytes (35.5% versus 59.9% for intact tails versus broken tails, respectively) and in a significant decrease in the number of one-pronuclear oocytes (15.6% versus 3.9%, respectively), which reflect oocyte activation without normal fertilization. Although the authors did not investigate the mechanism that accounts for these improvements, they speculated that tail damage induced changes in the sperm plasma membrane that facilitated biochemical changes necessary for decondensation and pronuclear formation from the sperm nucleus.

Palermo et al evaluated the effects on ICSI results of permanently crimping the sperm tail for immobilization compared with standard immobilization. Only a slight improvement in fertilization rates (69.9% vs. 73.4%; $p = 0.02$) and no improvement in pregnancy rates (42.3% vs. 45.5%; $p = $ NS) were observed in sperm processed from ejaculated semen samples. In contrast, significant differences in fertilization and pregnancy rates were observed in immature sperm retrieved from the epididymis of men with unreconstructable reproductive tract obstruction. Fertilization rates increased from 48% to 82% for fresh epididymal sperm ($p = 0.03$) and from 51% to 84% for frozen, thawed epididymal sperm ($p = 0.02$). Pregnancy rates increased from 51% to 82% and 19% to 75% for fresh and frozen epididymal sperm, respectively (Table 17.3). It was concluded that unlike spermatozoa from ejaculated specimens, spermatozoa retrieved from the epididymis have not undergone the final maturation processes that occur in the epididymis and vas deferens and therefore may require membrane manipulation, because they maybe resistant to leakage of sperm factors from the sperm cytoplasmic necessary to induce oocyte activation after intracytoplasmic injection. Alternatively, the membrane changes induced by aggressive immobilization could allow leakage of toxic material from the cytoplasmic droplet that is frequently found on immature sperm and that could adversely affect the fertilization process.

## Oocyte Activation and Intracytoplasmic Injection

The oocyte is stabilized using a holding pipette with the extruded polar body in the 6 o'clock or 12 o'clock position. The extruded polar body and associated degranulated area containing the oocyte nuclear material on its metaphase plate are thereby located away from the planned injection site. The aspirated spermatozoon is then injected into the oocyte cytoplasm with an injection pipette. A small amount of cytoplasm is withdrawn into the injecting pipette just prior to depositing the spermatozoon, to ensure that the injecting pipette is indeed within the cytoplasm. It is possible that the volume of ooplasm aspirated determines whether oocyte stimulation will occur during the microinjection procedure, a necessary step for efficient achievement of fertilization.

In a recent study, Tesarik and Sousa[32] reported improved fertilization and pregnancy rates with vigorous oocyte cytoplasm aspiration at the time of sperm injection compared with gentle aspiration. In this study, gentle (10 µm of cytoplasm aspirated) and vigorous (100 µm of cytoplasm aspirated) techniques of aspiration were directly compared in a group of 15 patients. Fertilization rates per oocyte and pregnancy rates were 38% and 20%, respectively, for the gentle aspiration group but 80% and 40% for the vigorous aspiration group. They then applied the vigorous aspiration technique for 100 consecutive patients and reported fertilization and clinical pregnancy rates of 87% and 52%, respectively. No increase in oocyte injury was noted after vigorous aspiration.

In the same study, calcium fluxes were measured by loading preinjection oocytes with a fluorescent calcium indicator. These oocytes were then subjected to ICSI with the gentle or vigorous technique. During manipulation of the oocytes, confocal images of the fluorescence emitted by the calcium indicator were recorded. Vigorous aspiration results in an additional peak of intracellular calcium levels, which were comparable to those with gentle aspiration and injection. The authors proposed that the additional intracellular calcium peak induced by vigorous cytoplasmic aspiration contributes to the improved fertilization rates observed after vigorous aspiration.

# Results of Assisted Reproductive Techniques

Over the past few years several large studies have been published that report fertilization and pregnancy rates for the various assisted reproductive techniques. One paradigm in which reliably poor sperm quality is routinely obtained is that in which sperm are retrieved from men with chronic reproductive tract obstruction, including bilateral congenital absence of the vas deferens (CAV). The low pregnancy rate with IVF alone using sperm of poor quality was illustrated in the sperm microaspiration retrieval and assisted reproductive technologies (SMART) study, published in 1994.[33] This study reported on 219 procedures performed at 22 centers across the United States. Half of the procedures were performed for the treatment of CAV. The overall clinical pregnancy rate for the 219 procedures performed was only 10%.

## PZD and SuZI Results

Pregnancy and fertilization rates for PZD and SuZI have been published on microsurgical epididymal sperm aspiration in combination with IVF alone, PZD, and SuZI.[24] In all cases, sperm were retrieved from the epididymis with the micropuncture technique previously described. Microsurgical epididymal sperm retrieval with PZD or SuZI resulted in fertilization and clinical pregnancy rates of 19% and 27%, respectively. This is a significant improvement over the 10% clinical pregnancy rate reported in the SMART study and appears to be attributable to the application of PZD and SuZI for these couples. Catt et al[34] reported comparable results using ejaculated sperm treated with SuZI in 141 couples with severe male factor infertility. They reported a fertilization rate per oocyte of 23% and a pregnancy rate per embryo transfer of 29%. Successful fertilization and pregnancies were even reported in cases of extreme male factor infertility. Lippi et al[35] reported a fertilization rate per oocyte of 57% and a clinical pregnancy rate per cycle of 9.4% in 213 cycles in which less than 50,000 total motile sperm were retrieved. Several investigators have attempted to correlate SuZI success with individual semen parameters. The results have been conflicting.[36–38] Although semen parameters may correlate with SuZI and PZD success, SuZI and PZD can be expected to improve fertilization and pregnancy rates over IVF alone in cases of moderate and severe male-factor infertility.

## ICSI Results

Preliminary reports from one of the largest studies[39] using IVF/ICSI indicate that in 150 couples who underwent 150 consecutive treatment cycles, 1409 oocytes were injected and 830 were successfully fertilized for a fertilization rate of 59%.[39] A total clinical pregnancy rate of 35% was achieved. The fertilization rate in this study was not influenced by the standard semen characteristics of concentration, motility, and strict criteria morphology. The fertilization and pregnancy rates from an updated study series are shown in Table 17.2.

In another large series, Palermo et al[29] reported on 227 couples treated with IVF/ICSI for failed IVF cycles or for severe male-factor infertility. Fertilization and pregnancy rates were evaluated relative to semen parameters and the origin of the semen samples. They reported successful fertilization in 1142/1923 (59%) metaphase II oocytes injected, and ongoing pregnancies in 84/227 (37%) couples. Neither semen quality nor the source of sperm (ejaculated, surgically retrieved, or electroejaculated) affected pregnancy rates. They concluded that IVF/ICSI offers fertilization and pregnancy rates comparable to those achieved with normal sperm quality in couples who have failed to achieve pregnancy on repeated IVF cycles or who have severe impairments in semen quality. In addition, the success of IVF/ICSI was independent of standard semen parameters (density, motility, and morphology).

Results with IVF/ICSI[25] in combination with microsurgical epididymal sperm retrieval show that microsurgical epididymal sperm retrieval with IVF/ICSI resulted in a 45% fertilization rate and a 52% clinical pregnancy rate, with an ongoing pregnancy rate of 48% per attempt at sperm and egg retrieval. These results, and the fact that very small numbers of sperm are needed for ICSI, indicate the use of ICSI exclusively over all other micromanipulation techniques for couples in whom sperm must be surgically retrieved.

## Discussion

Since the first report of a successful delivery from in vitro fertilization in 1983,[1] the advances in the field of assisted reproduction and micromanipulation have been truly dramatic. Perhaps the most exciting advances have been in the area of male-factor infertility. Couples who previously would have been offered donor insemination or adoption are now achieving pregnancies despite severe impairments in semen quality, the presence of only single numbers of sperm in the ejaculate, or unreconstructable reproductive tract obstruction. Techniques of micromanipulation that were revolutionary less than 5 years ago are now obsolete, replaced by even more successful methods. Even nonobstructive azoospermia due to maturation arrest or other impairments in germ cell maturation has been added to the list of treatable factors in male infertility because sperm can frequently be extracted directly from testicular parenchyma that is surgically biopsied. For patients without sperm in the testicular parenchyma, round spermatid injection[40] and round spermatid nuclear injection[41] are possible. Several important questions remain, however, with regard to these exciting discoveries: (1) What are the specific indications for IUI, IVF, and ICSI? Should IVF alone ever be used for male-factor infertility? (2) What are the reasons for ICSI failures that still represent over half of our attempts at achieving ongoing pregnancies? (3) Can we be certain that using severely impaired or less mature sperm will not result in significant birth defects or in genetic abnormalities that could affect the offspring in adolescence or adulthood? (4) What is the most cost-effective approach for the infertile couple with severely impaired semen parameters?

## Indications for Specific Assisted Reproductive Techniques (ARTs)

The indications for IUI, IVF, and ICSI are largely center-dependent. In general, IUI is reserved for couples who lack severe impairments in semen quality or in whom a known cervical factor exists. Some advocate that as long as the semen analysis reveals at least 4% morphologically normal forms by strict criteria, IUI should be used as a first-line therapy in male-factor infertility prior to proceeding with other more sophisticated ARTs.

IVF is indicated in couples with female-factor infertility as well as in some couples with male-factor infertility. Multiple studies have shown that IVF success is dependent on semen quality. Therefore, in couples with established male-factor infertility, only those with moderate impairments in sperm quality are considered candidates for IVF. Semen parameters that are unacceptable for success with IVF are defined as follows:

1. sperm concentration of less than 2 million,
2. motility less than 5%,
3. morphology of less than 4% normal forms by strict criteria.

Patients who meet these indications and who have not experienced a previous failed IVF attempt are considered candidates for ICSI. An additional indication for ICSI is documented failure to achieve fertilization with IVF regardless of the semen quality.

ICSI is so effective that it allows fertilization rates equivalent to those resulting from normal-appearing sperm. Therefore, it has been suggested that ICSI should be applied to all men, even those with mild male-factor infertility. However, there are potential long-term complications from ICSI that may not have been detected as yet because ICSI has only been in widespread use for 2 to 3 years. Therefore, caution is warranted before extending indications for ICSI beyond the most severe cases of male-factor infertility until the safety and efficacy of this treatment have been confirmed.

## Determinants of ICSI Success: Male and Female Factors

Palermo et al[42] reported in 1993 that success with ICSI is independent of the three basic semen parameters: sperm concentration, motility, and morphology. They did show, however, that extensive teratospermia did correlate with significantly lower embryo implantation rates than those achieved with less severe teratospermia.

These findings have not been corroborated by other studies. Cohen et al[43] reported no significant correlation between the fertilization, implantation, and the percentage of normal sperm forms. Nagy et al[44] reported high fertilization and pregnancy rates in 966 microinjected cycles despite cryptospermia, total asthenospermia, or total teratozoospermia. They concluded that the only absolute criterion for successful ICSI is the presence of at least one living spermatozoon per oocyte in the pellet of the treated semen sample. For patients with no motile sperm in the ejaculate, pregnancy rates were decreased to 12% per cycle. If no sperm were motile in the ejaculate and no motile sperm were obtained after processing, Nagy et al did not achieve any pregnancies in their patients, presumably because none of the sperm injected were viable. Similarly, Mansour et al[45] report that fertilization and pregnancy rates were not affected by semen parameters as long as injections were performed with morphologically well-shaped, live spermatozoa. These reports of fertilizations and pregnancies occurring independently of male factors argue for an examination of female factors that could account for ICSI failures.

Oehninger et al[46] implicated maternal factors as contributors to the failure to achieve an ongoing pregnancy after ICSI in a prospective clinical trial that correlated maternal age with ICSI outcome. A total of 92 couples were studied and 1163 oocytes were injected; a fertilization rate per oocyte of 61% was achieved. The overall ongoing pregnancy rate per cycle was 25% (26/102). Female age did not have an impact on fertilization rates but did affect pregnancy rates. The pregnancy rates were 49%, 23%, and 6% for couples for whom the maternal age was ≤34, 35 to 39, and ≥40 years, respectively (Table 17.4). The authors

TABLE 17.4. Fertilization and pregnancy rates from ICSI according to maternal age.[46]

| Age | Fertilization per oocyte (%) | Pregnancy per cycle (%) |
|---|---|---|
| ≤34 | 349/571 (61.1) | 17/49 (34.7) |
| 35 to 39 | 262/424 (61.8) | 8/36 (22.2) |
| ≥40 | 97/168 (57.7) | 1/17 (5.9) |

TABLE 17.5. Fertilization and pregnancy results of ICSI according to female age in 190 couples with severe male-factor infertility.[47]

| Maternal age | No. of eggs per retrieval | Fertilizations/ oocyte injected (%) | Pregnancies/ cycle (%) |
|---|---|---|---|
| 23 to 29 | 15.1 | 50 | 30 |
| 30 to 34 | 13.5 | 46 | 31 |
| 35 to 39 | 10.1 | 45 | 16 |
| 40 to 48 | 6.5 | 36 | 13 |

concluded that although ICSI has succeeded in treating many couples with severe male-factor infertility, female age may play a critical role in ICSI outcome.

Similarly, Sherins et al[47] evaluated fertilization and pregnancy results of ICSI according to female age in 190 couples with severe male-factor infertility who underwent 229 consecutive IVF cycles. They found a reduction in the number of eggs retrieved and fertilized in couples with female partners over age 40 (Table 17.5). In couples with female partners <40 years of age, the number of eggs per retrieval was 15.1, 13.5, and 10.1 for the age groups 23 to 29, 30 to 34, and 35 to 39, compared with 6.5 for the age group between 40 and 48 years. The fertilization rates were constant for the age group between 23 and 39 years (50%, 46%, and 45% for age groups 23 to 29, 30 to 34, and 35 to 39), whereas the fertilization rate was 36% for the age group 40 to 48 years. Pregnancy rates per cycle also declined with age, from 30% in the youngest age group to 13% in the oldest age group. The authors concluded that reductions in fertilization and pregnancy rates in their study could not be attributed to the severity of semen quality impairment but could be correlated with advanced maternal age.

## Effects on Birth Defect Rates

The bypass of natural barriers to fertilization, possible genetic defects in men with severe male infertility, and the use of severely abnormal sperm for intracytoplasmic sperm injection have engendered concern over the impact of ICSI on the genetic complement of the off-spring. Bonduelle et al[48] reported on a prospective study of 55 children born after subzonal insemination or intracytoplasmic sperm injection. The children underwent antenatal diagnosis and postnatal follow-up. A total of 55 children had been examined at the time of publication. One child had multiple congenital malformations and a second had quadriparesis for a major birth defect rate of 3.6%, which does not differ from the prevalence of major congenital malformations in the general population. Van Steirteghem[49] also reported no increase in the congenital malformation rate in their center when compared with the general population. Of 877 children born after ICSI procedures, 23 (2.6%) had major congenital malformations compared with 2.0% to 2.85% in the general population and 1.9% to 2.9% of children resulting from assisted reproductive techniques.

Sex chromosomal abnormalities have also been reported in ICSI cases. In't Veld et al[50] reported on 12 patients with ICSI pregnancies who underwent prenatal diagnosis for advanced maternal age. Three of the 12 women had twin pregnancies for a total of 15 diagnostic procedures by amniocentesis or chorionic villus sampling. A total of five chromosomal abnormalities were detected: two cases of XXY, one complex mosaic 45,X/46,X.dic(Y)(q11)/46.X.del(Y)(q11), and two cases of 45, XO. This high rate of sex chromosome abnormalities has not been corroborated by other studies. The Brussels group[51] reported on a total of 585 prenatal diagnoses performed in pregnancies established by ICSI. A total of six sex chromosome abnormalities (1.0%) were detected compared with 0.2% in the general population. Govaerts et al[52] reported on 55 karyotypes obtained by amniocentesis or chorionic villus sampling in pregnancies from ICSI and found no sex chromosome abnormalities. When sex chromosome abnormalities have been identified, it is unclear whether they are related to the ICSI procedure itself, mosaic Klinefelter's syndrome in the male partner, or can be ascribed to advanced maternal age. What is reassuring is that the rates of non–sex chromosomal abnormalities in the ICSI population published to date do not exceed the rates seen in the general

TABLE 17.6. Sex chromosome abnormalities reported in pregnancies established by intracytoplasmic sperm injection.

| | No. of sex chromosome abnormalities per prenatal diagnosstic procedure* | Percentage of sex chromosomal abnormalities detected | Sex chromosomal abnormalities detected | Maternal age |
|---|---|---|---|---|
| In't Veld et al[50] | 5/15 | 33 | 247,XXY 1 complex mosaic† 245,XO | Not given |
| Van Steirteghem[49] | 6/585 | 1.0 | 247,XXY | 25 to 32 |
| | | | 147,XXY | 25 to 32 |
| | | | 147,XXY | 25 to 32 |
| | | | 1 trisomy 21 | 41 |
| | | | 146,XX/47,XXX | 44 |

*In all studies prenatal diagnoses were made by amniocentesis or chorionic villus sampling.
†45 X/46 X.dic (Y) (qll)/46 X.del (Y) (qll).

population. These studies are summarized in Table 17.6.

The relationship of ICSI to sex chromosomal abnormalities in offspring may be related to the association between Y chromosomal abnormalities and severe male-factor infertility. Investigators[53,54] have reported that 10% to 15% of men with azoospermia or severe oligospermia will have deletions of 15,000 to 200,000 base pair lengths of the Y chromosome. At least one gene DAZ (deleted in azoospermia) is deleted in 13% of patients with nonobstructive azoospermia.

Although chromosomal abnormality rates thus far have not exceeded those in the general population, studies essential to a thorough and objective evaluation of the new technologies in assisted reproduction must continue. In addition to studying congenital malformations, analysis of the psychosocial impact of assisted reproduction on the children and parents is also critical to a thorough assessment of the repercussions of these new technologies. Genetic counseling, preimplantation genetic diagnosis, and state of the art prenatal diagnosis must also be available to couples enrolled in assisted reproductive programs. Genetic counseling should be available to all couples and should be mandatory for couples who meet the following criteria:

1. male-factor infertility due to congenital bilateral absence of the vas,

2. male or female partner with a karyotype abnormality,
3. female partner greater than 40 years old,
4. either partner with a genetic disease.

All couples undergoing micromanipulation procedures are strongly recommended to have a prenatal diagnosis with amniocentesis or chorionic villus sampling. The need for prenatal diagnosis is dependent on whether the couple would consider terminating the pregnancy if the results are abnormal. If the couple would carry a pregnancy to term regardless of the results of prenatal diagnosis, then the procedure of prenatal intervention would carry risks to the fetus without benefit and therefore cannot be required.

## Risks of ICSI

All couples for whom IVF with ICSI is recommended should be apprised of the risks associated with assisted reproductive procedures. Complications from ovarian stimulation, oocyte retrieval, and multifetal pregnancies have been reported.

One of the most significant risks associated with stimulation of the ovaries is the ovarian hyperstimulation syndrome (OHSS). This manifests itself as massive ovarian enlargement, peritoneal irritation due to follicular rupture or hemorrhage, ovarian torsion, ascites, pleural effusion, oliguria, electrolyte imbalance, hypercoagulability,[55] and sometimes death.[56] The syndrome occurs in the moderate form in 3% to 4% of the population and severe form in 0.1% to 0.2% of the population[57] undergoing ovarian hyperstimulation. Other reported complications of ovarian hyperstimulation are pituitary hemorrhage, endometriotic bloody ascites, and genital cancer.[58]

Complications of ovarian retrieval have been reported for transvaginal aspiration as well as for laparoscopic aspiration. Complications associated with transvaginal aspiration have been reported to occur in 0.3% to 3% of cases[58,59] and include bleeding, pelvic infections, and abdominal viscera perforation. Laparoscopic complications include hemorrhage, intestinal perforation, infection, and carbon dioxide embolism. The risks are no higher in ovarian retrieval procedures than in other laparoscopic applications.

Finally, pregnancies resulting from ovarian stimulation are at risk for spontaneous abortion, ectopic pregnancy, and multiple gestation. The rate of spontaneous abortions associated with assisted reproduction is approximately 25% and is attributed to advanced maternal age and an increased prevalence of chromosomal abnormalities, higher rates of pregnancy loss due to multiple gestations, and early recognition of these pregnancies due to close monitoring.[60] Ectopic pregnancies occur in 3% to 5.5% of patients and can be life threatening. The causes are usually pelvic adhesions and tubal damage from pelvic inflammatory disease or previous surgery.[61] Multifetal pregnancies occur in 10% of hMG stimulated cases,[62] 22% of cases of IVF with embryo transfer,[63] and 44% to 46% of IVF/ICSI cases.[29,46] Multifetal pregnancies are considered a complication of assisted reproductive techniques because of the associated increased incidence of preeclampsia, placenta previa, placental abruption, premature rupture of membranes, and postpartum hemorrhage.[64] Most importantly, multiple gestations are almost universally associated with prematurity and the associated complications to offspring, including cerebral palsy and intracranial hemorrhage with mental retardation or blindness. To prevent multifetal pregnancies

and their attendant complications, it is recommended that ovarian stimulation drugs be used with extreme caution and the number of embryos transferred be limited, based on maternal age.

## Cost-Effectiveness of ICSI

The cost of assisted reproductive technologies can be prohibitive without third-party insurance coverage. For this reason it is imperative that both male and female partners be evaluated prior to the application of assisted reproductive procedures, because specific treatment of male or female-factors may be more effective, less expensive, and carry fewer risks to the couple and offspring. In a comparison of the cost per successful live delivery from IVF/ICSI with the cost per successful live delivery with treatment of varicocele,[65] the most common treatable cause of male-factor infertility, the cost per delivery of IVF/ICSI was $89,091 compared with $26,268 for varicocelectomy. Therefore, there was a significant cost benefit to repairing a varicocele rather than initially performing IVF/ICSI. These results emphasize two other points: the value of a thorough examination and workup of the male partner, and the importance of pursuing treatable causes of infertility prior to pursuing assisted reproductive techniques as long as maternal age allows. If an initial specific intervention does not result in pregnancy, then assisted reproductive techniques may still be applied to further increase the chance of achieving a pregnancy.

# Conclusion

The field of assisted reproductive technology is growing rapidly. Already technologies that were revolutionary 5 years ago are obsolete. This sort of growth is likely to continue as more is learned about sperm and oocyte physiology and the biology of sperm-oocyte interactions. For this reason, it is important that continued investigations into the biology of sperm-egg interaction accompany the clinical application of these successful technologies.

There is a growing need for specific guidelines as to which couples will benefit from IUI and IVF initially and which should proceed directly to more invasive forms of ARTs, such as ICSI . The cost-effectiveness of each new technology must be rigorously tested so that the couple can be assured of maximal benefit at minimal risk and cost. Standardized reporting of fertilization and pregnancy rates by centers performing assisted reproductive techniques is essential. Despite the lack of a documented increase in birth defects after ARTs, there is an ongoing need for further surveillance of children born after application of these technologies. It is possible that the effects of ARTs may not be detectable until the children born have grown to the age where they attempt to have children. Continued studies of the children and parents of ARTs are essential to understanding the long-term impact of these extraordinary advances.

# References

1. Steptoe P, Edwards R. Pregnancy in an infertile patient after transfer of an embryo fertilized in vitro (letter). *Br Med J (Clin Res Ed)* 1983; 286:1351–1352.
2. Hiramoto Y. Microinjection of the live spermatozoa into sea urchin eggs. *Exp Cell Res* 1962; 27:416–426.
3. Uehara T, Yanagimachi R. Microsurgical injection of spermatozoa into hamster eggs with subsequent transformation of sperm nuclei into male pronuclei. *Biol Reprod* 1976; 15:467–470.
4. Thadani VM. A study of hetero-specific sperm-egg interactions in the rat, mouse, and deer mouse using in vitro fertilization and sperm injection. *J Exp Zool* 1980; 212:435–453.
5. Markert CL. Fertilization of mammalian eggs by sperm injection. *J Exp Zool* 1983; 228:195–201.
6. Gordon JW, Talansky BE. Assisted fertilization by zona drilling: a mouse model for correction of oligospermia. *J Exp Zool* 1986; 239:347–354.
7. Cummins JM, Yanagimachi R. Development of ability to penetrate the cumulus oophorus by hamster spermatozoa capacitated in vitro, in relation to the timing of the acrosome reaction. *Gamete Res* 1986; 15:187–212.
8. Talbot P, DiCarlantonio G, Zao P, et al. Motile cells lacking hyaluronidase can penetrate the hamster oocyte cumulus complex. *Am J Anat* 1985; 174:331.
9. Saling PM. How the egg regulates sperm function during gamete interaction: facts and fantasies. *Biol Reprod* 1991; 44:246–251.
10. Bleil JD. Sperm receptors of mammalian eggs. In: Wasserman PM, ed. *Elements of Mammalian Fertilization.* Boca Raton, FL: CRC Press; 1991; 1:133–151.
11. Syms AJ, Johnson AR, Lipshultz LI, et al. Studies on human spermatozoa with round head syndrome. *Fertil Steril* 1984; 42:431–435.
12. Aithem RJ, Kerr L, Bolton V, et al. Analysis of sperm function in globospermia: implications for the mechanism of sperm-zona interaction. *Fertil Steril* 1990; 54:701–707.
13. Dale B, Iaccarino M, Fortunato A, et al. A morphological and functional study of fusibility in round-headed spermatozoa in the human. *Fertil Steril* 1994; 61:336–340.
14. Ho PC, So WK, Chan YF, et al. Intrauterine insemination after ovarian stimulation as a treatment for subfertility because of subnormal semen: a prospective, randomized controlled study. *Fertil Steril* 1992; 58:995.
15. Horvath PN, Bohrer M, Sheldon RN, et al. The relationship of sperm parameters to cycle fecundity in superovulated women undergoing intrauterine insemination. *Fertil Steril* 1989; 52:288.
16. Sigman M. Assisted reproductive techniques and male infertility. *Urol Clin North Am* 1994; 21:509.
17. Wolf DB, Byrd W, Sandekar P, et al. Sperm concentrations and the fertilization of human eggs in vitro. *Biol Reprod* 1984; 31:837.
18. Kruger TF, Menkveld R, Stander FSH, et al. Sperm morphologic features as a prognostic factor in in vitro fertilization. *Fertil Steril* 1986; 46:1118.
19. Oehninger S, Acosta AA, Morshedi M, et al. Corrective measures and pregnancy outcome in in vitro fertilization in patients with severe sperm morphology abnormalities. *Fertil Steril* 1988; 50:283–287.
20. Schlegel PN. Techniques of assisted reproduction. In: Bahnson RR, ed. *Management of Urologic Disorders.* London: Mosby-Year Book Europe; 1994: 28.2.
21. Ng SC, Bongso A, Sathananthan AH, et al. Pregnancy after transfer of multiple sperm under the zona. *Lancet* 1988; 2:790.
22. Cohen J, Talansky BE, Malter H, et al. Microsurgical fertilization and teratospermia. *Hum Reprod* 1991; 6:118.

23. Cohen J. A review of clinical microsurgical fertilization. In: Cohen J, Malter HE, Talansky BE, Grifo J, eds. *Micromanipulation of Human Gametes and Embryos*. New York: Raven Press; 1992: 177.

24. Schlegel PN, Berkeley AS, Goldstein M, et al. Epididymal micropuncture with in vitro fertilization and oocyte micromanipulation for the treatment of unreconstructable obstructive azoospermia. *Fertil Steril* 1994; 61:895–901.

25. Schlegel PN, Palermo GD, Alikani M, et al. Micropuncture retrieval of epididymal sperm with in vitro fertilization: importance of in vitro micromanipulation techniques. *Urology* 1995; 46:238–241.

26. Craft IL, Khalifa Y, Boulos A, et al. Factors influencing the outcome of in vitro fertilization with percutaneous aspirated epididymal spermatozoa and intracytoplasmic sperm injection in azoospermic men. *Hum Reprod* 1995; 10:1791–1794.

27. Silber SJ, Van Steirteghem AC, Liu J, et al. High fertilization and pregnancy rate after intracytoplasmic sperm injection with spermatozoa obtained from testicle biopsy. *Hum Reprod* 1995; 10:148–152.

28. Bourne H, Watkins W, Spiers A, et al. Pregnancies after intracytoplasmic injection of sperm collected by fine needle biopsy of the testis. *Fertil Steril* 1995; 64:433–436.

29. Palermo GD, Cohen J, Alikani M, et al. Intracytoplasmic sperm injection: a novel treatment for all forms of male factor infertility. *Fertil Steril* 1995; 63:1231–1240.

30. Pickering SJ, Braude PR, Johnson MH, et al. Transient cooling to room temperature may cause irreversible disruption of the meiotic spindle in the human oocyte. *Fertil Steril* 1990; 54:102–108.

31. Gerris J, Mangelschots K, Royen EV, et al. ICSI and severe male factor infertility: breaking the sperm tail prior to injection. *Hum Reprod* 1995; 10:484–504.

32. Tesarik J, Sousa M. Key elements of a highly efficient intracytoplasmic sperm injection technique: $Ca^{2+}$ fluxes and oocyte cytoplasm dislocation. *Fertil Steril* 1995; 64:770–776.

33. The Sperm Microaspiration Retrieval Techniques Study Group. Results in the United States with microaspiration retrieval techniques and assisted reproductive technologies. *J Urol* 1994; 151:1255–1259.

34. Catt J, Krzyminska U, Tilia L, et al. Subzonal insertion of multiple sperm is a treatment for male factor infertility. *Fertil Steril* 1994; 61:118.

35. Lippi J, Mortimer D, Jansen PS. Sub-zonal insemination for extreme male factor infertility. *Hum Reprod* 1993; 8:908.

36. Sakkas D, Lacham O, Gianaroli L, et al. Subzonal sperm microinjection in cases of severe male factor infertility and repeated in vitro fertilization failure. *Fertil Steril* 1992; 57:1279.

37. Garrisi GJ, Chin AJ, Dolan PM, et al. Analysis of factors contributing to success in a program of micromanipulation-assisted fertilization. *Fertil Steril* 1993; 59:366.

38. Wolf JP, Ducot B, Kunstmann J, et al. Influence of semen parameters on outcome of subzonal insemination in the case of previous IVF failure. *Hum Reprod* 1992; 7:1407.

39. Van Steirteghem AC, Nagy Z, Joris H, et al. High fertilization and implantation rates after intracytoplasmic sperm injection. *Hum Reprod* 1993; 8:1061–1066.

40. Tesarik J, Mendoza C, Testart J. Viable embryos from injection of round spermatids into oocytes. *N Engl J Med* 1995; 333:525.

41. Sofikitis NV, Myagama I, Agapitos E, et al. Reproductive capacity of the nucleus of the male gamete after completion of meiosis. *J Assist Reprod Genet* 1994; 11:335–341.

42. Palermo G, Joris H, Derde MP, et al. Sperm charactericstics and outcome of human assisted fertilization by subzonal insemination and intracytoplasmic sperm injection. *Fertil Steril* 1993; 59:826–835.

43. Cohen J, Alikani M, Munne S, et al. Micromanipulation in clinical management of fertility disorders. *Sem in Reprod Endocrinol* 1994; 12:151–156.

44. Nagy ZP, Liu J, Joris H, et al. The result of intracytoplasmic sperm injection is not related to any of the three basic sperm parameters. *Hum Reprod* 1995; 10:1123–1129.

45. Mansour RT, Aboulghar MA, Serour GI, et al. The effect of sperm parameters on the outcome of intracytoplasmic sperm injection. *Fertil Steril* 1995; 64:982–986.

46. Oehninger S, Veeck L, Lanzendorf S, et al. Intracytoplasmic sperm injection: achievement of high pregnancy rates in couples with severe male factor infertility is dependent primarily on female and not male factors. *Fertil Steril* 1995; 64:977–981.

47. Sherins RJ, Thorsell LP, Dorfmann A, et al. Intracytoplasmic sperm injection facilitates fertilization even in the most severe forms of male

infertility: pregnancy outcome correlates with maternal age and number of eggs available. *Fertil Steril* 1995; 64:369–375.

48. Bonduelle M, Desmyttere S, Buysse A, et al. Prospective follow-up study of 55 children born after subzonal insemination and intracytoplasmic sperm injection. *Hum Reprod* 1994; 9:1765–1769.

49. Van Steirteghem AC. Breaching the zona pellucida: recent advances in micromanipulation. Presented at the annual meeting of the American Society for Reproductive Medicine, October 11, 1995, Seattle, WA.

50. In't Veld I, Brandenburg H, Verhoeff A, et al. Sex chromosomal abnormalities and intracytoplasmic sperm injection. *Lancet* 1995; 346: 773.

51. Liebaers I, Bonduelle M, Van Assche E, et al. Sex chromosome abnormalities after intracytoplasmic sperm injection. *Lancet* 1995; 346:1095.

52. Govaerts I, Englert Y, Vamos E, Rodesch F. Sex chromosome abnormalities after intracytoplasmic sperm injection. *Lancet* 1995; 346:1095–1096.

53. Ma K, Sharkey A, Kirsch E, et al. Towards the molecular localization of the AZF locus: mapping of microdeletions in azoospermic men with 14 subintervals of interval 6 of the human Y chromosome. *Hum Mol Genet* 1992; 1:29–33.

54. Vogt P, Chandley AC, Hargreave TB, et al. Microdeletions in interval 6 of the Y chromosome of males with idiopathic sterility point to disruption of AZF, a human spermatogenesis gene. *Hum Genet* 1992; 89:491–496.

55. Schenker JG, Weinstein D. Ovarian hyperstimulation syndrome: a current survey. *Fertil Steril* 1978; 30:255–268.

56. Mozes M, Bogowsky H, Anteby E, et al. Thromboembolic phenomena after ovarian stimulation with human menopausal gonadotrophins. *Lancet* 1965; 2:1213.

57. Bergh T, Lundkvist O. Clinical complications during in vitro fertilization treatment. *Hum Reprod* 1992; 7:625–626.

58. Schenker J, Ezra Y. Complications of assisted reproductive techniques. *Fertil Steril* 1994; 61:411–422.

59. Howe RS, Wheeler C, Mastroianni I Jr, et al. Pelvic infection after transvaginal ultrasound-guided ovum retrieval. *Fertil Steril* 1988; 49:726–728.

60. Ezra Y, Schenker JG. Appraisal of in vitro fertilization. *Eur J Obstet Gynecol Reprod Biol* 1993; 48:127–133.

61. Dubuisson JB, Aubriot FX, Mathieu I, et al. Risk factors for ectopic pregnancy in 556 pregnancies after in vitro fertilization: implications for preventive management. *Fertil Steril* 1991; 56:686–690.

62. March CM. Improved pregnancy rate with monitoring of gonadotropin therapy by three modalities. *Am J Obstet Gynecol* 1987; 156:1473–1479.

63. Seoud MA, Toner JP, Kruithoff C, et al. Outcome of twin, triplet, and quadruplet in vitro pregnancies: the Norfolk experience. *Fertil Steril* 1992; 57:825–834.

64. Seoud MA, Kruithoff C, Muasher SJ. Outcome of triplet and quadruplet pregnancies from in vitro fertilization. *Eur J Obstet Gynecol Reprod Biol* 1991; 41:79–84.

65. Schlegel PN. Is assisted reproduction the optimal treatment for varicocele-associated male infertility? A cost-effectiveness analysis. *Urology* 1997; 49.

66. Van Steirteghem A, Joris H, Liu J, et al. Evolution of intracytoplasmic injection (ICSI) results. *Fertil Steril* 1994; 62:S83.

67. Tsirigotis M, Yang D, Redgement CJ, et al. Assisted fertilization with intracytoplasmic sperm injection. *Fertil Steril* 1994; 62:781–785.

68. Payne D, Flaherty SP, Jeffrey R, et al. Successful treatment of severe male factor infertility in 100 consecutive cycles using intracytoplasmic sperm injection. *Hum Reprod* 1994; 11:2051–2057.

69. Harari O, Bourne H, McDonald M, et al. Intracytoplasmic sperm injection: a major advance in the management of severe male subfertility. *Fertil Steril* 1995; 64:360–368.

# 18
# Fertility Issues in the Patient with Testis Cancer

Dana A. Ohl and Jens Sonksen

In the past 20 years a marked improvement in the outlook for men with testis cancer has been achieved, aided by advances in imaging technologies, which now can better diagnose the presence or absence of metastatic disease, and refinements in surgical and anesthetic techniques for excision of difficult, persistent metastatic lesions. The most marked change, however, has come from the development of effective chemotherapy for the treatment of metastatic lesions. In the 1990s, it is expected that >95% of men with low-volume *metastatic* testicular cancer will survive their neoplasm.[1]

In a disease where survival is the rule rather than the exception it is necessary to confront quality-of-life issues. Most men who have had testis cancer do not suffer from nonurologic complications of their disease and treatment. However, because the site of the disease is also the site of sperm production, testis cancer brings a significant risk for infertility. The problem is amplified by the fact that the peak incidence of testis cancer is from age 20 to 40—the prime reproductive years.

When discussing fertility in the patient with testis cancer, several areas require consideration. First, subfertility may already exist prior to treatment. Treatment regimens, although effective in treating the cancer, may further damage fertility in survivors. Because there are a number of men who become completely infertile from testis cancer therapy, sperm banking before treatment needs to be discussed with patients prior to initiation of therapy.

## Preexisting Subfertility

A subfertile semen analysis following orchiectomy but prior to institution of radiation or chemotherapy is an indication of pretreatment subfertility. The problem appears to be due to some aspect of the disease itself, rather than to a simple postorchiectomy change, because semen quality is similar prior to and immediately after orchiectomy.[2]

Several investigators have verified that pretreatment subfertility is present in a large percentage of patients[2-8] (Table 18.1). Berthelsen[5] found a median sperm concentration of only 15 million per milliliter in 34 patients prior to initiation of radiation therapy or chemotherapy. Drasga[3] found an incidence of azoospermia prior to chemotherapy of 17%.

Loss of testicular tissue, as is seen with destruction by tumor or orchiectomy or both, is an obvious reason for decreased fertility. Men with a solitary testis have been found to have decreased fertility. Ferreira et al[9] found that half of men with a single testis had a sperm concentration below the World Health Organization (WHO) limit of adequacy (20 million per milliliter). Loss of effective volume of testicular tissue may also be seen in men with contralateral carcinoma in situ (CIS) (see below), but the 4% incidence of CIS in the contralateral testis does not fully explain the incidence of subfertility.

An argument against simple loss of testicular tissue as the reason for pretreatment subfertility is found in the series of Fossa et al.[10] In

TABLE 18.1. Selected published reports of pretreatment subfertility in testis cancer.

| Study | N | % with subfertile semen analysis |
|---|---|---|
| Drasga et al,[3] 1983 | 41 | 93% |
| Hendry et al,[4] 1983 | 208 | 73% |
| Fossa et al,[6] 1984 | 60 | 50% |
| Bouchot et al,[7] 1989 | 22 | 77% |

their group, 14 patients had pretreatment azoospermia, but follow-up 2 years later showed that seven patients had >10 million sperm per milliliter on semen analysis. This suggests that there is an active mechanism causing the subfertility that is related to the cancer.

Immunologic infertility has been suggested as a contributing cause of subfertility of testis cancer patients. Because growth of a testis tumor can compromise the integrity of the testis structure, systemic leakage of sperm-specific antigens that are usually sequestered in a protected immunologic environment may occur, causing the production of antisperm antibodies. In reports on the topic, investigators have noted an incidence of antisperm antibodies of 18% to 73% of men with testis cancer.[11-13] The argument against the importance of these data is that most series of pretreatment subfertility have focused on a decrease in the sperm *count*. Because antisperm antibodies are thought to cause infertility mainly via effects on sperm *function* and not sperm count, an immunologic cause does not adequately explain the pretreatment subfertility phenomenon. If antibodies are present, however, they may further compromise an already handicapped situation.

A few testis tumors produce human chorionic gonadotropin (HCG), which may lead to increased levels of estrogens[14,15] and decreased levels of follicle-stimulating hormone (FSH). This decrease may prevent quantitatively normal spermatogenesis. However, a minority of testis tumors produce markedly elevated levels of HCG, but this does not explain the changes in the semen in most patients.

There may be undefined factors, common to testis tumors and other cancers, that are active inhibitors of fertility. Men who have a recent diagnosis of cancer may not be able to produce their previous semen volume because of preoccupation with the diagnosis. Systemic effects of the cancer may lead to generalized dysfunctions, including disordered sperm production. Pretreatment subfertility has been seen in young men presenting with other neoplasms, such as Hodgkin's disease and others.[4,16]

## Testis Cancer and Related Conditions—A Common Origin?

A fascinating relationship exists between testis cancer and other conditions of the testis, including infertility, cryptorchidism, and contralateral carcinoma in situ. This raises the possibility that the development of testis cancer and these other conditions may have a common etiology.

Cryptorchidism represents a risk factor for both testis cancer and subfertility. The undescended testis is more likely to develop a neoplasm. However, the location/environment of the undescended testis is not the reason for the increased risk of neoplasm, in that testes brought down into the scrotum at an early age continue to exhibit an increased risk of neoplasm. Furthermore, in men with a history of cryptorchidism, the risk of the contralateral, normally descended testis developing a neoplasm is increased compared with the general population. These pieces of information suggest that the increased risk of developing a tumor appears to be predetermined and cannot be reduced to baseline by orchidopexy.

Similarly, there is not an environmental explanation for the subfertility seen in men who previously had an undescended testis. Orchidopexy prevents temperature-dependent spermatogenic failure, but does not allow fertility to equal that of the general population.[17] Men with a unilateral undescended testis at birth have a higher rate of infertility than the general population. These similarities support the possibility of a common causal factor between the infertility associated with cryptorchidism and the increased risk of testis cancer.

It has been suggested that abnormal early development of germ cells may be this common link. Abnormal germ cells can be detected by testicular biopsy early in life, particularly in undescended testes.[18-20] CIS may be seen in up to 3% of men with undescended testes and in 6% of men with a contralateral testis tumor.[21] More evidence of global testicular dysfunction at the cellular level was found by Berthelsen and Skakkebaek,[22] who saw severe pathophysiology in 24% of contralateral testes in men with cancer.

In men presenting for infertility evaluation, where the initial examination has not revealed a testis tumor, CIS is found in 0.4% to 1.1% of testis biopsies,[23-26] but was not found in any of 399 men aged 18 to 50 who were examined following unexpected sudden death.[27]

# Effects of Testis Cancer Treatment on Fertility

## Radiation Therapy

Radiation therapy is important in the treatment of testis cancer. Men presenting with clinical stage I seminoma experience a high cure rate when given 2500 to 3000 cGy to the retroperitoneum, thereby eradicating micrometastases in those with undetected spread. Direct radiation to the testis for biopsy proven CIS is also curative, but requires a much higher direct dose of 1400 cGy. Radiotherapy of bulky retroperitoneal metastatic seminoma has yielded to chemotherapy in modern treatment regimens, and radiation has no place in the nonradiosensitive nonseminomatous germ cell tumors.

In patients undergoing prophylactic retroperitoneal radiation for stage I seminoma, the testicular dose via intracorporal scatter is approximately 20 to 130 cGy.[5,28] In this dosage range temporary azoospermia usually results. In the higher dosage range (>1000 cGy), the germinal failure will usually be permanent. Thus, men being treated for contralateral carcinoma in situ with direct testicular doses of 1400 cGy can expect to be rendered permanently sterile.[29] Older series of higher level radiation for CIS (2000 cGy) showed that this

dosage range caused both permanent infertility and endocrine deficiencies, leading to lowering of the dosage in recent years.[30]

Berthelsen[5] found that two thirds of the men undergoing prophylactic radiotherapy for seminoma became azoospermic, and nearly 3.5 years were necessary to reach baseline sperm counts. Other investigators have found a more rapid recovery of less than 2 years.[31,32] In a more recent, small series, recovery to a normal sperm count in 1 year has been noted.[28]

About two thirds of the men who have previously undergone prophylactic radiotherapy for seminoma will succeed in fathering children.[33,34] Although physicians commonly urge caution on those attempting pregnancies after radiotherapy, for fear of teratogenic effects of the treatment carried by the sperm, there is little evidence that this occurs. No increased rate of congenital anomalies has been reported in the children of these men.[34,35]

## Chemotherapy

Chemotherapy has a central role in the treatment of metastatic testis cancer, but, as in other types of cancer, damage to sperm production may result from this treatment. This is because actively dividing cells, such as spermatogonia, are most affected by chemotherapeutic agents. Most men with combination chemotherapy for this disease will become azoospermic shortly after treatment initiations.[3]

Fortunately, most of these men will recover some degree of sperm production. The time to recovery of spermatogenesis varies in published reports, but all agree that full recovery takes at least 2 years and perhaps longer.[36-38] It is uncommon to recover sperm in the ejaculate of men who remain azoospermic 4 years following treatment. Despite return of sperm to the ejaculate, sperm production and reproductive efficiency may not be normal (Table 18.2).[3,39] Drasga et al[3] noted a 32% pregnancy rate at 4 years following chemotherapy treatment.

Suppression of spermatogenesis during chemotherapy treatment theoretically may lead to protection of the germinal epithelium via decreased spermatogonial cell division rate.

TABLE 18.2. Sperm counts in men treated with chemotherapy for testis cancer.

| Study | N | Time from treatment | % azoospermia | % oligospermia | % normal |
|---|---|---|---|---|---|
| Drasga et al,[3] 1983 | 41 | 4 years | 18 | 41 | 41 |
| Poirier et al,[39] 1992 | 21 | 2 years | 29 | 33 | 38 |

Animal studies created some initial excitement for this philosophy. However, human studies with medroxyprogesterone and luteinizing hormone–releasing hormone (LHRH) agonists have not produced beneficial protective effects, despite successful suppression of sperm production during treatment.[40–42]

## Retroperitoneal Lymphadenectomy

Retroperitoneal lymph node dissection (RPLND) may be indicated in the treatment of testis cancer, most commonly for stage I non-seminomatous tumors, where the false-negative rate of detection of metastases is about 20% to 25%, and in men with residual retroperitoneal masses following chemotherapy. This integral component of treatment may also impair fertility through neurogenic injury to ejaculation. The classic radical dissection had a high rate of anejaculation due to disruption of postganglionic sympathetic fibers responsible for seminal emission.[43,44]

Nerve-sparing RPLND has been developed in an attempt to circumvent this problem and has been quite successful. Different groups have utilized modification of dissection templates or dissection and freeing of the postganglionic fibers from the lymphatic tissue or both.[45–48] Nerve-sparing RPLND may not be appropriate in men with advanced tumors, in which a wider margin around tumor masses may be desirable, but in low-stage disease the newer techniques preserve ejaculatory function in nearly 100% of cases.[46,47] This preservation of ejaculation is reflected in a high pregnancy forecast rate in individuals treated with nerve-sparing RPLND (no chemotherapy) for their testis cancer. Of 53 such men attempting to initiate a pregnancy in one series, 43 (81%) were successful.[49]

In men who suffer ejaculatory dysfunction following RPLND, it is essential to evaluate for retrograde ejaculation. If retrograde ejaculation is found, the sperm may be retrieved and used for artificial insemination.[50,51] However, if ejaculatory dysfunction is found after RPLND, it is more likely to be total absence of seminal emission.[43] Sympathomimetic therapy (e.g., ephedrine, imipramine) may be initiated to convert a retrograde ejaculator into an antegrade ejaculator or to stimulate seminal emission in those where it is absent.[52–54]

Men with anemission due to RPLND may undergo rectal probe electroejaculation (EEJ) to retrieve sperm for assisted reproductive technologies (ART). EEJ is uniformly successful in inducing emission, but in a series of 24 patients at the University of Michigan, adequate numbers of sperm were found in only 21/24 (88%). The failures in this group were due to carcinoma in situ in the remaining testis (one patient) and germinal failure from chemotherapy (in the other two). Of couples who proceeded to intrauterine insemination, 37% achieved a pregnancy.[55]

## ART Procedures Following Testis Cancer Treatment

In the event that oligospermia persists after testis cancer treatment, introduction of ART is appropriate in an attempt to improve the odds of initiating a pregnancy with the suboptimal semen specimen. ART procedures include intrauterine insemination (IUI), in vitro fertilization (IVF), and intracytoplasmic sperm injection (ICSI). With ICSI, only a handful of viable sperm may be needed to cause a pregnancy.

Non-ICSI ART procedures that would be introduced in the posttestis cancer treatment still require the sperm to function normally and fertilize the oocyte spontaneously. With this requirement for normal sperm function with the lower-level ART procedures, it is reasonable that markedly injured sperm would not be successful in initiating a pregnancy, and the risk of congenital anomalies from pregnancies in this patient population should be similar to that seen in couples who obtain a spontaneous pregnancy following testis cancer treatment. The risk of anomalies in such spontaneous pregnancies (initiated by men treated for testis cancer) is no different from the rate seen in the general population.[56,57]

However, when considering the ICSI procedure, added caution may be indicated because fertilization will be possible for sperm that might normally be nonfunctional. If there is a common origin of testis cancer, infertility, and genital anomalies, the ICSI procedure might inadvertently pass this tendency to the male offspring.

## Sperm Banking in Testis Cancer

In past years, there was a fairly consistent opinion that sperm banking had little value in the majority of testis cancer patients who were facing surgery, radiation, or chemotherapy.[58–60] Pretreatment subfertility accounted for much of the lack of enthusiasm, because pretreatment sperm quality was such that initiation of a pregnancy following thawing was unlikely. However, a large component of the pessimistic opinion was the lack of effective methods of sperm handling and ART protocols that require fewer sperm.

Loss of sperm cell viability is a significant problem with semen preservation, and the initial freezing process is responsible for most of the cell death. Development of more effective cryoprotectants and freezing methodology has better optimized sperm survival after cryopreservation. A recent study suggests that young men with testicular neoplasms and lymphomas will have approximately 50% cell survival following thaw.[61] Stimulation with the methylxan-

thine derivatives, caffeine, 2-deoxyadenosine, and pentoxifylline may improve the postthaw motion characteristics in cancer patients.[62]

In cancer patients, a treatment delay may compromise the results. However, a delay is inevitable when initiating a program of sperm cryopreservation. The more rapid the specimens can be collected, the faster the cancer treatment can be given. Agarwal et al,[63] in a report of cancer patients facing additional therapy (36 with testicular cancer, 39 with Hodgkin's disease, and 20 with other neoplasms), found no difference in sperm quality in those with ejaculation intervals of <2 days, 2–3 days, or >3 days. Therefore, a daily frequency of collection for freezing seems optimal.

Pregnancies from cryopreserved sperm of cancer patients are not uncommon. In data collected from case reports and nine sperm banks, Sanger et al[64] reported 115 live births of children conceived by the use of cryopreserved sperm from cancer patients.

Different ART procedures have been utilized in attempting pregnancies with sperm from cancer patients. Artificial insemination of cryopreserved sperm from testis cancer and Hodgkin's disease patients gave a cumulative pregnancy rate of 45% through six cycles.[65] Khalifa et al[66] achieved four pregnancies in nine cycles of IVF using semen cryopreserved prior to cancer treatment. The sperm yield was only 0 to 4.2 million motile spermatozoa per patient, further underscoring the efficiency of IVF in initiating pregnancies with minimal numbers of viable sperm.[66] The ICSI procedure, which requires even fewer sperm, will be a viable option in many situations where the cryopreserved specimen is unsuitable even for standard IVF.

Because of advances in ART procedures and improvements in the cryopreservation process, sperm banking recommendations must now be revised. Sperm cryopreservation should be offered to all men with testis cancer who are facing treatment by chemotherapy, radiation therapy, or retroperitoneal lymphadenectomy.

## References

1. Horwich A, Norman A, Fisher C, et al. Primary chemotherapy for stage 11 nonseminomatous

germ cell tumors of the testis. *J Urol* 1994; 151:72–77.

2. Nijman JM, Schraffordt-Koops H, Kremer J, et al. Fertility and hormonal function in patients with a nonseminomatous tumor of the testis. *Arch Androl* 1985; 14:239–246.

3. Drasga RE, Einhorn LH, Williams SD, et al. Fertility after chemotherapy for testicular cancer. *J Clin Oncol* 1983; 1:179–183.

4. Hendry WF, Stedronska J, Jones CR, et al. Semen analysis in testicular cancer and Hodgkin's disease: pre- and post-treatment findings and implications for cryopreservation. *Br J Urol* 1983; 55:769–773.

5. Berthelsen JG. Sperm counts and serum follicle-stimulating hormone levels before and after radiotherapy and chemotherapy in men with testicular germ cell cancer. *Fertil Steril* 1984; 41:281–286.

6. Fossa SD, Abyholm T, Aakvaag A. Spermatogenesis and hormonal status after orchiectomy for cancer and before supplementary treatment. *Eur Urol* 1984; 10:173–177.

7. Bouchot O, Plougastel ML, Karam G, et al. [Sterility and tumors of the testis. Study of late exocrine and endocrine functions in stage I or IIA tumors]. *J Urol (Paris)* 1989; 95:367–371.

8. Fossa SD, Aabyholm T, Vespestad S, et al. Semen quality after treatment for testicular cancer. *Eur Urol* 1993; 23:172–176.

9. Ferreira U, Netto NRJ, Esteves SC, et al. Comparative study of the fertility potential of men with only one testis. *Scand J Urol Nephrol* 1991; 25:255–259.

10. Fossa SD, Theodorsen L, Norman N, et al. Recovery of impaired pretreatment spermatogenesis in testicular cancer. *Fertil Steril* 1990; 54:493–496.

11. Foster RS, Rubin LR, McNulty A, et al. Detection of antisperm-antibodies in patients with primary testicular cancer. *Int J Androl* 1991; 14:179–185.

12. Guazzieri S, Lembo A, Ferro G, et al. Sperm antibodies and infertility in patients with testicular cancer. *Urology* 1985; 26:139–142.

13. Hobarth K, Klingler HC, Maier U, et al. Incidence of antisperm antibodies in patients with carcinoma of the testis and in subfertile men with normogonadotropic oligoasthenoteratozoospermia. *Urol Int* 1994; 52:162–165.

14. Lefebvre H, Laquerriere A, Cleret JM, et al. A hCG-secreting testicular seminoma revealed by male infertility: mechanism of hCG-evoked endocrine disturbances. *Andrologia* 1993; 25:283–287.

15. Carroll PR, Whitmore WFJ, Herr HW, et al. Endocrine and exocrine profiles of men with testicular tumors before orchiectomy. *J Urol* 1987; 137:420–423.

16. Sharma RK, Tolentino MV, Thomas AJ, et al. Optimal dose and duration of exposure to artificial stimulants in cryopreserved human spermatozoa. *J Urol* 1996; 155:568–573.

17. Chilvers C, Dudley NE, Gough MH, et al. Undescended testis: the effect of treatment on subsequent risk of subfertility and malignancy. *J Pediatr Surg* 1986; 21:691–696.

18. Muller J, Skakkebaek NE, Nielsen OH, et al. Cryptorchidism and testis cancer. Atypical infantile germ cells followed by carcinoma in situ and invasive carcinoma in adulthood. *Cancer* 1984; 54:629–634.

19. Muller 1, Skakkebaek NE, Ritzen M, et al. Carcinoma in situ of the testis in children with 45,X/46,XY gonadal dysgenesis. *J Pediatr* 1985; 106:431–446.

20. Andres TL, Trainer TD, Leadbetter GW. Atypical germ cells preceding metachronous bilateral testicular tumors. *Urology* 1980; 15:307–309.

21. Daugaard G, Giwercman A, Skakkebaek NE. Should the other testis be biopsied? *Semin Urol* 1996; 14:8–12.

22. Berthelsen JG, Skakkebaek NE. Gonadal function in men with testis cancer. *Fertil Steril* 1983; 39:68–75.

23. Pryor JP, Cameron KM, Chilton CP, et al. Carcinoma in situ in testicular biopsies from men presenting with infertility. *Br J Urol* 1983; 55:780–784.

24. Skakkebaek NE. Carcinoma in situ of the testis: frequency and relationship to invasive germ cell tumours in infertile men. *Histopathology* 1978; 2:157–170.

25. Bettocchi C, Coker CB, Deacon J, et al. A review of testicular intratubular germ cell neoplasia in infertile men. *J Androl* 1994; 15:14S–16S.

26. Nistal M, Codesal J, Paniagua R. Carcinoma in situ of the testis in infertile men. A histological, immunocytochemical, and cytophotometric study of DNA content. *J Pathol* 1989; 159:205–210.

27. Giwercman A, Muller J, Skakkebaek NE. Prevalence of carcinoma in situ and other histopathological abnormalities in testes from 399 men who died suddenly and unexpectedly. *J Urol* 1991; 145:77–80.

28. Centola GM, Keller JW, Henzler M, et al. Effect of low-dose testicular irradiation on sperm count and fertility in patients with testicular seminoma. *J Androl* 1994; 15:608–613.

29. Littley MD, Shalet SM, Morgenstern GR, et al. Endocrine and reproductive dysfunction following fractionated total body irradiation in adults. *Q J Med* 1991; 78:265–274.

30. Giwercman A, von der Maase H, Berthelsen JG, et al. Localized irradiation of testes with carcinoma in situ: effects on Leydig cell function and eradication of malignant germ cells in 20 patients. *J Clin Endocrinol Metab* 1991; 73:596–603.

31. Brennemann W, Brensing KA, Leipner N, et al. Attempted protection of spermatogenesis from irradiation in patients with seminoma by D-tryptophan-6 luteinizing hormone releasing hormone. *Clin Invest* 1994; 72:838–842.

32. Fossa SD, Abyholm T, Normann N, et al. Post-treatment fertility in patients with testicular cancer. III. Influence of radiotherapy in seminoma patients. *Br J Urol* 1986; 58:315–319.

33. Bracken RB, Johnson DE. Sexual function and fecundity after treatment for testicular tumors. *Urology* 1976; 7:35–38.

34. Malas S, Levin V, Sur RK, et al. Fertility in patients treated with radiotherapy following orchidectomy for testicular seminoma. *Clin Oncol (R Coll Radiol)* 1994; 6:377–380.

35. Fossa SD, Almaas B, Jetne V, et al. Paternity after irradiation for testicular cancer. *Acta Radiol Oncol* 1986; 25:33–36.

36. Fossa SD, Ous S, Abyholm T, et al. Post-treatment fertility in patients with testicular cancer. II. Influence of cis-platin-based combination chemotherapy and of retroperitoneal surgery on hormone and sperm cell production. *Br J Urol* 1985; 57:210–214.

37. Johnson DH, Hainsworth JD, Linde RB, et al. Testicular function following combination chemotherapy with cisplatin, vinblastine, and bleomycin. *Med Pediatr Oncol* 1984; 12:233–238.

38. Kreuser ED, Harsch U, Hetzel WD, et al. Chronic gonadal toxicity in patients with testicular cancer after chemotherapy. *Eur J Cancer Clin Oncol* 1986; 22:289–294.

39. Poirier S, Einhorn LH, Rubin L. Evaluation of reproductive capacity in germ cell tumor patients following chemotherapy with cisplatin, VP-16 and bleomycin (meeting abstract). *Proc Annu Meet Am Soc Clin Oncol* 1992; A1313.

40. Fossa SD, Klepp O, Norman N. Lack of gonadal protection by medroxyprogesterone acetate-induced transient medical castration during chemotherapy for testicular cancer. *Br J Urol* 1988; 62:449–453.

41. Kreuser ED, Klingmuller D, Thiel E. The role of LHRH-analogues in protecting gonadal functions during chemotherapy and irradiation. *Eur Urol* 1993; 23:157–164.

42. Krause W, Pfluger KH. Treatment with the gonadotropin-releasing hormone agonist buserelin to protect spermatogenesis against cytotoxic treatment in young men. *Andrologia* 1989; 21:265–270.

43. Kedia KR, Markland C, Fraley EE. Sexual function following high retroperitoneal lymphadenectomy. *J Urol* 1975; 114:237–239.

44. Nijman JM, Schraffordt KH, Oldhoff J, et al. Sexual function after bilateral retroperitoneal lymph node dissection for nonseminomatous testicular cancer. *Arch Androl* 1987; 18:255–267.

45. Lange PH, Narayan P, Fraley EE. Fertility issues following therapy for testicular cancer. *Semin Urol* 1984; 2:264–274.

46. Jewett MAS, Kong YS, Goldberg SD, et al. Retroperitoneal lymphadenectomy for testis tumor with nerve sparing for ejaculation. *J Urol* 1988; 139:1220–1224.

47. Donohue JP, Foster RS, Rowland RG, et al. Nerve-sparing retroperitoneal lymphadenectomy with preservation of ejaculation. *J Urol* 1990; 144:287–291.

48. Weidner W, Zoller G, Sauerwein D, et al. A modified technique for nerve-sparing retroperitoneal lymph node dissection in stage II nonseminomatous germ cell tumors using intraoperative measurement of bladder neck pressure alterations following sympathetic nerve fiber electrostimulation. *Eur Urol* 1994; 26:67–70.

49. Foster RS, Bennett R, Bihrle R, et al. A preliminary report: postoperative fertility assessment in nerve-sparing RPLND patients. *Eur Urol* 1993; 23:165–167.

50. Ogura K, Nakamura K, Matsuda T, et al. [Successful artificial insemination in a patient with retrograde ejaculation following retroperitoneal lymph node dissection for testicular cancer: a case report]. *Hinyokika Kiyo* 1993; 39:373–376.

51. Umekawa T, Kiwamoto H, Iguchi M, et al. [AIH in male infertility due to retrograde ejaculation after retroperitoneal lymph node dissection]. *Nippon Hinyokika Gakkai Zasshi* 1991; 82:492–495.

52. Narayan P, Lange PH, Fraley EE. Ejaculation and fertility after extended retroperitoneal

lymph node dissection for testicular cancer. *J Urol* 1982; 127:685–688.

53. Brenner J, Vugrin D, Whitmore WFJ. Effect of treatment on fertility and sexual function in males with metastatic nonseminomatous germ cell tumors of testis. *Am J Clin Oncol* 1985; 8:178–182.

54. Fossa SD, Ous S, Abyholm T, et al. Post-treatment fertility in patients with testicular cancer. I. Influence of retroperitoneal lymph node dissection on ejaculatory potency. *Br J Urol* 1985; 57:204–209.

55. Ohl DA, Denil J, Bennett CJ, et al. Electroejaculation following retroperitoneal lymphadenectomy. *J Urol* 1991; 145:980–983.

56. Fried P, Steinfeld R, Casileth B, et al. Incidence of developmental handicaps among the offspring of men treated for testicular seminoma. *Int J Androl* 1987; 10:385–387.

57. Hansen PV, Glavind K, Panduro J, et al. Paternity in patients with testicular germ cell cancer: pretreatment and post-treatment findings. *Eur J Cancer* 1991; 27:1385–1389.

58. Bracken RB, Smith KD. Is semen cryopreservation helpful in testicular cancer? *Urology* 1980; 15:581–583.

59. Sanger WG, Armitage JO, Schmidt MA. Feasibility of semen cryopreservation in patients with malignant disease. *JAMA* 1980; 244:789–790.

60. Kolodziej FB, Katzorke T, Propping D. [Cryopreservation of human spermatozoa—evaluation of 93 semen depots]. *Andrologia* 1990; 22:164–170.

61. Ragni G, Caccamo AM, Dalla Serra A, et al. Computerized slow-staged freezing of semen from men with testicular tumors or Hodgkin's disease preserves sperm better than standard vapor freezing. *Fertil Steril* 1990; 53:1072–1075.

62. Sharma RK, Tolentino MV, Thomas AJ, et al. Optimal dose and duration of exposure to artificial stimulants in cryopreserved human spermatozoa. *J Urol* 1996; 155:568–573.

63. Agarwal A, Sidhu RK, Shekarriz M, et al. Optimum abstinence time for cryopreservation of semen in cancer patients. *J Urol* 1995; 154:86–88.

64. Sanger WG, Olson JH, Sherman JK. Semen cryobanking for men with cancer-criteria change. *Fertil Steril* 1992; 58:1024–1027.

65. Scammell GE, White N, Stedronska J, et al. Cryopreservation of semen in men with testicular tumor or Hodgkin's disease: results of artificial insemination of their partners. *Lancet* 1985; 2:31–32.

66. Khalifa E, Oehninger S, Acosta AA, et al. Successful fertilization and pregnancy outcome in in-vitro fertilization using cryopreserved/thawed spermatozoa from patients with malignant diseases. *Hum Reprod* 1992; 7:105–108.

# 19
# Infections and Infertility

Durwood E. Neal, Jr.

Genitourinary tract infections and other inflammatory conditions are known contributors to male-factor infertility.[1,2] Their effects are still not entirely understood, but there are strong associations. Because male-factor infertility accounts for 30% to 50% of infertility cases,[3] and genitourinary infections are ubiquitous, these associations are of great interest. Because these infections are both preventable and treatable, much study has been done in this field. Unfortunately, there is a paucity of confirmatory data on the etiology of the process and treatment efficacy. The difficulty in most of the research on the association between infection and infertility has been in proving the presence of a causal agent. Thus, it is problematic to assess the efficacy of any given treatment modality. In females, there is little doubt that early, aggressive antibiotic therapy is beneficial in preventing secondary tubular damage due to pelvic inflammatory disease.[4] Furthermore, localized infections in the vagina are known to limit fertility, and aggressive, curative treatment is beneficial to fertility rates.[5] The low incidence of symptoms and physical findings in the male proves to be daunting in the evaluation of treatment. When there is an absence of a proven causative organism, the results of any treatment may not be evaluable. When the final common pathway is pregnancy and the semen analysis is usually not definitive, one may be dealing simply with probabilities. It may be best to divide this discussion into infections versus noninfections; however, the line between these two is frequently indistinct.

## Bacterial Infections

Infection of the adnexal structures of the testicle is perhaps the most common anatomical location where bacteria are known to be responsible for infertility. Perhaps the prototypical bacterial infection associated with infertility is *Neisseria gonorrhoeae*.[6] This sexually transmitted organism causes a localized urethritis that may progress to prostatitis or epididymo-orchitis[7] and is usually diagnosed in the younger male. At its target sites, inflammation or abscesses may form, with the resultant tissue destruction and scar formation. The long-term outcome of untreated or incompletely treated infection is stricture of the urethra, which may predispose to other urinary tract infections. Additionally, infection of the epididymis can cause inflammatory and sclerotic changes that result in obstruction of the tubules and diminished semen quality.[8] Fortunately, this disease is usually symptomatic, leading to early therapy.[9] *Chlamydia trachomatis* causes a similar inflammatory reaction that often is not as exuberant, but may be as damaging, and is commonly referred to as nongonococcal urethritis (NGU). It is also more often associated with the young adult. In addition, this organism is more common than *N. gonorrhoeae* and thus possibly causes more cases of obstructive infertility than any other etiologic agent.[9] The paucity of symptomatology may lead to a lower number of confirmed cases. Epididymo-orchitis in the older male is more likely due to the usual uropathogens, specifically *Escherichia coli*,

*Staphylococcus saprophyticus*, and others. These may be related to other genitourinary tract abnormalities, such as benign prostatic hyperplasia, urethral stricture disease, urologic instrumentation/trauma, or others. When infection with these common uropathogens occurs in the younger individual, there is usually a congenital genitourinary anomaly that is present. Thus, it may be problematic to separate the effects on fertility status of the infection from those of the malformation.

Acute prostatitis is a relatively unusual infection at any age. The organisms are usually not sexually transmitted in the formal sense, but are pathogens that are commonly isolated from urinary tract infections in general, and only rarely are they due to *Neisseria* or *Chlamydia* species. The entire infectious process has not been extensively studied, but in a number of animal models intense inflammation with the resultant scarring occurs.[10,11] The inflammation may progress from acute to chronic, manifesting itself as recurrent urinary tract infections in the male with chronic bacterial prostatitis.[12] This process has not been clearly defined because of a lack of longitudinal data. Fibrosis in the prostate and ejaculatory ducts has also been documented in humans and is thought to be secondary to the host response to bacterial prostatitis. Recently, there have been reports of transurethral resection of the ejaculatory ducts, which resulted in pregnancies by patients whose ejaculatory duct obstruction was previously documented.[13,14] It was not determined to be consistent, however, that these patients had a confirmed history of prostatitis.

It is clear that the effects of prostatitis go beyond simple ductal obstruction. Infection has been shown to cause glandular secretory dysfunction as well.[15–19] A number of divalent cations are found in normal, healthy seminal plasma, and these are disordered in the setting of infection or inflammation. The most important of these, arguably, is zinc, which is critical for normal sperm function and motility. Bacterial infection greatly diminishes prostatic fluid zinc, and the levels may not recover after resolution of the infection. This has been shown not only in animal models of infection (nonhuman primate, dog),[15,16] but also in prostatic secre-

tions by men with a history of prostatitis.[17] Zinc is also the integral part of prostatic antibacterial factor, and low levels may pose an increased risk for recurrent infection.[20] In any case, there is a causal relationship between prostatic fluid zinc and fertility. Infection causes dysfunction in the acquisition or secretion of magnesium and other divalent cations as well, but their specific roles are not as well understood.[19]

The bacteria themselves may cause infertility by direct interaction with spermatozoa, resulting in toxicity and reduced seminal quality.[21–24] The bacteria have receptors on their surface that actually bind the sperm, resulting in agglutination or immobilization.[21,22] *E. coli* has been the organism that has been most extensively studied, and the receptors on the bacterial cell surface that facilitate bacterial binding to the uroepithelial cells at the time of incipient infection are the same that bind to spermatozoa. These same bacteria may be found in the perineum of female patients and thus may serve not only as a source of infection for the male but also as a risk to the sperm deposited in the vaginal vault. Both P-fimbriae (mannose-resistant) and type I fimbriae (mannose-sensitive) have been implicated in this process. Other bacterial appendages are involved as well, for motility, which may contribute to the transporting of bacteria into the ducts, and for binding to the urothelial or prostatic ductal cell membranes. Furthermore, bacteria secrete soluble substances into their local environment that can be toxic to spermatozoa. These substances may be more deleterious by their role in the initiation and perpetuation of the inflammatory process, rather than directly on sperm.[24] Many of these substances (endotoxin, bacterial enzymes) marshal the inflammatory response by aggregating leukocytes. These cells then secrete various bioactive cytokines that not only prolong and extend the inflammatory response but also are directly toxic to sperm.[25] Hydrogen peroxide, and probably all of the free radicals generated in this process, will injure and immobilize spermatozoa. It is difficult, if not impossible, to separate the effects of infection from the effects of inflammation, especially when there are limited culture data in many of the reported studies.

Other bacteria have been implicated in infection, the most common of which are *Chlamydia trachomatis* and *Ureaplasma urealyticum*.[26-29] There even appears to be evidence for direct interaction with sperm themselves,[30] but the major effects are mediated by the inflammatory process.[1,2,31] There is controversy over the significance of finding these organisms in the genitourinary tract. It has been problematic to prove causality, partly because 10% to 25% of patients are asymptomatic.[32] Furthermore, the organisms are difficult to culture because of their fastidious nature and specific growth requirements. Therefore, infection may be detected most efficiently using immunologic techniques, which provide secondary evidence of infection that does not prove concurrent infection, only exposure to the organism. Molecular biologic techniques are definitely more sensitive for infection, but may add a lack of specificity as well as their generally limited availability. This, however, will probably be a more important source of information in the future. The effects of *Chlamydia*, in any case, are perhaps more important in females, with the resultant pelvic inflammatory disease and fallopian tubular damage. The evidence for *Ureaplasma* or *Mycoplasma hominis* as a cause of reproductive failure is less compelling.[33] Implications for cause and effect exist, with a few authors finding that treatment of infection results in improved pregnancy rates as well as some improvement in the parameters of seminal quality.[34,35] Because these organisms may be found in fertile, asymptomatic males, and their rates of recovery are the same in fertile and infertile groups, their role in infertility is in question.[28] The only correlation with infection (or colonization) seems to be with the number of sexual partners. Conversely, others have found increased rates of *Ureaplasma* infection in infertile men. There are a few studies that have shown a direct interaction between *Ureaplasma* and sperm with resultant inactivation of sperm,[28,36] but translation to the clinical condition is difficult, especially because fertile couples may harbor the organism. Treatment specific for this organism has been determined, and some authors have reported facilitated pregnancy rates.[35,37] There is, perhaps, a host-organism interaction that in certain individuals impairs fertility but is not present in others. The final solution is still to be determined.

# Viruses

Viral infection of the genitourinary tract has been well studied in the paramyxovirus group, the etiologic agent of mumps. This disease afflicts young children and causes orchitis in approximately 20% of those infected. Of that group, the majority will suffer some degree of testicular atrophy, and almost 30% will develop contralateral orchitis.[38] Seminal quality is usually normal in the unilaterally infected person, but severe oligospermia is the usual result of bilateral disease. Presumably, this complication will continue its rapid decline because of the advent of an efficacious parenteral vaccine. Few other viruses are known to affect fertility. DNA virus groups, specifically cytomegalovirus (CMV) and herpes simplex virus (HSV), have been isolated from semen and the genitourinary tract, but no causality with diminished fertility has been demonstrated.[39,40] Their association with the other aforementioned sexually transmitted diseases is perhaps the most common deleterious effect.

Retroviruses, such as human immunodeficiency virus (HIV), the causal agent for acquired immunodeficiency syndrome (AIDS), and others, have been isolated from the genitourinary tract and from semen in particular.[41,42] The virus exists not only within the seminal leukocytes, but also in cell-free seminal plasma. It is found in higher concentrations when there is concurrent genital inflammation with increased leukocytospermia.[43] There is also a close association with concurrent CMV and HSV infections. There is no apparent detrimental effect on seminal quality or sperm itself that is separable from the systemic effects of the virus. There does not appear to be a direct association with infertility, although this may be difficult to study. It is perhaps more interesting from a viral transmission standpoint than from the infertility perspective. This is especially true now that a greater number of AIDS patients are desirous of fertility. The conditions under which transmission of HIV by semen occur have not been fully elucidated.

## Miscellaneous

There are numerous other infections that may affect seminal quality. The best studied of these is *Trichomonas vaginalis*, a sexually transmitted protozoan. It has been implicated in up to 5% of cases of NGU but may be found as an asymptomatic colonization.[44] The organism is motile by means of a flagellum and has been seen to attach to and immobilize sperm.[45] As such, the large numbers of organisms needed to drastically reduce the effective sperm count are never reached, but the concomitant inflammatory process may actually be more detrimental. Furthermore, the association with other sexually transmitted diseases adds to the risk.

Mycobacterial infections, while remaining relatively rare, may have devastating consequences in the genitourinary tract. The organisms rarely, if ever, are transmitted sexually, but are most commonly inhaled and then spread in a miliary fashion. Numerous cases of prostatitis, epididymo-orchitis, and other genital locations have been reported in the literature.[46] Treatment is usually curative, but the host response to the organism may cause fibrosis and subsequent obstruction. The damage to other organs, namely the kidney and ureter, is usually more dramatic and may greatly overshadow the effects on fertility, although vas deferens obstruction is common.

Fungal infections are perhaps more important in the female than in the male. Candidal balanoposthitis is perhaps the most common manifestation. Low levels of yeasts, usually *Candida albicans*, may be isolated from the penis and preputial areas, but no implication of diminished fertility has been made, except that yeasts, in general, bind and immobilize sperm.[47] Other fungi are known to infect the genitourinary tract, but are uncommon, except in the immunosuppressed population. There are few reports regarding these organisms and fertility. Prostatitis and epididymitis with *Cryptococcus neoformans*, *Histoplasma capsulatum*, *Blastomyces dermatitidis*, and *Coccidioides*

*immitis* have all been reported, as well as the many subspecies of *Candida*.[48] No data exist as to the effects on fertility, but that may be impossible to separate from the underlying disease process, which is usually present in patients with this type of infection.

## Diagnosis

### Urethritis

There are several ways to reliably diagnose urethritis. Symptoms may suffice, especially of dysuria or penile pain along with a urethral discharge. To ascertain the cause, a swab (cotton-tipped or alginate) is inserted into the urethra and the resultant sample is plated on the appropriate agar for culture (e.g., *Neisseria*), placed on a treated slide (*Chlamydia*), and placed in saline (*Trichomonas*). However, the high false-negative rate may make empiric therapy the most prudent course. Another method is to examine the initial urine for leukocytes and possibly culture the specimen. Ultimately, it may be problematic to precisely determine the source of inflammation in all circumstances.

## Prostatitis

The mainstay of diagnosis of male genitourinary tract infections has been the technique of collecting four urine specimens.[49] The initial urine, voided bladder 1 (VB1) is considered to be urethral in its origin. The midstream urine, voided bladder 2 (VB2) is used to document bladder or kidney infection. The patient then interrupts his stream and prostatic massage is performed. The expressed prostatic secretions (EPS) are collected either in a sterile container or on a glass slide or both for direct examination or staining. The postprostatic massage urine, voided bladder 3 (VB3) is then collected from the initial 15 to 50cc of urine expelled immediately after prostatic massage. All of the specimens are next examined under the microscope and cultured aerobically. Although this technique will usually differentiate the source of an infection, it is cumbersome and expensive. The cultured VB3, in many cases, will suffice to determine prostatic infection. Some authors have advocated culture of the ejaculate, which has proven to be predictive.[50] In any case, the number of organisms in the VB3 or semen should be at least 10 times the count in the midstream VB2 in order to localize the infection to the prostate.

The culture techniques are those considered to be routine for urinary microbiology. The most common finding is no organisms, but a variety of bacteria may be isolated, some of which are not usually considered to be uropathogens. The decision is easy when one isolates gram-negative rods or enterococci, and these should be treated aggressively. When organisms are found that are not usually considered to be uropathogens, treatment and outcomes may be confusing. Some researchers have implicated certain gram-positive cocci as causal agents in prostatitis, but the effect on fertility was not addressed.[51] Sometimes, quantitative leukocyte counts in the EPS or VB3 have been used in the diagnosis of prostatitis. However, these may be confusing as some white blood cells (WBCs) are normally present, and immature spermatozoa are almost identical to lymphocytes in appearance.[52] Arbitrary limits of normal numbers of WBCs in the prostatic fluid are the only measures of infection in some studies, thereby limiting the conclusions.

Nonbacterial prostatitis is distinguishable from chronic bacterial prostatitis by the findings of leukocytes in a negative bacterial culture. The symptoms are the same, but there is an absence of recurrent urinary tract infections, and patients have not been found to have fastidious organisms (*Chlamydia, Ureaplasma*), viruses, or other agents. There are a few reports of some commensal aerobes, but they are inconclusive. Most clinicians accept ≤5 WBC per high power field as normal.

Prostatodynia is distinguished from nonbacterial prostatitis by the absence of WBCs in the EPS. The symptoms are similar, but there may be subtle differences. The treatments are varied. This syndrome is also referred to by many other names, such as pelvic floor myalgia syndrome or prostatosis.

## Epididymitis

The differential diagnosis of epididymitis or epididymo-orchitis is that of the acutely painful scrotum, specifically torsion of the testis, appendicular torsion, acute hydrocele/hernia, trauma, or infection/inflammation. Differentiation among these entities may be difficult, and despite nuclear scans, color-flow Doppler ultrasound, and other techniques, surgery is often necessary in order to make the diagnosis, although clinical suspicion by history, physical examination, and urinalysis will typically suffice. On occasion, it may be advantageous to aspirate fluid from the epididymis or the resultant reactive hydrocele to determine the etiologic agent.

## Treatment

In all cases, the acute infectious process is treated with specific antibiotics. The treatment of gonorrhea has undergone a dramatic change in the past few years, from the combination of probenecid and procaine penicillin to intramuscular ceftriaxone to oral quinolones (ciprofloxacin, ofloxacin).[53] Similarly, the therapy for *Chlamydia* has changed, from 10 days of ofloxacin or doxycydine to a single dose of azithromycin.[53] *Ureaplasma* is treated in a similar fashion to *Chlamydia*.[53] Relapses are uncommon when compliance is assured. Reinfection seems the greater problem, so the partners must be treated. Trichomonas is typically treated with metronidazole as a single large dose, or it may be spread out over 7 days. Efficacy is high for both regimens. As with other forms of urethritis, the partner or partners should also be sought and treated.

The different syndromes of prostatitis are all treated according to the suspected cause as well as the specific syndrome. Acute bacterial prostatitis is treated with a broad-spectrum antibiotic by parenteral or oral means, depending on the clinical condition. Theoretically, the 5-fluoroquinolones have the advantage of concentrating within the prostatic glandular cells. This is perhaps less important in the setting of an acute inflammatory/infectious process, however, and probably any culture-specific antibiotic is appropriate. Therapy for 10 to 14 days, as is recommended for any acute urinary infection, should clear any simple acute prostatitis. Contrary to supposition, there is no evidence that 4 to 6 weeks of antibiotics is the optimal time course of treatment. Most of the research studies in this area have enhanced the longer treatment epochs, but no studies have been undertaken to define the ideal length of therapy. Consequently, most clinical studies on treatment are at least of 4 weeks' duration. Chronic bacterial prostatitis should probably be treated as a more deep-seated infection by a 4- to 8-week course of specific antibiotics that concentrate in the gland. The 5-fluoroquinolones concentrate in the prostate gland and may have this advantage in therapy. The culture result should be checked to determine sensitivity of the organism to the antibiotic selected.

Nonbacterial prostatitis has had myriad attempted treatment alternatives.[54,55] Because the precise cause remains an enigma, the therapies remain varied. It may be that this entity is actually not one disease but several, giving credence to the response to such varied therapeutic maneuvers. Antibiotics are empirically tried by many physicians, with varying results. The long-acting alpha-antagonists are used and have an acceptable efficacy.[55] No randomized placebo-controlled clinical trials have been accomplished in this area, although there have been numerous studies.

Antibiotics probably have a place in the treatment of some cases of nonbacterial prostatitis, but one should remember their potential toxicity to fertility.[56,57] Their action mechanism of some antibiotics, such as sulfa drugs, tetracycline derivatives, and nitrofurantoin, makes infertility very probable.[56] Others exert a detrimental effect on fertility by acting directly on the sperm themselves, causing decreased motility and diminished fertilizing capacity.[58] There are numerous reports of improved fertility after treatment with antibiotics, but these studies lack the proper controls.[35,37,58] It remains controversial as to whether empiric antibiotics should be instituted, but with significant numbers of leukocytes in the VB3 urine or EPS most clinicians would probably give a therapeutic trial of antimicrobials. The effects of antibiotics on spermatogenesis are well recognized but are also observed to be temporary. No studies have been done in situations where antibiotics are used in prophylactic doses. Although a dose-responsive curve might be assumed, this has not been shown to date.

Viral infections remain enigmatic with respect to their therapy, but the best treatment likely is prevention with vaccines. The treatment for fungal diseases has undergone a great deal of change in the past few years, with the development of highly effective oral agents of the imidazole class. These drugs are effective in most patients, but some, such as ketoconazole, with its depressive effects on steroidogenesis, may be injurious to spermatogenesis. The overall disease process itself may also be detrimental to fertility, or even the underlying condition that was predisposing to the fungal infection. Mycobacterial infections are still treated with the same agents as years ago, but the effects of the disease process itself may result in scarring and obstruction. No studies have been reported on the effects of antituberculous drugs.

## References

1. Hellstrom WJG, Neal DE Jr. Diagnosis and therapy of male genital tract infections. *Infertil Reprod Med Clin North Am* 1992; 3:399–411.
2. Bar-Chama N, Goluboff E, Fisch H. Infection and pyosphermia in male infertility. Is it really a problem? *Urol Clin North Am* 1994; 21:469–475.
3. Lipshultz LI, Howards SS. Evaluation of the subfertile man. *Semin Urol* 1984; 2:73.
4. Paavonen J. Chlamydia trachomatis in acute salpingitis. *Am J Obstet Gynecol* 1980; 138:957–960.
5. Rosenthal L. Spermagglutination by bacteria. *Proc Soc Exp Biol Med* 1977; 28:827–821.
6. Bowie WR. Nongonococcal urethritis. *Urol Clin North Am* 1984; 11:55–64.
7. Harnisch JP, Berger RE, Alexander ER. Etiology of acute epididymitis. *Lancet* 1977; 1:819–821.
8. Berger RE, Alexander ER, Harnisch JP, et al. Etiology, manifestations and therapy of acute epididymitis: prospective study of 50 cases. *J Urol* 1979; 121:750–754.

9. Handsfield HH, Lipman TO, Harnisch JB, et al. Asymptomatic gonorrhea in men: diagnosis, natural course, prevalence and significance. *N Engl J Med* 1974; 290:117–122.

10. Neal DE Jr, Dilworth JP, Kaack MB, et al. Experimental prostatitis in nonhuman primates: II. Ascending acute prostatitis. *Prostate* 1990; 17:233–239.

11. Nickel JC, Olson ME, Costerton JW. Rat model of experimental bacterial prostatitis. *Infection* 1991; 19:S126–130.

12. Blacklock NJ. The significance of the prostate in urinary tract infection in the male. *J R Naval Med Ser* 1970; 56:5–17.

13. Meacham RB, Hellerstein DK, Lipshultz LI. Evaluation and treatment of ejaculatory duct obstruction in the infertile male. *Fertil Steril* 1993; 59:393–397.

14. Weintraub MP, Demouy E, Hellstrom WJ. Newer modalities in the diagnosis and treatment of ejaculatory duct obstruction. *J Urol* 1993; 150:1150–1154.

15. Neal DE Jr, Kaack MB, Fussell EN, et al. Changes in seminal fluid zinc during experimental prostatitis. *Urol Res* 1993; 21:71–74.

16. Gowan LA, Barsanti JA, Brown J, et al. Effects of bacterial infection and castration on prostatic tissue zinc concentration in dogs. *Am J Vet Res* 1991; 52:1262–1265.

17. Krongrad A, Droller MJ. Zinc and the prostate. In: Paulson DF, ed. *Prostatic disorders*. Philadelphia: Lea and Febiger; 1989: 107–112.

18. Marmar JL, Katz S, Praiss DE, et al. Semen zinc levels in infertile and post-vasectomy patients and patients with prostatitis. *Fertil Steril* 1975; 26:1057–1060.

19. Gyorkey F, Min KW, Huff JA, et al. Zinc and magnesium in human prostate gland: normal, hyperplastic, and neoplastic. *Cancer Res* 1967; 27:1348–1352.

20. Fair WR, Couch J, Wehner N. Prostate antibacterial factor. *Urology* 1976; 7:169–173.

21. Monga M, Roberts JA. Sperm agglutination by bacteria: receptor-specific interactions. *J Androl* 1994; 15:151–156.

22. Fowler JE Jr. Infections of the male reproductive tract and infertility: a selected review. *J Androl* 1981; 3:121.

23. Roberts JA. Role of bacterial adherence in urinary tract infection. *Curr Opin Urol* 1992; 2:33–36.

24. Cohen J, Edwards R, Fehilly C, et al. In vitro fertilization: a treatment for male infertility. *Fertil Steril* 1985; 43:422–432.

25. Hill JA, Cohen J, Anderson DJ. The effects of lymphokines and monokines on sperm fertilizing ability in the zona-free hamster egg penetration test. *Am J Obstet Gynecol* 1989; 160:1154–1163.

26. Hellstrom WJG, Schacter J, Sweet RL, et al. Is there a role for *Chlamydia trachomatis* and genital mycoplasma in male infertility? *Fertil Steril* 1987; 48:337.

27. Friberg J. Mycoplasmas and ureaplasmas in infertility and abortion. *Fertil Steril* 1980; 33:351–359.

28. Harrison RG, DeLouvois J, Sweet RL. Is there a role for *Chlamydia trachomatis* and genital mycoplasma in male infertility? *Lancet* 1975; 1:605–607.

29. Greendale GA, Haas ST, Holbrook K, et al. The relationship of *Chlamydia trachomatis* infection and male infertility. *Am J Public Health* 1993; 83:996–1001.

30. Moskowitz MO, Mellinger BC. Sexually transmitted diseases and their relation to male infertility. *Urol Clin North Am* 1992; 19:35–44.

31. Wolff H, Neubert U, Zebhauser M, et al. *Chlamydia trachomatis* induces an inflammatory response in the male genital tract and is associated with altered semen quality. *Fertil Steril* 1991; 55:1017–1019.

32. Karam GH, Martin DH, Flotte TR, et al. Asymptomatic *Chlamydia trachomatis* infections among sexually active men. *J Infect Dis* 1986; 154:900–903.

33. Drach GW. Problems in diagnosis of bacterial prostatitis: gram-negative, gram-positive and mixed infections. *J Urol* 1974; 111:630.

34. Fowlkes DM, MacLeod J, O'Leary WM. T-mycoplasmas and human infertility: correlation of infection with alterations in seminal parameters. *Fertil Steril* 1975; 26:1212–1218.

35. Swenson CE, Toth A, O'Leary WM. *Ureaplasma urealyticum* and human infertility: the effect of antibiotic therapy on semen quality. *Fertil Steril* 1979; 31:660–665.

36. Busolo F, Zanchetta R. The effect of *Mycoplasma hominis* and *Ureaplasma urealyticum* on hamster egg in vitro penetration by human spermatozoa. *Fertil Steril* 1985; 43:110–114.

37. Toth A, Lesser ML, Brooks C, et al. Subsequent pregnancies among 161 couples treated for T-mycoplasma genital tract infection. *N Engl J Med* 1983; 308:505–507.

38. Riggs S, Sanford JP. Viral orchitis. *N Engl J Med* 1962; 266:990–993.

39. Litvin YS, Nagler H. Infertility and genito-urinary infections. *Infect Urol* 1992; 5:104–107.

40. Taub RG, Madden DL, Fuccillo DA, et al. The male as a reservoir of infection with cytomegalovirus, herpes and mycoplasma. *N Engl J Med* 1973; 289:697–698.

41. Krieger JN, Coombs RW, Collier AC, et al. Fertility parameters in men infected with human immunodeficiency virus. *J Infect Dis* 1991; 164:464–469.

42. Curran JW. The epidemiology and prevention of the acquired immunodeficiency syndrome. *Ann Intern Med* 1985; 103:657–662.

43. Mayer KH, Anderson DJ. Issue of the day. Heterosexual HIV transmission. *Infect Agents Dis* 1995; 4:273–284.

44. Holmes KK, Handsfield HH, Nang SP, et al. Etiology of nongonococcal urethritis. *N Engl J Med* 1975; 292:1199–1205.

45. Tuttle JF Jr, Holbrook TW, Derrick FC. Interference of human spermatozoal motility by *Trichomonas vaginalis. J Urol* 1977; 118:1024–1025.

46. Gow JG, Barbosa S. Genitourinary tuberculosis. A study of 1117 cases over a period of 34 years. *Br J Urol* 1984; 56:449–455.

47. Tuttle JF Jr, Bannister ER, Derrick FC. Interference of human spermatozoa agglutination by *Candida albicans. J Urol* 1977; 118:797–799.

48. Wise GJ, Silver DA. Fungal infections of the genitourinary system. *J Urol* 1993; 149:1377–1388.

49. Meares EM Jr, Stamey TA. Bacteriologic localization in bacterial prostatitis and urethritis. *Invest Urol* 1968; 5:492–503.

50. Mobley DF. Semen cultures in the diagnosis of bacterial prostatitis. *J Urol* 1975; 114:83–85.

51. Lowentritt JE, Kawahara K, Human LG, et al. Bacterial infection in prostatodynia. *J Urol* 1995; 154:1378–1382.

52. Morton RS. White cell counts in human semen. *Br J Vener Dis* 1968; 44:72–83.

53. Krieger JN. New sexually transmitted diseases treatment guidelines. *J Urol* 154:209–214.

54. Hellstrom WJG, Schmidt RA, Lue TF, et al. Neuromuscular dysfunction in nonbacterial prostatitis. *Urology* 1987; 10:183–188.

55. Neal DE Jr, Moon TD. Use of terazosin in prostatodynia and validation of a symptom score questionnaire. *Urology* 1994; 43:460–465.

56. Crotty KL, May R, Kulvicki A, et al. The effect of antimicrobial therapy on testicular aspirate flow cytometry. *J Urol* 1995; 153:835–838.

57. Schlegel PN, Chang TS, Marshall FF. Antibiotics: potential hazards to male infertility. *Fertil Steril* 1991; 55:235–242.

58. Quesada EM, Dukes CD, Deen CH, et al. Genital infection and sperm agglutinating antibodies in infertile men. *J Urol* 1968; 99:106–108.

# 20
# Gonadotoxicity

Suresh C. Sikka

"Each man in this room is half the man his grandfather was." These were the words recently quoted during a Congressional hearing reporting the startling and controversial finding that a serious decline in the quality and quantity of human spermatozoa has occurred over the past 50 years.[1] Another report from Scotland revealed that men born after 1970 had a sperm count 25% lower than those born before 1959—an average decline of 2.1% a year. The lower sperm count was also associated with poor semen quality.[2] In contrast, Olsen et al,[3] using several statistical models, found an actual increase in average sperm number. These data have led some scientists and environmentalists to believe that the human species is approaching a fertility crisis, but others think that the available data are insufficient to deduce worldwide conclusions.[4,5] Nevertheless, the topic of gonadotoxicity remains a real challenge and concern to almost everyone.

During the past 15 years, a dramatic increase in knowledge of male gonadal toxicity and subsequent changes in fertility has resulted from advances in the understanding of gonadal function and dysfunction. This has been made possible by many well-controlled clinical studies and basic scientific discoveries in the physiology, biochemistry, and molecular and cellular biology of the male reproductive system. Although any discussion of gonadal function and toxicity is of special relevance to man, much of this understanding has been obtained from research using animal species and various experimental models. Also, the increased risk of exposure to any environmental toxicant extends to both male and female.

## Background

Gonadotoxicity has recently been the subject of a number of reviews,[6,7] with myriad environmental agents now being classified as male reproductive toxicants. In the mid-1970s, it was determined that dibromochloropropane (DBCP) exposure impaired fertility in the absence of any other clinical signs of toxicity, suggesting that the male reproductive system was the most sensitive target organ. Reduced fertility, embryo/fetal loss, birth defects, childhood cancer, and other postnatal structural or functional problems were the most common outcomes from such exposures. However, the database for establishing safe exposure levels or risk assessment for such outcomes remains very limited. Declining semen quality is not the only indicator that the human testis is at risk. A marked increase in the incidence of testicular cancer in young men has been associated with other abnormalities (including undescended testis, Sertoli-cell–only pattern, and hypospadias), which cause poor testicular function and low fecundity rates.

The human male produces relatively fewer sperm on a daily basis compared with many of the animal species used for toxicity testing. A less dramatic decrease in sperm number or semen quality in humans can have serious consequences of reproductive potential. In fact, in many men over age 30, the lower daily sperm production rate already places them close to the subfertile or infertile range.[7,8] Decreased semen quality (low sperm number, motility, and structure) over the past 50 years has been attributed to environmental toxicants, many of which act as "estrogens."[9] This "estrogen hypothesis" has inspired a number of debates and serious investigations. Lists of such potential estrogenic chemicals continue to grow, although it is not known what exact levels and combinations of these chemicals may be hazardous to male reproductive functions. There is still not enough evidence to determine whether this decline in semen quality is geographically localized or is a global phenomenon. Certain synthetic chemicals termed "endocrine impostors" exert a variety of toxic effects on the gonads, fertility and sexual and reproductive function, in addition to behavioral and other effects. So far, 51 such hormone impostors referred to as "persistent organic pollutants" (POPs), have been identified, the most common of which are organochlorines (DDT, PCBs) and dioxins.[10–12] Unfortunately, there are no control populations for further evaluations of these widely distributed POPs.

Thus, the study of gonadotoxicity is an escalating concern not only to andrologists and reproductive biologists but also to environmentalists and the public at large.

# Development of Male Gonadal Components

The male gonads, a pair of testes, are the site of spermatogenesis and androgen production. Spermatozoa are the haploid germ cells responsible for fertilization and species propagation. There are paracrine and autocrine regulations in various compartments of testis that are under endocrine influences from the pituitary and hypothalamus. The testes develop abdominally at the renal level and descend into the scrotum. Each testis arises from a primitive gonad on the medial surface of the embryonic mesonephros. Primitive germ cells migrate to the medial surface from the yolk sac, cause the coelomic epithelial cells to proliferate, and form the sex cords that lead to the formation of major components of the testis.

## Seminiferous Tubules

The proliferation of the mesenchyme separates the sex cords from the underlying coelomic epithelium by the seventh week of fetal development. These sex cords become the seminiferous tubules that develop a lumen after birth.

## Rete Testis

During the fourth month, sex cords become U-shaped, and their ends anastomose to form the rete testis, which provides communication with the epididymis. The primordial sex cells are referred to as prespermatogonia and the epithelial cells of the sex cords as Sertoli cells.

## Sertoli Cells

These cells form a continuous and complete lining within the tubular wall and establish the blood-testis barrier by virtue of tight junctions. The luminal environment is both created and controlled by these Sertoli cells, also called "nurse cells." Thus, many irregularities of spermatogenesis due to gonadotoxicity may reflect changes in function of the Sertoli cell population, and not necessarily the pathology in the germ cells themselves. The differentiation of Sertoli cells and formation of a competent blood-testis barrier are essential to the establishment of spermatogenesis during puberty in all species.

## Leydig Cells

These cells are the site of testosterone production and arise from interstitial mesenchymal tissue between the tubules during the eighth week of human embryonic development.

## Establishment of Spermatogenesis

Extensive studies on spermatogenesis in the rodent testis have been carried out, but still very little is known about the details of these phenomena in primate and human testes. Spermatogenesis is a chronological process span-ning about 42 days in the mouse and 72 days in man. During this period, relatively undifferen-tiated spermatogonia, the immature germ cells, cyclically develop into highly specialized sper-matozoa. Spermatogonia undergo several mi-totic divisions to generate a large population of cells called primary spermatocytes, which pro-duce haploid germ cells by two meiotic cell divi-sions. Spermiogenesis is the transformation of spermatids into the elongated flagellar germ cells capable of motility. The release of mature germ cells is known as spermiation. The germ cells constitute the majority of testicular vol-ume, which can be appreciated easily as a smaller size if gonadal damage has occurred.

A significant characteristic of mitotic arrest is that the gonocyte becomes acutely sensitive to irradiation.[13] Low-dose irradiation may com-pletely eradicate germ cells while causing little damage to developing Sertoli cells, thus creat-ing Sertoli-cell–only testis in the rodent.

# Gonadotoxic Agents

Gonadotoxicity can be caused by any chemical, physical, or biologic agent that alters physi-ologic control processes and affects the normal functioning of the gonads. This can occur either by a direct chemical action of the agent or indi-rectly via the metabolic products formed during the reaction process. A potential gonadotoxic agent can interrupt the normal function of the male reproductive system at (1) any level of the hypothalamic-pituitary-gonadal axis, (2) di-rectly at the gonadal level, or (3) by altering posttesticular events, such as sperm motility or function or both. Any disruption of these events by toxicants may lead to hypogonadism, infer-tility, decreased libido/sexual function or all of these. The effect may be mild or severe, and the duration may vary from transient dysfunction to permanent gonadal damage.

## Environmental/Occupational Toxicants

The recent debate has focused on estrogenic environmental pollutants; however, certain heavy metals, agricultural chemicals, and indus-trial products have now been reported to alter the male reproductive axis, potentially influencing fertility. These toxicants have significant environmental consequences due to their multiple routes of exposure, their widespread presence in the environment, and their ability to bioaccumulate and resist biodegradation.

## Heavy Metals

Metals (e.g., lead, mercury, cadmium, alumi-num, cobalt, chromium, arsenic, lithium, and antimony) have been noted to exert adverse reproductive effects in human and experimen-tal animals.

More reports are available on lead-induced toxicity than any other heavy metal. Histori-cally, the fall of the Roman Empire has been attributed to lead poisoning.[14] Adverse effects on the reproductive capacity of men working in battery plants and exposed to toxic levels of lead have been reported.[15,16] In animals, lead exposure results in a dose-dependent suppression of serum testosterone and sper-matogenesis.[17] Although testicular biopsies reveal peritubular fibrosis, vacuolation, and oligospermia, suggesting that lead is a direct testicular toxicant,[18] recent mechanistic studies have revealed that lead exposure can disrupt the hormonal feedback mechanism at the hypothalamic-pituitary level.[19] Animal studies suggest that these effects can be reversed when lead is removed from the system. Such detailed evaluations in humans are not yet available.

Mercury exposure (during the manufacture of thermometers, thermostats, mercury vapor lamps, paint, electrical appliances, and in min-ing) can alter spermatogenesis and has been found to decrease fertility in experimental ani-mals.[20] Boron (extensively used in the manufac-ture of glass, cements, soaps, carpets, crockery, and leather products) has a major adverse re-productive effect on the testes and at the hypo-thalamic-pituitary axis in a manner similar to lead. Oligospermia and decreased libido were reported in men working in boric acid–produc-ing factories.[21] Polycyclic aromatic hydrocar-bons (PAHs) are another ubiquitous undefined

bases (primarily guanine via lipid peroxyl or alkoxyl radicals) or through covalent binding to malondialdehyde (MDA) resulting in strand breaks and cross-linking.[83] ROSs can also induce oxidation of critical sulfahydryl (SH) groups in proteins and DNA, which will alter spermatozoal structure and function with an increased susceptibility to attack by macrophages. Cellular damage is theoretically the result of an improper balance between ROS generation and intrinsic scavenging activities. The scavenging potential in gonads is normally maintained by adequate levels of superoxide dismutase (SOD), catalase, and probably glutathione (GSH) peroxidase and reductase. This balance can be referred to as oxidative stress status (OSS), and its assessment may play a critical role in monitoring gonadotoxicity and infertility (Fig. 20.1).

A situation in which there is a shift in this ROS balance toward pro-oxidants, because of either excess ROSs or diminished antioxidants, can be classified in terms of positive oxidative stress status.[76] There is at present no true ROS

detection method available that will evaluate this balance. However, assessment of OSS, or a similar paradigm when monitored more objectively, would be a good indicator of sperm damage caused by oxidative stress. Chronic asymptomatic genitourinary inflammation can be regarded as a condition with positive OSS, which may be the real cause of idiopathic infertility in such patients. GSH-peroxidase and GSH-reductase may directly act as antioxidant enzymes involved in the inhibition of sperm lipid peroxidation (LPO). A high reduced/oxidized glutathione ratio (GSH/GSSG) will help spermatozoa to combat oxidative insult. It seems that the role of these GSH enzymes and their associated mechanisms as related to biologic antioxidants in infertility is an important area for further development.[84] Although the therapeutic use of antioxidants appears attractive, clinicians need to be aware of exaggerated claims of antioxidant benefit by various commercial supplements for fertility purposes until proper multicenter clinical trials have been completed.

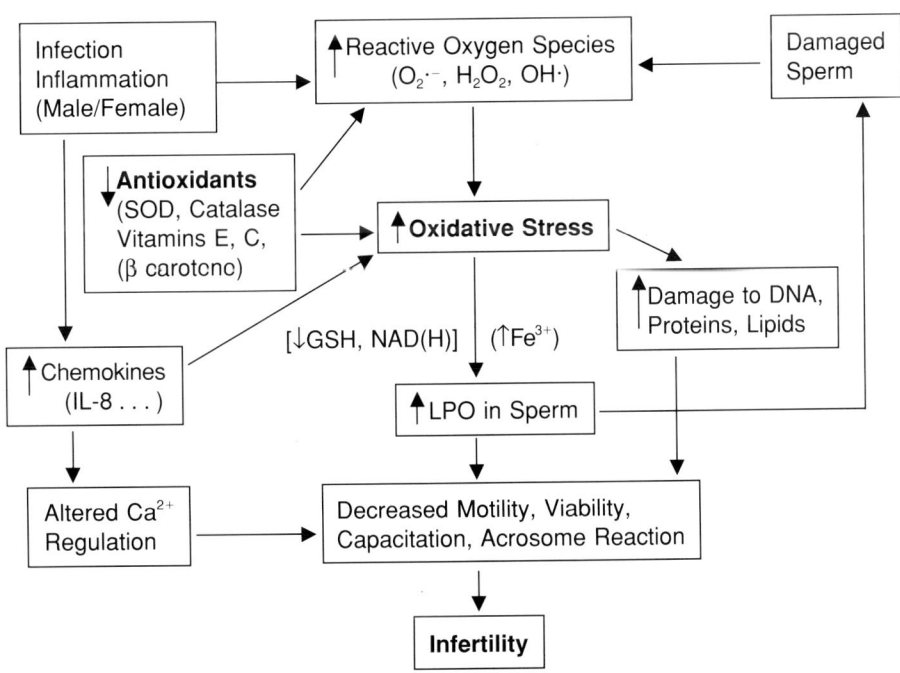

FIGURE 20.1. Scheme suggesting interacting mechanisms in the role of oxidative stress and antioxidants in male infertility. (From Sikka, R. and Hellstrom W. "Role of Oxidative Stress and Antioxidants in Male Infertility." *J Androl*: Nov–Dec 1995; 465.)

## Aging and Gonadotoxicity

Some forms of infertility are caused by age-related degenerative disorders of the testis, a problem that may be increasing in some industrialized societies as suggested by the reports of declining sperm population over the past two generations. Although the decline in sperm numbers is considered to be associated with male fetal, neonatal exposure or both to increased levels of environmental estrogens,[11,28] this idiopathic male infertility may also be explained as a form of premature or differential aging of the testis induced by ischemia and oxidative stress associated with a defective mitochondrial genome that controls oxidative phosphorylation.[66] The presence of retained cytoplasmic droplets on spermatozoa due to imperfect spermiation in the aging testis may be a sign of reduced fertility potential. It is known that LPO and midpiece anomalies are linked,[85] and that the increased rate of LPO and creatine kinase (CK) activity in immature sperm is due to incomplete cytoplasmic extrusion during terminal spermatogenesis.[86] In addition, Sertoli cell abnormalities in infertile men may well be central to the development of spermatogenic failure due to faulty spermiation and may be related to genetic defects, oxidative stress, or even aging of the gonads.

Decreased vascularity, increased spermatogenic failure, and reduced sperm output occur with senescence in a variety of animal species and in humans.[87] Germ cell degeneration with age starts with the spermatids and continues to completely sclerosed tubules consisting of thickened and highly collagenized tunica propria with myoid cells.[88] These may degenerate and be phagocytosed by Sertoli cells, resulting in lipid accumulations that increase progressively with age. A significant decrease in androgen and in Leydig cell number with a concurrent rise in serum follicle-stimulating hormone (FSH) and luteinizing hormone (LH) has been observed in the older population.[89,90] Increased levels of lipofuscin and lipids are seen intracellularly, suggesting mitochondrial dysfunction possibly compounded by oxidative stress in the older population.[91] These degenerative changes in gonads associated with an accumulation of lipofuscin pigment and multiple nuclei are considered to be due to ROS-induced lipid peroxidation with aging.[92] Most of these changes are strikingly similar to those seen in men with idiopathic testicular failure, probably due to induced gonadotoxicity. The differentiation between gonadal anomalies and posttesticular effects due to occupational exposures is difficult, and there is an obvious need to develop new methods for studying this problem.

# Assessment of Gonadotoxicity

Several methods are being evaluated for the assessment of the effects of toxicants on the male reproductive system. Essentially, any risk assessment usually has four components: (1) hazard identification, (2) dose-response assessment, (3) human-exposure assessment, and (4) risk characterization. The hazard identification and dose-response data are developed from experimental animal studies that may be supplemented with data from in vitro studies. This information is then extrapolated and integrated to characterize and assess the risk to the human population.

The most common approach to evaluate the effect of cytotoxic drugs on the testis has used testicular biopsy, semen analysis, and endocrine assessment of the hypothalamic-pituitary-testicular axis. Research on testicular toxicology has been advanced significantly by the introduction of in vitro testing systems. In vivo systems, however, are still essential parts of the risk assessment process, and they are unlikely to be eliminated entirely by in vitro models.

## In Vitro Systems

In vitro systems are uniquely suited to investigate specific cellular and molecular mechanisms in the testis and thus improve risk assessment.[93] These in vitro models can be used alone or in combination with each other to test hypotheses about testicular toxicity. An original toxicant, its metabolites, and the precursors or selective inhibitors can be individually administered to isolated cell types to evaluate specific toxicity mechanisms and to note the interaction of adjacent cell types. Numerous in vitro model systems are described in the literature, including Sertoli–germ cell cocultures,[94] Sertoli cell–enriched cultures,[95,96] germ cell–enriched cultures,[97] Leydig cell cultures,[98] Leydig-Sertoli cell cocultures,[99] and peritubular and tubular cell cultures.[100,101] These in vitro systems are the only way to directly compare human and animal responses and screen a class of compounds for new product development. Even though these in vitro systems are a valuable adjunct to the in vivo test system, they do not replace the in vivo data, because they cannot provide all the facts essential for hazard assessment. Moreover, certain dynamic changes associated with spermatogenesis are difficult to model in vitro. For example, the release of elongated spermatids by the Sertoli cells (spermiation), which is commonly inhibited by boric acid and methyl chloride, can only be studied at present by specific in vivo systems.

## In Vivo Systems

In vivo methods are important tools to study the integrated male reproductive system. The complete in vivo assessment of gonadotoxic response involves multigenerational studies, now required by most regulatory agencies. These multigenerational studies have a complex design, in part because testicular function and spermatogenesis are very complicated processes.[102] The spermatogenic cycle is highly organized throughout the testis. In the rat it requires 53 days. If a toxicant affects the immature spermatogonia, the effect may not be detectable as a change in mature sperm before 7 to 8 weeks. Effects on more mature germ cells would be detected sooner. To test the sensitivity of all stages of spermatogenesis, the exposure lasts the full duration of the cycle. This cannot be achieved in vitro because germ cell differentiation and the physical relationship of stages within the tubules are lost in cell culture systems. The germ cells are entirely dependent on the Sertoli cells for physical and biochemical support. Complicated endocrine and paracrine systems control Sertoli cells, Leydig cells, and germ cells. Besides the loss of paracrine inter-

actions, the altered metabolic activity of target or adjacent cells and the difficulty in isolating and testing certain spermatogenic stages are other significant limitations of in vitro assessment of gonadotoxicity.[93] In addition, for accurate identification of stage-specific lesions of the seminiferous epithelium, critical evaluation of morphologic structures is very important.[102] In vivo, germ cells are continuously dividing and differentiating. The staging of spermatogenesis, thus, has proven to be an extremely sensitive tool to identify even subtle toxicologic changes.

## Sperm Nuclear Integrity Assessment

Recent attention has been focused on assessments of sperm morphology and physiology as important end points in reproductive toxicology testing.[103] Structural stability of sperm nuclei varies by species and appears to be enhanced by the oxidation of protamine sulfhydryl to inter- and intramolecular disulfide bonds and is a function of the types of protamine present. Chemicals may disrupt the structural stability of sperm nuclei, which depend on their unique packaging either during spermatogenesis or sperm maturation. Decondensation of isolated sperm nuclei in vitro can be induced by exposure to disulfide reducing agents, and the time taken to induce extensive decondensation (assay end point) is considered to be inversely proportional to the stability of the sperm nucleus. This "sperm activation assay" is also useful in evaluation of some cases of unexplained infertility.[104] Human sperm decondenses most rapidly, followed by that of the mouse and of the hamster, but rat sperm nuclei show a slower decondensation.[105]

Other tests, such as the DNA stability assay or sperm chromatin structure assay (SCSA), use direct evaluation of sperm chromatin integrity and may provide information about genetic damage to sperm. A shift in DNA pattern (from double-stranded intact DNA to denatured single stranded) can be induced by a variety of mutagenic and chemical agents. Such changes can be evaluated by either dual-parameter DNA flow cytometry (SCSA)[106,107] or single-cell gel electrophoresis (Comet) assay, which uses fluorescence intensity measurements by microscopy and image analysis.[104,107] A shift in the DNA pattern can also be evaluated by acridine orange staining, or by flow cytometry. Double-stranded DNA is stained green, whereas single-stranded DNA is stained red. Animals exposed to known mutagens demonstrate increased amounts of single-stranded DNA, indicating an increase in genetic damage.[108–110]

Flow cytometry, although a very useful tool that permits rapid, objective assessment of a large number of cells, may not be readily available. Comet assay, when combined with centrifugal elutriation, can provide a useful in vitro model to study differences in metabolism and susceptibility of different testicular cell types to DNA damaging compounds.[108,111] Thus, new findings through these systems should lead to greater knowledge about why a chemical or class of chemicals can cause testicular toxicity.

# Conclusion

A variety of extraneous and internal factors can induce gonadotoxicity leading to poor sperm quality and male factor infertility. Unfortunately, a number of these influences (e.g., glandular infection, smoking, environmental toxicants that are mainly estrogenic chemicals, nutritional deficiencies, aging, ischemia, and oxidative stress) have been underestimated. Partial androgen insensitivity mainly due to altered androgen-to-estrogen balance may contribute to significant oligozoospermia. The role of chronic inflammation on the reproductive organs is not completely understood because it is asymptomatic and is difficult to demonstrate objectively. There is an urgent need to characterize all the factors involved and to develop reliable animal models of testicular disease. No major advances have been made for the medical management of poor sperm quality. The application of assisted reproductive techniques, such as intracytoplasmic sperm injection (ICSI) to male infertility, regardless of cause, does not necessarily treat the cause and may inadvertently pass on adverse genetic consequences. Clinicians should always attempt to identify the cause of a possible gonadotoxicity, assess the degree of risk to the patients being evaluated for infertility, and initiate a plan to control and prevent the exposure to others once an association between occupation/exposure and infertility has been established.

# References

1. Carlsen E, Giwercman A, Keiding N, et al. Evidence for decreasing quality of semen during past 50 years. *Br Med J* 1992; 305:609–613.
2. Brake A, Krause W. Decreasing quality of semen. *Br Med J* 1992; 305:1498–1503.
3. Olsen GW, Bodner KM, Ramlow JM, et al. Have sperm counts been reduced 50 percent in 50 years? A statistical model revisited. *Fertil Steril* 1995; 63:887–893.
4. Fisch H, Goluboff ET, Olson JH, et al. Semen analyses in 1283 men from the United States over a 25-year period: no decline in quality. *Fertil Steril* 1996; 65:1009–1014.
5. Paulsen CA, Berman NG. Data from men in greater Seattle area reveal no downward trend in semen quality: further evidence that deterioration of semen quality is not geographically uniform. *Fertil Steril* 1996; 65:1015–1020.
6. Kavlock RJ, Perreault SD. Multiple chemical exposure and risks of adverse reproductive function and outcome. In: Yang RSH, ed. *Toxicology of Chemical Mixtures: From Real Life Examples to Mechanisms of Toxicological Interactions.* Orlando, FL: Academic Press; 1994: 245–297.
7. Sokol RZ. Toxicants and infertility: identification and prevention. In: Whitehead ED, Nagler HM, eds. *Management of Impotence and Infertility.* Philadelphia: JB Lippincott; 1994: 380–389.
8. Schrader SM, Kanitz MH. Occupational hazards to male reproduction. In: Gold E, Schenker M, Lesley B, eds. *State of the Art Reviews in Occupational Medicine: Reproductive Hazards.* Philadelphia: Hanley and Belfus; 1994: 405–414.
9. Working PK. Male reproductive toxicity: comparison of the human to animal models. *Environ Health Perspect* 1988; 77:37–44.
10. Sharpe RM, Skakkebaek NE. Are estrogens involved in falling sperm counts and disorders of the male reproductive tract? *Lancet* 1993; 351:1392–1395.
11. Kelce WR, Stone CR, Laws SC, et al. Persistent DDT metabolite p,p′-DDE is a potent andro-

gen receptor antagonist. *Nature* 1995; 375:581–585.

12. Zenick H, Perrault S, Richards J. Paternally mediated development toxicity: implications for risk assessment and science policy. In: Mattison DR, Olshan AF, eds. *Male-Mediated Developmental Toxicity: Father's Exposure and Their Children's Health.* New York: Plenum Press; 1994: 85–292.

13. Mandl AM. The radiosensitivity of germ cells. *Biol Rev* 1964; 39:288–294.

14. Gilfillan SC. Lead poisoning and the fall of Rome. *J Occup Med* 1965; 7:53–60.

15. Lancranjan I, Popescu HI, Gavanescu O, et al. Reproductive ability of workmen occupationally exposed to lead. *Arch Environ Health* 1975; 30:396–399.

16. Winder C. Reproductive and chromosomal effects of occupational exposure to lead in males. *Reprod Toxicol* 1989; 3:221–233.

17. Foster WP, McMahon A, Young-Lai EV, et al. Reproductive endocrine effects of chronic lead exposure in the male cynomolgus monkey. *Reprod Toxicol* 1992; 7:203–209.

18. Braunstein GD, Dahlgren J, Loriaux DO. Hypogonadism in chronically lead poisoned men. *Infertility* 1978; 1:33–35.

19. Sokol RZ. Hormonal effects of lead acetate in the male rat: mechanism of action. *Biol Reprod* 1987; 37:1135–1138.

20. Barlow SM, Sullivan FM. *Reproductive Hazards of Industrial Chemicals.* London: Academic Press; 1982.

21. Weir RJ, Fisher RS. Toxicological studies on borox and boric acid. *Toxicol Appl Pharmacol* 1972; 23:251–264.

22. Georgellis A, Topari J, Veromaa T, et al. Inhibition of meiotic divisions of rat spermatocytes in vitro by polycyclic aromatic hydrocarbons. *Mutat Res* 1990; 231:125–135.

23. Friberg L, Piscator M, Nordberg GF, et al. *Cadmium in the Environment,* 2nd ed. Cleveland: CRC Press; 1974: 37–53.

24. Snow ET. Metal carcinogenesis: mechanistic implications. *Pharmacol Ther* 1992; 53:31–65.

25. Whorton MD, Krauss RM, Marshall S. Infertility in male pesticide workers. *Lancet* 1997; 2:1259–1261.

26. Mattison DR. The mechanisms of action of reproductive toxins. *Am J Industr Med* 1983; 4:65–79.

27. Lipschultz LT, Ross EC, Whorton MD, et al. DBCP and its effects on testicular function in man. *J Urol* 1980; 124:464–468.

28. Kelce WR, Monosson E, Gamcsik MP, et al. Environmental hormone disruptors: evidence that vinclozolin developmental toxicity is mediated by antiandrogenic metabolites. *Toxicol Appl Pharmacol* 1994; 126:276–285.

29. Chapin RE, White RD, Morgan KT, et al. Studies of lesions induced in the testis and epididymis of F-344 rats by inhaled methyl chloride. *Toxicol Appl Pharmacol* 1984; 76:328–343.

30. Schrader SM, Principles of male reproductive toxicology. In: Brooks SM, Gochfeld M, et al, eds. *Environmental Medicine.* St. Louis: Mosby; 1995: 95–100.

31. Stillman RJ, Rosenberg MJ, Sachs BP. Smoking and reproducton. *Fertil Steril* 1986; 46:545–550.

32. Lahdetie J. Cigarette smoking—a possible genotoxic hazard to male germ cells? *Int J Androl* 1987; 10:431–434.

33. Vine MF, Tse CJ, Hu PC, et al. Cigarette smoking and semen quality. *Fertil Steril* 1996; 65:835–842.

34. Chia SE, Ong CN, Tsakok FM. Effects of cigarette smoking on human semen quality. *Arch Androl* 1994; 33:163–168.

35. Zavos PM. Cigarette smoking and human reproduction: effects on female and male fecundity. *Infertility* 1989; 12:35–40.

36. Sofikitis N, Miyagawa I, Demitriadis D, et al. Effects of smoking on testicular function, semen quality and sperm fertilizing capacity. *J Urol* 1995; 154:1030–1034.

37. Klaiber EL, Broverman DM, Pokoly TB, et al. Interrelationships of cigarette smoking, testicular varicoceles, and seminal fluid indexes. *Fertil Steril* 1987; 47:481–486.

38. Kucheria K, Saxena R, Mohan D. Semen analysis in alcohol dependence syndrome. *Andrologia* 1985; 17:558–561.

39. Parazzini F, Marchini M, Tozzi L, et al. Risk factors for unexplained dyspermia in infertile men: a case-controlled study. *Arch Androl* 1993; 31:105–113.

40. Kolodny RC, Masters WH, Kolodner RM, et al. Depression of plasma testosterone levels after chronic intensive marijuana use. *N Engl J Med* 1974; 290:872–876.

41. Hembree WC, Nahas GG, Zeidenberg P, et al. Changes in human spermatozoa associated with high dose marijuana smoking. In: Nahas GG, Patton WDM, eds. *Marijuana: Biological Effects.* New York: Pergamon Press; 1979: 429–434.

42. Knuth UA, Maniera H, Nieschlag E. Anabolic steroids and semen parameters in body builders. *Fertil Steril* 1989; 52:1041–1047.

43. Jarow JP, Lipshultz LI. Anabolic steroid-induced hypogonadotropic hypogonadism. *Am J Sports Med* 1990; 18:429–431.

44. Schlegel PN, Chang TSK, Marshall FF. Antibiotics: potential hazards to male fertility. *Fertil Steril* 1991; 55:235–242.

45. Ericsson RJ, Baker VF. Binding of tetracycline to mammalian spermatozoa. *Nature* 1967; 214:403–407.

46. Shalet SM. Effects of cancer chemotherapy on gonadal function of patients. *Cancer Treat Rev* 1980; 7:141–152.

47. Spitz S. The histological effects of nitrogen mustards on human tumors and tissues. *Cancer* 1948; 1:383–388.

48. Meistrich ML. Quantitative correlation between testicular stem cell survival, sperm production, and fertility in mouse after treatment with different cytotoxic agents. *J Androl* 1982; 3:58–68.

49. Qiu J, Hales BF, Robaire B. Adverse effects of cyclophosphamide on progeny outcome can be mediated through post-testicular mechanisms in the rat. *Biol Riol Reprod* 1992; 46:926–931.

50. Trasler JM, Hales BF, Robaire B. A time course study of chronic paternal cyclophosphamide treatment of rats: effects on pregnancy outcome and the male reproductive and hematologic systems. *Biol Reprod* 1987; 37:317–326.

51. Sherins RJ, De Vita VT Jr. Effect of drug treatment for lymphoma on male reproductive capacity. *Ann Intern Med* 1973; 79:216–220.

52. Parvinen M, Lahdetie J, Parvinen L-M. Toxic and mutagenic influences on spermatogenesis. *Arch Toxicol Suppl* 1984; 7:147–150.

53. Oats RD, Lipshultz LI. Fertility and testicular function in patients after chemotherapy and radiotherapy. In: Lytton B, ed. *Advances in Urology*, Chicago: Mosby Year Book; 1989; 2:55–83.

54. Shalet SM. Effects of cancer chemotherapy on gonadal function of patients. *Cancer Treat Rev* 1980; 7:141–152.

55. Rowley MJ, Leach DR, Warner GA, et al. Effects of graded doses of ionizing radiation on the human testis. *Radiat Res* 1974; 59:665–668.

56. Ogilvy-Stuart Al, Shalet SM. Effect of radiation on the human reproductive system. *Environ Health Perspect* 1993; 101(suppl 2): 109–116.

57. Margalioth EJ, Navot D, Beyth Y. Diagnosis of drug related male infertility by zona-free hamster egg sperm penetration assay. *Lancet* 1985; 2:275–279.

58. Rivier C, Rivier J, Vale W. Antireproductive effects of a potent GnRH antagonist in the male rat. *Science* 1980; 210:93–95.

59. Sikka SC, Swerdloff RS, Rajfer J. In vitro inhibition of testosterone biosynthesis by ketoconazole. *Endocrinology* 1985; 116:1920–1925.

60. Bhasin S, Sikka SC, Fielder T, et al. Hormonal effects of ketoconazole in the male rat: mechanism of action. *Endocrinology* 1986; 118:1129–1132.

61. Rajfer J, Sikka SC, Lemmi C, Koyle MA. Cyclosporine inhibits testosterone biosynthesis in the rat testis. *Endocrinology* 1987; 121:586–589.

62. Seethalakshmi L, Flores C, Khauli RB, et al. Evaluation of the effect of cyclosporine toxicity on male reproduction and renal function. *Transplantation* 1990; 49:17–19.

63. Sikka SC, Bhasin S, Coy DC, et al. Effect of cyclosporine on hypothalamic-pituitary-gonadal axis in the male rat: mechanism of action. *Endocrinology* 1988; 123:1069–1074.

64. Agger P. Scrotal and testicular temperature: its relation to sperm count before and after operation for varicocele. *Fertil Steril* 1971; 22:286–297.

65. Robinson D, Rock J. Intrascrotal hyperthermia induced by scrotal insulation: effect on spermatogenesis. *Obstet Gynecol* 1967; 29:217–220.

66. Cummins JM, Jequier AM, Kan R. Molecular biology of human male infertility: links with aging, mitochondrial genetics and oxidative stress? *Mol Reprod Dev* 1994; 37:345–362.

67. Lemaire L, Heinlein UA. Detection of secreted and temporarily inducible heat shock responsive proteins in mouse testicular tissue. *Life Sci* 1991; 48:356–362.

68. Derrick FC Jr, Dahlberg B. Male genital infections and sperm viability. In: Hafez ESE, ed. *Human Semen and Fertility Regulation in Men.* Chicago: CV Mosby; 1976: 389–397.

69. Purvis K, Christiansen E. Male infertility: current concepts—trends in clinical practice. *Ann Med* 1992; 24:259–272.

70. Nikkanen V, Gronroos M, Suominen J, et al. Silent infections in male accessory genital organs and male infertility. *Andrologia* 1979; 11:236–241.

71. Ulstein M, Capell P, Holmes KK, et al. Nonsymptomatic genital tract infection and

male infertility. In: Hafez ESE, ed. *Human Se-men and Fertility Regulation in Men.* St Louis, MO: CV Mosby; 1976: 355–362.

72. Hellstrom WJG, Neal DE Jr. Diagnosis and therapy of male genital tract infections. In: Diamond MP, DeCherney, Overstreet JW, eds. *Infertility and Reproductive Medicine Clinics of North America.* Philadelphia: W.B. Saunders; 1992: 399–411.

73. Rajasekaran M, Hellstrom WJ, Naz RK, et al. Oxidative stress and interleukins in seminal plasma during leukocytospermia. *Fertil Steril* 1995; 64:166–171.

74. Rajasekaran M, Hellstrom WJ, Sikka SC. Quantitative assessment of cytokines (GRO$\alpha$ and IL-10) in human seminal plasma during genitourinary inflammation. *Am J Reprod Immunol* 1996; 36:90–95.

75. Aitken RJ, West KM, Buckingham DW. Leoukocyte infiltration into the human ejaculate and its association with semen quality, oxidative stress, and sperm function. *J Androl* 1994; 15:343–352.

76. Sikka SC, Rajasekaran M, Hellstrom WJG. Role of oxidative stress and antioxidants in male infertility. *J Androl* 1995; 16:464–468.

77. Hibbs JB Jr, Taintor RR, Vavrin Z, et al. Synthesis of NO from a terminal guanidine nitrogen atom of L-arginine: In: Moncada S, Higgs EA, eds. *Nitric Oxide from L-Arginine: A Bioregulator System.* Amsterdam: Elsevier; 1990:189–223.

78. Koppenol WH, Moreno JJ, Pryor WA, et al. Peroxynitrite, a cloaked oxidant formed by nitric oxide and superoxide. *Chem Res Toxicol* 1992; 5:834–842.

79. Rosselli M, Dubey RK, Imthurn B, et al. Effects of nitric oxide on human spermatozoa: evidence that nitric oxide decreases sperm motility and induces sperm toxicity. *Hum Reprod* 1995; 10:1786–1790.

80. Beckman JS, Beckman TW, Chen J, et al. Apparent hydroxyl radical production by peroxynitrite: implications for endothelial injury from nitric oxide and superoxide. *Proc Natl Acad Sci USA* 1990; 87:1620–1624.

81. Gagnon C, Iwasaki A, de Lamirande E, et al. Reactive oxygen species and human spermatozoa (review). *Ann N Y Acad Sci* 1991; 637:436–444.

82. Aitken RJ, Clarkson JS. Cellular basis of defective sperm function and its association with the genesis of reactive oxygen species by human spermatozoa. *J Reprod Fertil* 1987; 81:459–469.

83. Alvarez JG, Touchstone JC, Blasco L, et al. Spontaneous lipid peroxidation and production of hydrogen peroxide and superoxide in human spermatozoa. Superoxide dismutase as major enzyme protectant against oxygen toxicity. *J Androl* 1987; 8:338–348.

84. Lenzi A, Picardo M, Gandini L, et al. Glutathione treatment of dyspermia: effect on the lipoperoxidation process. *Hum Reprod* 1994; 9:2044–2050.

85. Rao B, Soufir JC, Martin M, et al. Lipid peroxidation in human spermatozoa as related to midpiece abnormalities and motility. *Gamete Res* 1989; 24:127–134.

86. Huszar G, Vigue L. Correlation between the rate of lipid peroxidation and cellular maturity as measured by creatine kinase activity in human spermatozoa. *J Androl* 1994; 15:71–77.

87. Johnson L. Evaluation of the human testis and its age-related dysfunction. *Prog Clin Biol Res* 1989; 302:35–67.

88. Paniagua R, Nistal M, Saez FJ. Ultrastructure of the aging human testis. *J Electron Microsc Tech* 1991; 19:241–260.

89. Neaves WB, Johnson L, Porter JC, et al. Leydig cell numbers, daily sperm production, and serum gonadotrophic levels in aging men. *J Clin Endocrinol Metab* 1984; 59:756–763.

90. Baker HWG, Hudson B. Changes in the pituitary-testicular axis with age. In: de Kretser DM, Burger HG, Hudson B, eds. *The Pituitary and Testis: Clinical and Experimental Studies.* Berlin: Springer-Verlag; 1983:71–184.

91. Kerr JB, de Kretser DM. Cyclic variations in Sertoli cell lipid content through the spermatogenic cycle in the rat. *J Reprod Fertil* 1975; 43:1–8.

92. Reichel W. Lipofuscin pigment accumulation and distribution in various organisms as a function of age. *J Gerontol* 1968; 23:145–153.

93. Lamb JC IV, Chapin RE. Testicular and germ cell toxicity: in vitro approaches. *Reprod Toxicol* 1993; 7:17–22.

94. Gray TJB. Testicular toxicity in vitro: Sertoli-germ cell co-cultures as a model system. *Food Chem Toxicol* 1986; 67:601–605.

95. Chapin RE, Gray TJB, Phelps JL, Dutton SL. The effects of mono-(2-ethylhexyl)phthalate on rat Sertoli cell-enriched primary cultures. *Toxicol Appl Pharmacol* 1988; 96:467–479.

96. Galdieri M. Ziparo E. Palombi F, et al. Pure Sertoli cell cultures; a new model for the study of somatic-germ cell interactions. *J Androl* 1981; 2:249–254.

97. Foster PMD, Lloyd SC, Prout MS. Toxicity and metabolism of 1,3-dinitrobenzene in rat testicular cell cultures. *Toxicol In Vitro* 1987; 1:31–37.

98. Ewing LL, Zirkin BR, Chubb C. Assessment of testicular testosterone production and Leydig cell structure. *Environ Health Perspect* 1981; 38:19–27.

99. Chapin RE, Phelps JL, Somkuti SG, et al. The interaction of Sertoli and Leydig cells in the testicular toxicity of tri-o-cresyl phosphate. *Toxicol Appl Pharmacol* 1990; 104:483–495.

100. Gray TJB. Application of in vitro systems in male reproductive toxicology. In: Lamb JC IV, Foster PMD, eds. *Physiology and Toxicology of Male Reproduction*. San Diego, CA: Academic Press; 1988; 10:25–253.

101. Chapin RE, Phelps J. Recent advances in testicular cell culture: implications for toxicology. *Toxicol In Vitro* 1990; 4/5:543–559.

102. Lamb JC IV. Design and use of multigeneration breeding studies for identification of reproductive toxicants. In: Working PK, ed. *Toxicology of the Male and Female Reproductive Systems*. San Diego, CA: Hemisphere; Bristol, PA; 1989: 173–184.

103. Darney SP. In vitro assessment of gamete integrity. In: Goldberg AM, ed. *Alternative Methods in Toxicology, vol. 8. In Vitro Toxicology: Mechanisms and New Toxicology*. New York: Ann Liebert; 1991: 63–75.

104. Brown DB, Hayes EJ, Uchida T, et al. Some cases of human male infertility are explained by abnormal in vitro human sperm activation. *Fertil Steril* 1995; 64:612–622.

105. Perrault SD, Barbee RR, Elstein KH, et al. Interspecies differences in the stability of mammalian sperm nuclei assessed in vivo by sperm microinjection and in vitro by flow cytometry. *Biol Reprod* 1988; 39:157–167.

106. Evenson DP. Flow cytometry evaluation of male germ cells. In: Yen A, ed. *Flow Cytometry: Advanced Research and Clinical Applications*. Boca Raton, FL: CRC Press; 1989; 1:218–246.

107. Evenson DP, Baier RK, Jost LK, et al. Toxicity of thiotepa on mouse spermatogenesis as determined by dual-parameter flow cytometry. *Toxicol Appl Pharmacol* 1986; 82:151–163.

108. Evenson DP, Jost L, Baier R, et al. Individuality of DNA denaturation patterns in human sperm as measured by the sperm chromatin structure assay. *Reprod Toxicol* 1991; 5:115–125.

109. Hoyt JA, Fisher LF, Swisher, DK. Short-term male reproductive toxicity study with sulfasalazine in the rat. *Reprod Toxicol* 1995; 9: 315–326.

110. Ulbrich B, Palmer AK. Detection of effects on male reproduction—a literature survey. *J Am Coll Toxicol* 1995; 14:293–327.

111. Zenick H, Clegg ED, Perrault SD, et al. Assessment of male reproductive toxicity—a risk assessment approach. In: Hayes WA, ed. *Principles and Methods of Toxicology*. New York: Raven Press; 1994: 937–988.

# 21
# Cryptorchidism and Infertility

Manoj Monga and Wayne J.G. Hellstrom

Cryptorchidism is a defect involving maldescent of the testicle. The aims of therapy for cryptorchidism include preservation of fertility, reduction in risk of malignancy, and alleviation of psychological stress. It was first described by Hunter[1] in 1841, who noted an association between maldescent and alterations in testicular function and fertility.

The incidence of cryptorchidism in the newborn is 2% to 5.8%; however, with spontaneous descent this incidence drops to 1% by the age of 3 months and 0.8% to 2.0% by the age of 1 year.[2–5] Up to 15% to 33% of cryptorchidism may be bilateral.[2,6–8] Prematurity, low birth weight, and multiple gestations (twins) are predisposing factors, with the increase in incidence correlating to the degree of prematurity. The incidence of cryptorchidism in premature infants is 30%; in infants under 1800 g, 69%; and in infants under 900 g, 100%.[6]

A family history of cryptorchidism may be present in 3.5% to 5%.[7] The incidence of cryptorchidism in siblings is 1% to 4% and in fathers of the patients 6%.[9] Mothers of children with cryptorchidism tend to have mild pituitary impairment manifested by short menses and delayed menarche.[9] A peak in incidence in children born from January through March and a nadir in incidence in children born between August and October have been attributed to effects of sunlight on maternal gonadotropin secretion during pregnancy.[6,9]

Associations with specific human leukocyte antigen (HLA) haplotypes support a congenital intrinsic defect.[5] Associated hypospadias may be present in 6% to 9% of cryptorchid patients.[8] Cryptorchidism is also associated with disorders of gonadotropin deficiency, such as Kallmann's, Prader-Labhart-Willi, and Laurence-Moon-Biedl syndromes. In addition, cryptorchidism is associated with neural tube defects, with incidences of 24% in sacral myelomeningocele and 50% when lesions are above L-2.[9] Cryptorchidism is also associated with disorders of the abdominal musculature, such as gastroschisis and prune belly syndrome.

## Embryology of Descent and Pathophysiology of Maldescent of the Testis

Attachment of the gubernaculum to the epididymis occurs at the eighth gestational week. By the 12th to 14th week of gestation, the testis migrates from the urogenital ridge to the level of the internal inguinal ring, where it waits to begin its transinguinal descent during the 26th to 28th week of gestation with associated gubernacular swelling and processus vaginalis extension into the scrotum. Testicular descent is believed to depend on an integration of factors: an increase in intraabdominal pressure, gubernacular tension, and the hormonal influence of high local concentrations of dihydrotestosterone. Because hormonal influence depends on an intact fetal hypothalamic-pituitary-testicular axis, aberrations in testicular descent may result from a deficiency in one or more of these factors. Mechanical obstruction of the inguinal canal is noted in only 9% of patients, but abnormal gubernacular attachments are noted in 83% to 93% of cryptorchid testes.[2,10]

Hormonal influence may also depend on müllerian-inhibiting factor, as the absence of androgen receptors in the testicular feminization syndrome does not preclude testicular descent, and transabdominal descent has been shown to fail in animals with persistent müllerian structures. Müllerian-inhibiting factor is produced by fetal Sertoli cells during the seventh to ninth week of pregnancy. The transabdominal descent during weeks 10 to 15 may depend on müllerian-inhibiting substance stimulation of gubernacular growth, and the transinguinal descent requires androgen-dependent stimulation of the genitofemoral nerve, which releases calcitonin gene-related peptide (CGRP) and causes cyclic adenosine monophosphate (cAMP)-dependent contraction and chemotactic migration of the gubernaculum.[2] Estrogen-induced cryptorchidism is accompanied by preservation of the müllerian duct structures and atrophy of the gubernaculum.[11]

The effects of cryptorchidism on subsequent fertility may be associated with alterations in hormonal-dependent transformations of the gonocyte. A surge of luteinizing hormone (LH) and follicle-stimulating hormone (FSH) during the first 60 to 90 days of life stimulates Leydig cell proliferation, which peaks at 3 months of age and results in a surge of testosterone. A transient perinatal period of hypogonadism due to blunting of this gonadotropin surge may be the primary hormonal defect in cryptorchidism. This would lead to understimulation of the fetal Leydig cells, with resultant Leydig cell hypoplasia and regression. Subsequently, a blockage of the normal surge of testosterone at this age would prevent transformation of the gonocytes into adult dark spermatogonia, the first postnatal maturational step in germ cell development, normally completed by 6 months.[2,12–14] An underlying endocrinopathy is supported by evidence of reduced Leydig cell and germ cell counts as well as by defective germ-cell maturation in the contralateral descended testis.[2]

The genitofemoral nerve may play an important role in transinguinal testicular migration. The genitofemoral nucleus (cremasteric nucleus) and nerve are sexually dimorphic structures under androgenic control.[15] With androgenic stimulation, there is an increase in substance P nociceptive and thermal afferents from the testes, serotonin thermal regulatory fibers, and myelinated motoneurons innervating the cremasteric muscle.[15] The genitofemoral nerve innervates the distalmost aspect of the gubernaculum. CGRP is secreted by the genitofemoral nerve and is known to cause rhythmic contractions of the tip of the gubernaculum.[15]

The genitofemoral nerve may act as a mediator between androgen stimulation and the gubernaculum, as transection of this nerve or division of the spinal cord above its origin (L1–2) inhibits testicular descent through the inguinal canal, inhibits formation of the processus vaginalis, and causes a decrease in testicular weight and degeneration of the seminiferous tubules.[6,11,15,16] These findings correspond to the clinical observation that patients with spina bifida with lesions above L3 have an unexpectedly high incidence of cryptorchidism.[11] The gubernaculum is insensitive to androgen stimulation following transection of the genitofemoral nerve. Capsaicin, a substance P inhibitor, increases the likelihood of flutamide-induced cryptorchidism and inhibits scrotal development.[2]

Malposition of the testis may result in sensory neural transmissions that may play a role in contralateral damage. Transection of the nerve in naturally unilateral cryptorchid rats was shown to protect the contralateral testis from atrophy and impaired spermatogenesis, and improved the fertility rate from 10% to 60%.[16]

Flutamide-induced cryptorchidism in the fetal rat is associated with reduction in the neural diameter and number of large and small myelinated fibers in the genitofemoral nerve. These changes correlate with cremasteric muscle atrophy.[15] It is believed that these changes are not the result of a direct antiandrogen effect on the neural tissue, but rather the gubernaculum or cremasteric muscle producing paracrine factors that modulate neuronal survival by retrograde transport back to the neuronal cell. Potential paracrine factors known to be androgen dependent that may play a role in this process include neurotrophic growth factor, epidermal growth factor (EGF), and CGRP. As EGF is involved in stabilization of wolffian duct structures, abnormal secretion may account for coexisting epididymal abnormalities.[15]

Although testicular absence (agenesis) may reflect the most severe form of cryptorchidism, it may be the end result of intrauterine testicular torsion of the spermatic cord.[17,18] Histologic findings in the contralateral descended partner of unilateral agenesis support the intrauterine torsion theory, as contralateral histologic changes found in other cases of cryptorchidism (decreases in Leydig cells, total germ cells, adult dark spermatogonia, and primary spermatocytes) are absent.[19]

The deleterious effects of cryptorchidism on the testis may reflect primary genetic or congenital defects, or may be secondary to hormonal, vascular, autoimmune, or temperature-sensitive alterations.

## Clinical Classification

When a testicle is not located in the scrotal compartment, it is necessary to differentiate between a true cryptorchid testicle and a retractile testis. The scrotal compartment of a retractile testis is normally developed and inverts during retraction of the gubernaculum. A retractile testis can easily be manually manipulated into the scrotum and will remain there for a short period of time after overstretching of the cremasteric muscle, before retracting into the canal as the cremasteric muscle regains its tone. This entity is considered benign, with no demonstrable effects on testicular function and no indication for intervention. Because the cremasteric reflex becomes active at 3 months of age, documentation of testicular position prior to this may assist in identifying retractile testes. The incidence of retractile testis in fertile men is 12%.[20] Careful examination will demonstrate that 66% to 80% of mal-located testicles are retractile in nature, but only 28% are truly cryptorchidic.[2,9,21]

A gliding testis, a testicle that lies below the external inguinal ring, can be manipulated into the upper scrotum but immediately returns to the superficial inguinal pouch upon release. The gliding testicle is associated with absence of the gubernaculum and with a partially patent processus vaginalis from the upper scrotum to the midgroin, allowing manual manipulation. By age 7, 24% of gliding testes demonstrate loss of volume, and histologic degeneration is evident.[6]

Cryptorchid testes may be canalicular (75%), intraabdominal (6–11%), ectopic (10–15%), or high-scrotal (8%).[7,8] Ectopic positions include perineal, femoral, and penopubic. The most common location for a cryptorchid testis is in the superficial inguinal pouch. The proportion of intraabdominal testes in bilateral cases is significantly higher (51%).[8] The cryptorchid testis may be nonpalpable in 5% to 28% of cases; however, preoperative physical observations with regard to testicular location do not correlate well with intraoperative findings.[2,8]

Testicular agenesis occurs in 49% to 88% of unilateral nonpalpable testes as compared with 5% of bilateral nonpalpable testes.[8,9] Contralateral compensatory hypertrophy, with a 2-cc testicular volume in boys aged 3 or older, may be a sensitive indicator of agenesis of the nonpalpable testis.[22] With bilateral nonpalpable testes, elevated basal gonadotropin levels in boys under the age of 9 and the lack of serum testosterone response to human chorionic gonadotropin (hCG) stimulation may also indicate testicular anorchia.[2,10] Elevated prepubertal serum gonadotropins can be considered confirmatory for bilateral anorchia; however, absence of response to hCG stimulation should not be considered proof of anorchia. Bilateral nonpalpable testes should undergo karyotype examination to exclude congenital adrenal hyperplasia or other intersex abnormalities.

## Association with Infertility

Cryptorchidism is a preexisting factor in 3% to 8% of infertile men and in 20% of men with azoospermia.[21,23] The incidence of infertility ranges from 10% to 20% in patients with uni-

lateral cryptorchidism to 40% to 80% in patients with bilateral cryptorchidism.[24]

Animal studies support an effect from
cryptorchidism on fertility, with primary
bilateral cryptorchidism preventing paternity.[25]
In congenital unilateral cryptorchid rats, the
fertility rate is only 0% to 10%, compared
with 100% in the control rats.[16,26] In the
congenital canine cryptorchid model, all bilateral cryptorchid animals were azoospermic,
and the total sperm count, sperm motility,
and percentage of normal sperm morphology
were diminished in the unilateral cryptorchid
animals.[27]

Analysis of any clinical series of cryptorchidism should evaluate the study population
for the inclusion of retractile testes, as these
spontaneously descend and have no bearing on
future fertility. Isolated cryptorchidism not associated with congenital syndromes accounts
for 80% to 90% of instances of undescended
testes.[28] Patients with congenital syndromes,
such as prune belly syndrome and intersex
patients, should also be excluded from
study populations, as the pathophysiology of
maldescent and infertility may be different
from isolated cryptorchidism, and outcomes
may be adversely affected. Cases of entrapped
testis following inguinal surgery (e.g., herniorraphy) may demonstrate atrophic intratubular
changes and should likewise be excluded from
a clinical series of true primary cryptorchid
testes.

Study populations should be stratified
according to testicular location, as the percentage of testicular tubules containing spermatogonia (tubule fertility index, TFI)
correlates with proximity to the scrotum.[21]
Some studies report no correlation between
testicular location and TFI or tubular diameter,
although a trend toward a lower TFI with
intraabdominal testes has been noted.[7] Study
patients selected from infertility clinics may
represent a biased population when compared
with a spectrum of cryptorchid patients
followed from childhood, and clinical series
often incorporate a heterogeneous population
based on type and timing of surgical
intervention.

## Subfertility

Sterility occurs in 100% of patients with untreated bilateral cryptorchid testes, and
subfertility occurs in 71% of patients with
untreated unilateral cryptorchid testes.[4]
Oligospermia (78–84%), azoospermia (6–
16%), and asthenospermia (46%) have been
reported in patients who underwent unilateral
orchiopexy after puberty.[4,20,29] The incidence of
azoospermia was higher than in the general infertile population (5–8%).[20] Orchiopexy performed during the prepubertal period may
result in severe oligospermia or azoospermia in
75% to 100% of bilateral cases and in 28% to
50% of unilateral cases.[4,30] No difference has
been found in semen parameters in boys who
underwent prepubertal unilateral orchiopexy
compared with orchiectomy.[30] Two studies on
fertile men with a history of orchiopexy for
cryptorchidism and who underwent unilateral
vasectomy for elective sterilization demonstrated that 69% of cryptorchid testes were
azoospermic.[5]

Clinical studies involving 561 men with
unilateral cryptorchidism and 281 men with
bilateral cryptorchidism demonstrated decreased sperm density in 49% of the patients
with unilateral disease and in 72% of the
patients with bilateral disease.[21] A report on
200 patients presenting to an infertility
clinic found oligoteratoasthenozoospermia in
all patients, regardless of mode of therapy;
however, this was a retrospective study with a
heterogeneous group of patients in terms of
testes location, mode of therapy, and timing of
therapy.[31] FSH levels were high in all patients,
possibly reflecting primary Sertoli cell
malfunction, but the mean age at time of intervention was 11 years, with 95% of the
orchiopexies being performed after the age of
4. Although these investigators advised post-
poning surgical treatment because semen quality was not improved in the orchiopexy groups,
the significant selection bias of these patients
presenting to an infertility clinic should be
noted, and management conclusions based
on these findings should most definitely be
reserved.

Other studies confirm that type of intervention (surgical/hormonal/both/neither) and age at intervention had no effect on subsequent azoospermia or oligospermia.[32] Oligospermia after either unilateral or bilateral orchiopexy occurred in 31%, and azoospermia occurred in 14% after unilateral orchiopexy and 42% after bilateral orchiopexy.[32] Some investigators report decreased percentages of viable sperm in addition to oligoteratoasthenospermia in cryptorchid patients being evaluated for infertility.[33] Others have reported normal semen production and normal fertility following orchiopexy.[5,34–37]

Paternity is a more valid index of fertility than semen parameters because 14% of normal fertile men have oligospermia.[5] The paternity rate in the normal population is 85%.[9] Paternity rates following orchiopexy for unilateral cryptorchidism are 71% to 92% (cumulative average 81%), and 43% to 62% (cumulative average 51%) following orchiopexy for bilateral cryptorchidism.[5] The paternity rates following prepubertal bilateral orchiopexy (30–80%) compare favorably to those of postpubertal orchiopexy (13%).[25]

## Effects on Germinal Epithelium

The cryptorchid testis is histologically normal at birth. Progressive seminiferous tubular atrophy and peritubular hyalinization, collagenization, and interstitial fibrosis occur in the cryptorchid testis within the first few months of life, with the resulting postpubertal testis being devoid of germ cells.[4,5] Seminiferous tubular length is decreased at puberty to 100 μm in the cryptorchid boy compared with 300 μm in normal boys.[9] A Sertoli-cell–only pattern may be demonstrated in 70% of adult cryptorchid testes.[38] Severe histologic changes (Sertoli cell only, maturational arrest) are seen in 81% of unilateral cryptorchid men presenting to infertility clinics.[23] These changes are believed to commence between the first and second years of life, with complete absence of germ cells being noted in cryptorchid testes in 5% of boys under the age of 1 and 38% of 2-year-olds.[4,6] Decreased germ cells are noted in

40% to 50% of contralateral descended testes after the age of 2.[6]

The normal mean spermatogonia-per-tubule ratio (S/T ratio, fertility index) is 4 at birth, 2 at age 1, and 1 from the age of 2 through 6.[9] In cryptorchid boys the S/T ratio begins at 4, but it drops to 0.3 by age 2 and remains low until puberty, with only 1% of cryptorchid boys having normal S/T ratios at age 1.[9] Low germ cell counts and tubule fertility indices on prepubertal biopsies at the time of orchiopexy correlate with subsequent abnormalities in semen parameters, adult testicular volume, and reduced fertility.[5,14] Studies demonstrated that 22% of 2-year-olds with unilateral cryptorchidism had absence of germ cells in the ipsilateral testis, while the remainder demonstrated germinal atrophy.[21] Decrease in total germ cell counts begin at the age of 1 year.[14] Impairment of germ cell maturation (frequency of Ad spermatogonia) and a decrease in germ cell counts correlate with testicular position, with abdominal testes demonstrating the most significant impairment.[9,39]

Histologic studies of infants under the age of 4 months demonstrate a significantly smaller proportion of cryptorchid testicles containing adult dark spermatogonia, but gonocyte counts remain higher than in the contralateral descended testis until 18 months.[12–14] This may represent a block in the transformation of gonocytes to adult dark spermatogonia in the cryptorchid testis, and as the untransformed gonocytes start to degenerate after the sixth month of life, a decrease in the total germ count would not be evident until the second year.[12,13] Adult dark spermatogonia have been reported in only 31% of cryptorchid testes compared with 95% of controls by 3 months of age.[12,14] The second postnatal maturational step in germ cell development, transformation of adult dark spermatogonia to primary spermatocytes at the age of 3, has also been shown to be defective in cryptorchid boys.[14,40] Testicular biopsies at the time of orchiopexy demonstrated presence of Ad spermatogonia in only 17% of cryptorchid testes compared with 64% of descended contralateral testes. Spermatocytes were present in 20% to 27% of descended testes, as compared with 0 to 0.6% of cryptorchid testes.[14,39]

Gonocyte maturation has been thought to be dependent on hCG stimulation of intra-testicular testosterone levels, but müllerian-inhibiting substance (MIS) is now believed to regulate the transformation of gonocytes to type-A spermatogonia.[41,42] MIS peaks between 4 and 12 months of age, coinciding with the timing of gonocyte transformation to type-A spermatogonia, but low levels of MIS have been documented in cryptorchid patients.[41,43]

## Effects on Sperm Nuclear Content and Organization

Chromosomal abnormalities have been identified in 14% of cryptorchid infertile men, with sex chromosome aneuploidy accounting for half of these.[44] The average DNA content of spermatogonia is significantly increased in cryptorchid and contralateral descended testes in children with unilateral or bilateral crytorchidism.[38] Hormonal stimulation during puberty results in a more pronounced increase in DNA content of adult cryptorchid men, and this finding is unaffected by orchiopexy.[38] The increased DNA content is not due to a high proliferative activity level, for autoradiographic studies demonstrate a decreased proliferative activity in cryptorchid testes.[38] Bilateral decreases in DNA synthesis noted in germ cells of unilateral cryptorchid boys suggest an intrinsic nuclear anomaly in the cryptorchid spermatogonia that blocks completion of DNA replication or mitosis.[38,45] This defect may account for the inability of spermatogonia to proliferate to spermatozoa and for the predisposition to malignant degeneration in cryptorchid testes and contralateral descended partners.[38]

Cryptorchidism results in a high degree of sperm nuclear instability because of a defect in histone replacement by protamines.[33] Somatic histones are normally replaced by protamines, basic sperm-specific nucleoproteins, during transformation of round spermatids into spermatozoa.[33] Stable condensation of the nucleoprotein complex relies on the formation of cross-linking disulfide bridges and inter-chelation of zinc into the chromatin during epididymal transit.[33] Chromatin condensation is required for successful oocyte penetration.[33] The adverse effects of cryptorchidism on this process are not altered by early orchiopexy or prevention of testicular atrophy by orchiopexy, and orchiectomy does not protect the contralateral testis from these alterations.[33] These findings are supported by evidence that sperm chromatin from cryptorchid patients is more susceptible to in situ denaturation.[46]

## Effects on Sertoli Cell Function

Sertoli cell vacuolation and dilatation have been noted in 2-year-old boys.[47] Numerous free ribosomes are evident in a fibrotic cytoplasm by ages 3 to 8.[45] There is no evidence of differences in DNA content in Sertoli cells.[38] Significant reductions in the number of Sertoli cells are evident at puberty, correlating to a higher anatomical testicular position.[9]

The Sertoli cell type Sf is thought to produce müllerian-inhibiting substance, which itself may play a crucial role in testicular descent.[6] Absence of Sf cells has been demonstrated as early as 2 weeks postnatally in the cryptorchid testis.[6] Other cryptorchid-induced alterations in the Sertoli cell include incomplete maturation at puberty, increase in lipid droplets, dilation of the smooth endoplasmic reticulum, and abnormal inter–Sertoli cell junctional complexes.[48]

Alterations and reduction in androgen binding protein may affect both the cryptorchid and contralateral descended testes.[6,48] Androgen-binding protein (ABP) production is bidirectional, secreted across the apical surface into the tubular lumen and across the basal surface of the Sertoli cell into the testicular fluid where it is transported into the systemic circulation.[49] Impairment of ABP secretion at both locations has been demonstrated in the primary and secondary cryptorchid animal models.[49]

## Effects on Leydig Cell Function

Testosterone levels in the blood of the cord and in peripheral circulation of cryptorchid newborns are comparable to those in normal infants.[28] Testosterone levels fall postnatally because of declining levels of maternal hCG then rise to 2 to 3 ng/ml during the second and third months of life in response to LH stimulation.[9,28] These changes correlate with a peak in fetal Leydig cell/tubule ratio at 3 to 4 months.[2]

Between the ages of 3 and 8 years in boys with cryptorchidism, collagen proliferation in the interstitium of the testis is significantly increased and disorderly, with thickening of the tunica propria. From ages 9 to 13, increased basement membrane thickening and Leydig cell atrophy, degeneration, and lack of differentiation and maturation are evident.[45] Electron microscopy has demonstrated decreased Leydig cell number and Leydig cell atrophy with irregular nuclei, diminished mitochondria, and smooth endoplasmic reticulum.[28,50]

There is an attenuation in this rise in testosterone in unilateral and bilateral cryptorchid boys to 50% of the levels attained in normal infants, unless spontaneous descent occurs within the first 4 months of life.[28] Leydig cell/tubule ratio peaks are lower and occur earlier.[2] Gonadotropin-releasing hormone (GnRH) stimulation tests demonstrate diminished release of LH in prepubertal cryptorchid boys.[28,51] Leydig cell stimulation tests using parenteral hCG demonstrate a normal tenfold increase in basal testosterone secretion.[28] These findings suggest that a defect in the hypothalamic-pituitary axis may result in an early hypoandrogenic state in cryptorchid infants. Small fetal Leydig cells with decreased cytoplasm and small irregular nuclei are found in cryptorchid infants under the age of 4 months, suggesting understimulation of the Leydig cells.[13] Hypoplasia of the Leydig cells is evident from the first month of life, representing the earliest postnatal histologic abnormality in the cryptorchid testis.[12] This early, transient hypogonadism may be the cause of the subsequent germinal deterioration.

Other clinical and experimental evidence suggests normal basal LH levels in cryptorchid infants, pointing to a primary Leydig cell dysfunction as a cause of lowered testosterone secretion.[28] Leydig cell dysfunction may be secondary to disruption of paracrine interactions with the damaged seminiferous tubules or with the Sertoli cell. There may be decreased activity in the heat-sensitive enzymes $\Delta^5$ 3β- and 17β-hydroxysteroid dehydrogenase, responsible for the conversion of dehydroepiandrosterone to testosterone.[28]

Androgen levels (testosterone, dihydrotestosterone, androstenedione, dihydroepiandrosterone) are normal at age 6 years and remain normal through puberty and adulthood.[28] Reports on Leydig cell response to hCG stimulation are variable, possibly due to differences in dosage of hCG, timing of administration, and timing of androgen measurement. Ideally, androgen levels should be measured 72 to 120 hours after hCG administration, and doses should be adjusted for body size. The Leydig cell response to hCG stimulation may be blunted and remain blunted in the early stage of puberty (Tanner stage 2), normalizing by midpuberty.[28] This suggests a defect in the hypothalamic-pituitary axis that leads to insufficient preparation of the Leydig cell to respond to hCG stimulation tests.

Reports on androgen function in the adult population are more controversial. Reported incidence of decreased plasma androgen and seminal acid phosphatase levels ranges from 4% to 100%, and histologic evidence of damage ranges from none to multivacuolated Leydig cells with large lipid droplets in 50% of the cell population to Leydig cell hyperplasia.[28] Leydig cell hyperplasia has been demonstrated in both the undescended and the scrotal testes of unilateral cryptorchid postpubertal men.[51] Cryptorchid patients do not demonstrate clinical signs of hypogonadism (normal secondary male hair distribution, libido, potency), indicating that a peripheral androgen deficit does not exist, even though a high intratesticular androgen concentration may not be maintained.[28]

## Elevated Testicular Temperature Theory

Most mammals, with the exception of elephants and whales, have a scrotum that maintains a testicular temperature 4.8°C lower than the core body temperature.[2] Detrimental effects of hyperthermia on semen quality and fertility have been demonstrated experimentally by increasing testicular temperature (applied heat, testicular insulation, electromagnetic or ultrasound exposure, modified athletic supporters), and clinically by pathophysiologic associations with cryptorchidism and varicocele.[25] External ice application to the scrotum has improved sperm production in men with oligospermia.[25]

Measurements of testicular temperature at the time of orchiopexy in prepubertal boys have demonstrated significantly higher temperatures in the cryptorchid testis (34.4°C) when compared with the contralateral descended testis (33.2°C), and this temperature declined through the inguinal canal down to the scrotum.[52]

Studies have shown that among infertile men with a history of cryptorchidism, 45% had scrotal hyperthermia following orchiopexy (>35.2°C), and this was associated with more severe impairment of spermatogenesis and a greater degree of testicular atrophy than cryptorchid infertile men with normal scrotal temperature.[20] Patients with right-sided cryptorchidism were more likely to have contralateral scrotal hyperthermia, and this was associated with a higher incidence of contralateral testicular volume loss than in patients with left-sided cryptorchidism.[20] High location of the testis was a risk factor for scrotal hyperthermia.

Chilling of the congenital intraabdominal cryptorchid testis in the boar by use of a cooling coil around the testicle demonstrated normal development and differentiation of the germinal epithelium, indicating that increased testicular temperature rather than congenital defect results in progressive failure of spermatogenesis.[25]

## Autoimmunization Theory

Some researchers suggest that the prepubertal human testis does not contain antigenic germ cell components, thus making an autoimmune cause of cryptorchid-induced testicular damage unlikely. After puberty, according to this theory, testicular hyperthermia may damage the blood-testis barrier, facilitating the passage of immunoreactive cells. However, others have demonstrated antisperm antibodies in 21% of boys with testicular pathology, including cryptorchidism, varicocele, testicular torsion, inguinal hernia, and trauma.[53] By use of an indirect immunobead assay, antisperm antibodies have been noted preoperatively in 25% of prepubertal boys (mean age 2.8 years) undergoing orchiopexy, 40% of boys undergoing herniorraphy, and 50% of boys undergoing hypospadias repair, compared with 4% of controls.[54] This suggests that the prepubertal testis may contain antigenic germ cell components, although it is unknown whether adult sperm share the antigenic epitopes expressed on the prepubertal germ cells. Cryptorchidism, inguinal hernia, and hypospadias may therefore be manifestations of a common hormonal abnormality that also causes a delayed maturation or incomplete formation of the blood-testis barrier.

Antisperm antibodies in serum and seminal fluid have been demonstrated by use of macroagglutination tests, immobilization tests, and indirect immunobead assays in 66% of cryptorchid infertile patients, compared with 3% in infertile patients without a history of cryptorchidism and 3% in patients with proven fertility.[24,54] Progressive sperm motility was significantly diminished and the degree of sperm agglutination was significantly higher in patients who tested positive for antisperm antibodies, indicating that they may contribute to reduced fertility. Immobilizing antibodies were more common (57%) than agglutinating antibodies (14%), with the sperm midpiece being the most common immunoglobulin binding site (73%). Patients who developed antisperm antibodies had undergone orchiopexy after puberty (mean age 14.2 years), unlike the younger patients who did not develop antisperm antibodies (mean age 8.6 years). This supports the theory that the prepubertal testis may lack antigenic properties. Reports on antisperm antibodies in cryptorchid adults demonstrate positive findings in 13% to 55%.[44]

## Epididymal Anatomical Abnormalities

Epididymal anomalies are commonly associated with cryptorchidism and should be considered when predicting the prognosis for fertility and when evaluating results following intervention, as subfertility may result from defective sperm transport despite preservation of the germinal epithelium by early orchiopexy. Some consider the epididymis to be the key factor in testicular descent, as the gubernaculum actually inserts into the epididymis, with the testicle being carried passively into the scrotum due to its epididymal attachments.[2] Epididymal abnormalities may be categorized as anomalies of ductal fusion (65%) and anomalies of ductal suspension (35%).[55] Epididymal abnormalities ranging from complete absence of the epididymis to abnormal attachment of the body of the epididymis occur in 36% to 87% of cryptorchid testes, while only 19% of the descended partners have coexisting epididymal abnormalities.[10,21,55] If a looped epididymis is considered normal (seen in 84% of descended testes), then epididymal abnormalities occur in only 17% to 21% of cryptorchid testes.[2]

Flimsy attachment of the caput epididymis to the testis is the most common anomaly.[55] The incidence of epididymal abnormalities is greatest if the testis is undescended with a complete hernia sac (75%), rather than ectopic (29%) or undescended with an incomplete hernia sac (16%).[21] The degree of epididymal dysmorphism corresponds to higher testicular position.[2]

A patent process vaginalis (concomitant inguinal hernia) is present in 50% to 89% of patients.[5,7,8] Epididymal dissociation is present in 78% to 90% of the cases with an open processus vaginalis, compared with 38% with a closed processus.[10,56] A spermatogonia-per-tubule index of 0 to 0.2 in 62% of these prepubertal patients suggests a more severe form of cryptorchidism, indicating that a patent processus vaginalis may be a poor prognosticator of future fertility.[56] Absence of spermatogonia was noted in 42% of these patients. Some suggest empiric postoperative therapy

with a luteinizing hormone–releasing hormone (LHRH)-analogue (buserelin) in these patients.[56]

## Experimental Effects on Epididymal Function

The normal loop configuration of the epididymis positions the cauda epididymis, the site of sperm storage, in a significantly cooler position than the adjacent testis.[57] An experimental cryptepididymal state can be created where the epididymis is positioned in the abdominal cavity while remaining attached to a normally functioning scrotal testis.[57] Epithelial function and subsequent spermatozoal maturation in the caput and corpus epididymis remain normal. Elevation of the cauda epididymis into the abdomen results in an immediate suppression of the sperm storage capacity of this structure, as reductions in length and diameter of the epididymal ducts in this segment result in an inappropriately rapid transit of spermatozoa.[57] Disruption of the cauda epithelium's water and ion transport mechanisms and protein synthesis patterns results in alterations in the composition of the cauda fluid. These changes are reflected by an increase in abnormal sperm morphology and a decrease in sperm motility. A cryptepididymal state may also affect the capacitation characteristics of the spermatozoa. These changes in cauda epithelium capacity and function can be reversed with return to a scrotal position, with subsequent improvement in sperm density and motility.[57]

## Secondary Cryptorchidism

Secondary cryptorchidism may occur following inguinal herniorraphy, and even though studies suggest that significant loss of germinal epithelium occurs after 5 years of entrapment, fertility is minimally affected, probably due to the presence of a normal contralateral testis.[58] The number of spermatogonia per tubule is higher in boys with secondary cryptorchidism than in those with primary cryptorchidism, probably because normal transformation of gonocytes to spermatogonia occurs in the secondary cryptorchid testis during the first months of life.[58] Collagenization of the peritubular connective tissue occurs. Semen analyses following orchiopexy of a secondary cryptorchid testis are significantly better than following primary cryptorchidism.[58]

## Management Considerations Affecting Fertility Outcome

### Age of Repair

A contemporary trend toward early intervention may improve subsequent fertility, but results from this approach are not yet available. Spontaneous descent of undescended testes occurs by 3 months of age.[2] Testicular volume loss is demonstrable by 6 months of age.[2] Currently, orchiopexy prior to the age of 2 years is accepted, but early intervention within the first 6 months of life may be needed and is commonly recommended.[5,8] Orchiopexy in the infant may be facilitated by a shorter inguinal canal and a comparatively larger vas deferens and scrotal sac.

Histologic studies support early intervention. Leydig cell and germ cell atrophy have been observed in 1-year-old boys.[59,60] In severe forms of cryptorchidism, spermatogonia-per-tubule indices (fertility index) are normal under the age of 1, but 62% of boys ranging from ages 1 to 7 years demonstrated decreased indices, and 42% demonstrated absence of spermatogonia, indicating that the testis is susceptible to damage during the early years of childhood.[10,56] In contrast, one study reports no significant relationship between tubular fertility index or tubular diameter and time of surgery, refuting the dictum that progressive deterioration occurs in the malpositioned testis.[7] However, a normal TFI was noted in cryptorchid patients at the age of 1.[7] The importance of differential germ cell counts (gonocyte, adult dark spermatogonia, primary spermatocyte) has been emphasized, as blockage of transformation of gonocytes into adult dark spermatogonia would not be evident on total germ cell count until age 2, even though the defect occurs at the age of 2 months.[14]

Paternity rates following prepubertal therapy are 65% to 80% for unilateral cryptorchidism and 50% to 60% for bilateral cryptorchidism.[4] Paternity rates following orchiopexy may be inversely related to the age at surgery, although orchiopexy in older patients may be of benefit in the presence of azoospermia if normal sized testes are palpated in the inguinal canal.[61]

Adults with nonpalpable testes should undergo exploration and orchiectomy if under the age of 50 years, but the risk of exploration may outweigh the benefit of prevention of testicular malignancy in men over the age of 32.[2]

### Hormonal Manipulation

Early studies using hCG stimulation reported testicular descent in 47% of inguinal testes and 20% of intraabdominal testes, with response rates increasing with age possibly due to an age-related increment in Leydig cells.[9,62] Children younger than 2 years show a poor response to hCG stimulation.[6,63] Native and synthetic LHRH analogues have been reported from European centers but are unavailable in the United States. Intranasal administration of LHRH results in 1% to 2% of the dose reaching the systemic circulation.[62] Testicular descent in response to LHRH ranges from 22% to 60%, with 80% success if combinations of hCG and LHRH analogues were used.[9] The premise for combination therapy is that LHRH-stimulated increases in LH result in development of a larger population of juvenile Leydig cells for hCG to act on. Relapse rates have been reported as 15% at 6 months and 23% at 2 years.[9]

The criticisms of the above studies were addressed in randomized, blinded, placebo-controlled studies that documented the effectiveness of LHRH-analogue therapy in stimulating testicular descent in prepubertal boys, using intranasal buserelin (20 mg per day, 28 days) in combination with hCG (1500 IU intramuscular once a week for 3 weeks).[10,39] Success in stimulation of testicular descent for single agents, buserelin (28%) and hCG (10%), was surpassed with combination of both agents (38%). However, fewer patients treated with buserelin in this study had intraabdominal testes (8%) as compared with those treated with placebo or orchiopexy (16% and 14% respectively). Also, orchiopexy was avoided in only 20% of the patients treated with buserelin, 9% of the patients treated with HCG, and 32% of the patients treated with both medications.[39]

Independent studies support these findings, with testicular descent and improved germ cell quality being induced with LHRH (1.2 mg per day, 28 days) in 11% and combination of LHRH and hCG (500 IU 3×/week, 3 weeks) in 38%.[64] Similar studies report that the successful testicular descent with GnRH treatment (0–8%) and hCG (14%) was no better than with placebo controls (3–9%), suggesting that hormonal therapy is useless for undescended testes.[62,63,65] In addition, relapse rates are high, for 62% of testicles that descend after LHRH and 44% that descend with combination therapy will reascend after 7 years of follow-up.[2]

The gliding testis may represent the best candidate for hormonal treatment of maldescent. Hormonal stimulation may help identify the retractile testis that can be managed nonoperatively. Testicular descent in response to hormonal therapy may have positive prognostic implications on subsequent fertility, as response to hormonal stimulation correlates with higher germ cell counts and more normal epididymal development.[2,10,21] Evaluation of fertility following hormonal therapy with hCG has suggested no significant difference compared with primary orchiopexy.[62] Fertility rates are higher for patients cured with hCG therapy (74%) as compared with those undergoing orchiopexy, due to unresponsiveness to hCG (51%), although some of the responders may represent retractile testes.[62]

Preoperative buserelin has been reported to stimulate significant increases in vas deferens and spermatic cord length and vascularity, resulting in lower orchiectomy rates at the time of orchiopexy (5%) than in patients who did not receive preoperative buserelin (17%).[10,62] HCG therapy (3000 IU 2×/week for 4 weeks) may help identify the presence and position of the nonpalpable testis and increase the vascular distribution, resulting in a more lax vascular

supply.[2,66] These changes may obviate the need for a Fowler-Stephens procedure.

Buserelin may have additional benefits in stimulating testicular and epididymal maturation. A closed processus vaginalis and normal epididymal morphology were more frequently observed if buserelin succeeded in stimulating testicular descent (73% and 63%, respectively), as compared with patients treated primarily with orchiopexy (5% and 10%, respectively).[10] Hormonal therapy is postulated to stimulate testosterone secretion, inducing epididymal development.[10] A patent processus vaginalis after hormonal therapy indicates a severe form of cryptorchidism, with 90% having epididymal abnormalities, and 42% demonstrating azoospermia.[56]

Buserelin also resulted in a higher number and better maturation index of germ cells.[39] Normal germ cell counts were noted in 82% of patients treated with buserelin as compared with 48% of those treated with placebo or primary orchiopexy.[39] HCG did not demonstrate an additional effect on germ cell number or maturation.[39] These changes in germ cell counts are stable beyond 6 months after discontinuation of therapy.[2] LHRH stimulation resulted also in an increase in Leydig cell size and endoplasmic reticulum.[6]

If an early transient hypogonadotropic hypogonadism accounts for inhibition of gonocyte transformation and subsequent germinal atrophy, early hormonal replacement during the first 60 to 90 days of life may be needed to protect the fertility potential of cryptorchid patients. Stimulation of the transformations of the gonocyte to adult dark spermatogonia (age 2 to 3 months) and the adult dark spermatogonia to primary spermatocytes (age 3) may require supplementation with exogenous gonadotropins.[12,40]

## Role of Laparoscopy

Laparoscopy is the most sensitive and specific localizing test for the nonpalpable testis, with an accuracy of 88% to 100%.[2] Laparoscopy, used in the presence of an impalpable testis, will be diagnostic in 50% to 81% of the cases when an intraabdominal testis is present (9–

77%, pooled data 36%) or blind-ending spermatic vessels above the internal inguinal ring are identified (6–86%, pooled data 44%).[2,17,67] The wide variation in results reported in different studies can be accounted for by patient selection—primarily the mean age studied, percentage of bilateral cryptorchidism, and the percentage of patients pretreated by hormonal manipulation. Absence of a testis is most common in a unilaterally impalpable testis in a patient preselected by preoperative hCG or LHRH-analogue therapy.

Laparoscopy is diagnostic in 48% to 75% of bilateral cryptorchid patients (13–17% blind-ending vessels and 35–58% intraabdominal testis) compared with 43% to 53% of unilateral cryptorchid patients (27–34% blind-ending vessels, 16–19% intraabdominal testis).[17,67] An argument could be supported favoring initial inguinal exploration in patients with unilateral cryptorchidism, followed by laparoscopy if the pathology is not identified.

Laparoscopy can also be used therapeutically to perform one-stage orchiopexy or to clip ligation of the spermatic vessels as a first stage of a Fowler-Stephens procedure or orchiectomy.

## Orchiopexy Technique

Extensive mobilization of the vas deferens may exert an adverse effect on fertility. Depletion of germ cells with shedding of germinal epithelium and arrest of spermatogenesis proportional to the degree of mobilization has been demonstrated in experimental models.[68] Additionally, denervation of the adrenergic supply to the vas deferens may result in a functional obstruction of sperm transport not related to anatomical obstruction of the vas deferens or ischemia of the testis, epididymis, or vas deferens.[68]

Suture fixation of the testis through the tunica albuginea may stimulate secondary testicular atrophy due to severe inflammatory changes and granulomatous reactions elicited by the suture.[69–71] A nonsutured dartos pouch provides adequate fixation with circumferential adherence, as well as preservation of normal spermatogenesis (94%) and minimal focal tubular atrophy (23%).[70] If suture fixation is deemed necessary, the least reactive sutures are synthetic monofilaments, such as nylon and polypropylene.[71] A consensus exists that if suture fixation is performed it should be through the tunica vaginalis rather than the tunica albuginea, with suture preference ranging from chromic to Vicryl to permanent.[2]

Microvascular and radiographic studies demonstrate the absence of adequate collateralization to perform a Fowler-Stephens orchiopexy in 13% of cases.[6] Testicular autotransplantation may improve results in a patient with a high undescended testis that may have inadequate collateral blood supply for a traditional Fowler-Stephens procedure.[2,70] Success rates after microvascular autotransplantation exceed 80%, compared with 50% to 80% for the conventional Fowler-Stephens procedure.[2] The testicular vessels are ligated near their origins, the testis mobilized on a wide strip of peritoneum, and a subdartos orchiopexy performed. An end-to-end microvascular anastomosis is then performed between the inferior epigastric vessels and the testicular vessels.[72] Palpable testes have been demonstrated in 96% of these patients, compared with an average reported success rate of 73% for a traditional Fowler-Stephens procedure. Histologic studies demonstrate Leydig cell development and preservation of germinal epithelium and tubular diameter with this technique.[72]

If the testis cannot be positioned in the scrotum at the time of orchiopexy, it can be wrapped in Silastic mesh for reexploration in 1 year, which will usually allow advancement into the scrotum.[9] If blind-ending vessels are encountered in the inguinal canal, the remnant nubbin should be excised, for viable germ cell tissue will be present in 6% to 13%.[2]

## Results with Medical Management of Oligospermia in Cryptorchid Patients

Few studies compare the results of empiric medical therapy of oligospermia based on cause within subsets of patients. One pharmacologic intervention studied is gonadotropin supplementation in patients with idiopathic hypogonadotropic hypogonadism (IHH). In clinical applications, human menopausal gonadotropin (hMG) simulates the biologic role of FSH, and hCG simulates the biologic role of LH.

Finkel et al[73] demonstrated that hCG alone was effective in treating oligospermia in men with postpubertal onset of IHH. The addition of hMG was required to improve sperm count in prepubertal IHH, but this combination therapy was not efficacious if a history of cryptorchidism existed. Cryptorchidism decreased the response rate to 17%.[74] Testicular response to hMG and hCG is attenuated in postpubertal IHH patients with a history of cryptorchidism, as evidenced by decreased improvement in testicular volume and spermatogenesis when compared with IHH patients without a history of cryptorchidism.[73] An initial testicular volume of less than 4 ml is a poor prognostic indicator of initiation of spermatogenesis with hormonal stimulation.[75] Other studies have demonstrated that spermatogenesis was stimulated in four of five men with oligospermia associated with cryptorchidism with the use of subcutaneous hMG (37.5 IU twice daily) and intramuscular hCG (5000–10,000 IU weekly, dose titrated to serum testosterone).[76] Pregnancies resulted from this therapy.

## Conclusion

Outcome analysis following surgery or hormonal manipulation is clouded, because the cryptorchid testis may be a dysgenetic organ and inherent defects may be irreversible. Also, abnormalities in epididymal structure and function may lead to subfertility even in the presence of adequate spermatogenesis. The only certainty is that the postpubertal cryptorchid testis will not produce sperm. Until more is known about the pathogenesis and optimal management of this condition, hormonal stimulation of spermatogenesis and assisted reproductive technology will continue their roles in the management of infertility.

Preservation of fertility relies on early orchiopexy, possibly with adjuvant hormonal stimulation, especially in cases of maturational delay of the testis and epididymis. Early hormonal stimulation to induce transformations of the gonocyte to adult dark spermatogonia to the primary spermatocyte may be necessary between the third month and third year of life. The key to increased knowledge of cryptorchidism is a long-term, critical evaluation of today's children who are undergoing early orchiopexy and hormonal stimulation.

## References

1. Hunter JA. A description of the situation of the testis in the fetus with its descent into the scrotum. In: Haswell JJ, ed. *Observations on Certain Parts of the Animal Economy.* New Orleans: 1841.
2. Rozanski TA, Bloom DA. The undescended testis: theory and management. *Urol Clin North Am* 1995; 22:107–118.
3. Hadziselimovic F. Examination and clinical findings in cryptorchid boys. In: Hadziselimovic F, ed. *Cryptorchidism, Management and Implications.* Berlin: Springer-Verlag; 1983; chapter 8.
4. Thompson ST. Preventable causes of male infertility. *World J Urol* 1993; 11:111–119.
5. Lee PA. Fertility in cryptorchidism: does treatment make a difference? *Endocrinol Metab Clin North Am* 1993; 22:479–490.
6. Gill B, Palmer LS. Cryptorchidism: the data to support early repair. *Probl Urol* 1994; 8:518–532.
7. Gracia J, Gonzalez N, Gomez ME, et al. Clinical and anatomopathological study of 2000 cryptorchid testes. *Br J Urol* 1995; 75:697–701.
8. Cendron M, Huff DS, Keating MA, et al. Anatomical morphological and volumetric analysis: a review of 759 cases of testicular maldescent. *J Urol* 1993; 149:570–573.
9. Palmer JM. The undescended testicle. *Endocrinol Metab Clin North Am* 1991; 20:231–240.
10. Bica DTG, Hadziselimovic F. The behavior of epididymis, processus vaginalis and testicular descent in cryptorchid boys treated with buserelin. *Eur J Pediatr* 1993; 152(suppl 2): S38–42.
11. Hutson JM, Beasley SW. Embryological controversies in testicular descent. *Semin Urol* 1988; 6:68–73.
12. Huff DS, Hadziselimovic F, Snyder HM, et al. Early postnatal testicular maldevelopment in cryptorchidism. *J Urol* 1991; 146:624–626.
13. Hadziselimovic F, Herzog B, Huff DS, et al. The morphometric histopathology of undescended

testes and testes associated with incarcerated inguinal hernia: a comparative study. *J Urol* 1991; 146:627–629.

14. Huff DS, Hadziselimovic F, Snyder HM, et al. Histologic maldevelopment of unilaterally cryptorchid testes and their descended partners. *Eur J Pediatr* 1993; 152(suppl 2):S-11–14.

15. Husmann DA, Boone TB, McPhaul MJ. Flutamide-induced testicular undescent in the rat is associated with alterations in genitofemoral nerve morphology. *J Urol* 1994; 151:509–513.

16. Patkowski D, Czernik J, Jelen M. Division of the genitofemoral nerve in unilateral cryptorchid rats. *J Pediatr Surg* 1994; 29:832–835.

17. Cortes D, Thorup JM, Lenz K, et al. Laparoscopy in 100 consecutive patients with 128 impalpable testes. *Br J Urol* 1995; 75:281–287.

18. Turek PJ, Ewalt DH, Snyder HM, et al. The absent cryptorchid testis: surgical findings and their implications for diagnosis and etiology. *J Urol* 1994; 151:718–721.

19. Huff DS, Wu HY, Snyder HM, et al. Evidence in favor of the mechanical (intrauterine torsion) theory over the endocrinopathy (cryptorchidism) theory in the pathogenesis of testicular agenesis. *J Urol* 1991; 146:630–631.

20. Mieusset R, Bujan L, Massat G, et al. Clinical and biological characteristics of infertile men with a history of cryptorchidism. *Hum Reprod* 1995; 10:613–619.

21. Roth DR, Lipshultz LI. Overview of cryptorchidism with emphasis on the human. In: Abney TO, Keel BA. eds. *The Cryptorchid Testis.* Boca Raton, FL: CRC Press; 1989: 1–14.

22. Koff SA. Does compensatory testicular enlargement predict monorchism? *J Urol* 1991; 146:632–633.

23. Tellaloglu S, Kadioglu A, Kilicaslan I, et al. Cryptorchidism: is orchidopexy always preventive treatment for infertility. *Acta Chir Hungarica* 1994; 34:195–201.

24. Urry RL, Carrell DT, Starr NT, et al. The incidence of antisperm antibodies in infertility patients with a history of cryptorchidism. *J Urol* 1994; 151:381–383.

25. Keel BA, Abney TO. Cryptorchid-induced changes in spermatogenesis and fertility. In: Abney TO, Keel BA, eds. *The Cryptorchid Testis.* Boca Raton, FL: CRC Press; 1989: 161–170.

26. Patkowski D, Czernik J, Jelen M. The natural course of cryptorchidism in rats and efficacy of orchidopexy or orchiedectomy in its treatment

before and after puberty. *J Pediatr Surg* 1992; 27:870–873.

27. Kawakami E, Tsutsui T, Saito S, et al. Changes in peripheral plasma lutenizing hormone and testosterone concentrations and semen quality in normal and cryptorchid dogs during sexual maturation. *Lab Anim Sci* 1995; 45:258–263.

28. Jockenhovel F, Swerdloff RS. Alterations in the steroidogenic capacity of Leydig cells in the cryptorchid testis. In: Abney TO, Keel BA, eds. *The Cryptorchid Testis.* Boca Raton, FL: CRC Press; 1989: 35–54.

29. Grasso M, Buonaguidi A, Lania C, et al. Postpubertal cryptorchidism: review and evaluation of the fertility. *Eur Urol* 1991; 20:126–128.

30. Okuyama A, Nonomura N, Nakamura M. Surgical management of undescended testis: retrospective study of potential fertility in 274 cases. *J Urol* 1989; 142:749–751.

31. Yavetz H, Harash B, Paz G, et al. Cryptorchidism: incidence and sperm quality in infertile men. *Andrologia* 1992; 24:293–297.

32. Chilvers C, Dudley NE, Gough MH, et al. Undescended testis: the effect of treatment on subsequent risk of subfertility and malignancy. *J Pediatr Surg* 1986; 21:691–696.

33. Foresta C, Zorzi M, Rossato M, et al. Sperm nuclear instability and staining with aniline blue: abnormal persistence of histones in spermatozoa in infertile men. *Int J Androl* 1992; 15:330–337.

34. Puri P, O'Donnell B. Semen analysis of patients who had orchiopexy at or after seven years of age. *Lancet* 1988; 2:1051–1052.

35. Lee PA, Bellinger MF, Songer NJ, et al. An epidemiologic study of paternity after cryptorchidism: initial results. *Eur J Pediatr* 1993; 152(suppl 2):S-25–27.

36. Fallon B, Kennedy TJ. Long-term follow-up of fertility in cryptorchid patients. *Urology* 1985; 25:502–504.

37. Gilhooly PE, Meyers F, Lattimer JK. Fertility prospects for children with cryptorchidism. *Am J Dis Child* 1984; 138:940–943.

38. Codesal J, Paniagua R, Queizan A, et al. Cytophotometric DNA quantification in human spermatogonia of cryptorchid testes. *J Urol* 1993; 149:382–385.

39. Bica DTG, Hadziselimovic F. Buserelin treatment of cryptorchidism: a randomized double-blind, placebo-controlled study. *J Urol* 1992; 148:617–621.

40. Huff DS, Hadziselimovic F, Snyder HM, et al. Postnatal testicular maldevelopment in unilateral cryptorchidism. *J Urol* 1989; 142:546–548.

41. Zhou B, Hutson JM. Human chorionic gonadotropin (hCG) fails to stimulate gonocyte differentiation in newborn mouse testes in organ culture. *J Urol* 1995; 153:501–505.

42. Haneji T, Nishimune Y. Hormones and the differentiation of type-A spermatogonia in mouse cryptorchid testes incubated in vitro. *J Endocrinol* 1982; 94:43–50.

43. Yamanaka J, Baker ML, Metcalfe SA, et al. Serum levels of müllerian-inhibiting substance in boys with cryptorchidism. *J Pediatr Surg* 1991; 26:621–623.

44. Tarter TH, Kogan SJ. Contralateral testicular disease after unilateral testicular injury: current concepts. *Semin Urol* 1988; 6:120–139.

45. Mininberg DT. Histopathology of the undescended testis. *Semin Urol* 1988; 6:74–78.

46. Foresta C, Indino M, Mioni R, et al. Evidence of sperm nuclear chromatin heterogeneity in excryptorchid subjects. *Andrologia* 1987; 19:148–152.

47. Gaudio E, Paggiarino D, Carpino F. Structural and ultrastructural modifications of cryptorchid human testes. *J Urol* 1984; 131:292–296.

48. Abney TO, Keel BA. Influence of cryptorchidism on Leydig cell function. In: Abney TO, Keel BA, eds. *The Cryptorchid Testis.* Boca Raton, FL: CRC Press; 1989; 93–118.

49. De Kretser DM, Risbridger GP. Changes in Sertoli cell structure and functions. In: Abney TO, Keel BA, eds. *The Cryptorchid Testis.* Boca Raton, FL: CRC Press; 1989: 119–132.

50. Hadziselimovic F. Histology and ultrastructure of normal and cryptorchid testes. In: Hadziselimovic F, ed. *Cryptorchidism, Management and Implications.* Berlin: Springer-Verlag; 1983: 35.

51. Gotoh M, Miyake K, Mitsuya H. Alterations in Leydig cell morphology. In: Abney TO, Keel BA, eds. *The Cryptorchid Testis.* Boca Raton, FL: CRC Press; 1989: 71–92.

52. Mieusset R, Fouda PJ, Vaysse P, et al. Increase in testicular temperature in case of cryptorchidism in boys. *Fertil Steril* 1993; 59:1319–1321.

53. Lenzi A, Gandini L, Lombardo F. Antisperm antibodies in young boys. *Andrologia* 1991; 23:233–235.

54. Mininberg DT, Chen ME, Witkin SS. Antisperm antibodies in cryptorchid boys. *Eur J Pediatr* 1993; 152(suppl 2):S-23–24.

55. Mollaeian M, Mehrabi V, Elahi B. Significance of epididymal and ductal anomalies associated with undescended testis: study in 652 cases. *Urology* 1994; 43:857–860.

56. Herzog B, Rosslein R, Hadziselimovic F. The role of the processus vaginalis in cryptorchidism. *Eur J Pediatr* 1993; 152(suppl 2):S-15–16.

57. Bedford JM. Effects of elevated temperature on the epididymis and testis: experimental studies. *Adv Exp Med Biol* 1991; 286:19–32.

58. Imthurn T, Hadziselimovic F, Herzog B. Impaired germ cells in secondary cryptorchid testis after herniotomy. *J Urol* 1995; 153:780–781.

59. Hadziselimovic F. Cryptorchidism. Ultrastructure of normal and cryptorchid testis development. *Adv Anat Embryol Cell Biol* 1977; 53:3–71.

60. Knecht H. Tubular structure and germ cell distribution of cryptorchid or normal testes in early childhood. *Beitr Pathol* 1976; 159:249–270.

61. Heaton ND, Davenport M, Pryor JP. Fertility after correction of bilateral undescended testes at the age of 23 years. *Br J Urol* 1993; 71:490–491.

62. DeMuinck Deiser-Schrama SMPF, Hazebroek FWJ. Hormonal treatment of cryptorchidism: role of pituitary gonadal axis. *Semin Urol* 1988; 6:84–95.

63. DeMuinck Keiser-Schrama SMPF, Hazebroek FWJ, Matroos AW, et al. Double-blind placebo controlled study of luteinizing-hormone-releasing-hormone nasal spray in treatment of undescended testes. *Lancet* 1986; 1:876–880.

64. Lala R, Matarazzo P, Chiabotto P, et al. Combined therapy with LHRH and HCG in cryptorchid infants. *Eur J Pediatr* 1993; 152(suppl 2):S-31–33.

65. Christiansen P, Muller J, Buhl S, et al. Treatment of cryptorchidism with human gonadotropin or gonadotropin-releasing hormone. A double-blind controlled study of 243 boys. *Horm Res* 1988; 30:187–192.

66. Gearhart JP, Jeffs RD. Diagnostic maneuvers in cryptorchidism. *Semin Urol* 1988; 6:79–83.

67. Diamond DA, Caldamone AA. The value of laparoscopy for 106 impalpable testes relative to clinical presentation. *J Urol* 1992; 148:632–634.

68. Smith EM, Dahms BB, Elder JS. Influence of vas deferens mobilization on rat fertility: implications regarding orchiopexy. *J Urol* 1993; 150:663–666.

69. Bergh A. Experimental models of cryptorchidism. In: Abney TO, Keel BA, eds. *The Cryptorchid Testis.* Boca Raton, FL: CRC Press; 1989: 15–34.

70. Bukowski TP, Wacksman J, Billmire DA, et al. Testicular autotransplantation: a 17-year review of an effective approach to the management of the intraabdominal testis. *J Urol* 1995; 154:558–561.

71. Bellinger MF, Abramowitz HB, Brantley S, et al. Orchiopexy: an experimental study of the effect of surgical technique on testicular histology. *J Urol* 1989; 142:553–555.

72. MacMahon RA, O'Brien BM, Aberdeen J, et al. Results of the use of autotransplantation of the intraabdominal testis using microsurgical vascular anastomosis. *J Pediatr Surg* 1980; 15:92–96.

73. Finkel DM, Phillips JL, Snyder PJ. Stimulation of spermatogenesis by gonadotropins in men with hypogonadotropic hypogonadism. *N Engl J Med* 1985; 313:651–655.

74. McLachlan RI, Finkel DM, Bremner WJ, et al. Serum inhibin concentrations before and during gonadotropin treatment in men with hypogonadotropic hypogonadism: physiological and clinical implications. *J Clin Endocrinol Metab* 1990; 70:1414–1419.

75. Kirk JMW, Savage MO, Grant DB, et al. Gonadal function and response to human chorionic and menopausal gonadotrophin therapy in male patients with idiopathic hypogonadotropic hypogonadism. *Clin Endocrinol* 1994; 41:57–63.

76. Jones TH, Darne JF. Self-administered subcutaneous human menopausal gonadotrophin for the stimulation of testicular growth and initiation of spermatogenesis in hypogonadotrophic hypogonadism. *Clin Endocrinol* 1993; 38:203–208.

# 22
# The Effects of Testicular Torsion on Fertility

Manoj Monga and Wayne J.G. Hellstrom

Testicular torsion occurs primarily in either the neonatal or the adolescent period of life. The yearly incidence of testicular torsion in men under 25 years of age is 1 in 4000, but the overall risk of developing a testicular torsion by age 25 is 1 in 160. Because the overall risk is so high, the potential to impact the fertility of many young men is great.[1,2] Neonatal torsion, which accounts for only 17% of testicular torsion, involves torsion of the testicle and surrounding tunica vaginalis (extravaginal torsion) and will not be discussed further in this chapter. In the intravaginal (postnatal) form of testicular torsion, the mechanism of injury involves contraction of the cremasteric fibers, which causes a rotatory force on the testicle around the axis of the spermatic cord while surrounded by a high-inserting tunica vaginalis.[3,4] This condition more commonly involves the left testicle.[4] The two peak incidences for intravaginal testicular torsion are ages 1 to 5 and 11 to 15.[4] Seasonal variations in occurrence of torsion favor the colder months.[4,5]

Testicular torsion is a true urologic emergency, requiring prompt diagnosis and surgical intervention. Testicular torsion, or torsion of the spermatic cord, causes compression of the spermatic vessels and impairs testicular blood flow. Preservation of testicular function requires timely detorsion and orchiopexy. Numerous clinical studies and animal investigations have attempted to elucidate the pathogenesis of testicular injury and long-term testicular dysfunction following testicular torsion, but the treatment of testicular torsion has remained relatively unchanged.

The standard of care dictates detorsion and contralateral orchiopexy within 6 hours of onset of symptoms, with orchiectomy if the testicle appears nonviable. Viability of the testicle is assessed by gross appearance or by demonstration of perfusion by incising the tunica albuginea.[1,3] Detorsion within 6 to 10 hours increases the chance of salvage but does not guarantee preservation of function.[6] Testicular injury may result from hypoxia during torsion or reperfusion injury following detorsion.[6]

Recent advances in imaging studies have improved early diagnosis and management of testicular torsion. The nuclear testicular scan remains the best preoperative test, with an accuracy of 88% or greater in diagnosing torsion.[3] Color-flow Doppler imaging can be equally successful in detecting absent perfusion (540° torsion) and even more sensitive in detecting reduced testicular flow due to a lesser degree of twisting (360° torsion).[7] Doppler contrast agents and power Doppler technology can improve the accuracy of this test.[7]

Despite prompt management, testicular torsion remains a known risk factor for infertility. This places testicular torsion in the cauldron of unilateral pathologies that mysteriously cause detriment to the contralateral testicle and lead to impaired spermatogenesis. Decreased sperm concentrations and increased follicle-stimulating hormone (FSH) levels have been demonstrated in men with loss of one testicle because of cryptorchidism, torsion, testicular cancer, or iatrogenic injury during herniorraphy, with no significant differences between groups based on etiology.[8]

# Clinical Studies

Clinical studies of testicular torsion have evaluated atrophy rates, fertility rates, histologic characteristics of the ipsilateral and contralateral testes, and evidence supporting an autoimmune phenomenon. Most studies agree that prepubertal men who experience torsion preserve fertility regardless of treatment modality, but postpubertal men are at greater risk for subsequent infertility, a risk correlated with duration of torsion.[9,10] Many studies combine prepubertal and postpubertal populations, which can produce variable results. Additionally, definitions of testicular atrophy and normal semen parameters may vary.[11] Histologic studies also vary in grading systems and techniques, with evaluations of semisections providing better testicular morphologic detail than paraffin embedment.[12,13] Some dysplastic lesions require ultrastructural histologic techniques, such as electron microscopy or semithin sectioning, for visualization.[14]

## Testicular Atrophy

The rate of secondary testicular atrophy following detorsion and orchiopexy may be as high as 68%.[15] A positive correlation between duration of torsion and percentage of atrophy has been demonstrated, because treatment delayed longer than 8 hours significantly increases the risk of testicular atrophy.[11,16] Long-term follow-up studies indicate a significant secondary atrophy rate if the duration of torsion exceeds 24 hours.[17] Torsion of less than 360° for up to 12 hours' duration is better tolerated.[17]

## Subfertility

The effect of testicular torsion on spermatogenesis was first documented in 1978 by Krarup,[15] who found a normal semen analysis on follow-up in only 1 of 19 patients. Up to 50% to 87% of men may experience abnormalities on semen analysis following unilateral torsion.[14,16,18,19] Abnormalities on semen analysis at long-term follow-up may include oligospermia (35–57% of patients), asthenospermia (53–56%), and abnormal morphology (39–69%).[8,14,20,21] Dimin-

ished paternity rates following unilateral testicular torsion have also been reported.[18,21]

Following testicular torsion, elevated luteinizing hormone (LH) and FSH levels may be present in subfertile men.[10,11,16,19,22] Anderson et al[22,23] found elevated FSH levels in 40% of patients with oligozoospermia. A supranormal response of FSH to human chorionic gonadotropin (HCG) stimulation has been seen in patients following unilateral testicular torsion.[10,18,21,23,24] This response correlates with the degree of oligospermia and reflects the abnormal spermatogenesis present in these patients.

Duration of torsion may correlate with the degree of abnormalities found on semen analysis and hormonal analysis, and fertility may be preserved in patients with early detorsion when compared with those who present late and require orchiectomy.[10,11,15,18] FSH levels were elevated in 22% of patients who underwent detorsion and orchiopexy, compared with 71% with delayed diagnosis and orchiectomy.[10] Other reports, however, have indicated no superiority in semen parameters of patients who underwent early detorsion and orchiopexy, and in the preservation of normal semen analyses for those who presented late and underwent orchiectomy.[16,21,23] Some reports dispute the deleterious effects of torsion on spermatogenesis and fertility.[9]

## Histologic Examination

Nistal et al[25] evaluated 109 biopsy and orchiectomy specimens from the acutely torsed testicles of postpubertal males and found that primary lesions, such as focal hypospermatogenesis, intratubular calcification, and Sertoli-cell–only tubules, were superimposed on lesions secondary to anoxia in only 14%.

Horica et al[26] reported preexisting testicular abnormalities in the contralateral testis of 7 of 7 patients with acute testicular torsion, and suggested these may represent congenital dysplasia or damage from recurrent intermittent testicular torsion. Hadziselimovic et al[13] reported preexisting testicular abnormalities ranging from abnormal spermatogenesis to Sertoli-cell–only syndrome in 53% of the contralateral testis by biopsy at time of unilateral torsion. In this report, the ratio of spermatogonia to seminiferous tubule was reduced in prepubertal boys, and in postpubertal men the number of late spermatids was diminished. Anderson et al[22,23] reported similar preexisting abnormalities in the contralateral testis of 57% to 65% of patients, finding evidence of partial maturation arrest in spermatogenesis (mainly in the late spermatid stage), which correlated well with subsequent oligospermia. All patients with normal contralateral histology had normal sperm concentrations on follow-up. Laor et al[27] reported maturational arrest, germ cell degeneration, tubular hyalinization, immature tubules, and focal basement membrane thickening in the contralateral testicle of 60% of patients. Hagen et al[14] reported preexisting congenital testicular dysplasia in 88% of contralateral testes biopsied at the time of torsion in 34 pubertal and postpubertal men. Other studies have reported contralateral histologic abnormalities only if duration of torsion exceeds 5 hours, suggestive of an acquired cause resulting from prolonged ipsilateral ischemia.[28]

Dominguez et al[12] evaluated testicular histology in the normal testis after prepubertal testicular torsion caused subsequent atrophy of the affected testis. He noted in 62.5% of the patients a range of germinal hypoplasia as graded by fertility tubular index, Sertoli cell index, and minimum tubular diameter. Although this study confirmed abnormal contralateral testicular histology, it is not possible to conclude whether these changes were a consequence of a congenital testicular dysgenesis or secondary to the effects of the contralateral torsion.

Two explanations proposed for the above histologic findings are a preexisting congenital testicular dysplasia or an acquired testicular defect because of the cumulative effects of repeated episodes of ischemia induced by subacute torsion.[20,29] Both testes may be progressively damaged by recurrent transient torsion, because the anatomical abnormality of the high tunica vaginalis insertion that predisposes to torsion is bilateral in most patients, and one third of these patients have a history of previous attacks of testicular pain.[2,20]

## Autoimmunization

The testis is an immunoprotected site, with multiple tight junctions between the Sertoli cells creating the blood-testis barrier that protects the luminal compartment and the germinal epithelium. Disruption of this barrier by the ischemic trauma of testicular torsion may lead to autosensitization of sperm and testis antigens.[20,30]

There is no strong evidence for induction of antisperm or antitesticular antibodies as the cause for subfertility or contralateral damage, for only 0% to 9% of patients have antisperm antibodies or sperm agglutinating and sperm-immobilizing activity in the seminal plasma or serum.[10,11,14,20-23] In long-term follow-up of patients with nonviable testes not removed during prepubertal torsion, Puri et al[9] did not document any evidence of sperm autoantibodies. They concluded that for autoimmunity to occur, there must be prior exposure of the host-to-sperm antigens, which does not occur until the onset of spermatogenesis at puberty. Zanchetta et al[31] reported an incidence of antisperm or antitesticular antibodies of only 18% in patients after testicular torsion. Sperm agglutinating and sperm-immobilizing activity were found in 22% of the sera from these patients.

Thomas et al[32] reported antisperm or antitesticular antibodies in eight of nine patients with torsion of greater than 6 hours' duration, and patients who underwent prompt orchiopexy or orchiectomy did not develop autoantibodies.

## Experimental Models

Contradictory findings may be related to differences in qualitative evaluations and experimental design.[3] Variables include animal species and strain, age of sexual development, and degree and duration of the torsion as well as timing of detorsion, orchiectomy, and outcome evaluation.

### Animal Selection

Becker and Turner[33] demonstrated that ipsilateral damage to testicular endocrine and exocrine function following testicular torsion requires a longer duration of ischemia to manifest in the prepubertal rat than in the adult counterpart. The effects of testicular torsion on the contralateral testicle may be different in preadolescent and adult animal models, and spermatogenesis in the prepubertal contralateral testicle may be more sensitive to the effects of ischemia than the postpubertal testicle.[33]

Testicular torsion in the rat, guinea pig, mouse, hamster, dog, and rabbit has been studied.[29] Even within species, there may be variability in the immunopathologic sequelae, based on the strain studied. For example, the Sprague-Dawley rat is considered a "low responder" strain with regard to antisperm antibody production. Using identical experimental designs, no evidence of antisperm antibody production or contralateral damage was identified in the Sprague-Dawley rat, but significant antisperm antibody titers and decreased contralateral seminiferous tubular diameter were identified in the Lewis and brown Norway inbred rat.[29]

### Experimental Technique

Experimental torsion does not result in complete absence of testicular blood flow. Torsion of 720° results in a reduction in testicular blood flow to 3% to 16% of control values, with variation within and between species accounting for the range of values.[6,34] This reduction in blood flow is highly variable, with up to 60% of animals showing no change in intraparenchymal blood flow as evidenced by dynamic enhanced magnetic resonance imaging (MRI) scan.[35] Sonda[36] demonstrated that torsion of 1080° to 1440° resulted in necrosis within several hours, a turn of 360° resulted in necrosis in 24 hours, and a half-turn of 180° resulted in necrosis in only 50% of testes at 48 hours. Becker and Turner[33] demonstrated no decrease in testis weight or daily sperm production in adult or prepubertal rats after 360° torsion of 4 hours' duration. Other variables affecting degree of ischemia include length and thickness of the spermatic cord and arterial and venous occlusion pressure.[35]

Toxic agents may be spread by way of the testicular circulation, because the effects on the contralateral testis may be observed only after experimental torsion, not after simple ligation of the testicular artery.[37] Ligation of the spermatic cord may not allow for autosensitization to sperm and testicular antigens.[9] This observation is supported by clinical success with procedures that ligate the spermatic vessels, such as the Palomo procedure for varicocele repair and the Fowler-Stephens orchiopexy.[38]

The surgical approach used may affect the ipsilateral or contralateral testicle. Becker and Turner[33] recommend a low abdominal approach to create experimental torsion, as scrotal surgery may cause a generalized inflammatory reaction that could affect the contralateral testis.

### Limitations

Experimental models are limited in how closely they can approximate the clinical entity. They cannot account for subclinical insults to the ipsilateral and contralateral testes that may occur prior to the clinical presentation as an acute torsion, because preexisting acquired or congenital abnormalities in ipsilateral or contralateral testes that are predisposed to torsion would not be present in the experimental model.

# Effects on Spermatogenesis

## Preadolescent Animal Models

### Ipsilateral and Contralateral Effects

Blank et al[39] demonstrated preservation of ipsilateral tubular and germinal cell architecture after a 6-hour torsion in the prepubertal rat; however, a 12-hour torsion resulted in significant degeneration. Costentino et al[40-42] demonstrated, histologically, a significant contralateral effect of ipsilateral testicular torsion in prepubertal rats (age 35 to 50 days), with significant effects on fertility, but only if the torsed testis was left untreated for 9 to 12 hours, suggesting that immunologic phenomena may account for the contralateral effect. Following testicular torsion with no intervention in prepubertal rats, Kamada et al[43] demonstrated decreased contralateral mean seminiferous tubular diameter, decreased percentage of haploid cells by flow cytometric DNA analysis, and decreased fertility rates. Becker and Turner[33] did not note any detrimental effects on the contralateral prepubertal testis after a 4-hour torsion, and they demonstrated that the ipsilateral prepubertal testis may be more refractory to short periods of ischemia (1 hour or less); however, after 2-hour and 4-hour torsion, testicular damage was similar to that seen in the adult rat model.

## Autoimmunization

Other studies of detorsion suggest there is no increased immunoactivity in the contralateral testis and no contralateral tubular damage. Normal contralateral testicular development, normal spermatogenesis, and fertility were noted after detorsion in prepubertal hamsters, suggesting that the lack of an immune response may be due to absence of mature spermatozoa.[44–46] Kogan[47] demonstrated no contralateral damage or increased lymphocytotoxic antibodies and active spermatogenesis in rats that had undergone prepubertal torsion, concluding that immature spermatogenic elements were not immunogenic.

## Reperfusion Injury

Saba et al[48] demonstrated that a 2-hour testicular torsion followed by detorsion results in a time-dependent reperfusion injury to the contralateral testis that is refractory to antioxidant therapy at the time of detorsion. Blank et al[39] demonstrated a significant reperfusion injury that was not mediated by iron-catalyzed hydroxyl radical formation or alterations in calcium homeostasis. In this study, histologic changes after 6-hour torsion correlated with duration of reperfusion. After greater than 12-hour torsion, histologic changes were more consistent with ischemic injury than with reperfusion injury, as demonstrated by disruption of the tubular basement membranes and loss of germinal cell cohesiveness with maintenance of nuclear chromatin and intracellular organization.

# Adult Animal Models

## Ipsilateral Effects

### Ischemic Injury

In 1955 Smith[49] demonstrated that spermatogonia were damaged after only 2 hours of torsion-induced ischemia and were eliminated after 6 hours of ischemia. Oettle and Harrison[50] demonstrated that testicular ischemia of increasing duration is associated with increasing severity of testicular damage, with minor effects on the seminiferous tubules resulting after only 10 minutes of ischemia. Carroll et al[51] performed DNA flow cytometric analysis on testicular fine needle aspirates to show that critical ipsilateral testicular ischemia occurred with increasing severity after 1 hour of torsion. Contralateral hypospermatogenesis did not appear to be a time-dependent phenomenon.

Intratesticular oxygen pressure measurements using polarographic microcatheter probes have demonstrated a significant ipsilateral drop in pressure within 5 minutes of a 720° torsion, with normalization within 25 minutes following detorsion.[52] There was no change in contralateral intratesticular oxygen pressures. Testicular blood flow following detorsion returns to normal within 1 hour, as revealed by dynamic enhanced MRI.[35] Testicular blood flow does not return to normal if torsion lasts longer than 4 hours.[53]

Bergh et al[54] and others[41,55] demonstrated a significant reduction in testicular weight after 1 hour of testicular ischemia, due to a decrease in total epithelial mass of the seminiferous tubule. The numbers of B-type spermatogonia and preleptotene and leptotene spermatocytes were most significantly reduced after 100 minutes of ischemia.[54] Turner and Brown[6] demonstrated that testicular torsion of 1 hour's duration affects testicular weight, microvasculature, histology, and daily sperm production even though bilateral testicular blood flow returns to baseline within 4 hours after detorsion. Testicular torsion of 30 minutes' duration does not significantly affect these parameters.[6,33] Seminiferous tubules are virtually depleted after a 1-hour torsion, with progressive damage following increased duration of torsion.[33] As testicular blood flow is restored by detorsion of the testicle, damage to the seminiferous epithelium results from either the initial short period of ischemia or the release of free radical oxygen species during reperfusion. Alternatively, a reactive hyperemia following detorsion may lead to an increase in oxygen tension and may cause degenerative changes in the oxygen-sensitive seminiferous epithelium.[54,56]

Carmignani et al[55] demonstrated that intravenous inosine treatment prevents the morphologic changes associated with short-term torsion, suggesting that testicular damage is related to ischemia-induced adenine nucleotide degradation.

### Reperfusion Injury

Bergh et al[54] demonstrated no protective effect from subsequent ipsilateral testicular damage when using the free oxygen radical scavengers superoxide dismutase and catalase, suggesting that reperfusion injury by oxygen radicals is an unlikely source of testicular damage. The low intratesticular temperature and oxygen tension may have provided protection from reperfusion-induced lipid peroxidation. However, this study utilized testicular artery ligation that results in global ischemia, but testicular damage due to partial ischemia from testicular torsion may depend more on reperfusion injury and be more responsive to free radical scavengers.[57]

When testicles are detorsed within 6 hours of torsion, reperfusion injury plays a significant role in damage. After 6 hours of torsion, the effects of ischemic injury predominate.[57–59] Akgur et al[58] demonstrated significant ipsilateral reperfusion injury following detorsion of 1- and 2-hour torsions. In another study, the administration of polyethylene glycol-superoxide dismutase 1 hour prior to detorsion of a 3-hour torsion did not alleviate the gross histologic damage noted 2 weeks later in the ipsilateral testicle.[60] The administration of allopurinol (a xanthase oxidase inhibitor) 30 minutes prior to detorsion can prevent the increase in ipsilateral reperfusion injury following detorsion if performed within 5 hours of torsion.[59] Akhter et al[61] demonstrated prevention of reperfusion injury by pretreatment with heparin, oxypurinol, and polyethylene glycol-superoxide dismutase when detorsion is performed within 4 hours of torsion.

## Contralateral Effects

### Evidence

Neither Turner et al[6,33,53,62] nor Costentino's group[40] have demonstrated contralateral effects of ipsilateral testicular torsion in adult animal models. In these studies, contralateral testis histology and weight, daily sperm production, epididymal sperm concentrations and motility, and testicular blood flow were not affected by ipsilateral torsion. Likewise, quantitative morphometry did not demonstrate any contralateral testicular damage 2 months after torsion or ligation of the testicular artery despite a 50% decrease in sperm concentration.[54,63,64] Numerous other investigators, using adult rat and guinea pig models, have demonstrated reversible contralateral tubular damage, spermatid and spermatocyte degeneration, and elimination of germ cells following ipsilateral torsion or testicular artery ligation. These findings have been associated with an increase in circulating antitesticular antibodies and alterations in the specificity of antibody binding to normal control testis and contralateral testis.[65–68] Some investigators found that impaired spermatogenesis and seminiferous tubular atrophy were reversible with time.[69]

### Autoimmunization

Harrison et al[66] demonstrated that an increase in cytotoxic antisperm antibodies as well as antibody deposition in the contralateral testis could be reproduced in normal animals by allografting of an ischemic testis or by injection of an ischemic testis homogenate. Kogan[47] demonstrated increased lymphocytotoxic antibody titers following adult rat torsion, which could be prevented by pretreatment with corticosteroids. Kearney et al[70] prevented autosensitization in the rat by the administration of adrenocorticotropic hormone. As reported by Anderson and Williamson,[20] immediate orchiectomy in lieu of detorsion or delayed orchiectomy may prevent formation of spermagglutinating antibodies. Other investigators, although documenting contralateral testis damage, have not indicated production of antisperm antibodies nor immunoglobulin deposition in the contralateral testis.[30,37,44,71] Ryan et al[72,73] reported an increase in antispermatozoal antibodies 1 week after acute torsion; however, these disappeared by 6 months, and at 1 month there was no evidence of tissue fixation of these autoantibodies in the contralateral testis.

Nagler et al[46,74] demonstrated, by use of histologic examination and flow cytometric evaluation of DNA histograms, that acquired contralateral testicular changes and diminished fertility rates are dependent on the timing of surgical intervention. Contralateral tubular disruption, decreased contralateral tubular diameter, and azoospermia can be prevented by orchiectomy or immunosuppression with a combination of antilymphocyte globulin and splenectomy, suggesting an immunologic mediation of the contralateral damage.[42,69,74] Gulmez et al demonstrated immunosuppression with prednisolone prevented contralateral testicular damage. Recently, investigators have demonstrated induction on mast cell infiltration into the interstitium of the contralateral testis 4 weeks after testicular torsion, reaching a plateau at 8 to 24 weeks posttorsion. In this study, no other histologic alterations were noted in the contralateral testes.[76]

Karaguzel and colleagues[77] designed an experiment to evaluate the role of the torsed testicle in contralateral damage. They performed a subepididymal orchiectomy on one side, then 2 weeks later torsed the remaining epididymis and spermatic cord for 24 hours. Subsequent evaluation of the contralateral testes demonstrated deterioration in mean seminiferous tubular diameters, although changes were not as pronounced as those produced by torsion of an intact testicle.

## Ischemic/Reperfusion Injury

Turner and Brown[6] did not find an alteration in contralateral testicular blood flow with unilateral torsion. Others have demonstrated an increase in contralateral testicular blood flow with torsion of greater than 9 hours, which they postulate may cause an increase in testicular temperature and oxygen tension and thereby disturb spermatogenesis.[78] This increase in contralateral blood flow may result from a humoral mediator, as sera from rats with testicular torsion injected into normal rats stimulated a similar response.

Tanyel et al[79] demonstrated a progressive decrease in contralateral testicular blood flow following 2-hour testicular torsion. Others, using electromagnetic and radioisotopic blood flow studies, have confirmed a decrease in contralateral testicular blood flow and increase in contralateral tissue hypoxia parameters (lactic acid and hypoxanthine).[57,58,79–81] Increased levels of lactic acid, hypoxanthine, and lipid peroxidation products have been demonstrated in both testes following unilateral torsion of 2 hours' duration, indicating a bilateral decrease in testicular perfusion.[57,58,81] Detorsion within 6 hours did not suppress these increases.[57] The contralateral levels were suppressed by chemical sympathectomy using guanethidine or dopamine hydrobromide, indicating that a reflex-activating sympathetic system is stimulated by changes in the ipsilateral testicle and results in vasospasm, decreased blood flow, and subsequent hypoxic damage in the contralateral testicle.[81]

In these studies, detorsion resulted in increased contralateral testicular blood flow, which could cause reperfusion injury by free oxygen radical formation during the conversion of hypoxanthine, an adenosine triphosphate degradation product, to uric acid.[57,59] These free oxygen radical species could then trigger peroxidation of lipids in the cell and mitochondrial membranes. Akgur et al[58] demonstrated significant increases in lipid peroxidation products in the ipsilateral testis but not in the contralateral testis following detorsion of 1- and 2-hour torsions. Choi et al[56] demonstrated significant alterations in contralateral testicular cellular metabolic parameters following torsion of greater than 8 hours. Decreases in adenosine triphosphate and total adenosine nucleotide content in testicular tissue occurred in the absence of gross histologic changes, indicating that these metabolic alterations may be utilized in assessment of subtle testicular damage.

## Effects on Leydig Cell Function

### Clinical

Those who have measured testosterone levels in clinical settings have not reported hypoandrogenic results.[8,10,11,16,22] Normal levels of LH have been reported in 86% of men following testicular torsion.[8] Other researchers noted elevated LH levels and supranormal LH response to gonadotropin-releasing hormone in patients with delayed torsion of greater than 8 hours that required orchiectomy.[10,11]

Zanchetta et al[31] reported antibodies reacting to Leydig cell cytoplasmic antigens in 9% of patients following testicular torsion. Hagen et al[14] reported tubular atrophy of the Leydig cells in the contralateral testis of pubertal and postpubertal patients, but did not report the frequency of this specific pathologic finding.

### Experimental

Loss of Sertoli cells has been demonstrated to occur after 2 hours of torsion, but Leydig cells are more resistant to ischemia.[62,82] Bergh et al[54] did not demonstrate any alteration in interstitial mass or Leydig cell size after 100 minutes of testicular ischemia in the rat. Smith[49] demonstrated that 8 hours of testicular torsion were required to impair the Leydig cell function in dogs, and 10 hours resulted in fibrotic replacement of these cells.

Becker and Turner[33] and Costentino et al[42] independently demonstrated posttorsion Leydig cell proliferation in the prepubertal testis Kamada et al[43] demonstrated Leydig cell proliferation in the contralateral prepubertal rat testis. Experimental torsion of 1080° with no corrective intervention in prepubertal rats did not result in significant changes in serum testosterone levels.[83] In adult rats, torsion of 1 hour's duration followed by detorsion did not alter the subsequent response to LH stimulation as measured by ipsilateral testicular venous testosterone levels; however, torsion of 2 hour's duration attenuated this response.[82] There was no change in contralateral Leydig cell response to LH stimulation. Basal ipsilateral testicular venous concentrations following 4-hour torsions were 15% to 20% of the pretorsion value in both the prepubertal and postpubertal rat.[33]

## Management Considerations

### Delayed Torsion

There is controversy about management of the delayed presentation of testicular torsion. If contralateral damage occurs due to reperfusion injury resulting from free radical formation in the ischemic testicle or autosensitization by antigens from the ischemic testis, then the nonviable testis should be removed without detorsion. In addition to the potential initiation of contralateral damage, by whatever means, the nonviable testis is a source of discomfort and possible secondary infection, or wound sloughing and delayed wound healing.[2,5] In normal rats, unilateral orchiectomy in and of itself has not affected spermatogenesis or serum testosterone levels.[43,83] In addition, there may be a threefold increase in the risk of testicular cancer following testicular torsion.[84]

Nonetheless, the grossly infarcted or nonviable testis may retain some Leydig cell function and spermatogenesis and may not pose a risk of infection, abscess, or wound dehiscence.[85] Puri et al[9] found normal contralateral testicular growth or compensatory hypertrophy and normal spermatogenesis and fertility in 18 men who underwent detorsion with replacement of nonviable testis in the scrotum during their prepubertal years, even though the nonviable testis atrophied completely on follow-up. Although there is a report of the salvage of a testicle that had remained torsed for 5 days, early orchiectomy is generally advised in the postpubertal man with a nonviable testis.[86]

### Contralateral fixation

A retrospective study of 31 patients managed by inguinal exploration and detorsion without fixation of the contralateral testis did not report any contralateral torsion.[4] Most authors recommend fixation of the contralateral testicle and report a 5% to 42% torsion rate of unfixed contralateral testicles.[15,87] Animal studies have shown that contralateral orchiopexy does not affect spermatogenesis.[74]

## Fixation Technique

Orchiopexy techniques include fixation, with or without eversion of the tunica vaginalis, and use of either absorbable or nonabsorbable suture.[1,3] Detorsion without suture fixation of the testicle may be adequate due to fixation to the scrotal wall by the inflammatory process, and some authors report no incidence of retorsion.[4] Eversion of the tunica vaginalis by Lord's plication or the Jaboulay technique[88] results in sufficient adhesion formation, rendering suture fixation unnecessary.[3,88] A nonsutured dartos pouch also provides adequate fixation with circumferential adherence, as well as preservation of normal spermatogenesis (94%) and minimal focal tubular atrophy (23%). Alternatively, nylon suture fixation may result in absent spermatogenesis (29%), tubular necrosis (29%), and tubular atrophy (58%).[85] These changes have been demonstrated in both prepubertal and postpubertal animal models.[85,89] In the prepubertal rat, suture fixation resulted in testicular atrophy and severe inflammatory changes associated with granulomatous reactions and absence of spermatogenesis.[89]

If suture fixation is deemed necessary, the least reactive sutures are synthetic monofilaments, such as nylon and polypropylene.[89,90] Fixation should be performed at three points, with care taken to avoid the lower pole of the testicle where numerous superfical arteries are located.[1] Suture fixation should be performed if the tunica albuginea is not placed in contact with the dartos muscle by eversion of the tunica vaginalis.[3]

## Conclusion

The literature reporting effects of testicular torsion on testis biology and male fertility is confusing and divergent. The question of how unilateral torsion results in subfertility remains unanswered. The hypothesis that appears to have the least contradictory evidence is that the contralateral testis must have a preexisting defect: congenital, acquired from previous subclinical insults, or a predisposition to free-oxygen radical injury during reperfusion of the torsed testicle.

The current management of testicular torsion in the acute presentation is with early detorsion and orchiopexy or orchiectomy if the testicle is nonviable. The management of subfertility resulting from testicular torsion may benefit from the assisted fertility techniques that have been applied generically to most forms of male factor infertility. Adjuvant antioxidant therapy, immunosuppressive therapy, and chemical sympathectomy during operative intervention for testicular torsion hold promise in minimizing future deleterious effects on testicular function.

## References

1. Popowitz SM, Nagler HM. Testicular torsion. In: Thomas AJ, Nagler HM, eds. *Atlas of Surgical Management of Male Infertility*. New York: Igaku-Shoin; 1995: 96–101.
2. Anderson JB, Williamson RCN. Testicular torsion in Bristol: a 25 year review. *Br J Surg* 1988; 75:988–992.
3. Smith-Harrison LI, Koontz WW. Torsion of the testis: changing concepts. In: *AUA Update Series*, Houston, TX. Lesson 32. 1990; vol. 9.
4. Mizrahi S, Shtamler B. Surgical approach and outcome in torsion of testis. *Urology* 1992; 39:52–54.
5. Williamson RCN. Torsion of the testis and allied conditions. *Br J Surg* 1976; 63:465–476.
6. Turner TT, Brown KJ. Spermatic cord torsion: loss of spermatogenesis despite return of blood flow. *Biol Reprod* 1993; 49:401–407.
7. Babcock DS. Which is the most sensitive study for testicular torsion in children—Doppler sonography or testicular nuclear scan? *AJR* 1995; 165:224.
8. Ferreira U, Netto NR, Esteves SC, et al. Comparative study of the fertility potential of men with only one testis. *Scand J Urol Nephrol* 1991; 25:255–259.
9. Puri P, Barton D, O'Donnell B. Prepubertal testicular torsion: subsequent fertility. *J Pediatr Surg* 1985; 20:598–601.
10. Anderson JB, Dunn JK, Lipshultz LI, et al. Semen quality and endocrine parameters after

acute testicular torsion. *J Urol* 1992; 147:1545–1550.

11. Brasso K, Andersen L, Kay L, et al. Testicular torsion: a follow-up study. *Scand J Urol Nephrol* 1993; 27:1–6.

12. Dominguez C, Verduch MM, Estornell F, et al. Histological study in contralateral testis of prepubertal children following unilateral testicular torsion. *Eur Urol* 1994; 26:160–163.

13. Hadziselimovic F, Snyder H, Duckett J, et al. Testicular histology in children with unilateral testicular torsion. *J Urol* 1986; 136:208–210.

14. Hagen P, Buchholz MM, Eigenmann J, et al. Testicular dysplasia causing disturbance of spermiogenesis in patients with unilateral torsion of the testes. *Urol Int* 1992; 49:154–157.

15. Krarup T. The testes after torsion. *Br J Urol* 1978; 50:43–46.

16. Bartsch G, Frank S, Marberger H, et al. Testicular torsion: late results with special regard to fertility and endocrine function. *J Urol* 1980; 124:375–378.

17. Tryfonas G, Violaki A, Tsikopoulos G, et al. Late postoperative results in males treated for testicular torsion during childhood. *J Pediatr Surg* 1994; 29:553–556.

18. Thomas WEG, Cooper MJ, Crane GA, et al. Testicular exocrine malfunction after torsion. *Lancet* 1984; 2:1357–1360.

19. Danner C, Frick J, Rovan E. Testicular function after torsion. *Int J Androl* 1982; 5:276.

20. Anderson JB, Williamson RCN. Fertility after torsion of the spermatic cord. *Br J Urol* 1990; 65:225–230.

21. Fraser I, Slater N, Tate C, et al. Testicular torsion does not cause autoimmunization in man. *Br J Surg* 1985; 72:237–238.

22. Anderson JB, Cooper MJ, Thomas WEG, et al. Impaired spermatogenesis in testes at risk of torsion. *Br J Surg* 1986; 73:847–849.

23. Anderson JB, Williamson RCN. The fate of the human testes following unilateral torsion of the spermatic cord. *Br J Urol* 1986; 506:698–704.

24. Fisch H, Laor E, Reid RE, et al. Gonadal dysfunction after testicular torsion: luteinizing hormone and follicle-stimulating hormone response to gonadotropin releasing hormone. *J Urol* 1988; 139:961–964.

25. Nistal M, Martinez C, Paniagua R. Primary testicular lesions in the twisted testis. *Fertil Steril* 1992; 57:381–386.

26. Horica CA, Hadziselimovic F, Kreutz G, et al. Ultrastructural studies of the contorted and contralateral testicle in unilateral testicular torsion. *Eur Urol* 1982; 8:358–362.

27. Laor E, Fitsch H, Tannenbaum S, et al. Unilateral testicular torsion: abnormal histological findings in the contralateral testis—cause or effect? *Br J Urol* 1990; 65:520–523.

28. Chakraborty J, Hikim APS, Jhunjhunwala JS. Quantitative evaluation of testicular biopsies from men with unilateral torsion of the spermatic cord. *Urology* 1985; 25:145–150.

29. Tarter TH, Kogan SJ. Contralateral testicular disease after unilateral testicular injury: current concepts. *Semin Urol* 1988; 6:120–139.

30. Wallace DMA, Gunter PA, Landon GV, et al. Sympathetic orchiopathia—an experimental and clinical study. *Br J Urol* 1982; 54:765–768.

31. Zanchetta R, Mastrogiacomo I, Graziotti P, et al. Autoantibodies against Leydig cells in patients after spermatic cord torsion. *Clin Exp Immunol* 1984; 55:49–57.

32. Thomas WEG, Anderson JB, Williamson RCN. Autoimmunization in testicular torsion. *Br J Surg* 1985; 72:672.

33. Becker EJ, Turner TT. Endocrine and exocrine effects of testicular torsion in the prepubertal and adult rat. *J Androl* 1995; 16:342–351.

34. Unluer SE, Ercan MT, Arkdas A. Testicular blood flow in experimental torsion and epididymo-orchitis measured by 13-Xe-clearance technique in rats. *Urol Res* 1984; 12:183–186.

35. Costabile RA, Choyke PL, Frank JA, et al. Variability of ischemia during spermatic cord torsion in the rat. *J Urol* 1994; 151:1070–1072.

36. Sonda LP. Experimental torsion of the spermatic cord. *Surg Forum* 1961; 12:12.

37. Cerasaro TS, Nachtsheim DA, Otero F, et al. The effect of testicular torsion on the contralateral testis and the production of antisperm antibodies in rabbits. *J Urol* 1984; 132:577–579.

38. Palamo A. Radical cure of varicocele by a new technique. *J Urol* 1949; 61:604–607.

39. Blank ML, O'Neill PJ, Steigman CK, et al. Reperfusion injury following testicular torsion and detorsion in prepubertal rats. *Urol Res* 1993; 21:389–393.

40. Heindel RM, Pakyz RE, Costentino MJ. Spermatic cord torsion: contralateral testicular degeneration at various ages in the rat. *J Androl* 1990; 11:506–513.

41. Costentino MJ, Rabinowitz R, Valvo JR, et al. The effect of prepubertal spermatic cord torsion on subsequent fertility in rats. *J Androl* 1984; 5:93–98.

42. Costentino MJ, Nishida M, Rabinowitz R, et al. Histological changes occurring in the contralateral testes of prepubertal rats subjected to vari-

ous durations of unilateral spermatic cord torsion. *J Urol* 1985; 133:906–911.

43. Kamada K, Takihara H, Shirataki S, et al. Flow cytometric DNA analysis demonstrates contralateral testicular deterioration in experimental unilateral testicular torsion of prepubertal rats. *Andrologia* 1993; 25:349–244.

44. Henderson JA, Smey P, Cohen MS, et al. The effect of unilateral testicular torsion on the contralateral testicle in the prepubertal Chinese hamster. *J Pediatr Surg* 1985; 20:592–597.

45. Nagler H. Experimental aspects of testicular torsion. *Dialog Pediatr Urol* 1985; 8:2–5.

46. Nagler HM, Deitch AD, de Vere White R. Testicular torsion: temporal consideration. *Fertil Steril* 1984; 42:257–262.

47. Kogan SJ. Experimental aspects of testicular torsion. *Dialog Pediatr Urol* 1985; 8:5–6.

48. Saba M, de Lamirande E, Gagnon C. The oxidative stress induced in rat testis following torsion/reperfusion: effects on contralateral testis and of scavengers. *J Urol* 1995; 153:427A(#795).

49. Smith GI. Cellular changes from graded testicular ischemia. *J Urol* 1955; 73:355–362.

50. Oettle AG, Harrison RG. The histological changes produced in the rat testis by temporary and permanent occlusion of the testicular artery. *J Pathol Bacteriol* 1954; 64:273–297.

51. Carroll T, Green D, Regan M, et al. Determination of testicular function using flow cytometry following testicular torsion. *J Urol* 1995; 153:427A(#794).

52. Klotz T, Homann HH, Mathers M, et al. Follow-up of contralateral intratesticular oxygen pressure in unilateral testicular torsion. *Urologe [A]* 1995; 34:143–145.

53. Turner TT. On unilateral testicular and epididymal torsion: no effect on the contralateral testis. *J Urol* 1987; 138:1285–1290.

54. Bergh A, Damber JE, Marklund SL. Morphologic changes induced by short-term ischemia in the rat testis are not affected by treatment with superoxide dismutase and catalase. *J Androl* 1988; 9:15–20.

55. Carmignani G, Tedde G, DeStefani S, et al. An experimental study of the effect of ischemia on testicular structure in the rat: efficacy of intravenous inosine. *J Androl* 1983; 4:378–386.

56. Choi H, Choo MS, Kim KM, et al. The alterations of cellular metabolism in the contralateral testis following spermatic cord torsion in rats. *J Urol* 1993; 150:577–580.

57. Akgur FM, Kilinc K, Tanyel FC, et al. Ipsilateral and contralateral testicular biochemical acute

changes after unilateral testicular torsion and detorsion. *Urology* 1994; 44:413–418.

58. Akgur FM, Kilinc K, Aktug T. Reperfusion injury after detorsion of unilateral testicular torsion. *Urol Res* 1993; 21:395–399.

59. Akgur FM, Kilinc K, Aktug T, et al. The effect of allopurinol pretreatment before detorting testicular torsion. *J Urol* 1994; 151:1715–1717.

60. Greenstein A, Smith-Harrison LI, Wakely PE, et al. The effect of polyethylene glycol-superoxide dismutase administration on histological damage following spermatic cord torsion. *J Urol* 1992; 148:639–641.

61. Akhter S, Sridher S, Katlowitz NM, et al. Immune response to testicular ischemia and reperfusion. *J Urol* 1990; 143:262A.

62. Turner TT. Acute experimental testicular torsion, no effect on contralateral testis. *J Androl* 1985; 6:65–72.

63. Janetshek G, Heilbronner R, Wachtner W, et al. Unilateral testicular disease: effect on the contralateral testis (morphometric study). *J Urol* 1987; 138:878–882.

64. Janetshek G, Schreckenbert F, Mikuz G, et al. Experimental testicular torsion: effect on endocrine and exocrine function and contralateral testicular histology. *Urol Res* 1988; 16:43–47.

65. Kaya M, Harrison RG. An analysis of the effect of ischaemia of testicular ultrastructure. *J Pathol* 1975; 117:105–117.

66. Harrison RG, Lewis-Jones DI, Moreno de Marval MJ, et al. Mechanism of damage to the contralateral testis in rats with an ischemic testis. *Lancet* 1981; 2:723–725.

67. Chakraborty J, Jhunjhunwala J, Nelson L, et al. Effects of unilateral torsion of the spermatic cord on the contralateral testis in human and guinea pig. *Arch Androl* 1980; 4:95–108.

68. Lewis-Jones DI, Moreno de Marval MJ, Harrison RG. Impairment of rat spermatogenesis following unilateral experimental ischemia. *Fertil Steril* 1982; 38:482–490.

69. York JP, Drago JR. Torsion and the contralateral testicle. *J Urol* 1985; 133:294–297.

70. Kearney SE, Lewis-Jones DI. Effect of ACTH on contralateral testicular damage and cytotoxic antisperm antibodies after unilateral testicular ischemia in the rat. *J Reprod Fertil* 1985; 75:531.

71. Saltzman N, Sadi M, Hoffer A, et al. Is autoimmune fertility a consequence of unilateral testicular ischemia? *J Urol* 1984; 131:162A.

72. Ryan PC, Fitzpatrick JM. Experimental testicular torsion: do spermatozoal autoantigens cause immunological activation? *World J Urol* 1986; 4:92–99.

73. Ryan PC, Whelan CA, Gaffney EF, et al. The effect of unilateral experimental testicular torsion on spermatogenesis and fertility. *Br J Urol* 62:359–366.

74. Nagler HM, de Vere White R. The effect of testicular torsion on the contralateral testis. *J Urol* 1982; 128:1343–1348.

75. Gulmez I, Karacagil M, Sade M, et al. Effect of testicular torsion on the contralateral testis and prevention of this effect by prednisolone. *Eur Urol* 1987; 13:340–343.

76. Qo S. Mast cell induction to the mouse testicular interstitium. *Jpn J Urol* 1994; 85:747–752.

77. Karaguzel G, Gedikoglu G, Tanyel FC, et al. Is ipsilateral testis mandatory for contralateral testicular deterioration encountered following spermatic cord torsion? *Urol Res* 1994; 22:115–117.

78. Melikoglu M, Guntekin E, Erkilic M, et al. Contralateral testicular blood flow in unilateral testicular torsion measured by the 133-Xe clearance technique. *Br J Urol* 1992; 69:633–635.

79. Tanyel FC, Buyukpamukcu N, Hicsonmez A. Contralateral testicular blood flow during unilateral testicular torsion. *Br J Urol* 1989; 63:522–524.

80. Kizilcan F, Bernay I, Tanyel FC, et al. Ipsilateral and contralateral blood flows during testicular torsion by 133-Xe clearance technique. *Int Urol Nephrol* 1992; 24:515–520.

81. Karaguzel G, Tanyel FC, Kilinc K, et al. The preventative role of chemical sympathectomy on contralateral testicular hypoxic parameters encountered during unilateral testicular torsion. *Br J Urol* 1994; 74:507–510.

82. Baker LA, Turner TT. Leydig cell function after experimental testicular torsion despite loss of spermatogenesis. *J Androl* 1995; 16:12–17.

83. Mauss J, Hackstedt G. The effect of unilateral orchidectomy and unilateral cryptorchidism on sperm output in the rat. *J Reprod Fertil* 1972; 30:289–292.

84. Chilvers CED, Pike MC, Peckham MJ. Torsion of the testis: a new risk factor for testicular cancer. *Br J Cancer* 1987; 55:105–106.

85. Bellinger MF, Abramowitz HB, Brantley S, et al. Orchiopexy: an experimental study of the effect of surgical technique on testicular histology. *J Urol* 1989; 142:553–555.

86. Klinger ME. Viable testicle five days after unreduced torsion of the spermatic cord. *NY State J Med* 1954; 54:1951.

87. Skoglund RW, McRoberts JW, Ragde H. Torsion of the spermatic cord: a review of the literature and an analysis of 70 new cases. *J Urol* 1970; 104:604–607.

88. Williamson RCN, Thomas WEG. Sympathetic orchidopathia. *Ann R Coll Surg Engl* 1984; 66:264–266.

89. Dixon TK, Ritchey ML, Boykin W, et al. Transparenchymal suture fixation and testicular histology in a prepubertal rat model. *J Urol* 1993; 149:1116–1118.

90. Bickerton MW, Duckett JW. Suture materials and wound healing. In: *AUA Update Series*, Houston, TX. Lesson 15. 1984; vol. 3.

# 23
# Office Evaluation of the Impotent Man

David F. Mobley and Neil Baum

With a plethora of diagnostic and treatment options, there is probably no area of urology that has more diversity in diagnosis and treatment than erectile dysfunction. There is no unanimity or consensus as to what should be done or what is the usual and customary approach. There is wide variation in how the impotent man is approached in different areas of the country, as well as from urologist to urologist within the same community. A workup may vary from obtaining a thorough history and physical examination to thousands of dollars' worth of laboratory work, assessment of sleep erections, and imaging studies that leave the patient with a probable diagnosis and no solution to his problem. Treatments vary from the far too common reassurance that the man is "over the hill" and his days of sexual intimacy are over, to the immediate recommendation of a surgical procedure that may still leave the patient without a useful erection. For many men, it is a total surprise that there is help, and that there is far more than reassurance available as a solution to this common, but often devastating, medical problem.

With the use of medical therapy as a first-line treatment for the management of men with benign prostatic hyperplasia (BPH), there are fewer prostate operations being performed. On the other hand, there are other medical problems that have replaced lower tract obstructive symptoms, and impotence is one of them. According to Dr. Irwin Goldstein,[1] associated with the Massachusetts Male Aging Study, there are 30 million American men who suffer from some degree of impotence. It is difficult to determine what the incidence really is, but probably between 20 and 30 million men suffer with erectile dysfunction (ED). With no more than 500,000 penile implants having been performed, perhaps fewer than 1 in 20 men who might benefit from treatment have been helped. With an increasing number of men in the over-55 age group, there will be an increasing number of men who have a problem of erectile dysfunction and need the assistance of a urologist. Fortunately, the taboo of discussing this problem with a physician has been lifted to some extent. However, many physicians are still very uncomfortable dealing with sexual issues, which is one of the reasons that reassurance is perhaps the most common "treatment." The news media provide numerous articles, information, and even advertisements on the treatment of impotence; therefore, more men are asking for help, or their partners are suggesting that they seek medical assistance for the problem that affects both of them.

## Before the First Visit

To enhance the impotent patient's first office visit, a well-trained, sensitive receptionist can inquire about the reason for the patient's appointment and can determine which information to send to the patient before the initial visit. If the receptionist identifies a sexual problem, the caller should be reassured immediately that he has contacted the proper specialist. A welcome-to-the-practice package should then be mailed to the potential patient. Include a letter and any other educational materials that might be helpful, for these will not only educate the patient but also reassure him that his sexual problem can almost certainly be solved. Consequently, the patient will arrive informed, optimistic, and enthusiastic.

## The Office Visit

The urologist's first interaction with the patient is vital to establishing rapport. At the first visit, the patient will probably be uncomfortable talking about a sensitive and personal topic such as impotence. He should be reassured that other men have been helped. Physicians should be aware that impotent patients may be discussing a subject that they find very difficult to talk about to a stranger. Many an impotent man will not share his feelings or his problem with his partner, his best friend, or even his clergyman. To most men, impotence is a terrible source of mental pain and discomfort, and the patient needs to quickly sense how comfortable the urologist is in discussing this topic and consequently be put at ease himself. The patient will also be judging the office staff as to their tact, concern, compassion, and willingness to be of help.

In the history-taking process, the physician needs to be aware that most men are considerably distressed about having a problem with potency and do not realize how common this problem is. Each patient may feel he is the only one with impotence. The anxiety and loss of self-esteem can result in depression that will affect other areas of a man's life—his libido, his job performance, and his interaction with others.

It is helpful to have the patient complete, before the first visit, a urologic questionnaire that includes questions about sexual performance. Alternately, the questionnaire can be returned on the second visit, so the patient's partner will have an opportunity to help him complete the form, because there are certain risk factors associated with ED that patients

TABLE 23.1. Risk factors associated with erectile dysfunction.

| |
|---|
| Age |
| Smoking |
| Alcohol abuse |
| Diabetes |
| Hypertension |
| Peripheral vascular disease |
| Medications associated with impotence |
|    Antihypertensives |
|    Thiazide diuretics |
|    $H_2$ blockers |
|    Tranquilizers |
|    Analgesics |
| Radical pelvic surgery |
| Neurologic disease |
|    Multiple sclerosis |
|    Spinal cord injury |
|    Stroke |
| Priapism |
| Conflict with partner |
| Recent divorce or death of spouse |
| Fear of failure (performance anxiety) |
| Endocrine disease |
|    Adrenal disorders |
|    Hyper/hypothyroidism |
|    Pituitary tumor |

Modified from Nadig.[5]

may momentarily forget about (Table 23.1). For most men older than 55 to 60 years, the history is straightforward, but it is often helpful to ask if there was a precise episode or event that brought him in for help. If he admits that his partner urged or coerced him to make the appointment, it may be necessary to include the partner and to be concerned about primary libido problems or marital discord as a source of the erectile failure. In this latter situation, it is important to determine how important his ED is to him and how motivated he is to find a solution to the problem.

During history-taking, open-ended questions beginning with "How" or "What" are helpful in establishing rapport. The partner may be included in the initial visit, but it may be more appropriate to include the partner at the second or subsequent visits when treatment options are discussed. This is often a moot point, however, because usually the couple will decide who shows up for which visits. Sometimes both of them are there for each discussion, and sometimes the treating urologist may never meet the partner until perhaps the day of surgery.

The physical examination includes an inspection of the general habitus, escutcheon, and external genitalia. A neurosensory examination includes a cremasteric reflex and pin prick/light touch discrimination. During the rectal examination, the bulbocavernosus reflex, sphincter tone, and the prostate gland must be evaluated, giving a measure of sacral root function. Examination of the external genitalia includes an assessment of the testes and appraisal of the corpora cavernosa for Peyronie's plaques.

The vascular system can be evaluated by palpating the pulses in the lower extremities. A simple noninvasive method of grossly determining the blood flow to the penis is to gently compress and quickly release the corporal body to observe how quickly blood returns to the penis.

The penile/brachial index has lost its initial popularity as an assessment of blood supply to the penis, but some urologists still prefer to use this technique or the nocturnal penile tumescence (NPT) test to differentiate organic from psychogenic impotence. Most patients can indicate whether they have nighttime erections, but such NPT studies can often show the degree of erection and duration and provide definite clues as to organicity of the condition. If the patient states he is aware of no erections at any time, the snap gauge® may serve as a good, simple, and inexpensive screening test. The sleep lab with simultaneous monitoring of the EEG for REM sleep is sometimes desirable if legal proof of erectile status is needed.

After the physical, if the patient is already aware of treatment options, it is very helpful to ask the patient, "What would be the ideal solution to your problem?" This question can be very insightful as to the patient's expectations and what solutions to recommend. The goal-directed impotence management devised by Dr. Tom Lue[2] can help the patient select the appropriate treatment (Table 23.2). This management system is based on the desires of the patient and is very effective in tailoring the treatment to the needs and wants of the patient.

If it is concluded that the problem is primarily psychogenic, e.g., premature ejaculation, abrupt onset associated with personal or occupational stress, or partner-specific impotence, then referral for sex therapy is appropriate. However, it is important to keep the patient's sensitivity in mind. A patient may not accept the idea that the problem is psychogenic and may require some proof before considering such a referral. In discussion with the patient, try to determine how he might react to an immediate referral to a sex therapist. Approach this area with a question like, "If your evaluation shows this to be a psychological problem, how would you feel about a referral to a specialist in this area?" When making a referral to a sex therapist, be certain that the patient is reassured that his problem does not require a pill, an injection, or an operation, but may be helped and even cured with a course of sex therapy. Strong encouragement and reinforcement of the benefits of sex therapy should be carefully laid out, for the term *sex therapy* can be intimidating to a patient. Prior to making a referral to a sex therapist, spend a few minutes to explain what the patient can expect to occur with this therapy. Occasionally, a patient will not respond adequately to sex therapy and will need additional urologic treatment. It is a good

TABLE 23.2. Patient's goal-directed management of impotence.

| |
|---|
| Group I (not interested in treatment)—No workup |
| Group II (only interested in oral medications or vacuum constriction devices) |
| Group III (interested in other treatment)—Proceed with workup |
| III-A (probably psychogenic)—Confirm with CIS* and refer for sex therapy |
| III-B (hormonal)—Trial of testosterone therapy of endocrine consultation |
| III-C (neurovascular)—Obtain neurologic consultation if neurogenic history; all others proceed to CIS* |
| Full erection—injection therapy or sex therapy |
| Full erection after manual stimulation—injection therapy |
| Partial erection—vacuum constriction device, injection therapy, or both |
| Poor or no response—proceed to prosthesis |

*CIS, combined intracavernous injection and stimulation test.

idea to encourage the patient to make a return appointment after he completes the prescribed therapy. Make him aware that he is welcome to return to the urologist at any point. The sex therapist should provide written communication to the referring urologist regarding the patient's progress.

Following the history and physical examination, a laboratory evaluation is tailored to the individual patient. This avoids the expense of a battery of tests that in many situations are not necessary. For example, if a patient has normal-sized testes and his libido is intact, it may be unnecessary to obtain a serum testosterone. On the other hand, a patient with a solitary testis that has become smaller after an episode of epididymo-orchitis may have a decreased serum testosterone. If the testosterone is found to be decreased or is at the lower limit of normal, then a serum prolactin should be obtained. Urinalysis should be done to check for glycosuria and infection. Glycosuria or a history of polyuria and polydypsia or both will require a workup for diabetes mellitus. If the patient has had no laboratory assessment within the past year to determine that he is not diabetic, some screening blood work should be obtained.

At the end of the first visit, a trial of yohimbine may be suggested. Most men will not improve with this medication, but some do. It is inexpensive, quite safe, and offers the patient a potentially easy treatment on the first visit. Two to three weeks of yohimbine (5.4 mg, three times daily) is an adequate trial, with a plan for a follow-up. Specific literature relative to the patient's other medical and urologic problems can be given at the end of the first visit.

The second visit reviews the lab work, any sleep erection testing that may have been done, results of yohimbine therapy if tried, any intervening sexual activity, and the patient's assessment of the information materials provided. If the patient has decided to try a vacuum device, the patient can review a video and be fitted on this second visit. Some physicians use "demo" models, others sell the devices, and others prescribe them for the patient to purchase at a pharmacy or medical supply company. If the

patient has selected injection therapy, there are a number of different options available. Because prostaglandin is now available with a prescription (Caverject), the patient may receive a demonstration of the technique of injection therapy.

The patient's consent must be obtained after the possible problems associated with the intracorporal injection have been discussed, such as priapism, corporal fibrosis, Peyronie's disease, and blood pressure changes. The patient is asked to schedule a date with his partner, so that intercourse can be attempted after the injection. Inject the patient's phallus with saline so he knows the proper technique, and send him home with one syringe of the urologist's choice of vasoactive drug(s). The patient should be instructed to call the office the following day to tell the nurse how the erection was rated on a 1 to 10 scale. Based on this rating, the physician can select the optimal dosage by starting with small dosages of prostaglandin ($PGE_1$), for example, and titrating to the appropriate or effective dose.

The initial dose is tailored to the history of the patient. For example, an older patient or one who has an obvious history of atherosclerosis, cerebrovascular accident (CVA), myocardial infarction (MI), or hypertension, might be started with 10 µg of $PGE_1$. A younger patient or one with suspected neurogenic impotence (e.g., spinal cord injury) should be started with a lower dose, i.e., 5 µg of $PGE_1$.

If the injection is given in the office, the patient can be either sent home or asked to wait. If no erection occurs after 20 minutes, another injection may be given, and repeated up to a total of 1 cc or a maximum of 20 µg of $PGE_1$. If small doses of vasoactive agents are used initially, the probability of trips to the emergency room are unlikely. Oral terbutiline, 5 mg tablets, can be prescribed in the event that the erection is sustained or the patient experiences severe penile pain. The dose can be repeated every 15 minutes until detumescence occurs or after a total of three tablets of terbutiline (15 mg). This oral therapy is effective in 20% to 30% of those who use it for priapism.[3,4] Pseudoephedrine is also effective for the relief of prolonged erections due to vasoactive

TABLE 23.3. Priapism treatment.

| | |
|---|---|
| Phenylephrine (1-cc vial, 10 mg/cc) | 0.5 cc |
| Saline, injectable | 9.5 cc |
| | Total 10 cc |

1. Inject 1 to 2 cc with a 27-gauge needle (repeat once)
2. If no detumescence, insert 19-gauge scalp vein needle into side of corpora cavernosum
3. Aspirate or squeeze trapped blood out of corpora
4. Slowly inject 0.5 to 1.0 cc of phenylephrine solution into the corpora
5. Observe for 15 to 20 minutes and reinject as needed
6. Wrap the penis in a compression bandage and maintain for several hours

agents. If oral therapy is not effective and the erection lasts longer than 4 hours, the patient should be seen immediately by the urologist or go to an emergency room for treatment by injection of a vasoconstrictor (phenylephrine [Table 23.3]), and irrigation of the corporal bodies if necessary. Phenylephrine should not be used in patients taking monoamine oxidase (MAO) inhibitors. When detumescence occurs, the corporal bodies should be compressed with an elastic bandage for several hours. Use of this technique will avoid the need for a cavernosal-spongiosum shunt.

If the patient does obtain a good erection with the original diagnostic injection and will accept this as a treatment modality, he should be given further detailed instruction by the urologist or a nurse or medical assistant or both regarding proper sterile technique and selection of the proper injection sites. The patient is cautioned to always use the smallest effective dose of medication, never to use it more than two to three times a week, to vary the injection sites on the shaft of the penis, and to gently compress the injection site for 1 to 2 minutes following the injection.

If the patient does not get an adequate erection with $PGE_1$, the problem is most likely vasculogenic, and the patient should be advised of the treatment options that are available to resolve his problem. The medical manufacturing and pharmaceutical companies have informational videos, or such videos can be made by the urologist with a video camera and a tripod. Whichever videos are used, provide the patient with a written summary after he has viewed the tape.

There are numerous advantages to using videos. The patient may take a copy home to watch or to show his partner about the test, procedure, or treatment. The urologist should document in the chart that the patient has seen the video, which helps provide medical-legal protection. An effective video can reduce the number of questions that the patient may ask.

## Summary

There are many changes occurring in the delivery of health care that are impacting the practice of urology. Certainly the days of being primarily transurethal resection of the prostate (TURP) doctors are past. The "three I's" (impotence, infertility, and incontinence) have now become important.

Incorporating the treatment of impotence will not usually require any significant additional equipment or staff. There are thousands of men suffering from impotence who need help from experts. To identify these men and educate them regarding the help that is available, an efficient and effective office evaluation is the critical first step.

## References

1. Goldstein I. Your erectile dysfunction patient load is due to boom. *Urology Times* December, 1994.
2. Lue T. Patient's goal-directed impotence management. *Urology Grand Rounds* 1989; 29.
3. Govier FE, Jonsson E, Kramer-Levine D. Oral terbutaline for the treatment of priapism. *J Urol* 1994; 151:878–879.
4. Lowe FC, Jarow JP. Letter to the editor. *J Urol* 1994; 153:163.
5. Nadig P. Office assessment of BPH, abnormal PSA/DRE and impotence using existing guidelines and proper CPT coding. AUA Postgraduate Course, San Francisco, 1994.

# 24
# Androgen Deficiency

Glenn R. Cunningham and Max Hirshkowitz

The classic belief is that androgen (of which testosterone is the major component) primarily mediates libido. Androgen deficiency has long been known to contribute to, but not necessarily be the sole underlying cause of, erectile failure. Clinical studies provide information for understanding the role of androgens in human sexual function. Loss of sexual drive and desire in association with hypogonadism has long been recognized, and self-reports have verified clinical observations.[1-3] The nocturnal penile tumescence study has provided a sensitive, objective, physiologic index for studying erectile capability and screening androgen deficiency.[4,5]

## Diagnosis

Androgen deficiency in individuals with delayed puberty is clinically apparent when severe androgen deficiency occurs in young adult males after puberty; the symptoms and physical signs usually make the diagnosis obvious. However, less severe deficiencies in adult men can be difficult to recognize even by an experienced andrologist.

A good laboratory measurement of testosterone (T) is essential for establishing the diagnosis of hypogonadism. The clinician must recognize factors that can cause erroneous interpretations of eugonadism or hypogonadism. Diurnal variations in T secretion cause higher levels in the early morning with the nadir occurring during the late afternoon and evening.

These diurnal variations tend to be reduced with aging.[6] T must be determined in a correctly timed blood specimen. Most normal ranges have been established using early morning samples. Moderate exercise acutely increases total and free T levels.[7] T is bound with high affinity to sex hormone–binding globulin (SHBG) and lower affinity to albumin. There is evidence that albumin-bound T, as well as free T, is available to peripheral tissues.[8-10] When alterations of SHBG are suspected (Table 24.1), it is important to request that the laboratory measures free T or non-SHBG-bound T. Studies suggest that a single plasma T level reliably reflects the annual mean T level.[11-13]

After the diagnosis of androgen deficiency has been established, it is useful to determine if it is caused by testicular, pituitary, or hypothalamic disease. Measurement of serum luteinizing hormone (LH) provides the most useful means for separating patients who have testicular disease from those who have pituitary or hypothalamic abnormality. LH levels are increased in patients who have primary testicular disease unless they also have concomitant pituitary or hypothalamic disease. A diagnosis of primary testicular failure may not require further evaluation. Measurement of serum prolactin is indicated in patients with normal or low serum LH levels. Hyperprolactinemia decreases T levels by decreasing gonadotropin-releasing hormone (GnRH) secretion. Values above 50 ng/ml require further assessment. Prolactin levels in excess of 200 ng/ml strongly suggest a prolactinoma, requiring further evaluation. Because low or inappropriately normal levels of LH are observed in patients with both pituitary and hypothalamic disease, differentiation requires considerably more evaluation and is beyond the scope of the present discussion. It is useful to separate hypogonadal states into those that are hypogonadotropic and those that are hypergonadotropic, congenital, or acquired (Table 24.2).

Studies suggest that 95% of hypogonadal men over 50 years of age have a secondary cause.[14] The large majority of these men will have an isolated gonadotropin deficiency. Because it is rare to find anatomic abnormalities on magnetic resonance imaging (MRI) scanning of the pituitary and hypothalamus, these patients should be evaluated by an endocrinologist. Anatomical imaging may not be warranted unless other pituitary hormone deficiencies are evident. One approach to evaluating such men is to administer the antiestrogen clomiphene citrate 50 mg two times a day for 7 or 10 days.[15] A 40% or greater increase in total T and a 100% increase in free T, with values in the normal range, will suggest a resetting of the factors that regulate GnRH and LH secretion.[13] Further endocrine evaluation may not be necessary in these patients. Abnormal T responses to clomiphene citrate are seen in healthy aged individuals;[16] therefore, abnormal responses may be seen in men with normal

TABLE 24.1. Conditions associated with alterations in serum SHBG levels or reduction of SHBG binding sites.

Increased levels of SHBG
 Newborn
 Aging (after the fifth decade)
 Low fat diet (<20 g/day)
 Hyperthyroidism
 Cirrhosis
 Estrogen
Decreased levels of SHBG
 Increased body mass index
 High fat diet (>100 g/day)
 Nephrotic syndrome
 Testosterone
Drugs that compete with T and DHT for binding sites
 Spironolactone
 Danazol
 19-nor progestins

TABLE 24.2. Causes of male hypogonadism.

Hypogonadotropic conditions
Congenital
 Delayed puberty
 Isolated deficiency of GnRH (with and without anosmia)
 Fertile eunuch syndrome
 Polymalformation syndromes (Prader-Labhart-Willi; Laurence-Moon-Biedl)
Acquired
 Isolated gonadotropin deficiency
  Aging
  Chronic illnesses (renal, liver)
  Drugs
  Idiopathic
  Obesity
  Sleep apnea
  Starvation
  Stress
 Associated with deficiency of multiple other pituitary hormones
  Autoimmune destruction of pituitary
  Head trauma
  Infection (tuberculosis, syphilis)
  Infiltrative diseases (sarcoidosis, hemochromatosis)
  Irradiation
  Metastatic tumors to the pituitary (breast, lung)
  Primary intracranial tumors (pituitary, craniopharyngioma, parameningioma, pinealoma)
  Surgery
Hypergonadotropic conditions
Congenital
 Abnormal LH
 Androgen resistance
 Bilateral cryptorchidism
 Enzymatic defects in testosterone synthesis
 Gonadal dysgenesis
 Klinefelter's syndrome
 Myotonic dystrophy
 Polyglandular failure syndrome
 Polymalformation syndrome (Laurence-Moon-Biedl)
 Vanishing testis syndrome
Acquired
 Aging
 Chronic illnesses (renal, liver)
 Drugs
 Idiopathic
 Irradiation
 Nonsurgical testicular trauma
 Orchiectomy or surgical trauma to testes
 Postinfection (viral, bacterial)
 Testicular torsion

MRI scans. Nevertheless, this approach provides reassurance when the response is normal, and it saves extensive evaluation for many men.

## Libido and Erectile Responsivity

Libido in hypogonadal men can be restored by T replacement therapy.[2,17] Clopper et al[18] treated gonadotropin-deficient hypopituitary male patients with T, gonadotropin, or a placebo in a crossover design. Sexual desire and ejaculatory frequency increased during T and gonadotropin administration.

Androgen sensitivity of sleep-related erections appears to differ from erections elicited by visually presented sexual stimuli (VSS). It is possible that very low T levels are needed to support VSS erectile function, but sleep-related erections have more linear effects across a broader range.[19-21] A recent study found VSS functional erections in 4 of 16 men castrated to treat prostatic cancer.[22] All patients were reportedly sexually active before castration. The men with normal VSS response had abnormally low, but significantly higher, T levels than those who did not achieve erections (1.125 vs. 0.628 pg/ml).

VSS erections also change as a function of age. Rowland et al[23] reported that age inversely correlates with maximum circumference increase during VSS, and there is age-related slowing in the time required to achieve maximal erection. This study did not find an age-related change in T.

## Erectile Capability

In assessment of sleep-related erections before and during T replacement in hypogonadal men, T treatment has consistently produced increased spontaneous nocturnal erections.[19,24] In sleep studies during and after androgen replacement, cessation of androgen replacement was associated with decreased spontaneous sleep-related erection frequency, magnitude, duration, and rigidity.[25]

## Other Effects

Testosterone affects many bodily systems in addition to altering libido and erectile function. The effects of androgen on skin and hair, external genitalia, accessory sex organs (including the prostate and testes), bone, skeletal muscle, lipids, and red blood cells are well recognized.

Androgen receptors have been identified in these sites by binding studies, immunohistochemistry, and in situ hybridization. Less well understood are the T-induced changes in fat distribution, vascular smooth muscle, and immune function. Because T is metabolized to both dihydrotestosterone (DHT) and to estradiol ($E_2$), many of the effects of T are mediated by these metabolites.

### Skin and Hair

Androgen has an effect on scrotal skin, sebaceous glands, and hair follicles. The increase in T levels at puberty is associated with an increase in rugation of scrotal skin. The skin becomes more oily because of the effects on the sebaceous glands. Acne is very common at this age, usually involving the face and back. Stimulation of hair follicles in the axillae, pubic area, beard area, chest, back, and extremities results in growth of terminal hair. The type I isoenzyme of 5α-reductase is the predominant enzyme in skin and hair follicles.[26] Activity is correlated with sensitivity of skin and hair follicles. Pubic, scrotal, and penile skin have higher levels of activity than skin from the trunk. The variation in hair patterns among racial groups is thought to be more related to local tissue factors than to differences in circulating levels of testosterone; 5α-reductase activity is reduced in Japanese and Chinese men when compared with Caucasian men, but the concentration and affinity of androgen receptors appears to be similar.[27,28] An acquired loss of T is associated with a slow reduction in hair growth and loss of androgen-sensitive hair. Although scalp hair is not androgen-dependent for growth, recession of the temporal hair line at puberty and development of male-pattern baldness are dependent on changes in normal levels of T, tissue 5α-reductase activity, and androgen receptors.

### External Genitalia

The external genitalia are developed by the 12th week of fetal growth. In addition to adequate levels of T and normally responsive androgen receptors, 5α-reductase activity must be present at this critical time for normal penile development. T is the more important androgen for spermatogenesis. Sertoli cells have follicle-stimulating hormone (FSH) and androgen receptors, and peritubular cells have androgen receptors. FSH and androgen act on these cells to support spermatogenesis.

When testicular T levels are severely reduced, spermatogenesis is impaired, and testicular volume is reduced. Usually, changes in the consistency of the testis are appreciated before changes in testicular volume are apparent.

## Accessory Sexual Organs

Development of normal male accessory sexual glands depends on DHT. This process is disrupted by defects in androgen receptors or 5α-reductase activity. Congenital deficiency of 5α-reductase type 2 results in a poorly developed prostate, with minimal growth of the prostate at puberty and impaired spermatogenesis. Conditions causing a T deficiency after puberty may result in a regression of prostate and seminal vesicle volume,[29,30] but androgen replacement can normalize the volume of the prostate and seminal vesicles. If T deficiency occurs after benign prostatic hyperplasia (BPH) has been established, regression in prostate volume is usually less remarkable.

## GH and IGF-I

Growth hormone (GH) and insulin-like growth factor-I (IGF-I) levels increase at puberty, and T deficiency reduces levels of GH and IGF-I levels. Androgen replacement therapy increases these parameters in individuals with primary hypogonadism or isolated hypogonadotropic hypogonadism.[31] GH and IGF-I levels can be reduced during treatment with T and the antiestrogen tamoxifen, indicating that they are mediated by conversion of T to $E_2$.[32] Consistent with this observation, T treatment of boys with delayed puberty increases GH and IGF-I levels. By contrast, these changes are not observed with DHT because DHT cannot be aromatized to estrogen.[33]

## Bone

The timing of puberty and the concomitant increase in T secretion are critical for the development of normal bone mass. Young adult men with delayed puberty have a decreased radial and spinal bone mineral density.[34] The reduction in peak bone mineral density is reportedly greater in males with hypogonadotropic hypogonadism[35] and possibly in individuals with Klinefelter's syndrome.[36] T treatment increases cortical and trabecular bone density in men with open epiphyses and cortical bone density in those with closed epiphyses.[37,38]

Evidence indicates the direct and indirect effects of estrogen acting via growth hormone and IGF-I are primarily responsible for the growth spurt and for epiphyseal closure.[39] Other factors may be operative at the level of bone. Open epiphyses and decreased bone mineral density of males in their mid-twenties who have estrogen resistance or aromatase deficiency underscore the importance of estrogen in bone development.[40,41] Individuals with androgen resistance have peak height velocity more similar to normal girls than boys.[42] Androgen receptors in osteoblasts mediate androgen effects.[43,44] T and DHT reduce interleukin-6 (IL-6) production by murine bone marrow-derived stromal cells. IL-6 may upregulate osteoclasts; thus, T or DHT and estrogen are important for bone maturation and bone mineralization.[45]

Acquired T deficiency is a cause of osteoporosis in men.[46,47] Treatment of aging men having metastatic prostate cancer with a long-acting GnRH agonist may also decrease bone mineralization.[48]

## Muscle

Muscle weakness is observed in men with both primary and secondary hypogonadism, but is reportedly more prevalent in men with secondary hypogonadism, which suggests that concurrent GH deficiency may be a contributing factor.[49] Puberty in the male is characterized by an increase in skeletal muscle mass and strength. When androgen is administered to prepubertal adolescents or to hypogonadal men, it causes nitrogen retention.[50,51] In one study, lean body mass increased in men aged 57 to 76 with low or borderline low total testosterone levels when they were treated with 100 mg of testosterone enanthate every week for 12 weeks.[52]

## Red Blood Cells

The increase in T at puberty coincides with increases in red blood cell counts and in hemoglobin and hematocrit levels.[53] Early studies using a bioassay for erythropoietin showed that androgen increases erythropoietin activity.[54] When hypogonadism was induced with a GnRH agonist in men with BPH, hemoglobin levels fell from 15.2 ± 0.9 to 14.1 ± 0.4 g/dl.[55] Levels returned to pretreatment values within 6 months after discontinuing the agonist. These changes were not accompanied by altered serum erythropoietin, indicating a direct androgen effect on red blood cell precursors. Combining erythropoietin and T has a synergistic effect on erythroid colony formation in human bone marrow cultures.[56] Thus, it is thought that androgen has a direct effect on stem cells to increase the number of erythropoietin-sensitive cells and an indirect effect mediated by increased erythropoietin levels, which stimulates the erythropoietin-sensitive red blood cell precursors.

## Immune System

Androgen deficiency and replacement effects on the immune system have not been studied extensively in humans. In rats castration causes increased thymus weight, and T reverses this effect.[57] This relationship is inhibited by antiandrogens but not by 5α-reductase inhibitors, and it does not require conversion of T to $E_2$.[58] The changes may be mediated indirectly by the thymic epithelial cells.

## Lipids

In men with hypogonadism, fat tends to be distributed more to the hips and thighs and less to the abdomen, suggesting sex steroids affect fat distribution and, perhaps, serum lipids. Recent studies in middle-aged, abdominally obese men show that androgen has marked effects on adipose metabolism.[59] T treatment of boys with delayed puberty causes a decrease in high-density lipoprotein (HDL) cholesterol levels without a significant change in low-density lipoprotein (LDL) cholesterol.[60] In a study involving prepubertal and early pubertal boys, human

chorionic gonadotropin (hCG) stimulation of T and estradiol secretion resulted in decreased lipoprotein lipase activity and increased hepatic lipase activity.[61] HDL cholesterol levels were positively correlated with lipoprotein lipase activity and negatively correlated with hepatic lipase activity.

Differences in T-induced effects on lipids in hypogonadal men have been reported. After controlling for age and body mass index (BMI), Oppenheim and colleagues[62] found that hypogonadal men had higher total cholesterol, LDL cholesterol, triglycerides levels, and a higher total cholesterol/HDL cholesterol ratio. HDL cholesterol levels were similar when compared with those of eugonadal men. When serum T was lowered acutely in normal men with a GnRH agonist, only HDL cholesterol levels increased.[63,64] This pattern reversed when the agonist was stopped. Chronic androgen replacement of hypopituitary men increased hepatic lipase without affecting lipoprotein lipase activity.[65] Serum apoproteins A-I and A-II were decreased. Castrating aged men with prostatic carcinoma increased total and LDL cholesterol and apoprotein B levels without affecting HDL cholesterol.[66] Most evidence indicates androgen deficiency is associated with an increase in total, LDL, and HDL cholesterol levels and replacement therapy tends to decrease each parameter, but the HDL/LDL cholesterol ratio tends to be reduced slightly by treatment.

## Vascular Endothelium and Smooth Muscle

Vascular endothelium and smooth muscle are involved in atherosclerosis, and sex steroid–induced factors may contribute to atherosclerosis. Plasma levels of endothelin, a potent vasoconstrictor produced by endothelial cells, are normally higher in men than women.[67] The difference is mediated by sex steroids because treatment of male-to-female transsexuals with ethinyl estradiol (0.1 mg/d) and cyproterone acetate, an antiandrogen, reduces endothelin levels, and treatment of female-to-male transsexuals with testosterone esters (250 mg every 2 weeks) increases endothelin levels.

Androgen induces proliferation of cultured smooth muscle cells when isolated from the rat aorta. These cells have androgen receptors and possess 5α-reductase activity.[68] The smooth muscle cells also possess estrogen receptors and exhibit aromatase activity.[69] It is probable that T and its metabolites DHT and $E_2$ have significant effects on endothelium and vascular smooth muscle in man.

# Benefits and Risks of Androgen Replacement

Traditionally, the benefits of androgen replacement therapy have focused on virilization and improving psychosocial well-being for the young hypogonadal male. Restoring libido and potency are the usual therapeutic goals in men with acquired androgen deficiency, but age must be considered when assessing the benefits and risks of androgen replacement (Table 24.3).

## Age 14 to 18 Years

Clinicians should be aggressive in providing androgen replacement to young men with hypogonadism. In addition to the psychosocial benefits (proper timing of virilization, voice deepening, and increasing skeletal muscle mass), normal bone mass requires adequate androgen and estrogen at a critical stage of development or the risk for developing osteoporosis and debilitating fractures's increased.

The major risk of androgen replacement in the young male is premature closure of the epiphyses and a reduction in the individual's potential height. This risk is readily managed by using lower doses of T while monitoring growth and bone age. As in normal puberty, transient gynecomastia and acne can occur. The theoretical risk of suppressing the hypothalamic-pituitary-testicular axis in boys can be managed with cyclical therapy: treat for 3 or 6 months, stop therapy for 3 months, and assess development and T levels to determine if endogenous hormone secretion has been activated. Fertility among boys with delayed puberty or men with permanent hypogonadotropic hypogonadism is not adversely affected.[70] Individuals with permanent GnRH or FSH and LH deficiency can undergo hormone replacement therapy when fertility is desired. T replacement in young hypogonadal males may produce a slight reduction in HDL/total cholesterol. Androgen replacement normalizes cholesterol levels to those found in eugonadal males.

TABLE 24.3. Benefits and risks of androgen replacement in males.

| Age | Benefits | Risks |
|---|---|---|
| 14–18 | Cause virilization<br>Improve psychosocial well-being<br>Increase skeletal muscle<br>Achieve normal bone mass | Premature closure of epiphyses and blunting of potential height<br>Cause gynecomastia<br>Decrease HDL:T cholesterol |
| >18–50 | Restore libido and potency<br>Preserve bone mass<br>Increase lean body mass<br>Improve strength<br>Improve physical stamina<br>Improve psychological well-being | Precipitate or worsen sleep apnea<br>Induce polycythemia<br>Facilitate development of BPH and/or prostate cancer<br>Cause gynecomastia<br>Decrease HDL:T cholesterol |
| >50 | Restore libido and potency<br>Preserve bone mass and prevent fractures<br>Increase lean body mass<br>Improve strength<br>Improve physical stamina<br>Improve psychological well-being | Precipitate or worsen sleep apnea<br>Induce polycythemia<br>Cause CVA<br>Exacerbate BPH and/or prostate cancer<br>Cause gynecomastia<br>Decrease HDL:T cholesterol |

## Age >18 to 50 Years

T treatment of androgen deficiency in >18- to 50-year-old men usually restores male hair patterns, heightens libido and potency, improves general well-being, increases energy and stamina, and enlarges the prostate. When hypogonadism occurs in an adult, treatment can retard the development of symptomatic osteoporosis and may increase cortical bone density.[71]

Androgen deficiency may be diagnosed in men with or predisposed to sleep-disordered breathing. Obesity in men is a strong risk factor for developing sleep apnea, and obese men frequently have low total and free T levels. Additionally, men with obstructive sleep apnea have lower serum T levels than men with primary snoring.[72] In patients where the low T level is related to sleep apnea, androgen replacement therapy may be unnecessary. Serum T correlates with oxygen saturation during overnight polysomnography. Hypogonadism associated with impaired respiration during sleep is usually secondary, perhaps due to a reduction in the bioactivity of LH.[73] Continuous positive airway pressure therapy reduces sleep apnea and increases plasma IGF-I, SHBG, and total T, but not free T levels.[74] Sleep apnea-related hypogonadism also may be reversed by uvulopalatopharyngoplasty.[72]

T replacement in androgen-deficient men can worsen or cause disordered breathing.[75,76] One proposed mechanism for androgen-induced sleep apnea points to increased sensitization to hypoxia (decreasing $pCO_2$ causes increased apnea). A direct effect of T on neuromuscular innervation of the upper airway is another possibility.[77] Hypoxia resulting from sleep apnea or chronic obstructive pulmonary disease stimulates erythropoietin-mediated erythropoiesis. Androgen can stimulate erythropoiesis both directly and indirectly by its effect on erythropoietin, but appropriate T replacement doses rarely lead to polycythemia in nonapneic >18- to 50-year-old men.[78]

Clinical prostate cancer and symptomatic BPH are very rare in this age group. Prostate size regresses in men who become hypogonadal before age 40.[30,79] Men who become hypo-gonadal before age 40 (perhaps age 50) and are not provided with replacement therapy are unlikely to develop either symptomatic BPH or prostate cancer. Autopsy studies reveal the beginnings of BPH in the prostates of men in their 30s, and the incidence increases with aging.[80] T appears necessary but not sufficient for developing clinical BPH. Similarly, latent prostate cancer may be found at autopsy of men in their thirties,[81] and it increases with age.[82] Androgen appears to promote cancer after a genetic mutation initiates it. No differences in serum T levels were found in men who were studied 5 to 15 years before the clinical diagnosis of BPH or prostate cancer was established.[83] At this time there is no evidence that hypogonadal men on appropriate doses of androgen have an increased prevalence of BPH or prostate cancer as compared with eugonadal men.

## Age >50 Years

T therapy in this age range improves well-being, increases libido and potency (in the absence of comorbid diseases that cause impotence), and increases muscle mass and strength. Changes noted in serum markers of bone activity also suggest a beneficial effect. However, T replacement in hypogonadal men over age 50 years may induce polycythemia, precipitate or worsen sleep apnea, or accelerate symptomatic BPH, clinical prostate cancer or both.[52,84,85]

Polycythemia can increase the viscosity of the blood and decrease cerebral blood flow.[86] Over age 50, polycythemia is also considered a significant risk factor for strokes, especially when underlying vascular disease exists. Risk increases further with androgen-induced elevations in endothelin and vascular smooth muscle and platelet thromboxane $A_2$ receptors.

Serum levels of total and free T at the time of diagnosis are similar to controls in patients with both BPH and prostate cancer.[87] However, androgen can exacerbate metastatic prostate cancer.[88,89] High-dose androgen regimens also have been associated with the development of clinical prostate cancer in a few young men.[90] Therapies directed at reducing intraprostatic T or DHT are partially effective in treating BPH and prostate cancer, which suggests that T should not be prescribed for patients with prostate cancer or symptomatic BPH.

Autopsy data reveal that the incidence of latent prostate cancer is similar throughout the world; however, clinical prostate cancer occurs less frequently in Japan and China.[82] The factors responsible for higher clinical prostate cancer prevalence in the United States and Western Europe are poorly understood. Diet is highly suspect, however. High-fat diets may prolong the metabolic clearance rates of T. Vegetarian diets can decrease T and increase SHBG, and may decrease free T.[91] Japanese and Chinese men appear to have less ability to convert T to DHT.[27,28] This could account for the difference in hair patterns and possibly differences in clinical prostate cancer and could provide a rationale for using a 5α-reductase inhibitor for chemoprevention or for using an androgen that could not be 5α-reduced for androgen replacement.

The true benefit/risk ratio for T therapy in men over age 50 is currently unknown. Effective prostate monitoring is essential when providing androgen replacement to men over the age of 50.

# Androgen Preparations and Doses

Clinicians now have a variety of approved T preparations from which to choose. T can be administered orally, transdermally, or parenterally. An acceptable androgen must effectively correct the symptoms and signs of androgen deficiency. The route of administration must be acceptable to the patient to promote long-term adherence. Pharmacodynamics must be predictable. The drug must be safe, and the delivery system should have minimal side effects. Reasonable costs will facilitate widespread acceptance.

To simulate normal physiology as much as possible, serum T levels should simulate physiologic levels. The daily T production rate in young adult males is 6 to 7 mg, but the metabolic clearance rate decreases in individuals after age 50, so adequate replacement therapy

TABLE 24.4. Androgen preparations.

| |
|---|
| Oral or sublingual |
|   Testosterone |
|   Methyl testosterone[a] |
|   Fluoxymesterone[a] |
|   Mesterolone[b] |
|   Testosterone undecanoate[b] |
| Parenteral |
|   Testosterone propionate[a] |
|   Testosterone cypionate[a] |
|   Testosterone enanthate[a] |
|   Testosterone phenylpropionate[b] |
|   Testosterone isocaproate[b] |
|   Testosterone decanote[b] |
|   Testosterone bucilate[c] |
| Transcutaneous |
|   Testosterone transdermal therapeutic system[a] |
|   Testosterone transdermal system (nonscrotal)[a] |
| Testosterone pellets |
|   Fused crystalline testosterone[a] |
|   Testosterone-poly (DL-lactide-co-glycolide) microspheres[c] |

[a] Available in the United States.
[b] Available outside of the United States.
[c] Experimental.

may not require more than 4 mg/day for older individuals. The efficiency of delivering this amount of androgen into the circulation varies greatly with the route of administration and the formulation (Table 24.4).

## Oral Preparations

Because orally administered T undergoes first-pass inactivation by the liver, this is the least efficient route for administering T. Chemical modifications of T have somewhat prolonged its biologic activity. The approved oral androgenic formulations in the United States include 17α-methyl testosterone and fluoxymesterone (9α-fluoro-11β-hydroxy-17α-methyl testosterone). Each can cause virilization if given in large enough doses (>40 mg/day). The serum half-life is short, and virilizing doses can cause serious hepatotoxicity. For these reasons most authorities favor other agents for androgen replacement. T analogues (norethandrolone, oxymetholone, and stanazol) are approved anabolic agents. Concerns relevant for 17α-methyl testosterone and fluoxymesterone also apply to androgen analogue use.

Two additional oral androgens are available outside of the United States. Mesterolone ($1\alpha$-methyl-$5\alpha$-androstan-$17\beta$-ol-3-one) is a weak androgen when given orally. Testosterone undecanoate is more popular. The 10 carbon chain at the $17\beta$ position enhances lipid solubility. When given in oleic oil, it is taken up by the intestinal lymphatics, bypassing the liver and thereby retarding its degradation, but the usual replacement dose is 40 mg qid. The relatively short serum half-life results in subnormal T levels at night. Nonetheless, virilization is possible, and restoration of libido and potency are well documented. Doses of testosterone undecanoate that provide adequate serum levels of T for the majority of the day also increase serum levels of DHT. This compound has had a good safety record for over 10 years,[92] and is the only oral androgen with an acceptable record of efficacy and safety.

## Transdermal Preparations

Two transdermal delivery systems for T have been approved in the United States and other countries. Gel formulation of both T and DHT are available in some parts of Europe. The transdermal delivery systems or gels provide the patient with control over his therapy and offer the theoretical advantage of simulating normal diurnal patterns with higher T or DHT levels or both in the morning.

The first transdermal delivery system approved in the United States was designed to deliver 4 to 6 mg of T into the circulation.[93] The system is replaced daily, but this system does not use agents that readily enhance T absorption through the skin. To deliver this amount of T, the system is applied to scrotal skin. The thinness of and the circulation to scrotal skin provide much greater absorption of T than when the system is applied to the torso or an extremity. Because scrotal skin exhibits considerable $5\alpha$-reductase activity, serum levels of DHT are increased above normal physiologic levels. More than 7 years' experience attests to a low incidence of topical and systemic side effects.[94] To enhance adherence to scotal skin, the patient must dry-shave the scrotum every 3 to 5 days.

Recently, a transdermal system that uses alcohol to enhance T penetration of the skin has been approved.[95] Two ($37 \text{ cm}^2$) patches are applied each 24 hours to the torso or extremities. Each system is designed to release 2.5 mg of T. Physiologic serum levels of T, DHT, and estradiol are achieved, and they persist for 24 hours. A small group of patients have been treated 4 years or more, and 94 patients have been studied for up to 3 years. Chronic skin irritation accounts for 5% discontinuation, and allergic contact dermatitis has caused an additional 4% to discontinue treatment.[96]

De Lignieres[97] reported the use of DHT-containing gel in 37 men 55 to 70 years of age, treated for 6 months to 5 years. Mean prostate size as measured by ultrasound decreased from $31.1 \pm 16.3$ g before treatment and $26.3 \pm 12.7$ g after a mean of 1.8 years of DHT treatment ($p < 0.01$). Topical application of this DHT gel to the penis of boys with micropenis has been reported to be beneficial, but some systemic effects were noted.[98]

## Parenteral Preparations of Testosterone

The length of the carbon chain that is esterified to testosterone at the $17\beta$ position and the vehicle in which the compound is administered will affect the rate of T release and clearance. Longer chain carbon esters are more lipophilic, thereby reducing the rate of release from the lipid vehicle. The lipid vehicle is important, as exemplified by studies in the rat.[99] The same dose of free T gave much more sustained serum levels of T when given in hydrogenated soybean oil as compared with liquid soybean oil.

Testosterone propionate contains only a 2 carbon ester. When 25 mg of testosterone propionate was administered in sesame oil to normal men, plasma levels of testosterone propionate were detectable within 3 hours, and low levels at 72 hours. Labeled T that was released from the testosterone propionate was detectable within 3 hours, and peak T levels of 11.5 and 14 ng/ml were achieved between 24 and 27 hours. The $t^{1}/_{2}$ was about 24 hours.

Testosterone cypionate and testosterone enanthate have received widespread clinical

**Editor's Comments:** The goal of testosterone (T) replacement therapy is to ameliorate the symptoms of T deficiency by establishing and maintaining stable physiologic concentrations of T, bioavailable testosterone, and the major metabolites, dihydrotestosterone (DHT) and estradiol. Because T replacement in hypogonadal men involves long-term treatment, therapeutic goals must be accomplished with minimal adverse effects.

Intramuscular administration of testosterone enanthate (TE) and testosterone cypionate (TC) has been a commonly used treatment for male hypogonadism, but often results in supraphysiologic T levels during the first few days after injection. These intermittent elevations of T may have physiological consequences.

Testosterone therapy can induce erythropoiesis and sleep apnea and can lead to polycythemia in some patients, particularly those >50 years of age. In these patients, polycythemia can increase blood viscosity and diminish cerebral flood flow, becoming a significant risk factor for stroke in patients with underlying vascular disease. Although the clinical significance to T-related increases in hemoglobin and hematocrit have been debated in medical literature, the temporal relationship between the administration of T and development of a thromboembolic event has not been definitively addressed in a well-designed clinical study. It is also important to note that in addition to the erythropoietic effects of T, normal prostatic development is known to be dependent on T and DHT, the principal androgens affecting the prostate. Therefore, important measurement of safety in patients receiving T treatment include effects on the prostate.

As the authors pointed out, therapeutic effects of different T treatments can vary according to age, the androgen preparation, and dose used. Transdermal delivery systems avoid the fluctuations in serum T concentrations and symptoms of hypogonadism associated with TE and TC treatment. Transdermal T provides physiologic serum T levels that mimic the normal circadian rhythm of endogenous T levels in healthy young men. In a recent study, as yet unpublished, comparing long-term treatment with a nonscrotal transdermal T system and TE, transdermal delivery did not lead to excessive stimulation of erythropoiesis as observed with TE treatment. Furthermore, the physiologic delivery of T by transdermal therapy was associated with PSA levels and increases in prostate size that were within normal ranges. However, periodic monitoring of hematocrit levels and prostate parameters is suggested for all patients who receive androgen therapy.

In summary, transdermal delivery systems can eliminate the spikes and deep troughs in serum T levels, thereby more closely simulating the normal physiological pattern. This mode of T administration may be less likely to induce sleep apnea and hematocrits >50% than standard doses of TE and TC administered by IM injection. However, the mechanisms for testosterone-induced polycythemia, especially in older men, are not well understood.

Wayne J.G. Hellstrom, M.D., F.A.C.S.
Editor

---

use for over four decades. The pharmacokinetics of these esters when given in oil are very similar.[100] Following a 200-mg injection of either testosterone cypionate or testosterone enanthate, serum total and free T levels are increased above the normal range for 1 to 5 days. They typically fall to subnormal levels by 14 days in men between 20 and 40 years of age.[101–103] Snyder and Lawrence[104] provided data indicating that 200 mg every 2 weeks or 300 mg every 3 weeks was preferable, a dose sufficient to suppress LH and the least frequent effective dosing schedule.[104] Reduced metabolic clearance rates will prolong the duration of action in men over age 50. Therefore, less frequent injections or a reduced dose should be given to these men.

## Testosterone Pellets

T also has been fused into crystalline pellets that are implanted subcutaneously with a trocar. Although this mode of delivering T has not received widespread popularity because it is a minor surgical procedure, it is available throughout the world. The pellets are available in 100- and 200-mg doses. The 200-mg capsule is estimated to release approximately 1.5 mg of T/day.[105] Implantation of a 600-mg dose provides serum levels of T that are within the normal range for 4 to 5 months, and a 1200 mg dose, after an initial high level, remains within the normal range for 6 months.

## Testosterone Preparations Under Development

Several T preparations are under clinical or preclinical evaluation or both. Testosterone bucilate is a longer-acting injectable ester. A single 600-mg injection was reported to increase the mean serum T + DHT into the low normal range for up to 12 weeks.[106] The 600-mg injection currently requires an injection volume

TABLE 24.5. Therapeutic guidelines for testosterone replacment therapy.

A.  Ages 14 to 18 years
   1. Give small doses of testosterone enanthate or cypionate ($75 mg/m^2$ month) for 3 to 6 months.[113] Experience with transdermal testosterone is limited in this age group.
   2. Gradually increase to $100–150 mg/m^2$/month of testosterone or cypionate. This will lead to a peak growth velocity approximately 1.5–2 years after the start of treatment. Axillary hair will develop approximately 1.5 years after the initiation of therapy. Larger doses of androgen can lead to premature epiphyseal closure and reduced ultimate height. Growth hormone is needed to achieve optimum effect.
   3. After complete virilization is achieved, adequate replacement can be maintained with oral testosterone undecanoate, transdermal testosterone, testosterone enanthate or cypionate, or testosterone pellets (see B.1.).
   4. Assess therapeutic and nadir serum total and free testosterone. Timing of sampling depends upon the route of administration and the preparation (see B.5.).
   5. Monitor virilization, height, weight, and growth velocity every 3 months; bone age and hematocrit should be obtained at 6-month intervals.
B.  Age >18 to 50 years
   1. Effective replacement therapy can be provided by oral testosterone undecanoate (40 mg qid or 80 mg bid), transdermal testosterone (4 or 6 mg scrotal system or two 2.5 mg nonscrotal systems every 24 hours), parenteral testosterone cypionate or enanthate (200 mg every 2 weeks or 300 mg every 3 weeks), or subcutaneous testosterone pellets (600 mg every 16 to 20 weeks).
   2. Perform digital rectal examination every 2 years after age 40 and yearly in men with a family history of prostate cancer. Those with a family history also should have an annual prostate specific antigen (PSA) test.
   3. Obtain baseline hematocrit prior to treatment, at 2 and 4 weeks, 3 months, and annually. An increase of >4% suggests chronic hypoxia or sleep apnea. Further evaluation is indicated.
   4. Measure serum triglycerides, total, HDL, and LDL cholesterol at baseline and 3 months.
   5. Assess serum total and free testosterone levels when they should be therapeutic (2 to 3 hours after oral testosterone undecanoate, 3 to 5 hours after application of a transdermal system, 3 to 5 days following an injection of testosterone enanthate or cypionate, and 1 to 2 weeks after implantation of testosterone pellets). Serum levels also should be obtained prior to the next dose to ensure that treatment is not excessive.
C.  Age >50 years
   1. Reduce the frequency of administration or the dose of testosterone cypionate or enanthate by 25–50% or use another delivery system that does not cause supraphysiologic levels of T. (The metabolic clearance rate of T decreases with age and the risks of sleep apnea, polycythema, and prostatic disease are increased.)
   2. Perform digital rectal examination every 6 months for first year and then yearly. After 60 years of age, patients should be examined every 3 months during the first year of therapy.
   3. Obtain baseline hematocrit prior to treatment, at 2 and 4 weeks, 3 months, and annually. An increase of >4% suggests chronic hypoxia or sleep apnea. Further evaluation is indicated.
   4. Measure serum triglycerides, total, HDL, and LDL cholesterol at baseline and 3 months.
   5. Assess therapeutic and nadir serum total and free testosterone levels (see B.5.).
   6. Measure prostate-specific antigen (PSA) before rectal examination at baseline and then yearly.
   7. Obtain transrectal ultrasound examination of the prostate and any time prostate pathology is suspected.

of 2.4 ml. If higher doses of testosterone bucilate provide somewhat higher serum levels of T, this formulation may be preferable for long-term replacement therapy. Microencapsulation of T into a biodegradable matrix composed of DL-lactide-co-glycolide also offers promise for prolonged release.[107] A single 630-mg injection increased levels of serum, total, and free T as well as of DHT and estradiol into the normal range for 10 to 11 weeks.[108] This dose was given as two 2.5-ml injections in an aqueous mixture.

A unique modality for delivery, T is provided by complexing T with 2-hydroxypropyl-β-cyclodextrin in a tablet and administering it sublingually.[109] T is quickly brought into solu-tion and absorbed through the oral mucosa, bypassing immediate degradation by the liver. The carrier is swallowed and subsequently di-gested. A 2.5-mg tablet will increase serum T levels within 20 minutes to approximately 30 nmol/l, and a 5.0-mg tablet will increase T levels to approximately 45 nmol/l.[110] Levels fall to approximately 10 nmol/l by 2 hours and reach baseline levels by 6 hours. Thus, it is nec-essary to administer the drug three times a day. Even though serum levels of T may be subnor-mal for part of the day and much of the night, patients report improvement in sexual motiva-tion and performance comparable to that in-duced by testosterone enanthate.

Animal studies with two other compounds

have suggested that they may be useful clinically. When testosterone undecanoate was administered parenterally to nonhuman primates, prolonged release was observed. A single 10 mg/kg dose of testosterone undecanoate in tea seed oil maintained serum T at supraphysiologic levels for 56 days and normal levels for an additional 56 days.[111] Undecanoate has a 10 carbon ester as compared with enanthate, which has a 6 carbon ester. The longer side chain gives undecanoate greater hydrophobicity. Seven-α-methyl-19 nor-testosterone has been proposed to provide anabolic effects with less effect on the prostate because it cannot be metabolized to a 5α-reduced androgen.[112] Whether this compound or others that follow this principle will prove effective and safe in hypogonadal men remains to be demonstrated.

## Summary

Variation in T delivery, depending on route of administration, dose, and frequency, will affect efficacy of T treatment. The risks of androgen replacement require that guidelines be established for monitoring potential side effects (Table 24.5). Appropriate dosing is the first step to preventing undesirable side effects. Age should be considered when deciding on dosage and the parameters to monitor.

## References

1. Davidson JM, Chen JJ, Crapo L, et al. Hormonal changes and sexual function in aging men. *J Clin Endocrinol Metab* 1983; 57:71–77.
2. Davidson JM, Camargo CA, Smith ER. Effects of androgen on sexual behavior in hypogonadal men. *J Clin Endocrinol Metab* 1979; 48:955–962.
3. Davidson JM, Kwan M, Greenleaf WJ. Hormonal replacement and sexuality in men. *Clin Endocrinol Metab* 1982; 11:599–623.
4. Cunningham GR, Karacan I, Ware JC, et al. The relationships between serum testosterone and prolactin levels and nocturnal penile tumescence (NPT) in impotent men. *J Androl* 1982; 3:241–247.
5. Fenwick PBC, Mercer S, Grant R, et al. Nocturnal penile tumescence and serum testosterone levels. *Arch Sex Behav* 1986; 15:13.
6. Plymate SR, Tenover JS, Bremner WJ. Circadian variation in testosterone, sex hormone-binding globulin, and calculated non-sex hormone-binding globulin bound testosterone in healthy young and elderly men. *J Androl* 1989; 10:366–371.
7. Murray FR, Cameron DF, Vogel RB, et al. The pituitary-testicular axis at rest and during moderate exercise in males with diabetes mellitus and normal sexual function. *J Androl* 1988; 9:197–206.
8. Manni A, Pardridge WM, Cefalu W, et al. Bioavailability of albumin-bound testosterone. *J Clin Endocrinol Metab* 1985; 61:705–710.
9. Ekins R. Measurement of free hormones in blood. *Endocr Rev* 1990; 11:5–46.
10. Mendel CM. The free hormone hypothesis distinction from the free hormone transport hypothesis. *J Androl* 1992; 13:107–116.
11. Goldzieher JW, Dozier TS, Smith KD, Steinberger E. Improving the diagnostic reliability of rapidly fluctuating plasma hormone levels by optimized multiple-sampling techniques. *J Clin Endocrinol Metab* 1976; 43:824.
12. Bain J, Langevin R, D'Costa M, Sanders RM, Hucker S. Serum pituitary and steroid hormone levels in the adult male: one value is as good as the mean of three. *Fertil Steril* 1988; 49:123–126.
13. Vermeulen A, Verdonck G. Representativeness of a single point plasma testosterone level for the long-term hormonal milieu in men. *J Clin Endocrinol Metab* 1992; 74:939–942.
14. Korenman SG, Morley JE, Mooradian AD, et al. Secondary hypogonadism in older men: its relation to impotence. *J Clin Endocrinol Metab* 1990; 71:963–969.
15. Guay AT, Bansal S, Hodge MB. Possible hypothalamic impotence. Male counterpart to hypothalamic amenorrhea? *Urology* 1991; 38:317–322.
16. Tenover JS. Effects of testosterone supplementation in the aging male. *J Clin Endocrinol Metab* 1992; 75:1092–1098.
17. Mulligan T, Schmitt B. Testosterone for erectile failure. *J Gen Intern Med* 1993; 8:517–521.
18. Clopper RR, Voorhess ML, MacGillivray MH, Lee PA, Mills B. Psychosexual behavior in hypopituitary men: a controlled comparison of gonadotropin and testosterone replacement. *Psychoneuroendocrinology* 1993; 18:149–161.
19. Bancroft J, Wu FCW. Changes in erectile responsiveness during androgen replacement therapy. *Arch Sex Behav* 1983; 12:59–66.
20. Eyal A, Ish-Shalom S, Hoch Z, Hochberg Z. Androgen therapy in hypogonadotrophic hypogonadism: time course of erectosexual functions. *Arch Androl* 1988; 20:163–169.
21. Carani C, Bancroft J, Granata A, et al. Testosterone and erectile function, nocturnal

penile tumescence and rigidity, and erectile response to usual erotic stimuli in hypogonadal men. *Psychoneuroendocrinology* 1992; 17:647–654.

22. Greenstein A, Plymate SR, Katz PG. Visually stimulated erection in castrated men. *J Urol* 1995; 153:650–652.

23. Rowland DL, Greenleaf WJ, Dorfman IJ, Davidson JM. Aging and sexual function in men. *Arch Sex Behav* 1993; 22:545–557.

24. O'Carroll R, Shapiro C, Bancroft J. Androgens, behaviour and nocturnal erection in hypogonadal men: the effects of varying the replacement dose. *Clin Endocrinol* 1985; 23:527–538.

25. Cunningham GR, Hirshkowitz M, Korenman SG, Karacan I. Testosterone replacement therapy and sleep-related erections in hypogonadal men. *J Clin Endocrinol Metab* 1990; 70:792–797.

26. Thigpen A-E, Silver RI, Guileyardo JM, et al. Tissue distribution and ontogeny of steroid 5α-reductase isozyme expression. *J Clin Invest* 1993; 92:903–910.

27. Ross RK, Bernstein L, Lobo RA, et al. 5-alpha-reductase activity and risk of prostate cancer among Japanese and US white and black males. *Lancet* 1992; 339:887–889.

28. Lookingbill DP, Demers LM, Wang C, et al. Clinical and biochemical parameters of androgen action in normal healthy Caucasian *versus* Chinese subjects. *J Clin Endocrinol Metab* 1991; 72:1242–1248.

29. Sasagawa I, Nakada T, Kazama T, et al. Volume change of the prostate and seminal vesicles in male hypogonadism after androgen replacement therapy. *Int Urol Nephrol* 1990; 22:279–284.

30. Behre HM, Bohmeyer J, Nieschlag E. Prostate volume in testosterone-treated and untreated hypogonadal men in comparison to age-matched normal controls. *Clin Endocrinol* 1994; 40:341–349.

31. Parker MW, Johanson AJ, Rogol AD, Kaiser DL, Blizzard RM. Effect of testosterone on somatomedin-C concentrations in prepubertal boys. *J Clin Endocrinol Metab* 1984; 58:87–90.

32. Weissbeger AJ, Ho KKY. Activation of the somatotropic axis by testosterone in adult males: evidence for the role of aromatization. *J Clin Endocrinol Metab* 1993; 76:1407–1412.

33. Keenan BS, Richards GE, Ponder SW. Androgen-stimulated pubertal growth: the effects of testosterone and dihydrotestosterone on growth hormone and insulin-like growth factor-I in the treatment of short stature and

delayed puberty. *J Clin Endocrinol Metab* 1993; 76:996–1001.

34. Finkelstein JS, Neer RM, Biller BMK, Crawford JD, Klibanski A. Osteopenia in men with a history of delayed puberty. *N Engl J Med* 1992; 326:600–604.

35. Finkelstein JS, Klibanski A, Neer RM, et al. Osteoporosis in men with idiopathic hypogonadotropic hypogonadism. *Ann Intern Med* 1987; 106:354–361.

36. Wong FH, Pun KK, Wang C. Loss of bone mass in patients with Klinefelter's syndrome despite sufficient testosterone replacement. *Osteoporosis Int* 1993; 3:3–7.

37. Finklestein JS, Klibanski A, Neer RM, et al. Increases in bone density during treatment of men with idiopathic hypogonadotropic hypogonadism. *J Clin Endocrinol Metab* 1989; 69:776–783.

38. Arisaka O, Arisaka M, Nakayama Y, Fujiwam S, Yabuta K. Effect of testosterone on bone density and bone metabolism in adolescent male hypogonadism. *Metabolism* 1995; 44:419–423.

39. Bourguignon J-P. Linear growth as a function of age at onset of puberty and sex steroid dosage: therapeutic implications. *Endocr Rev* 1988; 9:467–488.

40. Smith EP, Boyd J, Frank GR, et al. Estrogen resistance caused by a mutation in the estrogen-receptor gene in a man. *N Engl J Med* 1994; 331:1056–1061.

41. Morishima A, Grumbach MM, Simpson ER, Fisher C, Qin K. Aromatase deficiency in male and female siblings caused by a novel mutation and the physiological role of estrogens. *J Clin Endocrinol Metab* 1995; 80:3689–3698.

42. Zachman M, Prader A, Sobel EH, et al. Pubertal growth in patients with androgen insensitivity: indirect evidence for the importance of estrogens in pubertal growth of girls. *J Pediatr* 1986; 108:694–697.

43. Kasperk CH, Wergedal JE, Farley JR, et al. Androgens directly stimulate proliferation of bone cells in vitro. *Endocrinology* 1989; 124:1576–1578.

44. Kasperk C, Fitzsimmons R, Strong D. Studies of the mechanism by which androgens enhance mitogenesis and differentiation in bone cells. *J Clin Endocrinol Metab* 1990; 71:1322–1329.

45. Bellido T, Jilka RL, Boyce BF, et al. Regulation of interleukin-6, osteoclastogenesis, and bone mass by androgens. *J Clin Invest* 1995; 95:2886–2895.

46. Kelepouris N, Harper KD, Gannon F, Kaplan

FS, Haddad JG. Severe osteoporosis in men. *Ann Intern Med* 1995; 123:452–460.

47. Jackson JA, Riggs MW, Spiekerman AM. Testosterone deficiency as a risk factor for hip fractures in men: a case-control study. *Am J Med Sci* 1992; 304:4–8.

48. Goldray D, Weisman Y, Jaccard N, et al. Decreased bone density in elderly men treated with the gonadotropin-releasing hormone agonist decapeptyl (d-Trp$^6$-GnRH). *J Clin Endocrinol Metab* 1993; 76:288–290.

49. Chauhan AK, Katiyar BC, Misra S, Thacker AK, Singh NK. Muscle dysfunction in male hypogonadism. *Acta Neurol Scand* 1986; 73:466–471.

50. Kenyon AT, Knowlton K, Sandiford I, Koch FC, Lotwin G. A comparative study of the metabolic effects of testosterone propionate in normal men and women and in eunuchoidism. *Endocrinology* 1940; 26:26–45.

51. Sandiford I, Knowlton K, Kenyon AT. Basal heat production in hypogonadism in men and its increase by protracted treatment with testosterone propionate. *J Clin Endocrinol* 1941; 12:931–939.

52. Tenover JS. Effects of testosterone supplementation in the aging male. *J Clin Endocrinol Metab* 1992; 75:1092–1098.

53. Krabbe S, Christensen T, Worm J, Christiansen C, Transbol I. Relationship between haemoglobin and serum testosterone in normal children and adolescents and in boys with delayed puberty. *Acta Paediatr Scand* 1978; 67:655–658.

54. Alexanian R. Erythropoietin and erythropoiesis in anemic man following androgens. *Blood* 1969; 33:564–572.

55. Weber JP, Walsh PC, Peters CA, et al. Effect of reversible androgen deprivation on hemoglobin and serum immunoreactive erythropoietin in men. *Am J Hematol* 1991; 36:190–194.

56. Moriyama Y, Fisher JW. Effects of testosterone and erythropoietin on erythroid colony formation in human bone marrow cultures. *Blood* 1975; 45:665–670.

57. Aboudkhil S, Bureau JP, Garrelly L, et al. Effects of castration, depo-testosterone and cyproterone acetate on lymphocyte T subsets in mouse thymus and spleen. *Scand J Immunol* 1991; 34:647–653.

58. Kumar N, Shan L-X, Hardy MP, Bardin CW. Mechanism of androgen-induced thymolysis in rats. *Endocrinology* 1995; 136:4887–4893.

59. Marin P, Oden B, Bjorntorp P. Assimilation and mobilization of triglycerides in subcutaneous abdominal and femoral adipose tissue in vivo in men: effects of androgens. *J Clin Endocrinol Metab* 1995; 80:239–243.

60. Kirkland RT, Keenan BS, Probstfield JL, et al. Decrease in plasma high-density lipoprotein cholesterol levels at puberty in boys with delayed adolescence. *JAMA* 1987; 257:502–507.

61. Sorva R, Kuusi T, Dunkel L, et al. Effects of endogenous sex steroids on serum lipoproteins and postheparin plasma lipolytic enzymes. *J Clin Endocrinol Metab* 1988; 66:408–413.

62. Oppenheim DS, Greenspan SL, Zervas NT, Schoenfeld DA, Klibanski A. Elevated serum lipids in hypogonadal men with and without hyperprolactinemia. *Ann Intern Med* 1989; 111:288–292.

63. Goldberg RB, Rabin D, Alexander AN, et al. Suppression of plasma testosterone leads to an increase in serum total cholesterol and high density lipoprotein cholesterol and apolipoproteins A I and B. *J Clin Endocrinol Metab* 1985; 60:203.

64. Bagatell CJ, Knopp RH, Vale WW, Rivier JE, Brenmer WJ. Physiologic testosterone levels in normal men suppress high-density lipoprotein cholesterol levels. *Ann Intern Med* 1992; 116:967–973.

65. Sorva R, Kuusi T, Taskinen M-R, et al. Testosterone substitution increases the activity of lipoprotein lipase and hepatic lipase in hypogonadal males. *Atherosclerosis* 1988; 69:191–197.

66. Moorjani S, Dupont A, Labrie F, et al. Changes in plasma lipoproteins during various androgen suppression therapies in men with prostatic carcinoma: effects of orchiectomy, estrogen, and combination treatment with luteinizing hormone-releasing hormone and flutamide. *J Clin Endocrinol Metab* 1989; 66:314–322.

67. Polderman KH, Coen DA, Stehouwer A. Influence of sex hormones on plasma endothelin levels. *Ann Intern Med* 1993; 118:429–432.

68. Fujimoto R, Moiimoto I, Morita E, et al. Androgen receptors, 5 alpha-reductase activity and androgen-dependent proliferation of vascular smooth muscle cells. *J Steroid Biochem Mol Biol* 1994; 50:169–174.

69. Bayard F, Clamens S, Meggetto F, et al. Estrogen synthesis, estrogen metabolism, and functional estrogen receptors in rat arterial smooth muscle cells in culture. *Endocrinology* 1995; 136:1523–1529.

70. Burger HG, deKretser DM, Hudson B, et al. Effects of preceding androgen therapy on testicular response to human pituitary gonadotropin in hypogonadotropic hypogonadism: a study of three patients. *Fertil Steril* 1981; 35:64–68.

71. Greenspan SL, Oppenheim DS, Klibanski A. Importance of gonadal steroids to bone mass in

men with hyperprolactinemic hypogonadism. *Ann Intern Med* 1989; 110:526–531.

72. Santamaria JD, Prior JC, Fleetham JA. Reversible reproductive dysfuction in men with obstructive sleep apnea. *Clin Endocrinol* 1988; 28:461–470.

73. Wortsman J, Eagleton LE, Rosner W, Dufau ML. Mechanism for the hypotestosteronemia of the sleep apnea syndrome. *Am J Med Sci* 1987; 293:221–225.

74. Grunstein RR, Handelsman DJ, Lawrence SJ, et al. Neuroendocrine dysfunction in sleep apnea: reversal by continuous positive airways pressure therapy. *J Clin Endocrinol Metab* 1989; 68:352–358.

75. Matsumoto AM, Sandblom RE, Schoene RB, et al. Testosterone replacement in hypogonadal men: effects on obstructive sleep apnea, respiratory drives, and sleep. *Clin Endocrinol* 1985; 22:713–721.

76. Schneider BK, Pickett CK, Zwillich CW, et al. Influence of testosterone on breathing during sleep. *J Appl Physiol* 1986; 61:618–623.

77. Cistuli PA, Grunstein RR, Sullivan CE. Effect of testosterone administration on upper airway collapsibility during sleep. *Am J Respir Crit Care Med* 1994; 149:530–532.

78. Matsumoto AM. Effects of chronic testosterone administration in normal men: safety and efficacy of high dosage testosterone and parallel dose-dependent suppression of luteinizing hormone, follicle-stimulating hormone, and sperm production. *J Clin Endocrinol Metab* 1990; 70:282–287.

79. Woo JP, Gu FL. The prostate 41–75 years postcastration: an analysis of 26 eunuchs. *Chin Med J* 1987; 100:271–272.

80. Berry SJ, Coffey DS, Walsh PC, Ewing LL. The development of human benign prostatic hyperplasia with age. *J Urol* 1984; 132:474–478.

81. Sakr WA, Haas GP, Cassin BF, Pontes JE, Crissman JD. The frequency of carcinoma and intraepithelial neoplasia of the prostate in young male patients. *J Urol* 1993; 150:379–385.

82. Breslow N, Chang CW, Dhom G, et al. Latent carcinoma of prostate at autopsy in seven areas. *Int J Cancer* 1977; 20:680–688.

83. Carter HB, Pearson JD, Metter EJ, et al. Longitudinal evaluation of serum androgen levels in men with and without prostate cancer. *Prostate* 1995; 27:25–31.

84. Drinka PJ, Jochen AL, Cuisinier M. Polycythemia as a complication of testosterone replacement therapy in nursing home men with low testosterone levels. *J Am Geriatr Soc* 1995; 43:899–901.

85. Krauss DJ, Taub HA, Lantinga I-J, Dunsky MH, Kelly CM. Risks of blood volume changes in hypogonadal men treated with testosterone enanthate for erectile impotence. *J Urol* 1991; 146:1566–1570.

86. Semple Pd'A, Lowe GDO, Patterson J, et al. Comparison of cerebral blood flow after venesection of bronchitic secondary polycythaemic and primary polycythaemic patients. *Scott Med J* 1983; 28:332–337.

87. Anderson S-O, Adami H-O, Bergstrom R, Wide L. Serum pituitary and sex steroid hormone levels in the etiology of prostatic cancer—a population-based case control study. *Br J Cancer* 1993; 68:97–102.

88. Fowler JE Jr, Whitmore WF Jr. The response of metastatic adenocarcinoma of the prostate to exogenous testosterone. *J Urol* 1981; 126:372–375.

89. Manni A, Santen RJ, Boucher AE, et al. Androgen depletion and repletion as a means of potentiating the effect of cytotoxic chemotherapy in advanced prostate cancer. *J Steroid Biochem* 1987; 27:551–556.

90. Roberts JT, Essenhigh DM. Adenocarcinoma of prostate in 40-year-old body-builder. *Lancet* 1986; 2:742.

91. Hamalainen E, Adlercreutz H, Puska P, Pietinen P. Diet and serum sex hormones in healthy men. *J Steroid Biochem* 1984; 20:459–464.

92. Gooren LG. A ten-year safety study of the oral androgen testosterone undecanoate. *J Androl* 1994; 15:212–215.

93. Korenman SG, Viosca SP, Garza D, et al. Androgen therapy of hypogonadal men with transscrotal testosterone systems. *Am J Med* 1987; 83:471–478.

94. Cunningham GR, Snyder PJ, Atkinson LE. Testosterone transdermal delivery system. In: Bhasin S. et al, eds. *Pharmacology, Biology, and Clinical Application of Androgens.* New York: Wiley-Liss; 1996: 437–448.

95. Meikle AW, Mazer NA, Moellmer JF, et al. Enhanced transdermal delivery of testosterone across nonscrotal skin produces physiological concentrations of testosterone and its metabolites in hypogonadal men. *J Clin Endocrinol Metab* 1992; 74:623–628.

96. Meikle AW, Arver S, Dobs AS, Sanders SW, Mazer NA. ANDRODERM: A permeation enhanced non-scrotal testosterone transdermal system for the treatment of male hypo-

gonadism. In: Bhasin et al, eds. *Pharmacology, Biology, and Clinical Application of Androgens.* New York: Wiley-Liss; 1996: 449–457.

97. de Lignieres B. Transdermal dihydrotestosterone treatment of "andropause." *Ann Med* 1993; 25:235–241.

98. Choi SK, Han SW, Kim DH, de Lignieres B. Transdermal dihydrotestosterone therapy and its effects on patients with microphallus. *J Urol* 1993; 150:657–660.

99. Gerrity M, Freund M, Peterson RN, Falvo RE. The physiologic effects of testosterone in hydrogenated soybean oil vehicle as compared to free testosterone, testosterone propionate, and testosterone enanthate in a conventional oil vehicle. *J Androl* 1982; 3:221–226.

100. Schultel-Beerbuhl M, Nieschlag E. Comparison of testosterone, dihydrotestosterone, luteinizing hormone, and follicle-stimulating hormone in serum after injection of testosterone enanthate or testosterone cypionate. *Fertil Steril* 1980; 33:201–203.

101. Cunningham GR, Silverman V, Kohler PO. Gonadotropin suppression in normal males and males with 1° hypogonadism: evaluation of four androgens. *Int J Androl* 1978; (suppl 2, part 2):720–729.

102. Nankin HR. Hormone kinetics after intramuscular testosterone cypionate. *Fertil Steril* 1987; 47:1004–1009.

103. Sokal RZ, Palacios A, Campfield LA, et al. Comparison of the kinetics of injectable testosterone in eugonadal and hypogonadal men. *Fertil Steril* 1982; 37:425–430.

104. Snyder PJ, Lawrence DA. Treatment of male hypogonadism with testosterone enanthate. *J Clin Endocrinol Metab* 1980; 51:1335–1339.

105. Handelsman DJ, Conway AJ, Boylan LM. Pharmacokinetics and pharmacodynamics of testosterone pellets in man. *J Clin Endocrinol Metab* 1990; 71:216–222.

106. Behre HM, Nieschlag E. Testosterone bucilate (20-Aet-1) in hypogonadal men: pharmacokinetics and pharmacodynamics of the new long-acting androgen ester. *J Clin Endocrinol Metab* 1992; 75:1204–1210.

107. Burris AS, Ewing LL, Sherins RJ. Initial trial of slow-release testosterone microspheres in hypogonadal men. *Fertil Steril* 1988; 50:493–497.

108. Bhasin S, Swerdloff RS, Steiner B, et al. A biodegradable testosterone microcapsule formulation provides uniform eugonadal levels of testosterone for 10–11 weeks in hypogonadal men. *J Clin Endocrinol Metab* 1992; 74:75–83.

109. Stuenkel CA, Dudley RE, Yen SSC. Sublingual administration of testosterone-hydroxylpropyl-β-cyclodextrin inclusion complex stimulates episodic androgen release in hypogonadal men. *J Clin Endocrinol Metab* 1991; 72:1054–1059.

110. Salehian B, Wang C, Alexander G. Pharmacokinetics, bioefficacy, and safety of sublingual testosterone cyclodextrin in hypogonadal men: comparison to testosterone enanthate—a clinical research center study. *J Clin Endocrinol Metab* 1995; 80:3567–3575.

111. Partsch C-J, Weinbauer GF, Fang R, Nieschlag E. Injectable testosterone undecanoate has more favourable pharmacokinetics and pharmacodynamics than testosterone enanthate. *Eur J Endocrinol* 1995; 132:514–519.

112. Sundarin K, Kumar N, Bardin CW. 7 alpha-methyl-19-nortestosterone: an ideal androgen for replacement therapy. *Recent Prog Horm Res* 1994; 49:373–376.

113. Richman RA, Kirsh LR. Testosterone treatment in adolescent boys with constitutional delay in growth and development. *N Engl J Med* 1988; 319:1563–1567.

# 25
# Premature Ejaculation

Allen D. Seftel and Stanley E. Althof

Traditionally, the etiology of premature ejaculation, a prevalent male dysfunction, was believed to be psychological and was treated therefore with a variety of behavioral or other psychotherapeutic techniques. Pharmacotherapy for treatment of premature ejaculation is presently in its infancy; however, it offers urologists an additional option for medical management of this distressing condition.

## Historical Perspective

There is no consensus on the definition of premature ejaculation. Various studies have defined the dysfunction in terms of time from intromission to ejaculation, number of coital thrusts, partner satisfaction, and degree of voluntary control. The most recent set of criteria, published in the fourth edition of the American Psychiatric Association's *Diagnostic and Statistical Manual of Mental Disorders*,[1] delineates three criteria for premature ejaculation:

1. Persistent or recurrent ejaculation with minimal stimulation before, during, or shortly after penetration and before the person wishes it. The clinician must take into account factors that affect duration of the excitement phase, such as age, novelty of the sexual partner, or situation, and recent frequency of sexual activity.
2. The disturbance causes marked distress or interpersonal difficulty.
3. The premature ejaculation is not due exclusively to the direct effects of a substance (e.g., withdrawal from opioids).

To confirm a diagnosis of premature ejaculation, the clinician must make three additional determinations: first, whether the dysfunction is lifelong or acquired; second, whether it is of a generalized or specific type; and third, whether it is due to psychological or combined factors. Although this set of criteria employs a multidimensional definition using time and voluntary control, it provides few quantifiable points of reference. For instance, what is meant by minimal sexual stimulation and how quickly should ejaculation occur after penetration for it to be considered dysfunctional?

Individual, conjoint, and group psychotherapy approaches in combination with behavioral strategies such as stop-start or squeeze techniques have all been used to treat premature ejaculation.[2-9] It is now recognized that the initial posttreatment success rates ranging from 60% to 95%[7,10] were not sustainable; 3 years after treatment, success rates had dwindled to 25%.[11,12] These data suggest the failure of clinicians to develop long-term strategies that allow patients to maintain their initial therapeutic gains. It would be interesting to examine data on the efficacy of treatment where therapists employ periodic booster or maintenance sessions after the termination of the original treatment.

This psychological/behavioral approach to rapid ejaculation, which has been in ascendancy for over 20 years, has been challenged by studies that suggest that ejaculatory latency can be prolonged by clomipramine or the selective serotonin reuptake inhibitor drugs (SSRIs)—fluoxetine, sertraline, and paroxetine—without troubling side effects.[13-17]

# The Case Western Reserve University (CWRU) Experience with Clomipramine for Premature Ejaculation

## Urologists' Perspective

As the treatment of erectile dysfunction has become less surgical, urologists are faced with new challenges in the treatment of male sexual dysfunction. Pharmacotherapy for premature ejaculation is one such new frontier. Urologists must now become conversant and knowledgeable about the diagnosis and management of this dysfunction.

To this end, CWRU initiated a trial of clomipramine for those patients with primary, lifelong premature ejaculation. The selection process was a careful one. A sample questionnaire was given to potential patients (Table 25.1). Excluded were those patients who were suspected of secondary or acquired premature ejaculation or those patients with concomitant erectile dysfunction. Cursory psychosocial screening excluded patients with overt psychopathology. To date, 10 patients have been followed with an average follow-up of 1.5 years. Five of the patients were happily married, and the remaining five patients had a stable rela-

tionship with a solo partner. The subjects did not perceive that the dysfunction had a negative impact on the nonsexual relationship, although they were dissatisfied with the quality of their sexual life. Other patients not accepted in the study had unrealistic expectations that correction of premature ejaculation would lead to marital harmony. To date, 7 of 10 patients continue on pharmacotherapy and find it helpful and satisfying. The one treatment "failure" was due to the deterioration of the relationship rather than to the lack of efficacy of the drug. This therapy is not a substitute for marital counseling, should not be used for treatment of erectile dysfunction, and should not be offered to men contemplating new relationships who are concerned about their possible sexual performance (performance anxiety). The two other failures with clomipramine were middle-aged men, both married. One patient found the clomipramine of no help and was switched to paroxetine. A second patient tried oral clomipramine for 2 weeks, 25 mg qd for the first week and 25 mg qod for the second week; he developed headaches, nausea, and chest flushing and was switched to paroxetine. The remaining seven patients on long-term therapy have displayed good results. Two of the seven men have been maintained on an as-needed schedule as opposed to a more intensive regimen.

TABLE 25.1. Urologic history for premature ejaculation.

I.  Complaint and duration of complaint (self-described)
    a. When did it start—acquired or lifelong? If acquired, was there a precipitating event or life circumstance that was temporally related to the onset?
    b. Does the patient sense that he has voluntary control over the ejaculatory reflex even if it is rapid?
    c. What is the patient's attribution for the rapid ejaculation?
    d. What solutions has the patient undertaken to remedy the dysfunction?
    e. Are there other sexual dysfunctions present in the patient or partner?
    f. What is the quality of the nonsexual relationship?
II. Partner's assessment of ejaculation
    a. Is this a problem for her/him? How so?
    b. Is it viewed as a lifelong or acquired dysfunction?
    c. Have the patient and partner ever had successful intercourse?
    d. What is the quality of the nonsexual relationship?
    e. What is believed to be causing the problem?
III. Physician's assessment of mean latency
    a. With intercourse
    b. With manual/oral stimulation
    c. With masturbation

Patients with erectile dysfunction who have developed premature ejaculation secondarily are generally not helped by SSRI therapy. Anecdotal experience suggests that these patients' premature ejaculation will improve with treatment of the erectile dysfunction.

## Treatment Experience

Initially, these patients were treated with clomipramine, 25 mg qd. Early on, this regimen produced side effects for many of these men. Side effects included headache, hot flashes, nausea, vomiting, and fatigue. Subsequently, the oral therapy has been tailored to qod or twice a week or even to the day of anticipated intercourse. This has significantly reduced the incidence of side effects, appears to have reasonable efficacy, and is currently employed for all new patients.

## Side Effects

The side effects of clomipramine treatment are generally mild, dose-related, and tend to diminish over time. However, 5 out of 27 patients in the aforementioned study could not tolerate even low doses of clomipramine and would not consider switching to another drug.

## Patient Acceptance Rates

In carefully selected research populations the patient acceptance rate was over 79%. However, it appears that in less carefully selected samples the patient acceptance rate markedly drops to 52%. This treatment is likely to negative have a impact on nonphysician therapists who would lose potential therapy patients and slightly less likely to be negative for physician therapists who see patients for a medication-only treatment. The economics might benefit both the patient and third-party payers.

## Preliminary Guidelines for Patient Selection

The key to patient satisfaction lies in selecting appropriate candidates who have realistic expectations about treatment outcome. Based on limited clinical experience, guidelines have been developed, but further research needs to validate these as useful. The lifelong versus acquired classification or premature ejaculation may prove to be a useful marker for formulating treatment recommendations. The ideal candidate for drug therapy might be a man who is free of substance abuse, depression, and psychosis; capable of developing stable, satisfying nonsexual relationships; and with several years of sexual experience accompanied by a lifelong pattern of premature ejaculation. Drug therapy can also be considered for those patients who have not profited from competently conducted psychological treatment. In contrast, a history of acquired premature ejaculation should demand that the clinician be interested in the forces that generated the new symptom. Given a relatively recent onset and some degree of psychological involvement, men with premature ejaculation and couples affected by it might, in the long run, react better with behavioral or psychologic intervention.

## Sexual Experience Level

Pharmacologic treatment should not be a first line of consideration for the young or inexperienced male who in his first few sexual encounters experiences premature ejaculation. Reassurance and education are likely to be worthwhile, and it is hoped that in time such patients will develop increased confidence and learn to control ejaculation.

## Quality of the Nonsexual Relationship

Caution is warranted in offering drug therapy alone to men where the symptom clearly reflects intrapsychic or interpersonal conflict. Therapists must not lose sight of the time-honored dynamic maxim that symptoms exist for reasons. The correction of premature ejaculation may disrupt the individual's or couple's equilibrium. This caution is not simply a restatement of the psychoanalytic theory of symptom substitution, but is a concern based on experience where treatment in a small minority of cases resulted in destructive acting out.

# Other Pharmacologic Studies

## Clomipramine

Early studies suggesting that premature ejaculation can be controlled by drug therapy led researchers to conduct several additional trials.

Althof et al[18] conducted a double-blind, randomized, placebo-controlled study employing strict dosages in a carefully selected population to see if clomipramine was biologically and psychologically efficacious in delaying ejaculation. The results with 15 couples were that 25 mg of clomipramine increased ejaculatory latency 249%, and 50 mg of the drug increased time to orgasm by 517%. However, when the men discontinued the medication, the improvements vanished, and their ejaculatory latencies returned to baseline. Placebo administration (nonsignificantly) increased ejaculatory latency 30% over baseline. These results were consistent with prior studies conducted by Assalian[13] and Segraves et al.[15]

Psychosocially, there were significant improvements in male and female sexual satisfaction, male relationship satisfaction, and male psychological well-being. Three women partners who never achieved coital orgasm became orgasmic while their partners were taking medication. Six of ten women who commonly achieved orgasm reported that it occurred with greater frequency when their partners were taking the active drug.

Side effects were generally mild, dose-related, and tended to diminish with time. Dry mouth, constipation, and feeling "different" were the longest-lasting effects on 50 mg but were not generally clinically significant at 25 mg. Nausea, sleep disturbance, fatigue, and hot flashes were infrequently observed at 50 mg.

A second open-label study[19] was undertaken to determine: (1) whether prolonged treatment with clomipramine could lead to continued ejaculatory control upon discontinuation of the medication, (2) whether men can take the drug on less than a daily basis, and (3) the characteristics of those subjects who continue with pharmacologic treatment and those who drop out.

Of 37 men calling the CWRU Center, 27 (average age 45 years) agreed to treatment. They were begun on a daily regimen of 25 mg of clomipramine and asked to complete sexual and side effect logs on five coital experiences. Based on their self-report, medication was increased to 50 mg daily, 50 mg qod, 50 mg prn, decreased to 25 mg qod, 25 mg prn, or left unchanged. Each time the medication schedule was altered, subjects were asked to complete sexual and side effect logs on five more coital experiences. Each subject's dose continued to be adjusted upward or downward until some reasonable efficacy was achieved. Those subjects who could not tolerate the side effects of clomipramine or who failed to adequately respond were offered trials on fluoxetine or paroxetine. Subjects continued on medication for 7 months, at which point they were asked to take a 1-month drug holiday while reporting on ejaculatory latency and sexual satisfaction.

After 7 months, 14 men continued to take medication and 13 dropped out. The baseline of ejaculatory latencies of stayers was shorter than those of the dropouts (64 seconds vs. 81 seconds). The stayers' average estimated ejaculatory latencies on 25 mg was 403 seconds; the latencies of the dropouts averaged 206 seconds. Five of 13 dropouts reported no efficacy on 25 mg. All 14 stayers reported an improvement of at least 55 seconds. Equal numbers of dropouts and stayers reported side effects.

Sexual satisfaction scores at baseline were lower for stayers than for dropouts. However, on a daily dose of 25 mg the stayers' satisfaction levels had improved more than twofold, but the dropouts' levels had decreased (3.2 vs. 2.07). At 50 mg daily and 50 mg prn, satisfaction levels for the stayers increased to 3.8 and 4.2, respectively.

By 7 months, the 14 subjects were distributed among five medication schedules (in mg): 1–25 qd; 2–25 qod; 1–25 prn; 7–50 qd; 1–50 prn. Only 2 of 14 subjects were successful with taking the medication the day of intercourse; the other 12 required more intensive regimens.

Eleven of 14 men went on drug holiday, three by design at 7 months and eight by themselves at various intervals ranging from 2 to 7 months. None of the 4 men who went on holiday-by-design at 7 months were able to maintain the increases in ejaculatory latency. Two of the 4 men returned to baseline. The other 2 reported losing 25% to 50% of the ejaculatory gains. All the men who placed themselves on holiday returned to baseline ejaculatory latencies. This open-label trial confirmed our group's previous findings regarding the efficacy of clomipramine in the treatment of rapid ejaculation. However, 7 months of treatment did not bring about permanent gains in ejaculatory latency once treatment stopped. Only a minority of subjects had been able to delay ejaculation on less than a daily dose of medication. This suggests the need for lifelong use of oral therapy in treatment of premature ejaculation.

The results of this second study should be viewed as preliminary and interpreted with caution because of the small sample size, the lack of control groups, objective timing, or blinding of the investigators or subjects. The 48% dropout rate was believed due in part to failure to closely monitor the patients' progress. It is recommended that, initially, patients be followed at least monthly. Dropouts should be anticipated, because some patients unrealistically hope the medication will remedy relationship problems as well as cure premature ejaculation.

As a note of caution regarding the use of clomipramine, 1 study reported that a daily regimen of 75 mg of clomipramine taken for 3 months in a series of 11 depressed patients resulted in pathologic spermiograms in all patients in terms of volume, sperm motility, and sperm structure.[20] This important finding warrants replication and further research into the possible consequences of pharmacotherapy with clomipramine or other antidepressant medications or both on male fertility.

## Sertraline

In a double-blind, randomized placebo-controlled study, Mendels et al[21] reported that sertraline produced clinically and statistically significant improvements relative to placebo in time to ejaculation and number of successful attempts at intercourse. The average daily dose was 121 mg/day. Similarly, in an open-label trail, Swartz[22] reported on 10 patients who were prescribed either 25 or 50 mg of sertraline. The average ejaculatory delay was 20 minutes. Side effects were infrequent and consisted of transient anorexia and headaches.

## Paroxetine and Fluoxetine

Waldinger et al[17] studied the effect of paroxetine on ejaculation in a double-blind, placebo-controlled trial of men with premature ejaculation. The dose of paroxetine was increased from 20 to 40 mg after the first week. Successful outcomes were noted in most patients, and side effects were minimal. Presently, there are no double-blind placebo-controlled studies regarding the efficacy of fluoxetine in treating premature ejaculation; however, several anecdotal reports and clinical experience suggest that it may also be effective at doses ranging from 20 to 40 mg daily (S. Levine, personal communication, 1996).

## Conclusion

In sum, oral therapy for premature ejaculation is in its infancy. It is exciting to be able to provide such therapy for men suffering from this dysfunction. As with other oral therapies, clinical use will ultimately dictate the optimal drug dose as well as delineate the appropriate patient for treatment. An understanding of the psychobiology of the effects of the oral therapy is needed for researchers to better understand the ejaculation reflex arc and the central pathways that affect it, allowing better tailored therapy and the production of drugs with greater specificity.

## References

1. American Psychiatric Association. *Diagnostic and Statistical Manual of Mental Disorders.* 4th ed. Washington, DC: American Psychiatric Association; 1994.
2. Halvorsen J, Metz M. Sexual dysfunction. Part 1: classification, etiology, and pathogenesis. *J Am Board Fam Pract* 1992; 5:51–61.

3. Kaplan H. *Overcoming Premature Ejaculation.* New York: Bruner-Mazel; 1989.

4. Levine S. *Sexual Life: A Clinicians Guide.* New York: Plenum; 1992.

5. LoPiccolo J, LoPiccolo L. *Handbook of Sex Therapy.* New York: Plenum; 1978.

6. McCarthy B. Cognitive-behavioral strategies and techniques in the treatment of early ejaculation. In: Leiblum SR, Rosen R, eds. *Principles and Practice of Sex Therapy: Update for the 90's.* New York: Guilford; 1990.

7. Masters W, Johnson V. *Human Sexual Inadequacy.* Boston: Little, Brown; 1970.

8. St. Lawrence J, Madakasira S. Evaluation and treatment of premature ejaculation: a critical review. *Int J Psych* 1992; 22:77–97.

9. Semans J. Premature ejaculation: a new approach. *South Med J* 1956; 49:353–358.

10. Hawton K, Catalan J. Prognostic factors in sex therapy. *Behav Res Ther* 1986; 24:377–385.

11. Bancroft J, Coles L. Three years experience in a sexual problems clinic. *Br Med J* 1976; 1:1575–1577.

12. DeAmicus L, Goldberg D, LoPiccolo J, et al. Clinical follow-up of couples treated for sexual dysfunction. *Arch Sex Behav* 1985; 14:467–489.

13. Assalian P. Clomipramine in the treatment of premature ejaculation. *J Sex Res* 1988; 24:231–251.

14. Goodman RE. An assessment of clomipramine (Anafranil) in the treatment of premature ejaculation. *J Intern Med Res* 1980; 8(suppl3):53–59.

15. Segraves RT, Saran S, Segraves K, et al. Clomipramine versus placebo in the treatment of premature ejaculation: a pilot study. *J Sex Marital Ther* 1993; 19:198–200.

16. Kaplan P. The use of serotonergic uptake inhibitors in the treatment of premature ejaculation. *J Sex Marital Ther* 1995; 20:321–324.

17. Waldinger M, Hengeveld M, Zwinderman A. Paroxetine treatment of premature ejaculation: a double-blind randomized placebo-controlled study. *Am J Psychiatry* 1994; 151:1377–1379.

18. Althof S, Levine S, Corty E, et al. Clomipramine as a treatment for rapid ejaculation: a double-blind crossover trial of fifteen couples. *J Clin Psychiatry* (in press).

19. Althof S, Resnick K, Levine S, et al. Early experience with clomipramine for rapid ejaculation. Paper presented to the Annual Meeting of the American Urological Association, Las Vegas, Nevada, 1995.

20. Maier U, Koinig G. Andrological findings in young patients under long-term antidepressive therapy with clomipramine. *Psychopharmacology* 1994; 116:357–359.

21. Mendels J, Camera A, Sikes C. Sertraline treatment for premature ejaculation. *J Clin Psychopharmacol* 1995; 15:341–346.

22. Swartz D. Sertraline hydrochloride for premature ejaculation [abstract 471]. In: *Programs and Abstracts of the 89th Annual Meeting of the American Urological Association*, San Francisco, CA, 1994: 345A.

# 26
# The Normal Penis and Augmentation Surgery in Adult Males

Claudio Telöken

Phallus dimension—as evidenced by the increasing number of men seeking penis enlargement—is a growing concern. Some men request penis enlargement for functional reasons; however, the majority seek it for aesthetic purposes to reinforce a sexual "macho" image.

The penis in healthy human males varies greatly in size, so much so that the establishment of norms is difficult. It is universally accepted, however, that penile length needs to be sufficient for an individual to stand up to urinate, to allow penetration during sexual intercourse, and—from the social standpoint—to avoid embarrassment when seen by others.

The most important single predictor of adult penile size appears to be the initial length of the penis at birth.[1] The size of the foot or the diameter of the hand does not predict the penile length (unpublished data).

## The Normal Penis

### Development

Penile development in the human embryo occurs in three phases: (1) the genital tubercle phase, when the phallus appears as a hillock in the perineum; (2) the phallic phase, when the organ becomes progressively elongated and cylindrical, with the urethral groove extending to the tip; and (3) the last phase, when the urethral tube closes and the glans becomes demarcated by the formation of the coronal sulcus.[2]

During the first 3 months of life, the masculinizing process of the genitalia is initiated by human chorionic gonadotropin secreted by the placenta. From month 4 onward, the fetal pituitary gland takes over and begins to secrete luteinizing hormone and follicle-stimulating hormone in response to gonadotropin-releasing hormone produced by the hypothalamus. The final period of phallic growth occurs at puberty.[1,3]

### Anatomy

The normal penis is constructed of paired corpora cavernosa covered by double layers of a thick and dense elastic sheath of connective tissue, the tunica albuginea. The outer collagen bundles are oriented longitudinally and play an important role in determining the tunica's thickness and strength. The finer fibers of the inner layer are arranged circularly; they surround and penetrate each corpus separately and, by their junction in the median plane, form the septum of the penis. The circular bundles send off perpendicular projections, the intracavernous pillars, originating from around 6 o'clock and inserting into the tunica at the lateral walls of the cavernous bodies. They reinforce the tunica albuginea.[4] The corpora cavernosa make up the bulk of the penis and contain erectile tissue. They are incompletely separated by a layer of the tunica albuginea tissue, the septum.

The erectile bodies are surrounded by Buck's fascia that splits to contain the corpus spongiosun, which supports the urethra. Buck's fascia is the tough layer of elastic tissue immediately adjacent to the tunica albuginea.[5]

The corpus spongiosum lies in the ventral groove between the two corpora cavernosa. The tunica albuginea of the corpus spongiosum is thinner than the tunica of the corpora cavernosa, and there is less erectile tissue.

At its base, the penis is supported and suspended by two ligaments composed primarily of elastic fibers that are continuous with the fascia of the penis. The fundiform ligament is continuous with the lower end of the linea alba; then it splits into two lamina that surround the body of the penis and unite underneath it to fuse with the septa of the scrotum. The suspensory ligament, which is deep to the fundiform ligament, is triangular and is attached above the front of the pubic symphysis, and, below it, blends with the fascia of the penis on each side of the organ.[6] The septum becomes more complete toward the base of the penis, but the corpora become truly independent only as they split to form the crura attached to the inferior ramus of the pubis and ischium.

Longitudinally, the penis is divided into three portions. The root lies in the superficial perineal pouch and provides fixation and stability. The corpora diverge from each other to form the crura and gain attachment to the pubic arch of the ischia. Each crus is firmly adherent to the ramus of the ischia and is surrounded by the fibers of the ischiocavernous muscles. The body, which constitutes the major part, is composed of the three spongious erectile tissues completely covered by skin. The glans is the distal portion of the corpus spongiosum. The corpus spongiosum lacks both a rigid fibrous covering and intraspongiosal pillars. Their absence allows the urethra to function in a low-pressure milieu even during erection. The glans penis has only a minimal amount of fibrous tissue between the sinusoids and the superficial epidermis.[4]

## Size

Medical literature does not clearly define what constitutes normal penis length in the adult male. Therefore, what constitutes insufficient or inadequate penile size is still a controversial issue. Because no standard method of penile measurement has yet been developed, the accuracy of some reported data is questionable.

Although for some authors the flaccid-state measurement has been found to correlate closely with the length of the penis in the erect state,[7] there is evidence that relaxed or flaccid penile length varies excessively and this measurement is, therefore, not reproducible.[8]

Schonfeld and Beebe[9] evaluated several methods of measuring penile size and found a highly significant correlation between the fully stretched penile length and the erect length of the penis. The correlation between flaccid and erect length, as noted above, is not reliable enough to recommend using flaccid length to predict erect length. Wessells et al,[10] however, found that stretched length most closely predicted erect length. Using penis extensibility as a measurement appears to be a reliable, easy, and noninvasive test. Its correlation to erectile function suggests its significance.[11]

Penile length measurements in adults should be made with a full erection, which can be produced either by visual sexual stimulation (VSS) or intracavernous injection of vasoactive agents. The latter method seems to be more effective because general environmental conditions, such as inadequate room temperature, and anxiety, embarrassment, or fear accompanied by exacerbated adrenergic status can alter the length of the penis, thus preventing an accurate measurement. (Taking an objective measurement of the penis and showing the patient that his penis is within the mean of the healthy population may be enough to convince him that his phallus is normal and appropriate for intercourse, and he may withdraw his request for phalloplasty augmentation.)

Whether using the stretched penis or a fully erect one, the measurement should be taken using a rigid ruler. If using the stretched penis, the glans penis should be grasped firmly between the thumb and forefinger and the penis pulled to its full length. The distance is recorded along the dorsal aspect of the penis, from the symphysis pubis to the tip of the glans, disregarding the prepuce. The ruler should be pressed against the pubis, depressing the suprapubic fat as much as possible. If the penis is in full erection, the measurement should be made along the dorsum to the tip in the same way.

Lee et al[8] found the stretched penile length in normal adult males to be 13.3 cm ± 1.6 cm SD[7]; Wessells et al[10] demonstrated that mean flaccid penile length was 8 cm, mean flaccid circumference was 10 cm, and the new stretched length 11 cm. The mean erect length increased to 12.5 cm, and the mean erect circumference increased to 12.5 cm. The mean functional penile length (erect length and fat pad depth) was 16 cm.

Ros and colleagues[11] examined 150 potent Caucasian males after full erection was obtained following injection of intracavernous vasoactive agents. These men were chosen for the study because they had no penile size complaints and were very satisfied with their genitalia. Even the patients with the smallest penile length testified to feeling comfortable with the functional aspect as well as the aesthetic profile of their penises and denied any embarrassment about their penile size when seen by others. Penile lengths (from pubis to distal glans) as well as proximal and distal circumferences were obtained. The shortest and the longest penises measured 9 cm and 19 cm, respectively. The mean length was 14.5 cm. The mean proximal circumference was 11.92 cm, and the distal circumference was 11.05 cm.[11]

As to body type and its correlation to the size of the genitalia, it has been suggested that there is no direct correlation between somatic and skeletal development of phallic length.[12]

# Penile Abnormalities

## Micropenis, Webbed Penis, Buried Penis

The term *micropenis* describes a penis that is abnormally small, but otherwise perfectly formed, with the urethra opening at the tip of the glans. It is usually described in children as a penis that has a stretched length measuring less than 2.5 standard deviations below the mean.[6] True micropenis is rare, and is usually investi-

gated and treated during childhood or puberty. However, sometimes micropenis is not discovered until adulthood.

Mircopenis must be distinguished from the condition called *webbed penis*, in which the penis may be of normal size but is buried and enclosed by the skin of the scrotum.[13] In such cases, palpation of the corporeal bodies will confirm that they are well developed. An even more common source of confusion is a *buried penis*, in which the shaft lies hidden within an abundant mass of prepubic fat, often leaving only the prepuce protruding. The full length of the organ can be revealed simply by holding the fat back out of the way, allowing the penis to stand out.[7]

# Lengthening of the Penis

## Psychosocial Adjustment

Phalloplasty is medically necessary only in adults with uncorrected micropenis, webbed penis, buried penis, or other anatomical abnormalities, and bodily changes resulting from disease, injury, or other surgical procedures. Great misconceptions exist about the correlation between penile length and sexual adequacy.[14] Therefore, most people seeking augmentation phalloplasty probably do not need the procedure. For many patients, the desire for the operation is based on fantasies or lack of sex education about which factors in the male genitalia are responsible for female orgasm, what constitutes normal male genitalia, and what women's actual sexual expectations are.

Psychiatric or psychological consultation is imperative, because severely depressed, psychotic, or unrealistic patients definitely should not undergo penile augmentation surgery.

## Surgery

When indicated, penile lengthening can be obtained by partial detachment of the crura from the puboischial rami so that the proximal penile part of the corpora cavernosa can be advanced into the shaft.[15] The main objective is to release the proximal portions of the erectile bodies from their attachment to the widespread inferior pubic rami and to excise the dysgenetic scar tissue encountered during the dissection. Complete detachment of the corpora should be avoided, as it can cause devascularization of the corporal bodies.[16]

A second alternative for penis elongation is to incise the suspensory ligament and release the fundiform ligaments. The preferred incision is the V-Y flap. Excessive fat should be removed, while keeping adequate subcutaneous tissue to maintain a healthy blood supply. By pulling on the penis, the suspensory ligament is palpated and easily incised, as are the bands of the fundiform ligaments. The ligament is released 1 cm to each side of the midline of the pubis. The lower limit of the release is the inferior border of the pubis. The dissection should be kept directly on the periosteum to prevent injuring the dorsal bundle of nerves and vessels. The penis falls forward, gaining some length.[17] Reattachment of the ligament, which in the past was simply loosened, is mandatory to avoid penile shortening.[18] Before reattachment, the curve of the penis is pushed out, ensuring extra lengthening outside the pelvis. This technique was first used on a small farm child who had half of his penis bitten off by a pig.[19]

A good choice of suture for penis reattachment is 3–0 Prolene. This has a double function: to maintain penile advancement (penile length can retract after releasing the suspensory ligament) and to eliminate dead space between the dorsal corpora and the pubis. This space must be filled to prevent spontaneous reattachment of these structures and possible shortening of the penis. A roll of Gore-Tex can be used for this purpose.[20]

Although no incision is completely satisfactory for the mentioned approach, the most commonly used is the V-Y advancement flap. Several variations have been described to incise the suspensory ligament and release the fundiform ligament.[17–20] Longer incisions than this may deform the genitalia, resulting in dog-ear formation of the penis buried in the scrotum, paradoxically creating the appearance of a short penis.[18,20]

The M-plasty incision, another variation popularized in China, is placed in the suprapubic region, but it frequently causes hypertrophic scars.[21]

A large Z-plasty or a double Z-plasty in the pubic region is often used to advance the skin and concomitantly remove the suprapubic fat pad. This technique creates more reliable flaps with less noticeable scarring. The vertical limb of this incision is about 4 cm in length, and the distal end is just proximal to the penopubic junction. The resulting skin advancement is about 2 cm.[17]

Perineal insertion of a penile prosthesis is also a recommended treatment for an adult male with micropenis.[21] In selected cases, liposuction or formal excision of the prepubic fat pad will give a worthwhile improvement in penile appearance.[7]

Webbed scrotum (the scrotal sac extends well up onto the ventral shaft of the penis) can be easily corrected by a straightforward reconstructive procedure.

# Conclusion

Men seeking phalloplasty must be made aware of some caveats. Many of the studies on penile augmentation lack scientific methodology, sufficient sample size, or matched comparison populations. In addition, most results are anecdotal and follow-up data are often difficult to interpret. Moreover, a predictive index of successful management of penile length and data evaluating the gain in length from ligament release are still unavailable. The demand for penile aesthetic surgery is increasing, in spite of the limited medical knowledge and appropriate clinical trials to document its need and the best techniques to be used. This demand may be due in part to the social stigma attached to the small penis, promotion by the media of the "macho" male image, and the mystique surrounding sexual matters in general.

Patients seeking penile lengthening must be made aware that sometimes no gain is possible; reattachment of the penis after cutting the suspensory ligament can occasionally produce a shorter, not a longer, penis; and a 1-cm gain in length is considered a surgical success although neither self-esteem nor sexual performance may change as a result.

Finally, from the psychologic point of view, each case must be managed individually before surgery in order to avoid possible disappointment because of a less than spectacular outcome.

## References

1. Danish RK, Lee PA, Mazur T, et al. Micropenis. II. Hypogonadotropic hypogonadism. *Johns Hopkins Med J* 1980; 146:177–184.

2. Spaulding MH. The development of the external genitalia in human embryo. *Embryol Carnegie Inst* 1921; 143:67–73.

3. Kaplan SL, Brumbach NM, Aubert ML. The ontogenesis of pituitary hormones and hypothalamic factors in the human fetus: maturation of central nervous system regulation of anterior pituitary function. *Recent Prog Horm Res* 1976; 32:161–172.

4. Breeza A, Aboseif S, Lea TF. Anatomy of the penis. In: Montague DK, ed. *Atlas of the Urology Clinics of North America*. Philadelphia: W.B. Saunders; 1993: 1–8.

5. Devine CJ Jr, Jordan GH, Schlossberg SM. Surgery of the penis and urethra. In: Walsh PC, Retic AB, Stamey TA, et al, eds. *Campbell's Urology*. Philadelphia: W.B. Saunders; 1992: 2957–3032.

6. Tanagho EA. Anatomy of the lower urinary tract. In: Walsh PC, Retik AB, Stamey TA, et al, eds. *Campbell's Urology*, Philadelphia: W.B. Saunders; 1992: 40–69.

7. Aaronson IA. Micropenis: medical and surgical implications. *J Urol* 1994; 152:4–14.

8. Lee PA, Mazur T, Danish R, et al. Micropenis: I. Criteria, etiologies, and classification. *Johns Hopkins Med J* 1980; 146/147:156–163.

9. Schonfeld WA, Beebe GW. Normal growth and variation in the male genitalia from birth to maturity. *J Urol* 1942; 48:759–777.

10. Wessells H, Lue T, McAninch JW. The relationship between penile length in the flaccid and erect states: guidelines for penile lengthening? *J Urol* 1995; 153:374A, Abstr 582.

11. Ros C, Telöken C, Sogari P, et al. Caucasian penis: what is the normal size? *J Urol* 1994; 151:323A.

12. Masters WH, Johnson VE. The penis. In: *Human Sexual Response*. Boston: Little, Brown; 1996: 201–230.

13. Crawford BS. Buried penis. *Br J Plast Surg* 1977; 30:95–99.

14. Rivard DJ. Anatomy, physiology, and neurophysiology of male sexual function. In: Bennett AH, ed. *Management of Male Impotence*. Baltimore: Williams & Wilkins; 1982: 1–25.

15. Gearhart JP, Jeffs RD. Exstrophy of the bladder, epispadias, and other bladder anomalies. In: Walsh PC, Retik AB, Stamey TA, et al, eds. *Campbell's Urology*. Philadelphia: W.B. Saunders; 1992: 1772–1821.

16. Devine CJ Jr, Jordan GH, Schlossberg SM. Surgery of the penis and urethra. In: Walsh PC, Retik AB, Stamey TA, et al, eds. *Campbell's Urology*. Philadelphia: W.B. Saunders; 1992: 2957–3032.

17. Alter GJ. Augmentation phalloplasty. In: Melman A, ed. *Urological Clinics of North America*. Philadelphia, PA; W.B. Saunders Co. 1995; 4:887–902.

18. Roos H, Lissoos I. Penis lengthening. *Int J Aesthetic Restorative Surg* 1994; 2:89.

19. Long DC. Elongation of the penis. *Chung Hua Cheng Hsing Shoa Shang Wai Ko Tsa Chih* 1990; 6:17–19.

20. Alter GJ. Penis enhancement. *AUA Update Series* 1996; 15:94–99.

21. Burkholder GV, Newell ME. New surgical treatment for micropenis. *J Urol* 1983; 129:832–834.

# 27
# Color Duplex Doppler Ultrasound: Penile Blood Flow Study

Gregory A. Broderick

A recent estimate of the number of men in the United States suffering with complete erectile dysfunction is 10 to 20 million. When partial erectile dysfunction is included, the estimate jumps to 30 million.[1] Age-specific prevalence is estimated to be 5% at age 40, increasing to 15% to 25% by age 65. In clinical series, the ratio of organic to psychologic male sexual dysfunction also varies with age: 70% of patients under 35 years of age have a psychogenic cause, and 85% of patients over 50 years of age have organic impotence.[2] Patient accounts of coital frequency similarly vary with age: 75% of men in their seventh decade report having coitus once monthly, and 37% of patients 60 to 69 years old describe having weekly coitus.

Normative data on the prevalence of impotence in the community have only recently become available.[3] The Massachusetts Male Aging Study (MMAS) assessed the prevalence of impotence among 1290 men ranging in ages from 40 to 70 years. On a four-point scale, a complaint of impotence was offered by 51% of the men: 16% were minimally impotent, 25% were moderately impotent, and 10% were completely impotent. Diabetes, hypertension, and coronary artery disease were each associated with increased probability of impotence complaints; these risks were amplified by concurrent smoking. Complete impotence was more prevalent among men taking hypoglycemic medication, antihypertensive and cardiac drugs, and vasodilators. Normative community-based data clearly have established a relationship between aging and male sexual

dysfunction and, more importantly, have demonstrated the relationship to vascular risk factors.

Based on an appreciation of these vascular risk factors and other para-aging phenomena, urologists can usually direct patients toward therapy after obtaining a good sexual history and medical history, and performing a physical examination and basic blood tests. When diagnostic testing is indicated or desired, the penile blood flow study (PBFS), an intracavernous challenge of a vasoactive agent and assessment by color duplex Doppler ultrasound (CDDU), is the most reliable and least invasive means of screening for vasculogenic erectile dysfunction and efficiently selects patients who are candidates for invasive testing.[4-7] CDDU provides a detailed examination of the vascular anatomy of the penis and elucidates the dynamics of erection.

## Investigating Penile Blood Flow

Numerous diagnostic tests have been employed to evaluate penile hemodynamics: penile plethysmography, penile blood pressures, penile brachial index, duplex Doppler sonography, dynamic infusion cavernosometry/cavernosography, nuclear washout radiography, and color duplex Doppler ultrasound. In 1971 Gaskell[8] described a noninvasive test of penile arterial inflow using a photometer to quantify the absorption of light by the pigment oxyhemoglobin in the glans penis. An occlusive cuff at the base of the penis was slowly loosened, and the pressure at which oxyhemoglobin became measurable in the glans indicated the penile systolic blood pressure. Abelson[9] used the Doppler stethoscope to measure penile blood pressure in flaccidity and compared this value to systolic brachial pressure, yielding the penile-brachial index (PBI)—maximal systolic penile pressure divided by systolic brachial artery pressure. Michal et al[10] and Goldstein et al[11] modified the PBI test with a dynamic component by adding lower extremity and pelvic musculature exercises, with Doppler stethoscope auscultation made before and after exercise. A decrease in the ratio of penile systolic pressures (<0.15 mm Hg) was indicative of pelvic steal, or significant penile inflow disease. Subsequent reviews comparing the PBI to pharmacopenile angiography found PBI values from normal patients overlapped with those from impotent patients, and pressures were inadvertently obtained from the dorsal artery not reflecting the central cavernous arteries.[12]

Indisputably, arteriography provides the best anatomical information about the origin of the common penile arteries, but these data have been difficult to correlate with patient complaints and with erection dynamics.[13] Accurate penile angiography requires pharmacologically induced erection, as the vessels of the flaccid shaft are contracted and tortuous. High osmolality contrast agents are painful, may induce anaphylaxis, and may require intravenous sedative-anesthesia. Some centers use epidural or spinal anesthesia because of the additional benefit of reducing vasospasm.[14,15] Low osmolality contrast agents reduce angiographic morbidity but are more expensive.

The common penile artery typically arises from the third segment of the internal pudendal artery (IPA) as it passes through the urogenital diaphragm. The paired common penile arteries may originate from one internal pudendal artery or from an accessory internal pudendal artery. The accessory IPA may take origin from the hypogastric artery, remnant of the umbilical, ischial, or obturator arteries. An accessory IPA is more common on the right, but prevalence has been variably described from 4% to 70%. Therefore, performing selective internal pudendal arteriography (missing an accessory IPA) has an inherent false-positive rate for diagnosing penile inflow disease.[15-19] More importantly, deviations from paired common penile arteries have been documented in 50% of normally potent volunteers; unilateral absence or hypoplasia of a dorsal artery has been shown in up to 30% of volunteers.[14] Anatomic variation of intrapenile arterial anatomy appears to be the rule rather than the exception, such as unilateral or bilateral origin of the cavernous arteries, distal shaft communications between the dorsal and central cavernous arteries, and anastomoses between the corpus spongiosum and cavernous body.[20] The problem for the arteriographer has been twofold: how to differentiate congenital variations in penile arterial anatomy from acquired abnormalities, and how to correlate anatomical alterations in the pattern of vascular inflow with the patient's complaints of impotence. For the patient there remains the discomfort of the intraarterial contrast, exposure to ionizing radiation, risk of minor or severe dye reaction, and potential for endothelial cell and smooth muscle damage following ionic contrast agents. As a screening test, phalloarteriography is overly invasive and nonspecific of penile hemodynamics.[21]

## Penile Blood Flow Study

A PBFS consists of an intracavernous injection and visual rating of the subsequent erection; the test is the most commonly used diagnostic procedure for impotence. PBFS is simple, minimally invasive, and performed without monitoring equipment. A positive injection test in a neurologically normal patient implies psychogenic impotence, presumably excluding significant venous or arterial insufficiency.[22,23] All too often the penile response is suboptimal, leaving the clinician questioning whether the patient has severe arterial insufficiency, venous leakage, or high anxiety. A standard intracavernous test dosage has never been established for any agent; furthermore, a contemporary hemodynamic investigation suggests that a positive injection test is associated with normal veno-occlusion (low flow to maintain erection values of 0.5 to 3 ml per minute and minimal contrast medium or no contrast leakage during cavernosometry-cavernosography), but not necessarily with normal arterial function. In as many as 19% of patients the test may be a false negative. Despite the presence of an erection, there may be a significant disparity between the systemic and cavernous systolic arterial pressures, which can be correlated with abnormalities on pharmacopenile angiography. A normal PBFS indicates meeting or exceeding a threshold response for intracavernous pressure ($\geq 80\,mm\,Hg$), which may occur in the presence of a significant gradient between systemic systolic pressure and cavernous systolic pressure. A positive erection test only selects patients for home injection therapy; it does not rule out mild arterial insufficiency.[24]

In 1985 Lue et al[25] introduced the technique of high-resolution sonography and quantitative Doppler spectrum analysis to evaluate dynamic changes in cavernous arterial flow after intracorporal injection of papaverine. In July 1995 the Upjohn Company (Kalamazoo, Michigan) received Food and Drug Administration (FDA) approval to market injectable prostaglandin $E_1$ ($PGE_1$) (Caverject; Upjohn, Kalamazoo, Michigan) specifically for the diagnosis and treatment of male impotence. The demonstration that vasoactive injections could produce penile erection without benefit of psychic or tactile stimuli has revolutionized the diagnosis and treatment of erectile dysfunction by providing a direct test of end organ integrity and therapy specifically for vascular deficiency.

## CDDU Anatomy of the Penis

The human penis consists of three corpora—the paired corpora cavernosa and the ventral corpus spongiosum—which form the glans penis distally. The cavernous bodies share a fenestrated septum, which allows them to neurophysiologically function and pharmacologically respond as a single unit. The tunica albuginea of the corpora cavernosa in the flaccid state has a thickness of 2 to 3 mm. The tunica albuginea of the corpus spongiosum is much thinner than that of the corpora cavernosa. Each of the corporeal bodies is surrounded by a dense fascial structure, Buck's fascia. Additionally, Buck's fascia forms a thin, nonfenestrated septum between the corpora cavernosa and the corpus spongiosum. With real-time ultrasound the corpus cavernosum and spongiosum have a homogeneous medium echogenicity that is distinguished from the hyperechoic tunica albuginea and septum (Fig. 27.1, see color insert for parts B and C). The tunica albuginea should have uniform thickness and echogenicity; the subcutaneous tissues and Buck's fascia are not identifiable sonographically except by the location of the dorsal vascular bundle—paired dorsal arteries (DA) and deep dorsal vein complex (DDV) (Figs. 27.1B and 27.2B, see color insert). The proximal penis (crural bodies) is anchored to the inferior pubic bone. The penile bulb is surrounded by the bulbocavernosus (or bulbospongiosus) muscle. The crura and proximal part of the shaft are covered by the ischiocavernosus muscles. Although the pendulous penis is easily imaged from either the dorsal (Figs. 27.1 and 27.2) or ventral projection, the proximal third of the penis may be imaged in transverse or sagittal view only by scanning from the ventral penis or below the scrotum at the level of the perineum (Figs. 27.2C and 27.2D, see color insert). The urethral lumen will be compressed but can be imaged by retrograde filling with sterile gel or water.[26,27] The glans penis is covered with very thin and firmly adherent skin, has no fibrous sheath, and contains much connective tissue.

## Penile Inflow

The penis is supplied mainly by the internal pudendal artery. After giving off the perineal artery in Alcock's canal, it becomes the common penile artery. Branches of the penile artery consist of the bulbar, urethral (spongiosal), dorsal, and cavernous arteries. The cavernous artery penetrates the tunica albuginea and enters the crura of the corpora cavernosa along with the cavernous veins and cavernous nerves (Fig. 27.2D). The cavernous arteries are easily identified by their echogenic walls; in the flaccid state the arteries are tortuous and $\leq 0.5\,mm$ in diameter. With CDDU, low blood flows are visible, but detection of flow prior to injection of the vasodilator depends on the patient's level of sympathetic tone (anxiety) and is of no predictive value.[4,28] Cavernosal tissue is sponge-like and composed of a meshwork of interconnected cavernosal spaces that are lined by vascular endothelium and separated by trabeculae containing bundles of smooth muscle in a framework of collagen, elastin, and fibroblasts. The terminal helicine arteries are multiple muscular and corkscrew-shaped arteries (150 to 350 μm) that open directly into the cavernous spaces and act like resistance arteries. The corporal tissue becomes more hypoechoic (darker) as the sinusoids distend with blood, making the echogenic walls of the cavernous arteries more distinct sonographically (Fig. 27.1C). The dorsal artery enters the penis and continues distally beneath Buck's fascia between the centrally located deep dorsal vein(s) and the paired dorsal nerves (Fig. 27.1B). The urethral artery runs longitudinally through the corpus spongiosum lateral to the urethra (Fig. 27.2C). This supplies the corpus spongiosum, the urethral tissue, and the glans penis. The bulbar artery enters the bulb of the penis shortly after its origin and supplies blood to Cowper's gland and the proximal urethral bulb. Recently described anatomic variations of penile arterial supply include dorsal to cavernous, cavernous to cavernous, and cavernous to urethral collaterals, duplication of the cavernous artery, and unilateral absence of a dorsal artery.[14]

## Penile Outflow

Based on scanning electronic microscopy of vascular corrosion casts, Banya et al[29] suggested two circulatory routes in the human corpora. One route goes from the cavernous artery to capillary networks collected into the venular plexus just beneath the tunica albuginea; it is suggested that this route serves as a main circulatory pathway during the flaccid state. The

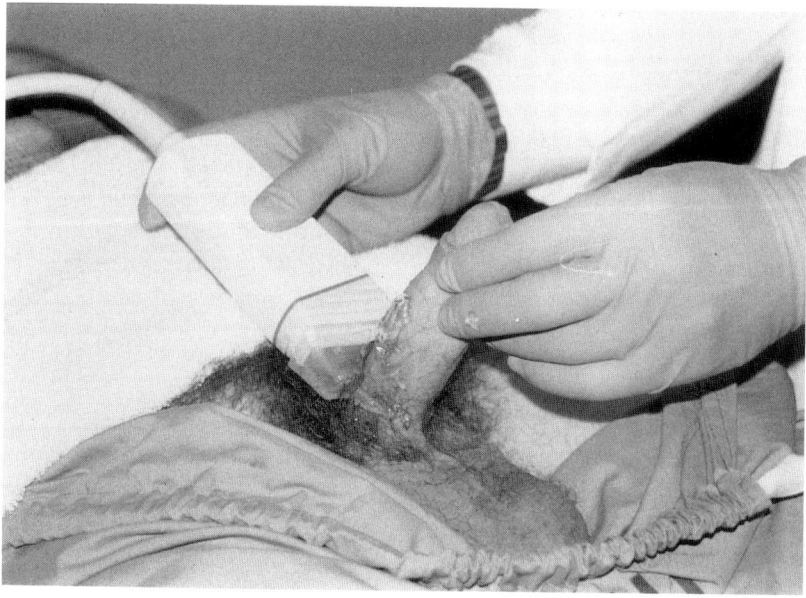

A

FIGURE 27.1. (A) The penis is held in the anatomic position of erection with the scanning probe in the transverse position. (B) Transverse color Doppler image following a 6-μg injection of PGE₁ reveals the normal vascular anatomy. RCA, right cavernous artery; LCA, left cavernous artery; DDV, deep dorsal vein; LDA, left dorsal artery; CS, corpus spongiosum. (C) Transverse image of right corporal body 5 minutes after injection of dilator. Helicine arterioles (red/blue) are seen with central sinusoids beginning to fill (arrows); note that blood distended sinusoids appear more hypoechoic than surrounding tissue. See color plate for parts B and C.

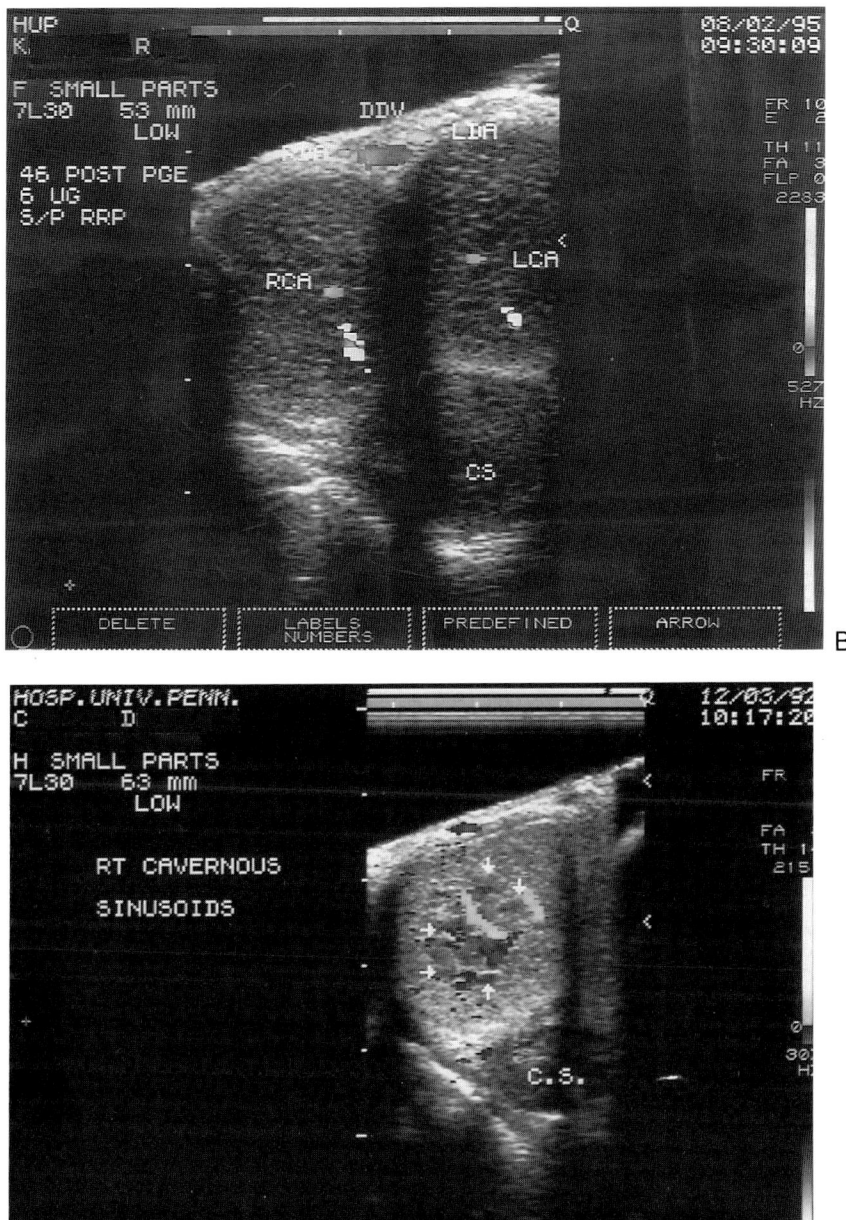

FIGURE 27.1. *Continued*

other route is through anastomoses from the cavernous artery, via the helicine arteries to the cavernae (sinusoids), which are then emptied into the postcavernous venules. This ultrastructural detail is not visualized sonographically.

There are three sets of veins draining the penis: the superficial, the intermediate, and the deep. The deep venous system drains both the corpora cavernosa and the corpus spongiosum. The postcavernous venules coalesce to form larger emissary veins that pierce the

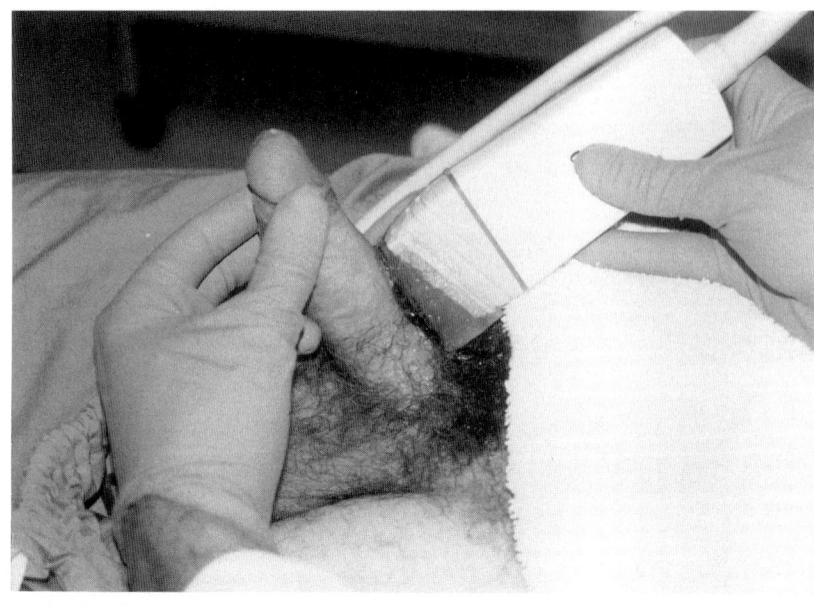

A

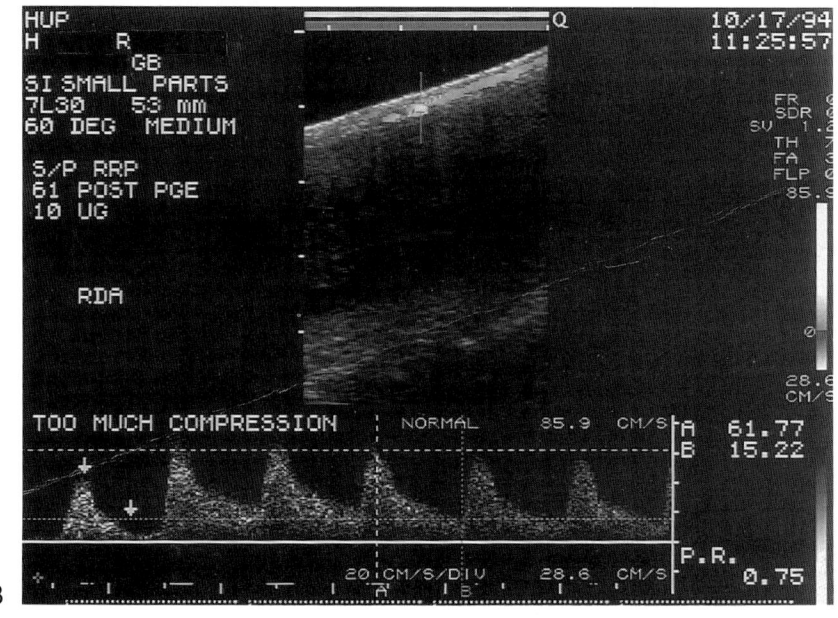

B

FIGURE 27.2. (A) Probe held in the sagittal position from the dorsum; note cushion of ultrasound gel between standoff wedge of transducer and penile shaft. (B) Sagittal view of right dorsal artery (RDA); too much compression (arrows) damps dorsal vascular flow and will alter both systolic and diastolic waveforms. (C) The pendulous penis may be scanned from the ventral aspect. This sagittal image shows the proximal bulb with the urethral artery (BUA) and right cavernous artery (RCA). Imaging of the urethral lumen is not possible unless the urethra is filled in a retrograde fashion with gel or water. See color plate. (D) Sagittal scanning below the scrotum (transperineal) reveals the origin of the right cavernous artery (RCA). See color plate for parts B, C, and D.

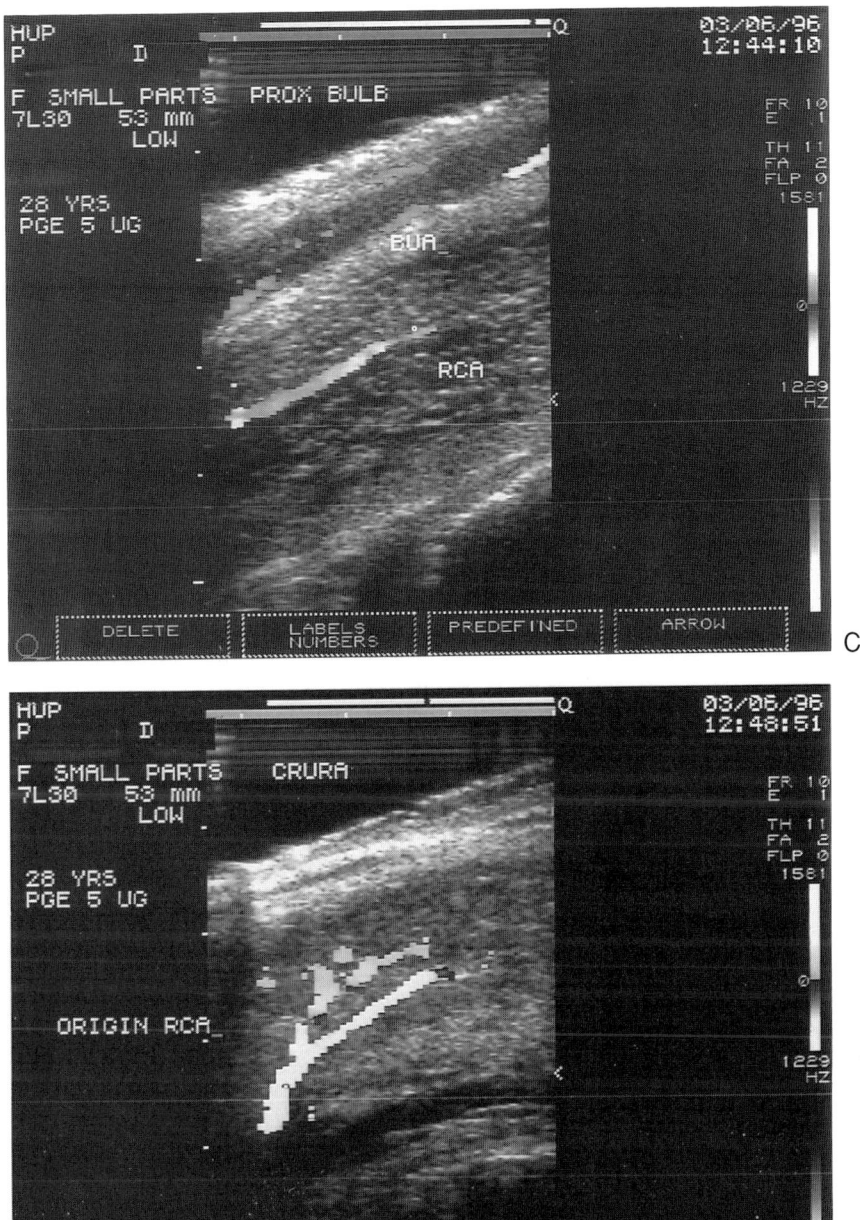

FIGURE 27.2. *Continued*

tunica albuginea. The emissary veins of the middle and distal penis join to form the circumflex veins, which empty into the deep dorsal vein (Fig. 27.1B). The emissary veins of the proximal penis form the cavernous vein, which empties into the internal pudendal vein (Fig. 27.3, see color insert for part A).

The intermediate set of veins is deep to Buck's fascia. Veins from the glans penis form a retrocoronal plexus that drains into the

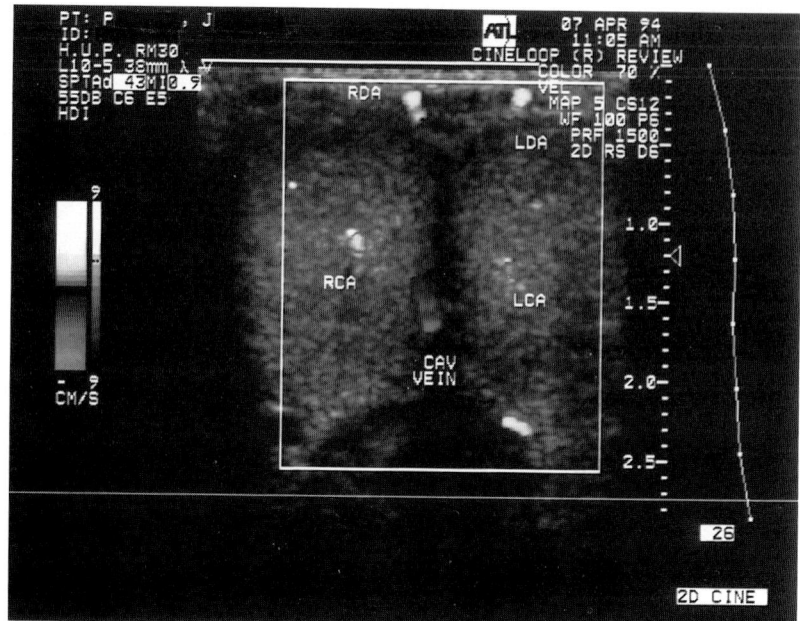

A

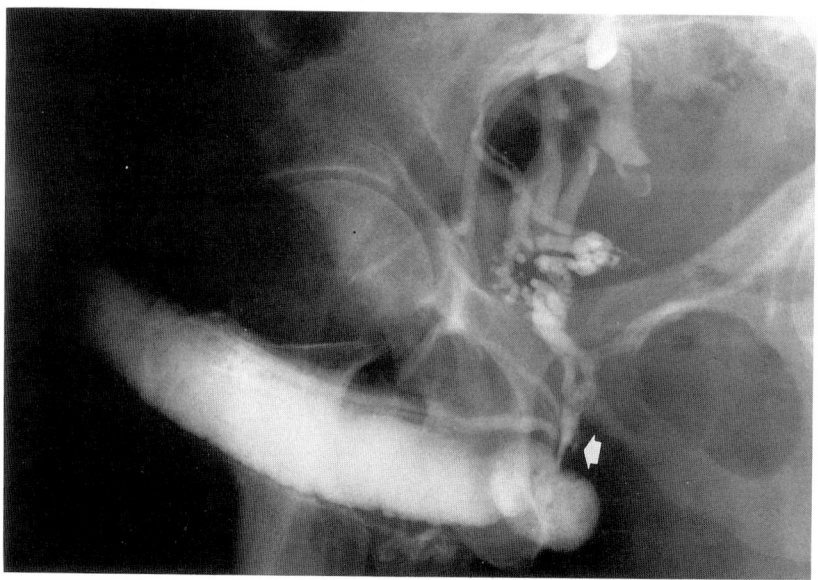

B

FIGURE 27.3. (A) Transverse scan of patient with severe veno-occlusive dysfunction revealing large cavernous vein. (B) Dynamic cavernosogram of the same patient showing leakage via the deep dorsal vein and prominent cavernous vein (arrowhead). See color plate for part A.

deep dorsal vein. The deep dorsal vein courses proximally in the midline between the two corpora cavernosa and empties into the periprostatic plexus. The superficial dorsal vein drains the skin and the subcutaneous tissue superficial to Buck's fascia. It drains into the superficial external pudendal vein.

## Erection Hemodynamics

Erection is a complex event regulated by the tone of smooth muscle composing the cavernous arterioles, venules, and sinusoids. Tumescence follows a decrease in corporal smooth muscle tension—decreasing arterial, arteriolar, and sinusoidal resistance. Decreasing resistance to arterial inflow bathes the cavernous tissues in highly oxygenated arterial blood. Venous outflow during erection is dynamically limited by distension of the sinusoids compressing the subtunical venular plexus against the inner layer of the tunica albuginea. The differential stretching of the two primary layers of the tunica albuginea during erection compresses the exiting emissary veins closed. The rigid penis is veno-occluded, in a low outflow state, with distended sinusoids and elevated intracorporal pressure. During rigid erection arterial inflows are paradoxically very low—by Doppler estimation 1.5 to 5.6 ml per minute, by phalloarteriography 4.7 ml per minute, by radioisotope study <5 ml per minute. Dynamic cavernosometry similarly reveals that with maximal smooth muscle relaxation rigid erection is associated with low flow to maintain values of 0.5 to 3 ml per minute.[24,25,30]

Detumescence and flaccidity are initiated and maintained by corporal smooth muscle contraction. Aboseif and Lue[31] and Andersson and Wagner[32] studied the dynamics of erection in several species and divided the progress from flaccidity to erection into distinct phases. In the flaccid phase, there is a dominant sympathetic influence, and the terminal arterioles and cavernous smooth muscles are contracted. Electrical activity recorded from the smooth muscle of the corpus cavernosum indicates that the smooth muscle cells are contracting. In the latent (filling) phase, parasympathetic nervous activity dominates, and there is an increased blood flow through the internal pudendal and cavernous arteries. Peripheral resistance is decreased due to dilatation of the cavernosal and helicine arteries. The penis elongates. In the tumescence phase, the intracavernous pressure increases rapidly. The compliance of the sinusoidal muscle is markedly enhanced, causing penile engorgement. In full erection the relaxed trabecular muscle expands and, together with the increased blood volume, compresses the plexus of subtunical venules, reducing venous outflow and increasing intracavernous pressure to 10 to 20 mm Hg below the systolic blood pressure. In the rigid erection phase cavernous pressure may increase well above the systolic pressure. As a consequence of voluntary or reflexogenic contraction of the ischiocaver-

nosus and bulbocavernosus muscles, suprasystolic pressures may be transiently achieved during pelvic thrusting.

Although the phases of erection documented in the laboratory in animals have correlates with human erectile responses during PBFS, there are variables in clinical testing, which may preclude full erection. In addition, the threshold dosage for a single agent or multiple agents to reliably promote complete smooth muscle relaxation has not been established. Available data on the minimal effective dosage of $PGE_1$ suggest 2 μg will produce erection in 38% of men with psychogenic impotence and in 20% of men with vasculogenic erectile dysfunction.[33] A pattern of spectral waveform progression on CDDU has been correlated with a normal rigid response during PBFS.[34] In the latent/filling phase when sinusoidal resistance is low (5 minutes) following injection, the waveform is characterized by high forward flow during diastole. As intrapenile pressure increases, diastolic velocities decrease. With full erection, the systolic waveforms will sharply peak and may be slightly less than during full tumescence; diastolic flow will be zero. In rigid erection, cavernous pressure will exceed systemic diastolic blood pressure and reversal of diastolic flow occurs. Similarly in the rigid erection phase the systolic waveform may be damped. The bulbocavernosus reflex may be stimulated by intermittent glans compression during examination.[4]

## Technique: Instruments

Since its introduction by Lue[25] in 1985, duplex Doppler penile sonography has proven an accurate and reproducible technique for evaluating erectile dysfunction. The addition of color has facilitated consistent detection of dorsal, cavernous, and urethral vessels. CDDU permits the rapid acquisition and measurement of small vessels in low-flow states.[35–37] High-frequency linear array transducers (5 to 10 MHz) provide the best images of the penis; the higher the frequency, the better the near field resolution. [All images in this discussion were retrieved from a 7.0-MHz linear transducer with standoff wedge (Siemens/ Quantum) or a 7.5-MHz linear array transducer (Bruel and Kjaer); these permit continuous color encoded gray-scale images during Doppler sampling. Others have reported adequate high-resolution penile imaging with (noncolor) gray-scale 13.5-MHz probes.[38]]

Color flow uses the imaging principles of pulsed Doppler; a pulse of ultrasound is emitted from the transducer, reflected back, and received. When the returning echo has a different frequency from the emitted frequency, a Doppler shift has occurred; ultrasound reflecting from a moving object (penile blood) causes a Doppler shift. Doppler frequency shift depends on several factors: frequency of the transducer, velocity of the moving object (penile blood), speed of sound through the medium (penile tissue), and angle between the Doppler beam and direction of blood flow. The blood flowing in a vessel that is approaching the transducer will produce echoes with a higher frequency than was emitted; blood flowing away produces a lower frequency. As blood flow velocities increase, Doppler shift increases. The Doppler shift is displayed on gray scale as a spectrum (waveform) or in CDDU as a two-dimensional color image. In CDDU the color display has an angle dependence just like the gray scale spectrum of the Doppler shift. If the vessel runs parallel to the skin surface, ultrasound scanning lines are perpendicular (90° Doppler angle) and will yield no Doppler shift and no color within the vessel. To correct this problem of physics, linear array transducers use phasing to steer the scan lines at a more appropriate angle or an angled standoff wedge on the end of the transducer to provide a nonperpendicular Doppler angle. The angled standoff wedge is acoustically neutral and is ideal for imaging penile vessels that are parallel to the skin. Arterial flow velocity determinations depend on the ultrasound beam–vessel angle; the optimal angle is 60°. The angle correction is set by the examiner. Because arterial flow velocities will be repeated several times after injecting the vasodilator, particular attention should be given to maintaining the same angle of insonation. Arterial velocity in the same vessel will be recorded at 20 cm/s,

25 cm/s, 31 cm/s, or 203 cm/s if the probe-vessel angle is altered from 30° to 45° to 55° to 85°, respectively.[39–43]

## Examining Protocol

The examination should be performed in a warm, darkened room, a secure setting essential to reduce anxiety and reduce sympathetic cavernous smooth muscle tone. The patient should be assured that no one will come walking in during his testing. He lies in the supine position; he need only disrobe from the waist down. His attention should be directed at the ultrasound monitor with periodic explanation of images displayed, such as, "You are going to see ultrasound views of your penile vessels; some of these run on the surface of the penis, and two are central arteries providing the pressure to your erection. When the Doppler is activated, the sound you hear will be blood flowing into your penis with each heartbeat."

The corporal bodies should be scanned in the transverse plane from base to tip to demonstrate normal anatomy (paired cavernous and dorsal arteries); the echotexture should be homogeneous; fibrotic processes are relatively hyperechoic in comparison (Fig. 27.4, see color insert). Peyronie's plaques will be denser than normal tunica; they may be visible as linear echogenic thickenings. If they cast an acoustic shadow like a renal stone, calcification should be suspected and plain radiographs taken following PBFS/CDDU. The penile vessels and flow velocities are assessed in the sagittal plane (parallel to the long axis of the penis). Vessels may be scanned from a dorsal or ventral approach (Fig. 27.2). Lateral scanning will demonstrate both cavernous vessels in the same image, with the hyperechoic septum in between both arteries (Fig. 27.5, see color insert). Cavernous-to-cavernous collaterals are only imaged in the sagittal projection from the lateral penis. These vessels are perforating the septum in more than 50% of men examined and are seen in patients with neurogenic and psychogenic impotence, suggesting a congenital origin. The dynamics of collateral flow are im-

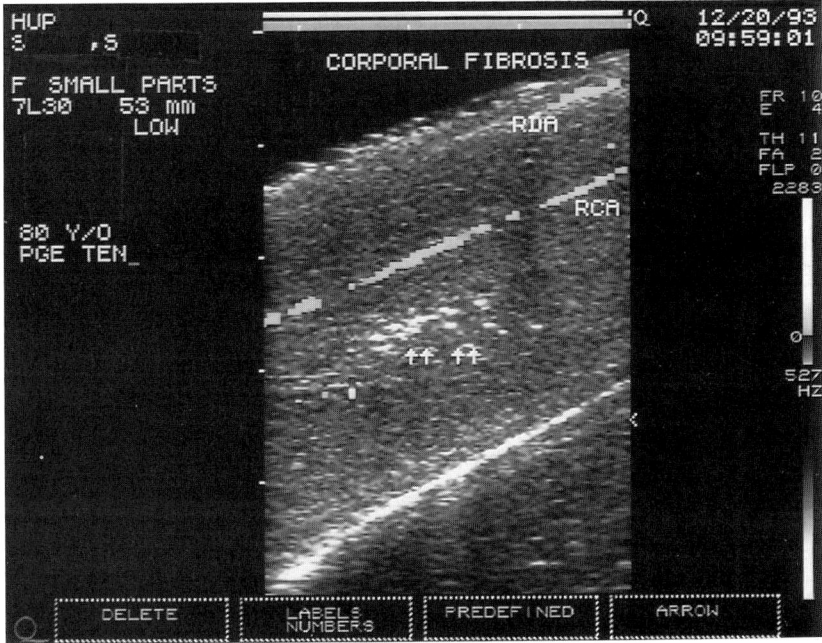

FIGURE 27.4. Corporal fibrosis (arrows) in an 80-year-old patient, sagittal scan; right dorsal artery (RDA) and right cavernous artery (RCA). See color plate.

portant; high flow collaterals ≥25 cm/s may supplement unilateral cavernous arterial insufficiency. A dorsal projection is required to image the dorsal artery and ipsilateral cavernous artery (Fig. 27.6, see color insert). Following vasodilation, dorsal-to-cavernous collaterals were recently demonstrated in 59% of men, but these were hemodynamically significant only in 15% of patients (≥25 cm/s).[44] The dorsal arteries are not subjected to intracorporal pressure changes of each progressive erection phase; therefore, antegrade diastolic flow persists even in well-sustained rigidity. During peak erection, dorsal systolic flow is maximal. Copious acoustic gel on the surface of the penis and a light touch of the probe apparatus are needed in order not to alter flow dynamics of dorsal vessels.

All four penile arteries should be scanned at least from the level of the penoscrotal junction to the glans. When there is asymmetry of cavernous flows (≥10 cm/s) or when collaterals are seen, the crura should be examined to determine if proximal inflow disease exists (prepenile) or if intracorporal stenosis has re-

sulted in decreased unilateral CDDU signal. If the patient's legs are abducted in a frog-leg position, the perineum can be scanned, revealing the entry of the cavernous arteries into the penis. This view is especially helpful when searching for arterial sinusoidal malformations causing high-flow priapism or if the patient develops a rapid rigidity.

Cavernous flow velocities will be highest at the perineum and distally will segmentally diminish. Several investigators[45,46] have confirmed that systolic velocities of the cavernous arteries vary significantly as a function of sampling location. Traditionally, arterial velocities are measured at the penoscrotal junction (proximal pendulous shaft), from either the ventral or lateral sagittal projections. If the penis has not become erect, it should be held upright by the glans; this is the anatomic position of erection and serves to straighten the course of the cavernous and dorsal arteries. Because the principal source of error in flow velocity determinations is incorrectly assigned Doppler angle, holding the shaft upright stretches the tortuous cavernous vessels and permits

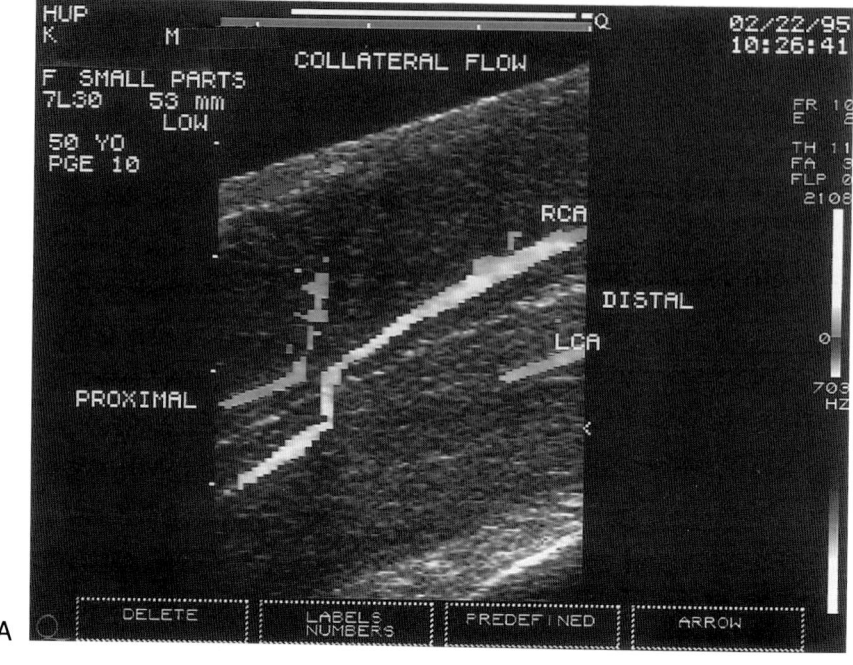

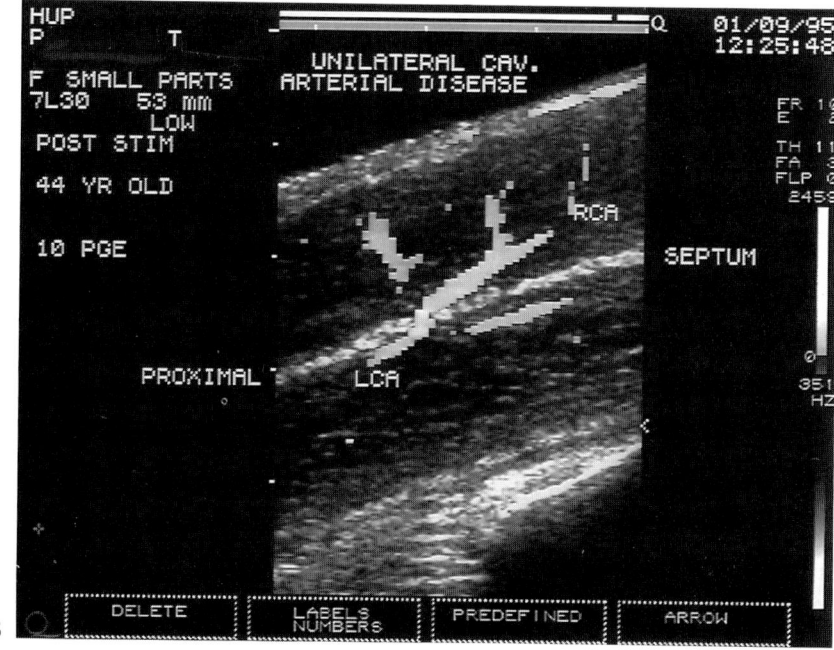

FIGURE 27.5. (A) Sagittal scan of cavernous artery collaterals, with distal right cavernous flow, supplemented by collateral. (B) Sagittal scan shows absence of right proximal inflow, with distal right cavernous flow depending on left collateral. See color plate.

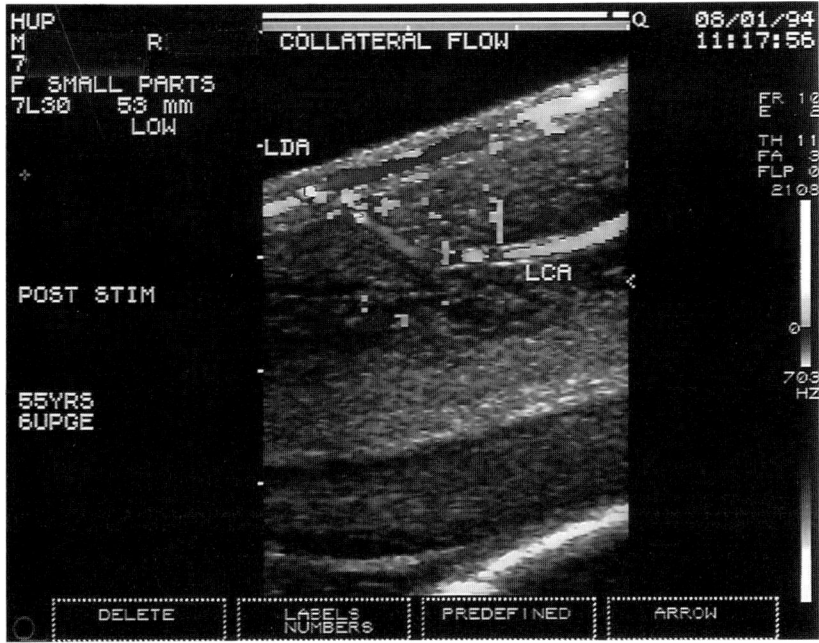

FIGURE 27.6. Left dorsal artery (LDA) to left cavernous artery (LCA) collateral, sagittal scan. See color plate.

consistent measurements with the probe-vessel Doppler angle remaining set (60°).

Timing is important. Arterial diameter and cavernous peak systolic velocities will maximize before rigid erection (maximal intracavernous pressure). Some investigators advocate continuous penile sampling for up to 30 minutes following penile injection.[47] Meuleman et al[48] found peak velocities highest 5 to 10 minutes following vasodilation. Fitzgerald et al[49] noted that 24% of patients tested did not reach maximum cavernous flow until 10 to 15 minutes after injection. If initial measurements are made at 5 to 10 minutes after injection and full or rigid erection waveforms are not seen, a period of privacy and self-stimulation will enhance the penile response in ≥70% of patients (Fig. 27.7, see color insert).[4] CDDU assessment is repeated immediately following self-stimulation, and notation is made of whether the response weakens or is sustained.[50] It is very useful to visually rate the erectile quality during Doppler assessment: inadequate, adequate, or unbending rigidity sustained for 20 minutes. Correlation of visual erection rating and Doppler parameters is an essential element in the

diagnostic process; although the Doppler parameters are distinctly different, tumescence without rigidity is characteristic of both severe veno-occlusive disease and arterial insufficiency. Finally, the patient should be questioned about whether the pharmacologic erection is similar, better, or worse than those he achieves at home.[38] If the answer to this question is "worse," then the patient is redosed to achieve maximal smooth muscle relaxation.[51] European investigators have recommended audiovisual sexual stimulation in lieu of or to supplement manual stimulation for PBFS.[52]

The choice of an intracavernous vasoactive agent for CDDU has not been standardized. The initial duplex Doppler studies[13,53,54] were performed following injection of 60 mg of papaverine. Trimix has been used recently in efforts to achieve maximal smooth muscle relaxation—0.2 ml of papaverine (6 mg), phentolamine (0.2 mg), and $PGE_1$ (2 µg).[38] $PGE_1$ (Caverject) is the only FDA-approved injectable for the treatment of erectile dysfunction. Of the currently used agents it is thought to have the greatest biocompatibility. $PGE_1$ is a corporal smooth muscle relaxant and has

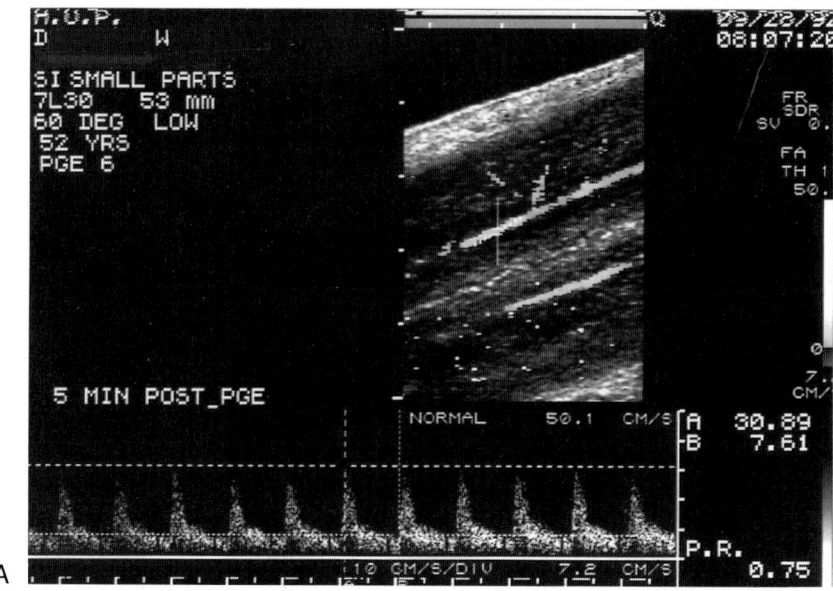

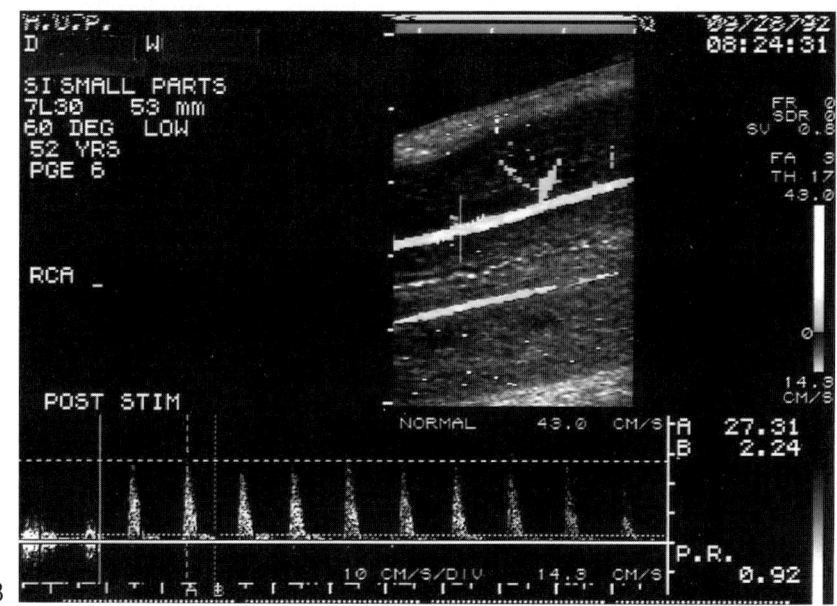

FIGURE 27.7. (A and B) Normal progression of Doppler waveform: response 5 minutes after penile injection of PGE$_1$ and response following privacy and self-stimulation; note minor decrease in peak systolic velocities from 30 to 27 cm/s and significant decrease in end diastolic velocities from 7 to 2 cm/s. See color plate.

antiadrenergic activity that may explain its efficacy in patients suffering high-anxiety psychogenic erectile dysfunction.[55-58] In a recent dose-finding study,[33] the median effective dosage was 5.0 µg in patients with vasculogenic dysfunction, producing a mean duration of erection of 37 minutes. Penile discomfort was noted in 34%, and prolonged erection (4 to 6 hours) in 5%. PGE$_1$ is highly effective with dosing of 6 µg for patients 50 to 60 years old and

10 µg for patients 60 to 70 years old when coupled with privacy and self-stimulation. With this regimen of age-specific dosing, <4% of patients develop persistent rigidity for 2 hours. Patients are successfully managed with direct corporal injection of the α-adrenergic phenylephrine (100 µg/cc, using 1 to 3 cc), if treated within 2 hours of their study.

## CDDU and Penile Inflow: Arterial Adequacy

The original parameter used to infer the integrity of penile circulation was cavernous peak systolic velocity (PSV). In efforts to further refine the diagnosis of cavernous inflow disease, Doppler parameters have been expanded: end diastolic arterial velocity (EDV, flow velocity measured during diastole immediately prior to takeoff of the systolic waveform), systolic rise time (in milliseconds from the start of systolic velocity to the maximum value),[28,59] and cavernous artery acceleration (peak flow velocity over systolic rise time).[60] Flow velocities should be measured 5 to 10 minutes after injection; a delay in response is typical in both the hypertensive and the anxious patient. A visual rating of erectile quality should be recorded each time a set of Doppler parameters is recorded.

Investigations have shown that cavernous arterial diameters normally decrease from proximal to distal and that measurement of cavernous arterial lumina actually exceeds ultrasound resolution of 7- to 10-MHz probes.[37,61–64] In the University of California–San Francisco (UCSF) series, normal subjects had a mean PSV of 34.8 cm/s and a mean arterial diameter of 0.89 mm.[43] In a study from Baylor University, normal volunteers had mean PSV of 40 cm/s and mean arterial diameter of 1.0 mm.[65] Normal volunteers at the Harvard Medical School study had mean PSV of 47 cm/s.[64] Each of these groups concurs that a peak systolic velocity <25 cm/s suggests severe arterial insufficiency. When penile angiography is compared with duplex Doppler examinations of the same patients, PSV <25 cm/s is consistently associated with severe arterial disease; in the Mayo Clinic

series PSV <25 cm/s had a sensitivity of 100% and specificity of 95% in selection of patients with abnormal pudendal arteriography[66] (Fig. 27.8, see color insert). A PSV of 35 cm/s or more is generally associated with a normal penile arteriogram.[66] The Mayo Clinic group has recommended that if there is a good clinical response to vasodilating injection, and bilateral peak systolic velocities are >30 cm/s with arterial dilation to 0.7 mm, arteriography should not be performed.[66] When PSV is compared with cavernous arterial systolic occlusion pressures (CASOP) generated during dynamic infusion cavernosometry, a PSV ≥25 cm/s predicts a normal CASOP with a sensitivity of 95% and specificity of 95%.[67] Asymmetry greater than 10 cm/s between right and left cavernous inflows is abnormal; if cavernous inflows are asymmetric or absent at the perineum, one should suspect prepenile (pudendal) arterial disease. Intrapenile arterial disease is evident when crural inflows are adequate and symmetric but asymmetry of R/L PSVs is noted in the pendulous penis. On CDDU, severe unilateral cavernous arterial insufficiency may be associated with reversal of systolic flow proximal to the entry of a collateral (Fig. 27.9, see color insert).

Schwartz et al[68] correlated progressive changes in Doppler spectral waveform pattern with increasing intracorporal pressure in potent volunteers stimulated with papaverine/phentolamine. Rigid erection was associated with intracorporal pressures ranging from 83 to 106 mm Hg. During tumescence both PSV and EDV increased, with corporal pressure ranging from 11 to 25 mm Hg. With rigidity, EDV approached 0, and diastolic flow reversed when intracorporal pressures reached 63 to 83 mm Hg. Planiol and Pourcelot[69] derived the index of vascular resistance from the Doppler spectrum: resistive index (RI) = PSV − EDV/PSV. The RI calculation is not directly dependent on the probe vessel angle; it does not matter that the Doppler angle is not ideal (60°). The value of RI depends on the resistance to arterial inflow, and in the context of corporal physiology this is a function of sympathetic tone in the flaccid state and of changing intracorporal pressure during the

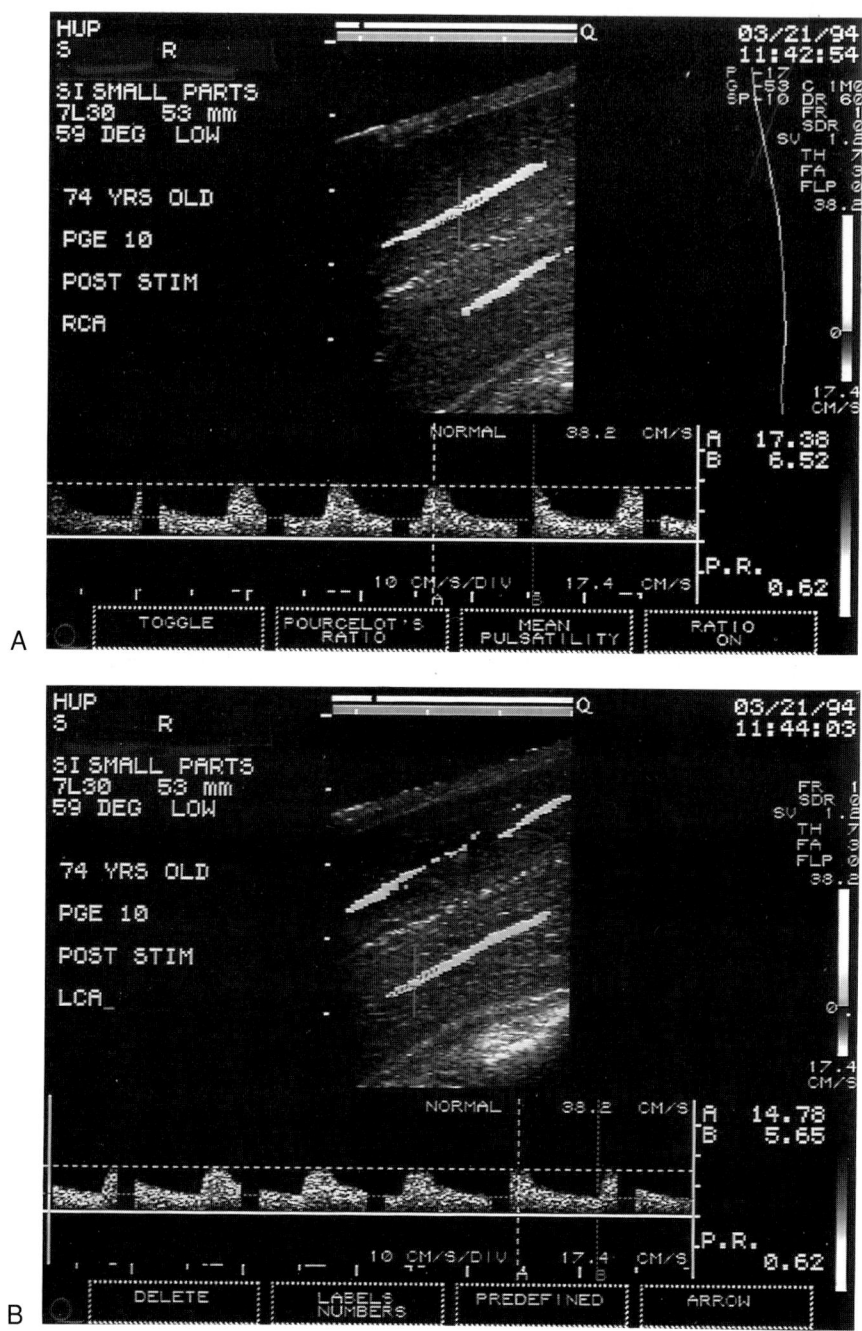

FIGURE 27.8. (A and B) Severe bilateral cavernous arterial insufficiency in 74-year-old patient, with peak systolic velocities <25 cm/s in each central artery (poststimulation responses). See color plate.

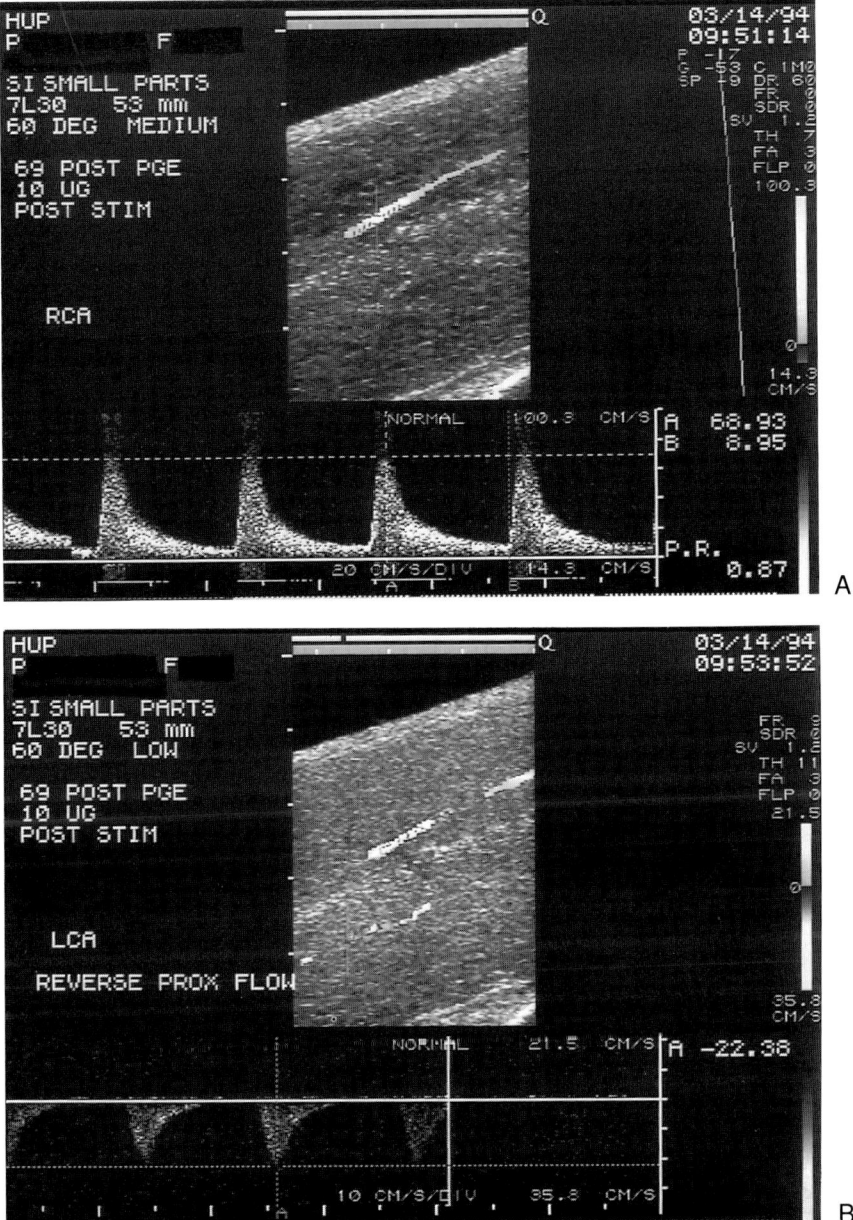

FIGURE 27.9. (A and B) Unilateral cavernous arterial insufficiency in left cavernous artery (LCA) with high peak systolic velocity in the right central artery, 68 cm/s. The direction of blood flow is actually reversed in the proximal LCA, because of RCA to LCA collateral. See color plate.

various phases of erection following either natural or pharmacologic smooth muscle relaxation. As penile pressure equals or exceeds diastolic systemic pressure, diastolic flow in the corpora will approach 0 and RI will approach a value of 1. During tumescence and until full rigidity, diastolic flow persists and the value for RI remains <1.0. The RI correlates very well with visual rating of erectile responses as both are descriptions of penile rigidity/pressure. Both EDV and RI are useful parameters in predicting adequacy of veno-occlusion.

# Presbyrectia: Age-Related Decrease in Erection

Age-related decreases in erectile function have long been evident in clinical series and have now been verified in normative community groups like the Massachusetts Male Aging Study.[70] Using computerized morphometry of penile biopsies, Wespes et al[71] observed an age-related decrease in smooth muscle content. Comparing young patients with penile curvature but hemodynamically adequate erections to elderly patients with erectile dysfunction, he found young patients (with penile curvature) have corpora cavernosa composed of 40% to 52% smooth muscle, patients with corporal veno-occlusive dysfunction have 19% to 36% smooth muscle, and patients with arterial impotence have 10% to 25% smooth muscle with collagen content correspondingly increased.

Recent research suggests that, in the aging man, decreasing number and duration of nocturnal erections may be related to corporal hypoxia from arterial or arteriolar insufficiency.[72-74] In a retrospective review of over 600 cases,[75] 106 instances were documented in patients of a variety of ages where intracavernous challenge with $PGE_1$ produced excellent, well-sustained rigidity of at least 20 minutes. These data suggest that cavernous arterial flow decreases with age, but normal corporal dynamics permit penile rigidity across a wide range of PSVs, and the technique of privacy and self-stimulation should permit safe and effective diagnostic dosing for the typical impotence patient with 10 µg of $PGE_1$. The RI parameter did not vary with age, suggesting the dynamics of veno-occlusion are the critical factor in the aging erectile response.

# CDDU and Penile Outflow: Documenting Veno-Occlusive Adequacy

Failure of the veno-occlusive mechanism is reflected in the Doppler spectral waveform of the cavernous artery. The suspicion of venous leakage is raised when the patient has an excellent arterial response to injected vasodilator ($\geq 30$ cm/s, PSV), with well-maintained EDV ($>3$ to 5 cm/s), accompanied by transient rigidity after self-stimulation.

Although the definitive criteria for CDDU-diagnosed venous leakage have not been agreed upon, the examiner should reliably be able to select patients for more invasive investigations (dynamic infusion cavernosometry and cavernosography) by observing waveform progression through each phase of erection. When the Doppler spectral waveform continues to exhibit forward diastolic flow despite peak systolic flow ($>30$ cm/s), a low-resistance state persists in the sinusoids and the patient may have venogenic impotence (Fig. 27.10, see color insert). The dorsal arteries are not subjected to the intracorporal pressure changes with each phase of erection, and well-sustained rigidity is associated with antegrade diastolic flow. Deep dorsal vein flow persists during rigid erection; DDV flows are a function of dorsal arterial flow to the glans and should not be interpreted as evidence of corporal venous leakage (Fig. 27.11, see color insert). When DDV flows are high, a pattern of respiratory venous variation may be detected (Fig. 27.12, see color insert). The primary veno-occlusive mechanism consists of passive compression of the subtunical venular plexus by the distended sinusoids. The secondary mechanism is the scissoring off of the emissary veins as they egress through the two layers of the tunica albuginea. Emissary veins unlike dorsal-artery to cavernous-artery collaterals are difficult to localize with CDDU, presumably because of their low flow state and easy compressibility (Fig. 27.13, see color insert).

# Priapism: CDDU Characteristics of Low Flow and High Flow

Priapism is a persistent erection that fails to subside after climax and is accompanied by penile pain and tenderness; it is an overfunction of a normal mechanism.[76] Traditionally, priapism has been categorized as primary (spontaneous-idiopathic) or secondary to specific pathologies: sickle cell disease, leukemia,

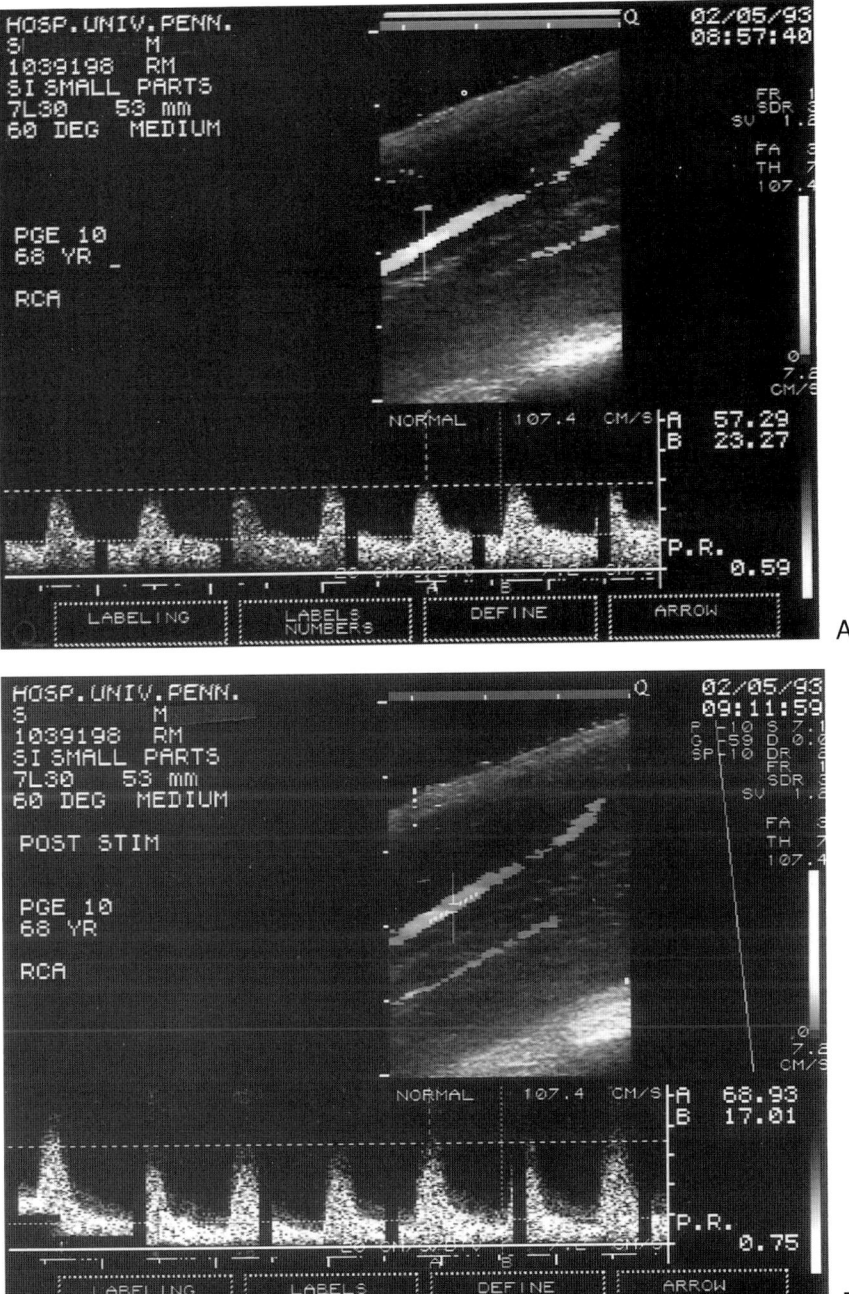

FIGURE 27.10. (A and B) An unequivocal diagnosis of cavernous venous occlusive disease based on ultrasound criteria can be given when cavernous arterial flows exceed 35 cm/s, end diastolic velocities remain high, and resistive index is low. This 68-year-old patient, following PGE$_1$ 10 μg and self-stimulation, has postinjection PSV of 57 cm/s and poststimulation PSV of 68 cm/s, EDV of 17 cm/s, and RI of 0.75. See color plate.

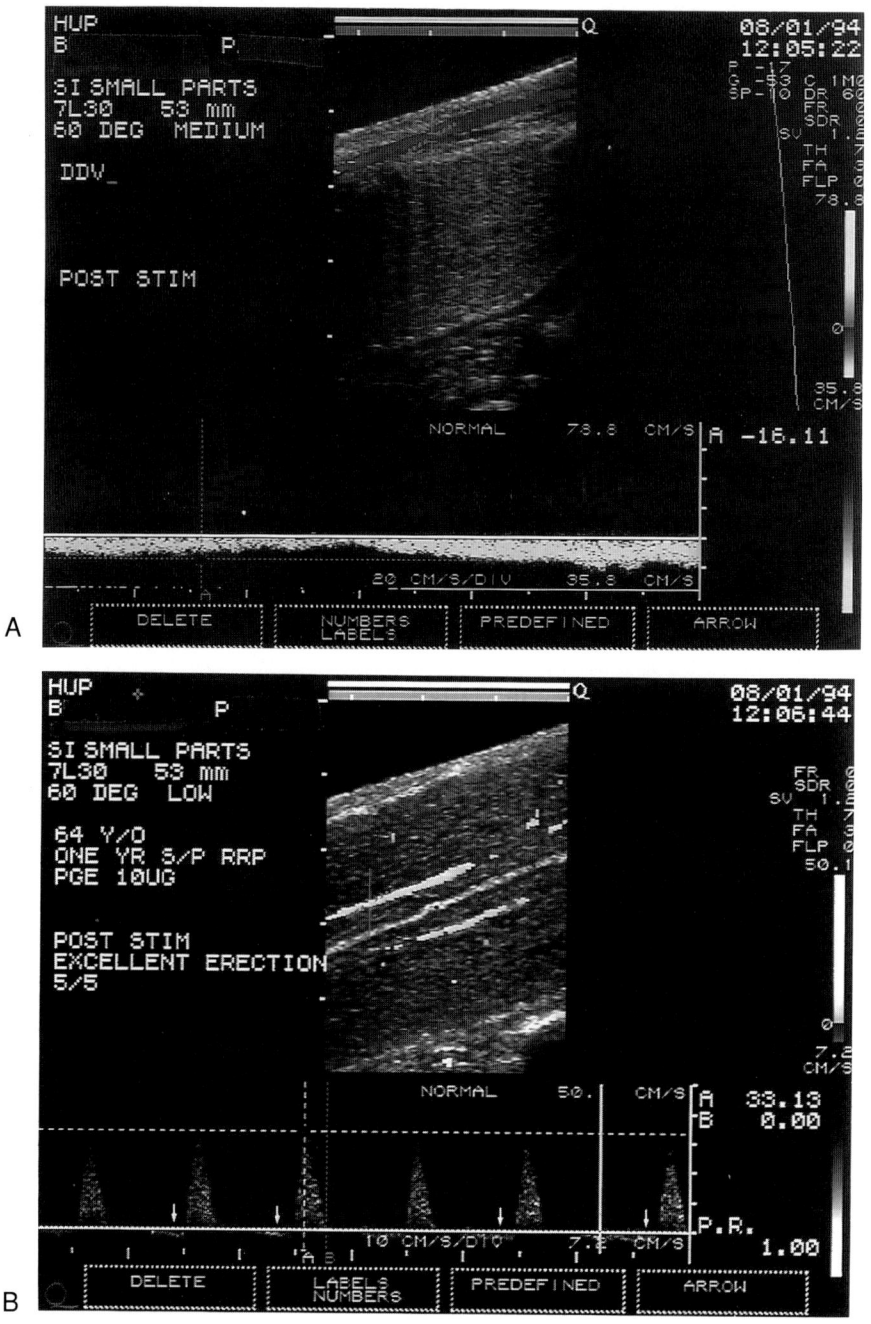

FIGURE 27.11. (A) Deep dorsal vein flow (DDV) persists during rigid erection. (B) Rigid erection following 10 μg of PGE$_1$, associated with PSV of 33 cm/s and reversal of diastolic flow; see arrows. See color plate.

fat emboli, malignant infiltration, neurologic injury, alcohol, and psychotropic drugs. With the increasing popularity of pharmacologic erection programs, iatrogenic or therapeutically induced prolonged erection has become the most common cause of priapism.[77] Functional classification is preferable, and more accurately describes the pathophysiology: high flow–arterial, versus low flow–ischemic.

Ischemic priapism is an obvious failure of the detumescence mechanism that may result from

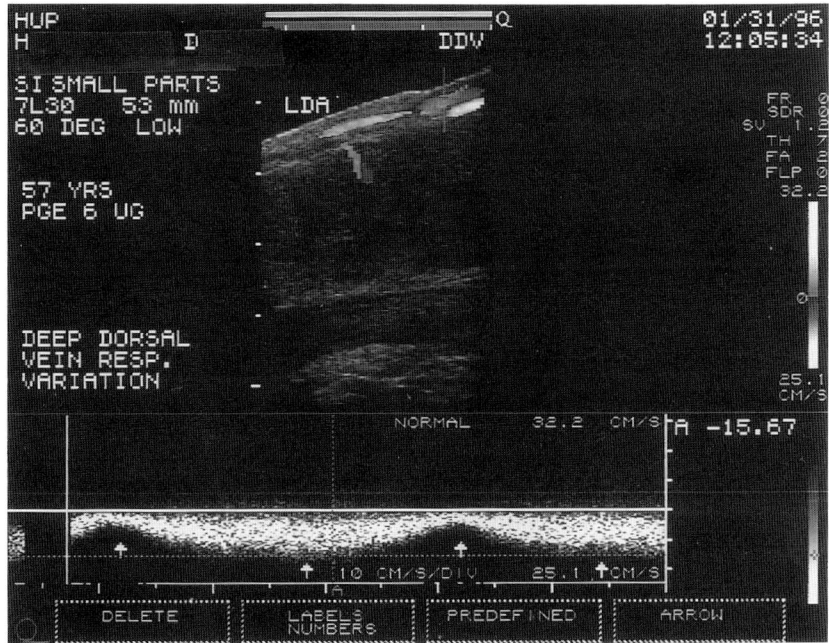

FIGURE 27.12. Respiratory variation in deep dorsal vein flow (DDV). See color plate.

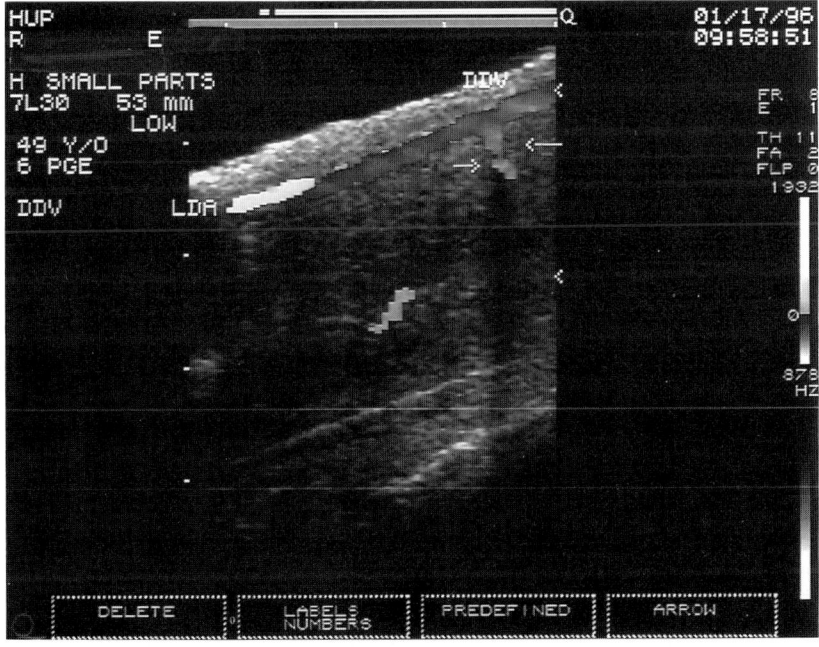

FIGURE 27.13. Emissary veins perforating the tunica albuginea are rarely seen because of their small size and low flow state (arrows). See color plate.

direct dysregulation of the cavernous-arterial-sinusoidal system through persistent stimulation of corporal relaxing factors, inhibition of neurotransmission normally terminating erection, or inactivation of the smooth muscle cellular cofactors that regulate corporal smooth muscle tone like an altered metabolic environment (hypoxia, hypercarbia, and acidity).[78]

Of the various causes of priapism only trauma has been attributed to "dysregulation" of inflow and production of high-flow priapism.[79,80] Hakim et al[81] demonstrated the utility and accuracy of duplex Doppler in the diagnosis and management of high-flow priapism when compared with selective internal pudendal arteriography. It is essential to establish the correct classification of priapism by aspiration of bright red blood from the corpora confirming high oxygen tension or dark venous blood suggesting "low flow" priapism. Remote corporal injury may be evident on CDDU by hyperechoic changes within the corpora, a nonspecific finding consistent with scar formation (Fig. 27.14, see color insert). Acute disruption

of the sinusoid architecture is evidenced by turbulent flow on CDDU, marking the site of arteriosinusoidal fistula (Fig. 27.15, see color insert). In the acute phase of injury, unregulated flow may be imaged without vasoactive injection. In follow-up, low-dosage vasoactive injection is needed. The crural bodies must be imaged from the ventrum (transperineum) by frog-legging the patient and lifting the scrotum.

## CDDU: Staging of Peyronie's Disease

Surgical staging of Peyronie's disease must address both penile form and function. The tunica albuginea and dorsal vascular complex are well imaged with CDDU. A standoff wedge increases near-field resolution, bringing plaques into view. The tunica albuginea is normally hyperechoic compared with the corpora proper (Fig. 27.16A, see color insert). As the corporal bodies distend with blood, the cavernous sinusoids become more hypoechoic, increasing the

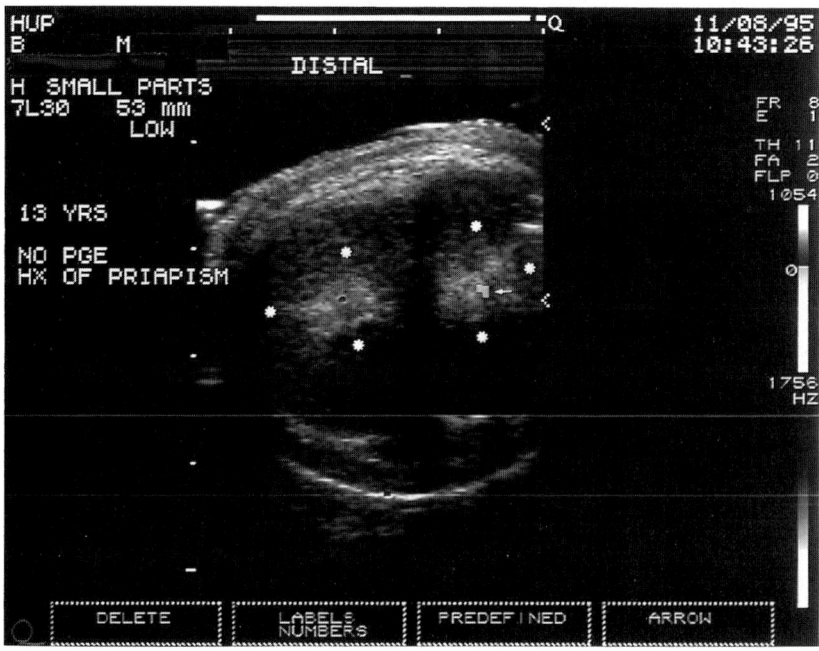

FIGURE 27.14. Transverse scan of 13-year-old boy with repeated episodes of sickle cell priapism: left cavernous arterial flow is present (arrow); cavernous tissues are hyperechoic consistent with central fibrosis (*). See color plate.

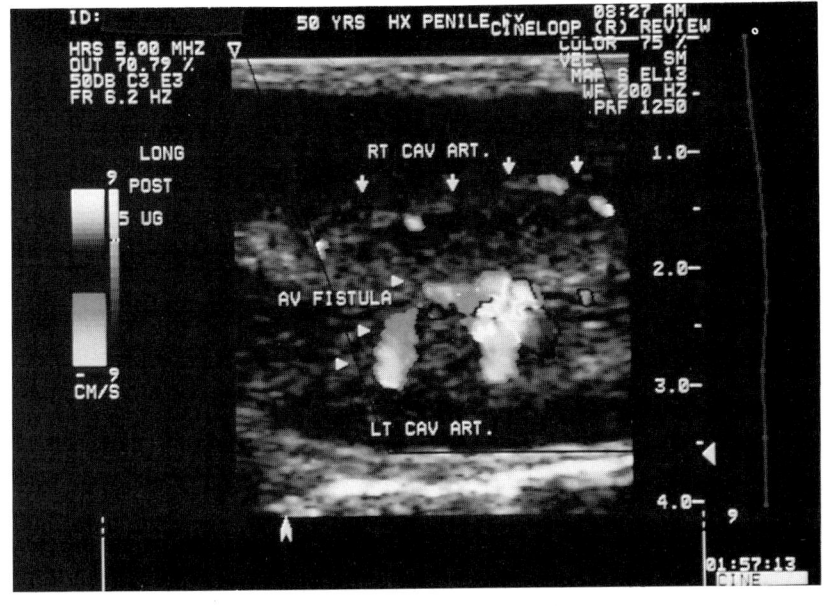

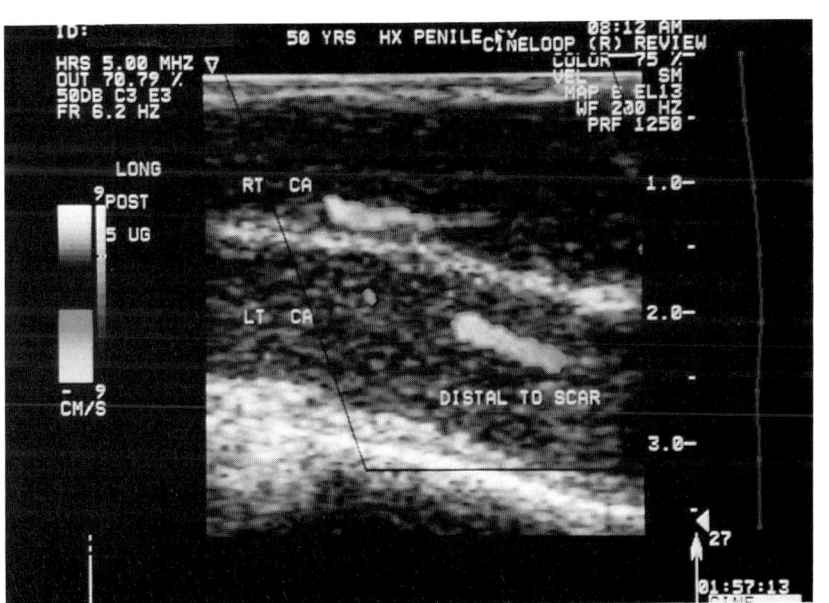

FIGURE 27.15. (A) Sagittal image of left cavernous sinusoidal fistula producing high-flow priapism; note turbulent flow. (B) Distal-to-site-of-trauma cavernous flows are more distinct. See color plate.

contrast between the tunica and corpora. Penile plaques are hyperechoic thickenings of the tunica albuginea. The typical dorsal plaque underlies the dorsal vasculature. Denser plaques cast an acoustical shadow (Fig. 27.16B, see color insert) and are well visualized in either the transverse or sagittal planes (Figs. 27.17A and Fig. 27.17B, see color insert). Although most plaques localize to the proximal and middle third of the pendulous shaft, distal plaques may exert minimal curvature even at the level of the corona. Circumferential narrowing of the corporal bodies by plaque results in an hourglass shape to the erection; the

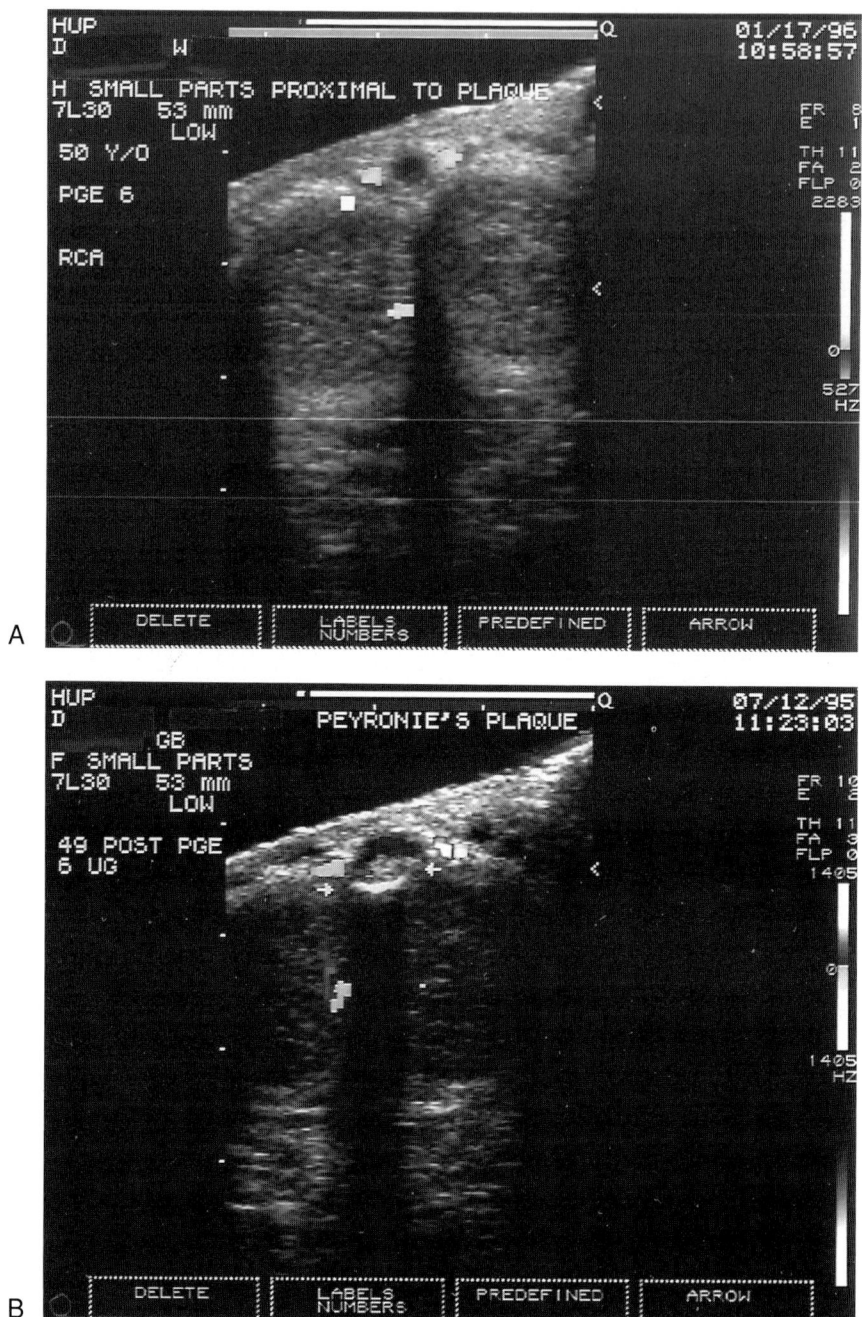

FIGURE 27.16. (A) Transverse scan proximal to plaque. (B) Transverse scan of Peyronie's plaque (arrows); note acoustic shadow below plaque. See color plate.

patient complains of "hinging" with erection. The sonographic correlate is a ring of thickened tunica. A similar, but focal, wedge is seen when penile deviation is lateral.

Septal fibrosis is the most technically challenging abnormality to demonstrate. If increased tissue density is discrete, hyperechoic aggregates within the septum are seen. More diffuse septal fibrosis is identified by scanning in a sagittal plane parallel to the septum; from this vantage point the denser septal fibers take on a veil-like appearance with posterior acoustical shadowing. In cases where acoustical shadowing is generated by dense plaques, plain radiographs should follow CDDU.

The most potentially useful preoperative staging information is the demonstration of collaterals from the dorsal vascular bundle. Dorsal artery collaterals diving downward through the tunica to anastomose with the ipsilateral cavernous artery may be in close proximity. Operative mobilization of the neurovascular

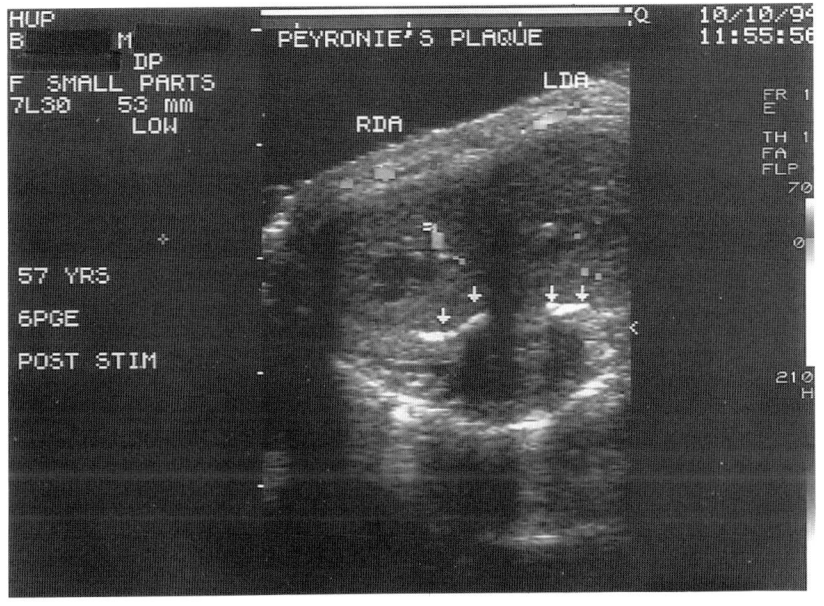

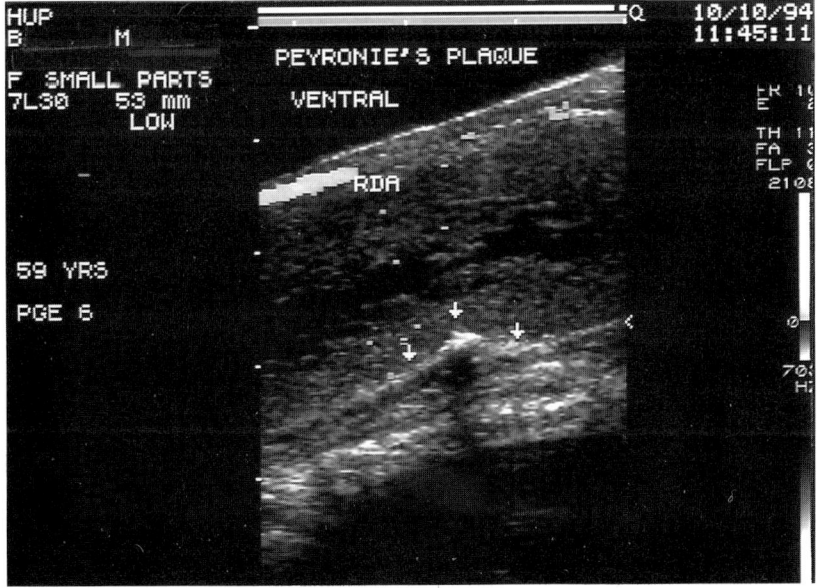

FIGURE 27.17. (A) Transverse scan of ventral Peyronie's plaque. (B) Sagittal scan of ventral plaque. (C) Home photograph. See color plate.

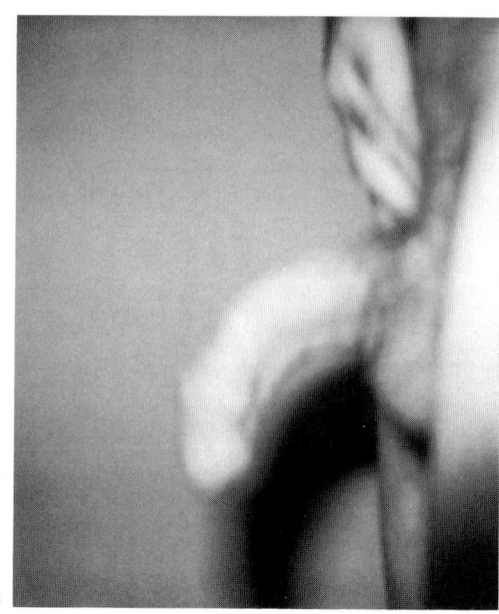

C

FIGURE 27.17. *Continued*

bundle for plaque excision in these cases would of necessity sacrifice the dorsal contribution to cavernous inflow. It is very difficult with current technology to image emissary veins despite the fact that these are ubiquitous[82] (Fig. 27.13). Experience with CDDU suggests high-resolution sonography provides a dynamic noninvasive vascular assessment of erectile function and can precisely localize penile plaques. Timing must take into account the dynamic phases of erection, the fact that penile pain may preempt complete smooth muscle relaxation, and the obstacle that severe penile deviations present to imaging. The plaque should be imaged at 5 to 10 minutes in the latent/tumescent phase while the penis may still be straightened by the examiner before rigidity (Fig. 27.17C, see color insert)

## Conclusion

When dynamic testing is required, CDDU is minimally invasive and adds no additional risk to a diagnostic challenge of intracavernous vasoactive agent, the traditional penile blood flow study. Doppler sonography is more accurate

than physical examination alone following penile injection and, unlike phalloarteriography, exposes anatomical abnormalities as well as corporal hemodynamics. An important question remains unanswered as to the adequate dosing in pharmacoerection testing: Should that dosage vary with age or vasculogenic risk factors? False-positive evaluations can be avoided by addition of the privacy and self-stimulation that enhance erectile responses with pharmacotesting in 70% of patients or by redosing to achieve maximal smooth muscle relaxation.

## References

1. Consensus development conference statement: impotence. National Institutes of Health. *JAMA* 1993; 270:83–90.
2. Mellinger B, Weiss J. Sexual dysfunction in the elderly male. *Am Urol Assoc Update Series* 1992; 11:146–152.
3. Feldman HA, Goldstein 1, Hatzichristou DG, et al. Impotence and its medical and psychosocial correlates: results of the Massachusetts Male Aging Study. *Int J Impotence Res* 1992; 4(suppl 2):AI7.
4. Broderick GA, Arger PA. Duplex doppler ultrasonography: noninvasive assessment of penile anatomy and function. *Semin Roentgenol* 1993; 28:43–56.
5. Landwehr P. Penile vessels: erectile dysfunction. In: Wolf K-J, Fobbe F, eds. *Color Duplex Sonography: Principles and Clinical Application.* Stuttgart: Thieme; 1995: 204–215.
6. Herbener TE, Seftel AD, Nehra A, et al. Penile ultrasound. *Semin Urol* 1994; 12:320–332.
7. King BF, Lewis RW, Mckusick MA. Radiologic evaluation of impotence. In: Bennett AH, ed. *Impotence.* Philadelphia: W.B. Saunders; 1994: 52–91.
8. Gaskell P. The importance of penile blood pressure in cases of impotence. *Can Med Assoc J* 1971; 105:104.
9. Abelson D. Diagnostic value of the penile pulse and blood pressure: a Doppler study of impotence in diabetics. *J Urol* 1975; 113:636.
10. Michal V, Kramer R, Pospichal J. External iliac "steal syndrome." *J Cardiovasc Surg* 1978; 19:355.
11. Goldstein I, Siroky MB, North RI, et al. Vasculogenic impotence: role of the pelvic steal test. *J Urol* 1982; 128:300.

12. Schwartz AN, Lowe MA, Ireton R, et al. A comparison of penile brachial index and angiography: evaluation of corpora cavernosa arterial inflow. *J Urol* 1990; 143:510.

13. Rajfer J, Canan V, Dorey FJ, et al. Correlation between penile angiography and duplex scanning of cavernous arteries in impotent men. *J Urol* 1990; 143:1128–1130.

14. Bahren W, Gall H, Scherb W, et al. Arterial anatomy and arteriographic diagnosis of arteriogenic impotence. *Cardiovasc Intervent Radiol* 1988; 11:195–210.

15. Bookstein JJ, Lange EV. Penile magnification pharmacoarteriography: details of intrapenile arterial anatomy. *AJR* 1987; 148:883.

16. Breza J, Aboseif SR, Orivs BR, et al. Detailed anatomy of penile neurovascular structures: surgical significance. *J Urol* 1989; 141:437–443.

17. Polascik TJ, Walsh PC. Radical retropubic prostatectomy: the influence of accessory pudendal arteries on the recovery of sexual function. *J Urol* 1995; 153:150–152.

18. Curet P, Grellet J, Perrin D, et al. Technical and anatomic factors in filling of distal portion of internal pudendal artery during arteriography. *Urology* 1987; 29:333.

19. Rosen MP, Greenfield AJ, Walker TG, et al. Arteriogenic impotence: findings in 195 impotent men examined with selective internal pudendal angiography. *Radiology* 1990; 174:1043.

20. Garibyan H, Lue TF. Anastomotic network between the dorsal and cavernous arteries in the penis. *J Urol* 1990; 143:221A.

21. Gall H, Bahren W, Scherb W, et al. Diagnostic accuracy of Doppler ultrasound technique of the penile arteries in correlation to selective arteriography. *Cardiovasc Intervent Radiol* 1988; 11:225.

22. Virag R, Frydman D, Legman M, et al. Intracavernous injection of papaverine as a diagnostic and therapeutic method in erectile failure. *Angiology* 1984; 35:79.

23. Lue TF. Impotence: a patient's goal directed approach to treatment. *World J Urol* 1990; 8:67.

24. Pescatori ES, Hatzichristou DG, Namburi S, et al. A positive intracavernous injection test implies normal veno-occlusive but not necessarily normal arterial function: a hemodynamic study. *J Urol* 1994; 151:1209–1216.

25. Lue TF, Hricak H, Marich KW, et al. Vasculogenic impotence evaluated by high resolution ultrasonography and pulsed Doppler spectrum analysis. *Radiology* 1985; 155:777.

26. McAninch JW, Laing FC, Jeffrey RB. Sonourethrography in the evaluation of urethral strictures. *J Urol* 1988; 139:294–297.

27. Benson CB, Doubilet PM, Richie JP. Sonography of the male genital tract. *AJR* 1989; 153:705–713.

28. Oates CP, Pickard PH, Powell PH, et al. The use of duplex ultrasound in the assessment of arterial supply to the penis in vasculogenic impotence. *J Urol* 1995; 153:354–357.

29. Banya Y, Ushiki, Takagane H, et al. Two circulatory routes within the human corpus cavernosum penis: a scanning electron microscopic study of corrosion casts. *J Urol* 1989; 979:883.

30. Bookstein JJ. Cavernosal venooclusive insufficiency in male impotence: evaluation of degree and location. *Radiology* 1987; 164:175.

31. Aboseif SR, Lue TF. Hemodynamics of penile erection. *Urol Clin North Am* 1988; 15:1–7.

32. Andersson K-E, Wagner G. Physiology of penile erection. *Physiol Rev* 1995; 75:191–223.

33. Linet OI, Ogrinc FG. Efficacy and safety of intracavernosal alprostadil in men with erectile dysfunction. *N Engl J Med* 1996; 334:873–877.

34. Schwartz AN, Wang KY, Mack LA, et al. Evaluation of normal erectile function with color flow Doppler sonography. *AJR* 1989; 153:1155–1160.

35. Quam JP, King BF, James EM, et al. Duplex and color Doppler monographic evaluation of vasculogenic impotence. *AJR* 1989; 153:1141–1147.

36. Paushter DM. Role of duplex sonography in the evaluation of sexual impotence. *AJR* 1989; 153:116.

37. Collins JP, Lewandowski BJ. Experience with intracorporeal injection of papaverine and duplex ultrasound scanning for the assessment of arteriogenic impotence. *Br J Urol* 1987; 59:84.

38. Herbner TE, Seftel AD, Nehra A et al. Penile ultrasound. *Semin Urol* 1994; 12:320–332.

39. Burns PN. Hemodynamics and interpretation of Doppler signals. In: Taylor KJW, Burns PN, Wells PNT, eds. *Clinical Applications of Doppler Ultrasound.* New York: Raven Press; 1987.

40. Burns PN. Physical principles of Doppler ultrasound and spectral analysis. *J Clin Ultrasound* 1987; 15:567–590.

41. Foley WD, Erickson SJ. Color Doppler flow imaging. *AJR* 1991; 156:3–13.

42. Merritt CR. Doppler color flow imaging. *J Clin Ultrasound* 1987; 15:591–597.

43. Broderick GA, Lue TF. The penile blood flow study: evaluation of vasculogenic impotence. In: Jonas U, Thon WF, Stief CG, eds. *Erectile Dysfunction*. Berlin, Heidelberg, New York: Springer-Verlag; 1991.

44. Wegner HEH, Andersen R, Knispel HH, et al. Evaluation of penile arteries with color coded duplex sonography: prevalence and possible therapeutic implications of connections between dorsal and cavernous arteries in impotent men. *J Urol* 1995; 153:1469–1471.

45. Paick JS, Won Lee S, Hyup Kim S. Doppler sonography of deep cavernosal artery of the penis: variation of peak systolic velocity according to sampling location. *Int J Impotence Res* 1994; 6:A34.

46. Chung WS, Park YY, Back SY. The effect of measurement location of the blood flow parameters on their values during Duplex sonography. *Int J Impotence Res* 1994; 6:A29.

47. Govier FE, Asase D, Hefty TR, et al. Timing of penile color flow duplex ultrasonography using a triple drug mixture. *J Urol* 1995; 153:1472–1475.

48. Meuleman EJH, Bemelmans BLH, Doesburg WH, et al. Penile pharmacological duplex ultrasonography: a dose effect study comparing papaverine, papaverine/phentolamine and PGE₁. *J Urol* 1992; 148:63.

49. Fitzgerald SW, Erickson SJ, Foley WD, et al. Color Doppler sonography in the evaluation of erectile dysfunction: patterns of temporal response to papaverine. *AJR* 1991; 157:331–336.

50. Lue TF, Donatucci CF. The combined intracavernous injection and stimulation test: diagnostic accuracy. *J Urol* 1992; 148:61–62.

51. Nehra A, Hakim LS, Abokar RA, et al. A new method of performing duplex Doppler ultrasonography: effect of re-dosing of vasoactive agents on hemodynamic parameters. *J Urol* 1995; 153:415A.

52. Montorsi F, Guazzoni G, Barbieri L, et al. The effect of intracorporeal injection plus genital and audiovisual sexual stimulation vs second injection on penile color Doppler sonography parameters. *J Urol* 1996; 155:536–540.

53. Lue TF, Hricak H, Marich KW, et al. Evaluation of arteriogenic impotence with intracorporeal injection of papaverine and the duplex ultrasound scanner. *Semin Urol* 1987; 3:43–48.

54. Fitzgerald SW, Krysiewicz S, Mellinger C. The role of imaging in the evaluation of impotence. *AJR* 1989; 53:1133–1139.

55. Ishii N, Watanabe H, Irisawa C, et al. Intracavernous injection of prostaglandin E₁ for the treatment of erectile impotence. *J Urol* 1989; 141:323–325.

56. Golub M, Zia P, Matsuno N, et al. Metabolism of prostaglandins, A-I and E-1 in men. *J Clin Invest* 1979; 59:1404.

57. Hamberg M. Biosynthesis of prostaglandin E₁ by human seminal vesicles. *Lipids* 1976; 11:249.

58. Hedquist P. PGE₁ and prostaglandin synthesis inhibitors of norepinephrine release from vascular tissue. In: Robinson HJ, Vane ER, eds. *Prostaglandin Synthetase Inhibitors*. New York: Raven Press; 1973: 303.

59. Meuleman EFJ, Bemelmans BLR, et al. Assessment of penile blood flow by duplex ultrasonography in 44 men with normal erectile potency in different phases of erection. *J Urol* 1992; 147:51–56.

60. Mellinger BC, Fried JJ, Vaughan ED. Papaverine induced penile blood flow acceleration in impotent men measured by duplex scanning. *J Urol* 1990; 144:897.

61. Lue TF, Tanagho EA. Physiology of erection and pharmacological management of impotence. *J Urol* 1987; 137:829.

62. Benson CB, Vickers MA. Sexual impotence caused by vascular disease: diagnosis with duplex sonography. *AJR* 1989; 153:1149.

63. Shabsigh R, Fishman IF, Quesada ET, et al. Evaluation of vasculogenic erectile impotence using penile duplex ultrasonography. *J Urol* 1989; 142:1469.

64. Benson CB, Aruny JE, Vickers MA. Correlation of duplex sonography with arteriography in patients with erectile dysfunction. *AJR* 1993; 160:71–73.

65. Shabsigh R, Fishman IJ, Shottland Y, et al. Comparison of penile duplex utrasonography with nocturnal penile tumescence monitoring for the evaluation of erectile impotence. *J Urol* 1990; 143:924.

66. Lewis RW, King BF. Dynamic color Doppler sonography in the evaluation of penile erectile disorders. *Int J Impotence Res* 1994; 6:A30.

67. Rhee E, Osborn A,Witt M. The correlation of cavernous systolic occlusion pressure with peak velocity flow using color duplex Doppler ultrasound. *J Urol* 1995; 153:358–360.

68. Schwartz AN, Lowe MA, Berger RE, et al. Assessment of normal and abnormal erectile function; color Doppler flow sonography vs. conventional techniques. *Radiol Sci North Am* 1991; 180:105–109.

69. Planiol T, Pourcelot L. Doppler effect study of the carotid circulation. In: de Vlieger M, White DN, McCready VR, eds. *Ultrasonics in Medicine.* Amsterdam: Excerpta Medica; 1974; 104–111.

70. Kaplan HS. The concept of presbyrectia. Int J Impotence Res 1989; 1:59.

71. Wespes E, deGoes PM, Schulman C. *Vascular impotence: focal or diffuse penile disease.* J Urol 1992; 148:1435–1436.

72. Kim N, Vardi Y, Padma-Nathan H, et al. Oxygen tension regulates the nitric oxide pathway. Physiological role in penile erection. *J Clin Invest* 1993; 91:3006–3012.

73. Saenz de Tejada I, Mooreland RB. Physiology of erection, pathophysiology of impotence, and implications of $PGE_1$ in the control of collagen synthesis in the corpus cavernosum. Proceedings of a Symposium, Kalamazoo, August 3–4, 1993. Excerpta Medica, pp. 3–16.

74. Levin RM, Hypolite JA, Broderick GA. Dissociation of basal and stimulated tonic contraction of the corpus cavernosum with intracellular calcium during hypoxia. *J Urol* 1995; 153:A405.

75. Broderick GA, Arger PA. Penile blood flow study: age specific references ranges. *J Urol* 1994; 151:A371.

76. Hinman F Jr. Priapism, reasons for failure of therapy. J Urol 1960; 83:420.

77. Broderick GA, Lue TF. Priapism and physiology of erection. *AUA Update Series* 1988; 7:225–232.

78. Broderick GA, Harkaway R. Pharmacologic erection: time-dependent changes in the corporal environment. *Int J Impotence Res* 1994; 6:9–16.

79. Witt MA, Goldstein I, Saenz de Tejada I, et al. Traumatic laceration of intracavernosal arteries: the pathophysiology of nonischemic, high flow arterial priapism. *J Urol* 1990; 143:129–132.

80. Walker TG, Gran PW, Goldstein I, et al. High-flow priapism: treatment with superselective transcatheter embolization. *Radiology* 1990; 174:1053–1054.

81. Hakim LS, Kulaksizoglu H, Mulligan R, et al. Evolving concepts in the diagnosis and treatment of arterial high flow priapism. *J Urol* 1996; 155:541–548.

82. Gasior BL, Levine FJ, Sowannesian A, et al. Plaque associated corporal veno-occlusive dysfunction in idiopathic Peyronie's disease: a pharmacocavernosometric and pharmacocavernosographic study. *World J Urol* 1990; 8:90.

# 28
# The Role of the Cavernosal Biopsy and Studies on Penile Innervation

Eric Wespes

## Cavernosal Biopsy

Erectile dysfunction may be caused by psychological problems, neurogenic dysfunction, hormonal alterations, or compromised penile blood flow. Better understanding of the erectile mechanism and the development of new investigative techniques have led to dramatic improvements in researchers' ability to recognize the etiology of impotence. Clinical investigations suggest that the majority of patients experiencing erectile impotence are impotent because of vascular abnormalities.

Intracavernous injection is a simple and reliable test to evaluate vasculogenic impotence. A positive test confirms adequate arterial inflow and a functional veno-oclusive mechanism but cannot distinguish neurogenic from psychogenic impotence. Nocturnal penile plethysmography may, therefore, help distinguish between these diagnoses.

Venous return can be evaluated in a number of ways. Duplex Doppler examination of the penile arteries studies the arterial inflow accurately during the intracavernosal vasoactive injection test. Pudendal arteriography is recommended only if a surgical procedure is being contemplated. In addition, pharmacocavernosometry-cavernosography allows determination of the flows necessary to induce and maintain an erection.[1]

However, a method to assess the intracavernous structural components is still lacking. The intracavernous components consist of bundles of smooth muscles, elastic fibers, collagen, and loose alveolar tissue with numerous arterioles and nerves. These structures are fundamental to the problem of impotence, and demonstration of their alterations could potentially prevent some candidates with a poor prognosis from undergoing reconstructive surgery.

The intracavernous components can be studied by biopsy of the cavernous bodies. Although biopsies can be obtained during surgery after the opening of the tunica albuginea, there is a simple, minimally invasive technique to obtain cavernous tissue for more detailed structural assessment of the impotent patient.[2] This biopsy is performed by first infiltrating approximately 1 ml of lidocaine into the skin of the penis in the balanopreputial groove dorsolaterally. With the Biopty gun (Bard Urological, Covington, Georgia), which has a spring trigger mechanism, the biopsy needle is introduced longitudinally through the tunica albuginea into the corpus cavernosum. With one hand, the surgeon maintains the penis in a stretched position, and with the other hand, fires the needle from an anterior to posterior direction. More than one pass of the needle may be necessary to obtain adequate tissue for study.

These Biopty gun needle biopsies compare favorably with surgical biopsies obtained during insertion of penile implants. Corpus cavernosum tissue is histologically identified, with representative intracavernous smooth muscle fibers, arteries, nerves, and collagen. Cavernous penile arterial Doppler analysis performed both before and after Biopty gun biopsies demonstrated no significant change in the cavernous blood flow or tissue substance.

With these needle biopsies, none of the patients reported pain or required any postoperative analgesia and no hematoma or significant bleeding was encountered.

Use of the Biopty gun to perform penile biopsy under local anesthesia is a simple and reliable method for obtaining sufficient tissue for histologic study. The selected site of the needle puncture is important. If the patient is circumcised, the balanopreputial groove is the preferred site because the glans mucosa of the penile skin adheres closely here to the tunica albuginea, making the development of a hematoma under the skin unlikely. The small puncture in the tunica albuginea at this point does not damage either the intracavernous artery (as demonstrated by Doppler analysis performed before and after puncture) or the urethra.

This procedure typically lasts less than 10 minutes, is cost-effective, and can be performed in the clinic under local anesthesia. Although no complications have been reported, the patient needs to be informed about possible bleeding, infection, or failure to obtain adequate tissue.

Immunohistochemistry studies employing antidesmin antibody measure the amount of smooth muscle cells in both potent and impotent patients. The range in normal patients is 40% to 52%.[3] The ratio of smooth muscle cells in patients with arterial and venous disease decreases, which is an important factor to consider in patients with documented arterial lesions.

Vascular impotence is a diffuse disease, as studies have shown a reduction of smooth muscle cells exists throughout the penis.[4] In patients with venous leakage, a significant correlation has been shown between the decrease in smooth muscle cells and the maintenance flow rates. Data reveal that the percentage of smooth muscle cells present in men with erectile dysfunction is the only prognostic factor for predicting the long-term outcome success of venous ligation surgery.[5] Surprisingly, neither the patient's age nor the maintenance flow rates

corresponded with the ultimate surgical success rate. Operating on impotent men who quantitate less than 29% smooth muscle cells on penile biopsy is not recommended.

Future applications employing the immunohistochemical staining and electron microscopy techniques will allow researchers to study the neurotransmitters present in the cavernous tissue obtained from impotent men undergoing penile biopsy.

## Penile Innervation

It is well appreciated that the qualitative state of erection is dependent on the balance between the inflow and outflow of blood in the penis. In the flaccid state, there is a high resistance to penile blood flow due to contraction of the helicine arteries and of the corporeal smooth muscle cells. It is well known that $\alpha$-adrenoceptor stimulation plays a significant role in this respect. Within the corpus cavernosum the $\alpha_1$-adrenoceptor is the functionally dominant subtype.[6] Indeed, in this tissue three subtypes of $\alpha_1$-adrenoceptor messenger RNA (mRNA) have recently been identified ($\alpha_{1A}$, $\alpha_{1B}$, $\alpha_{1C}$), with the $\alpha_{1A}$ and $\alpha_{1C}$ subtypes predominating.[7] However, it is reasonable to speculate that noradrenaline is not the only neurotransmitter involved in both long- and short-term maintenance of penile smooth muscle tone, but that nonadrenergic noncholinergic (NANC) factors are also contributory.

At flaccidity, the penile arterial tree and trabecular smooth musculature are contracted due to a tonic sympathetic discharge. In contrast, at tumescence, neurotransmitters induce relaxation of the arteries and intracavernous smooth muscles; this relaxation results in expansion of the sinusoidal spaces with a decrease in vascular resistance. At full rigidity, the expanded sinusoids compress the subtunical venular plexuses against the tunica albuginea and similarly compress the emissary veins.[1,8]

The smooth muscle cells of the corpus cavernosum relax and contract in a rapid and synchronous manner, and the electrical activity recorded in vivo in human cavernous bodies is well synchronized, as revealed by electromyographic studies.[9] This evidence suggests that intracavernous smooth muscle cells behave as a functional syncytium despite the presence of a heavily collagenous extracellular matrix that separates the cells.[10,11] A mechanism recently postulated involves gap junctions, by which local neural and hormonal stimulation can be rapidly propagated in corporeal tissue.[11] Gap junctions appear to provide an intercellular pathway for coordinated cellular activation and syncytial tissue contraction and relaxation.[5]

Stimulation of the pelvic (cholinergic) nerves decreases the saline infusion flow rates needed during dynamic infusion cavernosometry to induce and maintain an artificial erection. By contrast, stimulation of the hypogastric (adrenergic) nerves reduces penile tumescence induced by either electrical stimulation of the pelvic nerves or by vasoactive intracavernosal injection, but has no effect on the erection induced by saline infusion alone.[1]

Parasympathetic activity plays a significant role in penile erection, although existing data concerning the effects of acetylcholine and different muscarinic receptor antagonists are quite controversial and contradictory and suggest that other transmitters besides acetylcholine may be released from cholinergic nerves.[12] Thus, there are at least three mechanisms by which parasympathetic activity may contribute to penile smooth muscle relaxation: (1) the neuronal release of noradrenaline may be inhibited by stimulation of prejunctional muscarinic receptors, (2) endothelium-derived relaxant factors may be released through stimulation of postjunctional muscarinic receptors, and (3) NANC relaxing factors may be released directly from parasympathetic nerves.[6,7]

Acetylcholine can provoke mixed relaxing and contracting effects on human corpus cavernosum muscle strips. Acetylcholine causes relaxation of both rat and human corpus cavernosum muscle strips precontracted by field stimulation or noradrenaline.[13] Cholinergic nerves do not mediate corpus cavernosum relaxation via postjunctional muscarinic receptors, but presynaptically modulate noradrenaline release and likely influence nitric oxide (NO) release by endothelial cells.[14,15]

NO and vasodilators acting through NO (such as nitroglycerin, sodium nitroprusside, S-nitroso-N-acetylpenicillamine, and linsidomine, all of which cause concentration-dependent relaxation of the corpus cavernosum) have been shown to stimulate soluble guanylate cyclase and increase the tissue levels of cyclic guanosine monophosphate (GMP).[16–18]

Cyclic GMP is degraded intracellularly by different phosphodiesterases (PDEs), with three PDE isoenzymes localized to the human corpus cavernosum: PDE III (cyclic GMP–inhibited), PDE IV (cyclic adenosine monophosphate [AMP]–specific) and PDE V (cyclic GMP–specific). Spontaneous contractile activity and noradrenaline-induced contractions are opposed by different PDE inhibitors, with quazinone (PDE III inhibitor) being the most potent.

NO production appears to be dependent on oxygen tension. Electrically induced relaxations are progressively inhibited as a function of decreasing oxygen tension, especially at $pO_2$ values below 50 mm Hg and are markedly attenuated when oxygen tensions are similar to those measured in the flaccid state. This implies that the low oxygen tension recorded in the flaccid state is associated with a decrease in the activity of nitric oxide synthase (NOS), thereby reinforcing the mechanisms responsible for maintaining a high degree of penile smooth muscle tone.

Neuropeptides (NP) have been implicated in neurotransmitter (NT) activity regulating peripheral smooth muscle tissue, including those within blood vessels.[19] Blood flow regulation is important in controlling the mechanisms responsible for penile tumescence and detumescence. Vasoactive intestinal polypeptide (VIP) is a neuropeptide that has been isolated within the male urogenital tract. Combined morphologic and experimental data suggest that VIP plays a role in the regulation of intracavernous smooth muscle tone and the cavernous blood flow ultimately responsible for erection.

However, the relaxing effects of VIP in vitro and the identification of VIP and VIP-containing nerves in penile erectile tissues do

## Color Plate I

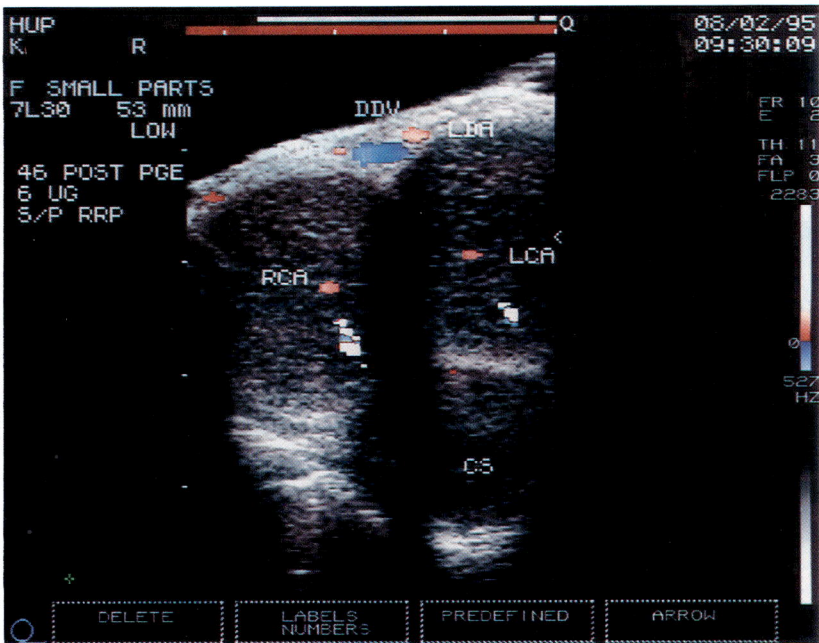

FIGURE 27.1.(B) Transverse color Doppler image following a 6-μg injection of PGE₁ reveals the normal vascular anatomy. RCA, right cavernous artery; LCA, left cavernous artery; DDV, deep dorsal vein; LDA, left dorsal artery; CS, corpus spongiosum.

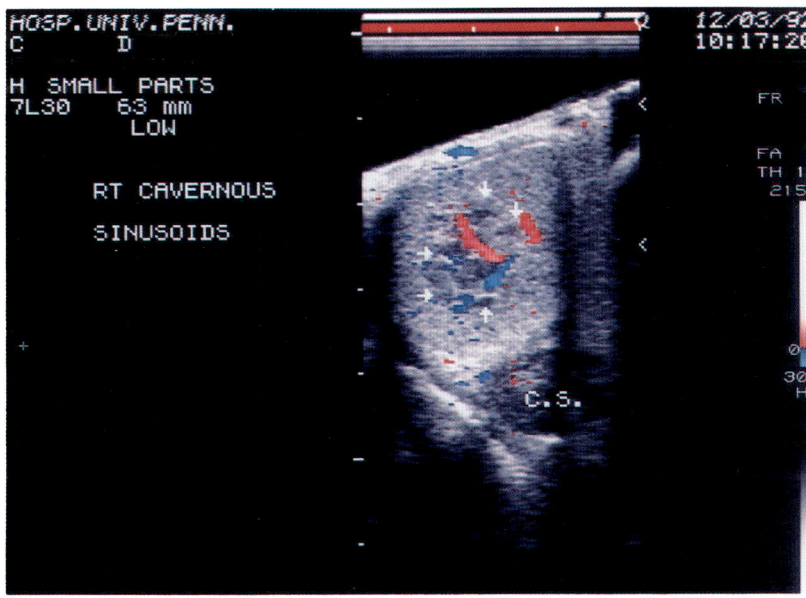

FIGURE 27.1.(C) Transverse image of right corporal body 5 minutes after injection of dilator. Helicine arterioles (red/blue) are seen with central sinusoids beginning to fill (arrows); note that blood distended sinusoids appear more hypoechoic than surrounding tissue.

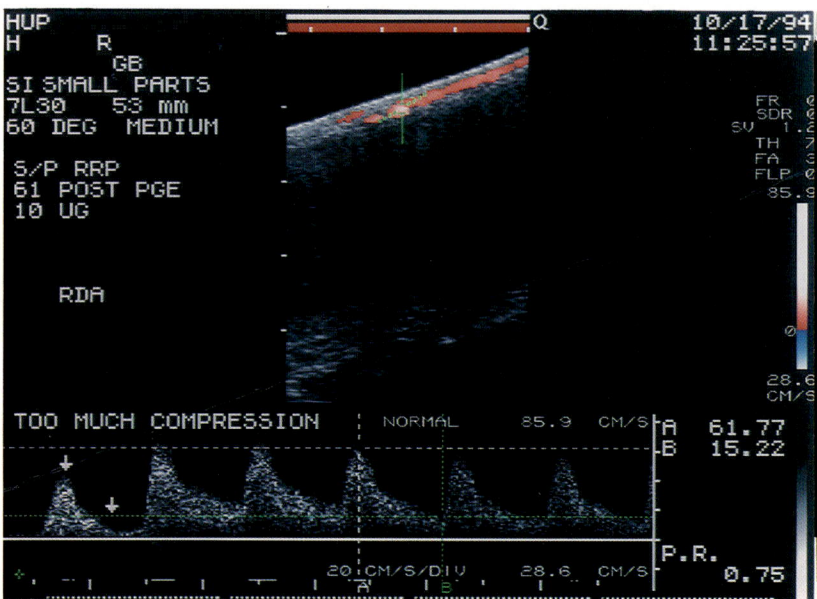

FIGURE 27.2.(B) Sagittal view of right dorsal artery (RDA); too much compression (arrows) dampens dorsal vascular flow and will alter both systolic and diastolic waveforms.

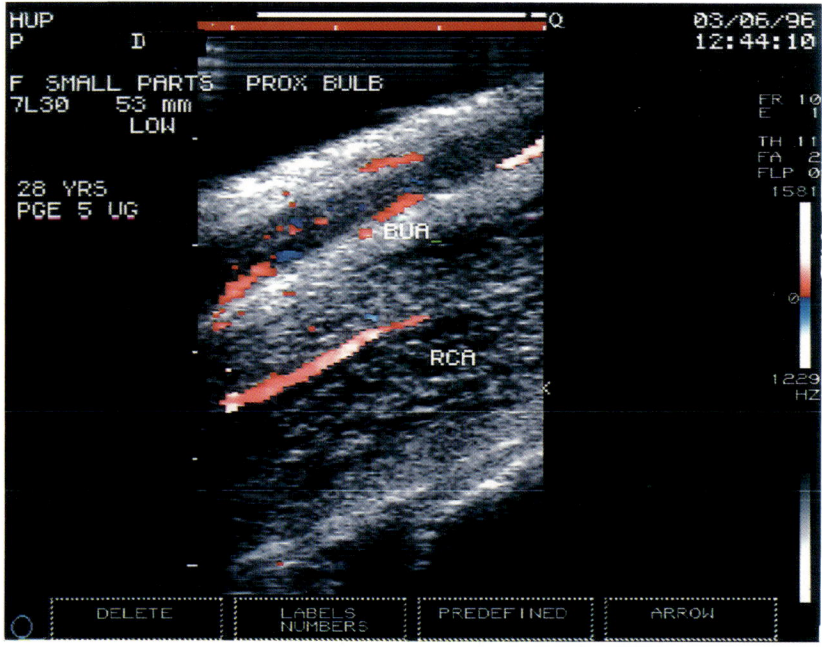

FIGURE 27.2.(C) The pendulous penis may be scanned from the ventral aspect. This sagittal image shows the proximal bulb with the urethral artery (BUA) and right cavernous artery (RCA). Imaging of the urethral lumen is not possible unless the urethra is filled in a retrograde fashion with gel or water.

Color Plate III

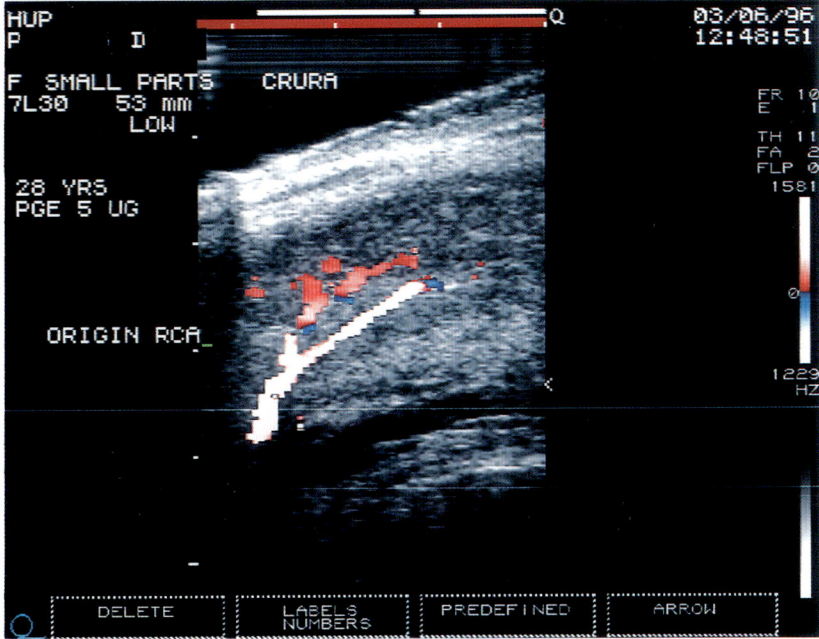

FIGURE 27.2.(D) Sagittal scanning below the scrotum (transperineal) reveals the origin of the right cavernous artery (RCA).

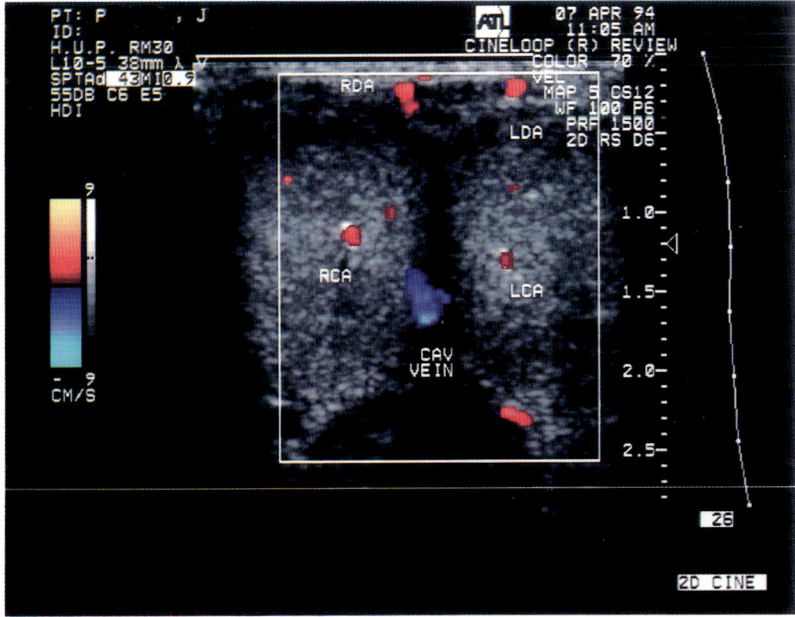

FIGURE 27.3.(A) Transverse scan of patient with severe veno-occlusive dysfunction revealing large cavernous vein.

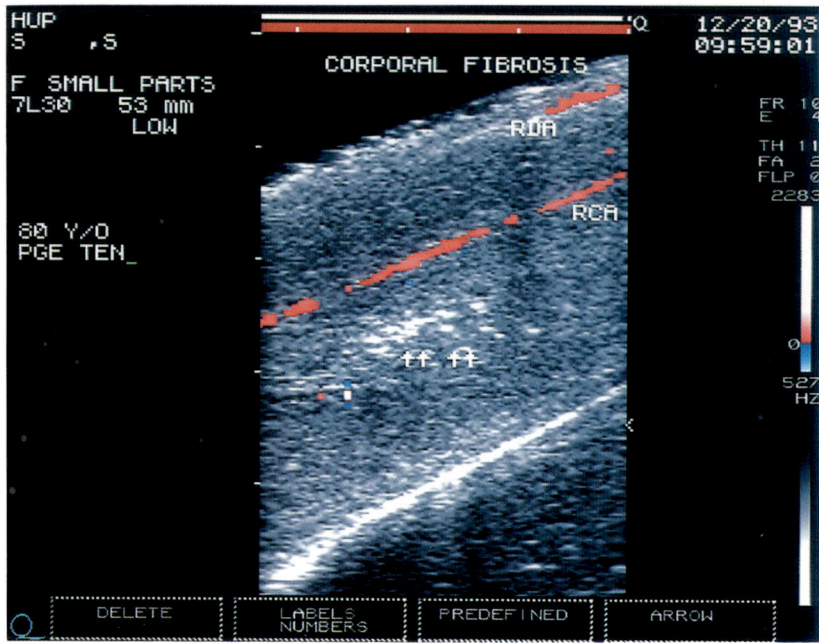

FIGURE 27.4. Corporal fibrosis (arrows) in an 80-year-old patient, sagittal scan; right dorsal artery (RDA) and right cavernous artery (RCA).

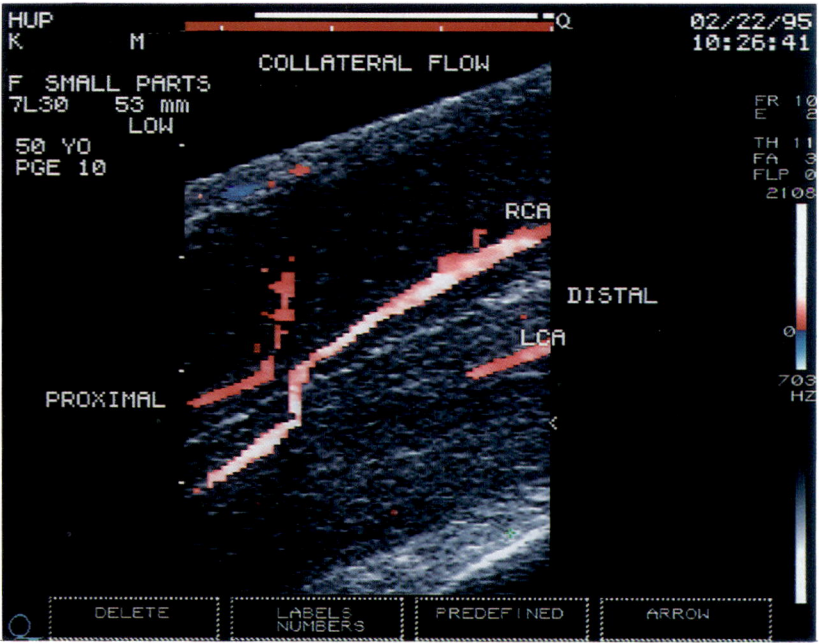

FIGURE 27.5.(A) Sagittal scan of cavernous artery collaterals, with distal right cavernous flow, supplemented by collateral.

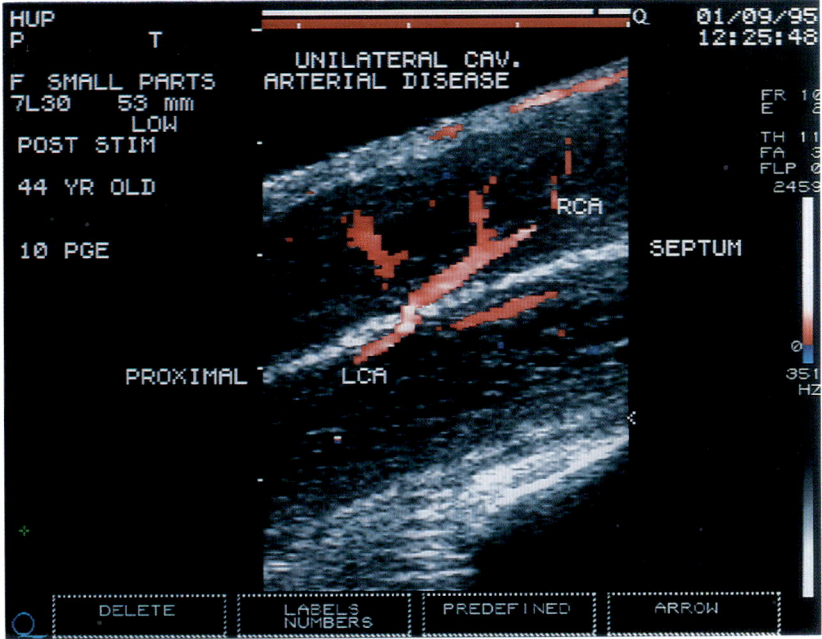

FIGURE 27.5.(B) Sagittal scan shows absence of right proximal inflow, with distal right cavernous flow depending on left collateral.

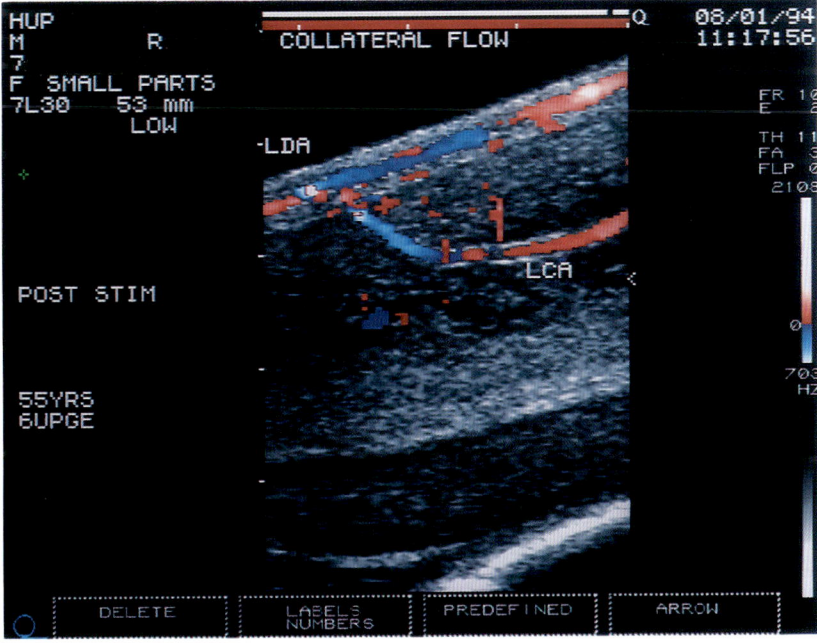

FIGURE 27.6. Left dorsal artery (LDA) to left cavernous artery (LCA) collateral, sagittal scan.

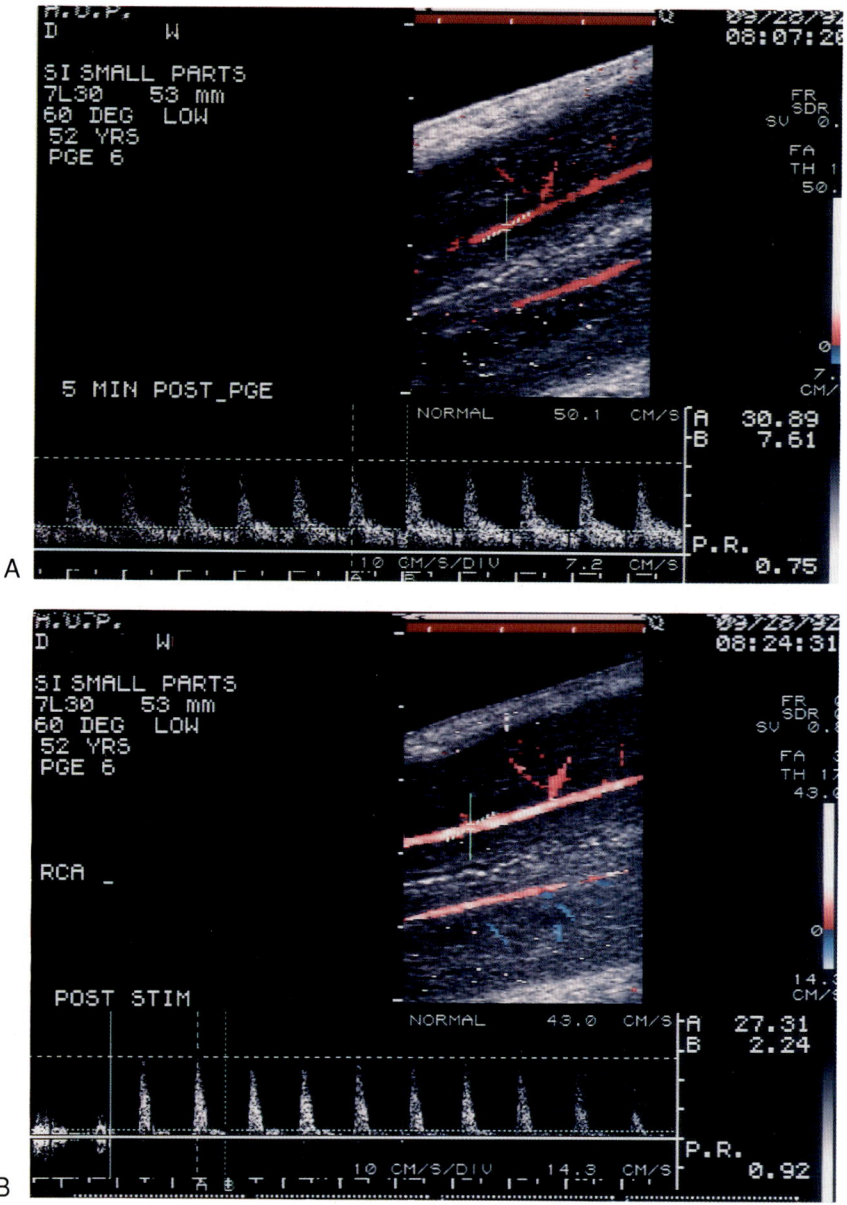

FIGURE 27.7. (A and B) Normal progression of Doppler waveform: response 5 minutes after penile injection of PGE₁ and response following privacy and self-stimulation; note minor decrease in peak systolic velocities from 30 to 27 cm/s and significant decrease in end diastolic velocities from 7 to 2 cm/s.

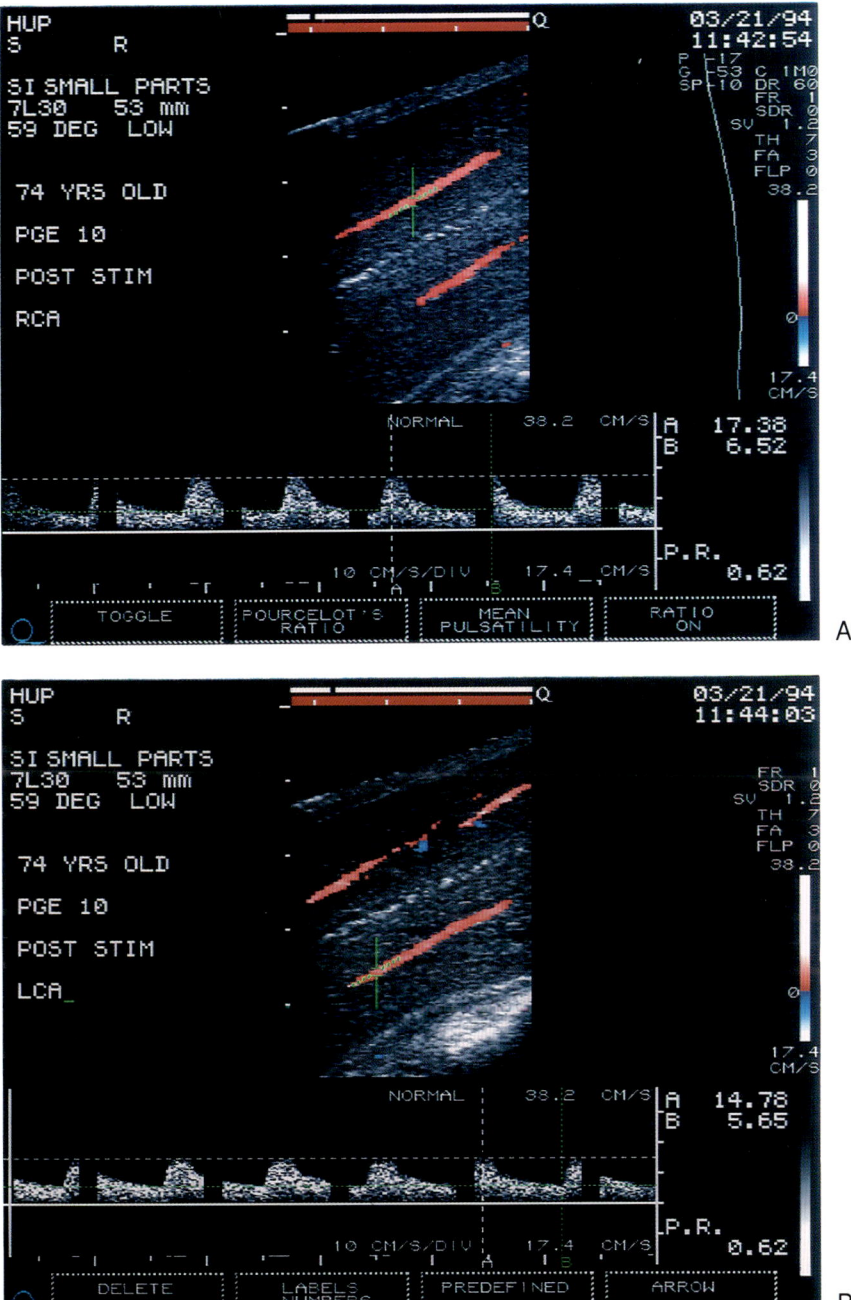

FIGURE 27.8. (A and B) Severe bilateral cavernous arterial insufficiency in 74-year-old patient, with peak systolic velocities <25 cm/s in each central artery (poststimulation responses).

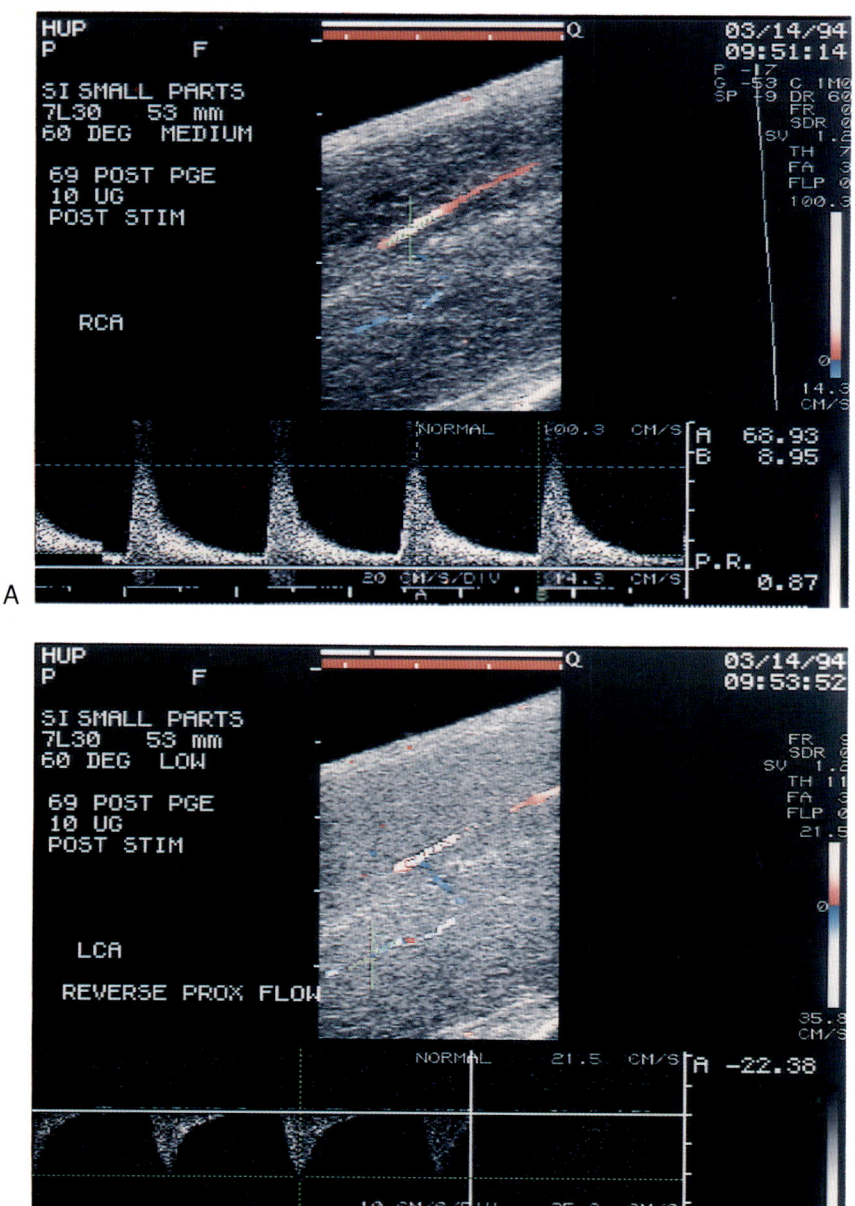

FIGURE 27.9. (A and B) Unilateral cavernous arterial insufficiency in left cavernous artery (LCA) with high peak systolic velocity in the right central artery, 68 cm/s. The direction of blood flow is actually reversed in the proximal LCA, because of RCA to LCA collateral.

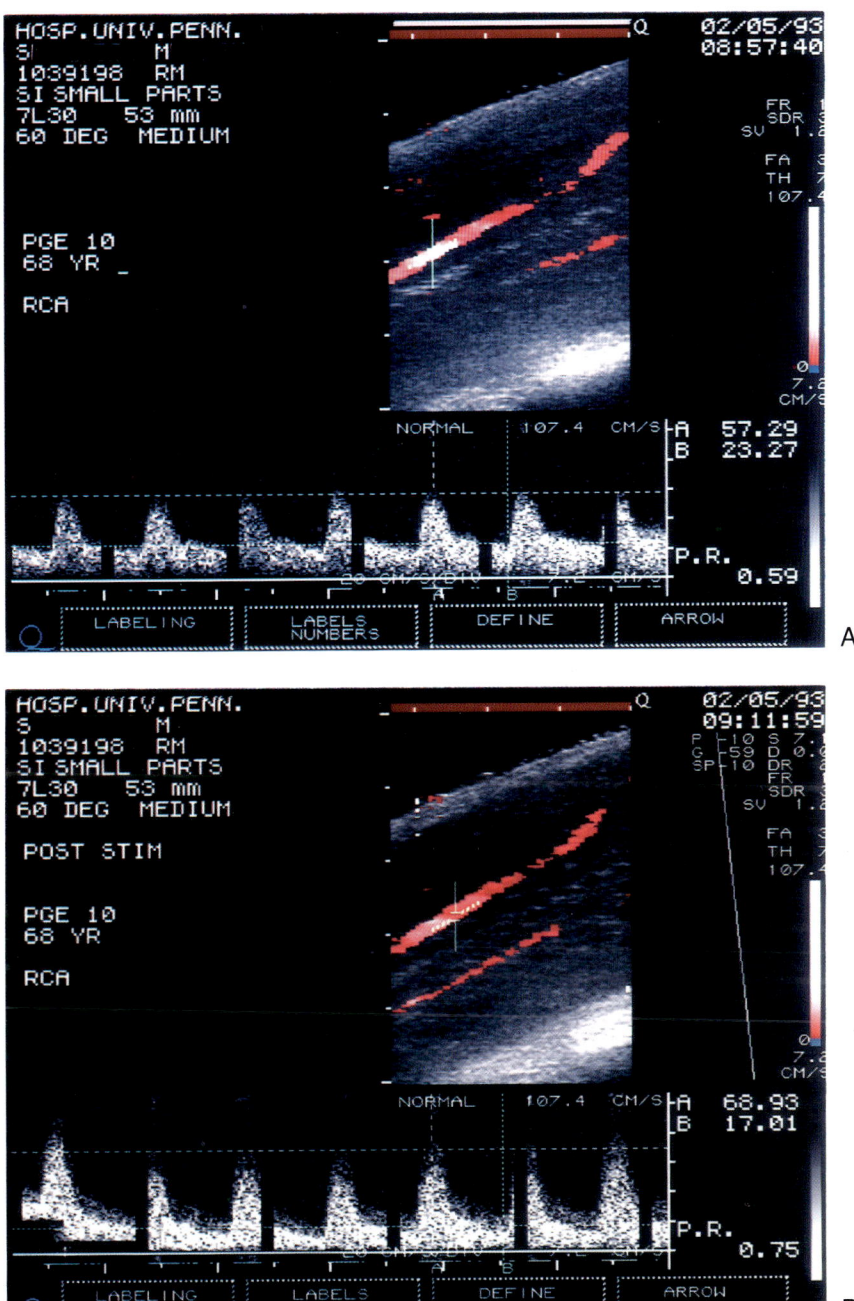

FIGURE 27.10. (A and B) An unequivocal diagnosis of cavernous venous occlusive disease based on ultrasound criteria can be given when cavernous arterial flows exceed 35 cm/s, end diastolic velocities remain high, and resistive index is low. This 68-year-old patient, following PGE$_1$ 10 µg and self-stimulation, has postinjection PSV of 57 cm/s and poststimulation PSV of 68 cm/s, EDV of 17 cm/s, and RI of 0.75.

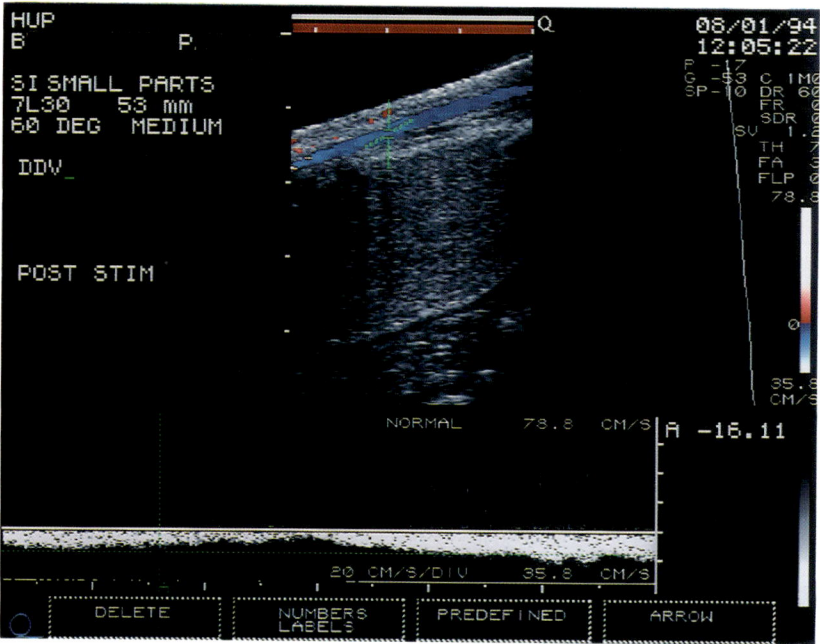

FIGURE 27.11.(A) Deep dorsal vein flow (DDV) persists during rigid erection.

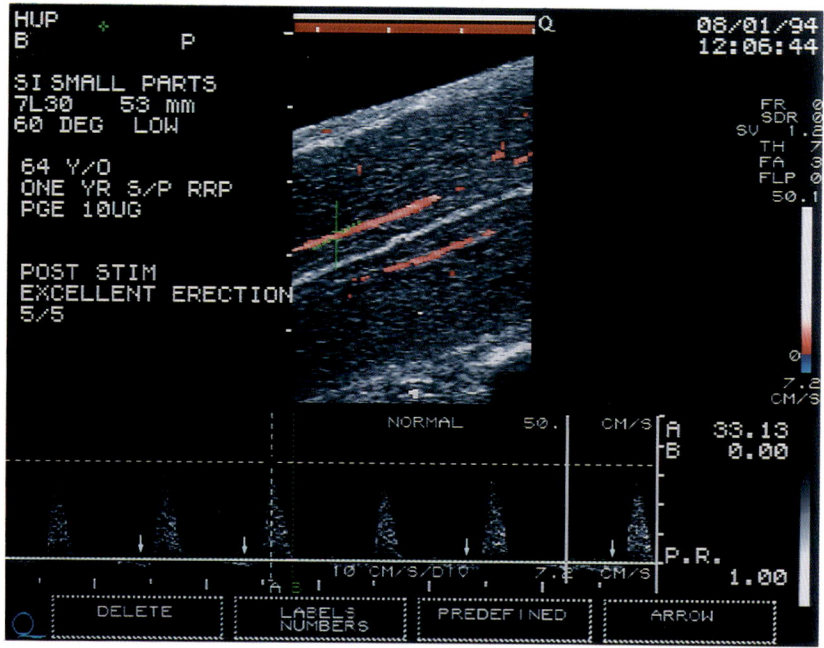

FIGURE 27.11.(B) Rigid erection following 10μg of PGE$_1$, associated with PSV of 33cm/s and reversal of diastolic flow; see arrows.

Color Plate XI

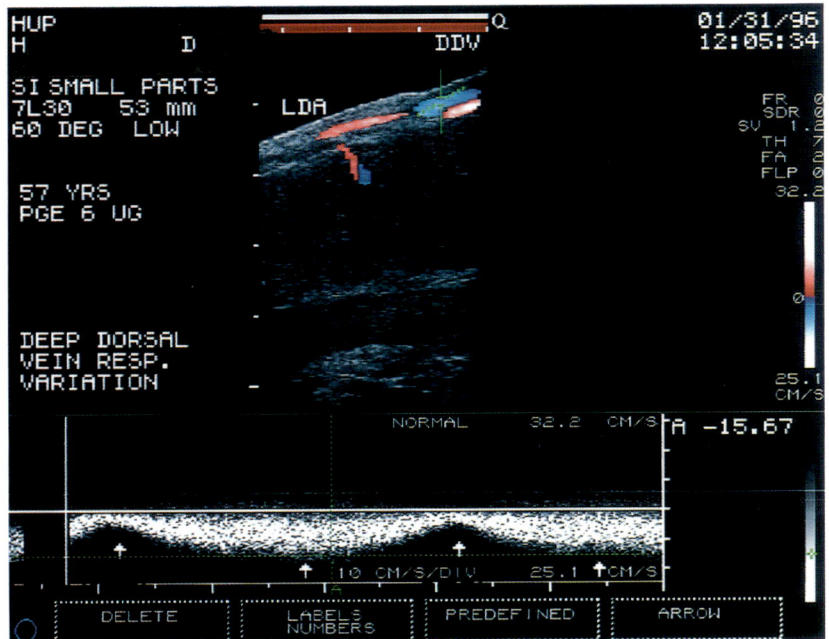

FIGURE 27.12. Respiratory variation in deep dorsal vein flow (DDV).

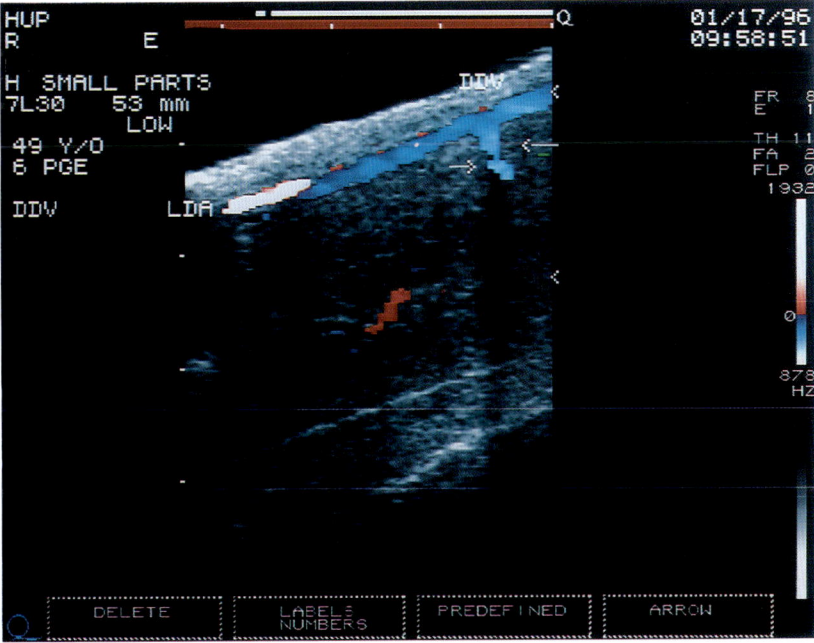

FIGURE 27.13. Emissary veins perforating the tunica albuginea are rarely seen because of their small size and low flow state (arrows).

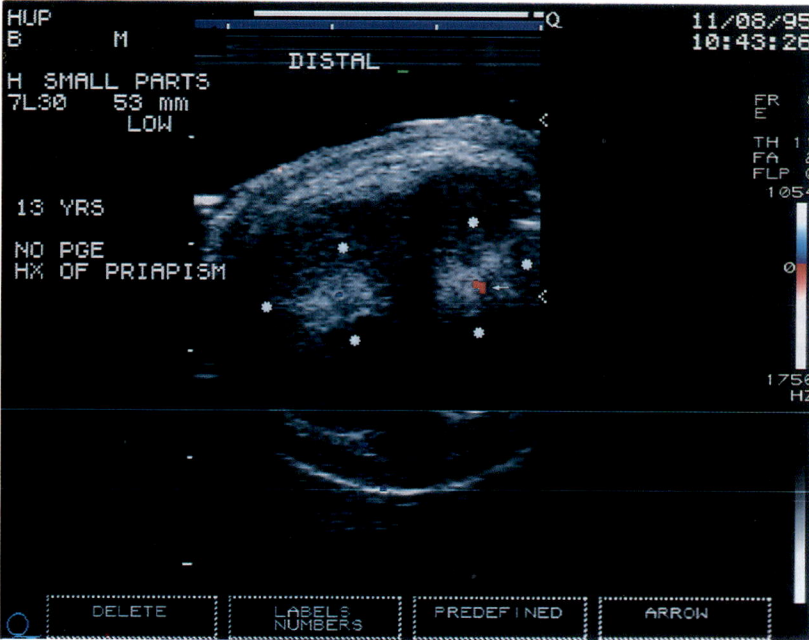

FIGURE 27.14. Transverse scan of 13-year-old boy with repeated episodes of sickle cell priapism: left cavernous arterial flow is present (arrow); cavernous tissues are hyperechoic consistent with central fibrosis (*).

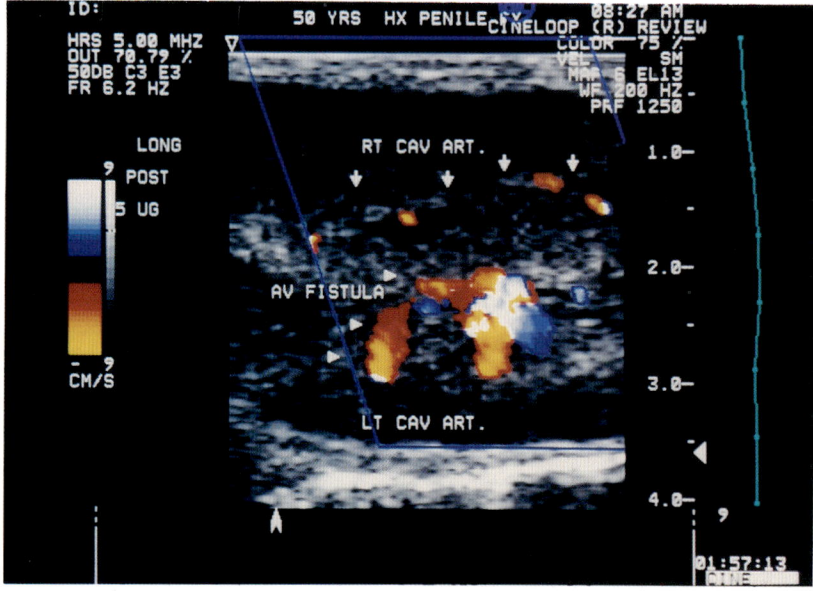

FIGURE 27.15.(A) Sagittal image of left cavernous sinusoidal fistula producing high-flow priapism; note turbulent flow.

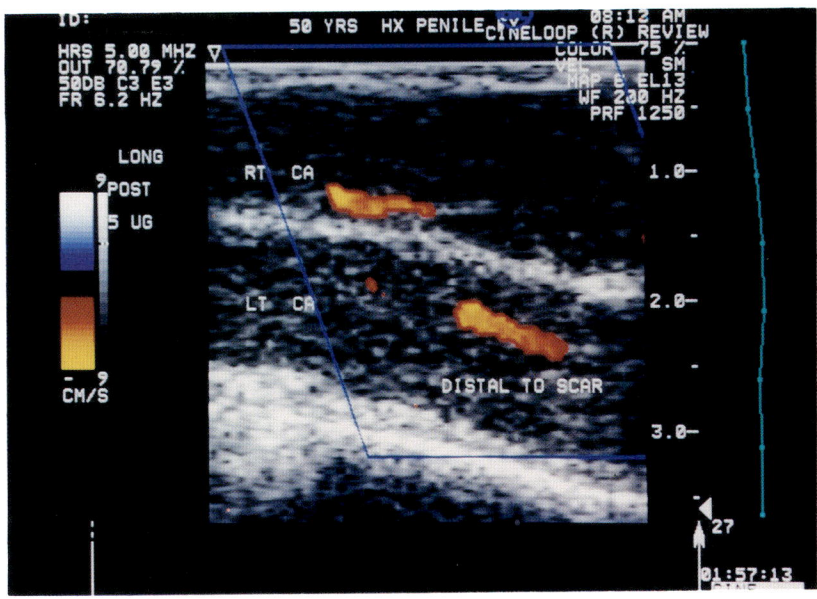

FIGURE 27.15.(B) Distal-to-site-of-trauma cavernous flows are more distinct.

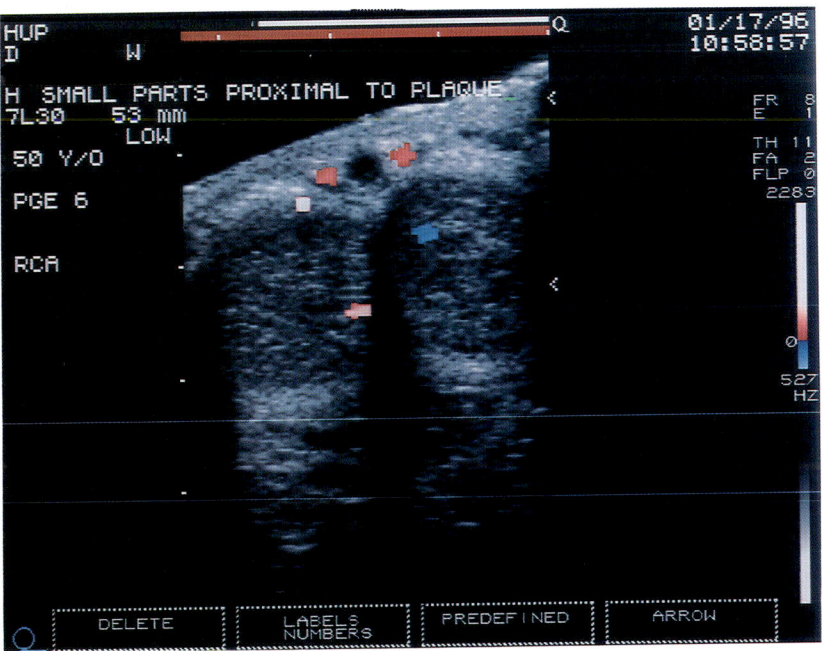

FIGURE 27.16.(A) Transverse scan proximal to plaque.

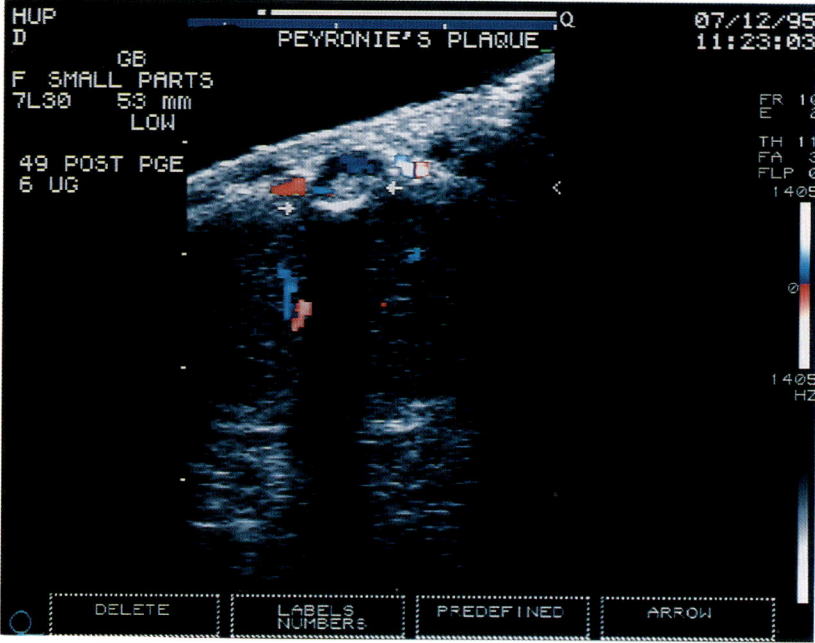

FIGURE 27.16.(B) Transverse scan of Peyronie's plaque (arrows); note acoustic shadow below plaque.

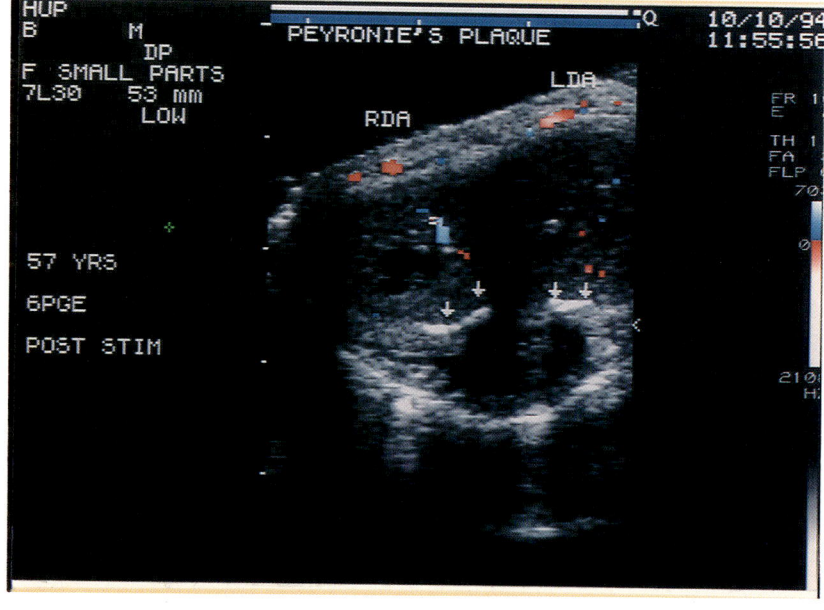

FIGURE 27.17.(A) Transverse scan of ventral Peyronie's plaque.

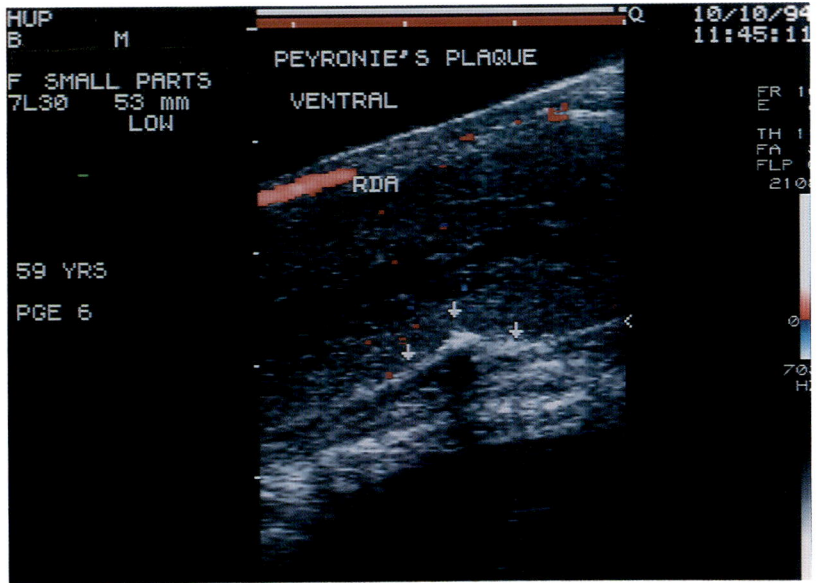

FIGURE 27.17.(B) Sagittal scan of ventral plaque.

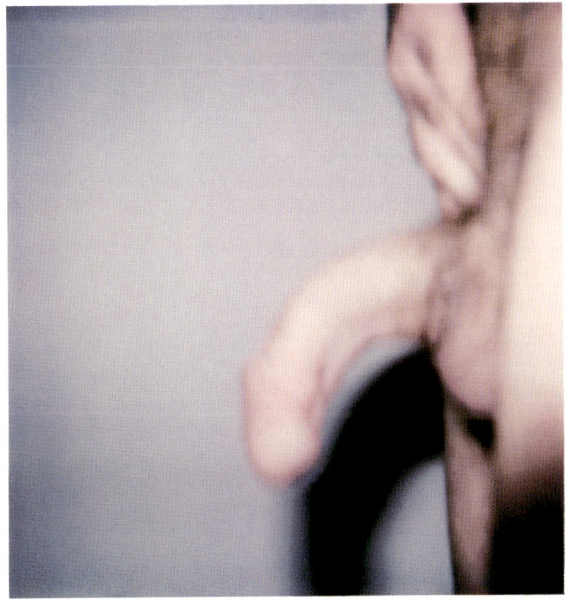

FIGURE 27.17.(C) Home photograph.

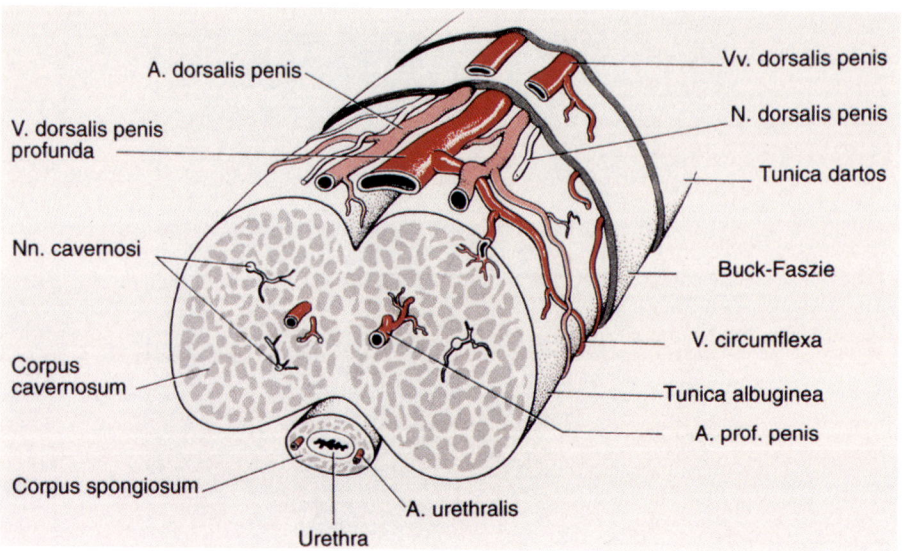

FIGURE. 32.1. Cross-section of penis. (From Alken P, Walz P eds., *Urologie*, VCH Verlagsgesellsc Weinheim, Germany, 1992.)

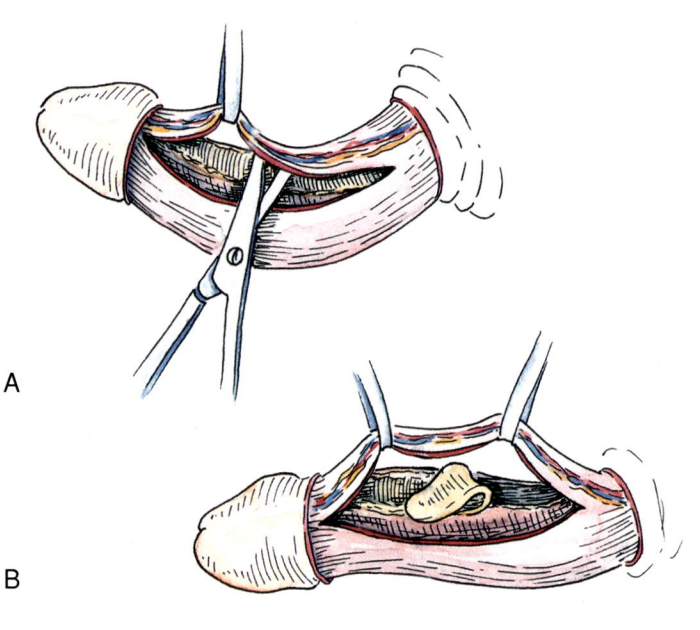

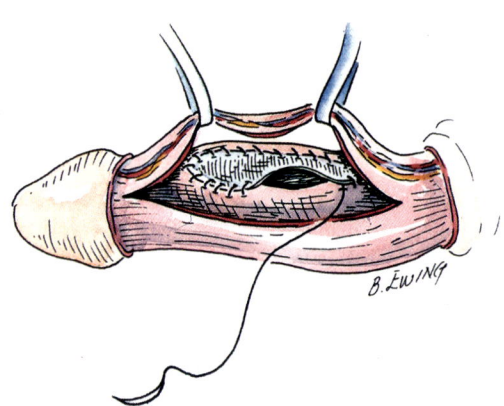

FIGURE 36.2. (A) To properly expose the frequently occurring dorsal plaques, Buck's fascia is entered laterally and carefully dissected underneath the neurovascular bundle. (B) The plaque is sharply excised with care taken not to damage any of the underlying erectile tissue. (C) A Silastic patch is fashioned slightly larger than the defect and sutured in a running 5-0 proline suture with knots placed under the dorsal vein complex.

not conclusively prove that this neuropeptide is of physiologic importance in penile erection. Evidence to support this contrary veiwpoint on VIP activity includes the finding that VIP antiserum nor α-chymotrypsin display neither change on the relaxation of cavernosal smooth muscle induced by electrical stimulation of penile nerves. These findings implicate the lack of neuronal release of VIP, at least in the in vitro situation described. Also, VIP did not produce penile erection when injected intracavernosally in healthy volunteers nor in impotent men.[20-24]

Adrenergic neural fibers and adrenergic receptors are present in the human corpus cavernosum and on cavernosal blood vessels. Immunohistochemical evidence of adrenergic nerve endings has been demonstrated in the penises of various animal species. Pharmacologic and receptor binding studies have demonstrated the presence of both α- and β-adrenergic receptors in the human corpus cavernosum, with the α-type largely outnumbering the β-type.

Inhibition of the sympathetic nervous system by phentolamine enhances the erectile response to electrical stimulation of the cavernous nerve. Phenylephrine injected intracavernously reduces the response to cavernous nerve stimulation.

In vitro, electrically induced contraction of corpus cavernosum and contractions induced by exogenous noradrenaline (NA) is readily blocked by prazosin, indicating that postjunctional α-adrenoreceptors probably mediate these phenomena. $\alpha_1$-Adrenoreceptors are involved in the contraction of the cavernous arteries. The contractile response to NA is mediated by a heterogeneous population of α-adrenoreceptor subtypes—$\alpha_{1A}$, $\alpha_{1B}$, and $\alpha_{1C}$, corresponding to three distinct genes expressed in the human corpus cavernosum. NA is recognized as the chief antierection agent. The importance of sympathetic nervous activity and α-adrenoreceptor function in the maintenance of penile flaccidity is universally accepted. Other vasoconstrictive peptide agents, such as endothelin, may also play a role in vasomotor tone.[25] Neuropeptide Y has been detected in the penis, but its role is more controversial.[26]

# Summary

Penile biopsy may become a helpful tool in the complete management of the impotent man. Definition and quantification of histologic abnormalities of the intracavernous structures will allow the clinician to decide on surgical reconstruction or a noninvasive approach.

The addition of immunohistochemical staining to penile biopsy techniques will allow researchers to appreciate penile innervation by identifying various neurotransmitters and provide a better understanding of neurogenic impotence.

# References

1. Lue T, Tanagho E. Physiology of erection and pharmacological management of impotence. *J Urol* 1987; 137:829–836.
2. Wespes E, Depierreux M, Schulman CC. Use of biopty gun for corpus cavernosum biopsies. *Eur Urol* 1990; 18:81–83.
3. Wespes E, Goes PM, Schiffmann S, et al. Computerized analysis of smooth muscle fibers in potent and impotent patients. *J Urol* 1991; 146:1015–1017.
4. Wespes E, Moreira de Goes P, Schulman CC. Vascular impotence: focal or diffuse penile disease. *J Urol* 1992; 149:1435–1436.
5. Wespes E, Moreira de Goes P, Sattar AA, et al. Objective criteria in the long-term evaluation of penile venous surgery. *J Urol* 1994; 152:889–890.
6. Andersson K-E, Holmquist F. Mechanisms for contraction and relaxation of human penile smooth muscle. *Int J Impotence Res* 1990; 2:209–225.
7. Giuliano FA, Rampin O, Benoit G, et al. Neural control of penile erection. In: Melman A, ed. *The Urologic Clinics of North America*. Philadelphia: W.B. Saunders; 1995; 22:747–766.
8. Wespes E, Schulman CC. Venous impotence: pathophysiology, diagnosis and treatment. *J Urol* 1993; 149:1238–1245.
9. Wagner G, Gerstenberg T, Levin RJ. Electrical activity of corpus cavernosum during flaccidity and erection of the human penis: a new diagnostic method? *J Urol* 1989; 142:723–725.
10. Christ GJ, Maayani S, Valcic M, et al. Pharmacological studies of human erectile tissue: characteristics of spontaneous contractions and alterations in α-adrenoceptor responsiveness

with age and disease in isolated tissues. *Br J Pharmacol* 1990; 101:375–381.

11. Christ GJ, Brink PR, Melman A, et al. The role of gap junctions and ion channels in the modulation of electrical and chemical signals in human corpus cavernosum smooth muscle. *Int J Impotence* 1993; 5:77–96.

12. Stief CG, Benard F, Bosch RJLH, et al. Acetylcholine as a possible neurotransmitter in penile erection. *J Urol* 1989; 14:1444–1448.

13. Hedlund H, Andersson K-E. Comparison of the responses to drugs acting on adrenoceptors and muscarinic receptors in human isolated corpus cavernosum and cavernous artery. *J Auton Pharmacol* 1985; 5:81–88.

14. Burnett AL, Tillman SL, Chana TSK, et al. Immunohistochemical localization of nitric oxide synthase in the autonomic innervation of the human penis. *J Urol* 1993; 150:73–76.

15. Furchgott RF, Zawadzki JV. The obligatory role of endothelial cells in the relaxation of arterial smooth muscle by acetylcholine. *Nature* 1980; 288:373–376.

16. Kim N, Azadzoi KM, Goldstein I, et al. A nitric oxide-like factor mediates nonadrenergic-noncholinergic neurogenic relaxation of penile corpus cavernosum smooth muscle. *J Clin Invest* 1991; 88:112–118.

17. Rajfer J, Aronson WJ, Bush PA, et al. Nitric oxide as a mediator of relaxation of the corpus cavernosum on response to nonadrenergic, noncholinergic neurotransmission. *N Engl J Med* 1992; 326:90–94.

18. Trigo-Rocha F, Aronson WJ, Hohenfellner M, et al. Nitric oxide and cGMP: mediators of pelvic

nerve-stimulated erection in dogs. *Am J Physiol* 1993; 264:H419–422.

19. Hedlund H, Andersson K-E. Effects of some peptides on isolated human penile erectile tissue and cavernous artery. *Acta Physiol Scand* 1985; 124:413–419.

20. Adaikan PG, Kottegoda SR, Ratnani SS. Is vasoactive intestinal polypeptide the principal transmitter involved in human penile erection? *J Urol* 1986; 135:638–640.

21. Gu J, Polak JM, Lazarides M, et al. Decrease of vasoactive intestinal polypeptide (VIP) in the penises from impotent men. *Lancet* 1994; 11:315–318.

22. Steers WD, McDonnell J, Benson GS. Anatomical localization and some pharmacological effects of vasoactive intestinal polypeptide in human and monkey corpus cavernosum. *J Urol* 1984; 132:1048–1093.

23. Sundler F. Relaxation of isolated human corpus spongiosum induced by vasoactive intestinal polypeptide, substance P, carbachol and electrical field stimulation. *World J Urol* 1983; 1:203–208.

24. Virag R, Ottesen B, Fahrenkrug J, et al. Vasoactive intestinal polypeptide release during penile erection in man. *Lancet* 1982; 2:1166.

25. Saenz de Tejada I, Goldstein I, Azadzoi K, et al. Role of endothelin, a novel vasoconstrictor peptide in the local control of penile smooth muscle. *J Urol* 1989; 141:222A.

26. Wespes E, Schiffman S, Gilloteaux J, et al. Study of neuropeptide Y-containing nerve fibers in the human penis. *Cell Tissue Res* 1988; 254:69–74.

# 29
# Priapism

Farhad Parivar and Tom F. Lue

The word *priapism* is derived from the name of Dionysus and Aphrodite's son Priapus, the Greek god of fertility, who was characterized as having an overzealous phallus. Priapism is a persistent and painful erection of the penis, not associated with sexual excitement and not subsiding after ejaculation. Priapism may either start de novo, follow a prolonged nocturnal erection, or occur after intercourse. Exactly how long an erection persists before it is considered priapism is not clear. Erections of more than 6 hours' duration have been considered priapism because blood gas studies show evidence of ischemia and acidosis after 4 to 6 hours and, therefore, potential damage may occur.[1,2]

Although priapism can occur in all age groups, including the newborn, there are peak incidences between the ages of 5 to 10 years and 20 to 50 years.[3] Most cases of priapism in the older age group are idiopathic, but in the younger groups it is most commonly associated with sickle cell disorder or malignancy.[4] The pathology always involves the corpora cavernosa, but in rare late cases it may involve the corpus spongiosum as well. Acute veno-occlusive priapism of more than 6 hours' duration is usually painful and secondary to ischemia. In contrast, arterial priapism is painless. Regardless of whether pain is present, ischemic priapism is considered a urologic emergency because if untreated, impotency may result. Ischemic changes take place within 6 hours, and, if untreated, variable degrees of fibrosis occur within 24 to 48 hours. It is of utmost importance for the patient who has

priapism for the first time to be referred to a urologist for prompt treatment. Patients who have a known cause with recurrent priapism usually can self-administer emergency treatment but will need to see a urologist if such a measure fails.

## Classification

Priapism can be classified as either primary or secondary (Table 29.1). Primary priapism occurs in up to 60% of all cases. This number includes all those patients in whom no etiologic factors can be identified. Priapism in these patients may follow a prolonged erection during intercourse or after a nocturnal erection. Depending on the underlying hemodynamic pathology, priapism can also be classified as high flow (nonischemic) or low flow (ischemic).[5] Arterial priapism and veno-occlusive priapism may be more appropriate terms for these two types.[6] By far, most etiologic factors cause a low-flow veno-occlusive type of priapism. High-flow priapism is usually traumatic in nature, with rupture of the cavernous artery.

## Anatomy

### Arterial Supply

The penis derives its blood supply from the penile artery, a terminal branch of the internal pudendal artery. The paired penile arteries

TABLE 29.1. Summary of etiologic factors for priapism.

| | |
|---|---|
| Primary: | Idiopathic |
| Secondary: | A. Hematologic |
| |     Sickle cell disease/trait |
| |     Thalassemia |
| |     Polycythemia |
| |     Leukemia |
| | B. Neoplastic |
| |     Prostate cancer |
| |     Sarcomas |
| |     Leukemias |
| |     Myelomas |
| |     Metastatic |
| | C. Traumatic |
| |     Pelvic, perineal, or penile |
| | D. Neurogenic |
| |     Spinal cord injuries |
| |     Spinal cord tumors |
| |     Multiple sclerosis |
| |     Spinal anesthesia |
| | E. Pharmacologic |
| |     Systemic |
| |       Chlorpromazine |
| |       Haloperidol |
| |       Trazodone |
| |       Methaquolone |
| |       Ethanol |
| |       Cannabis |
| |       Prazosin |
| |       Terbutaline |
| |       Heparin/warfarin |
| |       *TPN—>10% fat |
| |     Intracavernosal |
| |       Papaverine |
| |       Prostaglandin $E_1$ |
| |       Phentolamine |
| |       Drug combinations |

*TPN, total parenteral nutrition.

branch to form (1) the bulbourethral arteries, which supply the corpus spongiosum; (2) the dorsal artery of the penis, which supplies the penile and the glans; and (3) the cavernous artery, which is responsible for erection. The cavernosal artery on each side has helicine branches that supply the trabecular erectile tissue and the sinusoids. Some variations to the arterial supply do exist. Within the tunica of the corpus cavernosum, the sinusoids are interwoven with trabeculae of smooth muscle and supportive connective tissue. In the flaccid state, blood diffuses peripherally from the cen-

tral cavernosal artery, and the penile blood gas is similar to that of venous blood. During erection, because of increased arterial flow, the blood gas level is more like that of arterial blood.

## Venous Drainage

The venous drainage of the corpora cavernosa is through the emissary veins that traverse through the tunica albuginea of each corpus in a diagonal fashion. In the distal two thirds of the penis, emissary veins drain into circumflex veins along the shaft, which in turn drain into the deep dorsal vein of the penis beneath Buck's fascia. The latter traverses under the symphysis pubis to form the periprostatic venous plexus of Santorini. In the proximal one third of the corpora, emissary veins join to form two to five cavernous veins that exit the dorsomedial aspect of the penile hilum to form the pudendal vein and follow the course of the pudendal artery and nerves into the perineum.

## Nerve Supply

The penis is supplied by autonomic and somatic nerves. Somatic sensory nerves are mainly responsible for sensation in the penile skin. Somatic motor nerves are responsible for contraction of the bulbocavernosus and ischiocavernosus muscles. Motor stimuli to these two muscles travel through the pudendal nerve. Contraction of the ischiocavernosus muscle produces a more rigid erection phase by compressing the already engorged corpora cavernosa, thereby increasing intracavernosal pressure. Rhythmic contraction of the bulbocavernosus is responsible for seminal emission.

Parasympathetic nerve fibers to the penis arise from the second, third, and fourth sacral spinal cord segments forming the pelvic plexus. Branches of this plexus form the cavernous nerve that innervates the corpora cavernosa. Parasympathetic stimulation increases the blood flow to the penis, which results in distension of the sinusoidal spaces. This, in turn, causes compression of intermediary venules between the sinusoids and the tunica and subsequent compression of emissary veins. The resultant engorgement of the corpora is further enhanced by ischiocavernosus muscle contraction, raising intracavernosal pressure several hundred millimeters of mercury (mm Hg).

Sympathetic nerve fibers to the corpora arise from the T12-L2 spinal cord segments, forming the hypogastric plexus. Branches of this plexus merge with the pelvic plexus and join in with the cavernosal nerves. Sympathetic stimulation causes detumescence. Remembering the somatic and autonomic pathways is important when evaluating a patient for priapism.

## Pathophysiology

The final pathologic pathway of all etiologic factors of low-flow priapism is stasis of blood in the corpora cavernosa. This stasis results in low $pO_2$ and high $pCO_2$ within the corpora, causing edema of the cavernosal trabeculae and leading to further outflow obstruction. Additionally, low $pO_2$ and high $pCO_2$ and increased blood viscosity contribute further to venous stasis. One of the most intriguing aspects of penile blood is the lack of thrombosis, even after several days of priapism. This lack may be attributed to the very high fibrinolytic activity of cavernosal blood because it appears that local fibrinolysis takes place during prolonged erection.[7]

## Diagnosis

Diagnosis of priapism is usually based on findings during clinical examination. A thorough physical examination (rectal, abdominal, and neurologic) will reveal a turgid corpus cavernosum with a soft glans and corpus spongiosum. Chronic priapism and acute intermittent (stuttering) priapism may be more difficult to diagnose. Cavernosal blood gas measurement is an integral part of every examination. A blood gas level similar to that of venous blood is indicative of veno-occlusive disease; one similar to arterial blood, suggestive of arterial priapism. By definition, all priapisms start off as high flow and, therefore, an early

cavernosal gas measurement may be misleading. Technetium 99m ($^{99m}$Tc) scan has been advocated as a means of differentiating between high-uptake arterial priapism and low-uptake veno-occlusive priapism.[8] Cavernosography, another means of differentiating between the two types, demonstrates rapid drainage of the corpus cavernosum in the arterial type and venous stasis in the veno-occlusive type.[9] Once the diagnosis of high-flow priapism is made, use of selective arteriography to identify the site of the arterial pathology (usually a rupture) is effective. Arterial embolization of the site can be therapeutic.

## Treatment

The primary goal of all treatment modalities is to abort the erection as soon as possible, preventing permanent damage to the corpora that will lead to impotence; a secondary goal is to relieve pain. There is ample evidence that the risk of fibrosis and impotency increases with time. Generally, the incidence of impotence is less if the erection is aborted in less than 24 hours. Medical management should always be tried before resorting to surgery.

### Medical

#### High-Flow Priapism

In the early stage, ice packing may cause vasospasm and spontaneous thrombosis of the ruptured artery. Three reported cases of spontaneous resolution suggest that conservative treatment of high-flow priapism is advantageous.[10] However, most of the cases with delayed cavernous arterial rupture do not subside spontaneously, and arteriography and embolization of the internal pudendal artery are usually required.[11-13] Alternatively, injection of methylene blue to counteract the release of nitric oxide and embolization of the internal pudendal artery have been proposed by Steers and Selby.[14] One case of percutaneous autologus clot embolization of the arterial sinusoidal cavity was reported by Ilkay and Levine.[10]

## Low-Flow Priapism

Medical treatment is aimed at increasing venous outflow of the penis. The first line of treatment involves aspiration of the corpora and intracavernosal injection with an α-adrenergic agonist. Epinephrine, norepinephrine, and phenylephrine all have similar modes of action. Initial aspiration of old blood from the corpora via a 21-gauge butterfly needle is followed by injection of 250 to 500µg phenylephrine—a pure $\alpha_1$-adrenergic stimulant—every 5 minutes until detumescence takes place. The phenylephrine solution is made by mixing 10mg/ml of phenylephrine with 19ml of normal saline (500mcg/ml concentration). Irrigation with diluted α-adrenergic solution has also been described.[15,16] Alternatively, oral terbutaline has been shown to be effective in causing detumescence in some patients with prostaglandin-induced priapism. The response rate of up to 36% has been reported in patients treated with either 5 or 10mg of terbutaline as compared with only 12% with placebo.[17] However, in another study, terbutaline was found to

have no benefit over the placebo.[18] Nevertheless, intracavernous injection of an α-adrenergic agonist remains the most effective treatment for low-flow priapism. It is almost 100% effective if the priapism is treated within 12 hours of onset. Figure 29.1 shows the recommended algorithm for the medical management of priapism.

## Sickle Cell Disease

Sickle cell disorder accounts for approximately 28% of all cases of priapism. It is reported that 42% of all sickle cell adults and 64% of all sickle cell children eventually develop priapism. Treatment in these patients should be prompt and conservative as they often present with recurrent disease. The sickle cell patient should be treated by aggressive hydration, oxygenation, and metabolic alkalization to reduce further sickling. Supertransfusion and erythrophoresis should be used as second-line therapy. Irrigations and injections should be performed as soon as possible.

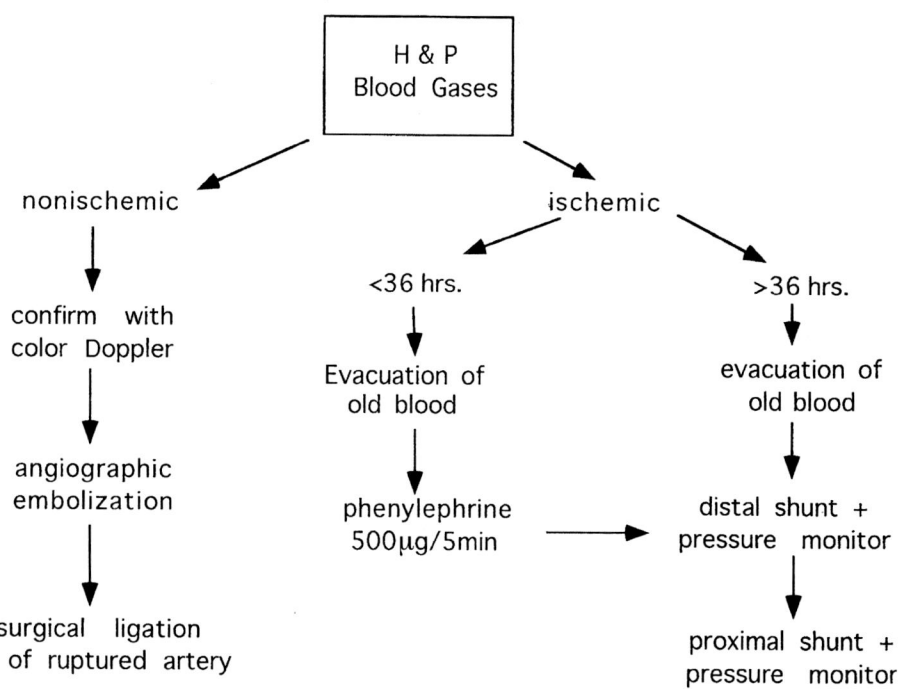

FIGURE 29.1. Algorithm for treatment of priapism.

TABLE 29.2. Distal shunts.

| | |
|---|---|
| Ebbehoj | 1974 |
| Winter | 1976 |
| Goulding | 1980 |
| Al-Ghorab | 1981 |
| Datta | 1986 |
| Kilinc | 1993 |
| Hashmat-Waterhouse | 1993 |

## Recurrent Priapism

Stuttering or recurrent priapism occurs often in patients with sickle cell traits or disease and in non-sickle patients with prior episodes. The mechanism is unknown, although alteration of the adrenoceptor or scarring of intra-cavernous venules may be partially responsible. For the sexually active patient, self-injection of an α-adrenergic agent such as phenylephrine 500 μg every 5 minutes usually results in detumescence. If sexual function is not a concern, a patient may use antiandrogen or a gonadotropin-releasing hormone (GnRH) agonist, which suppresses nocturnal penile erection and may be very useful in preventing its recurrence.[19,20]

## Surgical

### High-Flow Priapism

If the conservative and angiographic embolizations fail, surgical exploration and ligation of the ruptured artery will be necessary to avert the high-flow priapism secondary to arterial rupture.

### Low-Flow Priapism

The aim of all surgical procedures for veno-occlusive priapism is to divert the venous return from the corpus cavernosum into either the corpus spongiosum system that is unaffected by the priapism or into another nearby venous system. This is achieved by formation of a shunt between the two systems. Perform the shunts at either the distal shaft or the proximal shaft. Distal shunts are preferentially carried out first, as they are easier to perform and can be created under local anesthesia. Table 29.2 shows a sum-

mary of available choices. In the Ebbehoj shunt,[21] a window is made between the corpus cavernosum and the glans penis by percutaneously inserting a #11 blade at the coronal sulcus on each side. The Winter shunt[22] involves production of a communication between corpus cavernosum and glans using a Tru-Cut needle inserted through the glans. The Goulding shunt[23] achieves the same goal by removing a button of tunica albuginea of corpus cavernosum using a Kerrison rongeur inserted through an incision through the glans. The Datta shunt[24] uses a skin biopsy punch to achieve the same goal. In the Al-Ghorab shunt,[25] a transverse incision is made on the dorsum of the glans and the tips of both corpora are exposed, a 5 × 5 mm segment of corpora is excised, and the glans skin is closed. The Kilinc shunt[26] is an insertion of a specially made trocar with multiple side holes through the glans into the corpora. The corpora is then irrigated with saline. Intermittent compression of the shaft shunts the corporeal blood through the side holes to the glans. In the Hashmat-Waterhouse shunt, a #11 blade is percutaneously inserted in the glans, on both sides of the meatus, along the axis of the penis. The blade is advanced until it penetrates the tip of corpus cavernosum, producing a shunt between the two.

Proximal shunts may be performed as first-line surgical therapy in long-standing priapism or if a distal shunt has failed to resolve the problem. Table 29.3 summarizes the available proximal surgical options. These shunts require general or regional anesthesia.

In the Quackles shunt[27] (cavernoso-spongiosal), with the patient in lithotomy, the corpus spongiosum is identified at the level of the bulb through a perineal incision. Side-to-side anastomosis is performed between the spongy tissue and the opposing tunica albuginea of corpus cavernosum on one side. If

TABLE 29.3. Proximal shunts.

| | |
|---|---|
| Quackles (cavernoso-spongiosal) | 1964 |
| Grayhack (cavernoso-saphenous) | 1964 |
| Barry (cavernoso-dorsal vein) | 1976 |
| Odelowo (cavernoso-spongiosal) | 1988 |

priapism does not subside, the same procedure may be performed on the other side.

In the Grayhack shunt[28] (cavernoso-saphenous), the long saphenous vein in the groin is exposed. The distal end is tied off; the proximal end is rotated, transferring through a subcutaneous tunnel to the base of the penis where it must be anastomosed to the corpus cavernosum in an end-to-side fashion. If detumescence does not ensue, the same procedure should be performed on the opposite side.

In the Barry shunt[29] (cavernoso-dorsal vein), through a single incision at the base of the penis, the superficial dorsal vein is mobilized then tied off distally. The proximal end is anastomosed end-to-side, to the corpus cavernosum, diverting the venous drainage to the superficial system.

The Odelowo shunt[30] (cavernoso-spongiosal) uses the same principles as the Quackles, but the procedure is modified by interposition of a free venous patch (usually the saphenous vein)

at the anastomosis to prevent contracture and subsequent closure.

### Intraoperative Monitoring

The intracavernous pressure should be continuously monitored via an arterial line set up after the shunts are made.[31] If the intracavernous pressure remains below 40 mm Hg for more than 10 minutes, adequate shunting has been established and recurrence is unlikely (Fig. 29.2).

## Postoperative Care

Appropriate antibiotic coverage is essential if surgical treatment is undertaken. Infection of the corpora may have disastrous consequences. Compression dressings and blood pressure cuffs decrease venous drainage and may be counterproductive. However, occasional manual compression by the patient may help to

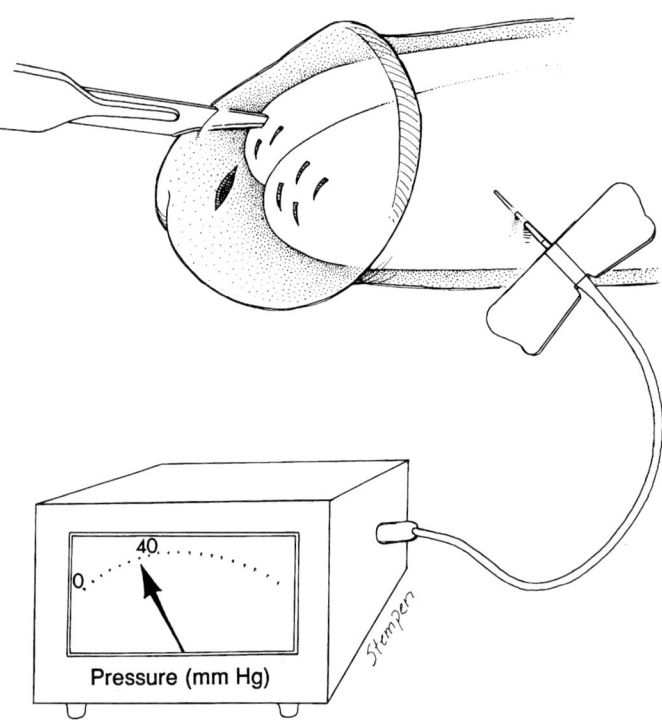

FIGURE 29.2. Continuous monitoring of intracavernous pressure using an arterial line while creating glanulo-cavernosal shunts using #11 blade.

reduce venous stasis in the corpora. After surgical shunting, the penis is in a state of temporary high-flow priapism because of reactive hyperemia from long-standing tissue anoxia. Additionally, edema of the corpora and penile skin may give the appearance of a rigid penis, but corporal blood gas measurement differentiates between high- and low-flow priapism.

## Complications

Untreated veno-occlusive priapism leads to corporeal fibrosis and impotence. The penis will have a permanent semirigid appearance. Complications of treatment can be classified as early and late. Early complications include bleeding, infection, and urethral injury. Bleeding from the glans penis after distal shunts is fairly common and is easily controlled by suturing of the puncture site or by gentle compression. Hematoma of the shaft after corporeal aspiration and irrigation is also common. Compression bandages should be avoided, for ice packs may be more useful to alleviate this problem. Infections are usually in the form of cellulitis. Strict asepsis should be followed when carrying out penile irrigations. Use of antibiotics is mandatory in order to avoid potentially disastrous complications that, if undiagnosed, may lead to abscess formation. Urethral injury is a rare complication but may lead to stricture or a urethrocutaneous fistula. Injury to the urethra can occur during needle aspiration and irrigation, performing distal shunts, or in more proximal cavernosospongiosal shunt procedures.

The most important late complication of priapism is impotence. Its incidence is directly related to the duration of priapism and to how aggressively it is treated. The overall impotence rate in men with priapism may be as high as 59%. Impotence may be either secondary to permanent fibrosis of the corpora or the consequence of surgical treatment. A persistent proximal or a distal shunt can lead to a venous leak-type impotence. If this is suspected, use of cavernosography can be diagnostic. High-flow arterial priapism has a better prognosis, with a reported impotence incidence of 20%.

## Conclusion

Priapism is an uncommon condition, and the low-flow type is considered a urologic emergency. Prompt treatment will avert permanent damage and preserve potency.

## References

1. Juenemann KP, Lue TF, Abozeid M, et al. Blood gas analysis in drug induced penile erections. *Urol Int* 1986; 41:207–211.
2. Broderick GA, Gordon D, Hypolite J, et al. Anoxia and corporal smooth muscle dysfunction: a model for ischemic priapism. *J Urol* 1994; 151:259–262.
3. Hashmat AI, Rehman JU. Priapism. In: Hashmat AI, Das S, eds. *The penis.* Philadelphia: Lea & Febiger, 1993: 219–243.
4. Tarry WF, Duckett JW Jr, McSnyder H III. Urologic complications of sickle cell disease in a pediatric population. *J Urol* 1987; 138:592–594.
5. Hauri D, Spycher M, Bruhlmann W. Erection and priapism: a new physiopathological concept. *Urol Int* 1983; 38:138–145.
6. Witt MA, Goldstein I, Saenz de Tejada I, et al. Traumatic laceration of intracavernosal arteries: the pathophysiology of nonischemic, high flow, arterial priapism. *J Urol* 1990; 143:129–132.
7. Rolle L, Bazzan M, Bellina M, et al. Coagulation and fibrinolytic activity of blood from corpus cavernosum. *Arch Ital Urol Nefrol Androl* 1991; 63:471–473.
8. Hashmat AI, Raju SI, Sing I, et al. $^{99m}$Tc penile scans—an investigative modality in priapism *Urol Radiol* 1989; 11:58–60.
9. Bruhlmann W, Pouliadis G, Hauri D, et al. A new concept of priapism based on the results of arteriography and cavernosography. *Urol Radiol* 1983; 5:31–36.
10. Ilkay AK, Levine LA. Conservative management of high-flow priapism. *Urology* 1995; 46: 419–424.
11. Walker TG, Grant PW, Goldstein I, et al. "High-flow" priapism: treatment with superselective transcatheter embolization. *Radiology* 1990; 174:1053–1054.
12. Ricciardi R Jr, Bhatt GM, Cynamon J, et al. Delayed high flow priapism: pathophysiology and management. *J Urol* 1993; 149:119–121.
13. Brock G, Breza J, Lue TF, et al. High flow priapism: a spectrum of disease. *J Urol* 1993; 150:968–971.

14. Steers WD, Selby JB Jr. Use of methylene blue and selective embolization of the pudendal artery for high flow priapism refractory to medical and surgical treatments [see comments]. *J Urol* 1991; 146:1361–1363.

15. Sidi AA. Vasoactive intracavernous pharmacotherapy. *Urol Clin North Am* 1988; 15:95–101.

16. Molina L, Bejany D, Lynne CM. Diluted epinephrine solution for the treatment of priapism. *J Urol* 1989; 141:1127–1128.

17. Lowe FC, Jarow JP. Placebo-controlled study of oral terbutaline and pseudoephedrine in management of prostaglandin $E_1$-induced prolonged erections. *Urology* 1993; 42:51–53.

18. Govier FE, Jonsson E, Kramer-Levien D. Oral terbutaline for the treatment of priapism. *J Urol* 1994; 151:878–879.

19. Levin LA, Guss SP. Gonadotropin-releasing hormone analogues in the treatment of sickle cell anemia-associated priapism. *J Urol* 1993; 150:475–477.

20. Steinberg J, Eyre RC. Management of recurrent priapism with epinephrine self-injection and gonadotropin-releasing hormone analogue. *J Urol* 1995; 153:152–153.

21. Ebbohoj J. A new operation for priapism. *Scand J Plast Reconstr Surg* 1974; 8:241–242.

22. Winter CC. Cure of idiopathic priapism: new procedure for creating fistulas between glans penis and corpora cavernosa. *Urology* 1976; 8:399.

23. Goulding FJ. Modification of cavernoglandular shunt for priapism. *Urology* 1980; 15:64.

24. Datta NS. A new technique for creation of a cavernoglandular shunt in the treatment of priapism. *J Urol* 1986; 136:602–603.

25. Wendel EF, Grayhack JT. Corpora cavernosaglans penis shunt for priapism. *Surg Gynecol Obstet* 1981; 153:586–588.

26. Kilinc M. A modified Winter procedure for priapism treatment with a new trocar. *Eur Urol* 1993; 24:118–119.

27. Quackles R. Cure of patient suffering from priapism by cavernospongiosal anastomosis. [French]. *Acta Urol Belg* 1964; 32:5–13.

28. Grayhack JT, McCullough W, O'Connor VJ. Venous bypass to control priapism. *Invest Urol* 1964; 1:509–513.

29. Barry JM. Priapism: treatment with corpus cavernosum to dorsal vein of penis shunts. *J Urol* 1976; 116:754–756.

30. Odelowo EO. A new caverno-spongiosum shunt with saphenous vein patch graft for established priapism. *Int Surg* 1988; 73:130–132.

31. Lue TF, Hellstrom WJG, McAninch JW, et al. Priapism: a refined approach to diagnosis and treatment. *J Urol* 1986; 136:104–108.

# 30
# Vacuum Constriction Devices

Joel L. Marmar

Vacuum constriction devices (VCDs) have been used for the nonsurgical management of erectile dysfunction for many years. Although the United States Patent Office has issued several patents to inventors of these devices since 1917, VCDs were prescribed cautiously for many years because the original devices were clumsy and utilized mouth suction for a vacuum, the pumps were rubber bulbs that were not reliable, and the constriction rings were crude arrangements of rubber bands.[1-3] There were few publications regarding either the safety of these devices or the effects of constriction on penile blood flow. Most clinicians were hesitant to recommend them because there were reports of surgery for penile incarceration from the rings.[4,5]

The basic VCD unit consists of a clear cylinder, a vacuum pump, and a rubber constriction ring (Fig. 30.1). After the application of lubricant, the open end of the cylinder is placed over the flaccid penis and compressed against the abdominal wall to create an airtight seal. Activation of the vacuum pump removes air from the cylinder and creates negative pressure. Blood, drawn into the penis, produces elongation and increased circumference. When maximum size and rigidity have been achieved, the rubber constrictor ring is guided off the back end of the cylinder to encircle the penis and is worn during intercourse to restrict venous drainage and to maintain rigidity. When the ring is removed, the erection usually declines rapidly.

At least seven companies now offer safe devices with improved features,[6] and the 1992 National Institutes of Health (NIH) Consensus Conference[7] listed the use of vacuum constriction devices among therapeutic options for men with erectile dysfunction. Recently, several new devices have been developed and approved by the U.S. Food and Drug Administration.

## Components of the Devices

### The Cylinder

The new cylinders are molded of clear plastic that permits observation of the penis during creation of the erection-like state. Because ecchymosis and petechia of the penis are potential complications, the patient can now observe the penis clearly during the application of the vacuum. If discoloration is noted, the negative pressure can be discontinued. Although some of the earlier models required special fitting and clinicians needed an inventory of sizes, most of the newer models have a rubber or plastic insert for the open end that may be sized to the patient. These inserts provide an excellent fit, and create an airtight seal against the abdominal wall to improve the effectiveness of the vacuum and to limit the undesirable effect of suctioning scrotal contents into the cylinder.

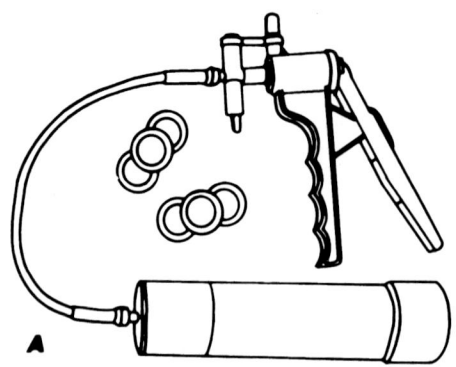
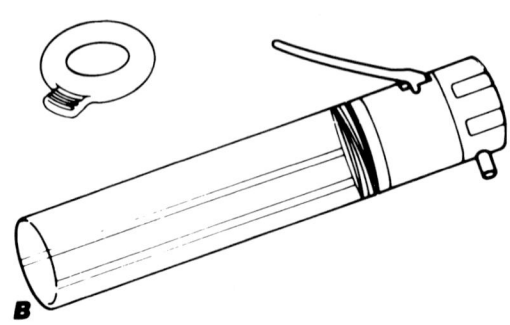

FIGURE 30.1. (A) Diagram of typical two-piece VCD with a cylinder and separate pump requiring two hands for operation. The rings have a central circle with two side loops constructed of a thinner rubber tubing (0.25 cm diameter). (B) Diagram of typical one-handed unit with the pump attached to the cylinder, some motorized. The "O" ring is constructed of thicker rubber tubing (0.5 cm diameter). (Reproduced by permission from Marmar et al.[17])

## The Pump

Some of the earlier devices used a piston syringe and a three-way stopcock or a rubber bulb to create the vacuum.[2,3] The newer devices utilize efficient vacuum pumps with governors or quick release valves that limit the negative pressure to −250 to −350 mm Hg. At these pressures, the vacuum-induced pain is minimized for most patients. Many of the new units still require two hands for operation because they consist of a separate pump and cylinder, but other models can be operated with one hand and some are motorized, a popular option according to patient surveys.[6]

## The Ring

In the past, combinations of rubber bands were used for constriction.[3] More recently, two new types of molded rings have become available in various sizes and degrees of firmness. The rings may be individually fitted for the patient by selecting one with an inner circumference approximately 2 cm less than the outer circumference of the flaccid penis. Some molded rings may have a central circle with two side loops for placement and removal. These rings are constructed of solid rubber tubing with a cross-sectional diameter of 0.25 cm and a durometer or hardness of about 55 in the resting position.

When stretched, the hardness increases to 65 to 70 durometer. Although this ring gives effective constriction, the hardness may be painful to some patients during the first few trials. Other models are constructed as simple "O" rings with a tab at one location. These are usually made of thicker rubber tubing with a cross-sectional diameter of 0.5 cm that compresses a greater surface area of the penis. The resting durometer of these thick rings is about 35 to 40, which increases to only 50 to 65 when stretched, which may be more comfortable for some patients.

## Clinical Application

Several investigators have utilized VCDs for patients with a variety of conditions (Table 30.1) and multiple risk factors (Table 30.2).[8–10] These reports suggest that VCD therapy may

TABLE 30.1. Potential categories for use of VCD.

| | |
|---|---|
| Arterial insufficency | Spinal cord injury |
| Venous leakage | Endocrine abnormalities |
| Hypertension | Peyronie's disease |
| Diabetes | Psychological causes |
| Post-radical prostatectomy | Prior therapy: implants, implant removals, oral medication and injections |

TABLE 30.2. Risk factors associated with patients who have used a VCD.

Medications—antihypertensives, muscle relaxants, sleeping pills
Smoking
Alcohol
Radiation therapy

be applicable for almost all patients who seek help for erectile dysfunction. Most manufacturers of VCDs warn against their use by patients with bleeding disorders, on anticoagulant therapy, or having a history of priapism. However, some investigators have used VCDs for these patients in selected situations.[9]

In addition, VCD therapy has been used in special situations. A VCD was used in association with unsuccessful injection therapy.[11] In this study, 21 of 22 men had a partial erection that was completed to full rigidity with a VCD following an intracavernous injection. These investigators recommended that such patients be taught both injection therapy and VCD therapy for a comprehensive approach to management. In another study,[9] a VCD was used to augment erections for four men with semirigid penile implants. Other investigators used VCDs on 11 patients after removal of penile implants, and 10 patients (91%) later achieved intercourse on a regular basis.[12]

The complications and complaints, minimal and transient in most cases, include penile petechia or ecchymosis, pain during application of the vacuum, pain with placement of the ring, limitations on the amount of antegrade ejaculate, coolness of the penis during constriction, and swiveling of the base of the penis with an erection-like state. Although these problems are unacceptable to some patients, they are usually self-limiting after repetitive use of the VCD.

In a few studies, there have been reports of severe complications with vacuum therapy related either to constriction or the vacuum. For example, skin necrosis was reported in a paraplegic male who utilized a VCD three times daily for 3 days.[13] After discontinuation of the VCD, the area healed with a hypertrophic scar. In other cases, uncontrolled vacuum re-sulted in extreme magnitudes of pulling force that were computed to be 10 times greater than those of a physiologic erection.[14,15] In these cases, the devices were used excessively: one patient developed a tear in the penis leading to a Peyronie's plaque,[14] and another patient developed a plaque as well as significant venous leakage.[15]

Although these devices seem safe for almost all patients, the potential for significant complications must be appreciated.

# Arterial Studies in Humans

VCDs maintain an erection-like state by acute corporal expansion, inflow of both arterial and venous blood, and limitations of venous outflow.[16] From an early report with VCDs, partial arterial occlusion caused the skin temperature to fall an average of 0.9°C (0.5° to 3.1°).[3] Although strain gauge plethysmography confirmed continuous blood flow into the penis during constriction, it was clear from these data that additional arterial flow studies were needed to evaluate the constriction process. In a separate study, pneumoplethysmography was used to evaluate pulse volume tracings before, during, and after constriction among 51 patients with varied diagnoses.[17] The patients were classified by their penile brachial index (PBI). A value less than 0.7 was consistent with arterial insufficiency. The pneumoplethysmo graph was easy to use, and the tracings were analyzed by established standards noted in Figure 30.2.[18] The amplitude of the pulse volume tracing was measured as the height of the tracing from the baseline to the highest peak. The crest time was measured from the base to the peak of the pulse wave in tenths of a second and compared with the time of the total cycle. The rate of rise of the ascending limb was calculated by drawing a parallel line to the most rapidly rising portion of the tracing to determine whether the ascending limb was rising abruptly.

While the constrictor ring was applied, the amplitude of the pulse volume tracing declined by 70% to 75% in each case, but continuous blood flow was demonstrated.[17] The decline in

## A. Normal        B. Abnormal

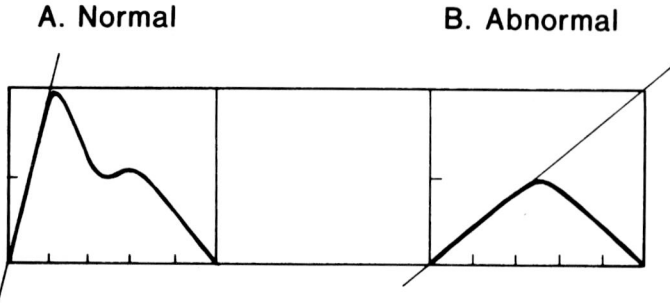

FIGURE 30.2. Normal and abnormal tracings with a pneumoplethysmograph. The amplitude is measured by the height of the tracing. The crest time is measured from the base to the peak of the pulse wave. A dichrotic notch is noted in the normal tracing on the down slope. The rate of rise of the tracing is noted by the angle of the ascending limb. (Reproduced by permission from Kedia.[18])

amplitude was influenced somewhat by the patient's position (Fig. 30.3). The greatest decline occurred while the patient was supine. Less decline in amplitude was noted when the patient stood upright or when he was positioned on the side. However, the crest time never exceeded 35% of the overall cycle and the rate of rise of the ascending limb remained abrupt in all positions. These findings confirm continuous blood flow in the different positions.

Within 60 seconds after removal of the constriction ring, the pulse volume tracings returned to baseline levels for all patients including 12 men with a PBI of less than 0.7.[17] Among 33 individuals with a PBI greater than 0.7, there was a transient rise in the pulse volume tracing over baseline levels within the first 10 seconds after removal of the ring. This finding suggests postischemic hyperemia, which is an expected response among men with normal vasculature.[19]

These findings suggest that the radial pressure produced by the constrictor ring probably exceeded the mean arterial pressure because the amplitude of the tracing declined. However, the radial constriction pressure from the ring did not exceed systolic blood pressure because the tracings were never reduced to a straight line. These data implied that VCDs were probably safe for most patients, but more specific studies were needed of cavernous artery flow.

In a recent report, a color Doppler duplex ultrasound was used for real-time imaging of arterial flow within the corpora cavernosa during vacuum-constriction erections.[20] The inner diameter of the cavernous artery and the cross-sectional areas of the cavernous bodies were measured in all patients before and after the use of the vacuum device. In most patients, it was difficult to localize the cavernosal arteries in the resting state. With the introduction of color, the arteries were identified, but the peak flow velocity was probably less than 9 to 12 cm/s, which was the threshold for flow detection by this instrument. After subatmospheric pressure, the cavernous arteries had a mean diameter of 1.5 mm, which is about three times wider than the nondilated vessel. After self-stimulation and the application of the cylinder, the arterial peak flow velocity was about 12 to 18 cm/s. This value was less than the arterial peak flow velocity of 38 cm/s following the injection of 20 μg of prostaglandin $E_1$. When the constriction ring was applied, the flow was not detectable, but again, the arteries were localized by color.

The long-term effects of chronic VCD usage on cavernous artery function were also evaluated by a Doppler duplex ultrasound.[21] Eighteen men (mean age 57.1) used a VCD over 6 months, and three had the diagnosis of partial arterial insufficiency. Each patient in the study had a baseline value following self-stimulation and the injection of 20 μg of prostaglandin $E_1$.

The mean arterial peak flow velocity was 22.8 cm/s for the right side and 18.7 cm/s for the left. After using the VCD for 6 months, the mean arterial peak flow velocity increased to 29.9 cm/s on the right side and 23.6 cm/s on the left. The differences were significant ($p < 0.1$–$0.03$). These results were comparable to the improved hemodynamic response or increased mean arterial flow after long-term treatment with intracavernous injections.[22]

A.    RESTING PULSE-VOLUME TRACING (5 MM/SEC AND 25 MM/SEC)

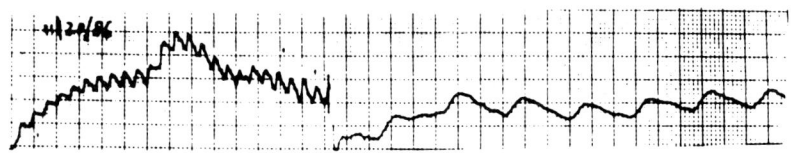

B.    FOLLOWING INJECTION, PARTIAL ERECTION (BUCKLING PRESSURE < 50MM HG)

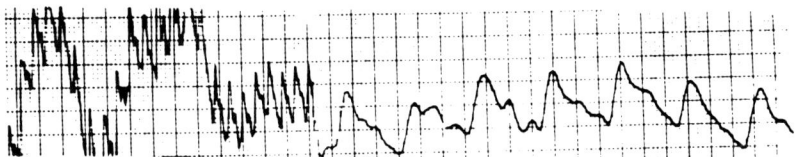

C.    FOLLOWING VCD, WITH CONSTRICTOR RING IN PLACE (LYING DOWN)

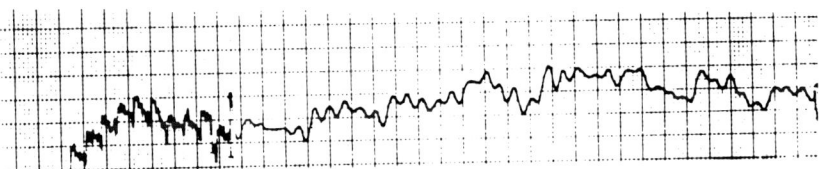

D.    FOLLOWING VCD, WITH CONSTRICTOR RING IN PLACE (STANDING UPRIGHT)

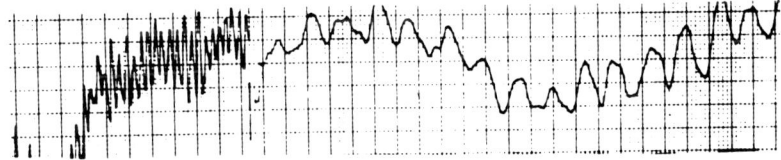

E.    CONSTRICTOR RING REMOVED

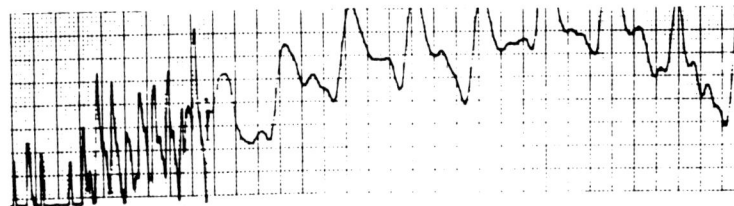

FIGURE 30.3. Pulse volume tracings using pneumoplethysmography. (A) Resting pulse volume tracing at 15 mm/s and 25 mm/s. (B) Tracing following intracavernous injection. (C) Tracing following application of a VCD with constriction ring in place (patient supine). (D) Tracing following application of a VCD with constriction ring in place (patient standing upright). (E) Constriction ring removed. (Reprinted with permission from Marmar et al.[11])

Some clinicians have reported that with chronic use, 20% to 30% of the VCD users may regain their own spontaneous erections.[8,9] These data and the arterial flow studies reported above suggest that the clinical use of a VCD is probably safe and that the repetitive stretching of the penile vascular bed appears to be a stimulus for improved flow.

## Venous Studies in Humans

It has been estimated that about 80% of men with vasculogenic impotence fail to store blood within the corpora during an erection because of venous leakage.[23] In addition, about 20% of men with normal erections may demonstrate venous leakage as well.[24] Although this condition may be confirmed with cavernosography/cavernosometry,[25,26] or suggested by end diastolic velocities greater than 5 cm/s with color Doppler duplex ultrasound,[27] management of venous leakage has been controversial. Surgery[28] and embolization[29] have been used, but the long-term results have been disappointing. Recently, patients with venous leakage have been classified into five groups, and all were given a trial with a rubber band around the penis during intercourse before recommending invasive therapy.[30] Constriction seemed reasonable for these men with venous leakage based on other clinical observations.

During constriction, it was apparent that venous congestion occurred during the application of a constriction ring. Superficial penile veins were dilated and the skin appeared dusky.[3] Doppler duplex ultrasonography noted an increase in the cross-sectional area of the penis during constriction,[20] and the circumference of the penis increased 3.4 to 4.3 cm after applying the device.[3] In addition, there was a mean increase in the circumference of 4.3 cm, which was greater than the increase in diameter of natural erections, estimated at 2.5 cm.[17] Xenon washout studies during constriction confirmed that in the flaccid state the clearance was 1.9 ml/minute compared with 0.27 ml/minute during constriction.[31] These findings demonstrated the effects of constriction on venous

drainage, but more specific measurements of corporal blood seemed important to investigate the safety of constriction.

In one study, a sample of corporal blood was obtained immediately after constriction and the mean $pCO_2$ was 39.9 mm Hg, which was between the mean arterial $pCO_2$ (37.7 mm Hg) and the mean venous $pCO_2$ (49.5 mm Hg).[32] Similar findings were noted for the mean $pO_2$ (mean arterial, 75.5 mm Hg; mean cavernous, 46.2 mm Hg; and mean venous, 32.1 mm Hg). From these data, it was computed that about 40% of the increased corporal blood was of venous origin after the application of the VCD. Despite this admixture, the mean corporal $O_2$ saturation was 79.2% during constriction versus 94.5% for arterial blood. This level of $O_2$ saturation seemed sufficient for oxygenation of the tissues because few long-term complications have been reported from constriction. However, most manufacturers continue to recommend a limit on constriction of 30 minutes. From these observations, it seemed reasonable to carry out studies involving constriction on men with venous leakage.

One such report utilized cavernosography, and documented venous leakage among 47 men who were unable to attain an erection sufficient for penetration.[33] These men were offered various treatment options and 29 patients (62%) chose a VCD. They completed questionnaires and 20 of 29 patients (69%) who used the device were satisfied, but there was no correlation with success and the severity of venous leakage. In a separate study on 31 men, infusion pharmacocavernosometry was used to document and quantify venous leakage.[34] After a 2-ml injection of papaverine (60 mg)/phentolamine mesylate (2 mg) or 20 μg prostaglandin $E_1$, an intravenous infusion was started to maintain an intracorporal pressure of 145 mm Hg. Severity of leakage was based on the maintenance infusion rate. A rate of less than 50 cc/min was mild leakage, 50 to 100 cc/min was moderate, and greater than 100 cc/min was severe. This group used a VCD and 18 (58%) were satisfied after a mean follow-up of 7.6 months. Again, there was no correlation with severity based on the infusion rate necessary to maintain an erection. These studies suggested that VCDs may be helpful for some men with venous leakage. To evaluate the use of the ring alone, 67 impotent men were studied (Marmar, unpublished data). Each patient was interviewed by a physician and told that the study was for men who achieved erection but who lost it before or during entry into the vagina. No other studies were performed on these men. It was hypothesized that many of these men had the potential for venous leakage as based on this symptom complex. Thirty controls, recruited for the study, stated that they had no history of erectile dysfunction. The patients and controls were to use a constriction ring (Fig. 30.4) with intercourse for 1 month and complete a questionnaire to evaluate the effect of the ring on penile firmness, sexual frequency, and their perception about the ring. There were four categories for penile firmness (none, soft, firm, very firm) and four categories for sexual frequency (once a week or more, twice a month, once a month, none).

Results of the questionnaires showed that there were 18 men who did not achieve an erection, and they were dropped from the study because they did not use the ring. The remaining 49 patients were classified as improved whenever there was a positive change to the next highest category for firmness or sexual frequency. Among the patient group, 41 of 49 (83.7%) reported improvement in at least one category: 25 of 41 (61%) noted improvement in the firmness of the erection and 37 of 41 (90.2%) noted increase in the frequency of intercourse. There were 8 of 49 patients (16.3%) who were considered unchanged. Although the controls were capable of satisfactory erections before the study, 27 of 30 (90%) described improved quality of the erections while using the ring.

Other information concerning perception of the rings was obtained from the questionnaires. Among the 41 patients who were improved with the use of the ring, 38 of 41 (92.7%) indicated that the rings led to improved sexual confidence, and 41 of 41 (100%) stated that they would recommend the ring for others. Even among the men who were unchanged by the use of the rings, 6 of 8 (75%) stated that they would recommend the rings for others, and 30 of 30 controls (100%) claimed that they would also recommend the ring.

These data suggest that the use of a constriction ring alone may benefit some men with erectile dysfunction, especially if there is a high probability of venous leakage or of losing erections before and during entry into the vagina.

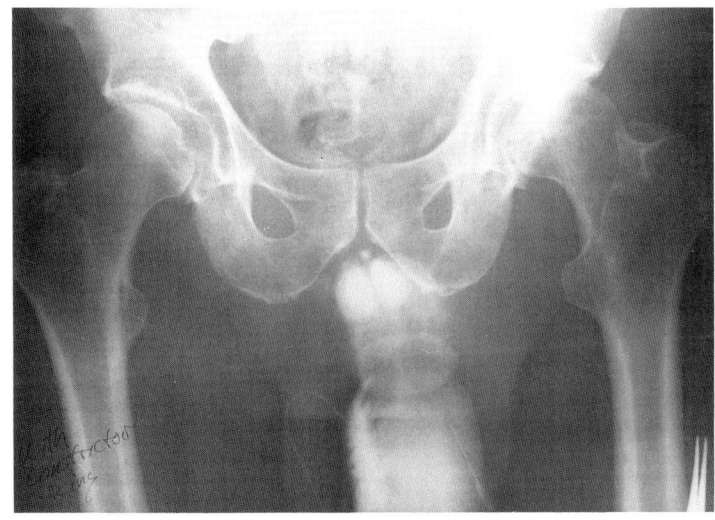

FIGURE 30.4. Cavernosography with a constriction ring at the base of the penis on a patient with previously documented venous leakage. Note compression of the venous drainage system.

## The Erection-Like State

When a VCD is used, it creates an "erection-like state." The penis is rigid distal to the ring, it swivels at its base, and it never achieves uplift or a 90° angle to the body. Although most patients who use a VCD achieve tumescence and intercourse, some men who discontinue its use complain about the erection-like state. Rigiscan studies indicated that tumescence of the penis does not always mean rigidity.[35]

In a sleep-lab setting, buckling pressures were measured with a tonometer to determine rigidity of nocturnal erections.[36] When buckling pressures were documented between 60 and 100 mm Hg, the rigidity was probably sufficient for vaginal penetration, and when the buckling pressures exceeded 100 mm Hg, the rigidity was certainly adequate. Rigiscan measurements express rigidity as the percentage of increase over the resting value.[37] A change of 70% at the base and the tip of the penis was suggested as sufficient for sexual intercourse.[37]

Both buckling pressures and Rigiscan monitoring have been used to evaluate rigidity following the application of a VCD. In one study, application of additional vacuum or placement of a second ring usually increased the buckling pressure to a level significant for vaginal penetration.[11] In another investigation, Rigiscan monitoring was used to determine rigidity of the erection-like state after the initial application of the VCD and again at 6 months.[32] The rigidity was directly correlated with the intracavernous pressure. Among this group of patients, the rigidity at the base was 80% to 90% while the intracavernous pressure was 80 to 100 mm Hg. In a study of 18 men with spinal cord injury, Rigiscan monitoring of the VCD noted that the base rigidity was 57% (range 30% to 80%),[38] as compared with Rigiscan measurements of 77% (range 30% to 100%) following a papaverine injection in the same men. Although the rigidity with the VCD was less than the rigidity with papaverine, 7 of these 18 men (39%) elected to use a VCD to achieve sexual intercourse. These data suggest that the rigidity created by an erection-like state is usually sufficient for vaginal penetration. Men who are displeased with the rigidity may require additional instruction on the use of the device and ring.

## The Workup

Most patients with erectile dysfunction use VCDs successfully with only minimal instruction, such as a demonstration in the doctor's office, a video from the manufacturer, or instruction from a company representative.[9] Although the VCD learning curve is short and the complications are usually minor, it is apparent that the workups have varied greatly between clinics.[10,32,39] Analysis of these reports suggests that only minimal testing may be needed before prescribing a VCD.

Each patient should have a baseline pulse volume tracing with pneumoplethysmography to estimate blood flow in the flaccid state. Doppler duplex ultrasonography is used by many clinics, but this system is expensive and not available in most urologists' offices. In contrast, pneumoplethysmography has proven to be a less expensive alternative that provides estimates of penile blood flow comparable to Doppler ultrasonography.[40]

After the baseline tracing, each patient receives 0.5 ml intracavernous injection of papaverine/phentolamine mesylate (30 mg/10 mg mixture). Another pulse volume tracing is repeated after 15 minutes and rigidity is estimated with a modified tonometer.[36] Rigiscan monitoring is used by some clinics, but it is expensive for routine office use.

Following this injection, patients can be categorized into three therapeutic groups: I, good response to penile injection; II, poor injection response, but completion of the erection by vacuum alone; and III, poor injection response with completion of the erection by VCD and constriction ring. A patient whose pulse volume tracings show a five- to sixfold increase in amplitude over the baseline and the buckling pressure exceeds 60 to 100 mm Hg is classified as group I and is started on home injection therapy with a VCD available as an alternative (Fig. 30.5). A poor injection response is considered group II, where pulse volume tracings have only a two- to fourfold increase in the

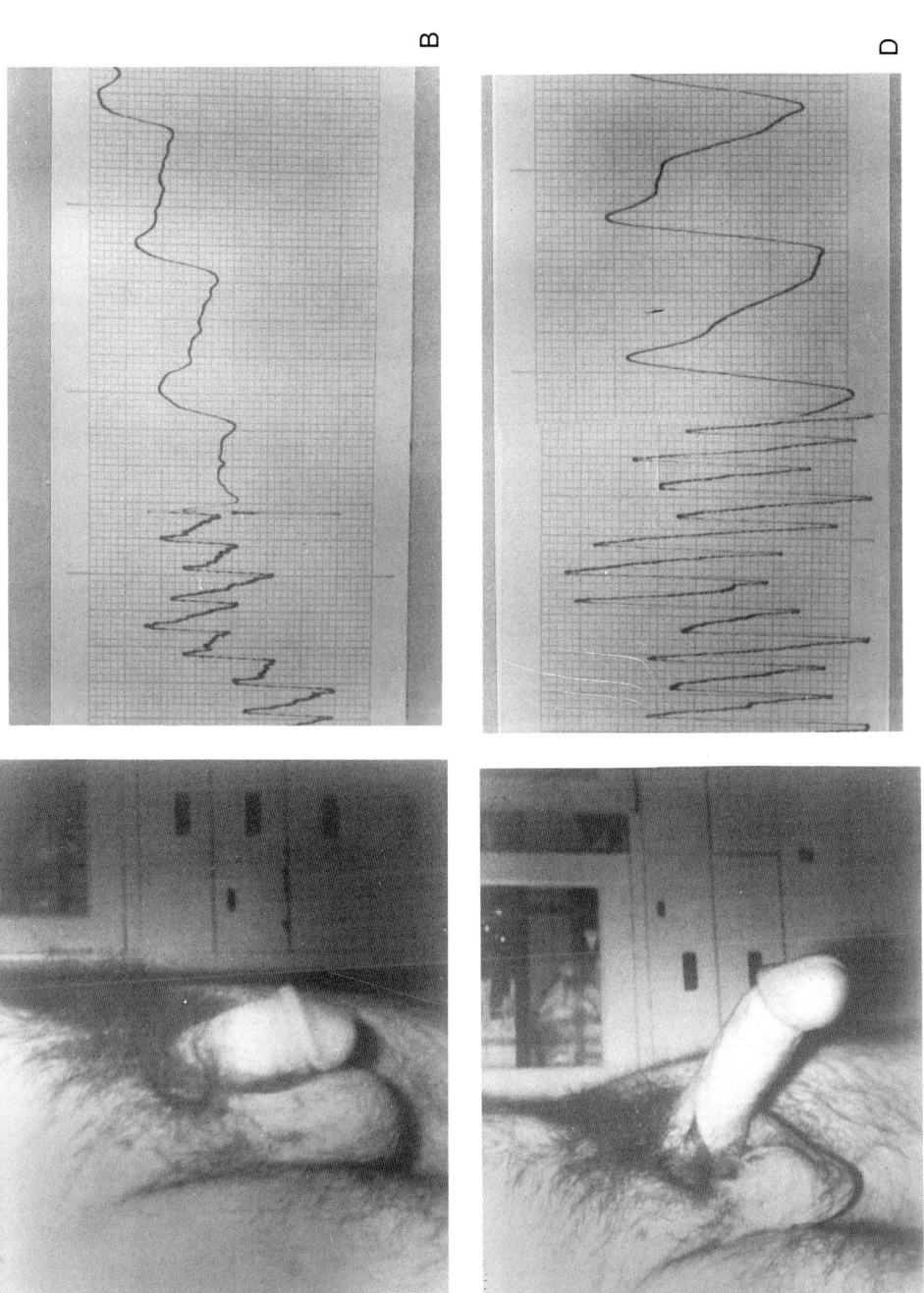

FIGURE 30.5. Group I patient—normal injection response. (A) Flaccid penis prior to injection. (B) Pulse volume tracing prior to injection. (C) Normal injection volume tracing in the flaccid state. (C) Normal injection response with rigidity and uplift. (D) Pulse volume tracing after normal injection response with at least a fivefold increase in the amplitude.

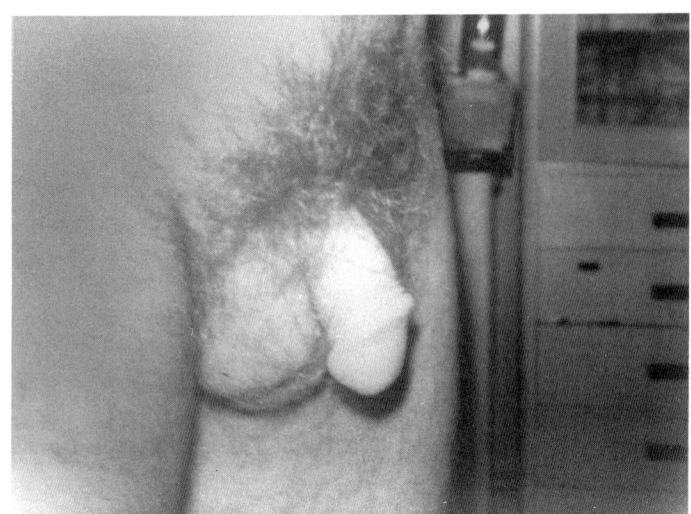

A

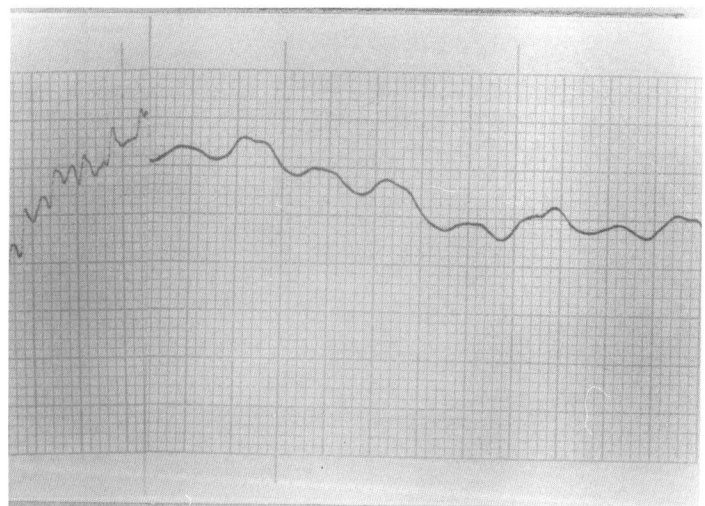

B

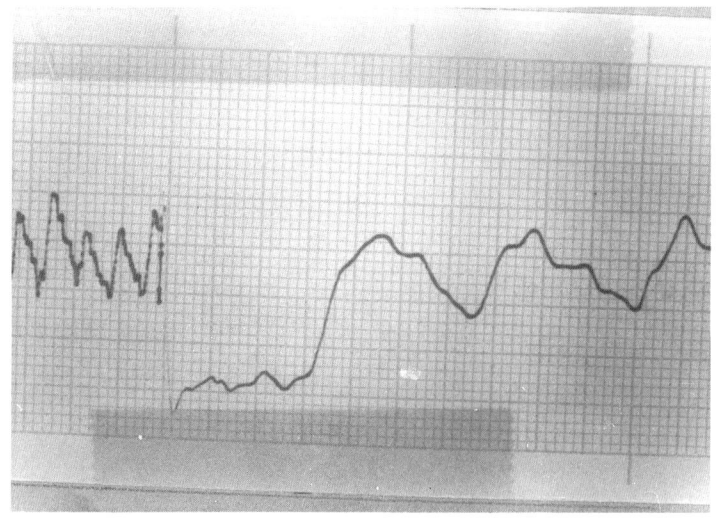

C

FIGURE 30.6. Group II patient—poor injection response, completion of the erection with a VCD alone. (A) Penis in the flaccid state. (B) Pulse volume tracing in the flaccid state with low amplitude. (C) Pulse volume tracing of partial response to a penile injection with only a three- or fourfold increase in amplitude. (D) Application of VCD. (E) Rigidity and uplift completed by vacuum alone.

FIGURE 30.6. *Continued*

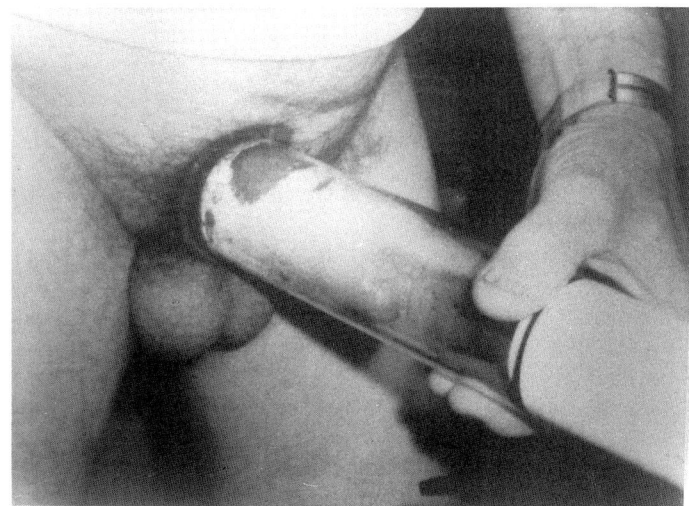

D

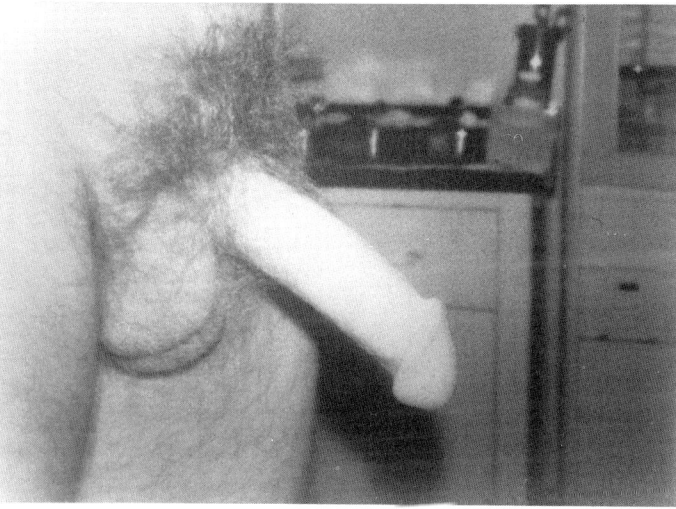

E

amplitude over baseline, and the buckling pressures are less than 60 mm Hg. In group II patients, a VCD should be immediately placed and a vacuum initiated. When the erection-like state appears, the VCD should be removed without placement of the ring. The erection will be completed and sustained by the vacuum alone (Fig. 30.6). In some patients, the VCD provides the necessary stimulus to complete the erection, comparable to observation of an erotic video to complete a partial erection following an intracavernous injection.[41] However, in clinical practice, a VCD seems more practical than the use of erotic films. Therefore, instruction with these devices should be included with the workup. Eventually, many of these group II men will be able to achieve satisfactory erections by the injection alone.

Group III is the category for patients with poor injection response, low amplitude on the pulse volume tracing, and inadequate buckling pressures (Fig. 30.7). A VCD alone may be tried on these men, but placement of the ring is required to complete and maintain the erection. This group should be managed with a combination of injections and vacuum constriction. With gravity cavernosometry,[42] men in this group may demonstrate possible venous leakage because the flow rate necessary to achieve a rigid erection by tonometry will exceed 60 to

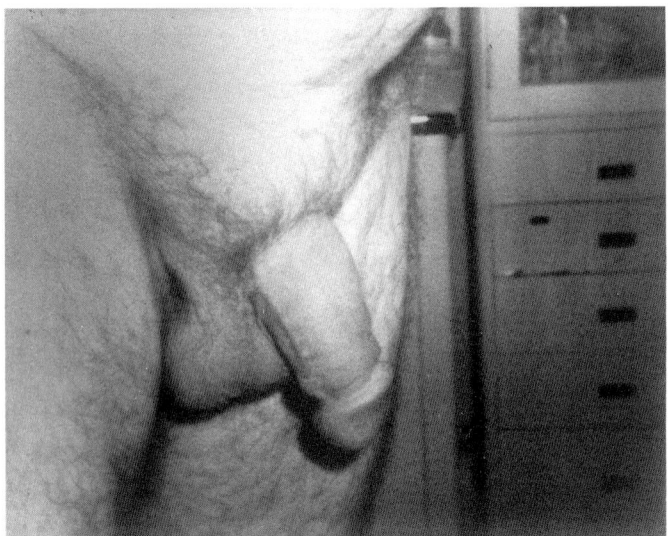

A

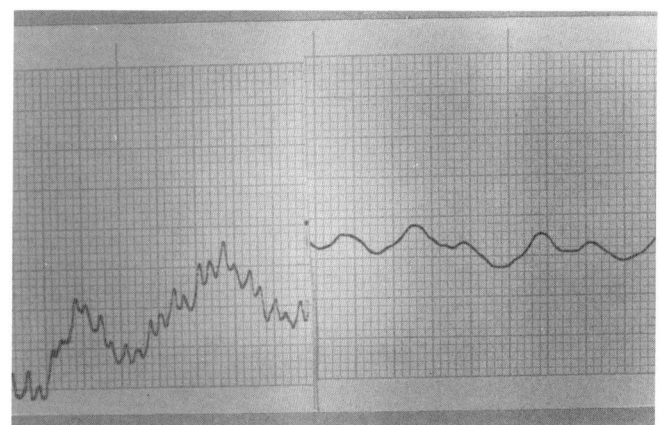

B

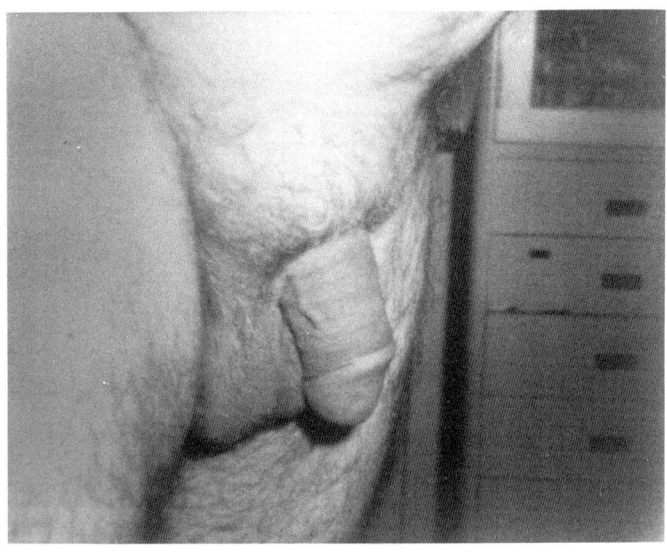

C

FIGURE 30.7. Group III patient—poor injection response. VCD and ring required to complete the erection. (A) Penis in the flaccid state. (B) Pulse volume tracing of the flaccid penis with low amplitude. (C) Partial injection response, tumescence but no rigidity and uplift. (D) Pulse volume tracing indicates partial response with three- to fourfold increase in amplitude. (E) Application of VCD. (F) Erection-like state completed as evidenced by tumescence and rigidity with the ring at the base of the penis.

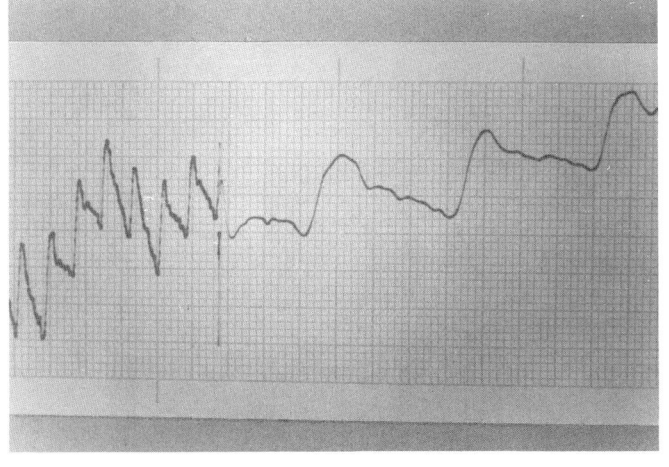

D

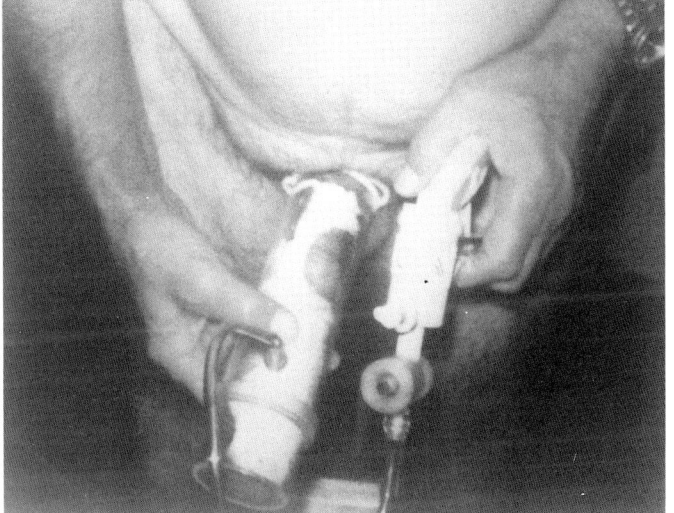

E

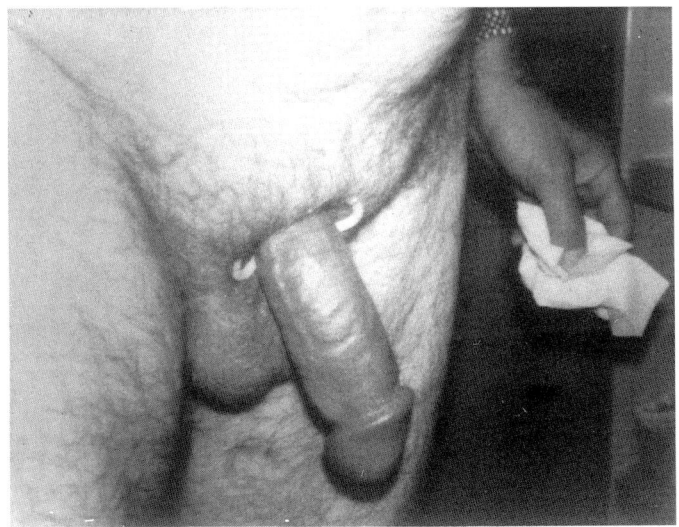

F

Figure 30.7. *Continued*

100 ml/m following an injection of papaverine/phentolamine mesylate. This limited workup is easy to complete and is cost-effective. Within two to three office visits, all patients can be started on a therapeutic program including intracavernous injections and VCD therapy.

## Patient Satisfaction

Because the VCD has become an option for treatment of erectile dysfunction, it is important for clinicians to have a better understanding of patient attitudes and satisfaction regarding the use of these devices. Greater knowledge in this area will help clinicians counsel patients who are considering a VCD and help salvage some patients who intend to drop out when problems arise. Studies suggest that many men are interested in the use of a VCD as an alternative to injections or implants.[8,10] The mean ages from several studies suggest that men who choose a VCD are between 57 to 65 years, which is comparable to the age group of men who choose intracavernous injection therapy.[3,8,10] Although in one study older men were reported to be less satisfied with the VCD than the younger patients,[3] older men in a stable relationship are more apt to use the VCD.

Overall, results from several series suggest that patient satisfaction with a VCD ranges between 67% to 92% among patients who had been sexually inactive for 6 months to greater than 10 years before the use of the VCD, 70% reported improvement in their self-image, 83% indicated a solid relationship with their partners, and 95% stated that they would recommend the device for others.[3,8–10,43,44]

In more recent studies, statistical methods have been used to evaluate patient satisfaction.[43] Studies show statistically significant differences in the following categories: (1) quality of erections and foreplay with vacuum device, (2) quality of erections in intercourse with the device, (3) frequency of intercourse attempts, (4) frequency of orgasm with intercourse, (5) sexual satisfaction, (6) quality of erections in foreplay without the device, and (7) quality of erections in intercourse without the device.[45,46]

There were no statistically significant differences over 6 months for frequency of feelings of sexual desire or frequency of masturbation. These data suggest that the use of a VCD for 6 months can significantly change sexual functioning. In addition, there is improvement regarding self-esteem in the sense of romantic and sexual attractiveness and improvement in social self-confidence, but levels of depression and anxiety are unchanged.

The partner's satisfaction was evaluated in several studies. In one report the male users rated the female partner's satisfaction.[8] The results of these questionnaires suggested that 86% of the females were satisfied by the appearance of the erection, and 87% were satisfied by performance. However, 11% of the men reported that their partners were dissatisfied by the coolness of the erection, the cause for discontinuance in some cases. In another study, 18 women who were sexual partners of VCD users rated their own responses, and this group showed statistically significant improvements in the level of arousal and foreplay with the device, frequency of intercourse attempts, frequency of masturbation, frequency of orgasm with intercourse, and sexual satisfaction.[45] There was no statistically significant increase in the group with regard to frequency of feeling of sexual desire. Nevertheless, like their spouses, the female partners also reported greater satisfaction with love making. After 6 months, the dropout rate with VCDs ranges between 19% to 36%.[3,8–10,43] Although this dropout rate seems comparable to those with intracavernous injections over the same length of follow-up, the reasons for VCD dropouts were reported as inadequate rigidity, pain with the vacuum or constriction ring, coolness of the penis, ecchymosis of the penis, or lack of ejaculation or both. With follow-up instruction and minor adjustments to the equipment, many of these patients may be rescued by VCD therapy. For example, patients may apply additional vacuum to increase rigidity or utilize two rings to improve firmness. Some dropouts simply lose interest or no longer have a stable relationship. On the positive side, some of the dropouts report that they regain spontaneous erections, a distinct advantage of VCD usage.

# Conclusion

During the past decade, the devices and rings have been improved and used on a variety of patients, and the one-time cost of the device is now relatively low compared with that of injection therapy or implants. In addition, physiologic studies on blood flow during constriction suggest that complications are minimal.

## References

1. Witherington R. Suction device therapy in the management of erectile dysfunction. *Urol Clin North Am* 1988; 15:123–128.
2. Aloui R, Lwaz J, Kokkidis J, et al. A new vacuum device as alternative treatment for impotence. *Br J Urol* 1992; 70:652–655.
3. Nadig PW, Ware JC, Blulmoff R. Noninvasive device to produce and maintain an erection-like state. *Urology* 1986; 27:126–131.
4. Snoy FJ, Wagner SA, Woodside JR, et al. Management of penile incarceration. *Urology* 1984; 24:18–20.
5. Stoller ML, Lue TF, McAninch JW. Constrictive penile band injury: anatomical and reconstructive considerations. *J Urol* 1987; 137:740–742.
6. Salvatore FT, Sharman GN, Hellstrom WJG. Vacuum constriction devices and the clinical urologist: an informed selection. *Urology* 1991; 38:323–327.
7. NIH Consensus Conference: Impotence. NIH Consensus Development Panel on Impotence (review). *JAMA* 1993; 83:270.
8. Cookson MS, Nadig PW. Long term results with vacuum constriction device. *J Urol* 1993; 149:290–294.
9. Sidi AA, Becher EF, Zhang G, et al. Patient acceptance of and satisfaction with an external negative pressure device for impotence. *J Urol* 1990; 144:1154–1156.
10. Vrijhof HJEJ, Delaere KPJ. Vacuum constriction devices in erectile dysfunction: acceptance and effectiveness in patients with impotence of organic or mixed etiology. *Br J Urol* 1994; 74:102–105.
11. Marmar JL, DeBenedictis TJ, Praiss DE. The use of a vacuum constrictor device to augment a partial erection following an intracavernous injection. *J Urol* 1988; 140:975–979.
12. Moul JW, McLeod DG. Negative pressure devices in the explanted penile prosthesis population. *J Urol* 1989; 142:729–731.
13. Meinhardt W, Kropman RF, Lycklama AAB, et al. Skin necrosis caused by use of negative pressure device for erectile impotence. *J Urol* 1990; 144:983.
14. Kim JH, Carson CC III. Development of Peyronie's disease with the use of a vacuum constriction device. *J Urol* 1993; 149:1314–1315.
15. Hakim LS, Munnariz RM, Kulaksizoglu H, et al. Vacuum erection associated impotence and Peyronie's disease. *J Urol* 1996; 155:534–535.
16. Diederichs W, Kaula NF, Lue TF, et al. The effect of subatmospheric pressure on the simian penis. *J Urol* 1989; 142:1087–1089.
17. Marmar JL, DeBenedictis TJ, Praiss DE. Penile plethysmography on impotent men using vacuum constrictor devices. *Urology* 1988; 32:198–203.
18. Kedia KR. Penile plethysmography useful in diagnosis of vasculogenic impotence. *Urology* 1983; 22:235–239.
19. Bell D, Lewis R, Kerstein MD. Hyperemic stress test in diagnosis of vasculogenic impotence. *Urology* 1983; 22:611.
20. Broderick GA, McGahan JP, Stone AR, et al. The hemodynamics of vacuum constriction erections: assessment by color Doppler ultrasound. *J Urol* 1992; 147:57–61.
21. Donataucci EF, Lue TF. The effect of chronic external vacuum device usage on cavernous artery function. *Int J Impotence Res* 1992; 4:149–155.
22. Marshall GA, Braze J, Lue TF. Improved hemodynamic response after long term intracavernous injection for impotence. *Urology* 1994; 43:844–848.
23. Rajfer J, Rosciszewski A, Mehringer M. Prevalence of venous leakage in impotent men. *J Urol* 1988; 140:69–71.
24. Fuchs AM, Mehringer CM, Rajfer J. Anatomy of penile venous drainage in potent and impotent men during cavernosography. *J Urol* 1989; 141:1353–1356.
25. Delcour C, Wespes E, Vandenbosch G, et al. Impotence: evaluation with cavernosography. *Radiology* 1986; 161:803–806.
26. Wespes E, Delcour C, Struyven J, et al. Pharmacocavernosometry-cavernosography in impotence. *Br J Urol* 1986; 58:429–433.
27. Meuleman EJ, Diemont WL. Investigation of erectile dysfunction. Diagnostic testing for vascular factors in erectile dysfunction. *Urol Clin North Am* 1995; 22:803–819.
28. Lewis RW. Venous surgery for impotence. *Urol Clin North Am* 1988; 15:115–121.

29. Bookstein JJ, Lurie AL. Selective penile venography: anatomical and hemodynamic observations. *J Urol* 1988; 740:55–60.

30. Lue TF. Treatment of venogenic impotence. In: Tanagho EA, Lue TF, McClure RD eds. *Contemporary Management of Impotence and Infertility*. Baltimore, MD: Williams & Wilkins; 1988: 175–177.

31. Katz PG, Haden HT, Mulligan T, et al. The effect of vacuum devices on penile hemodynamics. *J Urol* 1990; 143:55–56.

32. Bosshardt RJ, Farwerk R, Sikora R, et al. Objective measurement of the effectiveness, therapeutic success and dynamic mechanisms of the vacuum device. *Br J Urol* 1995; 75:786–791.

33. Blackard CE, Borkon WD, Lima JS, et al. Use of vacuum tumescence device for impotence secondary to venous leakage. *Urology* 1993; 41:225–230.

34. Kolletis PN, Lakin MM, Montague DK, et al. Efficacy of the vacuum constriction device in patients with corporeal venous occlusive dysfunction. *Urology* 1995; 46:856–858.

35. Wein AJ, Fishkin R, Carpinetio VL, et al. Expansion without significant rigidity during penile tumescence testing: a potential source of misinterpretation. *J Urol* 1981; 126:343–344.

36. Karacan I, Howell JW. Use of nocturnal penile tumescence in diagnosis of male erectile dysfunction. In: Tangho EA, Lue TF, McClure RD, eds. *Contemporary Management of Impotence and Infertility*. Baltimore, MD: Williams & Wilkins; 1988: 95–103.

37. Kessler WO. Nocturnal penile tumescence. *Urol Clin North Am* 1988; 15:81–86.

38. Chancellor MB, Rivas DA, Panzer DE, et al. Prospective comparison of topical minoxidil to vacuum constriction device and intracorporeal papaverine injection in treatment of erectile dysfunction due to spinal cord injury. *Urology* 1994; 43:365–369.

39. Broderick GA, Allen G, McClure RD. Vacuum tumescence devices: the role of papaverine in selection of patients. *J Urol* 1991; 145:284–286.

40. Dow JA, Gluck RW, Golimbu M, et al. Multiphase diagnostic evaluation of arteriogenic, venogenic and sinusoidogenic impotency. Value of noninvasive tests compared with penile duplex ultrasonography. *Urology* 1991; 38:402–407.

41. Montrosi F, Guazzoni G, Barbieri L, et al. The effect of intracorporeal injection plus genital and audio visual sexual stimulation versus second injection on penile color Doppler sonography parameters. *J Urol* 1996; 155:536–540.

42. Meuleman EJH, Wijkstra H, Doesburg WH, et al. Comparison of the diagnostic value of pump and gravity cavernosometry in the evaluation of the cavernous venoocclusive mechanism. *J Urol* 1991; 146:1266–1270.

43. Baltaci S, Aydos K, Kosar A, et al. Treating erectile dysfunction with a vacuum tumescence device: a retrospective analysis of acceptance and satisfaction. *Br J Urol* 1995; 76:757–760.

44. Witherington R. Vacuum constriction device for management of erectile dysfunction. *J Urol* 1989; 141:320–322.

45. Turner LA, Althof SE, Levine SB, et al. Treating erectile dysfunction with external vacuum devices: impact on sexual, psychological and marital functioning. *J Urol* 1990; 144:79–82.

46. Turner LA, Althof SE, Levine SB, et al. External vacuum devices in the treatment of erectile dysfunction: a one-year study of sexual and psychosocial impact. *J Sex Marital Ther* 1991; 17:81–93.

# 31
# Nitric Oxide and Other Neurotransmitters of the Corpus Cavernosum

Nestor F. Gonzalez-Cadavid and Jacob Rajfer

The physiology of erection comprises three distinct processes acting in concert: (1) increased arterial inflow, (2) active cavernosal smooth-muscle relaxation, and (3) decreased venous outflow. Cavernosal smooth-muscle relaxation appears to be the key event in a normal erection. Therefore, the cavernosal smooth muscle may be the critical site where erectile dysfunction begins.[1]

In a normal erection, the neural stimulation is transmitted to the penile tissues through the pelvic autonomic nerve fibers, the nervi erigentes. These nerves release three important neurotransmitters: (1) the sympathetic fibers release norepinephrine; (2) the parasympathetic fibers release acetylcholine; and (3) the nonadrenergic-noncholinergic (NANC) release nitric oxide (NO).

Evidence accumulated in the past 7 years shows that NO is the main mediator of penile erection in man and in experimental animals as well. It is considered the most likely NANC neurotransmitter released as a consequence of sexual stimulation triggering the relaxation of the corporal smooth muscle.

NO is synthesized in a variety of tissues and organs in a reaction where the amino acid L-arginine is converted into L-citrulline. The enzyme catalyzing this reaction is designated as nitric oxide synthase (NOS) and exists as three different isoforms: the constitutive neuronal and endothelial NOS (nNOS or NOS 1, and eNOS or NOS 3, respectively), and the inducible NOS (iNOS or NOS 2). Recent reviews have described the multiple roles of NO in biologic processes,[2-4] the features of NOS isoforms,[5] the potential therapeutic applications of NOS inhibitors,[6] and the physiopathologic significance of alterations of NO synthesis.[7] Other reviews have focused on the specific role of NO in the regulation of vascular tone,[8,9] neurotransmission,[10,11] and NO as the primary mediator of the erectile response in animal models and in in vitro systems.[12-15]

It is clear from the initial work carried out in the peripheral vascular tree, and confirmed in penile tissue, that NO released by NOS activation stimulates guanyl cyclase in the cavernosal smooth muscle, increasing cyclic guanosine monophosphate (cGMP), and thus reducing intracellular $Ca^{2+}$. This triggers smooth-muscle relaxation and blood inflow into the cavernosal cisternae, thereby eliciting penile erection.[1]

## Evidence of the Role of NO in Erection from In Vitro Studies on the Relaxation of Corpora Cavernosa Strips

The first demonstration that penile erection is mediated by NO generated in response to NANC neurotransmission was published in 1990.[16] This demonstration used electrical field stimulation (EFS) of isolated strips of rabbit corpus cavernosum in the presence of both guanethidine (an adrenergic neuronal blocker) and atropine (a muscarinic receptor blocker). The EFS-induced relaxation of the corporal smooth muscle was accompanied by an increase in nitrites and cGMP. Ignarro and colleagues[16] correctly inferred that this increase was due to NO synthesis that stimulated guanyl cyclase. Similarly, this outcome had previously been shown for vascular smooth muscle.

The blockade of the relaxation of the penile strips by NOS inhibitors, e.g., $N^G$-nitro-L-arginine (L-NOARG) or $N^G$-amino-L-arginine (L-NMMA), and the stereospecific reversal of this blockade by excess substrate (L-arginine) proved that NOS activity was necessary for this process. Additional support was obtained from the inhibition of the relaxation by oxyhemoglobin (NO scavenger) or methylene blue (guanyl cyclase inhibitor), and the independence from the cycloxygenase pathway was indicated by the lack of effect of indomethacin. This experimental paradigm was repeated in subsequent studies.

The rabbit penile strip preparation has been extensively used to further characterize the NO-dependence of corporal relaxation. EFS is not essential to induce this process, because L-phenylepinephrine–precontracted strips can be relaxed with acetylcholine. This effect can be abolished with L-NMMA, L-NOARG, methylene blue, or atropine, as expected from NO released from the corporal endothelium by acetylcholine. A nitrodonor, like sodium nitroprusside (SNP), directly relaxed the precontracted strips.[17] Hypoxia or endothelial damage blocked the NO-dependent relaxation mediated by acetylcholine,[18] but when EFS was applied, a functional endothelium was not necessary, thus confirming that NO may act in the penis both as a neurotransmitter and as a vasodilator released from the endothelium. The latter is in agreement with the previous demonstration in the vascular system[7-9] that NO is the main active component of EDRF (endothelium-derived relaxing factor).

Several groups have shown that the human corpora cavernosa reacts identically to the rabbit preparation,[18-21] and it has been proposed that NO or a closely related substance may act as the NANC neurotransmitter in the human corpus cavernosum smooth muscle. EFS evokes an atropine-resistant relaxation of guanethidine-treated human penile strips that can be inhibited by the sodium channel blocker tetrodotoxin and by NO-cascade inhibitors, reversed with L-arginine, and enhanced by a cGMP phosphodiesterase inhibitor. Comparing the relaxation of corporal cavernosal strips from both species,[22] a positive correlation was found between relaxation and cGMP formation.

These results support the hypothesis that endogenous NO is the principal mediator of penile erection caused by NANC stimulation, triggering a cGMP-mediated signal transduction mechanism. The role of the endothelium was ascertained by chemically removing it from rabbit corporal cavernosal strips, and comparing the response with the intact rabbit and human preparations.[23] The relaxation due to acetylcholine, bradykinin, and substance P is endothelium-dependent and due to NO release, whereas the relaxation due to papaverine and nitroprusside is endothelium-independent and that to vasoactive intestinal peptide (VIP) is only partially endothelium-dependent/NO-mediated. The EFS of rabbit cavernous smooth muscle in the presence or absence of muscarinic receptor blockade[24,25] showed that this receptor mediates a small fraction of the response. In the case of human corporal strips obtained from impotent patients with diabetes mellitus,[25] the relaxant effects by acetylcholine or EFS appeared to be significantly less than in strips from men who were nondiabetic and impotent.

The penile strip preparations have also been used to examine the modulation of the NO pathway, the relaxant response in relation to impotence risk factors, and other features, including the dose-curve relaxation effects of NO itself, NO donors, and a phosphodiesterase inhibitor.[26-28] Surprisingly, there was little correlation between the ability to release NO and the levels of cGMP or the relaxant efficacy. The active parts (ginsenosides) of a plant popularly used as an aphrodisiac have been shown to increase the acetylcholine- and EFS-induced relaxation in a process attenuated by NOS inhibitors and accompanied by the increase of cGMP.[29]

The relative contribution of NO, adrenergic, purinergic, and cholinergic stimulation in the relaxant response to EFS has recently been studied with rabbit corpus cavernosum strips.[30] It was concluded that virtually all the inhibitory effects of EFS relaxation could be explained by NO release. The NO-dependent relaxation has also been shown in strips of canine corpus cavernosum,[31] where neurogenic VIP and acetylcholine do not seem to participate in the regulation of penile muscle tone under the experimental conditions used for the study.

# Evidence for the Role of NO in Erection from the Study of the Erectile Response in Animal Models

The confirmation that NO is the mediator of penile erection in vivo derives from experiments in animal models, where the erectile response is elicited by EFS of the cavernosal nerve. NOS inhibitors are applied to determine to what extent the increase in intracavernosal pressure is attenuated. In some cases, the EFS response is compared with pharmacologically elicited erection. Using this approach, Holmquist et al[32] showed that in the rabbit intrapenile administration of L-NOARG abolished the EFS-induced erectile response, but the D-isomer had no effect. This indicated that penile erection triggered by stimulation of the cavernosal nerve is as dependent on the NO cascade as on the in vitro relaxation of cavernosal strips.

This finding was expanded in a series of papers in which essentially the same approach was used in the rat, an animal originally proposed as a model for the study of penile erection by Quinlan et al[33] as a substitute for rabbits, dogs, and cats. The cumbersome measurements of the erectile response by video imaging were replaced by the recording of the intracavernosal pressure, as in larger animals. This procedure was used to demonstrate that another NOS inhibitor, $N^\omega$-intro-L-arginine methyl ester (L-NAME), blocks the erectile response to EFS in a dose-dependent fashion,[34] and that L-arginine, but not D-arginine, partially prevents the erectile inhibition. The con-

tinuous intrajugular infusion of L-NOARG followed or not by L-arginine during EFS[35] replicated these results.

## EFS Response in the Rat Model

The fundamental role of the NO-cGMP cascade was shown in the rat model by the reduction of the EFS response caused by intracavernosal injection of methylene blue and by its stimulation elicited by cGMP.[36] Sodium nitroprusside caused a similar increase that was blocked by methylene blue. As expected, injection of a phosphodiesterase inhibitor, papaverine, that bypasses the NO-cGMP cascade elicited a corporal relaxation that was not affected by methylene blue. The cAMP pathway was shown not to contribute to the EFS response, because neither cAMP nor drugs that stimulate its synthesis induced an erectile response. These drugs included VIP, prostaglandin $E_1$ ($PGE_1$), and calcitonin gene-related peptide (CGRP). In rats whose cortical-spinal tract was interrupted by pithing[37] and nerve stimulation was sacral rather than cavernosal, the NO-dependence of the erectile response was confirmed by a dose-related inhibition by L-NAME, which did not affect the response to papaverine.

The dose-dependent inhibition of the EFS response by L-NAME has been used to assess how impotence risk factors affect NO-dependent erection.[38,39] The rat model of penile erection has been extensively characterized recently in terms of the EFS and pharmacologic parameters, including the study of a putative NANC sympathetic control different from norepinephrine.[40,41] Therefore, this animal is perhaps the most adequate laboratory model to study the mechanism of NO-dependent erectile response and the factors that affect its function.

## EFS Response in the Dog and Cat Models

The dog has also been used for EFS studies of the NO cascade. A NO donor (S-nitroso-N-acetylpenicillamine) induced a tumescence comparable to the one achieved by EFS, and the latter was blocked by L-NOARG and restored by L-arginine. The response was inhibited by methylene blue and enhanced by a phosphodiesterase inhibitor, as expected.[42] The destruction of the penile endothelium by intracavernosal injection of the detergent 3-[(3-cholamiclopropyl)-dimethylammonia]-1 propane sulfonate (CHAPS) abolished the response to acetylcholine but only partially inhibited the response to EFS. This indicates that the NOS contained in the cavernosal nerve plays a major role in penile erection and the endothelium is less important.[43] The significance of the NO-cGMP cascade previously shown in the rat was also confirmed in the dog, because intracavernosal cGMP was much more efficient than cyclic adenosine monophosphate (cAMP) in eliciting erection. N-ethylmalimide (an adenylate cyclase inhibitor) could not block the EFS response, whereas methylene blue was very effective. In contrast to the results in vitro, atropine reduced the EFS response, suggesting that cholinergic neuroeffectors complement the NANC NO neurotransmission. In cats, L-NAME blocks the acetylcholine-elicited penile erection, and NO donors are effective in inducing it.[44]

## Pharmacologic Agents

An alternative to the EFS approach, applied only in rats, is the use of a centrally evoked erection with pharmacologic agents. One widely used effector is apomorphine, which induces a dual response of erections and yawning.[45] Both of these effects produced by apomorphine (subcutaneous) or oxytocin (intracerebroventricular) were inhibited by L-NAME or L-NMMA, given either systemically or centrally,[46] suggesting the involvement of central NO in erection. The effects were located at the paraventricular nucleus of the hypothalamus by inducing an erectile response with N-methyl-D-aspartic acid (NMDA) and blocking with NOS inhibitors.[47] The apomorphine-induced model of erection has been compared with the EFS-induced model and found useful for the study of psychogenic

erectile reflexes.[48] However, because this is a centrally oriented approach, it is not focused on penile erectile physiology, and is therefore not adequate for studying NO involvement in the penis per se.

## Inhibition of NO Synthesis

The effects of the inhibition of NO synthesis by giving L-NAME systemically before tests of copulation, ex-copula genital reflexes, or sexual motivation/motor activity[49] seem to emphasize the direct role of NO in the penile erectile response over its putative participation in the central control of sexual behavior. Neither sexual motivation nor motor activity was affected, but copulation was clearly impaired, primarily by inhibiting erectile function. This study is the first direct proof of the role of NO in physiologic erection and also suggests that NO inhibits the sympathetic control of ejaculation, because L-NAME increased the number of seminal emissions and decreased their latency.

# Detection, Localization, and Function of NOS Isoforms in the Penis

The first demonstration of the presence of an NOS isoform in the penile corpora cavernosa was obtained simultaneously in the rabbit[50] and in the rat penis.[34] In both cases, NOS enzymatic activity was measured in the cytosol by the conversion of L-arginine into L-citrulline. It was shown to be $Ca^{2+}$-, reduced nicotinamide adenine dinucleotide phosphate (NADPH)-, and calmodulin-dependent, and abolished by NOS inhibitors. This is consistent with the presence of a constitutive NOS isoform.

At least a fraction of the penile constitutive NOS activity in the rat is the nNOS isoform, as shown by immunocytochemistry using antibodies directed against the rat cerebellar nNOS.[34] The nNOS protein was localized to penile neurons innervating the corpora cavernosa and neuronal plexuses in the adventitial layer of penile arteries, as well as in the urethra.

A similar conclusion was reached by NADPH diaphorase staining of the rat major pelvic ganglion (MPG), many axons of the cavernosal nerve, and terminals associated with various tissues of the penis.[51,52] The NADPH diaphorase staining colocalizes with NOS[52,53] and can be considered in most cases as a fair, but not absolute, indicator of NOS activity.

With diaphorase staining, it was possible to estimate that nearly all the postganglionic neurons in the MPG innervating the penis are NADPH diaphorase-positive. However, only one fifth of the penile neurons were immunoreactive against nNOS antibodies.[54] This suggests that either NADPH diaphorase staining may occur in non–NOS-containing nerves or that in the penis there are substantial amounts of NOS isoforms that do not cross-react with nNOS antibodies.

Similar conclusions regarding the predominance of NADPH diaphorase-positive nerves in the MPG were obtained by other groups,[55,56] and NOS was found to colocalize with VIP nerves in the rat MPG and penis.[57,58] By applying retrograde axonal techniques and NOS and choline acetyltransferase immunochemistry,[59] the NOS-containing neuronal populations were located within the lumbosacral spinal cord at the L5 to S2 segments of the sacral parasympathetic nucleus. The NANC NOS fibers in the cavernosal nerve regenerate after unilateral neurotomy,[60] supporting the view that unilateral nerve-sparing in humans may preserve erectile function.

The combination of NADPH diaphorase staining and immunocytochemistry allowed the confirmation that NO is the neuronal mediator of penile erection in man, because NOS was identified in discrete neuronal locations of the penis, including the pelvic plexus and the cavernous and dorsal nerves with their terminals.[61,62] NADPH diaphorase staining has been proposed as a diagnostic tool for neurogenic impotence due to cavernous nerve damage.[63] Using this technique, it was shown that NOS coexists in the human penis with VIP terminals in 40% of the cases, and to a lesser degree with tyrosine hydroxylase, an enzyme contained in catecholaminergic nerves.[64,65]

It appears that no publications report the immunocytochemical detection of NOS isoforms other than nNOS in the penis from any species. This is surprising, considering that the initial idea of NO being the mediator of penile erection stemmed from the role of NO present in EDRF as modulator of vascular tone and that an endothelium lining is spread throughout the corpora cavernosa. However, there are no claims on the visualization of either eNOS or iNOS in penile sections, despite the variety of specific polyclonal or monoclonal antibodies available.

It is clear, then, that NOS activity is detectable in the rat penile cytosol (arginine-citrulline conversion assay) and in situ in nerves and nerve terminals of the rat and human penis (NADPH diaphorase). In fact, nNOS is the only isoform so far visualized by immunocytochemistry in those locations in both species. By applying the original L-arginine/citrulline procedure used for rat cerebellum,[66] it was shown that the adult rat penis has a level of soluble L-NAME- and ethyleneglycotetraacetic acid (EGTA)-sensitive NOS activity[38,67] comparable to that found in the rabbit penis[50] and much higher than the one initially reported for the rat penis.[34] This was confirmed in several studies with three different strains of rats.[67–73]

Because the arginine/citrulline conversion assay does not discriminate between NOS isoforms, and because the immunocytochemical evidence on penile NOS is restricted to nNOS, the question of which other NOS isoforms are expressed in this organ was addressed by use of Western blot immunodetection. Using this assay with both polyclonal and monoclonal antibodies, a typical 150- to 160-kd nNOS band[39,68–76] can be detected in the rat penis and pelvic plexus cytosol. The Western blot technique demonstrated the eNOS species in both the cytosol and the particulate fractions as the expected 140-kd band, although only one of the monoclonal antibodies tested was effective.[71–75] This suggests that eNOS is a minor fraction of the total penile NOS. The iNOS isoform appears not to be expressed constitutively in the penis, because it is visualized only erratically in the rat penis cytosol as the typical 130-kd band.[74] It is indeed expressed in vitro in incubations of rat penile smooth muscle cells (RPSMC) and of pelvic plexus slices with iNOS inducers.[75]

No NOS isoforms have been reported in Northern blot analysis of penile tissue messenger RNA (mRNA), with the exception of iNOS mRNA in RPSMC induced in vitro.[77] They are, however, detectable by reverse transcription/polymerase chain reaction assays (Magee, Marquez, Garban et al., unpublished data). No NOS protein, mRNA, or enzyme activity data on human penile tissue have been published to date.

In the absence of functional direct assays, it is impossible to determine which NOS isoform is really the one responsible for penile erection. Although the evidence suggests that nNOS is the one involved in the triggering of the erectile process, the development of the first NOS-deficient transgenic mouse ("gene knockout" mice) seems to cast doubt on this hypothesis. The male animals whose nNOS gene is silenced by targeted disruption[78] are not only fertile, and therefore potent, but are even very sexually aggressive.[79]

Because the eNOS[80] and iNOS-deficient mice[81,82] are also potent, the reproduction of the knockout animals would appear to rule out all known NOS isoforms as major contributors to penile erection, contradicting the substantial experimental work that supports their role. However, two main arguments stand against the negative interpretation. First, it is likely that ancillary mechanisms may develop to compensate for the knockout gene, as it happens in most gene deficient mice when the disrupted gene is crucial for individual or species survival. In the case of the nNOS knockout, eNOS has been assumed to substitute for nNOS in the same neurons where both coexist,[83,84] or, alternatively, non-NO neurotransmitters and vasodilators may take over.[78] A second argument is that penile-specific variants of the known NOS isoforms may exist and differ in the gene regions used to target the disruption. Should this be the case, the penile specific NOS gene would remain operative in the currently available NOS-deficient mice.

## Impotence Risk Factors Affect the Regulation of Penile Erection and NOS Isoforms

Hypogonadism in man is associated with impotence assumed to result from a loss of libido rather than from the impairment of the erectile mechanism per se. The rat model of penile erection has provided a different interpretation that may be applicable to man.

Androgen depletion in the rat induced by castration for 1 week reduced the erectile response to EFS or to apomorphine, and these effects were prevented by testosterone (T)[35,67,76,85,86] or dihydrotestosterone (DHT)[67] administration. Although the castration-induced reduction is only 50%, when it is combined with the androgen-blocker flutamide the inhibition is nearly complete.[70,71] DHT appears to be the active androgen in maintaining erectile function, as shown by the inability of T in the presence of finasteride to prevent the castration-associated erectile dysfunction.[67]

Pituitary and adrenal factors are also essential. Hypophysectomy,[70,71] administration of a gonadotropin-releasing hormone (GnRH) antagonist,[70,71] and adrenalectomy[73] impair erection to different degrees. The combination of castration and adrenalectomy blocks the erectile response completely but can be partially prevented by replacement androgen or corticosteroid therapy or both.[73] The erectile response in the rat probably requires a low basal level of androgen receptor activation, because androgen receptor concentration is very low in the adult penis.[87] This would explain why residual amounts of serum androgens in castrated rats suffice to maintain half of the normal erection. Several constituents may exist in the erectile machinery with different degrees of androgen dependence. One is the bulbocavernosus and bulbospongiosus striated muscles that participate in the erectile response,[67,70,71] and another is penile NOS itself.

The obliteration of androgen and corticoid effects by androgen depletion, hypophysectomy, GnRH antagonist, or adrenalectomy considerably reduces penile NOS activity

TABLE 31.1. Control of penile erectile function and nitric oxide synthase by the gonadal/adrenal/pituitary/hypothalamic axis in the rat (one-week treatment).

| | | NOS | |
|---|---|---|---|
| Treatment | EFS Response | Activity | Content |
| Castration alone | ↓ | ↓ | = |
| Castration and flutamide | ↓↓ | ↓ | = |
| Castration and testosterone | = | = | |
| Castration and T and finasteride | ↓ | ↓ | |
| Castration and DHT | = | = | |
| Castration and estradiol | ↓↓ | ↓ | |
| Castration and EFS | NA | = | = |
| Hypophysectomy | ↓↓ | ↓↓ | = |
| GnRH antagonist | ↓ | ↓ | = |
| Adrenalectomy | ↓ | ↓ | = |
| Castration and adrenalectomy (C/A) | ↓↓ | ↓↓ | ↓ |
| C/A and DHT | =/↓ | | = |
| C/A and hydrocortisone and aldosterone | =/↓ | | = |
| C/A and hydrocortisone | =/↓ | | |
| C/A and aldosterone | =/↓ | | |

without significantly decreasing penile nNOS or eNOS content[69–71,73] by an as yet unidentified mechanism of enzyme activity control (Table 31.1). However, one study reported a castration-induced reduction of penile nNOS.[76] That NOS activity can be modulated in the penis was directly demonstrated in castrated rats by EFS of the cavernosal nerve, which is able by itself to stimulate penile NOS during the erectile response and raise the activity to levels found in the intact rat. This process resembles the activation of NO synthesis that is thought to occur upon sexual stimulation.[69] EFS of human penile corpus cavernosum and urethra in organ bath causes release of nitrites and nitrates derived from NO synthesis.[62]

It is likely that NOS enzyme activation in the penile tissue follows the pattern observed in other tissues or cells, due either to the opening of $Ca^{2+}$ channels increasing $Ca^{2+}$ binding at the calmodulin site or to dephosphorylation of an inactive phosphorylated NOS.[2–5,12] Alternatively, variations in the L-arginine substrate availability may also influence penile NOS activity. Long-term feeding of rats with L-arginine increases the EFS erectile response,[88] thus suggesting that local substrate concentration may become, in certain conditions, a rate-limiting step for NOS activity. Some of these factors may be involved in the negative control of NOS activity that can be observed in in vitro incubations of rat penile or pelvic plexus slices, or in induced RPSMC. In most cases, NOS remains inhibited, because nitrite synthesis is low and does not correlate with the amount of active NOS protein after tissue homogenization.[75]

An important factor in the modulation of penile NOS activity may be oxygen tension because NOS is an oxygenase. Intracavernosal blood $pO_2$ in the flaccid human penis is three- to fourfold lower than that in the erect stage. When these conditions were reproduced in organ bath of human corpora cavernosa strips, the EFS and acetylcholine NO-mediated responses (relaxation, cGMP synthesis, cytosol NOS activity) were inhibited by $O_2$ depletion and reverted by reoxygenation.[89] A subsequent study[90] showed that severe hypoxia of the type developed in the veno-occlusive priapism causes an increase of penile intracellular $Ca^{2+}$ and relaxation in rabbit corpora cavernosa strips, putatively due to inhibition of oxidative phosphorylation. Although this may apply to priapism, it does not address the question of the hypothetical NOS activation by $O^{2+}$ during physiologic erection.

TABLE 31.2. Effect of impotence risk factors on penile erectile function and nitric oxide synthase in the rat long-term conditions (2–25 months).

| Condition or Treatment | EFS Response | Penile Reflexes | NOS Activity | NOS Content |
|---|---|---|---|---|
| Aging, old | ↓ | | = | |
| Aging, old and T | = | | = | |
| Aging, old and DHT | = | | = | |
| Aging, very old | ↓↓ | | ↓↓ | |
| Diabetes Type I | = | ↓↓ | ↓↓ | ↓ |
| Diabetes Type II | = | ↓↓ | ↓↓ | ↓ |
| Passive smoking | ↑ | | ↓↓ | ↓ |
| Passive smoking and aging, old | ↑ | | ↓↓ | ↓ |
| Severe hypertension | ↓ | | | |

## Aging

Aging, another impotence-associated risk factor, has been found in the rat model[38] to be accompanied by a decrease in erectile response and, in very old animals only, by a reduction of penile NOS activity (Table 31.2). These changes occur in parallel with a reduction in the tissue compliance to vasoactive relaxant agents, in both old and very old rats; in the former group, the normal penile NO synthesis appears to be insufficient to compensate for the loss of penile compliance. No data are available on the content of penile nNOS and eNOS at these ages. Because aged rats are hypogonadal, a long-term administration of T and DHT was tested in old rats and shown to correct the decrease in erectile response.[39] However, this occurs without modifying penile NOS activity or nNOS content.

## Diabetes

Diabetes in man is a significant risk factor for erectile dysfunction. The spontaneously diabetic animals, BB and BBZ rats, are good models for diabetes type I and II, respectively. In both cases, hypogonadism and a severe loss of penile reflexes are present, but the erectile response to EFS is not affected.[68,74] This suggests a peripheral neuropathy in the penis occurring without compromise of the cavernosal nerve, accompanied by a depletion of both penile nNOS content and NOS activity, but not of VIP,[68,74] which suggests a selective loss of penile nerve terminals. Studies on the con-

tent of penile eNOS in the diabetic rats are in progress. However, a recent report on a chemically induced diabetes rat model (streptozotocin) claimed an increase in penile NOS activity.[91]

## Other Risk Factors

Chronic passive smoking[72] and radiation exposure,[92] two other conditions associated with impotence, were found in the rat model to be accompanied by a decrease of penile NOS activity. In the case of smoking, penile nNOS, but not eNOS or VIP, was reduced, suggesting a neuropathy similar to the one present in diabetes. The lack of effects on eNOS is probably related to the fact that the rat is refractory to vascular damage.[93] Surprisingly, despite the decrease in penile NOS and the severe hypertension, the EFS erectile response is not reduced by chronic passive smoking. This lack of reduction may be related to the development of NO-triggered (L-NAME–sensitive) ancillary vasodilator mechanisms in the penis during the long-term exposure to tobacco smoke. Severe hypertension impairs the erectile response in the spontaneously hypertensive (SHR) rat but moderate increase in blood pressure augments erectile response.[94]

The reduction of penile nNOS found in diabetes and smoking in the rat is likely to be a direct result of the loss of nerve terminals, but a downregulation of gene expression cannot be ruled out, despite the fact that nNOS was initially considered a "constitutive" enzyme. Recent evidence in other systems indicates that this is possible,[95,96] and suggests that upregulation of penile nNOS may occur under certain conditions. Should this be the case, it may provide a mechanism to compensate for penile nerve damage by increasing NO release from the spared nerves.

The experimental data accumulated on penile NOS in the rat model may not be directly applicable to the human and may even appear to conflict with clinical evidence in certain cases. It is necessary to investigate in men whether penile NOS is similarly affected by impotence risk factors, although the difficulty in obtaining penile tissue for analysis from adequate control subjects may be an impediment. The measurement of NO synthesis through a noninvasive procedure during erection would be an ideal approach. Unfortunately, the basal level of serum nitrites is high enough to hide the small changes that may occur in nitrite concentration in the corporal blood during the erectile response,[97] and NO chemical sensors are not sensitive enough to monitor NOS activity in the penis in situ.

## Therapy of Erectile Dysfunction Based on NO and Ancillary Penile Neurotransmitters

The NO-dependent cascade is the main functional pathway responsible for penile erection, and NO as the NANC neurotransmitter elicits this process. This conclusion is essentially based on the presence of the NO-relaxation mechanism in the human and animal corpora cavernosa, and particularly on the complete elimination of the erectile response in animals by NOS inhibitors. The latter blockade occurs in rats not only when L-NAME is given in acute doses but even after a long-term oral administration leading to sustained systemic hypertension (Moody, Rajfer, Gonzalez-Cadavid, unpublished data). Therefore, the release of NO from the penile nerve terminals must be a necessary condition for sexual stimulation to lead to cavernosal smooth-muscle relaxation, even if this involves other ancillary neurotransmitters.

Because non-NO neurotransmitters are present in the corpora cavernosa, they seem to fulfill a physiologic function, but it is reduced to a reinforcement of the NO-initiated erection while there is sufficient NO synthesis in the penis to maintain an erection. However, it is possible that under long-term conditions where NO synthesis is severely reduced, the ancillary neurotransmitters may start to play a more significant role in the development of compensatory mechanisms. This would include some of the impotence risk factors defined in the rat model and in the NOS knockout mice.

The identity of these ancillary neurotransmitters cannot be ascertained with the available evidence, but two stand as the most likely: VIP[98–105] and CGRP.[106–109] Considerable data are available on the presence of VIP and CGRP nerve fibers and on the measurable levels of these peptides in the human and the animal penis and on their relaxing effects on the corpora cavernosa both in vitro and in vivo. They act via the activation of the cAMP cascade and, at least in the case of CGRP and possibly VIP, may contribute to NO synthesis. However, their in vivo effects are partial and not very reproducible, and their contents in the penis do not correlate with erectile dysfunction. Their use as single vasodilators in the treatment of erectile dysfunction is not promising, and most trials have been limited to combination modalities with $PGE_1$ and other vasoactive agents.[103,108,109]

Relaxants, such as endothelial kinins,[110] are not neurotransmitters, and the same applies to the complex array of vasoconstrictors that regulate penile vascular tone, mainly endothelins.[111–113] Leaving aside acetylcholine, which triggers endothelial NO release, the other known penile neurotransmitters, such as norepinephrine,[111,114] act on $\alpha_1$-adrenergic receptors and control the detumescence. Although psychogenic impotence is probably associated with their hyperproduction, they are negative modulators of the erectile response not directly involved in its activation.

Therefore, the NO cascade appears to be the most logical target for a new therapy aimed at correcting erectile dysfunction through manipulation of the levels of penile neurotransmitters. Unfortunately, the approaches reported so far have focused mainly on the administration of NO-donors or cGMP. These are not novel concepts, because these drugs are vasoactive substances within the same category as the current ones in use (papaverine, $PGE_1$, phentolamine). Perhaps for this reason results have not shown a convincing improvement over the existing pharmacotherapy.

Two NO donors have been tested in humans: linsidomide chlorhydrate[113–116] and sodium nitroprusside.[119,120] The first compound (3-morpholinosidomine hydroaldehyde (SIN-1) was injected intracavernously in 63 patients, inducing a dose-dependent erectile response, with 46% of the patients experiencing a full erection and no side effects.[115] However, the overall result was not significantly better than with the papaverine/phentolamine mixture, except possibly for cost. The same conclusions were achieved in a larger study.[116] In one report focused on patients with venous leakage,[117] and in another with patients with erectile failure due to different causes,[118] SIN-1 was not superior to $PGE_1$. In the case of nitroprusside, the trial was discontinued because of severe hypotension and only mild penile tumescence.[119] In another study, nitroprusside was not better than $PGE_1$, except for absence of local pain and faster detumescence after orgasm.[120] It has also been tested in primates,[121–123] inducing a good erection with some systemic hypotension, and in dogs[123] and cats[104] with approximately the same results. However, in rats it is not very effective and induces hypotension.[123] The intracavernosal administration of cGMP to 15 patients induced an erection in 13 of the patients that was shorter than with the standard vasoactive mixture.[124]

In contrast to a conventional approach based on the direct administration of NO releasers or compounds downstream in the NO-cGMP cascade, the biologic modulation of the neurotransmission process itself may prove to be more physiologic and effective in the treatment of erectile dysfunction. The ultimate goal is to functionally modify the corpora cavernosa so that the neurotransmitters are synthesized physiologically during sexual stimulation rather than to depend on the direct intracorporeal injection of vasodilators, NO/cGMP-related or otherwise.

A simple alternative may be the stimulation of a diminished NOS activity by the administration of substrate or cofactors. This approach would be successful only if rate limiting in the corpora cavernosa, which may be the case under certain conditions. The investigation of how NOS activity is modulated in the penis will require biochemical and molecular biology studies that may eventually result in the discovery of either penile-specific NOS isoforms or regulatory factors. This is not implausible considering that the NO-cascade in the penis fulfills a fundamental role for the maintenance of the species that far exceeds the significance of individual survival. This approach, combined with procedures for local targeting to the penis, may achieve the objective of activating an inhibited or reduced penile NOS enzyme. The same rationale may be applied to the manipulation of non-NO penile relaxation pathways, in order to amplify the NO-mediated signal and counteract a possible loss of penile compliance in erectile dysfunction.[38]

*Acknowledgments.* Our work was funded in part with grants to N.G.C. from the Tobacco Related Disease Research Program, American Diabetes Association, American Federation of Aging Research, and Nirec, Inc.

# References

1. Saenz de Tejada I. Mechanisms for the regulation of penile smooth muscle contractility. In: Lue T, ed. *World Book of Impotence*. Nishimura, London: Smith Gordon; 1992: 264–292.

2. Moncada S, Higgs A. The L-arginine-nitric oxide pathway. *N Engl J Med* 1993; 329:2002–2012.

3. Lowenstein CHJ, Dinerman JL, Snyder SH. Nitric oxide: a physiologic messenger. *Ann Intern Med* 1994; 120:227–237.

4. Murad F. The nitric oxide-cyclic GMP signal transduction system for intracellular and intercellular communication. *Recent Prog Horm Res* 1994; 49:239–248.

5. Forsterman U, Closs EI, Pollock JS, et al. Nitric oxide isozymes. Characterization, purification, molecular cloning and functions. *Hypertension* 1994; 23:1121–1131.

6. Fukuto JM, Chaudhuri G. Inhibition of constitutive and inducible nitric oxide synthase: potential selective inhibition. *Annu Rev Pharmacol Ther* 1995; 35:165–194.

7. Gross SS, Wolin MS. Nitric oxide: pathophysiological mechanisms. *Annu Rev Physiol* 1995; 57:737–769.

8. Mehta JL. Endothelium, coronary vasodilation, and organic nitrates. *Am Heart J* 1995; 129:382–391.

9. Umans JG, Levy R. Nitric oxide in the regulation of blood flow and arterial pressure. *Annu Rev Physiol* 1995; 57:771–790.

10. Rand MJ, Li CG. Nitric oxide as a neurotransmitter in peripheral nerves: nature of transmitter and mechanism of transmission. *Annu Rev Physiol* 1995; 57:659–682.

11. Zhang J, Snyder SH. Nitric oxide in the nervous system. *Annu Rev Pharmacol Toxicol* 1995; 35:213–233.

12. Lugg J, Gonzalez-Cadavid NF, Rajfer J. The role of nitric oxide in erectile function. *J Androl* 1995; 16:2–6.

13. Giuliano FA, Rampin O, Benoit G, et al. Neural control of penile erection. *Urol Clin North Am* 1995; 22:747–766.

14. Burnett AL. Role of nitric oxide in the physiology of erection. *Biol Reprod* 1995; 52:485–489.

15. Burnett AL. Nitric oxide control of lower genitourinary tract functions: a review. *Urology* 1995; 45:1071–1083.

16. Ignarro LJ, Bush PA, Buga GM, et al. Nitric oxide and cyclic GMP formation upon electric field stimulation cause relaxation of corpus cavernosum smooth muscle. *Biochem Biophys Res Commun* 1990; 170:843–850.

17. Knispel HH, Goessl C, Beckmann R. Basal and acetylcholine-stimulated nitric oxide formation mediates relaxation of rabbit cavernous smooth muscle. *J Urol* 1991; 146:1429–1433.

18. Kim N, Azadzoi KM, Golstein I, et al. A nitric oxide-like factor mediates nonadrenergic-noncholinergic neurogenic relaxation of penile corpus cavernosum smooth muscle. *J Clin Invest* 1991; 88:112–118.

19. Pickard RS, Powell PH, Zar MA. The effect of inhibitors of nitric oxide biosynthesis and cyclic GMP formation on nerve-evoked relaxation of human cavernosal smooth muscle. *Br J Pharmacol* 1991; 104:755–759.

20. Holmquist F, Hedlund H, Andersson KE. L-N$^G$-nitro arginine inhibits non-adrenergic, non-cholinergic relaxation of human isolated corpus cavernosum. *Acta Physiol Scand* 1991; 141:441–442.

21. Rajfer J, Aronson WJ, Bush PA, et al. Nitric oxide as a mediator of relaxation of the corpus cavernosum in response to nonadrenergic, noncholinergic neurotransmission. *N Engl J Med* 1992; 326:90–94.

22. Bush PA, Aronson WJ, Buga GM, et al. Nitric oxide is a potent relaxant of human and rabbit corpus cavernosum. *J Urol* 1992; 147:1650–1655.

23. Azadzoi KM, Kim N, Brown ML, et al. Endothelium-derived nitric oxide and cyclooxygenase products modulate corpus cavernosum smooth muscle tone. *J Urol* 1992; 147:220–225.

24. Knispel HH, Goessl C, Beckmann R. Nitric oxide mediates neurogenic relaxation induced in rabbit cavernous smooth muscle by electric field stimulation. *Urology* 1992; 40:471–476.

25. Knispel HH, Goessl C, Beckmann R. Nitric oxide mediates relaxation in rabbit and human corpus cavernosum smooth muscle. *Urol Res* 1992; 20:253–257.

26. Kirkeby HJ, Svane D, Poulsen J, et al. Role of the L-arginine/nitric oxide pathway in relaxation of isolated human penile cavernous tissue and circumflex veins. *Acta Physiol Scand* 1993; 149:385–392.

27. Holmquist F, Fridstrand M, Hedlund H, et al. Actions of 3-morpholinsidomine (SIN-1) on rabbit isolated penile erectile tissue. *J Urol* 1993; 150:1310–1315.

28. Hedlund P, Holmquist F, Hedlund H, et al. Effects of nicorandil on human isolated corpus cavernosum and cavernous artery. *J Urol* 1994; 151:1107–1113.

29. Chen X, Lee TJ. Ginsenosides-induced nitric oxide-mediated relaxation of the rabbit corpus cavernosum. *Br J Pharmacol* 1995; 115:15–18.

30. Levin RM, Hypolite J, Broderick GA. Comparative studies on rabbit corpus cavernosal contraction and relaxation. An in vitro study. *J Androl* 1994; 15:36–40.

31. Hayashida H, Okamura T, Tomoyoshi T, et al. Neurogenic nitric oxide mediates relaxation of canine corpus cavernosum. *J Urol* 1966; 155:1122–1127.

32. Holmquist F, Stief CG, Jonas U, et al. Effects of the nitric oxide synthase inhibitor NG-nitro-L-arginine on the erectile response to cavernous

nerve stimulation in the rabbit. *Acta Physiol Scand* 1991; 143:299–304.

33. Quinlan DM, Nelson RJ, Partin AW, et al. The rat as a model for the study of penile erection. *J Urol* 1989; 141:656–661.

34. Burnett AL, Lowenstein CJ, Bredt D, et al. Nitric oxide: a physiologic mediator of penile erection. *Science* 1992; 257:401–403.

35. Mills TM, Wiedmeier VT, Stopper VS. Androgen maintenance of erectile function in the rat penis. *Biol Reprod* 1992; 46:3424–3428.

36. Martinez-Pineiro L, Trigo-Rocha F, Hsu GL, et al. Cyclic guanosine monophosphate mediates penile erection in the rat. *Eur Urol* 1993; 24:492–499.

37. Finberg JP, Levy S, Vardi Y. Inhibition of nerve stimulation-induced vasodilatation in corpora cavernosa of the pithed rat by blockade of nitric oxide synthase. *Br J Pharmacol* 1993; 108:1038–1042.

38. Garban H, Vernet D, Freedman A, et al. Effect of aging on nitric oxide-mediated penile erection in the rat. *Am J Physiol* 1995; 268:H467–H475.

39. Garban H, Marquez D, Cai L, et al. Restoration of normal penile erectile response in aged rats by long-term treatment with androgens. *Biol Reprod* 1995; 53:1365–1372.

40. Martinez-Piñeiro L, Brock G, Trigo Rocha F, et al. Rat model for the study of penile erection: pharmacologic and electrical stimulation parameters. *Eur Urol* 1994; 25:62–70.

41. Giuliano F, Bernabe J, Jardin A, et al. Antierectile role of the sympathetic nervous system in rats. *J Urol* 1993; 150:519–524.

42. Trigo-Rocha F, Aronson WJ, Hohenfellner M, et al. Nitric oxide and cGMP: mediators of pelvic nerve-stimulated erection in dogs. *Am J Physiol* 1993; 264:H419–H422.

43. Trigo-Rocha F, Hsu GL, Donatucci CF, et al. The role of cyclic adenosine monophosphate, cyclic guanosine monophosphate, endothelium and nonadrenergic, noncholinergic neurotransmission in canine penile erection. *J Urol* 1993; 149:872–877.

44. Wang R, Domer FR, Sikka SC, et al. Nitric oxide mediates penile erection in cats. *J Urol* 1994; 151:234–237.

45. Heaton JPW, Varrin SJ, Morales A. The characterization of a bioassay of erectile function in a rat model. *J Urol* 1991; 145:1099–1102.

46. Melis MR, Argiolas A. Nitric oxide synthase inhibitors prevent apomorphine- and oxytocin-induced penile erection and yawning in male rats. *Brain Res Bull* 1993; 32:71–74.

47. Melis MR, Stancampiano R, Argiolas A. Nitric oxide synthase inhibitors prevent N-methyl-D-aspartic acid-induced penile erection and yawning in male rats. *Neurosci Lett* 1994; 179:9–12.

48. Paick J-S, Lee SW. The neural mechanism of apomorphine-induced erection: an experimental study by comparison with electrostimulation-induced erection in the rat model. *J Urol* 1994; 152:2125–2128.

49. Hull EM, Lumley LA, Matuszewich L, et al. The roles of nitric oxide in sexual function of male rats. *Neuropharmacology* 1994; 33:1499–1504.

50. Bush PA, Gonzalez NE, Ignarro LJ. Biosynthesis of nitric oxide and citrulline from L-arginine by constitutive nitric oxide synthase present in rabbit corpus cavernosum. *Biochem Biophys Res Commun* 1992; 186:308–314.

51. Keast JR. A possible neural source of nitric oxide in the rat penis. *Neurosci Lett* 1992; 143:69–73.

52. McNeill DL, Papka RE, Harris CH. CGRP immunoreactivity and NADPH-diaphorase in afferent nerves of the rat penis. *Peptides* 1992; 13:1239–1246.

53. Alm P, Larsson B, Ekblad E, et al. Immunohistochemical localization of peripheral nitric oxide synthase-containing nerves using antibodies raised against synthesized C- and N-terminal fragments of a cloned enzyme from rat brain. *Acta Physiol Scand* 1993; 148:421–429.

54. Vizzard MA, Erdman SL, Forstermann U, et al. Differential distribution of nitric oxide synthase in neural pathways to the urogenital organs (urethra, penis, urinary bladder) of the rat. *Brain Res* 1994; 646:279–291.

55. Ding YQ, Wang YQ, Qin BZ, et al. The major pelvic ganglion is the main source of nitric oxide synthase-containing nerve fibers in penile erectile tissue of the rat. *Neurosci Lett* 1993; 164:187–189.

56. Schirar A, Giuliano F, Rampin O, et al. A large proportion of pelvic neurons innervating the corpora cavernosa of the rat penis exhibit NADPH-diaphorase activity. *Cell Tissue Res* 1994; 278:517–525.

57. Domoto T, Tsumori T. Co-localization of nitric oxide synthase and vasoactive intestinal peptide immunoreactivity in neurons of the major pelvic ganglion projecting to the rat rectum and penis. *Cell Tissue Res* 1994; 278:273–278.

58. Ding YQ, Takada M, Kaneko T, et al. Colocalization of vasoactive intestinal polypeptide and nitric oxide in penis-innervating neurons in the major pelvic ganglion of the rat. *Neurosci Res* 1995; 22:129–131.

59. Burnett AL, Saito S, Maguire MP, et al. Localization of nitric oxide synthase in spinal nuclei innervating pelvic ganglia. *J Urol* 1995; 153:212–217.

60. Carrier S, Zvara P, Nuñes L, et al. Regeneration of nitric oxide synthase-containing nerves after cavernous nerve neurotomy in the rat. *J Urol* 1995; 153:1722–1727.

61. Burnett AL, Tillman SL, Chang TS, et al. Immunohistochemical localization of nitric oxide synthase in the autonomic innervation of the human penis. *J Urol* 1993; 150:73–76.

62. Leone AM, Wiklund NP, Hokfelt T, et al. Release of nitric oxide by nerve stimulation in the human urogenital tract. *Neuroreport* 1994; 5:733–736.

63. Brock G, Nunes L, Padma-Nathan H, et al. Nitric oxide synthase: a new diagnostic tool for neurogenic impotence. *Urology* 1993; 42:412–417.

64. Tamura M, Kagawa S, Kimura K, et al. Coexistence of nitric oxide synthase, tyrosine hydroxylase and vasoactive intestinal polypeptide in human penile tissue. A triple histochemical and immunohistochemical study. *J Urol* 1995; 153:530–534.

65. Jen PYP, Dixon JS, Gearhart JP, et al. Nitric oxide synthase and tyrosine hydroxylase are colocalized in nerves supplying the postnatal human male genitourinary organs. *J Urol* 1966; 155:1117–1121.

66. Bredt DS, Snyder SH. Nitric oxide mediates glutamate-linked enhancement of cGMP levels in the cerebellum. *Proc Natl Acad Sci USA* 1989; 86:9030–9033.

67. Lugg J, Rajfer J, Gonzalez-Cadavid NF. Dihydrotestosterone is the active androgen in the maintenance of nitric oxide mediated penile erection in the rat. *Endocrinology* 1995; 136:1495–1501.

68. Vernet D, Cai L, Garban H, et al. Reduction of penile nitric oxide synthase in diabetic BB/WOR[dp] (type I) and BBZ/WOR[dp] (type II) rats with erectile dysfunction. *Endocrinology* 1995; 136:5709–5717.

69. Lugg J, Ng Ch, Rajfer J, et al. Cavernosal nerve stimulation reverses castration-induced decrease in rat penile nitric oxide synthase activity. *Am J Physiol* 1996; 271:354–361.

70. Penson DF, Ng Ch, Cai L, et al. Androgen dependence of neuronal nitric oxide synthase content and erectile function in the rat penis. In: Stamler J, Gross S, Moncada S, Higgs AE, eds. *The Biology of Nitric Oxide*. London: Portland Press; 1996.

71. Penson DF, Ng Ch, Cai L, et al. Androgen and pituitary control of penile nitric oxide synthase and erectile function in the rat. *Biol Reprod* 1996; 55:567–574.

72. Xie Y, Garban H, Ng Ch, et al. Effect of long-term passive smoking on erectile function and penile nitric oxide synthase in the rat. *J Urol* 1996.

73. Penson DF, Ng Ch, Rajfer J, et al. Adrenal control of erectile function and nitric oxide synthase in the rat penis. *J Urol* 1996; 155:617A (#1224).

74. Garban H, Murray FT, Said SI, et al. Normal erectile response to cavernosal nerve stimulation in diabetic BB rats with decreased penile nitric oxide synthase (NOS). 10th International Congress on Endocrinology, San Francisco, CA, 1996: 1–189.

75. Cai L, Murray FT, Rajfer J, et al. Glucose regulates the in vitro content of NOS isoforms in rat penile and pelvic plexus tissue. 10th International Congress on Endocrinology, San Francisco, CA, 1996: 3–854.

76. Chamness SL, Ricker JK, Crone CL, et al. The effect of androgen on nitric oxide synthase in the male reproductive tract of the rat. *Fertil Steril* 1995; 63:1101–1107.

77. Hung A, Vernet D, Rajavashisth T, et al. Expression of the inducible nitric oxide synthase in smooth muscle cells from the rat penile corpora cavernosa. *J Androl* 1995; 16:469–481.

78. Huang PL, Dawson TM, Bredt DS, et al. Targeted disruption of the neuronal nitric oxide synthase gene. *Cell* 1993; 75:1273–1286.

79. Nelson RJ, Demas GE, Huang PL, et al. Behavioral abnormalities in male mice lacking neuronal nitric oxide synthase. *Nature* 1995; 378:383–386.

80. Huang PL, Huang Z, Mashimo H, et al. Hypertension in mice lacking the gene for endothelial nitric oxide synthase. *Nature* 1995; 377:239–242.

81. Wei X-Q, Charles IG, Smith A, et al. Altered immune responses in mice lacking inducible nitric oxide synthase. *Nature* 1995; 375:408–411.

82. MacMicking JD, Nathan C, Hom G, et al. Altered responses to bacterial infection and en-

dotoxic shock in mice lacking inducible nitric oxide synthase. *Cell* 1995; 81:641–650.

83. Snyder SH. No endothelial NO. *Nature* 1995; 377:196–197.

84. O'Dell TJ, Huang PL, Dawson TM, et al. Endothelial NOS and the blockade of LTP by NOS inhibitors in mice lacking neuronal NOS. *Science* 1994; 265:542–546.

85. Mills TM, Stopper VS, Wiedmeier VT. Effects of castration and androgen replacement on the hemodynamics of penile erection in the rat. *Biol Reprod* 1994; 51:234–238.

86. Heaton JPW, Varrin SJ. Effects of castration and exogenous testosterone supplementation in an animal model of penile erection. *J Urol* 1994; 151:797–803.

87. Gonzalez-Cadavid NF, Rajfer J. Androgen receptors and penile growth during sexual maturation. In: Hussmann DA, ed. *Dialogues in Pediatric Urology,* 1996: 19:4–8.

88. Moody JA, Vernet D, Rajfer J, Gonzalez-Cadavid NF. Effects of the long-term oral administration of L-arginine on the rat erectile response. *J Urol* 1997 (abstract), in press.

89. Kim N, Vardi Y, Padma-Nathan H, et al. Oxygen tension regulates the nitric oxide pathway. Physiological role in penile erection. *J Clin Invest* 1993; 91:437–442.

90. Kim NN, Kim JJ, Hypolite J, et al. Altered contractibility of rabbit penile corpus cavernosum smooth muscle by hypoxia. *J Urol* 1996; 155:772–778.

91. Elabbady AA, Gagnon C, Hassouna MM, et al. Diabetes mellitus increases nitric oxide synthase in penises but not in major pelvic ganglia of rats. *Br J Urol* 1995; 76:196–202.

92. Carrier S, Hricak H, Lee SS, et al. Radiation-induced decrease in nitric oxide synthase–containing nerves in the rat penis. *Radiology* 1995; 195:95–99.

93. Turner J, McLennan PL, Abeywardena MY, et al. Absence of coronary or aortic atherosclerosis in rats having dietary lipid modified vulnerability to cardiac arrhythmias. *Atherosclerosis* 1990; 82:105–112.

94. Moody JA, Penson DF, Rajfer J, et al. Augmented erectile response to cavernosal nerve stimulation in the spontaneously hypertensive rat. *J Urol,* 1996: 618A, #1229.

95. Schaad NC, Vanacek J, Schulz PE. Photoneural regulation of rat pineal nitric oxide synthase. *J Neurochem* 1994; 62:2496–2499.

96. Verge VMK, Xu Z, Xu X-J, et al. Marked increase in nitric oxide synthase mRNA in rat dorsal root ganglia after peripheral axotomy: *in situ* hybridization and functional studies. *Proc Natl Acad Sci USA* 1994; 89:11617–11621.

97. Moriel EZ, González-Cadavid NF, Ignarro LJ, et al. Serum levels of nitric oxide metabolites do not increase during penile erection. *Urology* 1993; 42:551–554.

98. Ottessen B, Fahrenkrug J. Vasoactive intestinal polypeptide and other preprovasoactive intestinal polypeptide-derived peptides in the female and male genital tract: localization, biosynthesis, and functional and clinical significance. *Am J Obstet Gynecol* 1995; 172:1615–1631.

99. Hauser-Kronberger C, Hacker GW, Graf AH, et al. Neuropeptides in the human penis: an immunohistochemical study. *J Androl* 1994; 15:510–520.

100. Miller MA, Morgan RJ, Thompson CS, et al. Effects of papaverine and vasointestinal polypeptide on penile and vascular cAMP and cGMP in control and diabetic animals: an in vitro study. *Int J Impot Res* 1995; 7:91–100.

101. Yeh KH, Aoki H, Matsuzaka J, et al. Participation of vasoactive intestinal polypeptide (VIP) as a humoral mediator in the erectile response of canine corpus cavernosum penis. *J Androl* 1994; 15:187–193.

102. Takahashi Y, Aboseif SR, Benard F, et al. Effect of intracavernous simultaneous injection of acetylcholine and vasoactive intestinal polypeptide on canine penile erection. *J Urol* 1992; 148:446–448.

103. Gerstenberg TC, Metz P, Ottesen B, et al. Intracavernous self-injection with vasoactive intestinal polypeptide and phentolamine in the management of erectile failure. *J Urol* 1992; 147:1277–1279.

104. Wang R, Higuera TR, Sikka SC, et al. Penile erections induced by vasoactive intestinal peptide and sodium nitroprusside. *Urol Res* 1993; 21:75–78.

105. Pickard RS, Powell PH, Zar MA. Evidence against vasoactive intestinal polypeptide as the relaxant neurotransmitter in human cavernosal smooth muscle. *Br J Pharmacol* 1993; 108:497–500.

106. McNeill DL, Papka RE, Harris CH. CGRP immunoreactivity and NADPH-diaphorase in afferent nerves of the rat penis. *Peptides* 1992; 13:1239–1246.

107. Stief CG, Benard F, Bosch R, et al. Calcitonin gene-related peptide: possibly neurotransmit-

TABLE 32.2. Reported dosage.

| Drug | Minimum dose | Maximum dose | Usual dose range | Mean dose |
|---|---|---|---|---|
| Pap (mg) | 5 | 160 | 20–80 | 37.7 |
| Pap/Phen (mg) | 1.5/0.05 | 80/3 | 7.5/0.25–45/1.5 | 20.7/0.8 |
| $PGE_1$ (µg) | 1 | 100 | 5–40 | 14.8 |
| Pap/Phen/$PGE_1$ (mg/mg/µg) | 1.2/0.1/0.9 | 120/4/40 | 8/0.2/10–16/0.4/20 | 10.5/0.5/6.6 |

decreasing the calcium concentration, it exerts a myonolytic effect on smooth-muscle cells; relaxes all components of the penile erectile tissue, the deep penile artery, and the cavernous smooth musculature; and secondarily causes venous constriction.

To date, reports have been published on more than 6850 patients with more than 101,100 intracavernous papaverine injections[19,20,32–35] (Table 32.1). In 1982 Virag[1] successfully injected papaverine intracavernously, achieving a tumescence period of up to 2 hours. In his pilot study, he intracavernously administered injections of 80 mg papaverine to 30 patients. Three years later, his number of patients had risen to 227 men, and full rigidity was achieved by 26% of these patients. The first report on self-injection therapy also originated from this group of patients; 75% who demonstrated psychogenic or neurogenic impotence achieved a full erection with an injection dose of 26 mg papaverine. Reports have been provided on doses ranging from 5 to 160 mg (Table 32.2); the most common dose range was 20 to 80 mg with an average of 37.7 mg.[19,32–41] Review of the literature reveals an average success rate of 53.9% (Table 32.3). The lowest reported success rate was 14% and the highest was 100%.[19,32,33,35–41]

The most frequent negative side effect of intracavernous injection therapy with papaverine was prolonged erection (Table 32.4). During the pharmacotesting period, this was evaluated to be 7.4% per patient and 6.6% per injection,[36,38,39] and during the therapeutical administration period it decreased to 5.1% per patient and 0.5% per injection. Other common side effects, such as fibrosis-like changes within the erectile tissue (Table 32.5), were found in 6.2% of patients undergoing papaverine injection. Moreover, the dropout rate for intracavernous papaverine injection was 31.3% (Table 32.6).

## Papaverine/Phentolamine

Phentolamine evokes erection by blocking the α-adrenergic system and the erection-inhibiting effects of the sympathetic system. As it influences only the vascular side of the erectile tissue, patients with general vascular disease do not benefit from phentolamine injection. There is a distinct dose-dependent relationship between responder rate and the cause of erectile dysfunction. Moreover, single phentolamine administration does not usually induce a satisfactory erection response, regardless of the underlying organic disorder. Phentolamine was introduced by Domer et al[42] in 1978, and in 1985 Zorgniotti and Lefleur's[43] successful administration of a solution of 30 mg papaverine and 1 mg phentolamine was considered a breakthrough. Their success rate was 71.6% after injection of this mixed solution in 250 patients. Patient acceptance of autoinjection was excellent in this group—one sixth complained of inadequate erection when phentolamine was not included in the drug solution. Padma-

TABLE 32.3. Published success rates of intracorporeal pharmacotherapy.

| Drug | Average success (%) | Min. success (%) | Max. success (%) |
|---|---|---|---|
| Pap | 53.9 | 14 | 100 |
| Pap/Phen | 70.8 | 36.8 | 100 |
| $PGE_1$ | 73 | 40 | 100 |
| Pap/Phen/$PGE_1$ | 75.5 | 60.7 | 90.5 |

TABLE 32.4. Number of prolonged erections.

| Drug | Pharmacotesting (%) | | Therapy (%) | |
|------|-------------|---------------|-------------|---------------|
|      | Per patient | Per injection | Per patient | Per injection |
| Pap | 7.4 | 6.6 | 5.1 | 0.5 |
| Pap/Phen | 7.5 | No data | 7.7 | 0.4 |
| PGE$_1$ | 1.3 | No data | 1.1 | 0.06 |
| Pap/Phen/PGE$_1$ | 3.2 | No data | 1.8 | 0.1 |

Nathan et al[44–47] and Sidi et al[41,48] demonstrated a relationship between the responder rate and cause of erectile dysfunction, and in consequence it became possible to distinguish between vasculogenic and nonvasculogenic erectile failure.

During the latter half of the 1980s, the combination of papaverine and phentolamine became established as the most successful drug in intracavernous therapy. Reports have been made to date on more than 111,500 intracavernous injections of papaverine/phentolamine in more than 5950 patients undergoing this type of therapy (Table 32.1).[19,25,32,45,49,50]

The generally administered mixture and dosage ranges from 7.5 mg papaverine/0.25 mg phentolamine up to 45 mg papaverine/1.5 mg phentolamine (Table 32.2). Reports can be found on a minimum dose of 1.5 mg papaverine/0.05 mg phentolamine and a maximum dose of 80 mg papaverine/3 mg phentolamine.[19,27,35,37,45,49,50]

Full response (Table 32.3)—an erection adequate enough for sexual intercourse—has been reported in an average of 70.8% of cases[19,27,35,37,45,49,50] with a minimum success rate of 36.8%, and a maximum reported success rate of 100%.

Similar to papaverine hydrochloride, the most prevalent side effect with the combination papaverine/phentolamine is the risk of prolonged erections. These have been reported in up to 7.5% of patients during the testing period and in 7.7% of the patients and 0.4% per injection during autoinjection therapy.[45,49,50] Fibrosis of the corpora cavernosa has been reported in 6.9% of patients.

The average dropout rate with the papaverine/phentolamine combination (Table 32.6) was slightly lower at 27.5% than with papaverine monosubstance.[41,45]

## Prostaglandin E$_1$ (PGE$_1$)

Prostaglandin E$_1$ is a prostanoid. It exerts a stronger relaxing effect on human erectile muscles than most of the other substances in the prostanoid group. PGE$_1$ is rapidly inactivated in the human body—up to 80% in one single lung passage—and is excreted via the liver and kidneys. Prostaglandins affect various organs in different ways. In smooth-muscle cells, prostaglandin E$_1$ causes modulation of adenyl cyclase, thus evoking an increase in cAMP concentration with subsequent decrease of free calcium concentration, which results in the relaxation of muscle cells. In contrast, in adipose tissue prostaglandins cause the inhibition of cAMP.

PGE$_1$ also affects the vascular system. Here, it leads to venous constriction and relaxation of the arterioles, thus positively influencing arte-

TABLE 32.5. Reports on fibrosis-like changes.

| Drug | Fibrosis-like changes (%) |
|------|---------------------------|
| Pap | 6.2 |
| Pap/Phen | 6.9 |
| PGE$_1$ | 2.7 |
| Pap/Phen/PGE$_1$ | 2.3 |

TABLE 32.6. Reported dropout rates.

| Drug | Dropout rate (%) |
|------|------------------|
| Pap | 27 |
| Pap/Phen | 27.5 |
| PGE$_1$ | 42.3 |
| Pap/Phen/PGE$_1$ | 24.2 |

rial circulation. Prostaglandin $E_1$ was introduced by Ishii et al[51] at the 1986 World Meeting on Impotence. In 1988 Stackl et al[52] presented results from 210 patients screened for differential diagnosis of vasculogenic impotence. Of the 210 patients who were administered a test dosage of 20 μg $PGE_1$, 143 (68.1%) maintained an erection lasting 30 minutes to 7 hours (mean 2.3 hours); the remaining 67 patients were administered a 40 μg dose, and eight of those maintained an erection for a period of 30 minutes. The general dosage, prostaglandin dissolved in 1 to 2.5 ml of normal saline, varies from 5 to 40 μg.[19,24,32,33,36,38,39,48,49,52]

The success rate with prostaglandin injections (Table 32.3) is high, at an average of 73%,[19,24,32,33,36,38,39,48,49,52] and prolonged erections (Table 32.4) are rare: 1.3% in pharmacotesting and 1.1% during therapy.[8,31,36,38,39,49,52] Fibrosis-like changes occur in only 2.7%[8,52] (Table 32.5). Side effects of prostaglandin include a burning sensation during injection and pain during erection (Table 32.7). Painful sensations have been reported by 31.8% of patients undergoing pharmacotesting[14,24,29,32,39,49] and 15% of the patients undergoing intracavernous pharmacotherapy with prostaglandin.[8,40,52] The dropout rate of 42.3% (Table 32.6) with prostaglandin is markedly higher than with the papaverine/phentolamine combination, and the majority of these patients state that painful erections are the reason for their dropout.[29]

Nevertheless, prostaglandin is the most efficient drug in use today and has become accepted as the preferred agent in the pharmacotherapy of erectile dysfunction.

## Triple Drug

The "triple drug," a mixture of papaverine, phentolamine, and prostaglandin, is chiefly

TABLE 32.7. Painful erection.

| Drug | Pharmacotesting (%) | Therapy (%) |
|---|---|---|
| $PGE_1$ | 31.8 | 15 |
| Pap/Phen/$PGE_1$ | 20.6 | 2.9 |

used in the United States[48] (Table 32.1). Prolonged erections (Table 32.4) occurred in 3.25% of patients during pharmacotesting and 1.8% during pharmacotherapy. Fibrosis (Table 32.5) was observed in only 2.3%. Painful erections (Table 32.7) occurred in 20.6% of patients during pharmacotesting and in 2.9% during intracavernous therapy. Published data reveal the lowest dropout rate (Table 32.6) of all at 24.2%.

## Neurotransmitters

Calcitonin gene-related peptide (CGRP) (Table 32.8) is a neurotransmitter not capable of inducing an erection on its own. But a solution of 5 μg of CGRP and 20 μg of prostaglandin $E_1$ is reported to evoke full rigidity suitable for sexual intercourse.[20,24] Initial studies show that in 30% of the nonresponders to intracavernous therapy, success was achieved with the combination containing CGRP.

Vasoactive intestinal polypeptide (VIP) is another physiologic neurotransmitter that induces tumescence but not full rigidity. In Denmark, a solution of 30 μg VIP and 2 mg phentolamine is commonly used. Initial reports are encouraging, with success in almost 100% of patients.[10]

## Moxisylyte

Moxisylyte is a selective blocker of $\alpha_1$-receptors. Initial published data (Table 32.8) on approximately 500 patients and over 19,000

TABLE 32.8. Alternative drugs for intracavernous pharmacotherapy.

| Substance | Patients | Injections | Dose | Success (%) | Prolonged erections (%) | Fibrosis (%) |
|---|---|---|---|---|---|---|
| Moxisylyte (5) | 509 | 19,348 | 10–30 mg | 70 | 1 | 1.5 |
| NO-donors (2) | 630 | No data | Max. 1 mg | 34.7 | 0 | 0 |
| VIP/Phen (3) | 52 | 1,380 | 30 μg/0.5–2 mg | 100 | 0 | 0 |
| CGRP/$PGE_1$ | >36 | | 1–10 μg/2.5–20 μg | 86 | <1 | No data |

CGRP, calcitonin gene-related peptide; NO, nitric oxide; VIP, vasoactive intestinal peptide.

injections reveal a mean success in up to 70% with an optimal dosage of 10 to 30 mg. Prolonged erections were experienced by only 1% and fibrosis occurred in 1.5%.[7,8,11,28]

### NO Donors

The NO donors linsidomine, SIN-1, and nitroprusside natrium were introduced in 1992. Initial reports demonstrate a success rate of up to 65%, but this has not been reproduced in clinical practice. Presently, the reported dosage is 1 mg and the success rates are below 35% without any reports of prolonged erections or fibrosis of the erectile tissue.[5,6,9,12–19,21–23,25–27, 29–31]

## Drug Survey

The most objective way of reaching a conclusion as to which agent is the best to use clinically is to compare the application of various drugs in the same patient via the intracorporeal route. Such an intraindividually assessed drug survey (Table 32.9) allows direct evaluation of the advantages and drawbacks of each substance as compared with other agents.

In the reported surveys, only prostaglandin demonstrated a small prolonged erection rate and a low rate of painful erections (average approximately 15%).[32–34,36,38–40,49] The triple drug achieved the best success rate of all. Overall, no substantial difference was observed in the success rates of prostaglandin and papaverine/phentolamine.[49]

## Problems and Side Effects

### Dropout Rate

The dropout rate during intracavernous pharmacotherapy is considered high, ranging from 24.2% to 42.3% (Table 32.6).[29,41,45] This group consists of those patients who do not respond to any of the three drugs, those who are incapable of self-administration, and those who do not comply. In the prostaglandin group, the dropouts were usually those patients who experienced severe painful erections during pharmacotesting.[8,14,24,29,32,39,40,49,52]

## Short-Term Side Effects

The most relevant short-term side effect that needs to be emphasized to each patient is prolonged erection (Table 32.4). The exact interval between normal and prolonged (3 to 8 hours) erection has not yet been defined. From the clinically relevant pathophysiologic point of view, clear distinction must be made between high-flow and low-flow priapism. The pathophysiologic mechanism of high-flow priapism is triggered by an abnormal increase in arterial blood inflow as well as in venous outflow. The $pO_2$, $pCO_2$, and pH values will remain almost normal, and damage to erectile tissue will not occur. In general, high-flow priapism is found during the first 6 hours of prolonged erection after intracavernous injection with vasoactive agents. At a later stage of prolonged pharmacologic erection, the so-called low-flow priapism sets in with the circulation arrested. During this phase, pain caused by ischemia is experienced, and the degree of damage to the erectile tissue is time dependent. After 48 hours, the onset of fibrosis in the erectile tissue leads to permanent impairment of any future erectile function.

All urology units should be capable of treating the emergency of prolonged erection. In the case of high-flow priapism detected by duplex sonography less than 6 hours after intracavernous injection (revealing higher arterial blood flow in both cavernosal arteries, normal blood gas analysis, and absence of pain), vasoconstrictive agents need to be injected intracavernously. The most popular agents (Table 32.10) reported are metaraminol, epinephrine, and phenylephrine,[37,45,50] each of which can cause severe side effects—hypertensive crisis and cardiac arrhythmia have been described; less frequently, angina pectoris, pulmonary edema, and cardiovascular decompensation. The dosages used are 0.5 to 10 mg metaraminol, 0.001 to 0.3 mg epinephrine, or 0.02 to 0.5 mg phenylephrine. For low-flow priapism (reduced arterial inflow within the cavernosal arteries as detected by duplex sonography later than 6 hours after injection, acidic pH values, decreased $pO_2$ and increased $pCO_2$ in blood gas analysis, and accompanied by pain), therapy

TABLE 32.9. Drug survey: reported success rates.

| Author | Year | Papaverine (%) | Papaverine/phentolamine (%) |
|---|---|---|---|
| Porst | 1989 | 31.3 | 60.3 |
| Keogh et al | 1989 | 27 | 48 |
| Wetterauer et al | 1988 | 50 | 65 |
| Average | | 36.1 | 57.8 |

| Author | Year | Papaverine (%) | PGE$_1$ (%) |
|---|---|---|---|
| Kattan et al | 1991 | 14 | 64 |
| Liu et al | 1991 | 14.7 | 17.6 |
| Mahmoud et al | 1992 | 63.5 | 81 |
| Porst et al | 1989 | 31.3 | 72.3 |
| Sarsody et al | 1989 | 60 | 60 |
| Sogari et al | 1994 | 32.2 | 40.1 |
| Wang et al | 1994 | 65 | 85 |
| Average | | 38.8 | 60 |

| Author | Year | PGE$_1$ (%) | Papaverine/phentolamine (%) |
|---|---|---|---|
| Wetterauer et al | 1990 | 86 | 82 |
| Roy et al | 1990 | 62.5 | 79.2 |
| Floth et al | 1991 | 60.5 | 79.2 |
| Hanani et al | 1993 | 03.6 | 03.6 |
| Porst | 1989 | 72.3 | 60.3 |
| Schramek et al | 1991 | 22.2 | 66.7 |
| Waldhauser et al | 1988 | 91.6 | 50 |
| Average | | 56.9 | 57 |

| Author | Year | Triple drug (%) | Papaverine/phentolamine (%) |
|---|---|---|---|
| Hanani et al | 1993 | 60.7 | 03.6 |
| Schramek et al | 1991 | 88.9 | 66.7 |
| Average | | 74.8 | 35.15 |

| Author | Year | Triple drug (%) | PGE$_1$ (%) |
|---|---|---|---|
| Hanani et al | 1993 | 60.7 | 03.6 |
| Schramek et al | 1991 | 88.9 | 22.7 |
| Average | | 74.8 | 12.9 |

| Author | Year | SIN-1 (%) | PGE$_1$ (%) |
|---|---|---|---|
| Buvat et al | 1994 | 23 | 69.2 |
| Weiske | 1994 | 34.6 | 66.7 |
| Wegner et al | 1993 | 0 | 20 |
| Average | | 19.2 | 52 |

| Author | Year | Moxisylyte (%) | PGE$_1$ (%) |
|---|---|---|---|
| Buvat et al | 1994 | 7.7 | 69.2 |

| Author | Year | Papaverine/PGE$_1$ (%) | Papaverine/phentolamine (%) |
|---|---|---|---|
| Floth et al | 1991 | 77.5 | 57 |

| Author | Year | Papaverine/PGE$_1$ (%) | PGE1 (%) |
|---|---|---|---|
| Floth el al | 1991 | 77.5 | 60.5 |

| Author | Year | Papaverine/phentolamine (%) | PGE$_1$/CGRP (%) |
|---|---|---|---|
| Stief et al | 1991 | 64.3 | 78.6 |

| Author | Year | PGE$_1$ (%) | PGE$_1$/CGRP (%) |
|---|---|---|---|
| Stief et al | 1991 | 58.3 | 75 |

TABLE 32.10. Common treatment of prolonged erection.

| Reported substance | Reported doses | Reported side effects |
| --- | --- | --- |
| Metaraminol | 0.5–10 mg | Hypertensive crisis, cardiac arrhythmia, fluid in lung |
| Epinephrine | 0.001–0.3 mg | Hypertensive crisis, cardiac arrhythmia |
| Phenylephrine | 0.02–0.5 mg | Angina pectoris, headache, cardiac arrhythmia |

should include aspiration of the corpus cavernosum of up to 500 ml of blood until the erect penis becomes flaccid. Surgery should be performed only as a last resort, when the state of erection remains. An artificial shunt (e.g., Winter shunt) is made between the corpus cavernosum and corpus spongiosum.

General injection risks, such as infection and hematoma (2% to 10%), always exist but are easily reduced by correct application of hygenic injection techniques.

Prostaglandins can produce a painful erection that does not diminish with repeated use or with altered injection techniques. This complaint is usually encountered in the initial pharmacotesting group, as these patients usually drop out or elect not to enter intracavernosal pharmacologic therapy.

## Long-Term Side Effect

The long-term side effect of intracavernous pharmacotherapy is fibrosis or fibrosis-like changes in the erectile tissue. This is a drug- and injection-dependent disorder in 2.3% to 6.2% of affected patients.[8,45,52] After discontinuation of treatment, these changes usually reverse. The fibrotic lesions are hypothesized by some researchers to be related to the pH value of 2.8 to 3.8 of the drug used.

## Combination of Pharmacotherapy

Intracavernous pharmacotherapy is currently the most effective treatment for erectile failure, but its use is not limited to severe organic impotence. Psychogenic-impotent patients also may benefit from this type of treatment to initiate later spontaneous erections. However, in psychogenic- as in neurogenic-impotent patients, the therapist must use minimal doses of the drug. These psychogenic patients should be subject to pharmacotesting with a dose reduction of at least 50%.

## Future Research

The future of impotence research lies in improving pharmacotherapy. An ideal drug that renders the highest success rate, allows uncomplicated administration, and results in the lowest complication rate is yet to be identified. To date, prostaglandin is considered by most authorities to be the most effective agent. It must be noted, however, that data published on papaverine and phentolamine include long-term use of this combination of intracavernous injection. Hence, this makes direct comparison between papaverine (phentolamine) and prostaglandin more difficult, as past experience has demonstrated that the priapism rate decreases with the growing experience of the therapist.

## References

1. Virag R. Intracavernous injection of papaverine for erectile failure. *Lancet* 1982; 2:938.
2. Brindley GS. Cavernosal alpha-blockage: a new technique for investigating and treating erectile impotence. *Br J Psychiatry* 1983; 143:332–337.
3. Brindley GS. Pilot experiments on the actions of drugs injected into the human corpus cavernosum penis. *Br J Pharmacol* 1986; 87:495–500.
4. Brindley GS. Maintenance treatment of erectile impotence by cavernosal unstriated muscle relaxant injection. *Br J Psychiatry* 1986; 149:210–215.

5. Borges FD. A new approach to the pharmacologic treatment of impotency; Lecture at the 89th American Urology Association Congress, 1994, San Francisco. *J Urol* 1994; 151:474A.

6. Brock G, Breza J, Lue TF. Intracavernous sodium nitroprusside: inappropriate impotence treatment. *J Urol* 1993; 150:864–867.

7. Buvat J, Lemaire A, Buvat-Herbaut M, et al. Reduced rate of fibrotic nodules of the cavernous bodies following auto-intracavernous injections of moxisylyte compared to papaverine. *Int J Impotence Res* 1990; 2(suppl 2):299–300.

8. Buvat J, Lemaire A, Marcolin G, et al. Comparison of the two second generation drugs for intracavernosal injections moxisylyte and prostaglandin E$_1$. *Int J Impotence Res* 1994; 2(suppl):1–39.

9. Cavallini G. Minoxidil versus nitroglycerin: a prospective double-blind controlled trial in transcutaneous erection facilitation for organic impotence. *J Urol* 1991; 146:50–53.

10. Gerstenberg TC, Metz P, Ottesen B, et al. Intracavernous self-injection with vasoactive intestinal polypeptide and phentolamine in the management of erectile failure. *J Urol* 1992; 147:1277–1279.

11. Hermabessiere J, Condra, MC. Efficacy and tolerance of intracavernous injection of moxisylyte in patients with erectile dysfunction: a double-blind, placebo controlled study. *Prog Urol* 1995; 5:985–991.

12. Knispel HH, Wegner HEH. Effect of nitric oxide-donor, linsidominechlorhydrate treatment of human erectile dysfunction caused by venous leakage. *Urology* 1993; 42:409–411.

13. Lemaire A, Buvat J, Buvat-Herbaut M, et al. Erectile response to intracavernous injections of linsidomine in 38 impotent males. *Int J Impotence Res* 1994; 2(suppl).

14. Martinez-Pineiro L, Lopez-Tello J, Dorrego JMA, et al. Preliminary results of a comparative study with intracavernous sodium nitroprusside and prostaglandin E$_1$ in patients with erectile dysfunction. *J Urol* 1995; 153:1487–1490.

15. Martinez-Pineiro L, Tello JL, Dorrego JA, et al. Preliminary results of a comparative study with intracavernous sodium nitroprusside and prostaglandin E$_1$ in the diagnosis and treatment of penile erectile dysfunction. Lecture at the 89th American Urology Association Congress 1994, San Francisco. *J Urol* 1994; 151(suppl): 910A.

16. Meyhoff HH, Rosenkilde P, Bodker A. Non-invasive management of impotence with transcutaneous nitroglycerin. *Br J Urol* 1992; 69:88–90.

17. Nunez BD, Anderson DC. Nitroglycerin ointment in the treatment of impotence. *J Urol* 1993; 150:1241–1243.

18. Porst H. Effektivität und Hämodynamik von SIN-1 versus Prostaglandin E$_1$. Lecture at the 45th DGU Congress 1993, Wiesbaden. *Urologe [D]* 1993; 32(suppl).

19. Porst H. Ten years of experience with various vasoactive drugs—comparative studies in over 4000 patients. *Int J Impotence Res* 1994; 2(suppl):149D.

20. Schwarzer JU, Pickl U, Kropp W, et al. Schwellkörperautoinjektionstherapie mit calcitonin gene related peptide. Lecture at the 44th DGU Congress 1992, Munich. *Urologe [D]* 1992; 31(suppl).

21. Stief CG, Djamilian M, Krah H, et al. Die Verwendung des NO-Donors SIN-1 in der SKAT-Therapie der erektilen Dysfunktion. Lecture at the 44th DGU Congress 1992, Munich. *Urologe [D]* 1992; 31(suppl).

22. Stief CG, Holmquist F, Djamilian M, et al. Preliminary results with the nitric oxide donor linsidomine chlorhydrate in the treatment of human erectile dysfunction. *J Urol* 1992; 148:1437–1440.

23. Stief CG, Holmquist F, Krah H, et al. Preliminary results with the nitric oxide (NO) donor SIN-1 in the treatment of human erectile dysfunction. Lecture at the 87th American Urology Association Congress 1992, Washington DC. *J Urol* 1992; 147(suppl):205A.

24. Stief CG, Wetterauer U, Schaebsdau FH, et al. Calcitonin gene-related peptide: a possible role in human penile erection and its therapeutic application in impotent patients. *J Urol* 1991; 146:1010–1014.

25. Torres LO, Teloken, C, Da Ros CT, et al. Nitric oxide donor linsidomine does not produce full erection in men with corporeal veno-occlusive dysfunction. *Int J Impotence Res* 1994; 2(suppl):479.

26. Truss MC, Becker AJ, Djamilian MH, et al. Of the nitric oxide donor linsidomine chlorhydrate (SIN-1) in the diagnosis and treatment of erectile dysfunction. *Urology* 1994; 44:553–556.

27. Truss MC, Djamilian MH, Kuczyk M, et al. Follow up results of the nitric oxide donor linsidomine chlorhydrate in the diagnosis and treatment of erectile dysfunction. Lecture at the

89th American Urology Association Congress 1994, San Francisco. *J Urol* 1994; 151(suppl): 911A.

28. Virag R, Sussman H, Floresco J, et al. Late results on the treatment of neurogenic impotence by self-intracavernous injection of vasoactive drugs. *World J Urol* 1987; 5:166–170.

29. Wegner HEH, Knispel HH, Miller K. Prostaglandin E$_1$ versus SIN-1 versus SIN-1 and urapidil in erectile dysfunction: a double-blind cross-over trial. Lecture at the 89th American Urology Association Congress 1994, San Francisco. *J Urol* 1994; 151(suppl):912A.

30. Wegner HEH, Knispel HH. Effect of nitric oxide donor, linsidomine chlorhydrate in treatment of human erectile dysfunction caused by venous leakage. *Urology* 1993; 42:409–411.

31. Wegner HEH, Knispel HH, Klein R, et al. Prostaglandin E$_1$ versus linsidomine chlorhydrate in erectile dysfunction. *Urol Int* 1994; 53:214–216.

32. Sarosdy MF, Hudnall CH, Erickson DR, et al. A prospective double-blind trial of intracorporeal papaverine versus prostaglandin E$_1$ in the treatment of impotence. *J Urol* 1989; 141:551–553.

33. Sogari PR, Da Ros CT, Teloken C, et al. Comparison of papaverine hydrochloride versus prostaglandin E$_1$ in pharmacological erection test. *Int J Impotence* 1994; 6:D110.

34. Wang CJ, Wu CC, Huang CH, et al. A comparative study with intracavernous injection of prostaglandin E$_1$ versus papaverine for the diagnostic assessment of erectile impotence. *Int J Impotence* 1994; 6:146D.

35. Wetterauer U, Stief CG, Sommerkamp H. Increased efficacy in the induction of an erection with a combination of intracavernosal papaverine and phentolamine as compared with papaverine alone. Lecture at the 83rd American Urology Association Congress, 1988. *J Urol* 1988; 139:(suppl):495A.

36. Kattan S, Collins JP, Mohr D. Double-blind, cross-over study comparing prostaglandin E$_1$ and papaverine in patients with vasculogenic impotence. *Urology* 1991; 37:516–518.

37. Keogh EJ, Watter GR, Earrle CM, et al. Treatment of impotence by intrapenile injections. A comparison of papaverine versus papaverine and phentolamine: a double-blind, crossover trial. *J Urol* 1989; 142:726–728.

38. Liu LC, Wu CC, Liu LH, et al. Comparison of the effects of papaverine versus prostaglandin E$_1$ on penile blood flow by color duplex sonography. *Eur Urol* 1991; 19:49–53.

39. Mahmoud KZ, El Dakhli MR, Fahmi IM, et al. Comparative value of prostaglandin E$_1$ and papaverine in treatment of erectile failure: double-blind crossover study among Egyptian patients. *J Urol* 1992; 147:623–626.

40. Porst H. Prostaglandin E$_1$ bei erektiler Dysfunktion. *Urologe [D]* 1989; 28:94–98.

41. Sidi AA, Cameron JS, Dykstra DD, et al. Vasoactive intracavernous pharmacotherapy for the treatment of erectile impotence in men with spinal cord injury. *J Urol* 1987; 138:539–542.

42. Domer FR, Wessler G, Brown RL, et al. Involvement of the sympathetic nervous system in the urinary bladder internal sphincter and in penile erection in the anesthetized cat. *Invest Urol* 1978; 15:404–407.

43. Zorgniotti AW, Lefleur RS. Auto-injection of the corpus cavernosum with a vasoactive drug combination for vasculogenic impotence. *J Urol* 1985; 133:39–41.

44. Padma-Nathan H, Bennett A, Gesundheit N, et al. Vivus-Muse Study Group. Treatment of erectile dysfunction by the medicated urethral system for erection. Lecture at the 90th American Urology Association Congress 1995, Las Vegas. *J Urol* 1995; 153:975A.

45. Padma-Nathan H, Goldstein I, Payton T, et al. Intracavernosal pharmacotherapy: the pharmacologic erection program. *World J Urol* 1987; 5:160–165.

46. Padma-Nathan H, Keller T, Poppiti R. Hemodynamic effects of intraurethral alprostadil: the medicated urethral system for erection. Lecture at the 89th American Urology Association Congress 1994, San Francisco. *J Urol* 1994; 151:469A.

47. Padma-Nathan H, Keller T, Proppiti R, et al. Hemodynamic effects of intraurethral alprostadil: the medicated urethral system for erection. *Int J Imp Res* 1994; 6(suppl 1):42A.

48. Padma-Nathan H. The efficacy and synergy of polypharmacotherapy in primary and salvage therapy of vasculogenic erectile dysfunction. *Int J Impotence Res* 1990; 2(suppl 2):257–258.

48. Sidi AA, Chen KK. Clinical experience with vasoactive intracavernous pharmacotherapy for treatment of impotence. *World J Urol* 1987; 5:156–159.

49. Floth A, Schramek P. Intracavernous injection of prostaglandin E$_1$ in combination with papaverine: enhanced effectiveness in comparison with papaverine plus phentolamine and prostaglandin E$_1$ alone. *J Urol* 1991; 145:56–59.

50. Sidi A, Cameron JS, Duffy LM, Lange PH. Intracavernous drug-induced erections in the

management of male erectile dysfunction: experience with 100 patients. *J Urol* 1986; 135:704–706.

51. Ishii N, Watanabe H, Irisawa C, et al. Therapeutic trial with prostaglandin E₁ for organic impotence. In: *Proceedings of the Fifth Conference on Vasculogenic Impotence and Corpus Cavernosum Revascularization*. Second World Meeting on Impotence. Prague: International Society for Impotence Research (ISIR); 1986; 11:2.

52. Stackl W, Hasun R, Marberger M. Intracavernous injection of prostaglandin E₁ in impotent men. *J Urol* 1988; 140:66–68.

# 33
# Oral, Transdermal, and Transurethral Therapies for Erectile Dysfunction

Paul C. Doherty

With the advent of the first Food and Drug Administration (FDA)-approved drug for the treatment of impotence, a formulation of alprostadil [synthetic prostaglandin $E_1$ ($PGE_1$)] for intracavernosal injection (Caverject, Pharmacia-Upjohn), the treatment of erectile dysfunction has entered a new era. Although injection therapy is considered the standard of pharmacologic therapies for the induction of erection, many men would prefer not to undertake this procedure. Other less invasive therapies, were they readily available, would be far more likely to be used both because of the lack of aversion to these treatments and the lack of pain, bruising, and fibrosis that have been associated with intracavernosal injection regardless of the drug employed.[1]

Currently, there are few alternatives for men seeking a solution for their erectile problems. Available forms of treatment include psychological counseling, vacuum constriction devices, intracavernosal injections, vascular surgery, or penile prostheses. Each of the treatment modalities suffers serious drawbacks, including lack of long-term efficacy data, high dropout rates, and high levels of invasiveness.[2] Oral therapies, such as yohimbine, are also routinely attempted but offer little benefit.[3] Clearly there is more than sufficient need for new therapies in the treatment of erectile dysfunction. This is true not only on the basis of patient preferences but also because not all causes of erectile dysfunction warrant invasive techniques.

Advances in diagnosis and treatment have led to a total reassessment of the factors underlying erectile dysfunction. At the time of publication of the breakthrough findings of Masters and Johnson,[4] it was believed that nearly all cases of impotence were psychogenic in origin. Currently, nearly the opposite view is held, and recent reviews of the field suggest that as many as 90% of all cases of erectile dysfunction have an organic basis.[5] Although this viewpoint appears reliable, it may be influenced by the population of patients referred to the specialists currently treating the majority of cases of erectile dysfunction.[6,7] Furthermore, these numbers do not necessarily represent the profile of patients who are most likely to seek treatment for erectile dysfunction. For example, whether referring to Kinsey et al[8] or to more recent studies,[9,10] it is clear that the prevalence of erectile dysfunction increases with age (Fig. 33.1). Most men with erectile dysfunction are over the age of 60 and represent the population with the highest degree of organic factors as a cause of their disease. Yet, these men are among the least likely to seek treatment. In fact, it is men in their 40s and 50s who most often seek professional help in dealing with erectile problems.[11-14] Moreover, these men are more likely to have psychogenic factors as a primary cause of their problems. Recent studies from several urology-based, multidisciplinary clinics suggest that primary psychogenic dysfunction may occur in as many as 30% to 40% of all patients actively seeking treatment.[11,12,15-18] In many of these patients, invasive therapies

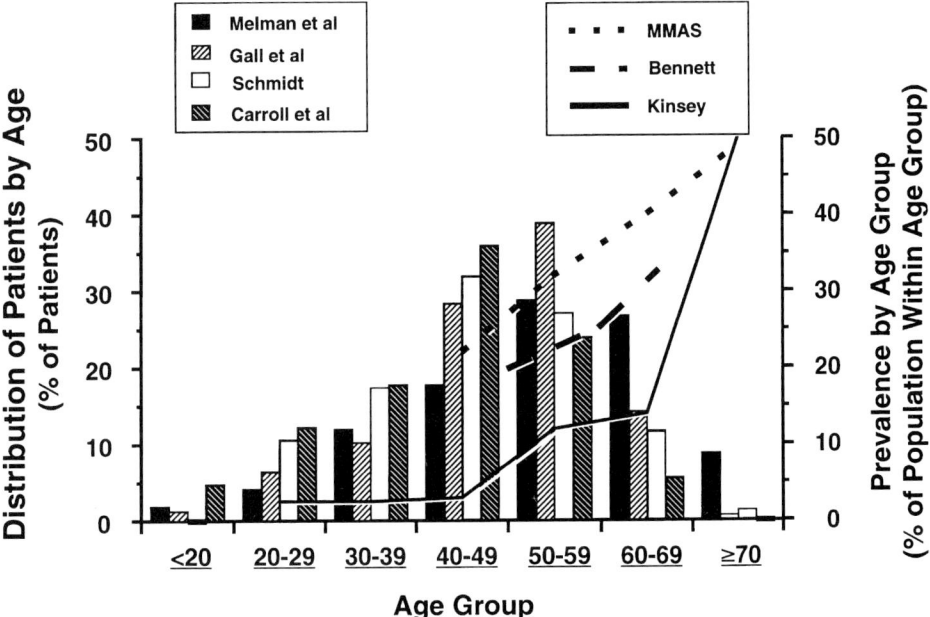

FIGURE 33.1. Age distribution of erectile dysfunction patients versus prevalence per age group. The histogram (left axis) illustrates the age distribution of patients seeking treatment for erectile dysfunction at four separate treatment centers.[11–14] The highest numbers of patients in each of these groups are in their 40s or 50s and the percentage seeking treatment declines rapidly for men in their 60s and beyond. In contrast, the prevalence of erectile dysfunction within the age groups of 60 and above increases dramatically regardless of whether the data come from studies by Kinsey[8] (solid line) or more recent studies like the Massachusetts Male Aging Study (MMAS)[9] (dotted line) or from a recent Gallup Poll (dashed line; Bennett[10]).

should be avoided except in cases of intractable dysfunction.

The reasons why the vast majority of men with erectile dysfunction do not currently seek treatment are not fully known. One possibility is that the current cadre of men in their 60s and beyond are more accepting of the idea that impotence is a natural sequela of the aging process. Clearly such attitudes will change. Baby boomers, the people who have lived through the so-called sexual revolution, will probably be more demanding of treatment than were the generations that preceded them. Other factors, including a decline in general health, death of a partner, or lack of availability of a partner, may also play a role.[17] It is highly probable, however, that the single most important factor contributing to the discrepancy between the prevalence of erectile dysfunction per age group and the likelihood that an individual will seek treatment is the lack of acceptance of the current treatment modalities.

What is it, then, that patients with erectile dysfunction are looking for? A safe, effective, minimally invasive therapy that could be administered just prior to sexual activity and produce a rigid erection with minimal risk of priapism would be highly desirable. It is also generally believed that among the pharmacologic approaches, oral therapy would be the most widely accepted form of treatment. This is followed by topical therapies and injections. The physical approaches also range in patient acceptance with level of invasiveness from vacuum constriction devices to vascular surgery and penile implants. Psychological counseling should be a part of nearly every couple's treatment regimen, as most forms of organic impotence are likely to involve an underlying psychogenic component.[2]

TABLE 33.1. Agents examined for ability to treat erectile dysfunction by oral administration.

| Drug | Trade name | Activity | Site of action | References |
|------|-----------|----------|---------------|-----------|
| Yohimbine | Yocon | $\alpha_2$-Adrenergic antagonist | CNS | 29,31–34 |
| Delequamine | — | $\alpha_2$-Adrenergic antagonist | CNS | 41–43 |
| Fluparoxan | — | $\alpha_2$-Adrenergic antagonist | CNS | 44 |
| Atipamezole | — | $\alpha_2$-Adrenergic antagonist | CNS | 45 |
| Idazoxan | — | $\alpha_2$-Adrenergic antagonist | CNS | 49 |
| Phentolamine | Regitine | $\alpha_1/\alpha_2$-Adrenergic antagonist | Penis | 51,53,54 |
| Naloxone | Narcan | $\mu$-Opiate antagonist | CNS | 35 |
| Naltrexone | ReVia | $\mu$-Opiate antagonist | CNS | 60,63,64,66 |
| Nalmefene | Revex | $\mu$-Opiate antagonist | CNS | 65 |
| Apomorphine | — | $D_1/D_2$ Dopamine agonist | CNS | 70,71,90 |
| Bromocriptine | Parlodel | $D_2$ Dopamine agonist | CNS | 83–85 |
| Quinelorane | — | $D_2/D_3$ Dopamine agonist | CNS | 87–89 |
| Chlorpromazine | Thorazine | Dopamine receptor blocker, anticholinergic agent $\alpha_1$-adrenergic antagonist, 5-HT antagonist | Both | 92,93 |
| Trazodone | Desyrel | 5-HT reuptake inhibitor, $\alpha_1$-adrenergic antagonist, 5-HT$_{2C}$ agonist | Both | 98–100 |
| Ketanserin | Sufrexal | 5-HT$_{2A}$ antagonist, $\alpha_1$-adrenergic antagonist | Both | 101,106 |
| Fluoxetine | Prozac | 5-HT reuptake inhibitor | CNS | 91,107,108 |
| Sildenafil (UK-92,480) | Viagra | Type V PDE inhibitor | Penis | 113 |
| Pentoxifylline | Trental | Nonspecific PDE inhibitor | Penis | 114,115 |

PDE, phosphodiesterase.

## Oral Therapies

The search for agents to increase desire or potency has occurred throughout recorded history, but serious investigation has been limited to the latter half of this century. Newer developments in oral therapies and topical approaches have taken a more direct approach of targeting delivery of agents that act within the erectile bodies of the penis.[19–21] Surprisingly, the locus of action of most oral therapies has been the central nervous system (Table 33.1). Mechanisms include blockade of $\alpha_2$-adrenergic receptors, opiate receptors, or serotonin receptors, and stimulation of specific subtypes of dopamine and serotonin receptors.[15,22]

## $\alpha$-Adrenergic Antagonists

### Yohimbine

Yohimbine, an $\alpha_2$-adrenergic antagonist, is among the agents whose action is thought to occur primarily within the CNS. Its effects are mediated through blockade of presynaptic $\alpha_2$-autoreceptors, leading to an increased release of norepinephrine in the brain and increased arousal. It has previously been used as part of the Afrodex formulation.[23] A resurgence of interest in yohimbine has occurred in the past 15 years as the result of basic and clinical research findings in the early 1980s demonstrating that yohimbine administration could improve the level of sexual activity of male rats[24–26] and increase erectile response in some men with impotence.[27,28]

These early reports were followed by more extensive investigations of the effects of yohimbine in men with various forms of erectile dysfunction. In men with psychogenic dysfunction, yohimbine appears to have the most beneficial effect.[29,30] In men with more severe forms of erectile dysfunction, yohimbine does produce subjective improvement, but in carefully controlled, double-blind clinical trials, the effects of yohimbine seldom reach significance.[31,32] Occasionally, statistical significance is observed but in surrogate end points rather than in the critical outcome of the trial.[33,34] Significant increases in erectile response have been seen when yohimbine has been combined with other drugs, specifically naloxone[35] and trazodone,[36] but not in tests of nocturnal penile tumescence[28] or in response to visual erotic stimuli.[37]

Yohimbine is generally administered in doses of 5.4 mg tid. It is taken chronically and effects are observed only after several weeks of treatment.[3] It has been suggested, however, that yohimbine may have greater beneficial effects when taken over several hours prior to anticipated sexual interactions.[34]

## Delequamine, Fluparoxan, and Idazoxan

Although believed to be largely ineffective, yohimbine is often prescribed for men who prefer not to proceed to intracavernosal injection therapy.[32] However, yohimbine treatment does appear to be useful in reversing various forms of sexual dysfunction associated with antidepressant treatment.[38,39] The relative success with yohimbine has led to the development of several more specific drugs. Delequamine, a highly specific and potent $\alpha_2$-antagonist,[40] has been shown to have some benefit in the erectile response of normal young volunteers in response to erotic ideation and visual erotic stimuli[41] as well as in erections during sleep.[42] In contrast, in men with psychogenic erectile dysfunction, little effect could be seen. In men below the age of 46, some response was seen to erotic stimuli. No beneficial effects could be obtained in an older group of men, however.[43] Fluparoxan, another $\alpha_2$-antagonist first developed as an antidepressant, was found to have little or no effect on erectile response in studies similar to those conducted for delequamine. This drug did appear to have beneficial effects on the level of sexual desire.[44]

Neither of these agents was routinely tested in animal models of erectile response. However, several other $\alpha_2$-adrenergic antagonists, including yohimbine, idazoxan, and atipamezole, have been shown to induce erections in several animal species.[24–26,45] The mechanism of action of each of these drugs involves interactions with presynaptic $\alpha_2$-receptors in the CNS. The effect of yohimbine may also include interactions with serotonin receptors.[24,26] Other possible mechanisms include increases in systemic blood pressure,[46] which might have beneficial effects on blood flow to the penis in some individuals, and interactions with postjunctional $\alpha_2$-receptors on the smooth muscle in the penis.[47,48] It is worth noting, however, that idazoxan, a more highly specific $\alpha_2$-antagonist than yohimbine, has been reported to have little effect on erection after the first week when given orally in a trial lasting several weeks,[49] and to have no effect when directly injected into the penis.[50]

## Phentolamine

In addition to the specific $\alpha_2$-antagonists, it has also been suggested that oral or buccal formulations of phentolamine may be effective in treating men with erectile dysfunction. The use of phentolamine, a compound that possesses antagonist activity for both the $\alpha_1$- and $\alpha_2$-adrenergic receptor subtypes, was first shown by Brindley[50] to have activity in inducing erections after intracavernosal injection. Gwinup[51] first reported on the possible use of oral phentolamine as a therapy for impotence. Shortly thereafter, Zorgniotti,[52] who first proposed that phentolamine be used in combination with papaverine for intracavernosal injection, successfully demonstrated the value of this approach in a small placebo-controlled trial.[53] A buccal formulation of this compound is being developed by the Zonagen Corporation for use in erectile dysfunction. In recent reports, its efficacy was approximately equivalent to the previously reported efficacy of yohimbine.[54] Buccal phentolamine targets pre- and postjunctional $\alpha$-adrenergic receptors in the penis. Unlike yohimbine, it has no central effects as it does not easily penetrate the blood-brain barrier.[55] Its use may be limited to men with psychogenic dysfunction; phentolamine when injected directly into the penis has benefit to normal controls but has little effect in men with organic causes for erectile dysfunction.[50,56]

# Opiate Antagonists

Changes in levels of endogenous opiates within the central nervous system have been proposed as an underlying cause of sexual dysfunction. This has been suspected on the basis of the effects of heroin and morphine addiction on sexual function. During drug administration, addicts are known to have reduced sexual desire, erectile dysfunction, and ejaculatory incompetence; during withdrawal, spontaneous erections and ejaculation are commonly seen.[57,58] Initial interest in the relationship between opiate antagonists and erectile function occurred after reports of increased erections following naltrexone administration in a group of rhesus macaques during toxicologic testing[59] as well as in a group of human volunteers.[60] Opiate antagonists also increase the number of erections observed after maximal doses of the mixed $D_1/D_2$ dopamine (DA) receptor agonists apomorphine[61] and N-n-propyl-norapomorphine.[62] Charney et al[35] have reported that naloxone, when coadministered with the $\alpha_2$-adrenergic antagonist yohimbine, produces erections in male volunteers lasting for 2 to 4 hours. The effect was reliably elicited when the two drugs were given together but seldom observed when each was given alone.

In contrast to the apparent lack of effect of naloxone on erection when administered as a single agent, the success of naltrexone may be due to its higher potency and longer duration of action. In one study, naltrexone (25 or 50 mg/day) restored erectile function in six impotent men.[63] In another, 50 mg/day of naltrexone for 13 days in an open label study caused increased morning erections and frequency of intercourse in a group of men with idiopathic erectile dysfunction.[64] However, acute administration of nalmefene to a group of men with organic impotence was without effect on nocturnal penile tumescence despite significant changes in food intake and serum gonadotropin levels in the treated individuals.[65]

Rather than implying a lack of efficacy of opiate antagonists on erectile function in men with organic dysfunction, the latter results may indicate that patients with milder forms of erectile dysfunction may best benefit from this form of therapy. Furthermore, the results of this study suggest that hormonal changes associated with the use of opiate antagonists may not contribute to the effects of these drugs on erectile response and that prolonged administration may be necessary for efficacy. A recent clinical study supports these ideas. In a placebo-controlled, double-blind trial of 50 mg of naltrexone once daily, men with idiopathic erectile dysfunction reported significant increases in the frequency of morning erections.[66] No significant side effects of the treatment were observed, and no changes in serum hormone levels occurred between the placebo and naltrexone treated groups. Despite the increase in morning erections, the effects of naltrexone on frequency of sexual intercourse were not significant. More potent and selective antagonists for the $\mu$-opiate receptor may result in better efficacy; however, little work is being done to explore this possibility.

# Dopamine Agonists

Since the first reports of hypersexuality in patients with Parkinson's disease on L-dopa therapy,[67] dopamine and dopamine receptor agonists have been thought to increase sexual motivation and desire. However, data from the past 20 years now suggest that administration of dopamine receptor agonists can stimulate erections without affecting sexual drive. For example, administration of apomorphine increases the occurrence of spontaneous erections in rats,[68] rhesus monkeys,[69] and men.[37,70,71] Moreover, there appears to be a high degree of correlation in the ability of dopamine agonists to induce erections across these species. Thus, the animal models have proven useful in the development of tools for the diagnosis and treatment of erectile dysfunction.[72,73]

Initial observation of erections in men after apomorphine treatment were made by researchers while studying the effects of this mixed $D_1/D_2$ dopamine receptor agonist on endocrine function in men with chronic alcoholism.[74] These findings have been confirmed in several follow-up studies. Apomorphine when administered by subcutaneous injection produces erections in normal men[37,70,75] and in men with psychogenic erectile dysfunction[71,76] without altering sexual motivation. Side effects include yawning, nausea, and hypotension, and occur with such frequency that the usefulness of this approach has been questioned.[71] Moreover, the reliability of the response appears to differ from one administration to the next.[77]

Several other dopamine agonists have also been examined for their potential as erectogenic agents. The specific $D_2$ dopamine agonist, bromocriptine (Parlodel), has largely been used for the treatment of impotence associated with hyperprolactinemia.[78–80] However, this drug has been reported to increase spontaneous erections in rats when given acutely[81] and to improve erectile response in both normal and hyperprolactinemic rats when given daily over a 2-week period.[82] Lal and coworkers[83] have reported successful treatment of a small group of men with erectile dysfunction with bromocriptine. The men were first screened for their response to acute apomorphine administration. If this proved successful, then the men were placed on chronic treatment with bromocriptine and most showed improvement in sexual function. The use of bromocriptine in nonhyperprolactinemic impotent men has been examined previously and showed little success.[84,85] However, it is believed that the response to apomorphine may provide a method to screen for patients who are best able to respond to this form of therapy. Improvements in serum prolactin levels were seen in the men who responded well to bromocriptine.[83]

Another highly potent $D_2/D_3$ dopamine receptor agonist, quinelorane, has also been examined in various forms of sexual dysfunction in large-scale clinical trials. Quinelorane has been shown to increase levels of sexual activity in adult male rats[86] and to increase the display of spontaneous erections through interactions with dopamine receptors within the central nervous system.[87,88] The effects of chronic oral administration of quinelorane have been examined in men with erectile dysfunction. Although this approach was found to have benefit in women with hypoactive sexual desire, chronic treatment with quinelorane was not associated with improved erectile response in the men.[89] It is not clear whether the lack of a significant outcome in this trial was due to the chronic dosing regimen used to reduce nausea associated with administration of dopamine agonists.

A buccal formulation of apomorphine has recently been developed that appears to address many of the shortcomings associated with subcutaneous administration of dopamine agonists while still achieving the rapid increases in plasma drug levels that appear to be necessary for the erectile response. In one study, 60% to 70% of men receiving the buccal apomorphine formulation were able to achieve erections sufficient for intercourse without debilitating side effects.[90] This approach appears promising and late-stage clinical trials are now being performed.

# Antidepressants and Other Psychotropic Drugs

Reports of priapism have been associated with the use of a number of psychotropic agents;[91–94] among these, trazodone (Desyrel) has been most frequently reported. Trazodone is an atypical antidepressant. The precise mechanism of its antidepressant activity is unclear but may include blockade of serotonin (5-HT) reuptake mechanisms or antagonism of 5-HT$_{2A}$ receptors. Some of its effects may also be attributable to formation of an active metabolite, m-chlorophenylpiperazine, which is a 5-HT$_{2C}$ receptor agonist. Stimulation of 5-HT$_{2C}$ receptors increases erectile response in several animal species.[95–97] In addition, trazodone has a significant activity as an $\alpha_1$-adrenergic antagonist.

Use of trazodone in treating erectile dysfunction has appeared in several reports in the literature. It has been suggested as a single oral agent[98,99] or in combination with other drugs like yohimbine[36] and moxisylyte.[100] Positive results have been achieved with doses of 50mg three times daily.[101] Others have suggested efficacy with higher doses (up to 150mg at bedtime) with few adverse events, including drowsiness and sedation.[21]

Priapism associated with trazodone use has been clearly related to its $\alpha_1$-adrenergic blocking activity.[102,103] This is best illustrated by its ability to delay detumescence in sleep lab studies.[104] Its activity in treatment of erectile dysfunction may be due to some of its other activities, however. The effects of trazodone on penile erection appear to involve activity in the CNS rather than direct effects in the corpora cavernosa.[105] This activity is probably not related to blockade of $5\text{-HT}_{2A}$ or $\alpha_1$-receptors, because ketanserin, which is an antagonist at both of these receptor subtypes, is far less effective[101] and has seldom been associated with priapism.[106] It is far more likely that the effects of trazodone on erection involve its ability to block serotonin reuptake or to stimulate of $5\text{-HT}_{2C}$ receptors. Fluoxetine (Prozac), another serotonin reuptake inhibitor, has been associated with prolonged erections[91,107] and return of erectile response in elderly men.[108]

## Phosphodiesterase Inhibitors

Given the efficacy of papaverine by intracavernosal injection, the potential role of phosphodiesterase inhibitors in treating erectile dysfunction should not be underestimated. Phosphodiesterases are a class of intracellular enzymes involved in the metabolism of second messenger cyclic nucleotides, cyclic adenosine monophosphate (cAMP), and cyclic guanosine monophosphate (cGMP). Of the seven major families of phosphodiesterases, three are readily found in the corpora cavernosa.[109–112] These are type III, the cAMP-specific cGMP-inhibitable form; type IV, the high-affinity, high-specificity cAMP-specific form; and type V, the cGMP-specific form. Much attention has recently been given to the type V isoform. It is believed to be found in high concentrations in the erectile tissue of the penis relative to other areas of the body, and its coexistence with the type III isoform, the cGMP-inhibitable enzyme, suggests the potential for interactions between cAMP- and cGMP-dependent processes in the penis (Fig. 33.2).[109] This would activate a number of processes that occur in response to binding of these cyclic nucleotides to specific protein kinases, including blockade of $Ca^{2+}$ entry into the cell and increased activity of adenosine triphosphate (ATP)-dependent

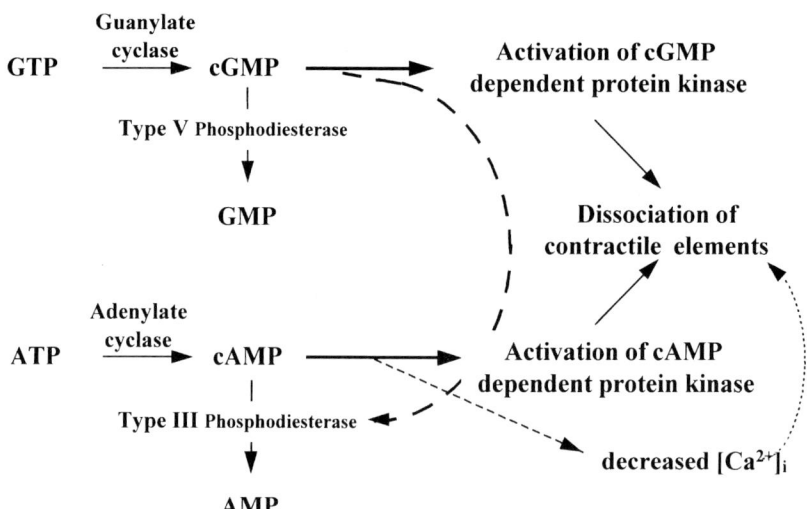

FIGURE 33.2. Potential interactions between the guanylate and adenylate cyclase systems in the smooth muscle of the corpora cavernosa: action of type V phosphodiesterase (PDE) inhibitors. Phosphodiesterases metabolize the activated second messengers cyclic adenosine monophosphate (cAMP) and cyclic guanosine monophosphate into the corresponding low energy 5'-monophosphates. The coexistence of the type III isoform (the cGMP-inhibited cAMP-specific PDE) with the type V isoform (cGMP-specific PDE) suggests the potential for a type V PDE inhibitor to increase the activity of both cGMP- and cAMP-dependent systems.

$K^+$ channels. Several large pharmaceutical firms have recently announced their interest in developing such compounds for the treatment of erectile dysfunction. The aim of such studies would be to develop an oral agent that acts specifically in the corpora cavernosa to increase the likelihood of erection.

This is a very promising approach but it may not be without limitations. Each of the isoforms of the enzyme is found in various sites throughout the body, including the vast majority of the cardiovascular system. Furthermore, inhibition of these enzymes does not initiate erection but rather enhances the erectile response or increases the duration of erection. This may mean that such treatment will be limited to men with milder (psychogenic) forms of erectile dysfunction,[113] as it is likely that doses necessary to treat men with moderate to severe dysfunction would be accompanied by increased side effects. In addition, recent evidence suggests that the type III[111] and type IV[109] isoforms may also serve as targets for the development of new approaches to the treatment of erectile dysfunction.

Pentoxifylline, a nonspecific phosphodiesterase inhibitor, has been used in the treatment of erectile dysfunction in men with arterial insufficiency.[114] Here the effect of the phosphodiesterase inhibitor appears to be on the fluidity of red blood cell membranes rather than on the vascular smooth muscle in the penis. The increased blood flow that occurs can be sufficient to help initiate and maintain an erection in men with claudication and vascular insufficiency.[115] It has not found application in erectile dysfunction of other etiologies.

# Topical Approaches

## Transdermal Therapies

Transdermal administration of vasoactive drugs has been investigated as an alternative to intracavernosal injection for the treatment of erectile dysfunction. Although intracavernosal injection is highly effective, it is extremely aversive and can be associated with patient dropout rates as high as 74%.[116–118] To date, five types of topical formulations have been investigated: nitroglycerin ointments, transdermal nitroglycerin patches, minoxidil ointments and creams, papaverine-containing ointments, and alprostadil-containing ointments.

## Nitroglycerin Ointment

Two studies from the Department of Urology at Queen's University in Canada demonstrate that although topical nitroglycerin administration can increase the level of blood flow into the penis and in some instances cause penile enlargement (tumescence), it does so without producing rigid erections.[119,120] When a nitroglycerin ointment was applied to the penis and the patients were allowed to view erotic films, 18 of the 26 impotent men demonstrated increased penile tumescence. However, the level of tumescence observed was on average 36% less than the maximum erectile response recorded from the same impotent patients during two nights of nocturnal erection evaluation. Only three of the 26 impotent men had erections superior to their maximal nocturnal erectile response. Doppler blood flow studies performed on an additional group of 20 patients, using the same formulation but without visual erotic stimuli, showed seven men with increased arterial flow rates, but only three with increased tumescence and none with rigid erections.[119] Similar results were obtained in a study of 140 impotent men. Again, increases in penile blood flow were observed, but only five of the 140 subjects reported any change in tumescence or rigidity after administration of the nitroglycerin paste.[120]

## Transdermal Nitroglycerin Patches

Nitroglycerin patches were first suggested as a therapy for erectile dysfunction by Talley and Crawley.[121] This report also suggested the potential side effects of this treatment for both the patient and his partner. A recent open-label trial of the nitroglycerin patch in 52 impotent men also demonstrates the potential drawbacks of this treatment.[122] Only a very small, statistically nonsignificant proportion of men achieved rigid erections (4/52) and successful intercourse

(3/52). In contrast, all of the men reported headaches despite pretreatment with analgesics. Despite the apparent lack of efficacy, several reports have suggested potential applications of nitroglycerin patches in men with neurogenic (spinal cord injury) or psychogenic dysfunction.[123–125]

## Minoxidil

The results of several recently published studies of topical administration of the vasodilator minoxidil are contradictory. Chancellor et al[126] compared topical minoxidil to intracavernosal papaverine injection and application of a vacuum constriction device. All subjects were spinal cord injury patients with lesions at the mid-thoracic region. These men were capable only of brief reflex erections in response to physical manipulation. To control for the possible influence of physical stimulation, minoxidil was applied to the glans penis using an aerosol spray. All patients responded to both intracavernosal papaverine injection and to a vacuum constriction device with rigid erections. The response to minoxidil did not differ from baseline either in the objective (strain gauge recordings of circumference and rigidity) or subjective (patient and physician scoring of the erection) measures that were taken. Similar results were obtained in a study of men with various causes of their erectile dysfunction.[127] Only two of 21 men showed improvement with the 2% minoxidil solution. Cavallini[128] has reported that topical minoxidil is better than both a nitroglycerin cream and placebo in increasing arterial blood flow rates in the penis. Strain gauge recordings of penile circumference and rigidity were also obtained. The results show a significant increase over placebo; however, the levels of rigidity reported fall well below accepted values for an erection that is satisfactory for sexual intercourse.[126]

## Papaverine and Alprostadil Ointments

Topical administration of a papaverine containing ointment increased the diameter of the cavernous artery, but only three of the 17 patients reported erections of sufficient rigidity for intercourse.[129] Neither significant increases in flow velocities nor erections were achieved, however. In a similar study using transdermal alprostadil, significant increases in both arterial diameter and peak systolic flow rates were observed.[130] Two patients reported erections lasting 3 and 12 minutes after drug administration; however, the remaining eight patients had no response.

# Transurethral Therapy

The greatest impediment to diffusion of drug into the erectile bodies after topical administration is not the stratified squamous epithelium of the skin, which can be overcome with penetration enhancers; rather, it is the tunica albuginea, a fibrous sheath that surrounds each of the erectile bodies. Recently, a novel approach to topical delivery of drugs for erectile dysfunction, transurethral drug delivery, has been described.[131–135] Like transdermal delivery, it relies on local administration of a vasoactive agent to achieve an erectile response. It differs from transdermal application in that it allows transfer of drugs from the urethra directly to the corpora cavernosa. Wolfson and colleagues[131] described the intraurethral administration of an ointment containing prostaglandin $E_2$. Rigid erections were achieved by 30% of patients, and overall 70% showed some degree of improvement. Intraurethral administration of capsaicin has also been shown to increase tumescence and rigidity.[135] The investigators ascribed their results to reflexive release of vasorelaxant neuromodulators in the corpora cavernosa after stimulation of capsaicin-sensitive sensory afferents in the urethra and did not consider the possibility of transfer of the pungent irritant from the urethra to the erectile bodies.

A formulation of alprostadil for transurethral delivery has been developed by VIVUS, Inc.[132–134] MUSE, the medicated urethral system for erection, consists of a small semisolid pellet of alprostadil in a plastic applicator. The stem tip of the applicator is inserted approximately $1^1/_4$ inches (30mm) into the urethra, and the drug is deposited by depressing a button at the opposite end. Results from several double-blind, placebo-controlled trials have shown transurethral delivery of alprostadil to be equally effective in men with moderate to severe erectile dysfunction associated with cardiovascular disease, diabetes, postsurgical and pelvic trauma, and with other organic causes of erectile dysfunction, such as high blood pressure medications and smoking.[133] In an early dose-ranging study, 70% of patients achieved intercourse with at least one dose of intraurethral alprostadil or alprostadil plus prazosin.[132]

The onset of erection after intraurethral application of alprostadil is similar to that observed with intracavernosal injection. This was examined in a Doppler ultrasound study that demonstrated that arterial flow rates and diameters in the cavernosal artery are the same 15 minutes after intracavernosal injection of $10\mu g$ or transurethral delivery of $500\mu g$ of $PGE_1$.[134] End diastolic flows were higher 15 minutes after application of intraurethral $PGE_1$, probably as a result of slight differences in onset of the peak erectile response between direct application of the drug into the corpora cavernosa and uptake of the drug from the urethra.

Although it is not yet fully proven, preferential transport of drug from the corpus spongiosum to the corpora cavernosa is the most likely explanation of the effects of intraurethral drug administration. The venous drainage of the more distal ends of the corpus spongiosum occurs largely through periurethral veins on the dorsolateral aspect of the urethra (Fig. 33.3). These veins also receive direct input from ventral portions of the corpora cavernosa on each side.[136] After intraurethral administration, drug is taken up by the urethral mucosa and diffuses into the corpus spongiosum. Direct transport of drug from the corpus spongiosum to the corpora cavernosa is most likely to occur through the periurethral veins and their tributaries. Transport is then enhanced by the hemodynamic gradient created by increased blood flow and tumescence in the corpus spongiosum.

Interconnections between the corpus spongiosum and the corpora cavernosa have been described previously. In one study, 25% of men with veno-occlusive dysfunction displayed the presence of radiopaque material in the corpus spongiosum after injection of contrast media into the corpus cavernosum.[137] Conversely, injections of contrast materials into the

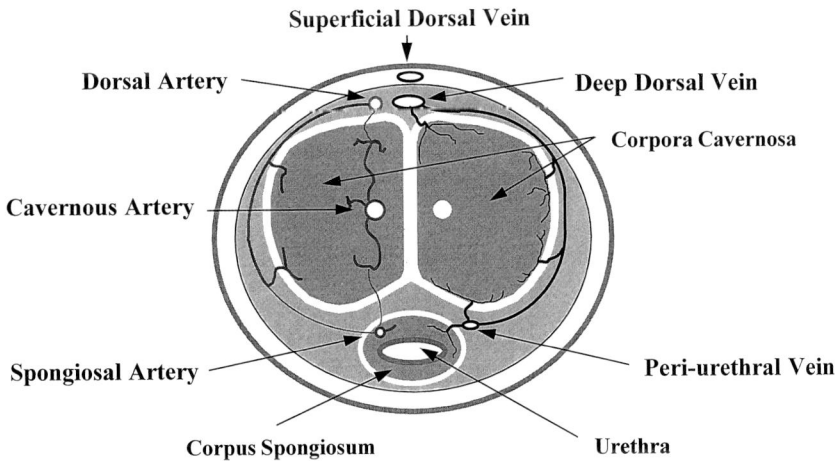

FIGURE 33.3. Cross-section of penis demonstrating vascular interconnections between the corpus spongiosum and corpora cavernosa. Anastomoses and collaterals can be found between the dorsal, cavernous and spongiosal arteries throughout the length of the penis (left side of illustration). The periure- thral veins, besides receiving tributaries from the corpus spongiosum, may also receive small veins that drain the ventral aspects of the corpora cavernosa.[136] The latter vessels would appear to be the most likely route of transfer of drug from the corpus spongiosum to the corpora cavernosa (see text).

corpus spongiosum and glans led to visualization of the corpora cavernosa.[138] Diffuse hyperemia and vascular interconnections between the erectile bodies were also noted in the Doppler studies performed after transurethral alprostadil administration.[134].

Transurethral delivery of alprostadil appears to be a safe, easy-to-administer, minimally invasive therapy that, like intracavernosal injection, is effective in most forms of erectile dysfunction. Because the drug is applied and acts locally, there is less potential of side effects than with either the transdermal or oral routes, due to lower systemic drug levels. It is a promising alternative to intracavernosal injection therapy.

## Summary and Conclusions

The availability of Caverject will bring a new level of understanding of erectile dysfunction much in the same way that advances in diagnosis and treatment in the 1980s did. This will include better approximations of the number of affected patients and the proportion of these men who are truly willing to engage in therapy. To date, only the most highly motivated individuals have sought the experimental therapies available. Nevertheless, this drug probably will not reach the total population in need of therapy. Efforts to provide alternative approaches, including many oral and topical therapies, have been disappointing. Future therapies, including transurethral drug delivery and oral administration of buccal apomorphine or specific phosphodiesterase inhibitors, appear more promising but await the outcome of the drug approval process. It appears, though, that several forms of approved therapies will soon be available to satisfy the demands of all the couples wishing to continue an active sex life.

## References

1. Krane RJ. Impotence. *J Urol* 1995; 153:1841–1842,
2. NIH Consensus Conference. Impotence. *JAMA* 1993; 270:83–90.
3. Yohimbine for male sexual dysfunction. *Med Lett Drugs Ther* 1994; 36:115–116.
4. Masters WH, Johnson VE. *Human Sexual Inadequacy.* Boston: Little, Brown; 1970.
5. Carrier S, Brock G, Kour NW, Lue TF. Pathophysiology of erectile dysfunction. *Urology* 1993; 42:468–481.
6. Donatucci CF, Lue TF. Erectile dysfunction in men under 40: etiology and treatment choice. *Int J Impot Res* 1993; 5:97–103.
7. Spark RF, White RA, Connolly PB. Impotence is not always psychogenic: newer insights into hypothalamic-pituitary gonadal dysfunction. *JAMA* 1980; 243:750–755.
8. Kinsey AC, Pomeroy WB, Martine CE. *Sexual Behavior in the Human Male.* Philadelphia: W.B. Saunders; 1948.
9. Feldman HA, Goldstein I, Hatzichristou DG, et al. Impotence and its medical and psychosocial correlates: results of the Massachusetts Male Aging Study. *J Urol* 1994; 151:54–61.
10. Bennett AH. Preface. In: Bennett AH, ed. *Impotence, Diagnosis and Management of Erectile Dysfunction.* Philadelphia: W.B. Saunders; 1994.
11. Melman A, Tiefer L, Pedersen R. Evaluation of first 406 patients in urology department based Center for Male Sexual Dysfunction. *Urology* 1988; 32:6–10.
12. Gall H, Bahren W, Holzki G, et al. Results of multidisciplinary assessment of patients with erectile dysfunction. *Hautarzt* 1990; 41:353–359.
13. Schmidt CW Jr. Common male sexual disorders: impotence and premature ejaculation. In: Meyer JK, Schmidt CW Jr, Wise TN, eds. *Clinical Management of Sexual Disorders.* 2nd ed. Washington, DC: American Psychiatric Association; 1986: 173–187.
14. Carroll JL, Ellis DJ, Bagley DH. Age-related changes in hormones in impotent men. Jefferson Sexual Function Center. *Urology* 1990; 36:42–46.
15. Foreman MM, Doherty PC. Experimental approaches for the development of pharmacological therapies for erectile dysfunction. In: Riley AJ, Peet M, Wilson CA, eds. *Sexual Pharmacology.* New York: Oxford University Press; 1993: 87–113.
16. Ellis LR, Nellans RE, Kramer-Levien DJ, et al. Evaluation of the first 300 patients treated at an outpatient center for male sexual dysfunction. *West J Med* 1987; 147:296–300.
17. Porst H. The rationale for prostaglandin E₁ (alpha-alprostadil) in the management of male

impotence. *Adv Prostaglandin Thromboxane Leukotriene Res* 1995; 23:539–544.

18. Virag R, Shoukry K, Floresco J, et al. Intracavernous self-injection of vasoactive drugs in the treatment of impotence: 8-year experience with 615 cases. *J Urol* 1991; 145:287–292.

19. Morales A. Nonsurgical management options in impotence. *Hosp Pract* 1993; 28:15–16, 19–20, 23–24.

20. Morales A, Johnston B, Heaton JPW, et al. Oral androgens in the treatment of hypogonadal impotent men. *J Urol* 1994; 152:1115–1118.

21. Montorsi F, Guazzoni G, Rigatti P, et al. Pharmacological management of erectile dysfunction. *Drugs* 1995; 50:465–479.

22. Foreman MM, Wernicke JF. Approaches for the development of oral drug therapies for erectile dysfunction. *Semin Urol* 1990; 8:107–112.

23. Afrodex and impotence. *Med Lett Drugs Ther* 1968; 10:97–98.

24. Smith ER, Lee RL, Schnur SL, et al. Alpha$_2$-adrenoceptor antagonists and male sexual behavior: I. Mating behavior. *Physiol Behav* 1987; 41:7–14.

25. Clark JT, Smith ER, Davidson JM. Enhancement of sexual motivation in male rats by yohimbine. *Science* 1984; 225:847–849.

26. Smith ER, Lee RL, Schnur SL, et al. Alpha$_2$-adrenoceptor antagonists and male sexual behavior: II. Erectile and ejaculatory reflexes. *Physiol Behav* 1987; 41:15–19.

27. Morales A, Surridge DH, Marshall PG. Yohimbine for treatment of impotence in diabetes. *N Engl J Med* 1981; 305:1221.

28. Buffum J. Pharmacosexology update: yohimbine and sexual function. *J Psychoactive Drugs* 1985; 17:131–132.

29. Reid K, Surridge DH, Morales A, et al. Double-blind trial of yohimbine in treatment of psychogenic impotence. *Lancet* 1987; 2:421–423.

30. Riley AJ. Yohimbine in the treatment of erectile disorder. *Br J Clin Pract* 1994; 48:133–136.

31. Morales A, Condra M, Owen JA, et al. Is yohimbine effective in the treatment of organic impotence? Results of a controlled trial. *J Urol* 1987; 137:1168–1172.

32. Sonda LP, Mazo R, Chancellor MB. The role of yohimbine for the treatment of erectile impotence. *J Sex Marital Ther* 1990; 16:15–21.

33. Riley AJ. Double blind placebo trial of yohimbine hydrochloride in the treatment of

erection inadequacy. *Sexual Marital Ther* 1996; 4:17–26.

34. Susset JG, Tessier CD, Wincze J, et al. Effect of yohimbine hydrochloride on erectile impotence: a double-blind study. *J Urol* 1989; 141:1360–1363.

35. Charney DS, Heninger GR. Alpha 2-adrenergic and opiate receptor blockade. Synergistic effects on anxiety in healthy subjects. *Arch Gen Psychiatry* 1986; 43:1037–1041.

36. Montorsi F, Strambi LF, Guazzoni G, et al. Effect of yohimbine-trazodone on psychogenic impotence: a randomized, double-blind, placebo-controlled study. *Urology* 1994; 44: 732–736.

37. Danjou P, Alexandre L, Warot D, et al. Assessment of erectogenic properties of apomorphine and yohimbine in man. *Br J Clin Pharmacol* 1988; 26:733–739.

38. Hollander E, McCarley A. Yohimbine treatment of sexual side effects induced by serotonin reuptake blockers. *J Clin Psychiatry* 1992; 53:207–209.

39. Jacobsen FM. Fluoxetine-induced sexual dysfunction and an open trial of yohimbine. *J Clin Psychiatry* 1992; 53:119–122.

40. Brown CM, MacKinnon AC, Redfern WS, et al. The pharmacology of RS-15385-197, a potent and selective α$_2$-adrenoceptor antagonist. *Br J Pharmacol* 1993; 108:516–525.

41. Munoz M, Bancroft J, Turner M. Evaluating the effects of an alpha-2 adrenoceptor antagonist on erectile function in the human male. 1. The erectile response to erotic stimuli in volunteers. *Psychopharmacology (Berl)* 1994; 115:463–470.

42. Bancroft J, Munoz M, Beard M, et al. The effects of a new alpha-2 adrenoceptor antagonist on sleep and nocturnal penile tumescence in normal male volunteers and men with erectile dysfunction. *Psychosom Med* 1995; 57:345–356.

43. Munoz M, Bancroft J, Beard M. Evaluating the effects of an alpha-2 adrenoceptor antagonist on erectile function in the human male. 2. The erectile response to erotic stimuli in men with erectile dysfunction, in relation to age and in comparison with normal volunteers. *Psychopharmacology (Berl)* 1994; 115:471–477.

44. Riley AJ. Alpha adrenoceptors and human sexual function. In: Bancroft J ed. *The Pharmacology of Sexual Function and Dysfunction.* New York: Excerpta Medica; 1995: 307–322.

45. Linnankoski I, Gronroos M, Carlson S, et al. Increased sexual behavior in male Macaca

arctoides monkeys produced by atipamezole, a selective alpha 2-adrenoceptor antagonist. *Pharmacol Biochem Behav* 1992; 42:197–200.

46. Grossman E, Rosenthal T, Peleg E, et al. Oral yohimbine increases blood pressure and sympathetic nervous outflow in hypertensive patients. *J Cardiovasc Pharmacol* 1993; 22:22–26.

47. Kirkeby HJ, Forman A, Sorensen S, et al. Alpha-adrenoceptor function in isolated penile circumflex veins from potent and impotent men. *J Urol* 1989; 142:1369–1371.

48. Steers WD, McConnell J, Benson GS. Some pharmacologic effects of yohimbine on human and rabbit penis. *J Urol* 1984; 131:799–802.

49. Haslam M. A trial of idazoxan and yohimbine in erectile dysfunction. *J Sex Marital Ther* 1996; 7:261–266.

50. Brindley GS. Pilot experiments on the actions of drugs injected into the human corpus cavernosum penis. *Br J Pharmacol* 1986; 87:495–500.

51. Gwinup G. Oral phentolamine in nonspecific erectile insufficiency. *Ann Intern Med* 1988; 109:162–163.

52. Zorgniotti AW, Lefleur RS. Auto-injection of the corpus cavernosum with a vasoactive drug combination for vasculogenic impotence. *J Urol* 1985; 133:39–41.

53. Zorgniotti AW. Experience with buccal phentolamine mesylate for impotence. *Int J Impot Res* 1994; 6:37–41.

54. Wagner G, Lacy S, Lewis R, et al. Buccal phentolamine. A pilot trial for male erectile dysfunction at three separate clinics. *Int J Impot Res* 1994; 6:D78.

55. Nordling J, Meyhoff HH, Hald T. Sympatholytic effect on striated urethral sphincter. A peripheral or central nervous system effect? *Scand J Urol Nephrol* 1981; 15:173–180.

56. Blum MD, Bahnson RR, Porter TN, et al. Effect of local alpha-adrenergic blockade on human penile erection. *J Urol* 1985; 134:479–481.

57. Mirin SM, Meyer RE, Mendelson JH, et al. Opiate use and sexual function. *Am J Psychiatry* 1980; 137:909–915.

58. Smith DE, Moser C, Wesson DR, et al. A clinical guide to the diagnosis and treatment of heroin-related sexual dysfunction. *J Psychoactive Drugs* 1982; 14:91–99.

59. Braude MC, Morrison JM. Preclinical toxicity studies of naltrexone. *NIDA Res Monogr* 1976; 9:16–26.

60. Mendelson JH, Ellingboe J, Keuhnle JC, et al. Effects of naltrexone on mood and neuroendocrine function in normal adult males. *Psychoneuroendocrinology* 1978; 3:231–236.

61. Berendsen HH, Gower AJ. Opiate-androgen interactions in drug-induced yawning and penile erections in the rat. *Neuroendocrinology* 1986; 42:185–190.

62. Ferrari F, Baggio G. Potentiation of the aphrodisiac effect of *N-n*-propyl-norapomorphine by naloxone. *Eur J Pharmacol* 1982; 81:321–326.

63. Goldstein JA. Erectile function and naltrexone. *Ann Intern Med* 1996; 105:799–801.

64. Fabbri A, Jannini EA, Gnessi L, et al. Endorphins in male impotence: evidence for naltrexone stimulation of erectile activity in patient therapy. *Psychoneuroendocrinology* 1989; 14:103–111.

65. Billington CJ, Shafer RB, Morley JE. Effects of opioid blockade with nalmefene in older impotent men. *Life Sci* 1990; 47:799–805.

66. Brennemann W, Stitz B, Van Ahlen H, et al. Treatment of idiopathic erectile dysfunction in men with the opiate antagonist naltrexone—a double-blind study. *J Androl* 1993; 14:407–410.

67. Barbeau A. L-dopa therapy in Parkinson's disease: a critical review of nine years' experience. *Can Med Assoc J* 1969; 101:59–68.

68. Gower AJ, Berendsen HG, Princen MM, et al. The yawning-penile erection syndrome as a model for putative dopamine autoreceptor activity. *Eur J Pharmacol* 1984; 103: 81–89.

69. Pomerantz SM. Apomorphine facilitates male sexual behavior of rhesus monkeys. *Pharmacol Biochem Behav* 1990; 35:659–664.

70. Lal S, Tesfaye Y, Thavundayil JX, et al. Apomorphine: clinical studies on erectile impotence and yawning. *Prog Neuropsychopharmacol Biol Psychiatry* 1989; 13:329–339.

71. Segraves RT, Bari M, Segraves K, et al. Effect of apomorphine on penile tumescence in men with psychogenic impotence. *J Urol* 1991; 145:1174–1175.

72. Doherty PC, Wilser PA. Effects of opiate antagonists on quinpirole-induced penile erection and yawning in the male rat. *Soc Neurosci Abstr* 1992; 18:659.

73. Heaton JP, Varrin SJ, Morales A. The characterization of a bio-assay of erectile function in a rat model. *J Urol* 1991; 145:1099–1102.

74. Lal S, De la Vega CE. Apomorphine and psychopathology. *J Neurol Neurosurg Psychiatry* 1975; 38:722–726.

75. Lal S, Ackman D, Thavundayil JX, et al. Effect of apomorphine, a dopamine receptor agonist, on penile tumescence in normal subjects. *Prog Neuropsychopharmacol Biol Psychiatry* 1984: 8:695–699.

76. Lal S, Laryea E, Thavundayil JX, et al. Apomorphine-induced penile tumescence in impotent patients—preliminary findings. *Prog Neuropsychopharmacol Biol Psychiatry* 1987; 11:235–242.

77. Murphy M. The pharmacology of erection and erectile dysfunction. In: Gregoire A, Pryor JP eds. *Impotence: An Integrated Approach to Clinical Practice.* New York: Churchill Livingstone; 1996: 55–77.

78. Carter JN, Tyson JE, Tolis G, et al. Prolactin-secreting tumors and hypogonadism in 22 men. *N Engl J Med* 1978; 299:847–852.

79. Buvat J, Lemaire A, Buvat-Herbaut M, et al. Hyperprolactinemia and sexual function in men. *Horm Res* 1985; 22:196–203.

80. Franks S, Jacobs HS. Hyperprolactinaemia. *Clin Endocrinol Metab* 1983; 12:641–668.

81. Ahlenius S, Engel J, Larsson K, et al. Effects of pergolide and bromocriptine on male rat sexual behavior. *J Neural Trans* 1982; 54:165–170.

82. Doherty PC, Bartke A, Smith MS. Differential effects of bromocriptine treatment on LH release and copulatory behavior in hyperprolactinemic male rats. *Horm Behav* 1981; 15:436–450.

83. Lal S, Kiely ME, Thavundayil JX, et al. Effect of bromocriptine in patients with apomorphine-responsive erectile impotence: an open study. *J Psychiatry Neurosci* 1991; 16:262–266.

84. Ambrosi B, Bara R, Travaglini P, et al. Study of the effects of bromocriptine on sexual impotence. *Clin Endocrinol (Oxf)* 1977; 7:417–421.

85. Pierini AA, Nusimovich B. Male diabetic sexual impotence: effects of dopaminergic agents. *Arch Androl* 1981; 6:347–350.

86. Foreman MM, Hall JL. Effects of $D_2$-dopaminergic receptor stimulation on male rats sexual behavior. *J Neural Trans* 1987; 68:153–170.

87. Doherty PC, Wisler PA. Stimulatory effects of quinelorane on yawning and penile erection in the rat. *Life Sci* 1994; 54:507–514.

88. Pomerantz SM. Quinelorane (LY163502), a D2 dopamine receptor agonist, acts centrally to facilitate penile erections of male rhesus monkeys. *Pharmacol Biochem Behav* 1991; 39: 123–128.

89. Foreman MM. Disorders of sexual response: pioneering new pharmaceutical and therapeutic opportunities. *Exp Opin Invest Drugs* 1995; 4:621–636.

90. Heaton JP, Morales A, Adams MA. Recovery of erectile function by the oral administration of apomorphine. *Urology* 1995; 45:200–206.

91. Murray MJ, Hooberman D. Fluoxetine and prolonged erection. *Am J Psychiatry* 1993; 150:167–168.

92. Seftel AD, Saenz de Tejada I, Szetela B, et al. Clozapine-associated priapism: a case report. *J Urol* 1992; 147:146–148.

93. Dawson-Butterworth K. Priapism and phenothiazines. *Br Med J* 1970; 4:118.

94. Raskin DE. Trazodone and priapism. *Am J Psychiatry* 1985; 142:142–143.

95. Szele FG, Murphy DL, Garrick NA. Effects of fenfluramine, m-chlorophenylpiperazine, and other serotonin-related agonists and antagonists on penile erections in non-human primates. *Life Sci* 1988; 43:1297–1303.

96. Berendsen HH, Jenck F, Broekkamp CL. Involvement of 5-HT1C-receptors in drug-induced penile erections in rats. *Psychopharmacology (Berl)* 1990; 101:57–61.

97. Steers WD, de Groat WC. Effects of m-chlorophenylpiperazine on penile and bladder function in rats. *Am J Physiol* 1989; 257:R1441–1449.

98. Adaikan PG, Ng SC, Chan C, et al. Oral trazodone in the treatment of total secondary impotence in a diabetic patient. *Br J Urol* 1991; 68:212–213.

99. Lance R, Albo M, Costabile RA, et al. Oral trazodone as empirical therapy for erectile dysfunction: a retrospective review. *Urology* 1995; 46:117–120.

100. Bondil P. The combination of oral trazodone-moxisylyte: diagnostic and therapeutic value in impotence. Report of 110 cases. *Prog Urol* 1992; 2:671–674.

101. Kurt U, Ozkardes H, Altug U, et al. The efficacy of antiserotoninergic agents in the treatment of erectile dysfunction. *J Urol* 1994; 152:407–409.

102. Abber JC, Lue TF, Luo JA, et al. Priapism induced by chlorpromazine and trazodone: mechanism of action. *J Urol* 1987; 137:1039–1042.

103. Saenz de Tejada I, Ware JC, Blanco R, et al. Pathophysiology of prolonged penile erection associated with trazodone use. *J Urol* 1991; 145:60–64.

104. Ware JC, Rose FV, McBrayer RH. The acute effects of nefazodone, trazodone and buspirone on sleep and sleep-related penile tumescence in normal subjects. *Sleep* 1994; 17:544–550.

105. Azadzoi KM, Payton T, Krane RJ, et al. Effects of intracavernosal trazodone hydrochloride: animal and human studies. *J Urol* 1990; 144:1277–1282.

106. Horby-Petersen J, Nielsen FC, Schmidt PF. Penile tumescence after injection of a serotonin antagonist (ketanserin). *Br J Urol* 1988; 62:277–278.

107. Power-Smith P. Beneficial sexual side-effects from fluoxetine. *Br J Psychiatry* 1994; 164:249–250.

108. Smith DM, Levitte SS. Association of fluoxetine and return of sexual potency in three elderly men. *J Clin Psychiatry* 1993; 54:317–319.

109. Sparwasser C, Drescher P, Will JA, et al. Smooth muscle tone regulation in rabbit cavernosal and spongiosal tissue by cyclic AMP- and cyclic GMP-dependent mechanisms. *J Urol* 1994; 152:2159–2163.

110. Trigo-Rocha F, Hsu GL, Donatucci CF, et al. Intracellular mechanism of penile erection in monkeys. *Neurourol Urodyn* 1994; 13:71–80.

111. Stief CG, Uckert S, Truss MC, et al. Cyclic nucleotide phosphodiesterase (PDE) isoenzymes in human cavernous smooth muscle: characterization and functional effects of PDE-inhibitors in vitro and in vivo. *Int J Impotence Res* 1995; 7:6.

112. Knispel HH, Gerhardus T, Beckmann R, et al. Relaxant effects of phosphodiesterase (PDE) inhibitors on rabbit corpus cavernosum smooth muscle. *Int J Impotence Res* 1995; 7:13.

113. Boolell M, Gepi-Attee S, Gingell C, et al. UK-92,480, a new oral treatment for erectile dysfunction. A double-blind, placebo controlled crossover study demonstrating dose response with Rigiscan and efficacy with outpatient diary. *J Urol* 1996; 155:495A.

114. Korenman SG, Viosca SP. Treatment of vasculogenic sexual dysfunction with pentoxifylline. *J Am Geriatr Soc* 1993; 41:363–366.

115. Allenby KS, Burris JF, Mroczek WJ. Pentoxifylline in the treatment of vascular impotence—case reports. *Angiology* 1991; 42:418–420.

116. Althof SE, Turner LA, Levine SB, et al. Sexual, psychological, and marital impact of self-injection of papaverine and phentolamine: a long-term prospective study. *J Sex Marital Ther* 1991; 17:101–112.

117. Turner LA, Althof SE, Levine SB, et al. Twelve-month comparison of two treatments for erectile dysfunction: self-injection versus external vacuum devices. *Urology* 1992; 39:139–144.

118. Irwin MB, Kata EJ. High attrition rate with intracavernous injection of prostaglandin E$_1$ for impotency. *Urology* 1994; 43:84–87.

119. Owen JA, Saunders F, Harris C, et al. Topical nitroglycerin: a potential treatment for impotence. *J Urol* 1989; 141:546–548.

120. Heaton JP, Morales A, Owen J, et al. Topical glyceryltrinitrate causes measurable penile arterial dilation in impotent men. *J Urol* 1990; 143:729–731.

121. Talley JD, Crawley IS. Transdermal nitrate, penile erection, and spousal headache. *Ann Intern Med* 1985; 103:804.

122. Nunez BD, Anderson DC Jr. Nitroglycerin ointment in the treatment of impotence. *J Urol* 1993; 150:1241–1243.

123. Sonksen J, Biering-Sorensen F. Transcutaneous nitroglycerin in the treatment of erectile dysfunction in spinal cord injured. *Paraplegia* 1992; 30:554–557.

124. Claes H, Baert L. Transcutaneous nitroglycerin therapy in the treatment of impotence. Urol Int 1989; 44:309–312.

125. Meyhoff HH, Rosenkilde P, Bodker A. Non-invasive management of impotence with transcutaneous nitroglycerin. *Br J Urol* 1992; 69:88–90.

126. Chancellor MB, Rivas DA, Panzer DE, et al. Prospective comparison of topical minoxidil to vaccum constriction device and intracorporeal papaverine injection in treatment of erectile dysfunction due to spinal cord injury. *Urology* 1994; 43:365–369.

127. Radomski SB, Herschorn S, Rangaswamy S. Topical minoxidil in the treatment of male erectile dysfunction. *J Urol* 1994; 151:1225–1226.

128. Cavallini G. Minoxidil versus nitroglycerin: a prospective double-blind controlled trial in transcutaneous erection facilitation for organic impotence. *J Urol* 1991; 146:50–53.

129. Kim ED, el-Rashidy R, McVary KT. Papaverine topical gel for treatment of erectile dysfunction. *J Urol* 1995; 153:361–365.

130. Kim ED, McVary KT. Topical prostaglandin-E$_1$ for the treatment of erectile dysfunction. *J Urol* 1995; 153:1828–1830.

131. Wolfson B, Pickett S, Scott NE, et al. Intraurethral prostaglandin E-2 cream: a possible alternative treatment for erectile dysfunction. *Urology* 1993; 42:73–75.

132. Padma-Nathan H, Bennett A, Gesundheit N, et al. Treatment of erectile dysfunction by the medicated urethral system for erection (MUSE). *J Urol* 1995; 153:472A.

133. Padma-Nathan H, Auerbach SM, Barada JH, et al. Multicenter double-blind, placebo-controlled trial of transurethral alprostadil in men with chronic erectile dysfunciton. *J Urol* 1996; 155:496A.

134. Padma-Nathan H, Keller T, Poppiti R, et al. Hemodynamic effects of intraurethral alprostadil: The Medicated Urethral System for Erection (MUSE). *J Urol* 1994; 151:345A.

135. Lazzeri M, Barbanti G, Beneforti P, et al. Intraurethrally infused capsaicin induces penile erection in humans. *Scand J Urol Nephrol* 1994; 28:409–412.

136. Lue TF. Physiology of erection and pathophysiology of impotence. In: Walsh PC, Retik AB, Stamey TA, Vaughan JED, eds. *Campbell's Urology*. Philadelphia: W.B. Saunders; 1992: 709–728.

137. Fuchs AM, Mehringer CM, Rajfer J. Anatomy of penile venous drainage in potent and impotent men during cavernosography. *J Urol* 1989; 141:1353–1356.

138. Vardi Y. Corporal response to intra-spongiosal injection of vasoactive drugs. *Int J Impotence Res* 1995; 7:8.

# 34
# Psychological Aspects of Erectile Dysfunction

Stanley E. Althof and Stephen B. Levine

Traditionally, the urologist and the mental health specialist have referred patients to one another on an as-needed basis. Therapists were not well acquainted with the medical factors causing erectile dysfunction, and urologists overlooked psychological forces that contributed to the dysfunction. Increasingly, there is a trend toward the establishment of multidisciplinary teams where urologists and mental health clinicians can work in tandem to address the complex interplay of biology and psychology.[1]

## Historical Perspective

In the early 1980s, mental health clinicians concerned themselves with the diagnosis and treatment of psychogenic erectile dysfunction.[2-4] This limited role was a logical outgrowth of the binary model of understanding erectile dysfunction as either organic or psychogenic. When fewer options were available, the rules were straightforward. Patients with psychogenic difficulties were referred for psychotherapy, those deficient in testosterone received hormone replacement, and those with other organic conditions were offered penile prostheses. There was generally no second line of treatment for psychogenic patients who did not recover with psychotherapy. Similarly, if a prosthesis failed or the patient with an organic dysfunction declined the implant, no other forms of treatment were available.

In the mid-1980s and early 1990s, five noninvasive, reversible, relatively safe treatment options were introduced: (1) self-injection therapy; (2) vacuum tumescence therapy; (3) transurethral treatment, (4) topical medications, and (5) oral medications.[5-11] These developments compounded the decision tree, and the previously simple binary treatment algorithm was no longer viable. Although a third category, mixed erectile dysfunction, was developed to account for patients who failed to fit neatly into the binary model, the creation of this etiologic category did not do justice to the complexity underlying the etiologic and motivational aspects of erectile dysfunction.

## Manifestations of Psychological Resistance

Follow-up studies on the new treatment alternatives began reporting that, irrespective of the etiology of the dysfunction, a sizable minority, and in some studies, a majority, of patients failed to use the prescribed interventions or dropped out of treatment.[12,13] These reports introduced the urologist to the psychological concept of resistance: patients who were offered efficacious treatments mysteriously were unable to use them. Although these studies focused on efficacy, side effects, and aesthetic preferences, the explanations did not seem to do justice to the riddle of why couples could not use these treatments. The early manifestations of resistance could be seen in the time it took for some men to present themselves for evaluation. Typically, between 6 months and 2 years passed before men were seen, because they were embarrassed, ashamed, or denied having a problem. During this time, the couple's sexual equilibrium[14] insidiously transformed itself from a pleasurable weekly or biweekly phenomenon into a hurried and frustrating attempt once every couple of months. Couples became more emotionally distant and expressions of affectionate holding and touching dwindled. A few couples continued to make love via manual or oral pleasuring, but frequently couples held to the mantra, "If you can't get the job done, why start." Urologists incorrectly assumed that by giving men injections, vacuum pumps, or oral medications that the couple's sexual equilibrium could easily be transformed to the predysfunction pattern. What became clear ultimately was that it is often necessary to undo the psychological response to the dysfunction before a prescribed intervention can be smoothly integrated into a couple's infrequent love life.

Another common response to erectile dysfunction was the development of acquired rapid ejaculation. This occurred because men had no confidence in the reliability of their erection. Using a football analogy, they developed a 2-minute offense, predicated on the strategy of hurry up and ejaculate before the erection is lost. And it was not uncommon for men to report having a significantly lowered sexual drive. Obviously, any combination of these dysfunctions made for a less than memorable sexual experience for the man and his partner.

With the advent of newer treatment options, the role of the mental health clinician has evolved from assisting with diagnosis and treatment of psychogenic erectile dysfunction to (1) working through responses and resistances in the motivational domain, (2) rehabilitating the sexual equilibrium, and (3) decreasing the performance anxiety that interferes with couples resuming a regular sexual life. This expanded role calls for a more collaborative relationship between the therapist and urologist where they work as a team to help patients function at the optimal level consistent with physical and psychological limitations.

## The Interactive Model

An interactive model was developed to understand the complex interplay of psychological and medical factors.[15-17] This model captures the ever-changing influences of biology and psychological life. Regardless of the precipitating causes, time brings changes in both domains. This model encompasses not only the psychological impact that the dysfunction has on the man and his partner's sexual equilibrium but also the fluctuating influence of his disease states.

This interactive model enables stepwise treatment recommendations. For instance, a couple might first be referred for time-limited psychological counseling to help pave the way for a future medical intervention. The model also explains the failure of treatments for biologic problems that ignore the psychological contributions; for example, a sizable percentage of men with penile prostheses never use the devices for intercourse. The following vignette illustrates how the coexistence of organic and psychologic factors may create a therapeutic impasse.

Mr. B., a 59-year-old married man with a 3-year history of insulin-dependent diabetes and medication-controlled hypertension, had been unable to achieve or maintain rigid erections for 18 months. Penile-brachial index (PBI), biothesiometry, and nocturnal penile tumescence (NPT) were abnormal. He met criteria for a major depressive disorder secondary to marital discord. Shortly after the onset of the dysfunction the couple began to avoid lovemaking.

Mr. B. was pleased to learn that a vacuum pump might restore his erectile capacity. He had some difficulty learning how to manipulate the device but mastered it with the support of the urologic nurse.

Mrs. B. would not accept that her husband's dysfunction was in part due to physical illness and medication. She believed he was dysfunctional because he was neither in love with nor attracted to her. She demanded that he achieve an erection without the vacuum pump in order to prove his devotion to her.

The situation was further complicated by Mr. B.'s alternating need to please his wife and his passive expressions of hostility. This couple could not integrate the vacuum pump into their lovemaking until the psychological/marital conflicts lessened.

# Contemporary Understanding of Psychogenic Erectile Dysfunction

The fourth edition of the *Diagnostic and Statistical Manual* of the American Psychiatric Association[18] offers the following criteria set for male erectile dysfunction (diagnosis no. 302.72):

A. Persistent or recurrent inability to attain or to maintain until completion of the sexual activity an adequate erection.
B. The disturbance causes marked distress or interpersonal difficulty.
C. The erectile dysfunction is not better accounted for by another Axis I disorder and is not due exclusively to the direct physiologic effects of a substance or a general medical condition.

The clinician is required to make three determinations: (1) lifelong dysfunction versus acquired, (2) generalized or situational type, and (3) caused by psychological or combined factors. Psychogenic erectile dysfunction comes in two forms, lifelong or acquired. This important distinction has implications not only for the modality in which the patient is to be treated but also for the underlying etiologic causes.

There are several distinct psychotherapy possibilities: individual therapy for one or both partners, conjoint or couples treatment, separate group psychotherapies for one or both partners, or a combination of the above. If the erectile dysfunction is lifelong—that is, there has never been a period in the man's life where he has been able to achieve or maintain good-quality erections for intercourse—individual therapy is generally recommended, based on the assumption that lifelong erectile dysfunction is a developmental failure rather than an interpersonal problem. Individual treatment lends itself to the intensive exploration of early life events and allows understanding of and working through the obstacles that inhibit the establishing of a comfortable sexual self. Lifelong impotence is often the end result of unre-

solved gender identity, sexual orientation, or paraphilic conflicts. These issues are more difficult to explore and resolve in couples or group treatment. Not only does the presence of others dilute the focus, but patients are often reluctant to share these concerns with others.

However, when a man with lifelong dysfunction has limited capacity for psychological reflectiveness, is markedly inarticulate, and/or is estranged from his emotional life, individual treatment is ill-advised. In these situations, the partner is asked to join the therapy as an adjunct therapist. She is often aware of his family events or can help the patient more readily talk about aspects of himself that might otherwise remain obscured in individual treatment.

Conjoint treatment is recommended for patients with acquired erectile dysfunction but viable relationships. Acquired dysfunctions suggest that the patient has successfully traversed developmental hurdles to establish a comfortable sexual self. Moreover, the symptom is generally rooted in the present or recent past; it is not simply an outgrowth of early childhood issues. The dysfunction often represents the couple's shared solution to some aspect of their relationship.

The exceptions to the guideline of conjoint treatment for acquired erectile dysfunction are in the case of the single man without a partner, the single man with an uncommitted partner, and the couple whose relationship has deteriorated so much that they cannot productively work with one another. Obviously, the man without a partner will be seen in individual treatment. Years ago, there were some therapists who would have demanded that the patient should first become involved with a partner and then seek treatment. Although the lack of involvement in a relationship does present clear limitations for therapy, the patient can benefit nonetheless. The stickier decision is how to determine whether a single man has a "committed" partner. Meeting with each partner alone is helpful in deciding how committed the partners are to one another. The therapist should attempt to see dysfunctional couples in a conjoint format first, but employ more structure than usual. If this proves unworkable, one or both can be referred for individual treatment.

# Goals of Psychotherapy for Psychogenic Erectile Dysfunction

Psychotherapy aims to restore a man's potency to the optimal level possible, given the limits of physical well-being and life circumstances. Treatment seeks to overcome the psychological barriers that preclude mutual sexual satisfaction. To accomplish these goals, the patient(s) and therapist embark on an intrapsychic and interpersonal journey to discover and demystify the meaning of the dysfunction. On this journey the psychosomatic symptom of impotence is transformed into cognitive and emotional experience. The therapist understands the patient's symptom as a metaphor that contains a compromised solution to one of life's dilemmas.

Psychogenically impotent men often feel puzzled, disgraced, weakened, and frightened. They have lost hope and confidence, and wonder "Why me?" Their perceived failure is attributed to physical illness, psychological concerns, interpersonal disturbance, or religious retribution. Although urologists frequently treat psychogenic erectile dysfunction as though it were a single entity, mental health professionals understand that psychogenic erectile dysfunction is actually a symptom of some underlying enigma to be overcome by understanding responses to difficult life dilemmas, integrating previously unacknowledged feelings, seeking new solutions to old problems, increasing communication, surmounting the barriers to intimacy, and restoring sexual confidence.

Although the enigmas vary, most cases have a metaphor in common; psychogenic erectile dysfunction is a message that tells the man's body not to cooperate with intercourse. The symptom is almost always a partial enigma to the man because he cannot allow himself to understand how his social or psychological dilemmas affect his potency.

Psychogenic erectile dysfunction is usually generated by the resonating interaction of emotional forces from three time periods: the present (performance anxiety), the recent past (the life events that precede the onset of the symptom), and childhood (developmental vulnerabilities from childhood and adolescent years).

Performance anxiety, the factor in the present, serves the man as a distraction from other feelings he may be having about making love in general and about making love to his particular partner. The recently dysfunctional man typically does not appreciate the significance of the life changes from the recent past that preceded his problem. He is either unsure of or denies the emotional meaning of these events. He fails to realize that his symptom is the result of these events and his responses to them. He focuses on his loss of sexual confidence (a frequently used phrase for performance anxiety) as the cause of his problem; he remains befuddled about how he originally fell into its pernicious trap. The trap, however, diminishes the frequency of lovemaking.

Part of the mystery of the psychogenic problem derives from events of long ago. Intercourse acquires meanings that derive from experiences much earlier in life. Therapists tend to describe these meanings with assorted jargon, such as failed tasks of psychological development, impairments in sexual identity, vulnerabilities of the self-system, oedipal issues, abuse, social learning difficulties, pregenital fixations, transference. Whatever terminology therapists prefer, the words refer to childhood processes.

The concept of resonation of forces from three time spheres provides a scheme for understanding generic varieties of psychogenic erectile dysfunction, but a scheme is only a skeletal outline of the process of symptom generation and maintenance. The mental health professional's work is to add the flesh by noting the extent of performance anxiety, pinpointing the precipitating events, and defining their emotional meanings. This is how therapy is conducted.

# Usual Precipitants of Acquired Psychogenic Erectile Dysfunction

Because new onset erectile dysfunction arises under diverse social and psychological circumstances, each case has a common component: the man's feelings during sexual foreplay interfere with arousal. The man may not recognize the emotional significance of the recent changes in his social situation or may fail to comprehend its relevance to his potency. The emotions associated with the impotence-triggering event soon are amplified by its similarities to past developmental experiences. Making love creates a confrontation with his private emotional truths. Performance anxiety, which usually begins after one or two erectile failures, enables him to avoid focusing on the dysfunction. Men are vulnerable to the development of this symptom to the degree to which they are characterized by the expectation that they ought to be able to perform sexually regardless of social circumstances and by the inability to quickly experience and understand their emotions.

## Relationship Deterioration

The self-declaration of impotence in the face of alienation, mutual hostility, lack of psychological intimacy, and partner unreceptivity is a testimony to the man's expectation that he and his penis ought to be able to function under any conditions. Such optimism is not warranted even though the patient may emphasize that in his last marriage he was able to have intercourse even when divorcing. It is reasonable for the clinician to presume that such a man's impotence involves some of the following: resentment, loneliness, confusion as to who is correct about the couple's unresolved differences, guilt over his role in their troubles, reaction to his partner's unreceptivity and anger, fear of abandonment, and helplessness to end their downward spiral.

## Divorce

Many divorcing and divorced men are surprised by their unreliable erections. Initially, they cannot relate an erection problem to bitterness, guilt, or uncertainty of future attachment. They expect their penises to operate autonomously. It is reasonable for the clinician to presume that such a man's impotence involves some of the following: continuing love for his divorced wife, fear of his rage at other women, doubt about his lovability, concern about his ability to love again, despair over his children's pain and alienation, wariness that a new partner will eventually turn into an impossible person as his wife did, and guilt over some dishonesty with new partners.

## Death of Spouse

Most widowers are at least in their 50s. Feelings about resuming a sexual life with a new partner are influenced by many factors, such as the duration and quality of the marriage, the cause of his wife's death, and his own health. Because there are partners readily available to physically healthy widowers, some men use dating as a distraction from being home alone and from other inevitably difficult aspects of grief. It is reasonable for the clinician to presume that the impotence of recent widowers involves some of the following: unresolved grief, guilt about impulses to have multiple partners, sense that he belongs only to his deceased wife, confusion about his new freedom, and discomfort about his children's and friends' reactions to his dating in general or to a specific woman he dates.

## Vocational Failure

Vocational adequacy is central to the self-identity and self-esteem of most men. Vocational failure or threatened vocational failure can create feelings of despair, uncertainty, anxiety, unworthiness, and guilt that may be most apparent when he attempts to make love. "I don't feel worthy of her any longer," may lurk behind the recent impotence of a man with an employment problem.

## Loss of Personal or Spousal Health

Psychogenic potency problems are common after major health events, such as myocardial infarction, open heart surgery, stroke, and cancer. Fear of death during sexual activity or the heightened awareness caused by a recent close call with death may be most apparent to the man during lovemaking. The partner's reactions to a man's illness and new health status may not be completely resolved and can create a subtle sexual unreceptivity that triggers erectile failure and performance anxiety. Conversely, the deterioration of his partner's health may lead to erectile impairment because of new perceptions of his partner's condition.

# Conclusion

With the advent of the newer reversible, relatively safe treatment alternatives for erectile dysfunction, the role of the mental health clinician has grown from diagnosing and treating patients with clearly psychogenic erectile dysfunction to helping patients overcome resistances that have precluded their using new treatment options. In this expanded role, the mental health clinician works in tandem with the urologist to sort through the often unspoken, unseen resistances that develop as the consequence of an erectile dysfunction and may require interdisciplinary intervention by which the medical as well as the psychological factors that preclude satisfactory lovemaking can be addressed.

## References

1. Althof SE, Seftel AD. The evaluation and treatment of erectile dysfunction. In: Levine SB, ed. *Psychiatric Clinics of North America.* Philadelphia: W.B. Saunders; 1995: 171–192.
2. Rosen RC, Leiblum SR. Erectile disorders: an overview of historical trends and clinical perspectives. In: Rosen RC, Leiblum SR, eds. *Erectile Disorders: Assessment and Treatment.* New York: Guilford; 1992: 3–26.
3. Althof SE. Psychogenic impotence: Treatment of men and couples. In: Leiblum SR, Rosen RC, eds. *Principles and Practice of Sex Therapy; Update for the 1990s.* New York: Guilford; 1989: 237–268.
4. Levine SB, Althof SE. The pathogenesis of psychogenic impotence. *J Sex Education Ther* 1991; 17(4):251–266.
5. Virag R, Frydman D, Legman M, et al. Intracavernous injection of papaverine as a diagnostic and therapeutic method in erectile failure. *J Urol* 1984; 138:52–54.
6. Brindley GS. Maintenance treatment of erectile impotence by cavernosal unstriated muscle relaxant injection. *Br J Psychiatry* 1986; 149:210–215.
7. Althof SE, Turner LA. Self injection therapy and external vacuum devices in the treatment of erectile dysfunction. In: Rosen RC, Leiblum SR, eds. *Erectile Disorders: Assessment and Treatment.* New York: Guilford; 1992: 283–312.
8. Nadig P, Ware J, Blumoff R. Noninvasive device to produce and maintain an erection-like state. *Urology* 1986; 27:126–131.
9. Witherington R. Vacuum tumescence device for management of erectile impotence. *J Urol* 1989; 141:320–322.
10. Morales A, Condra M, Owen J, et al. Oral and transcutaneous pharmacologic agents in the treatment of impotence. *Urol Clin North Am* 1988; 15(1):87–93.
11. Cavallini G. Minoxidil versus nitroglycerin: a prospective double-blind controlled trial in transcutaneous erection facilitation for organic impotence. *J Urol* 1991; 146:50–53.
12. Althof SE, Turner LA, Levine SB, et al. Why do so many people drop out from autoinjection therapy for impotence? *J Sex Marital Ther* 1989; 15:121–129.
13. Sidi A, Pratap R, Chen K. Patient acceptance of and satisfaction with vasoactive intracavernous pharmacotherapy for impotence. *J Urol* 1988; 140:293–294.
14. Levine SB. *Sex is Not Simple.* Columbus, OH: Psychological Publishing; 1988.
15. LoPiccolo J. Postmodern sex therapy for erectile failure. In: Rosen RC, Leiblum SR, eds. *Erectile Disorders: Assessment and Treatment.* New York: Guilford; 1992: 171–197.
16. Schnarf D. *Constructing the Sexual Crucible.* New York: Norton; 1990.
17. Levine S. *Clinical Life, a Clinician's Guide.* New York: Plenum; 1992.
18. American Psychiatric Association. *DSM-IV: Diagnostic and Statistical Manual.* 4th ed. Washington, DC: American Psychiatric Press; 1994.

# 35
# Peyronie's Disease and Its Medical Management

Laurance A. Levine and Lev Elterman

Plastic induration of the penis, referred to as Peyronie's disease, was described in 1743 by the French physician François de la Peyronie[1] when he reported on three patients with scar tissue that resulted in an upward curvature of the penis during erection. This fibrous inelastic scar involving the tunica albuginea of the corpora cavernosa is the distinguishing characteristic of this disease. The typical symptoms include a palpable scar (frequently referred to as a Peyronie's plaque), on the shaft of the penis, complaints of pain and abnormal curvature during erection, and difficulty with coitus because of the deformity or diminished rigidity or both. This condition often leads to unsatisfactory sexual performance and profound psychological trauma.[2]

Peyronie's disease affects males primarily between the ages of 40 and 60.[3] Prevalence of the disease is reported to be between 0.3% and 1% but may be higher because of such factors as limited physician reporting and patient embarrassment.[3,4] It has been reported that patients may delay seeking medical advice for up to 15 months.[5] The leading cause for seeking medical attention is painful erections, even though it is not the most consistent or common symptom. In men with Peyronie's disease, a palpable plaque occurs in 78% to 100% of the patients, curvature of the penis during erection in 52% to 100%, and pain in 70%.[6–8] Although plaque length is usually between 1.5 cm to 2 cm, it may range from a few millimeters to the entire length of the penis shaft.[8] The most frequent plaque location is in the dorsal

midshaft.[9–11] Because malignant degeneration of this condition has not been demonstrated, it is important to reassure men with Peyronie's disease of its benign nature.

Although de la Peyronie believed the causes for plaque formation and subsequent curvature of the penis were sexual abuse and sexually transmitted infections, it was not until 1966 that Smith[8] performed one of the first systematic pathologic studies of Peyronie's disease. His review of 26 cases documented scar formation in the space between the tunica albuginea and cavernosal tissue. Histologically, a chronic perivascular infiltrate with damage to small blood vessels was observed. Smith proposed that as the disease progressed, the infiltrate became less cellular, deposition of collagen fibers occurred, and areas of perivascular scarring and plaque formation resulted. Smith considered Peyronie's disease as primarily an inflammatory disease, but as noted by Roddy and Goldstein,[12] it is now believed that the inflammatory infiltrate is the result of injury rather than the cause of disease.

## Physiology of Trauma

Although the etiology of Peyronie's disease is unclear, the mechanical injury theory, as proposed by Devine et al,[13] describes a mechanism for the initiation of a Peyronie's plaque, based on the observation that most plaques are located either on the dorsal or ventral surface and are always associated with the septum of the corpora cavernosa. The tunica albuginea is composed of two layers, a longitudinal outer layer and an inner circular layer. The septal fibers interweave with the inner circular layer, and when pressure is placed on the erect penis, stress upon the septal fibers is transmitted to the tunica fibers. In a genetically predisposed population of men, where there may be a decrease in fiber elasticity, the pressure may result in delamination or fracture of the circular fibers within the tunica albuginea. In men with Peyronie's disease, it has been demonstrated that there is a qualitative and quantitative reduction of elastin production within the tunica albuginea.[13-15] This decrease in elasticity, which results in less tolerance to stress and ultimate injury, may be a possible predisposing factor to Peyronie's disease.

Following injury, the process of wound healing occurs with fibroblast proliferation and extracellular matrix deposition. It is at this point that the balance between scar formation and scar remodeling is lost in the patient with Peyronie's disease. The scar or extracellular matrix formation exceeds the degradation because of abnormal fibroblast activity or an altered remodeling process or both. Peyronie's disease may therefore be considered a disorder of wound healing, much like a hypertrophic scar or keloid, where the mechanical injury acts as the epigenetic factor activating the disease.[16]

## Natural History

The pathophysiology of the clinical deformity associated with plaque formation in Peyronie's disease is based on the mechanical properties of the plaque and the anatomy of the tunica albuginea. In 1993 Gelbard[17] described the conjoined corpora as a stack of hoop or ring elements that elongate during erection. In the normal state, these hoop-like elements move apart in parallel planes until the rigidity of a straight erect penis is achieved. In a patient with Peyronie's disease, the scar tissue restricts parallel displacement of the rings during erection and a bend results around the inelastic segment. With age, the decreasing elasticity of the tunica albuginea and subse-

quent loss of extensibility will gradually lessen the bend because of the decreasing separation of the free ends of the rings, which may explain the gradual resolution of Peyronie's disease in some patients.

In 1970 Williams and Thomas[17] referred to the natural evolution of Peyronie's disease as a process of "gradual resolution." In their study, 21 patients were followed for an average of 4 years without any medical treatment. Six patients demonstrated complete resolution of symptoms (29%), 10 improved so that sexual intercourse was possible (48%), and five remained unchanged (24%). Later studies were less optimistic and suggested that the natural history of Peyronie's disease remains unclear.[18,19]

In 1990 Gelbard et al[2] reported on the largest long-term study of the natural history of Peyronie's disease. In this study, 97 patients with a duration of disease ranging from 3 months to 8 years were characterized on the basis of disease duration, age, plaque size, penile deformity, ability to engage in coitus, and psychological effects. The study found that 40% of these patients experienced no change in penile curvature or sexual function during the observation period; the curve became worse in 40%; and the pain resolved in 94%. A negative psychological effect of this disorder was detected in 77% of patients at presentation. The most important finding with regard to the natural history of Peyronie's disease was that only 13% of these patients experienced complete resolution, 47% remained with little or no change, and 40% progressed with larger plaques, further penile deformity, or both.

In a recent unpublished review of over 300 men with Peyronie's disease, fewer than 10% had noted a functionally significant spontaneous improvement in penile curvature. Therefore, patients with Peyronie's disease should not be encouraged to believe that the problem will resolve on its own. On the other hand, those men who are not sexually compromised by the penile deformity and are not experiencing painful erections can be encouraged to continue sexual activity and will not require treatment.

# Medical Management

In spite of various treatment options, Peyronie's disease has remained a therapeutic dilemma for the practicing urologist. Peyronie advocated use of Barège spa water and mercurial ointments. In the 1800s iodine, arsenic, and camphor were used. More recently, different modes of energy transfer, including orthovoltage radiation, ultrasound, shortwave diathermy, laser therapy, and shock wave lithotripsy, have been used to treat this disease.[20–22] These methods have never found wide acceptance in the United States and are not recommended at this time.

The use of oral agents for the treatment of Peyronie's disease began in 1948. Scott and Scardino[23] reported on treatment of 23 patients with vitamin E, a tocopherol with antioxidant properties, but the study did not compare the effect of the treatment with the natural history of the disease. Use of vitamin E has continued and, over time, has become widely accepted because of its mild side effects and low cost, despite the lack of a controlled study showing its benefits.

In 1959 Zarafonetis and Horrax[24] studied potassium aminobenzoate (Potaba) as a systemic therapy agent. This substance is classified as "possibly effective" by the Food and Drug Administration for the treatment of Peyronie's disease, scleroderma, dermatomyositis, linear scleroderma, and pemfigus. The mechanism of action is not well understood. It has been suggested that Potaba increases utilization of oxygen by tissues and increases activity of monoamine oxidase, which decreases concentration of serotonin, a substance thought to be responsible for fibrogenesis. Based on its unsubstantiated mode of action, relatively high cost, and side effects (including gastrointestinal intolerance), which often result in noncompliance, enthusiasm for the use of Potaba is cautiously guarded.

Ralph et al[25] described experience with oral tamoxifen in 1992.[25] This preliminary study showed encouraging results in patients with recently acquired (less than 4 months) Peyronie's disease. The regimen included 20 mg of tamoxifen twice a day for 3 months. Eighty percent of patients reported an improvement in pain, 35% showed decrease in deformity, and 34% experienced plaque shrinkage. It has been suggested that tamoxifen facilitates the release of transforming growth factor-β (TGF-β) from fibroblasts.[26] TGF-β has been shown to play a central role in regulating immune response, inflammation, and tissue repair by deactivating macrophages and T lymphocytes. Tamoxifen results in a reduced inflammatory response and, therefore, diminished angiogenesis and fibrogenesis.[27] Tamoxifen, however, is difficult to recommend because long-term results, side effects, and larger cohorts are not available, yet this type of therapy is particularly interesting in light of better understanding of scar formation.

The use of procarbazine (Natulan) has brought rather disappointing results. This cytotoxic alkylating agent was commonly used for treatment of Hodgkin's lymphoma. In spite of the initial favorable reports in patients with Dupuytren's contractures, studies have not shown a benefit in men with Peyronie's disease. Theoretically, procarbazine should inhibit proliferation of rapidly dividing fibroblasts, but studies have suggested there is no value in the use of this toxic agent.[28,29]

Oral colchicine therapy was recently reported in a noncontrolled study by Akkus et al.[30] This agent is known to induce collagenase activity and decrease collagen synthesis.[31–34] Colchicine acts in four ways: (1) it binds to tubulin and causes it to depolymerize and, subsequently, inhibits mobility and adhesion of leukocytes; (2) it inhibits cell mitosis by disrupting the spindle fibers; (3) it blocks the lipoxygenase pathway of arachidonic acid metabolism, thus diminishing chemotaxis and inflammatory response; and (4) it interferes with transcellular movement of protocollagen. Akkus et al recommended an initial dose of 0.6 to 1.2 mg daily during the first week of treatment followed by a gradual increase to 2.4 mg over 3 to 5 months. Although not qualified further, penile curvature was slightly improved in two (11%) and markedly improved in five (26%) of the 19 patients. Seven of nine patients with painful erections reported significant relief. The palpable plaque disappeared in two and decreased in size in 10 patients. The investigators also performed ultrasound on five patients and noted a decrease of approximately 50% in plaque size.

Based on anti-inflammatory properties, as well as decreased collagen synthesis by unclear mechanisms, steroids have been employed as an intralesional therapy for Peyronie's disease.[35,36] In 1954 Winter and Khanna[37] published their results on the use of mechanically aided injection (Dermo-jet) of dexamethasone. Although a decrease was reported in both plaque size and pain during intercourse, no statistical difference was evident in comparison with the natural history of the disease. In 1980 Williams and Green[19] described the use of intralesional triamcinolone, a long-acting glucocorticoid with low solubility, which theoretically produces maximal local action with minimal systemic side effects. After the initiation of therapy, 33% of the 45 patients noticed marked improvement. Patients under the age of 50 with small, firm, discrete plaques were reported as more likely to respond to triamcinolone treatment. This treatment has also been shown to benefit Dupuytren's contractures and hypertrophic scars.[38,39]

Treatment of Peyronie's disease with intralesional steroids should be initiated with extreme caution because of local side effects and the inconsistent pattern of improvement in well-established curvature. Although steroids are known to suppress fibroblast production of collagen, this effect is unpredictable and may result in local tissue atrophy. In at least one unreported case, a patient developed adrenal insufficiency because of excessive use of steroid injections. In addition, steroid injections make surgery more complicated because of the difficulty in subsequent separation of tissue planes between Buck's fascia and the tunica albuginea.

Another hormone used in the intralesional treatment is parathyroid hormone (PTH).[40] The rationale for using PTH in Peyronie's patients is based on reports of increased production of a collagenolytic factor in bone by this hormone.[41] It has been suggested that injection of PTH into the plaque may depress collagen synthesis and promote collagen degradation. However, the use of PTH has not been further substantiated.

Purified clostridial collagenase was studied in vitro with surgically excised Peyronie's plaques by Gelbard et al[42] in 1982. In 1993 results of the only double-blind study of any type of medical therapy for Peyronie's disease were published.[43] In this study of 49 men, a statistically significant improvement in plaque size was found following collagenase treatment as compared to placebo control. The patients were stratified according to the severity of their disease, and a modified Kelâmi system was used for classification.[44] Category 1 patients had a bend of 30° or less, or a palpable plaque of less than 2 cm or both. Category 2 patients displayed 30° to 60° of angulation or a palpable plaque between 2 and 4 cm or both. Category 3 patients had greater than 60° of penile bending or greater than a 4 cm plaque or both. The researchers used vacuum chamber photography to document the degree of angulation. Patients in category 1 received 6000 units of purified clostridial collagenase, patients in category 2 received 10,000 units, and patients in category 3 received 14,000 units. The category 1 patients responded best to the treatment (100% noted some improvement), followed by category 2 (36%) and category 3 (13%). Maximal angular improvement observed ranged from 15° to 20°, which was acceptable only in category 1 patients. In more severe cases, change in curvature was detectable but not clinically significant. No side effects were noted by the authors. Currently, this mode of therapy is a promising option for mild-to-moderate degrees of Peyronie's disease and is being evaluated in an FDA-approved multicenter study.

Orgotein, an anti-inflammatory metalloprotein with pronounced superoxide dismutase activity, has been studied in Europe.[45–48] The drug was delivered intralesionally, decreasing the plaque size and increasing sexual function. Other investigators delivered orgotein via ionophoresis.[47] Orgotein is not available in the United States and was recently restricted for intralesional use in Germany because of a severe toxicity profile.

The calcium antagonist verapamil was first reported as an intralesional therapy in 1994.[16]

Intralesional injection of verapamil results in (1) rapid resolution of pain, (2) modest improvement of penile deformity, (3) improved rigidity or sexual performance in approximately 75% or both, and (4) no acute or chronic side effects. Verapamil therapy should be offered early in the course of the disease to prevent further progression and to reduce the tethering of the plaque. In addition, verapamil intralesional therapy should be offered if penile pain or deformity is present at the time of initial examination. The rationale for use of verapamil comes from the experiments that demonstrated that exocytosis of extracellular matrix molecules (including collagen, fibronectin, and glycosaminoglycans—the primary components of a Peyronie's plaque) is a calcium ion–dependent process.[49] When fibroblasts were exposed to antitubular agents and calcium antagonists in vitro, a change in cell shape was noted, and this morphogenic change resulted in an altered protein secretion phenotype, manifested by increased extracellular matrix collagenase secretion as well as decreased collagen and fibronectin synthesis and secretion.[50] Similar changes have been seen when fibroblasts have been exposed in vitro to other agents, such as colchicine, tamoxifen, and interferon.

Currently, 46 Peyronie's patients are participating in a nonrandomized, non–placebo-controlled phase II study of verapamil. Ten mg of verapamil diluted to 10 ml with saline is injected every 2 weeks for 6 months. The maximum dose of 10 mg was chosen because of the optimal response demonstrated in the previous study as well as the limited cardiovascular risk following intravenous injection of 10 mg as suggested by pharmaceutical industry safety data. The mean age and disease duration were 51 years and 17.2 months, respectively. Fifty-nine percent of these 46 men had unsuccessful prior oral therapy and 61% had painful erections. Only 26% were fully potent prior to therapy and 48% had erections sufficient for intercourse.

To date, 27 men have completed therapy. Subjectively, 96% (26/27) had rapid resolution of pain. Penile deformity improved in 85% (23/27), with improved distal rigidity in 74% (20/27) and increased sexual performance in 89%

(24/27). Objective evaluation included pre- and posttreatment duplex ultrasound, which demonstrated a decreased curvature in 61% (14/23) with a mean decrease of 22° (range 10–40°), no change in duplex ultrasound parameters, and no significant change in plaque volume.

Topical β-aminopropionitrile, a potent collagen cross-link inhibitor, has been employed in patients with Peyronie's disease.[51] β-Aminopropionitrile irreversibly binds to lysil oxidase, an enzyme responsible for the cross-linking of collagen fibrils, and prevents normal collagen fibrogenesis. A 4-week course of twice a day topical application brought only subjective improvement in three patients. No changes in plaque diameter were noted by ultrasonography or penile deformity following intracorporal infusion.

The potential use of interferons as intralesional therapy for Peyronie's disease was demonstrated in a 1991 study in which fibroblasts from Peyronie's plaques were cultured in the presence of interferons alpha-2B, beta-Ser17, and gamma.[52] The rationale for interferon therapy originates from studies illustrating similar fibroblast activity in Peyronie's plaque, keloid scars, and scleroderma.[53,54] In these cases, fibroblasts are activated and produce excessive amounts of extracellular matrix components, including collagen, glycosaminoglycans, and fibronectin. In vitro studies indicate that interferons normalize the activity of fibroblasts derived from patients with scleroderma and keloids.[53–55] In fibroblasts derived from Peyronie's plaques, the addition of interferons decreased the rate of proliferation in a dose-dependent fashion, decreased the production of extracellular collagen, and increased the production of collagenase. Interferon-gamma increased the production of fibronectin and glycosaminoglycans. These in vitro results suggest the potential of interferons as an in vivo treatment for Peyronie's disease.

Overall, therapeutic advances in Peyronie's disease have not resulted in a reliable cure, primarily because of incomplete understanding of the basic pathophysiology of this disease. Recent advances in the understanding of wound healing disorders may offer new therapies, such as the injection of calcium antagonists. The responses of cultured fibroblasts to colchicine, vinblastine, interferons, and to the calcium antagonists, verapamil, and nifedipine, suggest that through medical therapy some common primary cellular metabolic events may be altered in Peyronie's plaques. Ultimately, a multimodality therapy, such as verapamil with collagenase, and possible oral therapy may be indicated as a nonoperative approach and allow stabilization or improvement of the Peyronie's deformity. In advanced cases that do not respond to conservative therapy, surgery may offer considerable relief.

## References

1. de La Peyronie F. Sur quelques obstacles qui s'opposent a l'éjaculation naturelle de la semence. *Mem de l'Acad Roy de Chir* 1743; 1:425–434.
2. Gelbard MK, Dorey F, James K. The natural history of Peyronie's disease. *J Urol* 1990; 144:1376–1379.
3. Lindsay MB, Schain DM, Grambsch P, et al. The incidence of Peyronie's disease in Rochester, Minnesota, 1950 through 1984. *J Urol* 1991; 146:1007–1009.
4. Vorstman B, Lockhart J. Peyronie's disease. *Probl Urol* 1987; 1:507.
5. Hinman F. Etiologic factors in Peyronie's disease. *Urol Int* 1980; 35:407–413.
6. Mira JG. Is it worthwhile to treat Peyronie's disease. *Urology* 1980; 16:1–6.
7. Williams JL, Thomas GG. The natural history of Peyronie's disease. *J Urol* 1970; 103:75–76.
8. Smith BH. Peyronie's disease. *Am J Clin Pathol* 1966; 45:670–678.
9. Somers KD, Sismour EN, Wright GL, et al. Isolation and characterization of collagen in Peyronie's disease. *J Urol* 1989; 141:629–631.
10. Helvie WW, Ochsner SF. Radiation therapy in Peyronie's disease. *South Med J* 1972; 65:1192–1196.
11. Blandy JP. Penis and scrotum. In: John Blandy, ed. *Urology*, vol. 2. Oxford: Blackwell; 1976: 1049–1095.
12. Roddy MT, Goldstein I. Peyronie's disease. Part I. *AUA Update Series* 1991; 10.
13. Devine CJ, Sommers KD, Wright GL Jr, et al. A working model for the genesis of Peyronie's disease derived from its pathobiology. *J Urol* 1988; 139(part 2):286A, abstract 495.
14. Iacono F, Barva S, De Rosa G, et al. Microstructural disorders of tunica albuginea in patients affected by Peyronie's disease with or without erection dysfunction. *J Urol* 1993; 150:1806–1809.
15. Akkus E, Carrier S, Rahman J, et al. Structural alterations in the tunica albuginea: relevance to Peyronie's disease and impotence. *Int J Impotence* 1994; Res 6(suppl 1):D206.
16. Levine LA, Merrick PF, Lee RC. Intralesional verapamil injection for the treatment of Peyronie's disease. *J Urol* 1994; 151:1522–1524.
17. Gelbard M. Peyronie's disease. In: Hashmat AI, Das S, eds. *The Penis*. Malvern: Lea & Febiger; 1993:244–625.
18. Furlow WL, Swenson HE, Lee RE. Peyronie's disease: a study of its natural history and treatment with orthovoltage radiotherapy. *J Urol* 1975; 114:69–71.
19. Williams G, Green NA. The nonsurgical treatment of Peyronie's disease. *Br J Urol* 1980; 52:392–395.
20. Mazo VE. Nov metod za lschenie na bolestta na Peironi. *Khirurgiia (Sofiia)* 1989; 42(4):30–31.
21. Bellorofonte C, Ruoppolo M, Tura M, et al. Possibilita di impiego del litotritore piezoelettrico nel trattamento delle fibrosi cavernose gravi. *Arch Ital Urol Netrol Androl* 1989; 61: 417–422.
22. Frank IN, Scott WW. The ultrasonic treatment of Peyronie's dieseease. *J Urol* 1971; 106:83–87.
23. Scott WW, Scardino PL. A new concept in the treatment of Peyronie's disease. *South Med J* 1948; 41:173–177.
24. Zarafonetis CJD, Horrax TM. Treatment of Peyronie's disease with Potaba. *J Urol* 1959; 81:770–772.
25. Ralph DJ, Brooks MD, Battazzo GF, et al. The treatment of Peyronie's disease with tamoxifen. *Br J Urol* 1992; 70:648–651.
26. Colletta AA, Wakefield LM, Howell FV, et al. Anti-oestrogens induce the secretion of active transforming growth factor beta from human fetal fibroblasts. *Br J Cancer* 1990; 62:405–409.
27. Wahl SM, McCartney-Francis N, Mergenhagen SE. Inflammatory and immunomodulatory roles of TGF-β. *Immunol Today* 1989; 10:258–261.
28. Oosterlinck W, Renders G. Treatment of Peyronie's disease with procarbazine. *Br J Urol* 1975; 47:219–220.
29. Morgan RJ, Pryor JP. Procarbazine (Natulan) in the treatment of Peyronie's disease. *Br J Urol* 1978; 50:111–113.

30. Akkus E, Carrier S, Rehman J, et al. Is colchicine effective in Peyronie's disease? A pilot study. *Urology* 1994; 44:291–295.

31. Kershenobich D, Vargas F, Garsia-Tsao G, et al. Colchicine in the treatment of cirrhosis of the liver. *N Engl J Med* 1988; 318:1709–1713.

32. Diegelmann RF, Peterkofsky B. Inhibition of collagen secretion from bone and cultured fibroblasts by microtubular disruptive drugs. *Proc Natl Acad Sci USA* 1972; 69:892–896.

33. Ehrlich HP, Bornstein P. Microtubules in transcellular movement of procollagen. *Nature* 1972; 238:257–260.

34. Harris ED Jr, Krane SM. Effects of colchicine on collagenase in culture of rheumatoid synovium. *Arthritis Rheum* 1971; 14:669–684.

35. Tearsley GH. Peyronie's disease: the new approach. *J Urol* 1954; 105:523.

36. Bodner H, Howard AH, Kaplan JH. Peyronie's disease: cortisone-hyaluronidase-hydrocortisone therapy. *J Urol* 1954; 134:400.

37. Winter CC, Khanna R. Peyronie's disease: results with dermo-jet injection of dexamethasone. *J Urol* 1954; 72:400–403.

38. Pentland AP, Anderson TF. Plantar fibromatosis responds to intralesional steroids. *J Am Acad Dermatol* 1985; 2:212–214.

39. Uitto J, Santa-Cruz DJ, Eisen AZ, et al. Chromomycosis. Successful treatment with 5-fluorocytosine. *J Cutan Pathol* 1979; 6:77–84.

40. Morales A, Bruce AW. The treatment of Peyronie's disease with parathyroid hormone. *J Urol* 1975; 114:901–902.

41. Walker DG, Lapiere CM, Gross J. A collagenolytic factor in rat bone promoted by parathyroid extract. *Biochem Biophys Res Commun* 1964; 15:397.

42. Gelbard MK, Walsh R, Kaufman JJ. Collagenase for Peyronie's disease experimental studies. *Urol Res* 1982; 10:135–140.

43. Gelbard MK, James N, Riach P, et al. Collagenase versus placebo in the treatment of Peyronie's disease: a double blind study. *J Urol* 1993; 149:397–402.

44. Kelâmi A. Classification of congenital and acquired penile deviation. *Urol Int* 1983; 38:229–233.

45. Gustafson H, Johansson B, Edsmyr F. Peyronie's disease: experience of local treatment with Orgotein. *Eur Urol* 1981; 7:346–348.

46. Bartsch C, Menander-Huber KB, Huber W, et al. Orgotein, a new drug for the treatment of Peyronie's disease. *Eur J Rheumatol Inflamm* 1981; 4:250–259.

47. Verges J, Chateau A. Nouveau traitement dela maladie La Peyronie: la superoxyde desmutase par ionisations. Comparaison avec une serie ancienne classique. *Ann Urol (Paris)* 1988; 22:143–144.

48. Primus G. Orgotein in the treatment of plastic induration of the penis (Peyronie's) disease. *Int Urol Nephrol* 1993; 25:169–172.

49. Kelly RB. Pathways of protein secretion in eukariots. *Science* 1985; 230:25–32.

50. Aggeler J, Frisch SM, Werb Z. Changes in cell shape correlate with collagenase gene expression in rabbit synovial fibroblasts. *J Cell Biol* 1984; 98:1662–1671.

51. Gelbard M, Lindler A, Chvapil M, et al. Topical beta-aminopropionitrile in the treatment of Peyronie's disease. *J Urol* 1983; 129:746–748.

52. Duncan MR, Berman B, Nseyo UO. Regulation of the proliferation and biosynthetic activities of cultured human Peyronie's disease fibroblasts by interferons-alpha, -beta and -gamma. *Scand J Urol Nephrol* 1991; 25:89–94.

53. Berman R, Duncan MR. Short-term keloid treatment in vivo with human interferon-alpha$_{2b}$ results in a selective and persistent normalization of keloidal fibroblast collagen, glycosaminoglycan and collagenase production in vitro. *J Am Acad Dermatol* 1989; 21:694–702.

54. Duncan MR, Berman B. Persistence of a reduced-collagen producing phenotype in cultured scleroderma fibroblasts after short-term exposure to interferons. *J Clin Invest* 1987; 79:1318–1324.

55. Kahari V-M, Heino J, Vuorio T, et al. Interferon-alpha and interferon-gamma reduce excessive collagen synthesis and procollagen mRNA levels of scleroderma fibroblasts in culture. *Biochem Biophys Acta* 1988; 968:45–50.

# 36
# Treatment of Peyronie's Disease

Wayne J.G. Hellstrom and Wesley W. Bryan

Peyronie's disease is a nonmalignant idiopathic disorder named in honor of the noted French surgeon François Gigot de la Peyronie. The disease is characterized by the formation of an inelastic scar or plaque located within the tunica albuginea of the corpora cavernosa. Depending on the location of this fibrotic process, the plaque may result in dorsal, ventral, or lateral curvature of the penis secondary to shortening of the involved region of tunica albuginea.[1] Circumferential plaques may result in narrowing or bottlenecking of the shaft and resultant decreased rigidity distal to the area of disease.[2] Variable degrees of penile curvature, decreased penile rigidity, and a palpable plaque are the most common presenting clinical signs of Peyronie's disease. Painful erections are commonly encountered early in this condition but generally resolve with time once the progression of the disease has been established. Many men complain of difficulty with intromission, which in itself can be an extremely psychologically damaging condition.[3]

The exact etiology of this disease remains unknown and the pathogenesis is poorly understood. The majority of men with Peyronie's disease are in their fifth to sixth decade of life and most afflicted men are of Northern European descent.[4] This has led some researchers to believe there is a genetic predisposition. Repeated microtrauma, vitamin deficiencies, and autoimmune vasculitides are among the other purported causes, but no single unified theory has been successfully confirmed. Peyronie's disease is sometimes associated with other fibrosing diseases, such as Dupuytren's contracture, tymphanosclerosis, and Ledderhose's disease of the plantar fascia. The natural progression of Peyronie's disease is variable, with the active phase of the disease usually lasting anywhere from 6 to 18 months.[4] Occasionally, the disease regresses spontaneously and the associated symptoms resolve completely. Most patients, however, continue to be affected with symptoms and may then seek medical or surgical intervention. Because this condition is not associated with malignant degeneration, only those patients who complain of erectile difficulties and are motivated in correction of the problem need to be offered therapy. There are several pharmaceutical alternatives, each reported to have varying degrees of success. Oral therapies include colchicine, Potaba, vitamin E, and tamoxifen. Most of the investigations reported with these agents have not been well controlled or blinded, hence the results are suspect. Furthermore, most of these studies have not taken into account the variable progression of the disease, nor the spontaneous resolution occurring in some individuals.

When an interval of time or medical management or both has failed to improve function, surgical intervention may then be considered. An important caveat is that discussion of surgical options with both the patient and his partner should occur only after a thorough assessment of his sexual function or dysfunction. The treating urologist must recognize that with the many surgical options, no single surgical procedure is ideal. Each patient's treatment should include a surgical plan individualized for his particular need.

## Preoperative Evaluation

A thorough evaluation, which includes a detailed sexual, erectile, and psychological history, is necessary and, ultimately, very helpful in the complete care and understanding of Peyronie's patients. Important information includes any past penile trauma, the presence of impotence prior to the discovery of Peyronie's disease, and antecedent therapies employed. These and the time course of the condition have important implications on future surgical decisions. Home Polaroid photos may assist in assessing the degree of curvature. During the initial physical examination, it is helpful to manually extend the penis and palpate carefully for the length, thickness, and width of any plaque(s).[3] In-office intracorporal injection of a vasoactive agent, such as prostaglandin $E_1$ (PGE$_1$), is extremely useful to further delineate the clinical pathology in each case. Basic x-rays and xeroradiography are mentioned for historical interest but are not practical in present day clinical practice. Ultrasound measurement of the plaque dimensions has been promoted, but the actual anatomical information obtained from this study is not overly beneficial in patient care. Lopez and Jarrow[5] reported that ultrasound examination revealed evidence of a Peyronie's plaque in only 39% and plaques were manually palpable in 94% of patients diagnosed with Peyronie's disease. Hence, routine physical examination with palpation of the plaque is the optimal clinical approach for diagnosis.

In contrast, for vascular evaluation of patients with Peyronie's, duplex Doppler sonography has been strongly recommended, especially with patients who complain of erectile dysfunction. Montorsi et al[6] promote the use of color Doppler sonography as the most important diagnostic test for any Peyronie's disease patient who is about to undergo surgical correction. The existence of impotence secondary to vascular irregularities caused by

Peyronie's disease is generally different from other vascular causes of impotence and as such may be approached differently.

Several criteria have been established by authorities in the field with reference to which patients should be considered for surgical intervention:

1. Peyronie's disease should be beyond the acute inflammatory phase and have been present for a minimum of one year. (The exception is the presence of a calcified plaque.)
2. Disease activity (progression of deformity or sexual dysfunction, or both) should have been stable and unchanged for at least 3 months.
3. Difficulty with coitus or intromission is evident.[3,7]

It has been clearly shown that surgical correction alone for the resolution of pain rarely benefits the afflicted patient. Continuing with a course of conservative medical management for erectile pain over an extended period of time has better reported results.[3,8]

## The Nesbit Procedure

In 1965 Nesbit[9] described a procedure to correct congenital curvature of the phallus. Of interest, his original case reports did not document Peyronie's disease, as no evidence of fibrosis or plaques was noted in any of his patients. The procedure, though, became widely used in the surgical treatment of Peyronie's disease and is still popular today.

Typically, a circumcising incision is made approximately 1 cm proximal to the corona, and the penis is degloved to its base. An artificial erection is then induced, usually with an infusion of isotonic saline through a butterfly needle into one corpora cavernosum. The artificial erection allows the surgeon to view the site of maximum concavity and estimate the degree of penile curvature. This point is marked and Buck's fascia is then incised longitudinally to expose the tunica albuginea. Careful dissection is accomplished so as not to disturb the dorsal neurovascular bundle. A single ellipse of tunica albuginea, 0.5 to 1.0 cm in width and half the circumference of the corpora, is excised at that point on the opposite side of that of the maximum curvature. Depending on the degree of curvature, more than one ellipsoid may need to be excised to completely correct the deformity. Closure of the defect(s) is made with a nonabsorbable atraumatic suture. Pryor and Fitzpatrick[10] recommend a no. 1 nonabsorbable monofilament synthetic suture, and the subcutaneous tissues and skin are reapproximated. Patients who are uncircumcised are advised to have a concurrent circumcision.[7-11] With the Nesbit procedure, it should be noted that no attempt is made to remove the fibrotic plaque of Peyronie's disease.

As with any other penile intervention there are certain associated complications, including urethral injury, numbness of the glans and penile shaft, hematoma, wound infection, urinary retention, and phimosis. An inevitable outcome of the Nesbit procedure is shortening of the penis, but some reports suggest that this is no worse than the shortening originally caused by the disease. Bailey et al[7] reported that 17 of 179 patients who had the Nesbit operation commented on penile shortening, but none were sexually inactive secondary to this expected outcome. Overcorrection, a complication seen with a number of surgical treatments for Peyronie's disease, can be repaired after the Nesbit procedure by removing another smaller ellipsoid of corpora on the opposite side from the initial excision. Additionally, there have been reports that up to 30% of ellipsoid excisions have postoperative bleeding and anesthesia of the glans from nerve-vessel injuries.[11] The Nesbit procedure has also been associated with scar-tissue formation within the corpora cavernosa, resulting in erectile dysfunction. The procedure also places the corpus spongiosum in danger of injury.[12] On a positive note, however, Pryor and Fitzpatrick[10] reported that 20 of 23 patients had total correction of their penile deformity and resumed satisfactory coitus without any complications following the Nesbit operation.[10]

# Modified Nesbit and Plication Procedures

In the mid-1980s, several modifications of the Nesbit procedure were introduced. Essed and Schroeder[13] proposed a variation that did not excise an ellipse of tunica albuginea. Instead, they inserted wound hooks into Buck's fascia so that the penis straightened completely when the hooks were pulled crosswise. By this maneuver, the points of insertion are approximated, marked with sterile ink, and opposed with nonabsorbable 3-0 sutures. Sutures are placed approximately 2 mm apart. Tying of the sutures causes reeving of the penis on the side contralateral to the plaque.[13] This procedure allows straightening of the penis without the excision of tunica albuginea.

Similar to the Nesbit operation, plication procedures do cause penile shortening. Nooter et al[14] reported that eight of 23 patients who underwent the above procedure for congenital curvature of the penis complained of penile shortening. None, though, experienced sexual difficulty. Of 33 patients with acquired penile curvature (30 with Peyronie's disease), 18 were noted with penile shortening and two who underwent a second plication procedure were unable to have satisfactory intercourse because of the penile shortening. Another complication associated with the plication procedure when using nonabsorbable suture is that the permanent suture knots and sharply cut suture ends are palpable under the penile skin and cause irritation, suture granulomas, and extreme discomfort to the patient.[15] Unfortunately, if absorbable suture material is used, recurrence of the deformity is likely. Mufti et al[8] suggest that this problem may be circumvented by cutting the knot ends as short as possible and carefully covering them with Buck's fascia. Overall, the plication-type procedure for Peyronie's disease has been well established and is recommended as a relatively simple, safe, and effective method to treat congenital and acquired penile curvature.[8,11,14]

Another modification of the Nesbit procedure as reported by Lemberger et al[16] involves making a longitudinal incision on the tunica albuginea opposite the plaque or point of maximum curvature and closing the incision transversely with 0 Dexon sutures. A similar incision and closure may be required on the other corpora if the direction of curvature is still not rectified. In the Lemberger report deformities in 18 of 19 patients were completely corrected, and 15 were able to have satisfactory coitus, whereas only three had been able to have sexual intercourse prior to this surgery. A similar modification was introduced in 1973 by Saalfeld et al.[17] Their 10 years' experience was reported by Sassine et al.[12] This procedure consisted of exposing the tunica albuginea, inducing an artificial erection, and then making a longitudinal incision on the longer portion of the tunica albuginea. The maximum length of the incision was only 1 cm. If more correction were needed, a second or additional incisions would be made. By restricting the tunical incisions to 1 cm, this ensured that no sequestering of tunica would occur and that an even closure could be accomplished. Of the patients who underwent this modified corporoplasty, 95% reported cosmetic and functional satisfaction.[12,15,17] Complications did occur, however, with this procedure, with Udall[18] reporting penile narrowing as the major postoperative problem associated with the modified corporoplasty. Yachia[15] circumvented this problem by also using a longitudinal incision closed horizontally but using Allis clamps to artificially straighten the penis before making the incision. This maneuver removed much of the guesswork from the procedure.

Mufti et al[8] reported a retrospective study comparing outcome of correction of the three modified corporoplasty procedures: correction with the Nesbit procedure, correction by longitudinal incision and transverse closure of the corpora, and correction by corporeal plication alone. This report concluded that there was no significant difference in the success rates of these three approaches. They also concluded that there was no difference in outcome when using either polypropylene or polyglycolic acid suture material when closing or plicating. Furthermore, they recommended the corporeal plication procedure because it was simpler, less

time-consuming, and did not require the incision or excision of tunica albuginea.

The modified Nesbit and corporoplasty procedures have worked well with congenital curvature of the penis, yet many experts suggest that the curvature secondary to severe Peyronie's disease may be better treated with other approaches. Extensive Peyronie's plaques need plaque excision and grafting or, at least, incision of the large plaques to accomplish better outcomes.

## Plaque Excision and Autologous Graft Replacement

Devine and Horton[19] have stated that the Nesbit operation was not adequate for the "major bend" seen in the majority of their patients. Devine and Horton[20] first introduced their surgical approach for refractory cases of Peyronie's disease in 1974. In their procedure, modified as recently as 1991, an autologous dermal graft is employed to correct the deficit created in the tunica albuginea by the excision of the Peyronie's plaque. As the majority of Peyronie's plaques are located dorsally along the septum of the penis, Devine and Horton's technique utilizes a circumcising degloving incision. The dorsal vein is then excised after mobilizing it between the distal trifurcation and the suspensory ligament. Buck's fascia is then elevated from the tunica albuginea beginning in the midline and directed laterally under both neurovascular bundles. The dissection is extended proximally and distally beyond the extent of the plaque. An artificial erection is then induced to define the axis of curvature. At this point, the plaque's borders are outlined and the plaque is excised. Careful attention is taken so as not to injure the erectile tissue beneath the fibrotic tunical plaque. A further modification of their original procedure is to make multiple small, stellate incisions at the edges of the defect to release any stress.

Characteristically, the dermal graft is harvested over the anterior superior iliac crest by use of a dermatome. The epidermis is shaved at 16/1000 of an inch. The graft is incised, leaving a "rim" of dermis for final closure of the graft site. Fat is removed simultaneously as the graft is excised. The dermal graft with its fat side facing downward is then carefully positioned into the defect. Fine Polydioxamone Synthetic (PDS) suture is used to suture the graft in place. Devine also suggests that interdigitating the dermal graft into the stellated incision allows for the penis to elongate and prevents a circular scar contracture. He also sutures the midline of the graft to the septum when a dorsal corporotomy defect has been made. A second artificial erection is induced to observe the straightening of the penis. Buck's fascia is then reapproximated. A small suction drain is utilized to prevent hematoma formation before the skin is reapproximated.[19–21]

After the procedure, the patient is not permitted to have an erection for at least 2 weeks. Wild et al[22] recommend maintenance doses of diazepam and amyl nitrite pearls, which are inhaled should erections occur. Between 2 and 6 weeks, the patient and his sexual partner are encouraged to gently massage the erect penis so that the skin does not adhere to the graft. The Devine report refers to this as both physical and sexual therapy. After 6 weeks, patients are allowed to resume intercourse.[21]

In a report of 50 patients by Wild et al,[22] 84% of the patients noted their curvature and pain were completely resolved with the dermal graft procedure; 70% reported satisfactory results. Hicks et al[23] also reported similar results with a series using the dermal graft. Seventy-five percent of these patients reported a return to normal sexual activity without residual curvature or pain.

Naturally, there are problems associated with the dermal graft technique. Devine and Horton based the use of dermis on canine research that showed it to be the one autologous tissue that did not contract and scar. Their study was carried out for only 12 weeks. Bystrom and Norberg,[24] though, reported that in a similar canine model, contraction and scarring occurred 16 weeks postoperatively. Melman and Holland[25] contradicted the usefulness of the dermal graft in the surgical treatment of Peyronie's disease. In their study, all of the patients who were treated with the dermal graft procedure become impotent postoperatively despite technically excellent surgical results. They suggested continual corporeal scarring and internal vascular damage as the cause. Similarly, Pryor and Fitzpatrick[10] also reported poor results with the dermal graft.

Postoperative impotence following the placement of a dermal graft has been reported in 12% to 100% of patients. The mechanism of this remains somewhat controversial. Recently, Dalkin and Carter[26] reported on three patients who became impotent after undergoing dermal grafting for Peyronie's disease. Color Doppler studies revealed a venous leak in each of these three patients, which suggested a possible role for prophylactic ligation of the dorsal vein in patients undergoing dermal grafting. Jordan[27] recently stated that it is customary in his practice to perform a complete vein dissection, excision, and ligation on the pendulous portion of the penis to prevent the possible graft-induced veno-occlusive dysfunction. He noted that this has helped decrease the incidence of postoperative impotence in dermal grafted patients.

Other types of autologous grafts have been used to correct the defect of plaque excision. Some of the most recent research involves the use of temporalis fascia, deep dorsal vein, and saphenous vein as graft materials. Preliminary studies show encouraging results with these autologous tissues.[28,29] Unfortunately, all autologous tissues do require a second surgical incision for harvesting.

## Plaque Excision/Incision and Synthetic Graft Replacement

Because of the reported complications of dermal grafts, a number of investigators began to explore the use of synthetic materials. In 1982 Lowe et al[30] reported on four patients with severe Peyronie's disease who had undergone plaque excision and insertion of a graft made of Dacron, an inert material used in vascular surgery for over 20 years. The material is readily available and does not require any pregraft preparation as with dermal and other nonsynthetic graft materials. Using a method similar to the ones described earlier in this chapter, the corporeal plaque was removed along with a rim of normal corporeal tissue. Next, the easy-to-use Dacron graft was trimmed to the approximate size and sutured into place with 4-0 nonabsorbable suture. All of these patients reported excellent results. One patient developed a wound infection, had his Dacron graft saved, and ultimately did well.

Dacron grafts and other synthetic materials have certain advantages over autologous tissues. Specifically, the dermal and temporalis fascia grafts require a disfiguring second incision, and the graft requires meticulous preparation to remove fat and other connective tissues. With dermal grafts the fate of adnexal glands and hair follicles causes concern. Occasionally, inclusion cysts have developed after placement of dermal grafts.[30] Dacron is extremely easy to manipulate and has demonstrated an ability to expand during the erectile state but to maintain good tensile strength. It is also pliable, readily available, and reasonably inexpensive.

Nonetheless, it is important to mention that Dacron and other synthetic graft materials are foreign bodies, and as such they have the potential for infection, allergic reaction, and particle shedding. There already have been reports of particle shedding from genitourinary devices manufactured of silicone.[31,32] Notwithstanding, most clinical reports on cases employing Dacron, Dexon mesh, and Gore-Tex have been promising.[30,33–35]

Bazeed et al[34] used Dexon mesh in dogs, and histologic studies performed at 6 months showed complete healing of the tunica albuginea without cavernous tissue involvement. Dexon mesh fibers hypothetically serve as a scaffold for the growing collagen fibers. Schiffman et al[33] in a study of four patients, reported excellent results with Dacron grafts and all of the patients were potent postoperatively. Ganabathi et al[35] recently reported on 16 men with Peyronie's disease who had their plaques incised and had placement of polytetrafluoroethylene (Gore-Tex) grafts. All 16 men were potent subsequent to the procedure and maintained sexual relations postoperatively.

At Tulane University Medical Center, clinical experience with Silastic sheeting 0.01′ with open Dacron mesh borders (Mentor Corp., Goleta, CA) has been excellent (Table 36.1). Men with Peyronie's disease who present to the Sexual Dysfunction Clinic routinely complete a questionnaire and undergo a full medical history and examination (Fig. 36.1). This includes palpation of the full extent of the plaque and a carefully documented description of the penile deformity after an office injection with a vasoactive agent. If initial conservative therapy does not resolve the Peyronie's plaque and surgery is being considered, diagnostic evaluation with duplex Doppler is performed. Surgical alternatives are then considered and discussed with the patient and his partner. It is important to make sure that both patient and sexual partner have realistic expectations of the surgery and that it is emphasized that the primary goal of this surgery is to straighten the penis enough for the resumption of normal intercourse.

If Doppler studies reveal vascular causes of impotence, such as arterial insufficiency or significant venous leakage or both, concurrent placement of a penile prosthesis is recommended. In some cases, penile curvature straightens with just the placement of a prosthesis. In other cases, manual cracking or molding of the plaque over the prosthesis allows for correction of the penile curvature.[36]

The surgical approach is similar to that previously described. A circumcision-degloving incision is made for distal and midshaft plaques. A penoscrotal or infrapubic incision can be used

TABLE 36.1. Surgery on Peyronie's disease at Tulane University Medical Center, 1988–1996.

| Procedure | No. of patients |
|---|---|
| Prosthesis and Silastic patch | 18 |
| (1 distal erosion of single malleable rod) | |
| Prosthesis only: manual fracturing of plaque | 10 |
| (1 perimeatal ulceration) | |
| (1 10° curvature, originally 40°) | |
| (1 patient lost single rod) | |
| Excision and Silastic patch | 16 |
| (15° and 20° curvature, both originally 90°) | |
| (1 postoperative erectile pain) | |
| (1 failure, 130° curve, 70° retained) | |
| Total | 44 |
| (Mean age 55, range 29 to 71) | |

FIGURE 36.1. Patient with typical Peyronie's disease, 90° curvature to the right.

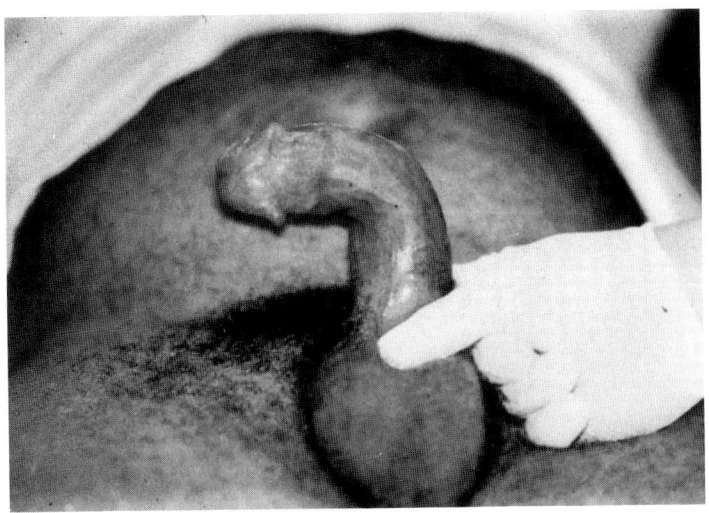

for more proximal plaques or when implanting prostheses. The more frequently occurring dorsal plaques (62% in the Tulane University Medical Center study) may be excised either by entering Buck's fascia laterally and dissecting underneath the neurovascular bundles (Fig. 36.2A, see color insert) or by removing the deep dorsal vein, carefully moving the neurovascular bundle laterally, and dissecting underneath the bundle along the tunical surface. The former approach is generally more versatile and is easier to perform.

The plaque is then sharply excised, with care taken not to damage any of the underlying erectile tissue (Fig. 36.2B, see color insert). A Silastic patch is then fashioned slightly larger than the defect and sutured in a running 5-0 proline suture with the knots placed under the dorsal vein complex (Figs. 36.2C, see color insert, and 36.3). This prevents a bothersome palpable suture end. If a prosthesis has not been implanted, an artificial erection can be created to confirm the desired result. Buck's fascia is then reapproximated to prevent hematoma formation, and the circumcision skin is closed with 4-0 chromic before a taut Coban dressing is applied. Because the Silastic material is a foreign body, it is critical that strict sterile technique must be followed. Intravenous antibiotics (vancomycin and Ciprofloxin) and a Foley catheter are discontinued the following morning be-

fore discharge. The light pressure dressing (Coban) is removed in approximately 3 days, and oral Ciprofloxin is continued for a week.

In a recent review of 44 patients surgically treated for Peyronie's disease (mean age 55 years, range 29 to 71), tabulated results were excellent. Thirty-eight percent of the patients had experienced erectile pain during the course of their disease. The mean duration of symptoms prior to surgery was 27 months (range, 6 months to 7 years). Sixty-two percent of patients had a dorsal plaque: 22% were ventral, 11% were lateral, and 5% were circumferential. Twenty five patients (60%) reported preoperative erectile dysfunction. Duplex Doppler screening revealed that 28 men had vascular causes for their impotence: ten with arterial insufficiency, five with venous leak, and two with mixed vascular problems. Seventy-four percent of the overall patient group were unable to have sexual intercourse because of their disease. The majority of patients—many of them treated conservatively by outside urologists—had received some form of failed medical therapy for their disease, e.g., vitamin E, Potaba, steroids, tamoxifen, and/or x-ray therapy. Two patients reported penile fractures in their past genitourinary history.

Among the 44 patients surgically treated, 16 patients had plaque excision and placement of a Silastic patch only, and 18 had an excision/

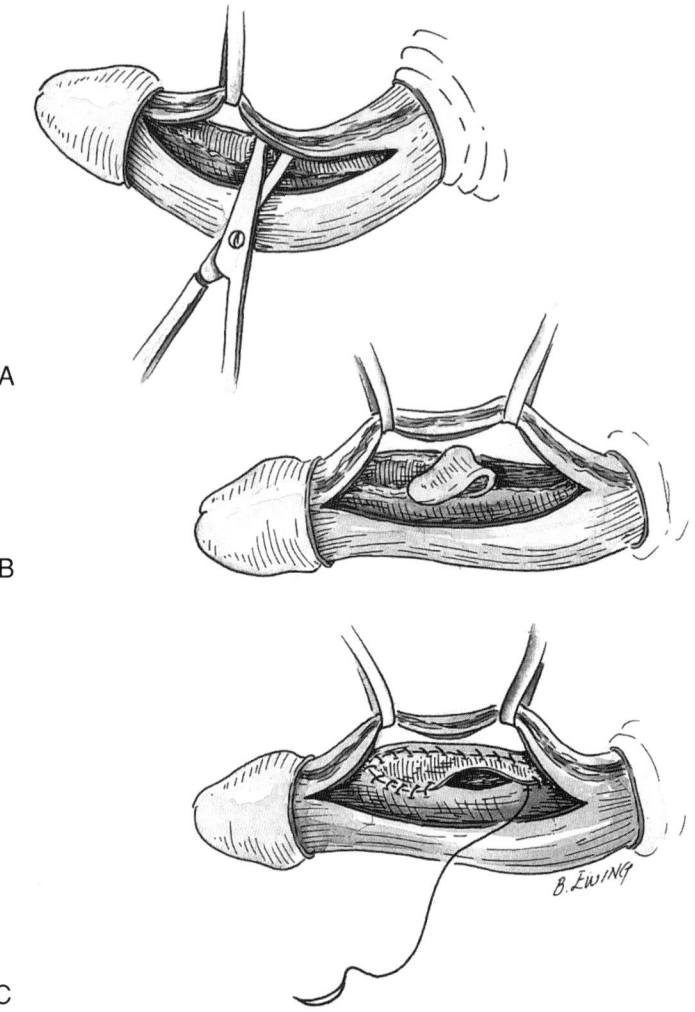

A

B

C

FIGURE 36.2. (A) To properly expose the frequently occurring dorsal plaques, Buck's fascia is entered laterally and carefully dissected underneath the neurovascular bundle. (B) The plaque is sharply excised with care taken not to damage any of the underlying erectile tissue. (C) A Silastic patch is fashioned slightly larger than the defect and sutured in a running 5-0 proline suture with knots placed under the dorsal vein complex. See color plate.

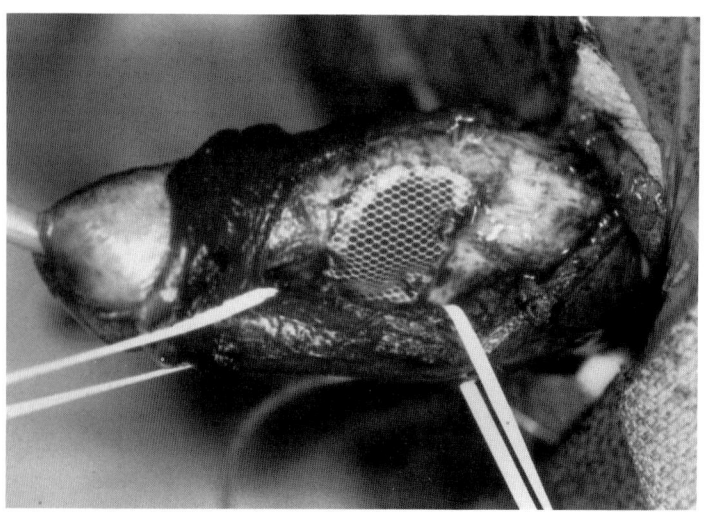

FIGURE 36.3. Intraoperative view of Silastic patch sutured in place.

incision of the plaque and implantation of a penile prosthesis. Of the 16 patients who underwent plaque excision and placement of a Silastic patch, 11 reported excellent results with no postoperative curvature or impotence. Two individuals had retained curvature of 15° and 20° (originally both were 90°) but were able to have intercouse postoperatively. Another patient had a 5° retained curve and was also able to have sexual intercourse postoperatively but complained of postoperative erectile pain. One patient in this group was impotent after surgical treatment, although his penile curvature was resolved. Seventeen of the 18 (94.4%) patients who received a penile implant and Silastic sheeting reported excellent results with no postoperative impotence or curvature. One patient had urethral erosion of a single distal malleable rod but has subsequently had this replaced and now has normal function. An additional 10 men (not included here) consented to prosthesis, excision, and Silastic patch grafting, and obtained adequate penile straightening by prosthesis implantation alone. Among these 10, eight (80%) reported excellent results with no postoperative curvature or impotence. One had a perimeatal ulceration that had to be repaired, and another continued to have a 10° curve (originally 40°), but both men were ultimately able to have intercourse postoperatively.

Overall, 42 out of the study's 44 patients have been able to resume normal sexual relations. In a mean follow-up of longer than 1 year, there have been no infections, no sensory deficits of the glans penis, and no prosthesis malfunctions reported. When it becomes necessary to use a graft to repair a defect left by either excision or incision of a plaque, Silastic sheeting, in our experience, is the most reliable, easy-to-use, and cost-effective material available to the urologist. Mentor, however, has withdrawn their Silastic sheeting material because of concerns about future litigation involving silicone. Fortunately, ABT Corporation (Silverdale, Washington) distributes a comparable product in sheets (8″ × 6″ × 0.01″). The cost is approximately $30 per sheet.

# Penile Implants and the Treatment of Peyronie's Disease

It has become common practice to consider a penile implant for men with Peyronie's disease and erectile dysfunction. Penile prosthesis implantation sometimes straightens the curvature without the need for incision or excision of the plaque. In a study of 138 patients with Peyronie's disease, Wilson and Delk[36] were successful in straightening the penile curvature simply by implanting an inflatable penile prosthesis and manually modeling the erect penis. Eighty-six percent (118) of their group did not need further surgical correction, such as plaque excision. In another recent study performed by Eigner et al,[37] 88% of their patients whose Peyronie's disease was treated with penile implantation reported normal intercourse.

The procedure for implantation of a penile prosthesis and the subsequent manual modeling or "cracking" of the penis is a relatively simple one. The prosthesis is placed in the usual fashion. If using an inflatable prosthesis, the surgeon closes the corporotomies and places the reservoir in its final position. Prior to placement of the pump in the scrotum, the device is inflated to its maximum capacity and the tubing between the cylinders and the pump is clamped with rubber-shod clamps, which allows a view of the erect penis and its curvature. The placement of the rubber-shod clamps prevents damage to the pump during the modeling of the penis, because excessive pressures may be generated during penile bending and can be transmitted to the pump if the clamps are not in place. Once the device is fully inflated, the penis is bent in the opposite direction of the curvature and held in that position for approximately 90 seconds. This results in the fracturing of the plaque. Surgeons utilizing this procedure report feeling the plaque "pop" or hearing audible "cracking" sounds. After 90 seconds of pressure on the penis, tension is released, the penis has straightened, and more fluid should be pumped into the cylinders. If significant curvature remains, the above process can be repeated. If penile straightening does not occur after several attempts of manually modeling the penis, it may become necessary to perform a plaque excision or incision. If surgical plaque manipulation becomes necessary, extreme caution must be used to prevent damage to the implanted device.[36–39]

This rather simplistic procedure is not perfect for all men with Peyronie's disease. Penile implants should never be placed in men who have normal erectile function. Only patients who are impotent or flaccid distal to their Peyronie's plaque should be considered as candidates for penile implants. Berger[2] suggests the option of a penile implant when it is necessary to make a very complex repair, including a larger graft. He indicates, though, that the patient may accept a simpler and safer shortening procedure. Nonetheless, a thorough workup with Doppler studies should be performed prior to considering any penile implantation.

Many different types of prosthesis are available, and most of these can be used in the treatment of Peyronie's disease. An exception is the AMS Ultrex inflatable prosthesis, which has been reported to have a tendency to form aneurysms and bulge out through the weakness created in the tunica albuginea from plaque excision.[2] Penile implants carry the same risks of infection found with other foreign materials that are placed in the body. On top of that risk, manual modeling of the penis increases the risk of urethral and glandular injury to the penis. Distal urethral laceration and urethral ulceration have been reported as complications of this procedure.[36,37] Great care must be taken to protect the urethra and the implanted device while bending the penis.

## Conclusion

There is no single, perfect surgical treatment of Peyronie's disease. Each surgical procedure presented has favorable outcomes and associated complications and risks that must be weighed by both patient and urologist. It is important that each patient with Peyronie's disease be treated as an individual and, as such, his surgical treatment should be customized to his condition and desires. Realistic expectations should be understood by the urologist as well as by the patient and his sexual partner. Today, many of the above surgical procedures can be modified or combined or both to better serve our patients. Careful understanding of each of the procedures, outcomes, and complications will enable the urologist to optimally treat Peyronie's disease.

## References

1. Schlossberg SM, Devine CJ Jr. Treatment of Peyronie's disease. In: Whitehead ED, Nagler HM eds. *Impotence and Infertility*. Philadelphia: J.B. Lippincott; 1994: 133–151.
2. Berger RE. Remodeling for Peyronie's disease with implants. *Contemp Urol* 1995; 7:45–49.
3. Roddy TM, Goldstein I, Devine CJ Jr. Peyronie's disease. Part II. *AUA Update Series* 1991; 10:10–15.
4. Viljoen IM, Goedhals L, Doman MJ. Peyronie's disease—a perspective on the disease and the long term results of radiotherapy. *S Afr Med J* 1993; 83:19–20.
5. Lopez JA, Jarrow JP. Duplex ultrasound findings in men with Peyronie's disease. *Mol Radiol* 1991; 12:199–202.
6. Montorsi F, Guizanni G, Bergamaschi F, et al. Vascular abnormalities in Peyronie's disease: the role of color Doppler sonography. *J Urol* 1994; 151:373–375.
7. Bailey MJ, Yande S, Walmsley B, et al. Surgery for Peyronie's disease. *Br J Urol* 1985; 57:746–749.
8. Mufti GR, Aitchison M, Bramwell SP, et al. Corporeal plication for surgical correction of Peyronie's disease. *J Urol* 1990; 144:281–283.
9. Nesbit RM. Congenital curvature of the phallus: report of three cases with description of corrective operation. *J Urol* 1965; 93:230–232.
10. Pryor JP, Fitzpatrick JM. A new approach to the correction of the penile deformity in Peyronie's disease. *J Urol* 1979; 122:622–623.
11. Erpenbach K, Rothe H, Derschum W. The penile plication procedure: an alternative method for straightening penile deviation. *J Urol* 1991; 146:1276–1278.
12. Sassine AM, Wespes E, Schulman CC. Modified corporoplasty for penile curvature: 10 years' experience. *Urology* 1994; 44:419–421.
13. Essed E, Schroeder FH. New surgical treatment for Peyronie's disease. *Urology* 1985; 25:582–587.

14. Nooter RI, Bosch JLHR, Schröder FH. Peyronie's disease and congenital penile curvature: long-term results of operative treatment with the plication procedure. *Br J Urol* 1994; 74:497–500.
15. Yachia D. Letter to the editor re: corporeal plication for surgical correction of Peyronie's disease. *J Urol* 1993; 149:869.
16. Lemberger RJ, Bishop MC, Bailey CP. Nesbit's operation for Peyronie's disease. *Br J Urol* 1984; 56:721–723.
17. Saalfeld J, Erlich RM, Gross JM, et al. Congenital curvature of the penis: successful results with variations in corporoplasty. *J Urol* 1973; 109:64–65.
18. Udall DA. Correction of three types of congenital curvatures of the penis, including the first reported case of dorsal curvature. *J Urol* 1980; 124:50–52.
19. Devine CJ Jr, Horton CE. Peyronie's disease. *Clin Plast Surg* 1988; 15:405–409.
20. Devine CJ Jr, Horton CE. Surgical treatment of Peyronie's disease with a dermal graft. *J Urol* 1974; 111:44–49.
21. Devine CJ Jr, Jordan GH, Schlossberg SM, et al. Surgical treatment of patients with Peyronie's disease. In: Smith PH, Pavone-Macaluso P eds. *Urological Oncology: Reconstructive Surgery, Organ Conservation, and Restoration of Function.* New York: Wiley-Liss; 1991: 359–364.
22. Wild RM, Devine CJ Jr, Horton CE. Dermal graft repair of Peyronie's disease: survey of 50 patients. *J Urol* 1979; 121:47–50.
23. Hicks CC, O'Brien DP III, Bostwick J III, et al. Experience with the Horton-Devine dermal graft in the treatment of Peyronie's disease. *J Urol* 1978; 119:504–506.
24. Bystrom J, Norberg KA. Free autogenous grafts into the penile cavernous tissue: an experimental study in dogs. *Urol Res* 1975; 3:145–148.
25. Melman A, Holland TF. Evaluation of the dermal graft inlay technique for the surgical treatment of Peyronie's disease. *J Urol* 1978; 120:421–422.
26. Dalkin B, Carter MF. Venogenic impotence following dermal graft repair for Peyronie's disease. *J Urol* 1991; 146:849–851.
27. Jordan GH. Letter to the editor re: venogenic impotence following dermal graft repair for Peyronie's disease. *J Urol* 1992; 148:1266.
28. Gelbard MK, Hayden B. Expanding contractures of the albuginea due to Peyronie's disease with temporalis fascia free grafts. *J Urol* 1991; 145:772–776.
29. Brock G, Nunes L, von Heyden B, et al. Can a venous patch graft be a substitute for the tunica albuginea of the penis? *J Urol* 1993; 150:1306–1309.
30. Lowe DH, Ho PC, Parsons CL, et al. Surgical treatment of Peyronie's disease with Dacron graft. *Urology* 1982; 19:609–610.
31. Barret DM, O'Sullivan DC, Malizia AA, et al. Particle shedding and migration from silicone genitourinary prosthetic devices. *J Urol* 1991; 146:319–322.
32. Fishman IF, Flores FN. Retrospective review of pelvic lymph nodes in patients with previously implanted silicone penile prosthesis. *J. Urol* 1993; 149:569A.
33. Schiffman ZJ, Gursel EO, Laor E. Use of Dacron patch graft in Peyronie's disease. *Urology* 1985; 25:(1)38–40.
34. Bazeed MA, Thüroff JW, Schmidt RA, et al. New surgical procedure for management of Peyronie's disease. *Urology* 1983; 21: 501–504.
35. Ganabathi K, Dmochowski R, Zimmern PE, et al. Peyronie's disease: surgical treatment based on penile rigidity. *J Urol* 1995; 153:662–666.
36. Wilson SK, Delk JR. A new treatment for Peyronie's disease: modeling the penis over an inflatable penile prosthesis. *J Urol* 1994; 152:1121–1123.
37. Eigner EB, Kabalin JN, Kessler R. Penile implants in the treatment of Peyronie's disease. *J Urol* 1991; 145:69–72.
38. Subini L. Surgical treatment of Peyronie's disease using penile implants: survey of 69 patients. *J Urol* 1984; 132:47–50.
39. Carson CC, Hodge GB, Anderson EE. Penile prosthesis in Peyronie's disease. *Br J Urol* 1983; 55:417–421.

# 37
# Total Phallic Construction and Penile Reconstruction

Gerald H. Jordan, Steven M. Schlossberg, and David A. Gilbert

The term *phallus* originates from the Greek word meaning "penis-like," or "primordial penis." Thus, any manmade creation of a "penis" is correctly, by definition, a phallus. The reproductive function, combined with the need for a urethra, makes penile reconstruction and phallic construction challenging. Ideally, each should be done in a single stage that is reliably reproducible. The phallus or reconstructed penis should have both tactile and erogenous sensibility created or maintained. The organ must be created with a competent neourethra that will allow voiding while standing. In most patients, there are concerns about subsequent capacity for insertion of a prosthetic stiffener to allow for successful intercourse. The phallus must be aesthetically acceptable to both patient and partner, and in the case of prepubertal phallic construction the phallus must grow so that it will have an acceptable adult size. Modern tissue transfer and reconstructive surgical and microsurgical techniques allow achievement of these objectives; however, they have yet to be achieved in a single-stage procedure.

Between 1917 and 1920, surgeons employed the tubed pedicle delay flap for upper extremity reconstruction.[1-3] This technology, however, was not utilized for phallic construction until 1936.[4] Initially, phallic construction was completed in several stages over a period as long as 5 months. Use of the tube-in-a-tube, pedicle delay technique of phallic construction in the transgender patient and in children with aphallia was reported in 1920 by Gillies.[3] He later expanded the technology into the trauma patients of World War II. His technique involved expansion of the tubed pedicle delay flap concept to incorporate a second inner tube that was meant to be either a urethra, which was seldom done, or a pocket to allow the insertion of a baculum. The abdominal pedicle tube-in-a-tube delay flap remained popular well into the 1970s. This technique, however, produced a phallus that was severely limited both functionally and aesthetically.

Laub et al[5] and Puckett and Montie[6] modified the lower abdominal tubed flap technique by creating a phallus based on the midline structures of the lower abdomen and vascularized by an abdominal branch of the superficial external pudendal artery. At a second stage, a sensible urethra and "glans" cap are added. This technique provided the transition from the use of tubed pedicle delay flaps with a random blood supply to axiocutaneous, local, and musculocutaneous flaps based on predictable vasculature; however, they were insensible and severely limited, both functionally and aesthetically.[7,8]

In 1978 Puckett and Montie[9] reported on creation of a phallus from a groin flap. Initially, they used tubed delay technology. However, their description of the first microsurgical free tissue transfer phalloplasty introduced revolutionary changes. The techniques of Chang and Hwang,[10] credited with the initial use of the forearm flap for phallic construction, and Koshima et al[11] allowed for microcoaptation of the forearm cuticular nerves to recipient nerves after the flap was transferred, unlike Puckett's procedure in which the phallus was insensible.

This microsurgical free forearm flap has become the mainstay of modern phallic construction (Fig. 37.1). The forearm tissues are thin, pliable, nonhirsute in many patients, and have a predictable vascular supply. The flaps can be tailored to the patient's needs, and the presence of sensory nerves in the forearm flap allows creation of a phallus that has both tactile protective sensibility as well as erogenous sensibility. A number of flap designs have been described, based on the forearm flap. The Chang flap is elevated on the radial artery of the nondominant forearm (Fig. 37.1A). A portion of the flap is incorporated as a urethral tube. In the Caucasian population, in whom the forearm tends to be thicker, there have been problems with ischemic stenosis of the urethral portion of the flap. By its very design, the urethral portion is far displaced on the cuticular vascular territory. Farrow et al[12] modified the forearm flap design and, with their cricket bat design, departed from the "skin island wrap concept"[13] (Fig. 37.1B). In this design, the neourethra and shaft are both centered over the vascular pedicle, and the urethral tubed portion is essentially flipped into the shaft portion. The particular advantage of this design is the ease with which the distal portion of the flap, the neourethra, can be adjusted in length to best accommodate to the native urethra. A drawback of this design is that in the transsexual population, the phallic length can be somewhat limited. However, in the trauma patient and in pediatric cases, the flap has produced excellent results. Biemer[14] described a further modification of the forearm flap (Fig. 37.1C). His modification centers the skin that is to be used for urethral reconstruction, and the flap includes a portion of the radial bone that is carried on the vessel. The concept is that the bone will provide suitable rigidity for intercourse; in practice, however, the bone significantly reabsorbs. Although the Biemer design has the inherent advantage of centering the urethra into the most reliable portion of the flap, the shaft will have two suture lines, but the urethra can be extended, if necessary, and the glansplasty modification originally used by

Puckett can be combined with the Biemer flap for an excellent cosmetic result.

All of these modifications were based on the radial artery. In 1984 Louvie et al[15] reported use of the relatively hairless ulnar forearm flap for reconstruction in the head and neck. The paucity of hair on the ulnar forearm, combined with the longer ulnar vascular pedicle, made this donor site equally suitable for penile reconstruction and for phallic construction and is now the recommended procedure.[16]

## Surgical Technique

The flap vasculature as well as the recipient vasculature are assessed in detail in each patient. If there is any history that would suggest that the deep inferior epigastric artery or the proposed recipient vessel might not be patent, abdominal angiography is performed. Likewise, any questions regarding the patency of the palmar arch or either of the forearm arteries must be clarified by either duplex Doppler study or nondominant forearm angiography or both.

The surgery itself is performed by a team led by a reconstructive plastic surgeon and a reconstructive urologist. One portion of the team begins the dissection of the forearm flap. The dissection is begun deep to the brachial fascia and carried to the level of the ulnar neurovascular bundle (Fig. 37.2). The ulnar nerve is not disturbed. The dissection of the superficial plane between the two antebrachial layers is quickest and easiest. Most importantly, dissection of that plane allows for an additional tissue layer between the eventual donor site coverage and the underlying nerves and tendons of the ulnar forearm. The full-thickness skin grafts provide both better cosmetic results as well as better functional results (Fig. 37.3). The basilic and cephalic veins are carefully elevated with the flap and are designated for use in the venous anastomosis, along with the venae comitantes of the ulnar pedicle. The lateral and medial antebrachial cutaneous nerves, which tend to run close to the cephalic and basilic veins, are carefully preserved and elevated for later coaptation to either the dorsal

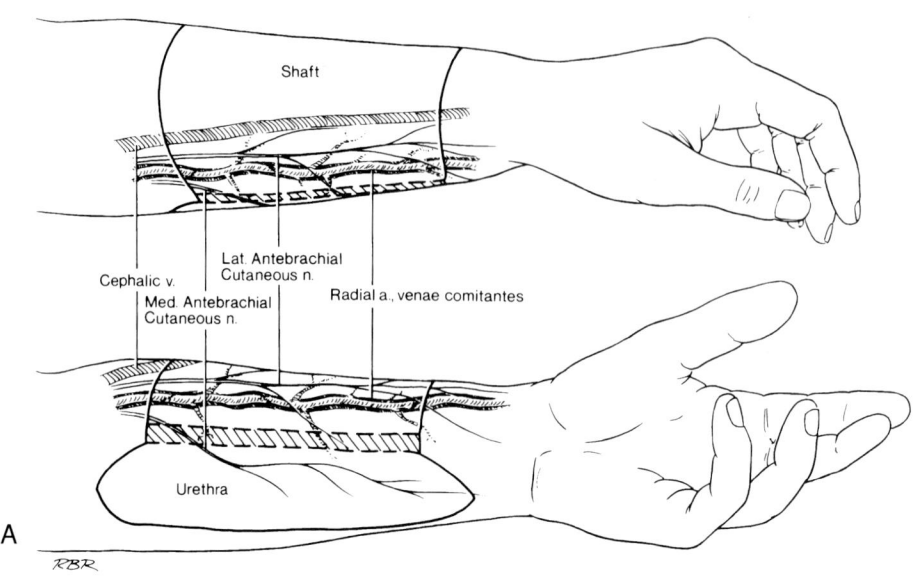

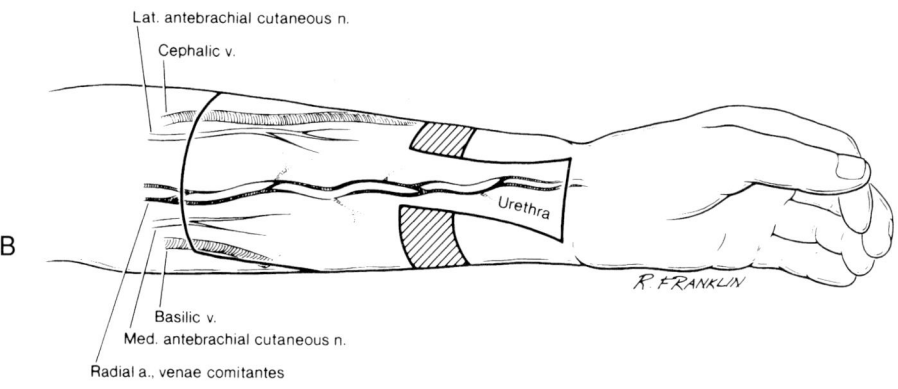

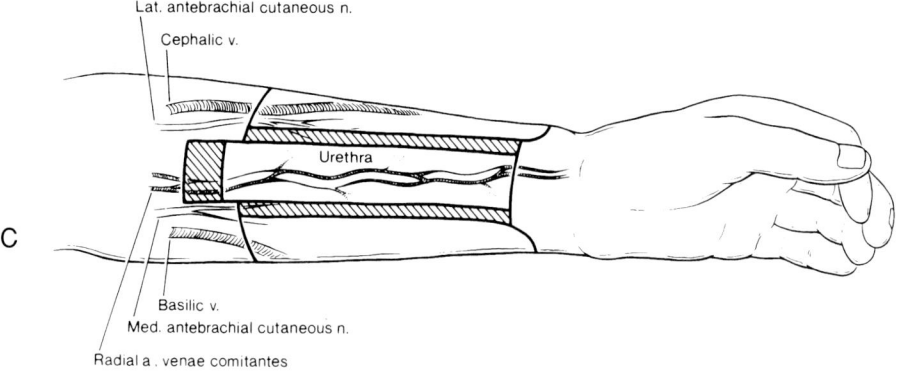

FIGURE 37.1. Various schema of forearm flaps for phallic construction. (A) "Chinese" flap. (B) "Cricket bat" flap. (C) Biemer flap.

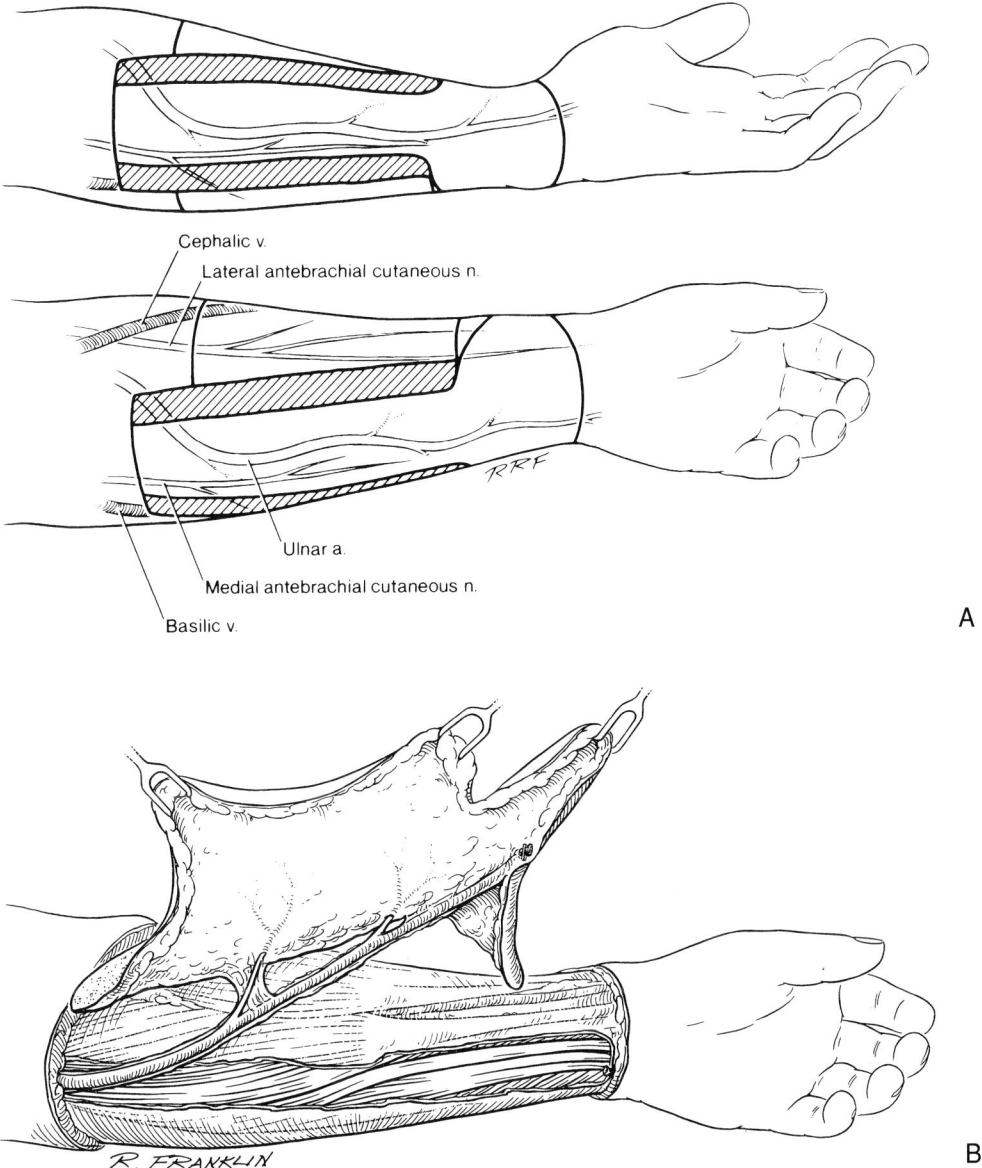

Cephalic v.
Lateral antebrachial cutaneous n.

Ulnar a.
Medial antebrachial cutaneous n.
Basilic v.

A

B

FIGURE 37.2. (A) Ulnar forearm flap for phallic construction. The midsection of the flap/urethral section is centered over the path of the ulnar artery. The shaft coverage is lateral to the de-epithelialized strips, and the glans extension shown is contiguous with the urethral strip. (B) The flap is elevated, leaving the deep lamina of superficial fascia on the forearm. The superficial lamina is carried with the flap.

nerves of the penis or, in the case of the transsexual patient, to the dorsal clitoral nerves.

Once the flap is dissected and elevated, it is configured into its eventual phallic shape; the flap remains perfused on the forearm during this portion of the procedure. The neourethra is thus created by tubing the central portion of the flap (Fig. 37.4). The outer skin paddles are then closed around the neourethra (Fig. 37.5), and the neoglans is turned over the distal shaft (Fig. 37.6). The phallus is now ready for transfer to the area of the perineum.

Meanwhile, the other portion of the team will have prepared the recipient site. The base

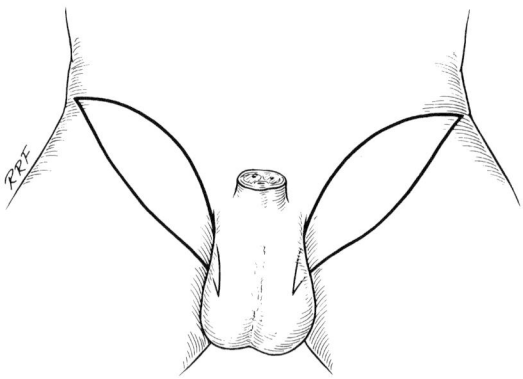

FIGURE 37.3. Area of donor site for full-thickness skin grafts used for donor site closure.

of the penis or the clitoris has been dissected, the dorsal penile nerves or clitoral nerves located. The urethra has been dissected and readied for the spatulated anastomosis to the flap neourethra. In most patients, the deep inferior epigastric vessels will have been dissected and transposed to the area of the phallus and the saphenous vein dissected in the nondominant leg to allow for an additional venous anastomosis (Fig. 37.7). In some patients, particularly those with massive pelvic trauma or patients with exstrophy/epispadias, the deep inferior epigastric vessels are not reliable, requiring that recipient vessels be created by dissecting the

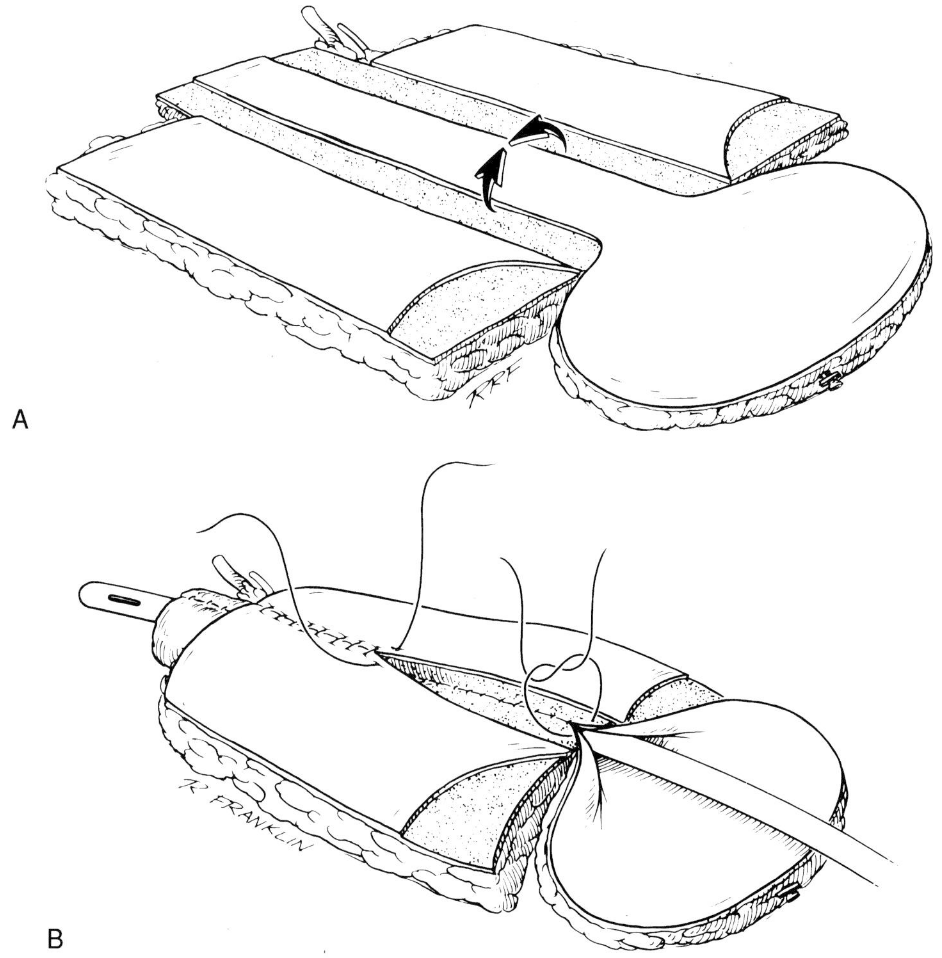

A

B

FIGURE 37.4. (A) Configuration of the ulnar forearm flap showing the de-epithelialized areas; the urethra is tubed as shown. Urethral tubularization has been completed; the shaft coverage islands are now being sutured. The glans extension has not been "flipped" proximally.

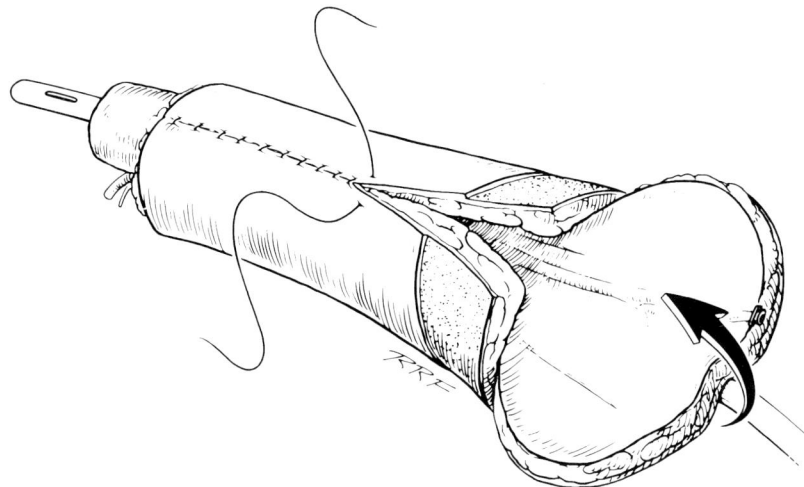

FIGURE 37.5. Shaft coverage is complete. The glans paddle extension is "flipped" proximally to achieve glans definition.

saphenous vein, allowing for a saphenous interposition vein graft between the femoral artery and the flap artery. The saphenous vein is the principal venous recipient vessel. The flap is next detached from the forearm and transferred. Anastomosis to the vessels is quickly accomplished, followed by a spatulated anastomosis to the urethra. Nerve coaptation is performed last.

In the case of the transsexual patient, a bipedicle flap is elevated and transposed be-

neath the phallus, not only creating bulk for a neoscrotum but also, and more importantly, providing a broad coverage over the area of the anastomosis. A gracilis muscle flap, from the nondominant leg, is usually dissected and transferred to the flap base to provide additional coverage and vascularity in the area of the urethral anastomosis (Fig. 37.8). The urethra is stented, and the patient's urine is diverted with a suprapubic cystostomy tube. The flap donor site (Fig. 37.9) is then covered with full-

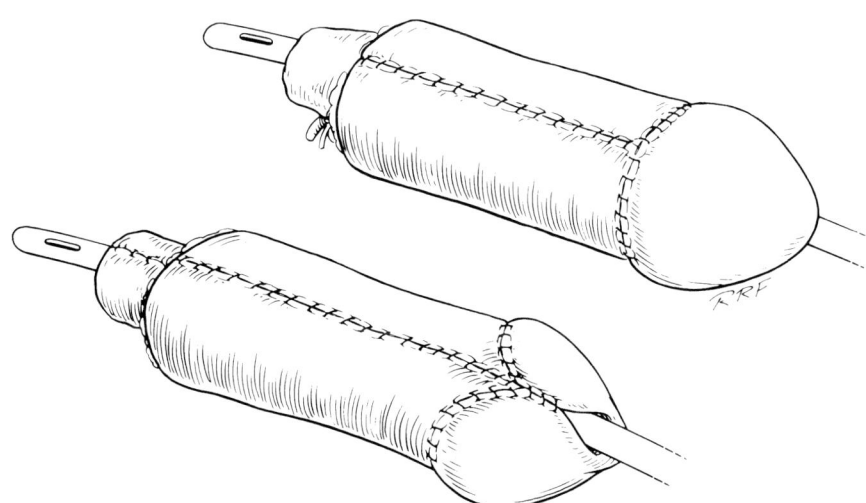

FIGURE 37.6. The appearance of the phallus as it is ready for transfer to the area of the perineum.

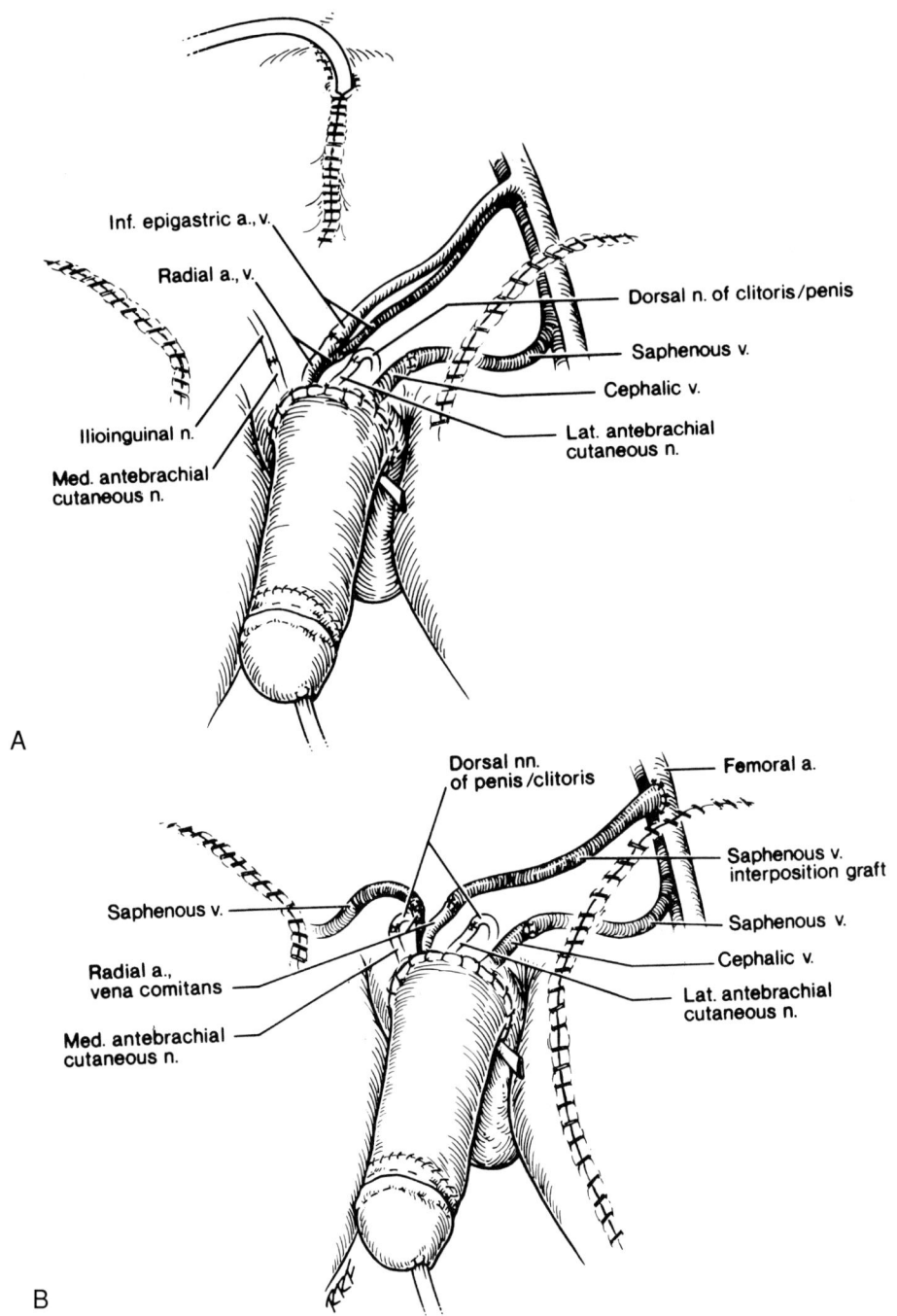

FIGURE 37.7. The various recipient vessels utilized. (A) The deep inferior epigastric artery and vena comitans is mobilized to the area of the phallus. Additional venous drainage is via mobilization of the saphenous vein, usually in the nondominant leg. (B) In patients in which the deep inferior epigastric vessels are found to be unreliable, a saphenous vein is vigorously dissected, allowing for a saphenous vein interposition graft between the femoral artery and the radial or ulnar artery in the flap. Drainage is then via the saphenous veins, usually dissected bilaterally.

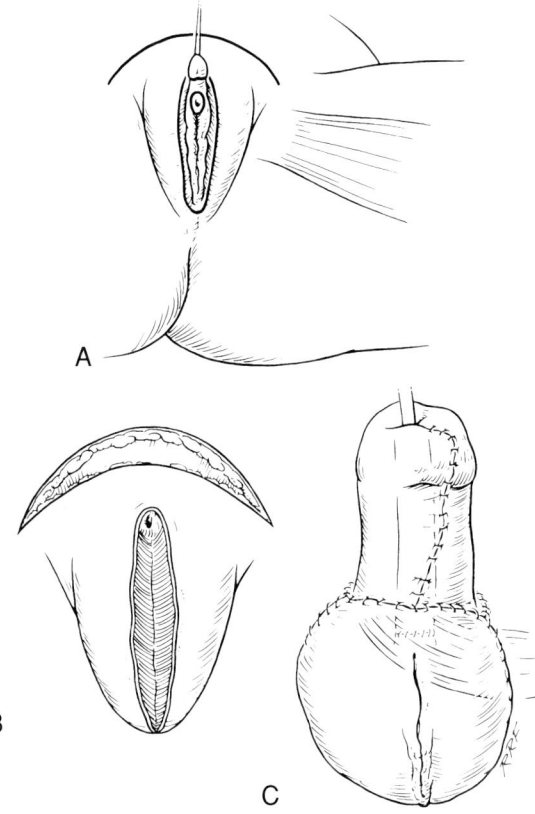

A

C

FIGURE 37.8. The bipedicle flap and gracilis flap transposition. (A) The flap is marked at the proposed site of the phallus. (B) The flap is elevated; in the case of the transsexual patient, the midline labial tissues are excised. (C) Gracilis muscle is transposed to the area of the urethral anastomosis. The bipedicle flap adds bulk in the area of the scrotum and also allows for correct male positioning of the phallus.

thickness skin grafts taken from either the inguinal crease or the redundancy of tissue over the iliac crest (Fig. 37.3).

The patient is placed on an air bed and transferred to the intensive care unit for close vascular monitoring, usually for 24 to 36 hours, and then transferred to a stepdown environment. Patients are kept at bed rest for approximately 7 days before being ambulated and placed in a whirlpool to begin cleaning up the wounds. Patients are generally discharged between 10 and 14 days. A voiding trial with contrast is performed on the 25th to 28th postoperative day, with the suprapubic cystostomy tube removed shortly thereafter. Patients are then assessed at 6 weeks, 3 months, and 6 months. At 6 months, flap sensibility should be developing well, although patients often notice sensation in the penis as early as 3 months postoperatively. At 6 months, the urethra is assessed with either flexible endoscopy or contrast studies or both. If there is any question about flap sensibility, biothesiometry can be performed.

Achieving predictable phallic rigidity is as challenging as the phallic construction itself. For prosthetic placement, an important factor is the presence of sensation that offers protection in the neophallus against pressure, necrosis, and sheer forces. Prosthetic placement should be considered only after the phallus regains sensibility and after a period of a year, at which point the urethral result is felt to be durable.

Prosthetic implants have been incorporated into phallic constructions by use of various techniques. Wahle and Mulcahy[17] reported wrapping the prosthesis with muscle and covering the phallus with skin grafts, although there

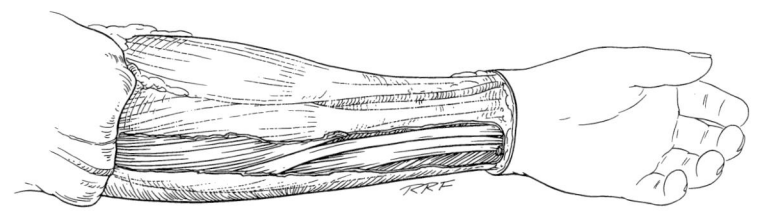

FIGURE 37.9. The appearance of the forearm donor after transfer of the flap.

is a high rate of migration and infection. In the 1970s, Puckett and Montie[9] reported on the insertion of a single cylinder of an inflatable penile prosthesis into a phallus created from a groin flap. Nonetheless, complications associated with the implantation of prosthetic implants in the phallus have led many centers to restrict such procedures.

Of three different penile prostheses used in phalloplasty patients over the past 10 years—the DuraPhase articulated prosthesis (Dacomed), the Uniflate 1000 (Surgitek), and the AMS-700 CX prosthesis (American Medi-

cal Systems)—the Uniflate has been removed from the market. Until recent years, only a single cylinder was routinely placed; however, there is improved stability by placing two cylinders, and the vast majority of phallic flaps easily accept two cylinders.

The prosthesis is placed into a neotunica created from Gore-Tex graft tailored and applied to the cylinder rod (Fig. 37.10). In patients with proximal corporal remnants, the Gore-Tex lead is anastomosed to the corporal remnant with Gore-Tex sutures. In the transgender patient or in the patient without corporal remnants, the

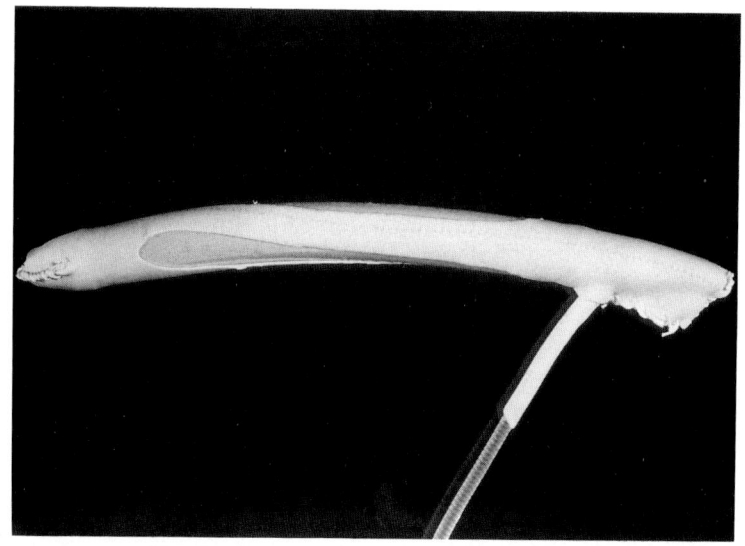

A

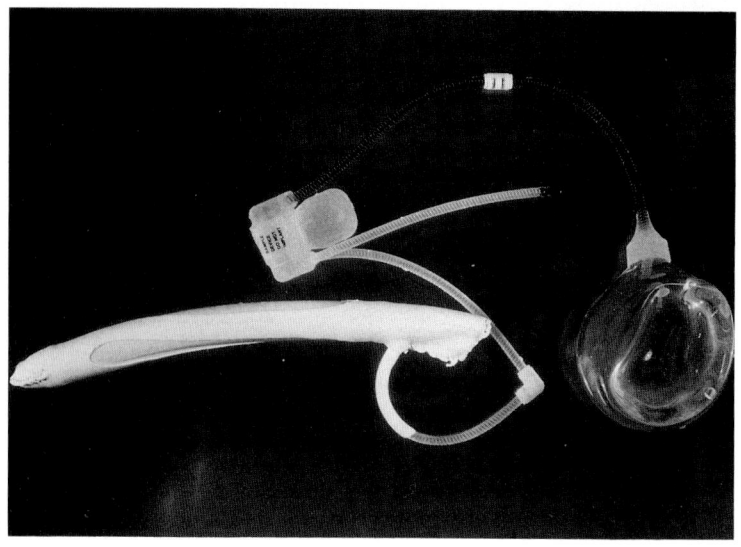

B

FIGURE 37.10. Photo showing a hydraulic cylinder, encased in a Gore-Tex "neocorporal body." A 14-mm Gore-Tex graft is used and 3-0 Gore-Tex suture is used. (A) magnified and (B) routine views).

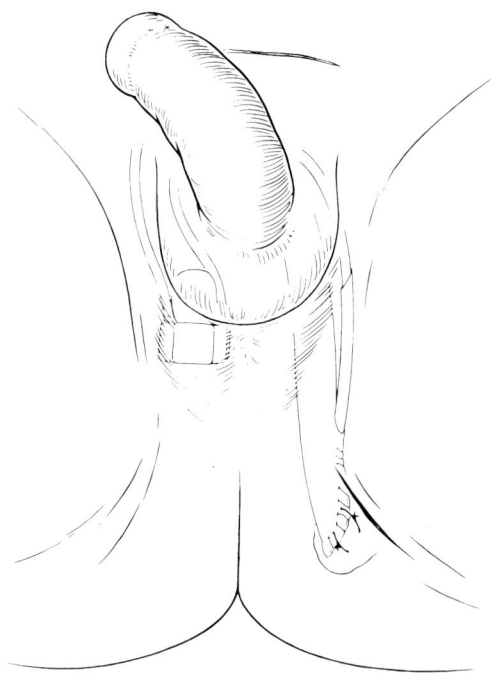

FIGURE 37.11. The proximal end of the Gore-Tex "neocorporal body" is fixed to the inferior pubic ramus. The figure shows use of a single cylinder; however, two cylinders can be used. Dilation of flap is achieved via the infrapubic transverse incision.

base of the cylinder/rod is enclosed within the Gore-Tex near the tunica, and the neotunical sleeve is attached to the periosteum of the inferior ramus of the pubis, using Gore-Tex suture (Fig. 37.11). This provides a firm base for the neocorporal bodies without migration of the devices.

Centers have reported common factors in failure, migration, erosion, and infection.[18] In a recent review of patients between 1982 and 1983 undergoing prosthetic placement after phalloplasty, four of eight patients required removal of the prosthesis because of infection.[19] Subsequent identification of technical factors significantly improved results. In the early patients, implantation had been accompanied by opening the flap ventrally and essentially unfolding it. This allowed for debulking, but even with drainage there was significant incidence of hematomas, seromas, and ensuing infection. More recently, the recommended technique is

to use a transverse suprapubic incision and dilate the flap, as opposed to creating an incision on the phallic shaft (Fig. 37.11). Small suction drains are placed for 48 hours, and the patient is admitted to the hospital for at least 72 hours of broad-spectrum intravenous antibiotics (nafcillin or vancomycin and tobramycin).

## Summary

Phallic constructive/reconstructive surgery has progressed significantly from its beginnings in Russia. Urethral construction continues to be a challenge; however, the incidence of strictures and fistulas is markedly less with the use of the gracilis flap and the bipedicle flap. Cosmetic results are now considered excellent and prosthetic placement represents the standard of care for creating rigidity for intercourse, although that continues to be a topic of great debate as the search continues for a procedure that can utilize autogenous tissues for rigidity. The future of phallic construction and penile reconstruction depends on continued close cooperation between reconstructive urologists and reconstructive plastic surgeons.

## References

1. Filatov VP. Plastika na Kruglom stebl. *Vestnik Oftal* 1917, 4–5.149.
2. Ganzer H. Weichteilplastik des gesichts bei kieferschussverletzunger. *Dtsch Monatschr Zahnh* 1917; 35:348.
3. Gillies HD. The tubed pedicle in plastic surgery. *NY State J Med* 1920; 20:404.
4. Bogoraz NA. Plastic restoration of the penis. *Sov Khir* 1936.
5. Laub DR, Eicher W, Laub DR II, et al. Penis construction in female-to-male transsexuals. In: Eicher W, Kubli F, Herms V. eds. *Plastic Surgery.* New York: Springer-Verlag, 1989.
6. Puckett CL, Montie JE. Construction of male genitalia in the transsexual using a tubed groin flap and a hydraulic inflation device. *Plast Reconstr Surg* 1978; 61:523–529.
7. Orticochea M. A new method of total reconstruction of the penis. *Br J Plast Surg* 1972; 25:347–366.

8. Horton CE, McCraw JB, Gilbert DA, et al. Phallic construction with genital sensation. In: *Transactions of IPRS*, vol. 7. Presented at International Congress of Plastic Surgery, 1983, Montreal, Canada.

9. Puckett CL, Montie JE. Construction of the male genitalia in the transsexual using a tubed groin flap for the penis and a hydraulic inflative device. *Plast Reconstr Surg* 1978; 61:523.

10. Chang TS, Hwang HY. Forearm flap in one-stage reconstruction of the penis. *Plast Reconstr Surg* 1984; 74:251.

11. Koshima I, Tai T, Yamansaki M. One stage reconstruction of the penis using an innervated radial forearm osteocutaneous flap. *J Reconstr Microsurg* 1986; 3:19.

12. Farrow GA, Boyd JB, Semple JL. Total reconstruction of a penis employing the "cricket bat flap" single stage forearm free graft. *AUA Today* 1990; 3(2).

13. Semple JL, Boyd JB, et al. The "cricket bat" flap. A one-stage free forearm phalloplasty. *Plast Reconstr Surg* 1988; 88:514.

14. Biemer E. Penile construction by the radial arm flap. *Clin Plast Surg* 1988; 15:425.

15. Louvie MJ, Duncan GM, Glasson DW. The ulnar artery forearm flap. *Br Plast Surg* 1984; 37:486.

16. Gilbert DA, Schlossberg SM, Jordan GH. Ulnar forearm phallic construction and penile reconstruction. *Microsurgery* 1995; 16(5):314–321.

17. Wahle GR, Mulcahy JJ. Ventral penile approach in unitary component penile prosthesis placement. *J Urol* 1993; 149:537–588.

18. Levin LA, Gottlieb J, et al. A new design for sensate functional total phallic construction. *J Urol* 1992; 147:289A.

19. Jordan GH, Alter GI, Gilbert DA, et al. Penile prosthesis implants in total phalloplasty. *J Urol* 1994; IS2:410–414.

# 38
# Venous Surgery for Impotence

Ronald W. Lewis

Venous occlusion has been clearly established as a necessary phase of the erectile cycle, particularly for the establishment of full rigidity. This veno-occlusion is dependent on the expansion of the intracorporeal spaces due to increased arterial inflow and relaxation of the sinus smooth muscle.[1,2] More recently, in a study of the tunica albuginea in men with penile veno-occlusive disorders, disruption of the normal elastic fiber arrangement has been reported, suggesting a causal relationship.[3]

There is no general agreement that surgery for elimination of veins on the outer surface of the tunica albuginea is effective or even reasonable for male erectile dysfunction.[4,5] The results of surgery directed at veno-occlusive disease are highly variable, and comparison between different surgical approaches is bound to produce interpretation problems.

## Background

Ebbehoj and Wagner[6] are credited with the introduction of diagnostic dynamic cavernosography techniques in surgical correction of abnormal drainage of the cavernous tissue. In 1982 Virag[7] reported successful treatment in six impotent males with deep dorsal vein ligation. In the 1980s, several series were reported of penile venous occlusive surgery for impotence.[8–12]

## Anatomy and Physiology of the Venous Drainage of the Corpora Cavernosa

Investigations into the hemodynamics of erection in animal models have clearly established the importance of veno-occlusion in the erectile process.[13] In man, following tumescence, rigidity is produced by the subtunical venous plexus being compressed by the expansion of the corpora cavernosa sinus tissue against the elastic, but firm, tunica albuginea. In addition, the linear expansion of the elastic corpora cavernosa further decreases venous outflow by increasing the oblique passage of the emissary veins through the tunica albuginea. Venous drainage from the cavernous bodies can occur through one or a combination of three different pathways: the superficial, intermediate, and the deep venous systems (Fig. 38.1). Multiple subcutaneous veins and some venous connections from the intermediate or deep system drain into the superficial dorsal vein, which subsequently drains into either the right or left saphenous venous system via the external pudendal vein. The intermediate drainage system consists of one or two deep dorsal veins that receive tributaries from the retrocoronal plexus with subsequent drainage from the emissary veins along the shaft of the penis or from circumflex veins, the usual route of emissary

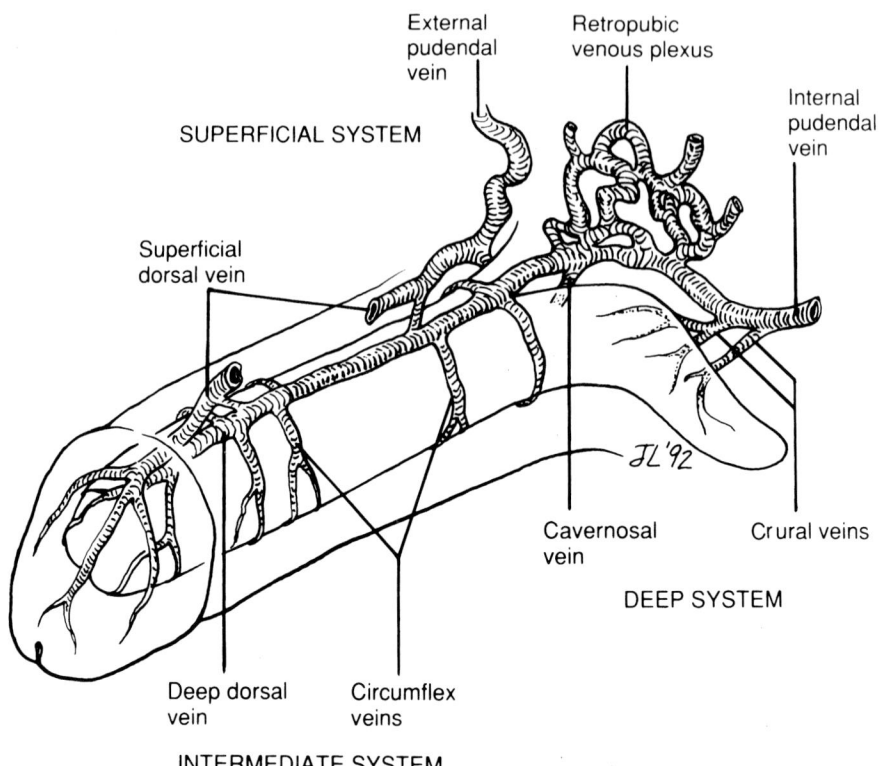

FIGURE 38.1. Schematic drawing of venous drainage of the corpora cavernosa. The superficial system drains the corporus cavernosum only by tributaries that connect between the intermediate and superficial dorsal vein. (From Lewis,[23] with permission.)

venous drainage from the corpora cavernosa. The deep dorsal vein that lies beneath Buck's fascia in the dorsal midline of the penis eventually drains into the preprostatic (retropubic) plexus or the internal pudendal veins, with ultimate drainage into the internal iliac vein. The deep drainage system of the corpora cavernosa consists of cavernosal veins draining into the internal pudendal vein, often with communications to the preprostatic retropubic plexus or crural veins draining into the internal pudendal veins or both.

## Pathophysiology of Veno-Occlusive Dysfunction

Faulty veno-occlusive function may be associated with iatrogenic damage to the tunica albuginea of the corpora cavernosa following treatment of priapism when shunts are created between the spongiosum and the cavernosum, or with urethrotomy for penile strictures.[6,14] Neovascularity, resulting in abnormal veno-occlusive dysfunction, is rarely found in patients with certain isolated diseases that affect the elastic properties of the tunica albuginea, such as inflammation secondary to stricture disease or Peyronie's disease.[13] There may be some congenital or rare abnormal drainage into the superficial drainage system.[14–17] Runoff into the deep dorsal vein and cavernosal venous system is often found in patients with veno-occlusive dysfunction on pharmacocavernosography[18,19] (Table 38.1). Crural veins, often seen on pharmacocavernosography, are rarely the only source of venous drainage, except in normal patients who obtain a full rigid erection.

The venous occlusion is very much dependent on relaxation of normal sinus smooth

TABLE 38.1. Site of venous leakage in veno-occlusive dysfunction.

| Site of leakage | Aboseif et al[17] | | Shabsigh et al[18] | | Fuchs et al[19] | |
|---|---|---|---|---|---|---|
| | No. of patients | % | No. of patients | % | No. of patients | % |
| Superficial system only | 6 | 6 | — | — | — | — |
| Intermediate system only | 8 | 9 | 8 | 18 | 6 | 17 |
| Deep system only | 16 | 17 | — | — | 9 | 25 |
| Cavernous veins only | 15 | 16 | | | | |
| Crural veins only | 1 | 1 | | | | |
| Superficial and intermediate systems | 11 | 12 | 6* | 13 | 8 | 22 |
| Intermediate and deep systems | 23 | 24 | 14 | 30 | 9 | 25 |
| Deep dorsal vein and cavernous veins | 7 | 7 | — | — | — | — |
| Deep dorsal vein, cavernosal veins, and glans/spongiosum | — | — | 17 | 37 | — | — |
| Deep system and spongiosum | — | — | — | — | 2 | 5.5 |
| All three systems | 24 | 25 | 1 | 2 | 2 | 5.5 |
| Total patients | 96 | | 46 | | 36 | |

*Leakage through deep dorsal vein and glans/spongiosum.

muscle. Although it is not yet possible to diagnose pathology of the sinus smooth muscle, it is very probable that patients having minimal functional disease of the smooth muscle would benefit from venous surgery. Wespes et al,[20] in their work with the quantification of smooth muscle in the cavernous tissue, show some promise in helping sort this out. In 12 of 23 patients responding with normal erections after venous surgery, all had greater than 29% smooth muscle cells of all the tissue cells present, but all nonresponders had less smooth muscle composition. There may be progressive venous sclerosis in surgically resistant veno-occlusive disorders.[21]

## Diagnosis of Venogenic Impotence

Veno-occlusive dysfunction can be found in cases of primary and secondary impotence. A patient may describe brief rigid erections with an inability to maintain adequate rigidity or may complain of soft erections insufficient for penetration. Studies of nocturnal penile tumescence (NPT) usually show REM-associated erections with normal tumescence (circumference changes), but the rigidity of the erection is deficient in degree or duration or both. The patient diagnosed with significant veno-

occlusive dysfunction is unable to achieve a rigid erection after intracavernosal smooth-muscle relaxant injections, or he achieves a rapid, rigid erection and early detumescence within 10 to 20 minutes. Use of tobacco by a patient must be eliminated before consideration of venogenic surgery, because nicotine can affect normal veno-occlusive function.

The two most accurate diagnostic tests for the diagnosis of veno-occlusive erectile dysfunction are maintenance flow rates on infusion cavernosometry and the plateau pressure on gravity cavernosometry after the injection of a smooth-muscle relaxing intracavernous agent[22,23] (Table 38.2). Either a maintenance flow rate of <15 to 20 ml/min or a plateau pressure on gravity pharmacocavernosometry of >60 mm Hg is indicative of an adequate veno-occlusive mechanism.[22,23] Some researchers consider these maintenance flow rates as above normal, perhaps an error in measurement caused by incomplete relaxation of intracavernous smooth muscle during testing.[4,24,25]

Color duplex Doppler ultrasonography of the deep penile arteries of the penis following injection of smooth-muscle relaxants, at doses high enough to produce maximal smooth-muscle relaxation, can also be used to rule out a faulty veno-occlusive mechanism.[26] In the presence of a normal arterial peak systolic velocity

TABLE 38.2. Technique of cavernosometry/caverno-sography.

---

Place two 19-gauge needles into each corpus cavernosum (obliquely, toward patient's head), without anesthesia, laterally along shaft of penis under sterile conditions.

Connect one needle for pressure measurement via a transducer connected to a physiologic recorder or monitor.

Connect other needle to an infusion roller pump for infusion of heparinized saline solution (1000 units/1000 ml)—prewarmed to body temperature.

Record baseline pressure.

Infuse fluid at 50 ml/minute increments until full erection occurs (90–100 mm Hg), then decrease flow to obtain flow rate needed to maintain erection (do not infuse above 300 ml/minute).

Inject through needle pharmacologic agent (usually 45 mg of papaverine and 2.5 mg of phentolamine).

Record baseline pressure 10 minutes later.

Obtain plateau pressure from gravity flow of saline without using flow pump.

Repeat flow study obtaining flow rate to maintain erection (do not infuse above 150 ml/minute).

Inject 30% diatrozoate or iothalomate meglumine (60 ml full strength or 120 ml 50% dilution with saline) at same rate as last maintenance flow rate and obtain cine, fluoroscopic images, or spot static x-ray images (AP and oblique) for cavernosography.

---

of 30 cm/sec or greater, if the end diastolic velocity is 0 or a negative value, then the veno-occlusive mechanism is considered intact.[27]

# Treatment of Venogenic Impotence

A patient with veno-occlusive disorder will rarely respond to pharmacologic injection therapy with vasoactive agents. However, a combination of pharmacologic injection therapy with a venous constriction system or the use of a vacuum device may be used.[28,29] Criteria for recommending surgery for a veno-occlusive disorder consist of the following: (1) short-duration erections or tumescence, with sexual stimulation; (2) failure to maintain or obtain an erection, with intracavernous injections on multiple trials with different agents with sexual stimulation; (3) normal cavernous arteries as evaluated by color duplex Doppler studies or by the second phase of dynamic infu-sion cavernosometry and cavernosonography (DICC); (4) determination of a faulty veno-occlusive mechanism as determined by infusion pump or gravity cavernosometry; (5) location of the site of venous leakage from the corpora cavernosa on pharmacocavernosography; (6) no medical contraindication for surgery; and (7) complete elimination of tobacco use. After presentation of alternative therapeutic choices, it is unusual for a patient who meets all these criteria to agree to a procedure with a long-term success rate of only 40% to 50%.

For deep penile vein dissection and ligation, the anterior scrotal peripenile incision is preferred (Fig. 38.2). It is necessary to have complete dissection and ligation of all the veins demonstrated on pharmacocavernoso-nography. This procedure includes a careful dissection, with ligation of all emissary and circumflex veins feeding into a deep dorsal vein, beginning approximately 1 cm from the glans, where the dorsal vein is made up of several different tributaries (Fig. 38.3). It is important to keep the vein dissection in the dorsal midline, because the nerves and arteries tend to lie in the immediate lateral positions. Ligate any communication allowing for drainage from the corpora cavernosa to the superficial system as seen on preoperative cavernosography (Fig. 38.4). All ligatures placed on the penile shaft veins should be absorbable. Inspect the junction of the corpora cavernosa to the spongiosum carefully and ligate any communications between the circumflex veins and the spongiosum veins. Take down the fundiform and suspensory ligaments in order to reach the deep venous drainage at the base of the penis (Fig. 38.5). If there is a question about whether a vessel exposed at surgery is an artery or vein, the use of a handheld intraoperative Doppler probe may be beneficial. Injection of indigo carmine intracavernously following a smooth muscle relaxant will help delineate veins for dissection (Fig. 38.6). Similarly, control pharmacocavernosometry can be used intraoperatively to demonstrate adequate venous dissection (Fig. 38.7).

Reform the suspensory ligament by fixation of the deep midline dorsal penis to the infrapubic periosteum of the pubic bone. Drain

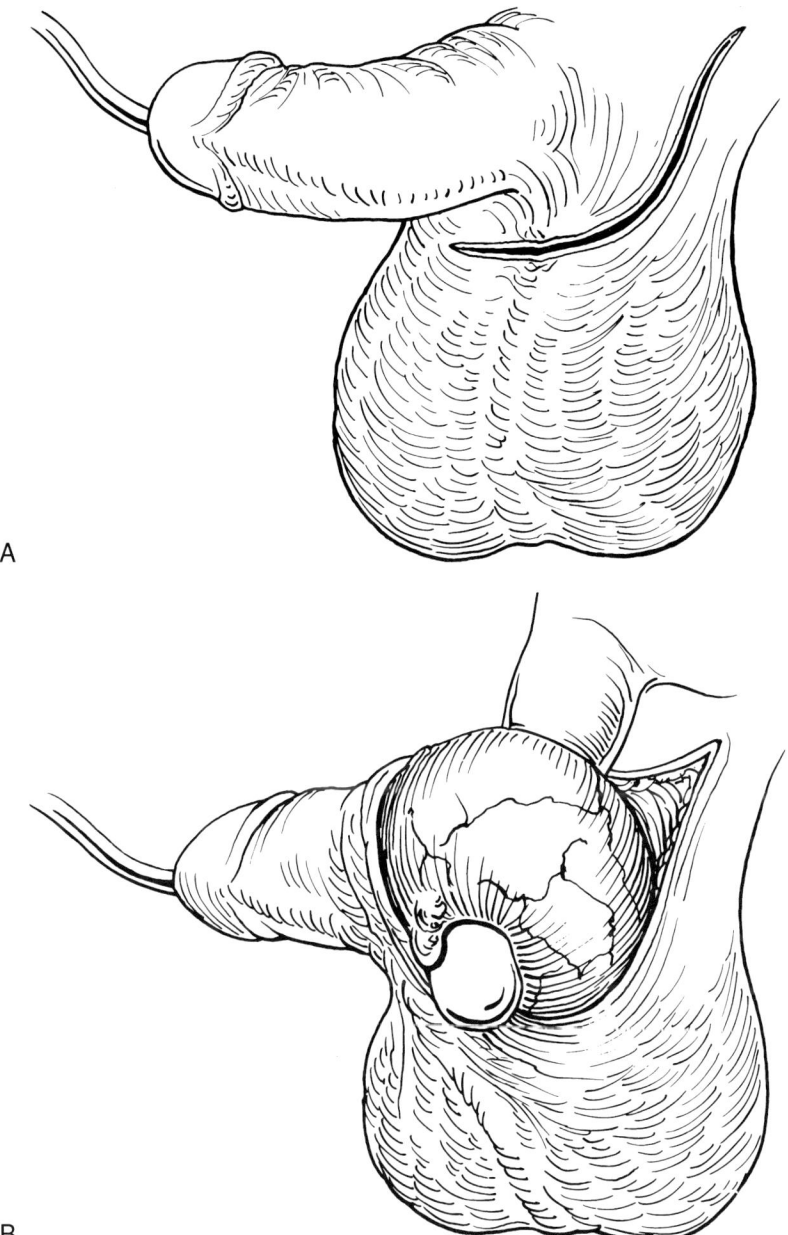

A

B

FIGURE 38.2. (A) The preferred anterior scrotal peripenile incision for veno-occlusive surgery. (From Lewis,[23] with permission.) (B) The complete shaft of the penis can be everted into this wound for exposure of the superficial veins and deep veins that are to be dissected. (From Lewis,[23] with permission.)

this infrapubic area with a small, round, fenestrated suction-type drain through a separate stab wound into the suprapubic region. Gently wrap the penis with a self-adherent elastic dressing, and leave a urethral catheter in overnight. The drain will function as a surgical drain and should be removed 1 to 2 days postoperatively. Resumption of sexual activities usually begins approximately 6 weeks after surgery.

The procedure is performed under general intubated or spinal anesthesia. Arrange the patient in the supine position, with the legs

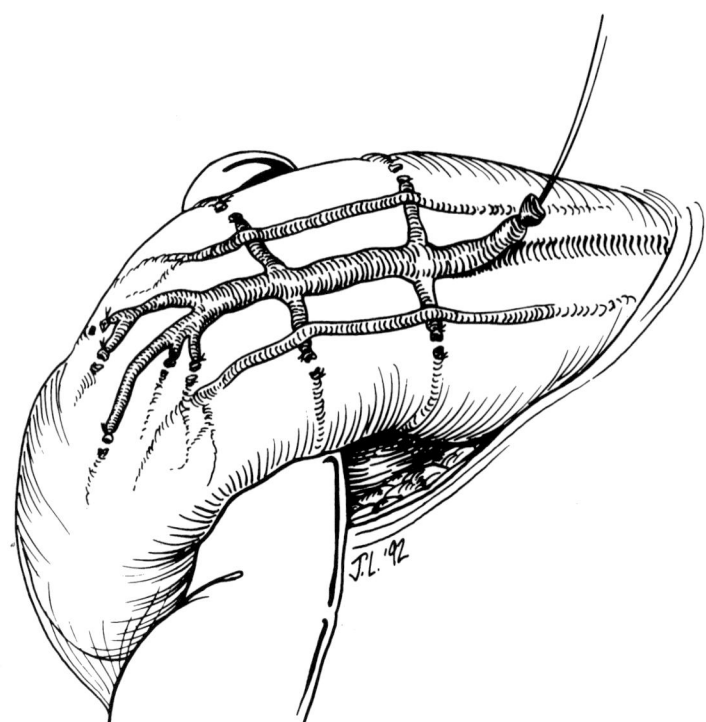

FIGURE 38.3. Dissection of the deep dorsal vein of the penis. For the sake of illustration, the Buck's fascia is not in place over the arteries that lie just laterally to the midline deep dorsal vein. The circumflex veins are ligated or divided and coagulated near junctional connections to the veins from the corpus spongiosum. (From Lewis,[23] with permission.)

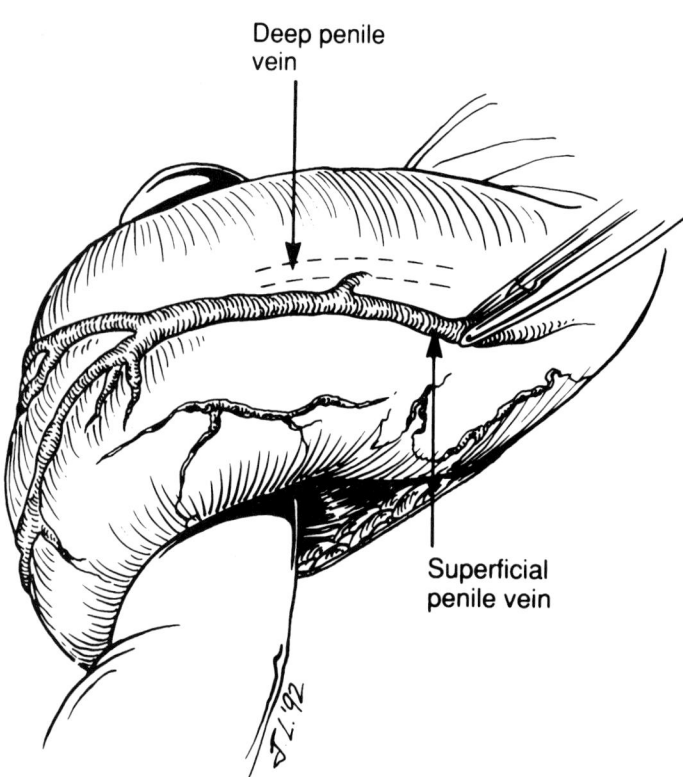

Deep penile vein

Superficial penile vein

FIGURE 38.4. On first eversion of the penis, the connections between the deep penile vein and the superficial penile vein are divided between ligatures of absorbable suture. (From Lewis,[23] with permission.)

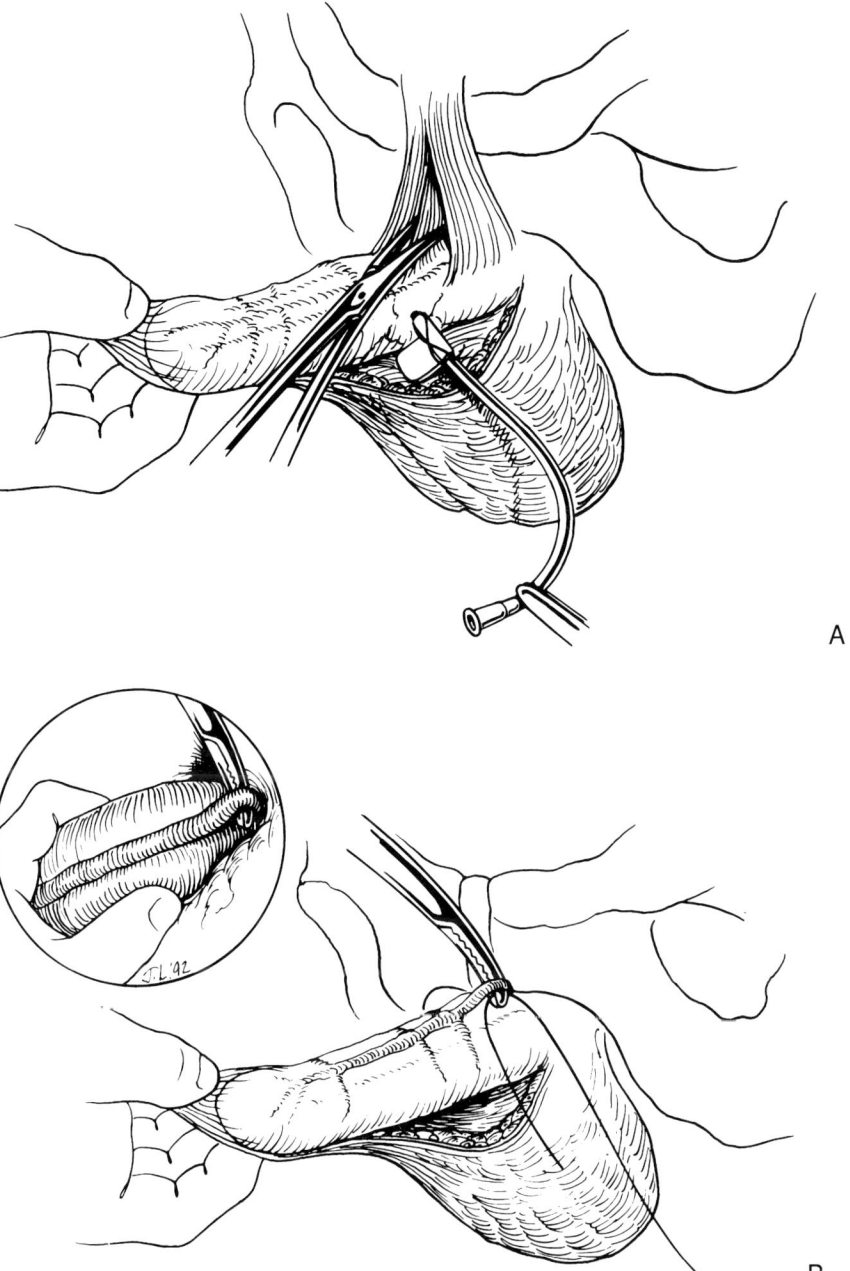

A

B

FIGURE 38.5. (A) The suspensory ligament and fundiform ligament are taken down completely. Note that a 19-gauge or butterfly needle has been sutured into the lateral surface of the corpora cavernosa for injection of indigo carmine blue to demonstrate effluxing veins from the corporal tissue and also for control cavernosometry at the end of a dissection. (From Lewis,[23] with permission.) (B) Ligation of the deep dorsal vein in the infrapubic region. This is difficult to show in illustration. The bony pelvis has been illustrated to demonstrate that it is an infrapubic position. The inset shows that the dissection is deep in the infrapubic region. (From Lewis,[23] with permission.)

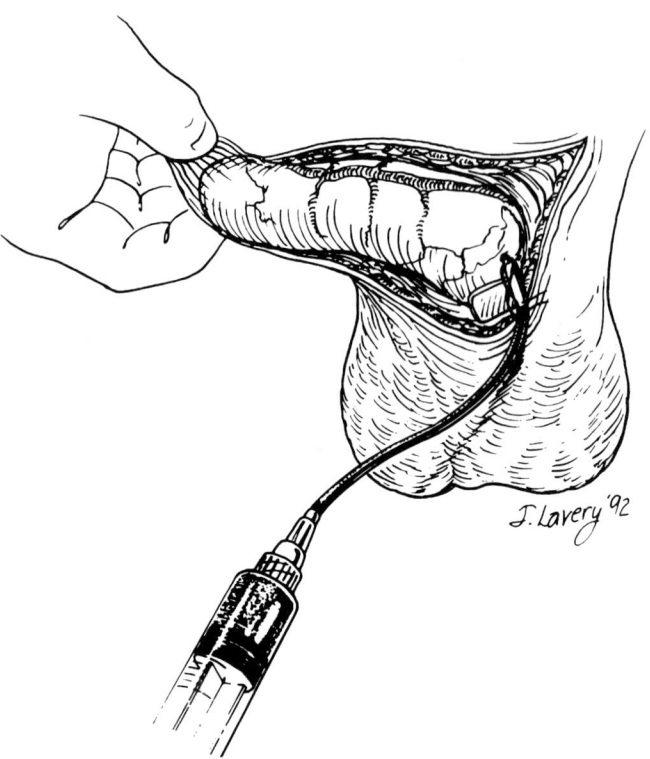

FIGURE 38.6. Injection of indigo carmine into the corpora to demonstrate effluxing veins that can aid in the dissection. (From Lewis,[23] with permission.)

slightly abducted, or in a dorsal lithotomy position. Surgical loupe magnification may be utilized during vein dissection, but it is not necessary. However, a lighted suction device is helpful for illumination of the deep infrapubic region during the deep vein dissection. Any use of electrocoagulation along the penile shaft during veno-occlusive surgery should be per-

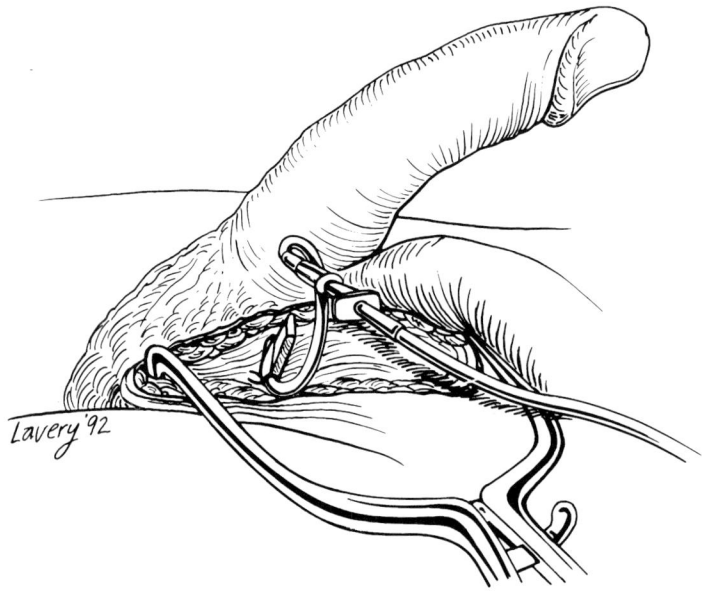

FIGURE 38.7. Controlled cavernosometry being performed after the vein dissection has been accomplished to demonstrate that the erection can be maintained with a low flow rate. (From Lewis,[23] with permission.)

formed with a bipolar unit to avoid possible transmission of the current to arteries and nerves along the penile shaft that could result in subsequent damage to these vessels.

Crural plication is suggested by some surgeons in addition to surgical correction of veno-occlusive dysfunction. This can be performed along the lateral surface of the tunica albuginea in the crural region of the corpora using the anterior scrotal incision, once the penile base has been dissected away from the pubis and the deep infrapubic region. A perineal incision also may be used to reach crural veins or in cases where a crural plication or banding is entertained, but this should be a secondary procedure[11] and only rarely as a primary operative procedure for veno-occlusive dysfunction.

Complications of veno-occlusive surgery include penile edema, which is quite common but appears to be less so with the use of a lightly applied elastic dressing the first day after surgery and with the use of the fenestrated drain 24 to 48 hours after the surgical approach.

Ecchymoses and bruising of the penile shaft and scrotum are not unusual or debilitating. Penile numbness or hypothesia, particularly of the glans region, can be seen in many patients. The penile sensation usually returns 12 to 18 months after surgery if no major penile sensory nerve has been significantly injured. Scar entrapment of the base of the penis can occur in approximately 20% of the patients. One of the facts that must be presented to the patient concerning penile veno-occlusive surgery is that there may be some penile shortening from scar entrapment. Moderate-to-severe scarring may require subsequent scar release by use of relaxing Z-plasty or scrotal flap coverage.

# Results of Veno-Occlusive Surgery for Erectile Dysfunction

Published studies that provide adequate data allow the impotence surgeon to make accurate statements about long-term results (Table 38.3).

TABLE 38.3. Results of surgery for veno-occlusive sexual dysfunction.

| Study (years of study) | No. of patients | Excellent | Improved | Immediate success/later failure | Failures | Average follow-up (months) |
|---|---|---|---|---|---|---|
| Lewis–Tulane Series (1981–1987)[10] | 49 | 12 (24%) | 12 (24%) | 8 (16%) | 17 (35%) | 15 |
| Wespes et al (1982–1986)[30] | 67[a] | 31 (46%) | 16 (24%) | | 20 (30%) | 24 |
| Donatucci and Lue (1986–1988)[31] | 100 | 44 (44%) | 24 (24%) | | 32 (32%) | 12–50 |
| Bondil et al (1981–1988)[32] | 60 | 25 (42%)[b] | | | 35 (58%) | 22 |
| Lunglmayr et al (1984–1986)[33] | 29 | 9 (31%)[b] | | | 10 (34.5%) | To 24 |
| Weidner et al[34] | | | | | | |
| (1985–1987) | 51 | 28 (55%) | | 8 (16%)[c] | 15 (29%)[c] | 12 |
| (1988–1989) | 40 | 24 (60%) | | 11 (27.5%)[c] | 5 (12.5%)[c] | 12 |
| Gilbert et al (1985–1990)[35] | 134 | 26 (19.4%) | 47 (35.1%) | | 61 (45.5%) | 12.9 |
| Lewis–Mayo Series[36] | | | | | | |
| (1987–1988) | 28 | 7 (25%) | 4 (14%) | 8 (29%) | 9 (32%) | 48 |
| (1988–1989) | 32 | 9 (28%) | 13 (41%) | 5 (15.6%) | 5 (15.6%) | 24 |
| Knoll et al (1987–1989)[37] | 41 | 19 (46%) | Unknown | Unknown | 22 (54%) | 28 |
| Kropman et al (1987–1989)[38] | 20 | 6 (30%) | 4 (20%) | 8 (40%) | 2 (10%) | 15 |
| Rossman et al (1985–1988)[39] | 16 | 2 (12.5%) | 2 (12.5%) | 10 (62.5%) | 2 (12.5%) | Unknown |
| Claes and Baert (1987–1989)[40] | 72 | 30 (41.7%) | 23 (31.9%) | | 19 (26.4%) | >12 |
| Montague et al (1988–1990)[41] | 18 | 11 (61%) | | 6 (33%) | 1 (6%) | 24 |
| Freedman et al (1986–1991)[42] | 46 | 11 (24%) | 8 (17%) | 23 (50%) | 4 (9%) | 31–33 |
| Stief et al (1989–1992)[43] | 77 | 31 (40.3%)[d] | 8 (10.4%) | — | 38 (49.4%) | 6 |

[a] There were 67 patient questionnaire responses to 105 letters sent.
[b] Series reported as excellent or improved as a group, not in each individual category.
[c] Seventeen of 39 are now able to achieve erection with pharmacologic agent injection.
[d] Four of 31 when followed for extended period (18.5 months) needed pharmacotherapy to obtain an erection.

In summary, the long-term success rate of 50% to 60% is less than optimal. One can surmise that perhaps 20% to 25% of patients who undergo venous ligation surgery, and who are initially unable to obtain a rigid erection with pharmacological erection therapy, may be converted to the ability to obtain erections.

Four possible mechanisms may account for failure of veno-occlusive surgery. A major fault in some of the earlier series reported was the lack of diagnosis of concomitant arterial disease. Newer diagnostic techniques, such as color duplex Doppler ultrasonography, have eliminated this problem to some extent. Many series reported failure from inadequate dissection of all of the draining veins seen on cavernosography. Veno-occlusive surgery must be performed in a very meticulous manner, and only very careful, complete dissection will ensure success. Common to all types of venous surgery, venous collateral circulation is probably a major source of failure of veno-occlusive surgery and is probably a major reason for those patients who show an initial success but later fail. Perhaps the greatest reason for failure is the presence of moderate-to-severe sinus smooth muscle disease. In the presence of this sinus smooth muscle disease, the cavernous tissue is probably no longer able to fully expand, and venous surgery directed at runoff above the tunica albuginea would not improve the intracavernosal state under these circumstances.

## Summary

There are few patients who are serious candidates for veno-occlusive surgery. The choice of surgery for these patients must be through a highly selective process. It is imperative that each patient be informed not only of the failure rates but also of the alternative treatments available.

## References

1. Wespes E, Schulman C. Venous impotence: pathophysiology, diagnosis and treatment. *J Urol* 1993; 149:1238–1245.
2. Carrier S, Brock G, Kour NW, et al. Pathophysiology of erectile dysfunction. *Urology* 1993; 42:468–481.
3. Gentile V, Modesti A, LaPera G, et al. Ultrastructural and immunohistochemical characterization of tunica albuginea in Peyronie's disease and veno-occlusive dysfunction. *J Androl* 1996; 17:96–103.
4. Nehra A, Moreland R, Saenz de Tejada I, et al. What is venous leak and why is there limited success with venous leak surgery in patients with vasculogenic impotence associated with vascular risk factors? A correlation of clinical, histological, molecular, and engineering aspects of corporal veno-occlusion. *J Urol* 1995; 153:471A(Abst 972).
5. Lewis RW. Venogenic impotence: is there a future? *Curr Opin Urol* 1994; 4:340–342.
6. Ebbehoj J, Wagner G. Insufficient penile erection due to abnormal drainage of cavernous bodies. *Urology* 1979; 13:507–509.
7. Virag R. Revascularization of the penis. In: Bennett AH ed. *Management of Male Impotence.* Baltimore: Williams & Wilkins; 1982: 219–233.
8. Wespes E, Schulman CC. Venous leakage, surgical treatment of a curable cause of impotence. *J Urol* 1985; 133:796–798.
9. Lewis RW, Puyau FA, Bell DP. Another surgical approach for vasculogenic impotence. *J Urol* 1986; 136:1210–1212.
10. Lewis, RW. Venous surgery for impotence. *Urol Clin North Am* 1988; 15:115–121.
11. Treiber V, Gilbert P. Venous surgery in erectile dysfunction: a critical report of 116 patients. *Urology* 1989; 34:22–27.
12. Lewis RW. Diagnosis and management of corporal veno-occlusive dysfunction. *Semin Urol* 1990; 8:113–123.
13. Lewis RW. Venous ligation surgery for venous leakage. *Int J Impotence Res* 1990; 2:1–19.
14. Puyau FA, Lewis RW, Balkin P, et al. Dynamic corpus cavernosography: effect of papaverine injection. *Radiology* 1987; 164:179–182.
15. Lewis RW, Puyau FA. Procedures for decreasing venous drainage. *Semin Urol* 1986; 4:263–272.
16. Stief CG, Gall H, Scherb W, et al. Erectile dysfunction due to ectopic penile vein. *Urology* 1988; 31:300–303.
17. Aboseif SR, Breza J, Lue TF, et al. Penile venous drainage in erectile dysfunction: anatomical, radiological and functional considerations. *Br J Urol* 1989; 64:183–190.
18. Shabsigh R, Fishman IJ, Toombs BD, et al. Venous leaks: anatomical and physiological observations. *J Urol* 1991; 146:1260–1265.

19. Fuchs A, Mehringer CM, Rajfer J. Anatomy of penile venous drainage in potent and impotent men during cavernosography. *J Urol* 1989; 141:1353–1356.

20. Wespes E, deGoes PM, Saltar AA, et al. Objective criteria in the long-term evaluation of penile venous surgery. *J Urol* 1994; 152:888–890.

21. Hirsch M, Lubetsky R, Goldman H, et al. Dorsal vein sclerosis as a predictor of outcome in penile venous ligation surgery. *J Urol* 1993; 150:1810–1813.

22. Meuleman EJH, Wijkstra H, Doesburg WH, et al. Comparison of the diagnostic value of gravity- and pump-cavernosometry in the evaluation of the cavernous veno-occlusive mechanism. *J Urol* 1991; 146:1266–1271.

23. Lewis RW. Venous surgery in the patient with erectile dysfunction. *Atlas Urol Clin North Am* 1993; 1:21–38.

24. Pescatori ES, Hatzichristou DG, Hamburi S, et al. A positive intracavernous injection test implies normal veno-occlusive but not necessarily normal arterial function: a hemodynamic study. *J Urol* 1994; 151:1209–1216.

25. Udelson D, Hatzichristou DG, Saenz Tejada I, et al. A new methodology of pharmacocavernosography which enables hemodynamic analysis under conditions of known corporal smooth muscle relaxation. *J Urol* 1994; 151:320A(Abst 370).

26. Nehra A, Hakim LS, Abobakr RA, et al. A new method of performing duplex Doppler ultrasonography: the effect of re-dosing of vasoactive agents on hemodynamic parameters. *J Urol* 1995; 153:332A(Abst 415).

27. King BF, Lewis RW, McKusilk MA. Radiological evaluation of impotence. In: Bennett AH ed. *Impotence—Diagnosis and Management of Erectile Dysfunction*. Philadelphia: W.B. Saunders, 1994: 52–91.

28. Blackard CE, Borkon WD, Lima JS, et al. Use of vacuum tumescence device for impotence secondary to venous leakage. *Urology* 1993, 41:225–229.

29. Lanigan D, Roobottom C, Choa RG. A modified papaverine test and the use of venous constriction in erectile dysfunction. *Int J Impotence Res* 1993; 5:119–122.

30. Wespes E, Delcour L, Prejzerowicz L, et al. Long term follow-up of operation for venous leakage. In: *Proceedings of Sixth Biennial International Symposium for Corpora Cavernosum Revascularization and Third Biennial World Meeting on Impotence*. Boston: International Society of Impotence Research; 1988: 193.

31. Donatucci CF, Lue TF. Venous surgery: Are we kidding ourselves? In: Lue TF ed. *World Book of Impotence*. London: Smith-Gordon; 1992: 221–227.

32. Bondil P, Schauvliege T, Nguyen Qui JL. Venocavernous leakage: considerations in 60 operated cases. In: *Proceedings of Sixth Biennial Corpora Cavernosum Revascularization and Third Biennial World Meeting on Impotence*. Boston: International Society of Impotence Research; 1988: 189.

33. Lunglmayr G, Nachtigall M, Gindl K. Long-term results of deep dorsal penile vein transection in venous impotence. *Eur Urol* 1988; 15:209–212.

34. Weidner W, Weiske WH, Rudnick J, et al. Venous surgery in veno-occlusive dysfunction: long-time results after deep dorsal vein resection. *Urol Int* 1992; 49:24–28.

35. Gilbert P, Sparwasser C, Beckert R, et al. Venous surgery in erectile dysfunction. The role of dorsal-penile-vein ligation and spongiosolysis for impotence. *Urol Int* 1992; 49:40–47.

36. Lewis RW. Venous ligation for venogenic impotence. In: Whitehead ED, Nagler HM eds. *Management of Impotence and Infertility*. Philadelphia: J.B. Lippincott; 1992: 73–92.

37. Knoll LD, Furlow WL, Benson RC. Penile venous ligation surgery for the management of cavernosal venous leakage. *Urol Int* 1992; 49:33–39.

38. Kropman RF, Nijeholt AABL, Giespers AGM, et al. Results of deep penile vein resection in impotence caused by venous leakage. *Int J Impotence Res* 1990; 2:29–34.

39. Rossman B, Mieza M, Melman A. Penile vein ligation for corporeal incompetence: an evaluation of short-term and long-term results. *J Urol* 1990; 144:679–682.

40. Claes H, Baert L. Cavernosometry and penile vein resection in corporeal incompetence: an evaluation of short-term and long-term results. *Int J Impotence Res* 1991; 3:129.

41. Montague DK, Angermeier KW, Lakin M, et al. Penile venous ligation in 18 patients with 1 to 3 years of follow-up. *J Urol* 1993; 149:306–307.

42. Freedman AL, Neto FC, Rajfer J. Long-term results of penile vein ligation for impotence from venous leakage. *J Urol* 1993; 149:1301–1303.

43. Stief CG, Djamilan M, Truss MC, et al. Prognostic factors for the postoperative outcome of penile venous surgery for venogenic erectile dysfunction. *J Urol* 1994; 151:880–883.

# 39
# Arterial Surgery for Erectile Dysfunction: Microvascular Arterial Bypass

John Mulhall and Irwin Goldstein

Erectile dysfunction is the consistent change in the rigidity or sustaining capability of the penile erection that interferes with satisfactory sexual intercourse. Epidemiology studies have revealed that 52% of men age 40 to 70 years have self-reported minimal (17%), moderate (25%), and complete (10%) forms of impotence.[1] Nonsurgical treatment options include psychological, endocrinologic, neurologic, and pharmacologic interventions. Surgical options consist primarily of penile prosthesis insertion and penile microvascular arterial bypass. Surgery for corporal veno-occlusive dysfunction remains controversial, is used in very limited cases, and is associated with poor long-term success.

The overall goal of penile microvascular arterial bypass surgery for impotence is to provide an alternative arterial pathway beyond obstructive arterial lesions in the hypogastric-cavernous arterial bed (Fig. 39.1). The specific objective of the surgery is to increase the cavernosal arterial perfusion pressure and blood inflow in patients with vasculogenic erectile dysfunction secondary to pure arterial insufficiency. A successful surgical result will yield improved erectile hemodynamics during sexual stimulation, that is, a more rigid (increased arterial perfusion pressure), and more spontaneous (increased arterial inflow) penile erection.[2–4] The primary clinical motivation for this form of impotence surgery is the desire of the impotent patient to achieve restored natural erectile function without the need for external or internal mechanical de-

vices or for intracavernosal injections of vasoactive agents.

## Historical Perspectives

In 1973 Michal et al[5] reported penile arterial bypass surgery for impotence using the inferior epigastric artery as the neoarterial inflow source and the corpora cavernosa or dorsal artery as the recipient vessels. In the early 1980s, Virag et al[6,7] described the use of the deep dorsal vein as a recipient arterialized vein graft in impotent men. Since then, a variety of surgical techniques involving artery-artery, artery-vein, or combinations of vascular anastomoses have been developed.[5–24]

Erectile hemodynamics differ from those of other vascular organs. Arterial bypass surgery to the cavernosal artery is different from arterial bypass surgery to the coronary, renal, lower limb, or cerebral systems. In the penis, erectile function is dependent not only on arterial inflow and perfusion but also on the development of adequate venous outflow resistance. The other systems are not dependent on the creation of venous outflow resistance.

Microvascular arterial bypass surgery should be restricted to those patients with vasculogenic impotence secondary to pure arterial insufficiency. There is no physiologic basis for improvement of corporal venoocclusion through arterial bypass surgery. Recent research has revealed varying degrees of corporal fibrosis as the underlying pathophy-

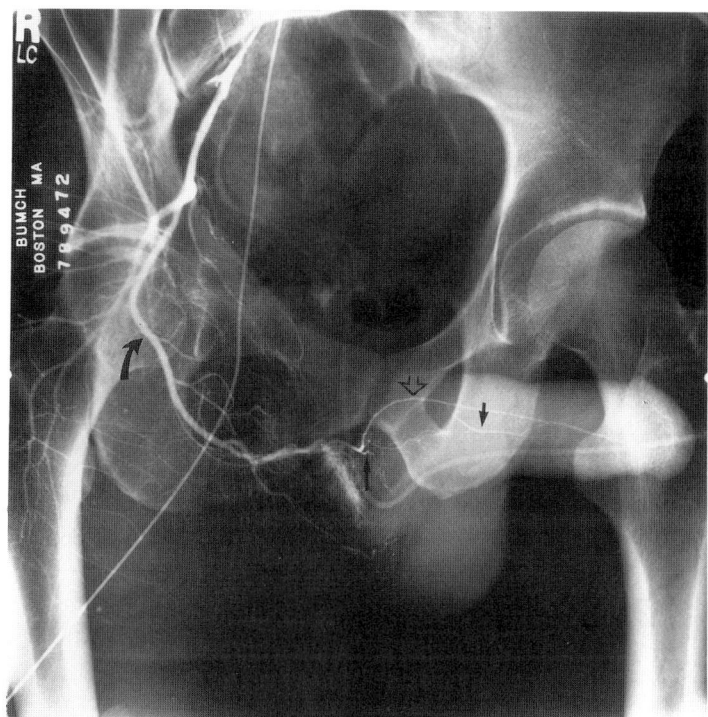

FIGURE 39.1. Selective internal pudendal arteriogram demonstrating the internal pudendal artery (curved arrow) and its terminal branches, the dorsal artery (open arrow), and the cavernosal artery (long arrow), which is occluded following perineal trauma in this patient. There is a communicating branch passing from the dorsal artery to the corpus cavernosum (small arrow), which acts as the neoarterial conduit following inferior epigastric to dorsal artery anastomosis.

siology of corporal veno-occlusive dysfunction.[25] This intracavernosal pathology for venous leakage eliminates the possibility of surgically improving outflow resistance in afflicted patients.

A single arterial bypass procedure is not applicable to all patients with pure arteriogenic impotence. The objective of the arterial bypass surgery, to increase the cavernosal arterial perfusion pressure and blood inflow to the erectile tissue, is best achieved by designing the vascular reconstruction to the individual's specific arteriographic findings. Radiology has confirmed the existence of arterial occlusive disease within the hypogastric-cavernous arterial bed previously only suspected by history and erectile function testing and has identified the location of communicating arterial pathways from the dorsal penile to the cavernosal artery to justify an anastomosis of the inferior epigastric artery to the dorsal penile artery.[8,26–28] If the dorsal artery does not communicate with the cavernosal artery, an anastomosis could be made to a deep dorsal vein segment; however, the long-term prognosis of dorsal vein arterialization is not as favorable as that associated with artery-artery anastomoses.

The surgical technique should consist of modern endothelium-sparing vascular and microvascular surgical principles similar to those applied for occlusive disease within other peripheral vascular beds.[29–38] There must not be any mechanical trauma to the donor or recipient arteries due to twisting or excessive stretching. Neither should there be any thermal changes due to electrocautery, exposure to cold irrigants, or drying from exposure to air. Ischemia resulting from compression or excessive adventitial dissection must also be avoided. Such arterial injuries may induce endothelial dysfunction that will result in arterial occlusive pathology and anastomotic failure.

## Patient Selection

Only patients with pure cavernosal artery insufficiency are considered candidates for microvascular arterial bypass surgery. Patients with concomitant veno-occlusive dysfunction are not considered to have a surgically treatable disorder.

## Clinical Criteria

Young men with impotence secondary to blunt pelvic or perineal trauma without neurologic or endocrinologic factors are the ideal candidates for this surgery (Figs. 39.2 and 39.3).[11,16,21,39–41] Their history includes (1) a strong libido, (2) a consistent reduction in erectile rigidity during sexual activity, (3) increased erection rigidity during morning erections, (4) variable sustaining capability with the best maintenance of the rigidity during early morning erections, and (5) poor spontaneity of erections taking much effort and excessive time to achieve the poorly rigid erectile response.

Patients without a pathologic basis for venous leakage may provide a history of frequently losing their erection during preparatory sexual stimulation prior to or soon after penetration. This may be confusing to the clinician, as this response, generally indicative of venous leakage, is the result of the increased sympathetic nervous system response associated with anxiety resulting from the delayed partially rigid erection. Such patients characteristically possess an ability to achieve a more rigid, longer-lasting erection upon awakening in the morning. It is likely that the frustration

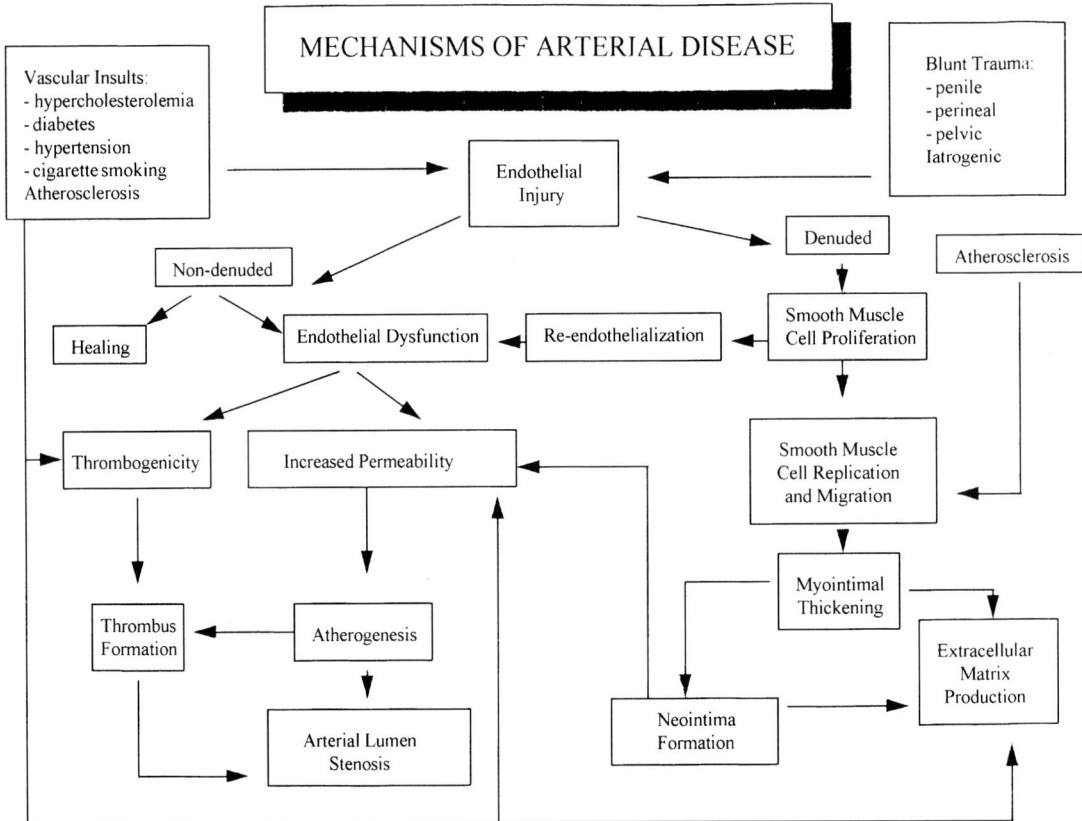

FIGURE 39.2. Mechanisms of arterial disease. Vascular endothelial damage is central to the development of arterial obstruction.

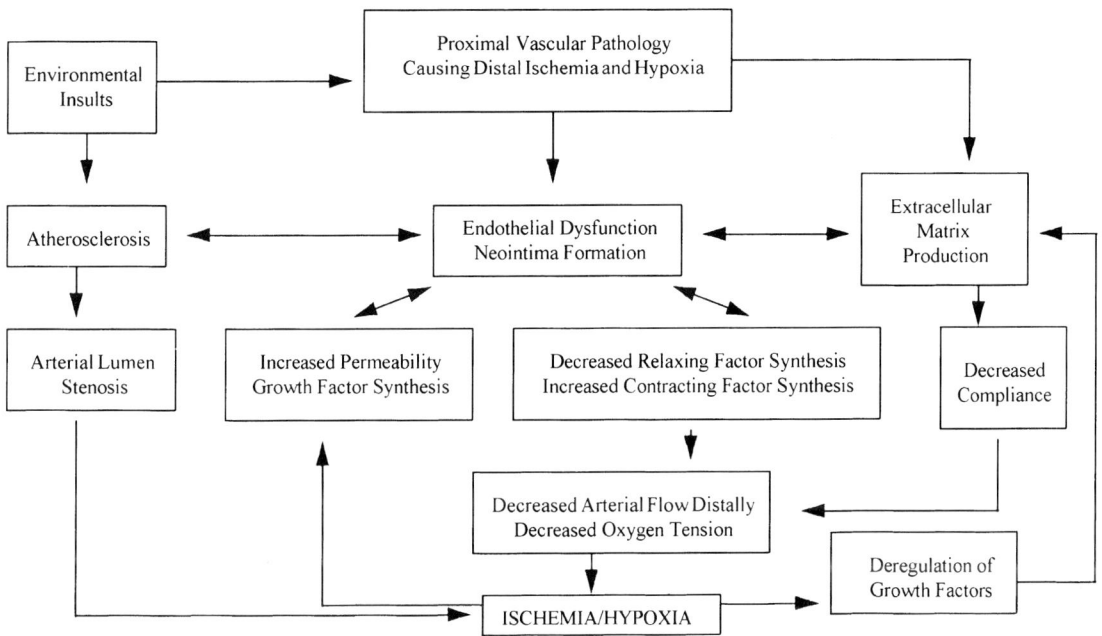

FIGURE 39.3. Mechanism of the development of distal arterial disease resulting from proximal arterial obstruction. The major factors involved are hypoxia, deregulation of growth factors and neointimal formation.

associated with the slowly developing erection is not appreciated with the nocturnal erection because the latter occurs during sleep. The increased ability to sustain the morning erection may reflect the fact that such patients have normal corporal veno-occlusive function if their trabecular smooth muscle is completely relaxed. Patients with pure arteriogenic impotence have also been labeled as having "failure-to-fill" or "cavernosal artery insufficiency" erectile dysfunction.[11]

Patients with systemic atherosclerotic disease or arterial occlusive disease secondary to atherosclerotic vascular risk factors, such as aging, hypertension, cigarette smoking, diabetes mellitus, and hypercholesterolemia, are not ideal candidates for microvascular arterial bypass surgery.[7,30,42–44] These patients have gener-

alized vascular disease and commonly have associated corporal veno-occlusive dysfunction with abnormal compliance of the erectile tissue. This may be secondary to an excess ratio of collagen to trabecular smooth muscle, dysfunctional endothelium, or abnormalities of the tunica albuginea preventing adequate elongation and compression of the subtunical venules despite complete smooth muscle relaxations.[30,45] It is, therefore, unusual for patients with atherosclerotic vascular risk factors to meet the strict selection criteria.

## Hemodynamic Criteria

The ideal candidates for penile revascularization surgery, those that have normal corporal veno-occlusive function and arterial obstruction within the hypogastric-cavernous arterial bed (failure-to-fill or cavernosal artery insufficiency), may exhibit a long-lasting erection of varying rigidity quality (depending on the magnitude of the cavernosal artery occlusion pressure) following office intracavernosal injection testing. A positive (rigid) office intracavernosal injection test may exist in the presence of clinically significant arterial insufficiency.[46] In a recent study, Pescatori et al[46] demonstrated that 19% of patients with positive office intracavernosal injection tests and rigid erectile response were found to have abnormal gradients between the cavernosal and the brachial artery systolic occlusion pressure, some even exceeding 80 mm Hg.

What is the basis for abnormal cavernosal arterial hemodynamics and arterial occlusive disease in the presence of a positive injection test? The answer lies in the relationships among (1) the systemic systolic arterial blood pressure (peak pressure in an individual), (2) the cavernosal systolic arterial blood pressure (actual cavernosal pressure), and (3) the threshold cavernosal systolic arterial blood pressure (prerequisite cavernosal pressure to achieve a positive injection test in a low-outflow state). Ideally, there should be no gradient between the systemic and cavernosal systolic arterial blood pressure values. The systemic systolic arterial blood pressure should be transferred without energy loss to the cavernosal artery via an intact hypogastric-cavernous arterial bed. This peak pressure should then be transferred to the closed outlet erectile chamber through relaxed helicine arterioles. If a systemic-cavernosal systolic arterial blood pressure gradient is identified, this reflects the presence of pressure energy loss, that is, arterial inflow occlusive disease within the hypogastric-cavernous arterial bed. As long as a threshold cavernosal pressure is achieved in a low-outflow state, a positive injection test will result, independent of any difference between systemic (peak) and cavernosal (actual) systolic arterial blood pressure. The positive injection test is, at worst, a threshold erectile response, and it may or may not indicate the maximum erection response as determined by the systemic pressure in an individual case.

Duplex ultrasonography and dynamic infusion pharmacocavernosometry and pharmacocaverno-sography are the most reliable tests for examination of the hemodynamic status of the erectile mechanism.[47] In particular, the pharmacocavernosometry procedure has the capability to evaluate the arterial as well as the corporal veno-occlusive function at the same time, in addition to providing an accurate assessment of the completeness of vasoactive agent-induced smooth muscle relaxation.

The first phase of the pharmacocavernosometry study records the penile volume (circumference), the equilibrium intracavernosal pressure responses, and the time from injection to the intracavernosal equilibrium pressure following intracavernosal vasoactive agent administration. In a normal study (with a normal systemic blood pressure of 120/80 mm Hg), the volume maximizes first (usually at 50 mm Hg), the intracavernosal pressure approaches the mean systemic arterial blood pressure (90 mm Hg), and the time to equilibrium pressure is less than 8 minutes.

The patient must achieve a pharmacologically induced erectile response similar to that in the privacy of his own bedroom, the so-called best-quality erection. Visual sexual stimulation or self-stimulation may be helpful for the patient to overcome sympathetic inhibition associated with anxiety in the test setting. When the best-quality erection is not achieved, pharmacocavernosometric evidence of incomplete smooth muscle relaxation exists, as revealed by observing a nonlinear relationship with intracavernosal pressure and flow-to-maintain or by observing a nonconstant value for venous outflow resistance. After the administration of a second or third dose of intracavernosal vasoactive agent, observation of a linear relationship between pressure and flow and constant venous outflow resistance has been shown to represent complete smooth muscle relaxation and achievement of the best-quality erection response.

During pharmacocavernosometry, organic vascular pathology is suspected when the intracavernosal pressure response is significantly lower than the mean systemic arterial blood pressure under conditions of complete smooth muscle relaxation. Normal veno-occlusion is consistent with flow-to-maintain values of 3 ml/min or less.

Venous outflow resistance is directly related to the time of pressure decay and is inversely related to the capacitor function, that is, the ability to store pressure energy in the penis. Veno-occlusive resistance may be additionally assessed by recording over a period of time intracavernosal pressure decay from an initial suprasystolic pressure. The intracavernosal pressure decay may be recorded from a suprasystolic pressure of 150 mm Hg over a 30-second period. Normal corporal veno-occlusive function has been associated with an intra-cavernosal pressure decay of less than 45 mm Hg in a period of 30 seconds.

Cavernosal artery integrity is determined during phase 3 of pharmacocavernosometry by recording cavernosal artery systolic occlusion pressure. The advantage of determining this arterial function study at this phase of the test is that the corporal smooth muscle relaxation status is known. Patients who achieve an equilibrium pressure approximating the mean systemic arterial blood pressure have been found to have cavernosal artery systolic occlusion pressures approximating the brachial artery systolic occlusion pressures. Patients with arteriogenic impotence reveal cavernosal artery systolic occlusion pressures at least 35 mm Hg lower than the simultaneously determined brachial artery systolic occlusion pressure.

Pharmacocavernosography, an anatomical study of the venous system draining the corporal bodies during erection, is performed at intracavernosal pressures of 90 mm Hg to confirm the findings of cavernosometry and to provide anatomical information of corporal veno-occlusive dysfunction. Normal corporal veno-occlusive function is associated with minimal or absent venous drainage. This procedure is indicated for patients in whom the diagnosis of venous leak based on pharmacocavernosometry is equivocal (especially at equilibrium pressures ranging from 40 to 60 mm Hg) and in those cases in which a radiographic localization of venous leakage is desired.

Further evaluation with selective internal pudendal pharmacoarteriography is indicated for candidates with pure arterial vasculogenic impotence who wish to undergo microvascular penile arterial bypass surgery.[27] Such impotent patients will demonstrate on invasive hemodynamic testing (1) abnormal equilibrium intracavernosal pressure, (2) normal corporal veno-occlusive function, and (3) abnormal pressure gradients between brachial and cavernosal arteries systolic occlusion pressures. The anatomical pattern of arterial occlusive disease during subsequent pharmacoarteriography will direct the surgeon to select the appropriate microvascular surgical procedures.[22]

## Arteriographic Criteria

Arterial blood flow to the corpora cavernosa is usually from the right and left cavernosal arteries, and terminal branches of the hypogastric-cavernous arterial bed. Multiple muscular, corkscrew-shaped arteries, the helicine arterioles, branch off the cavernosal arteries and open directly into the lacunar spaces. Increased arterial blood flow to the lacunar spaces may be achieved by increasing the flow in the cavernosal arteries through their communications with the proximal dorsal arteries.[16]

Selective arteriography is the present method for obtaining the anatomical information necessary for surgical strategy making.[26–28] The pattern (Fig. 39.1) of arterial occlusive disease involves bilateral occlusive lesions that are (1) focal in nature and proximal to the cavernosal artery in the internal pudendal or common penile artery prior to the bifurcation to dorsal penile and cavernosal arteries or (2) focal in nature in the cavernosal artery but proximal to an arterial communication from the dorsal penile artery to the cavernosal artery. Patients with such lesions may be considered for one or two anastomoses of the inferior epigastric artery to the dorsal penile artery(ies). The rationale for this surgical procedure is to increase perfusion pressure and inflow to the cavernosal arteries either retrograde through the proximal dorsal penile arteries or through distal dorsal penile artery branches that communicate to the cavernosal artery.

# Operative Technique

The vascular principles used in microvascular arterial bypass surgery for impotence are similar to those vascular and microvascular principles used in arterial bypass procedures for occlusive disease in other vascular beds.[10,19,23,48] Long-term bypass patency is based on four microvascular principles: (1) prevention of ischemic, mechanical, or thermal injury to the vascular endothelium of the donor or recipient vascular structures; (2) transmission of systolic neoarterial inflow pressures and flow; (3) technically accurate arterial anastomoses; and (4) low recipient vascular outflow resistances.

The prevention of endothelial injury is critical during surgical preparation of the vessels for anastomoses, using technically sound "no touch" techniques in order to improve long-term vascular patency. The presence of healthy vascular endothelium is essential. The endothelium releases numerous endothelium-derived relaxing factors, which act not only as potent vasodilators but also as strong inhibitors of platelet adhesion and aggregations.[10,19,23,48]

The integrity of the donor and recipient vessels prior to the anastomoses is of paramount concern as well, because the donor vessels provide transmission of the systemic blood pressure and the recipient vessels provide low-resistance outflow runoff. Histomorphologic analyses reveal that preexisting atherosclerotic lesions exist in over 50% of the dorsal penile arteries.[34] Although present, such preexisting lesions were rarely identified in the inferior epigastric artery or the deep dorsal vein. Vascular risk factors did not per se predict the quality of the vessels. These data reinforce the use of the inferior epigastric artery as the neoarterial pathway and support the concept of using multiple neoarterial anastomoses and not necessarily relying on one pathway to achieve the goals of increased cavernosal arterial perfusion and blood inflow.[11]

The goal of the microvascular arterial bypass procedure is to increase cavernosal arterial perfusion pressure and inflow using the branched inferior epigastric artery as the donor artery with bilateral anastomoses to the dorsal penile arteries.

## Inguinoscrotal Incision

Prior to the commencement of the operation, the patient is placed in the supine position, and a Foley catheter under sterile conditions is placed and left to closed drainage throughout the procedure. The preoperative arteriogram is reviewed, and the best quality inferior epigastric artery is selected. The site of the curvilinear inguinoscrotal incision is usually on the contralateral side of the anticipated incision for the inferior epigastric harvest. This site avoids two incisions on the same side of the body and allows for easier transfer of the inferior epigastric artery.

The inguinoscrotal skin incision is made two finger breadths from the base of the penis (Fig. 39.4). The uppermost aspect of the inguinal incision is at a plane consistent with the ventral aspect of the stretched penis. The lowermost aspect of the incision passes to the midline scrotal raphe. The advantages of this incision are that it offers excellent proximal and distal expo-

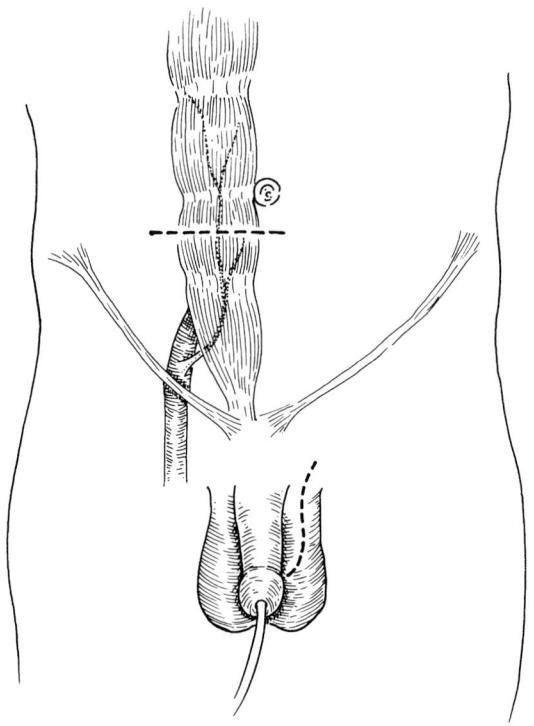

FIGURE 39.4. Incisions used for penile revascularization. The incisions are placed on opposite sides of the body.

FIGURE 39.5. Ligaments of the penis. Preservation of the suspensory and fundiform ligaments is important, as they contain sensory nerves for penile sensation and their preservation is necessary to maintain penile length.

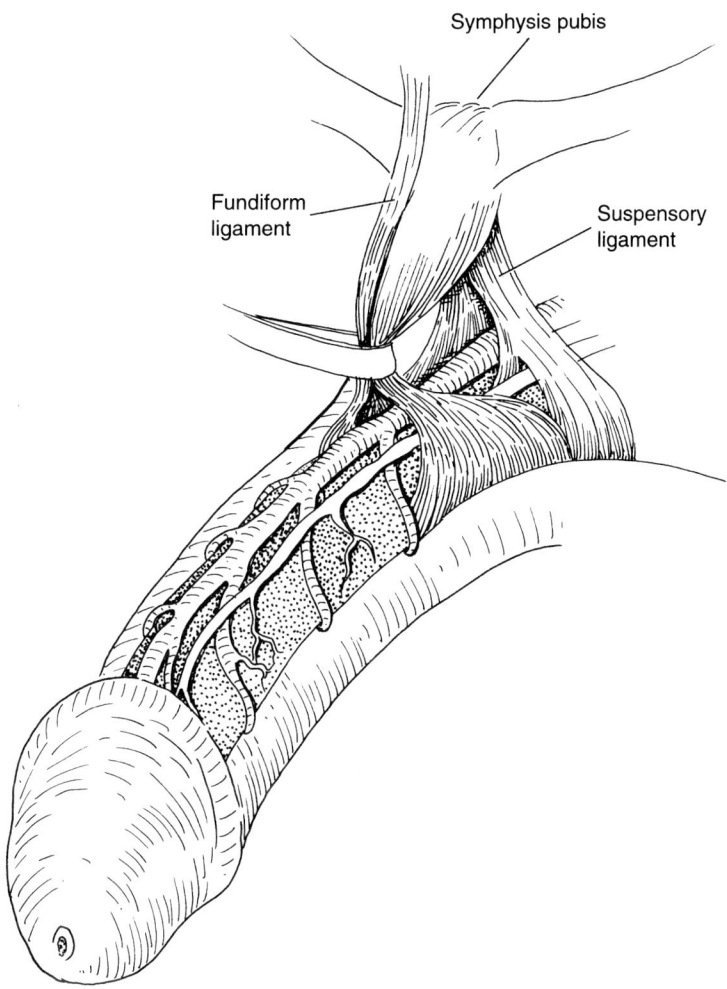

Symphysis pubis

Fundiform ligament

Suspensory ligament

sure of the penile neurovascular bundle, the ability to preserve the fundiform and suspensory ligaments, and the absence of unsightly postoperative scars on the penile shaft or at the base of the penis. Use of the Scott retractor with its elastic hooks maximizes operative exposure of the penis with a minimum of assistance.

## Preservation of the Penile Ligaments

The ipsilateral tunica albuginea is subsequently identified at the midpenile shaft. Blunt finger dissection along the tunica albuginea is performed in a distal direction deep to the spermatic cord structures along the lateral aspect of the penile shaft, avoiding injury to the fundi-

form ligament (Fig. 39.5). The penis is then inverted through the skin incision by carefully pushing the glans in fully. The penis must not be expanded during this maneuver. If a partial erection is present, intracavernosal adrenergic agents (100μg phenylephrine) should be administered. Blunt finger dissection around the distal penile shaft enables a plane to be established between Buck's fascia and Colles' fascia, and a Penrose drain is secured in this plane.

## Preparation of the Recipient Dorsal Arteries

Exposure of the neurovascular bundle and, in particular, the right and left dorsal penile arteries is now performed. Isolation of the dorsal penile arteries for such arterial bypass surgery requires limited dissection at this stage in the procedure; thus ischemic, mechanical, and thermal trauma to the dorsal penile arteries should be minimized. At all times during this vascular surgery, maximal smooth muscle relaxation is desired to decrease iatrogenic endothelial damage. The temperature of the operating room, the use of room temperature irrigating solution, and even the skin incision can induce vasoconstriction, spasm, and possible endothelial cell damage. Topical papaverine hydrochloride irrigation preserves endothelial and smooth muscle cell morphology during dorsal artery preparation, and its frequent use is encouraged. For intraluminal irrigation, use a dilute papaverine, heparin, and electrolytic solution. This solution has been demonstrated to inhibit the early development of myointimal proliferative lesions during surgical preparation.

The right and left dorsal penile arteries are identified first in the midpenile shaft. Their course is followed proximally underneath the fundiform ligament, with care taken to leave the fundiform ligament intact. A fenestration is fashioned in the fundiform ligament proximally, usually near the junction of the fundiform and suspensory ligaments at a location where the pendulous penile shaft becomes fixed proximally. Blunt dissection is performed under the proximal aspect of the fundiform ligament above the pubic bone toward the external ring. This dissection enables the inferior epigastric artery to pass from its abdominal location to the appropriate location in the penis while simultaneously preserving the fundiform ligament.

## Harvesting of the Inferior Epigastric Artery

The inguinoscrotal incision is temporarily closed with staples. A unilateral transverse abdominal incision provides excellent operative exposure of the inferior epigastric artery and heals with a more cosmetic scar as compared with those observed with previously used paramedian skin incisions (Fig. 39.4). The start-

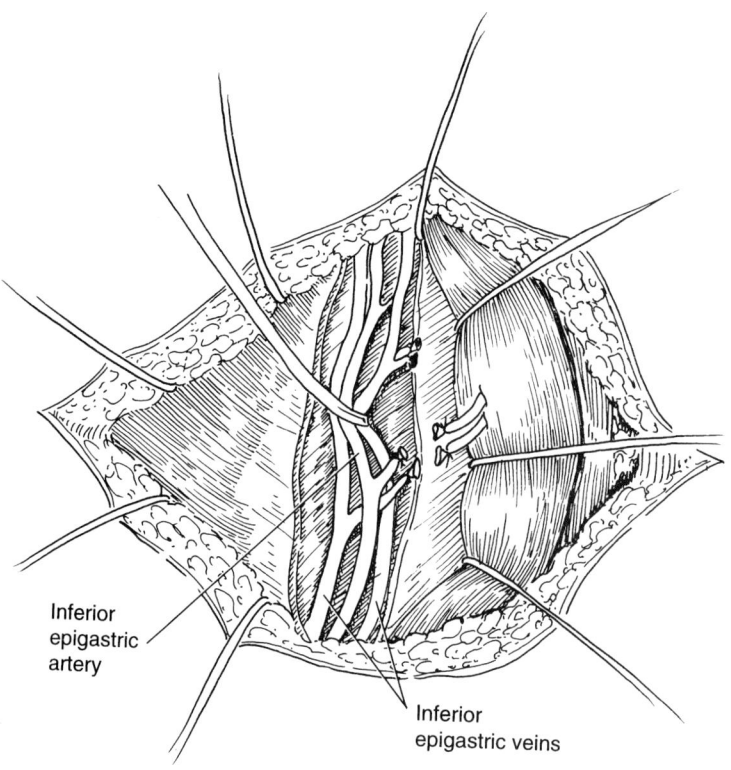

Inferior epigastric artery

Inferior epigastric veins

FIGURE 39.6. Inferior epigastric artery dissection. The artery is dissected carefully with its accompanying veins en bloc to avoid arterial intimal damage.

ing point of the incision is approximately five eighths of the total distance from the pubic bone to the umbilicus and extends laterally along the skin lines for approximately four finger breadths. The rectus fascia is incised vertically, and the rectus muscle is reflected medially. The junction between the rectus muscle and underlying preperitoneal fat is identified. The inferior epigastric artery and its two accompanying veins are located at this anatomical plane (Fig. 39.6). The Scott retractor is again used to maximize operative exposure. It is critical to harvest an inferior epigastric artery of appropriate length so that there will be no tension on any microvascular anastomosis. Application of topical papaverine is used on the inferior epigastric artery throughout the dissection. Thermal injury is avoided by use of low-current microbipolar cautery set at the minimum level necessary for adequate coagulation. The vasa vasorum blood supply is preserved by dissecting the artery en bloc with its surrounding veins and fat.

The transfer route of the neoarterial inflow source is prepared from the abdominal perspective prior to transacting the vessel distally (Fig. 39.7). (The penile transfer route has previously been dissected.) The temporary scrotal staples are removed and the penis is reinverted. The internal ring is identified lateral to the origin of the inferior epigastric artery in the pelvis. Using blunt finger dissection through the inguinal canal, the finger is passed through the internal ring and through the external ring to the previously fashioned defect between the fundiform and suspensory ligaments at the base of the penis. A Penrose drain is passed to protect the transfer route.

The donor vascular bundle is transected distally between two ligaclips and is carefully inspected for any proximal bleeding points. A long, fine, right-angled vascular instrument is carefully passed from the fenestration between the fundiform and suspensory ligaments to the internal inguinal ring. The instrument may grasp the distal vascular bundle. The inferior epigastric vascular bundle is transferred to the base of the penis. It should be briskly pulsating and of adequate length. The origin of the inferior epigastric artery should be inspected for

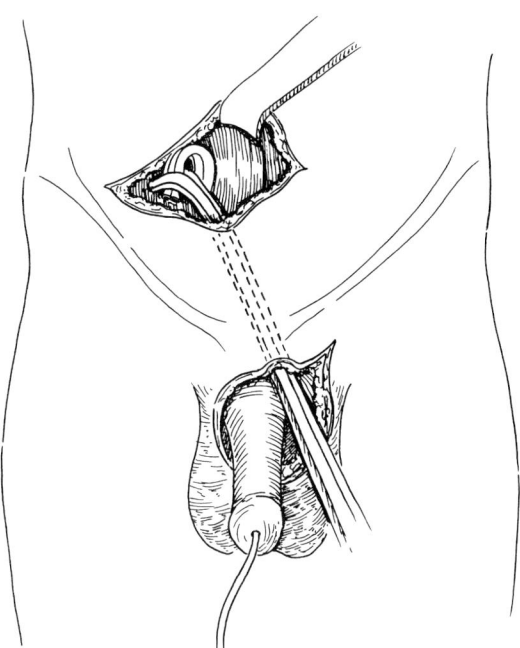

FIGURE 39.7. Inferior epigastric artery transfer. Transfer is accomplished via the inguinal canal. Care is taken to avoid twisting or kinking of the artery upon transfer.

kinking or twisting. If no further vascular bundle adjustments need be made, the abdominal incision may be closed in layers.

## Microvascular Anastomoses

A Scott retractor and the associated elastic hooks are used on the inguinal scrotal incision and the fenestration of the fundiform ligament to gain exposure of the proximal dorsal neurovascular bundle. The pulsating inferior epigastric artery is placed against the recipient dorsal penile arteries and a convenient location is selected for the vascular anastomoses. The anastomoses are created based on the arteriographic findings. An end-to-side anastomosis is best under conditions where dorsal penile artery communications exist to the cavernosal artery in both proximal and distal directions (Fig. 39.8). An end-to-side anastomosis protects arterial blood flow in the distal direction to the glans penis, and ligation of both dorsal penile arteries to perform bilateral

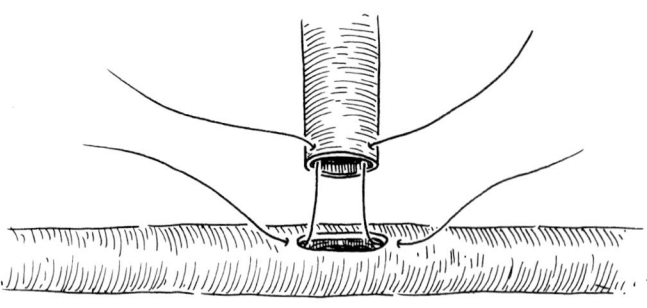

FIGURE 39.8. End-to-side anastomosis. The most commonly used anastomosis is the end-to-side variety.

End-to-side

proximal end-to-end anastomoses does not cause ischemic injury to the glans penis.

The appropriate dorsal penile artery segment is freed from its attachments to the tunica albuginea. Vascular hemostasis of this segment of the dorsal penile artery may be achieved with either gold-plated (low pressure) aneurysm vascular clamps or vessel loops under minimal tension for the minimal of operating time. The only location where the adventitia must be carefully removed is at the site of the vascular anastomosis, that is, the distal end of the inferior epigastric artery and the selected region of the dorsal penile artery, in order to avoid causing subsequent thrombosis. If segments of adventitia enter the anastomosis, patency of the anastomosis will be in jeopardy, as adventitia activates clotting factors from the extrinisic clotting system. The remaining adventitia should be preserved in the vessels as the vasa vasorum provide a nutritional role to the vessel wall. The preservation of the adventitia is additionally important in terms of vessel innervation.

Under microscopic control at 5 to 10× magnification, a 10-0 suture (single-armed, 100 μm/149° curved needle) is placed along the longitudinal axis of the dorsal penile artery in a 1-mm

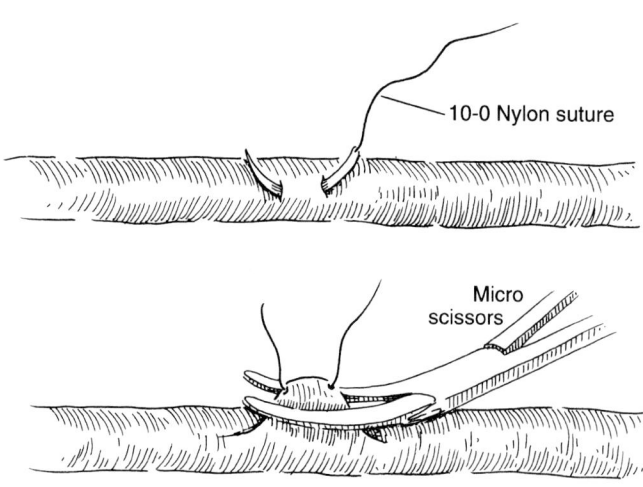

10-0 Nylon suture

Micro scissors

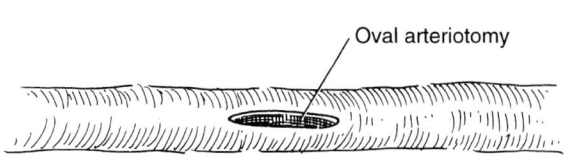

Oval arteriotomy

FIGURE 39.9. Arteriotomy. A 10-0 nylon suture is placed in the longitudinal axis of the dorsal penile artery and elevated. Microsurgical scissors are used to excise a segment of arterial wall resulting in an elliptical defect ready for the anastomosis.

segment in the region of the intended anastomosis (Fig. 39.9). After placing tension on the suture, an oval section of the artery wall is excised with a curved microscissors, resulting in a 1.2- to 1.5-mm horizontal arteriotomy. A plastic colored background material will aid in vessel visualization under the microscope. A temporary 2F Silastic stent is placed within the arteriotomy for clearer definition of the vessel lumen.

An end-to-side anastomosis is performed between the inferior epigastric artery and the dorsal artery, using interrupted 10-0 nylon sutures under the 5 to 10× magnification. The sutures are placed initially at each apex of the anastomosis and then subsequently three to five interrupted sutures are placed into each side wall. All sutures used to complete the anastomosis are inserted equidistant from each other to avoid an uneven anastomosis (Fig. 39.10). If a temporary vascular stent is used, it is removed following placement of all sutures; the sutures of one wall are tied, and the opposite side sutures are left temporarily untied. The use of a temporary vascular stent enables careful inspection of the vessel back wall. Following release of the temporary occluding vascular clamps (or vessel loops) on the dorsal penile artery, the anastomosed segment should reveal arterial pulsations along its length and retrograde in the inferior epigastric artery. Such an observation implies a patent anastomosis. At this time, the inferior epigastric artery-plated aneurysm clamp may be removed. The intensity of the arterial pulsations in the anastomosis usually increases. After hemostasis has been achieved and correct instrument and sponge counts are assured, closure of the inguinoscrotal incision may begin in routine fashion. The Foley catheter is left to closed-system gravity drainage overnight.

Modifications of the above-described procedure may be utilized. The most common alternative arterial anastomosis is an end-to-end anastomosis between the inferior epigastric artery and the ligated proximal end of the dorsal penile artery. Depending on the site of the arterial communication from the dorsal penile artery to the cavernosal artery, the end-to-end anastomosis may also be anastomosed to the distal ligated end of the dorsal penile artery. It is most common to anastomose the opposite dorsal penile artery to the inferior epigastric artery. This can be done with an appropriately sized distal branch of the inferior epigastric artery end-to-side as previously described, or an arteriotomy may be placed in the inferior epigastric artery for an end-to-side anastomosis to either the proximal end (most common) or distal end (least common) depending on the arteriographic findings.

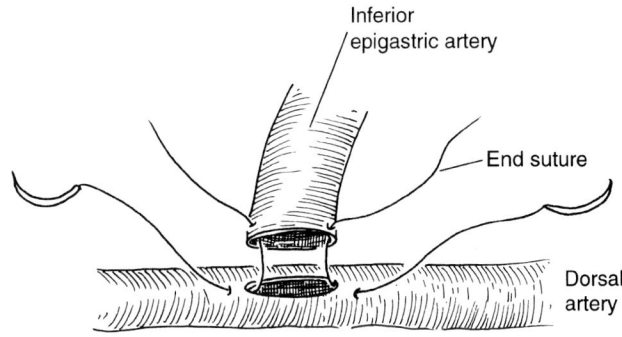

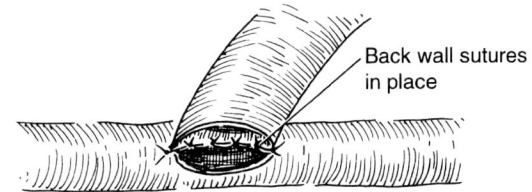

FIGURE 39.10. Anastomotic technique. (A) The end sutures of 10-0 nylon are placed first. (B) Each side is then anastomosed using interrupted sutures. Care is taken to place these sutures equidistantly and to avoid damage to the back wall of the vessel. A temporary Silastic stent is used to prevent luminal occlusion.

*Complications*

Following coitus, masturbation, or trauma in the region of the anastomosis in the first few postoperative weeks, mechanical disruption of the microvascular anastomosis and subsequent uncontrolled arterial hemorrhage may occur. Abstention from sexual activities involving the erect penis is recommended until 6 weeks postoperation.

Other complications include penile pain and diminished penile sensation from injury to the nearby dorsal nerve. Loss of compliance of the suspensory and fundiform ligaments postoperatively may lead to diminished penile length. Preserving the two ligaments markedly minimizes those complications.

Failed arterial anastomoses and non–newonset veno-occlusive dysfunction have been found to explain postoperative failure in patients with normal preoperative corporal venoocclusion. Failure of the microvascular arterial bypass may be due to problems of inadequate arterial inflow, technical errors of the microvascular anastomosis, or inadequate arterial runoff. Poor arterial runoff may be the result of preexisting vascular pathology, obstructing valves, or the development of vascular pathology, such as myointimal proliferative lesions within the recipient vessels.

# Results

In the recent literature there has been reported a variable success rate following penile revascularization, ranging from 30% to 74% (Table 39.1). A problem in interpreting these data is that there is no standardization of the definition of success following this operation. Success has been variably defined by questionnaire, patient interview, and hemodynamic evaluation. Furthermore, the patient populations have been heterogeneous, with varying numbers of patients with venogenic impotence. Use of dorsal vein arterialization seems to offer success rates inferior to procedures using pure arterial anastomoses. To evaluate this operation as a valid management strategy, analysis of prospective patient outcomes is essential. Because the goal of the operation is to restore natural, spontaneously occurring erections without the aid of any internal or external means to young men with erectile dysfunction, much research needs to be conducted to identify the reasons why a significant number of men fail to respond to revascularization of the penis.

# Conclusion

In patients with pure arteriogenic impotence who had an increased equilibrium pressure postoperatively, there is a correlation with their subjective improvement in erectile function. Patients with corporal veno-occlusive dysfunction should not be considered candidates for microvascular arterial bypass surgery.

Young men with pure arteriogenic impotence, and potentially many years of sexuality ahead of them, desire the natural restoration of their normal erectile function. To help them achieve this goal, marked improvements in diagnosis and surgical technique, founded on sophisticated hemodynamic testing and

TABLE 39.1. Major penile revascularization studies.

| Author | Ax | Operation | No. of patients | Success Rate (%) | Follow-up (months) |
|---|---|---|---|---|---|
| DePalma (1995) | A | DA,DDV | 23 | 30 | 36 |
| Vardi (1995) | A,V | DA,DDV | 30 | 73 | 16 |
| Melman (1994) | A,V | DA,DDV | 23 | 39 | 35 |
| Altwein (1994) | A,V | DA,DDV | 125 | 38 | 23 |
| Fitch (1994) | A,V | DA,DDV | 70 | 53 | 20 |

A, arteriogenic; DA, dorsal artery anastomosis; DDV, dorsal vein arterialization; V, venogenic.

sound vascular and microvascular principles, have been made. Strict patient selection criteria and more accurate and detailed diagnostic evaluation based on contemporary knowledge of erectile physiology enable more accurate decisions concerning hemodynamic integrity.

In microvascular arterial bypass surgery, each case should be treated individually, according to the arteriographic findings. Because the goal is to increase the arterial perfusion pressure and blood inflow to the erectile tissue, the best opportunity to achieve this goal is to individualize the new blood inflow pathways. To this end, it is best to use the least invasive technique that will allow maximal transmission of systemic blood pressure to the cavernous bodies through the most anatomically accessible available pathway.

## References

1. Goldstein I, Hatzichristou DG. Epidemiology of impotence. In: Bennett A, ed. *Impotence: Diagnosis and Management of Erectile Dysfunction.* Philadelphia: W.B. Saunders; 1994: 1–17.
2. Zorgniotti AW, Lizza EF. Complications of penile revascularization. In: Zorgniotti AW, Lizza EF, eds. *Diagnosis and Management of Impotence.* Philadelphia: B.C. Decker; 1991.
3. Junemann KP, Persson-Junemann C, Alken P. Pathophysiology of erectile dysfunction. *Semin Urol* 1990; 8:80–93.
4. Frohrib DA, Goldstein I, Payton TR, et al. Characterization of penile erectile states using external computer-based monitoring. *J Biomech Eng* 1987; 109:110–113.
5. Michal V, Kramar R, Popischal J, et al. Direct arterial anastomosis on corporal cavernosa penis in therapy of erectile dysfunction. *Rozhl Chir* 1973; 52:587–590.
6. Virag R, Zwang G, Dermange H, et al. Vasculogenic impotence: a review of 92 cases with 54 surgical operations. *Vasc Surg* 1981; 121:774–777.
7. Virag R, Bouilly P, Frydaman D. Is impotence an arterial disorder? A study of arterial risk factors in 400 impotent men. *Lancet* 1985; 1:181–184.
8. Levine FJ, Greenfield AJ, Goldstein I. Arteriographically-determined occlusive disease within the hypogastric-cavernous bed in impo-

tent patients following blunt perineal and pelvic trauma. *J Urol* 1990; 144:1147–1151.
9. Corso JD, Shamma AR, Meng RL. In-situ saphenous vein bypass. In: Bergan JJ, ed. *Arterial Surgery; New Diagnostic and Operative Techniques.* Orlando, FL: Grune & Stratton; 1988: 507–522.
10. Shaw WW. Microvascular surgery. In: Haimovichi H, ed. *Vascular Surgery: Principles and Techniques.* Norwalk: Appleton-Century–Crofts; 1988: 289–308.
11. Hatzichristou DG, Goldstein I. Arterial bypass surgery for impotence. *Curr Opin Urol* 1991; 1:144–148.
12. Michal V, Kramer R, Popischal J. Femoropudendal bypass, internal iliac thrombendarterectomy and direct arterial anastomosis to the cavernous body in the treatment of erectile impotence. *Bull Soc Int Chir* 1974; 33:341–345.
13. McDougal WS, Jeffrey RF. Microscopic penile revascularization. *J Urol* 1983; 129:517–521.
14. MacGregor RJ, Konnack JW. Treatment of vasculogenic erectile dysfunction by direct anastomosis of the inferior epigastric artery to the central artery of the corpus cavernosum. *J Urol* 1982; 131:542–545.
15. Sharlip I. Retrograde revascularization of the dorsal penile artery for arteriogenic erectile dysfunction. *J Urol* 1984; 1312:232A.
16. Crespo F, Soltanik E, Bove D. Treatment of vasculogenic sexual impotence by revascularizing cavernous and/or dorsal arteries using microvascular techniques. *Urology* 1982; 20:271–275.
17. Furlow WL, Fisher J, Knoll LD. Penile revascularization: experience with deep dorsal vein arterialization: the Furlow-Fisher modification with 27 patients. Presented at the Sixth Biennial Meeting on Corpus Cavernosum Revascularization and Third Biennal World Meeting on Impotence, Boston: International Society of Impotence Research, 1988.
18. Balko A, Malhotra CM, Wincze JP. Deep penile vein arterialization for arterial and venous impotence. *Arch Surg* 1986; 121:774–777.
19. Bennett AH, Rivard DJ, Blanc RP, et al. Reconstructive surgery for vasculogenic impotence. *J Urol* 1986; 136:599–602.
20. Hauri D. A new operative technique in vasculogenic erectile dysfunction. *World J Urol* 1986; 4:237–249.
21. Bergamini TM, Towne JB, Bandyc DF, et al. Experience with in-situ saphenous vein bypasses

during 1981–1989: determinants of long-term patency. *J Vasc Surg* 1991; 13:137–149.

22. Guity A, Young PH, Fisher VW. In search of the "perfect" anastomosis. *Microsurgery* 1990; 11:5–11.

23. Siemionow M. Evaluation of different microsurgical techniques for arterial anastomosis of vessels of diameter less than one millimeter. *J Reconstr Surg* 1987; 3:333–340.

24. Wespes E, Corbusier A, Delcour C, et al. Deep dorsal vein arterialization in vascular impotence. *Br J Urol* 1989; 64:535–540.

25. Wespes E, deGoes PM, Saltar AA, et al. Objective criteria in the long-term evaluation of penile venous surgery. *J Urol* 1994; 152:888–890.

26. Sharlip I. Penile arteriography in impotence after pelvic trauma. *J Urol* 1981; 126:477–479.

27. Rosen MP, Greenfield AJ, Walker TG, et al. Arteriogenic impotence: findings in 195 impotent men examined with selective internal pudendal angiography. *Radiology* 1990; 174: 1043–1048.

28. Lurie AL, Bookstein JJ, Kessler WO. Angiography of post-traumatic impotence. *Cardiovasc Intervent Radiol* 1988; 11:232–236.

29. Shiokawa Y, Fazlur Rahman M, Ishii Y, et al. The rate of reendothelialization correlates inversely with the degree of the following intimal thickening in vein grafts: electron microscopic and immunohistochemical studies. *Virchows Arch [A]* 1989; 415:225–235.

30. Saenz de Tejada I, Goldstein I, Azadzoi K, et al. Impaired neurogenic and endothelium-mediated relaxation of penile smooth muscle from diabetic men with impotence. *N Engl Med J* 1989; 320:1025–1030.

31. Pabst TSI, Flanigan DP, Buchbinde D. Reduced intimal injury to canine arteries with controlled application of vessel loops. *J Surg Res* 1989; 47:235–241.

32. Machiarelli G, Familiari G, Caggiati M, et al. Arterial repair after microvascular anastomosis: scanning and transmission electron microscopy study. *Acta Anat* 1991; 140:8–16.

33. Lue TF. Functional evaluation of penile arteries with papaverine. In: Tanagho EA, Lue TF, McClure RD, eds. Contemporary Management of Impotence and Infertility. Baltimore: Williams & Wilkins; 1988: 57–64.

34. Kalan JM, Roberts WC. Morphologic findings in saphenous veins used as coronary artery bypass conduits for longer than 1 year: necropsy analysis of 53 patients, 123 saphenous veins and 1865 five-millimeter segments of veins. *Am J Heart* 1990; 119:1164–1184.

35. Hirsch GM, Karnovsky MJ. Inhibition of vein graft intimal proliferative lesions in the rat by heparin. *Am J Pathol* 1991; 139:581–587.

36. Hayashi K, Takamizawa K, Nakamura T, et al. Effects of elastase on the stiffness and elastic properties of arterial walls in cholesterol-fed rabbits. *Atherosclerosis* 1987; 66:259–267.

37. Corson JD, Leather RP, Balko A, et al. Relationship between vasovasorum and blood flow to vein bypass endothelial morphology. *Arch Surg* 1985; 120:386–388.

38. Bush HL, Jakubowski JA, Curl R, et al. The natural history of endothelial structure and function in arterialized vein grafts. *J Vasc Surg* 1986; 3:204–215.

39. Barada JH, Bennett AH. Penile revascularization: where do we stand? *Int J Impotence Res* 1990; 2:79–84.

40. Lewis RW. Arteriovenous surgeries: do they make any sense? In: Lue TF, ed. *World Book of Impotence*. London: Smith-Gordon; 1992: 199.

41. Sohn M, Sikora R, Bohndorf K, et al. Selective microsurgery in arteriogenic erectile failure. *World J Urol* 1990; 8:104–107.

42. Rosen MP, Greenfield AJ, Walker TG, et al. Cigarette smoking as an independent risk factor for atherosclerosis in the hypogastric-cavernous bed of men with arteriogenic impotence. *J Urol* 1991; 145:759–763.

43. Lehman TP, Jacobs JA. Etiology of diabetic impotence. *J Urol* 1983; 129:291–294.

44. Ruzbarsky V, Michal V. Morphologic changes in the arterial bed of the penis with aging: relationship to the pathogenesis of impotence. *Invest Urol* 1977; 15:194–199.

45. Saenz de Tejada I, Moroukian P, Tessier J, et al. The trabecular smooth muscle modulates the capacitor function of the penis: studies on a rabbit model. *Am J Physiol* 1991; 260:H1590–1595.

46. Pescatori ES, Hatzichristou DG, Namburi S, et al. A positive intracavernosal injection test implies normal venoocclusive function but not necessarily normal arterial function: a hemodynamic study. *J Urol* 1994; 151:1209–1216.

47. Krane RJ, Goldstein I, Saenz de Tejada I. Impotence. *N Engl J Med* 1989; 321:1648–1659.

48. Levine FJ, Goldstein I. Vascular reconstructive surgery in the management of erectile dysfunction. *Int J Impotence Res* 1990; 2:59–78.

# 40
# Penile Prosthesis Implantation: Pearls, Pitfalls, and Perils

Steven K. Wilson

Penile prosthetic implants have been available for a quarter century. Early in the 1970s paired semirigid devices and multicomponent inflatable implants were first reported in the medical literature.[1-3] Initially, the malleable paired devices were much more popular with implanting surgeons because of lower cost, easier surgical implantation, and better mechanical reliability. The early inflatable devices were plagued with recurrent mechanical breakdown that necessitated multiple revision operations.[4,5] Devices from several different companies have come and gone in the marketplace. The devices that remain have become remarkably dependable mechanically. In fact, some authorities believe the inflatable devices are now more mechanically reliable than the human factor.[6] In fact, revision surgery may be more likely for hematoma, infection, patient dissatisfaction, or physician error than for mechanical breakdown.

Beginning in 1990, the pendulum has swung, and there are now more inflatable implants used annually than malleable devices. This is a reflection of higher patient satisfaction with inflatable implants and physician acknowledgment of vastly improved mechanical reliability. Today the impotent male has a choice of several malleable and positionable prostheses and six inflatable ones. There are important advantages and disadvantages to each model.

## Semirigid, Malleable, and Positionable Prostheses

Semirigid prostheses are manufactured in many countries (e.g., the United States, Germany, France, Hungary, Argentina, Taiwan). These semirigid prostheses are usually a variation of the original Small-Carrion model, which has been marketed in the United States for over two decades. The concept of impotence correction is the same with all models. Paired rods in the corpora cavernosa provide mild tumescence and moderate rigidity to allow vaginal penetration. Length and girth of the penis are unchanged in flaccidity and in "erection." For this reason, concealment is sometimes a problem. Although the original Small-Carrion required a large inventory of sizes, the newer models feature bases that can be trimmed and have "add-on" rear tip extenders. These features are an advantage because the number of prostheses required to fit all patients is markedly decreased. Some of the prostheses are so adaptable that only the two diameters are required to be carried in inventory. Some implants are quite stiff, others are so pliable that they are labeled "soft" (Subrini, France). Mechanical reliability has been excellent, but erosion in patients with diabetes or with spinal cord injury has been reported in long-term follow-up.[7,8]

529

Malleable prostheses are manufactured in Germany and the United States. They are an improvement over semirigid models because of better concealment. The outer material is usually silicone, and malleability is provided by a twisted wire of a material such as silver or stainless steel. Implantation is the same simple procedure as with semirigid models. The popular models available include the Jonas, the AMS 600, Mentor Malleable, and the Mentor Acu-Form. Implanting physicians perceive comparable advantages and disadvantages to these models, but patients (who receive only one model) are fairly happy with the result from any of the semirigid models. The model of choice in most countries is usually based on price. Mechanical reliability has been excellent with all devices. Nonhydraulic implants also have the advantage for use in patients with abnormalities of corporal tunica albuginea. A simple implantation will suffice in these patients, whereas corporal reconstruction and possible grafting with synthetic materials may be necessary with inflatable models.

A malleable device that deserves special mention is the Dura II by Dacomed. Introduced in 1992, the design of this implant features polyethylene segments strung on cable. The wire is under constant tension and the beads articulate upon it, providing superior malleability and improved positionability. This device is considerably more expensive than any of the above-mentioned malleable models. Mechanical reliability[9] has been improved over the previous Omniphase and Duraphase.

# Implantation of Semirigid and Malleable Prostheses

The surgical procedure of implantation of semirigid and malleable devices can be done through a variety of incisions. Originally, the perineal incision was advocated, but proximity to the rectum caused it to fall into disfavor. The infrapubic incision can be used, but is usually reserved for inflatable implants. Today, the most popular surgical approaches for paired rod insertion are the penoscrotal and subcoronal.

## Pearls, Pitfalls, and Perils

### The Penoscrotal Incision

Most authorities believe this is the best all-around incision because it provides superior access to the proximal corpora cavernosa should fibrosis be encountered. It also avoids the possibility of dorsal nerve injury, because the nerves run dorsally and the incision is on the undersurface of the penis. Urethral injury is possible but correctable with this incision. The disadvantage of this approach is that it requires a very long corporotomy to manipulate the flexible prosthesis into the corpora.

### The Subcoronal Incision

For routine implantation of malleable and positionable prostheses, use the subcoronal incision. It is the quickest because the surgery is straightforward, and the implant insertion requires only a small corporotomy. Minimal bending of the prosthesis during insertion into the corpora is necessary when compared with the penoscrotal approach. The incision is not recommended in patients who are uncircumcised, as prolonged preputial edema and incision sensitivity can result. Some authorities believe coincident circumcision with prosthesis insertion increases infection risk,[10] although this has not been the case in one large series of implants.[11] If there is a suspicion of Peyronie's disease or corporal fibrosis, another approach should be used, because crural dilatation of fibrotic corpora can be difficult from such a distal incision. Make the skin, dartos, and Buck's fascia incisions in a circumferential manner, and the corporal incisions should be at right angles to avoid the dorsal nerves and to facilitate prosthesis insertion (Fig. 40.1).

### Surgical Technique

Dilatation of the corpora should begin with size 10 or 11 Hegar or Brooks dilators and proceed to size 14. Only rarely is it not possible to dilate to size 14. It is not advisable to use smaller dilators than 10 or 11 to initiate dilatation because the risk of crural rupture or urethral perforation is increased. In most men, the surgeon should strive to achieve size 14 dilatation,

FIGURE 40.1. The circumferential subcoronal incision with longitudinal corporotomy.

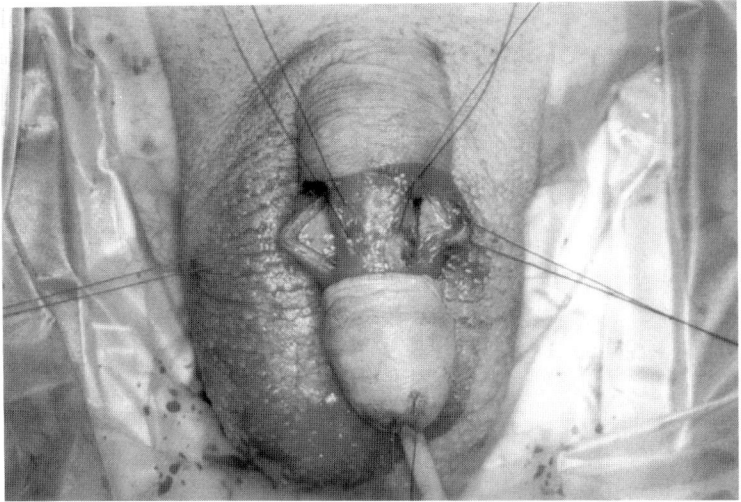

because the 11 mm diameter prosthesis gives unsatisfactory tumescence after a period of time. Patients may complain of diminished quality of erection a year or so after implantation of the 11 mm diameter prosthesis, for the corpora may have stretched in a tissue-expander effect of the semirigid prosthesis and the erection may have become floppy. Similar experience has been noted with self-contained prostheses.

Some men of small stature (e.g., Asians) may require a downsized diameter, and the AMS 600M is marketed in a 9-mm diameter for this purpose. The implanting surgeon should remember the function of the penis is to swell in tumescence, but even the small penis has considerable capacity for expansion. In a series of over 100 implants performed on Japanese, Thai, Korean, Chinese, Vietnamese, and Laotians, it was usually possible to dilate to 12 mm and frequently to 13 or 14 mm. This dilatation makes possible the use of size 11 to 13 mm diameter prostheses, although there may be difficulty in dilatation proximal rather than distal in these smaller patients, as the crura may be quite stenotic.

### Prosthesis Length

While maximizing the implant's girth, the surgeon should take care not to oversize the length of malleable (or inflatable) devices. A leading

cause of revision of malleable devices is pain and poor flexibility created by implantation of an overly long prosthesis. Undersizing the device by 0.5 cm may avoid these troublesome problems. Patients are happier when the surgeon concentrates on implanting a prosthesis of maximum girth rather than striving to implant the longest rod. The same caveat applies for inflatable implant cylinders.

## Self-Contained Inflatable Penile Prostheses

This prosthesis consists of paired hydraulic cylinders that are implanted in a manner similar to the semirigids and malleables. Several (Surgitek Flexiflate I and II, AMS Hydroflex) have come and gone from the marketplace since the introduction of Hydroflex in 1985. Presently, only the Dynaflex (Fig. 40.2) by American Medical Systems is available commercially. To cycle this device, it is necessary to pump the end of each cylinder by squeezing the penis immediately proximal to the glans. Fluid is transferred from a small reservoir in the base of the cylinder to a nondistensible central compartment. Filling of this compartment causes rigidity of the cylinder, which is almost as good as a rod. Girth enhancement is negligible. To deflate the prosthesis, it is necessary to flex the

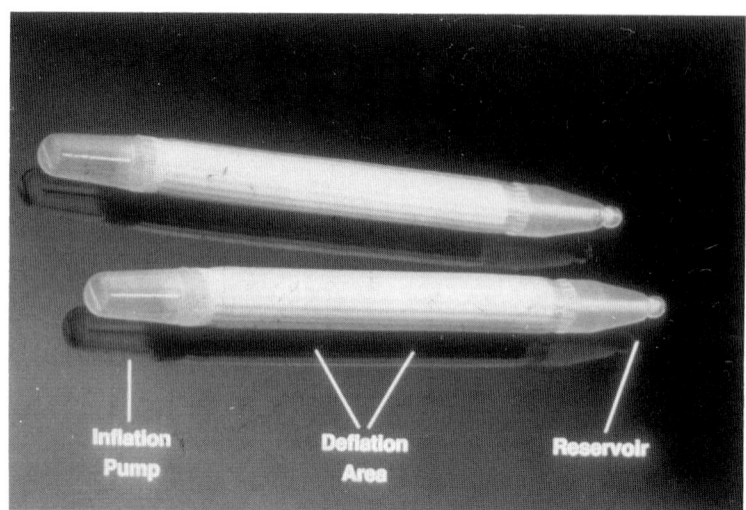

Figure 40.2. AMS Dynaflex.

penis for 12 seconds. After release the fluid flows from the central chamber to the reservoir, resulting in flaccidity better than with semirigid rods but inferior to multicomponent inflatables. Dynaflex prostheses come in two diameters: 11 mm and 13 mm. Device length is marked in 2-cm increments from 14 to 22. Adjustment between the lengths is possible by the addition of 0.5 cm rear tip extenders that are snap-on silicone spheres.

## Pearls, Pitfalls, and Perils

### Self-Contained Prostheses

Clinical research for both the Hydroflex and Dynaflex created enthusiasm about the concept of these "liquid rods" because of simple implantation, minimal morbidity, and mechanical reliability. Of 300 patients who were followed closely for many years, some who had been satisfied initially began returning with complaints of deteriorated erections. The implant that initially had excellent tumescence and rigidity had become floppy. The implant that initially was properly sized appeared now to be too short for the cavernosa and to have inadequate girth for tumescence. Patient dissatisfaction, particularly prevalent in well-endowed males, has caused disuse of the 11-mm device.[12]

### Tissue Space Expansion

The self-contained implants have an inherent rigidity that causes an increase in the intercavernosal measurements and a widening of the flaccid girth. The implant acts as a tissue expander and the result is a floppy, nonrigid erection. Over 50% of the patients in the above-mentioned series have now received three-piece inflatables.[12] Confirming the tissue expansion effect is the fascinating finding that the intercorporal measurements have increased an average of 2.7 cm, which results in a considerably longer replacement prosthesis.

### Replacement Prostheses

An important point needs to be made about the choice of replacement prostheses for self-contained prostheses that have failed mechanically or have created patient dissatisfaction. Deflation of self-contained prostheses requires flexion of the cylinders. Over time, the tunica albuginea overlying the site of flexion apparently becomes weakened. Small aneurysms may have developed at the base of the penis (where flexion was performed to effect deflation) after replacement of self-contained prostheses by three-piece inflatables (Fig. 40.3). It is advisable to use a replacement prosthesis with cylinder expansion controlled by a

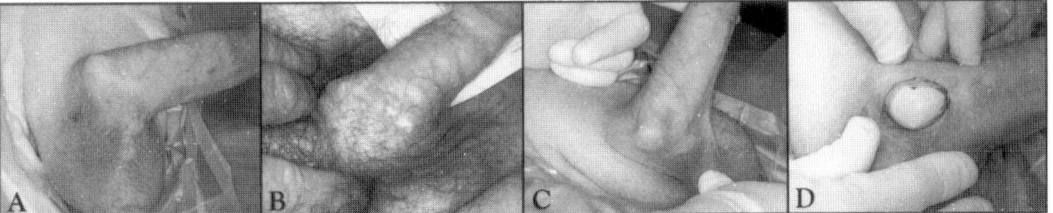

FIGURE 40.3. Aneurysm development (1–2 years) following replacement of self-contained prosthesis with three-piece inflatable. (A) AMS 700 CX replace Hydroflex. (B) Mentor Alpha I replace Dynaflex. (C and D) AMS 700 Ultrex replace Hydroflex.

nondistensible fabric wrap of the cylinder, e.g., the AMS CX. Use of the AMS Ultrex or the Mentor Alpha may promote the development of these penile deformities because of cylinder lengthening in the former and tunical dependent expansion in the latter.

### Prepubic Recession

Although the self-contained prosthesis is no longer a first-line implant, the inherent semirigidity of these devices may be helpful in the patient with prepubic recession who has developed a large prepubic fat pad with resultant penile recession. The Dynaflex or the new Ambicor is the ideal prosthesis for such a patient. After implantation, the patient is pleased to see his penis outside the plane of his body. The patient should be advised of the possibility of intercavernosal tissue expansion and that it may be necessary to substitute a three-piece prosthesis in the future. These individuals with the "hidden" penis are usually quite pleased to have developed enough stretching to make this necessary.

## Two-Piece Prostheses

Two-piece prostheses actually consist of three pieces—two cylinders and one pump. There are two presently on the market, one from each of the major American manufacturers. The Mentor Mark II prosthesis (Fig. 40.4) consists of two Bioflex (a polyurethane polymer) cylinders preconnected to a textured pump/reservoir. The cylinders are identical to the cylinders in the Mentor Alpha I, a three-piece inflatable

marketed with a separate pump and reservoir. Mentor Corporation also manufactures breast prostheses, and they have incorporated some of this technology into the Mark II. Two features of this technology transfer are a port for future repeated transcrotal addition of fluid and a textured reservoir to decrease the incidence of excessive periprosthetic capsule formation that may have prohibited full deflation.[13] The Mark II features cylinder lengths of 12 to 22 cm in 2-cm increments with rear tip extenders to fill in the gaps. There are two tubing lengths to allow infrapubic or the shorter penoscrotal implantation. Although some have reported good results with infrapubic incision,[14] most Mark II prostheses are placed through the penoscrotal approach.

## Pearls, Pitfalls, and Perils

### The Mentor Mark II

This prosthesis is available to assist surgeons who wish to place an inflatable prosthesis but who are reluctant to use a traditional three-piece because of insecurity regarding reservoir placement. It is useful in those patients in whom radiation or surgery or both may have obliterated the retropubic space. Unfortunately, many occasional implanters utilize the implant preferentially to avoid the dreaded blind reservoir placement necessary with a three-piece implant placed penoscrotally. The problems with the prosthesis revolve around the reservoir capacity. The reservoir holds 25 cc but the pump can only deliver 15 cc to the cylinders to achieve erection. The Bioflex cylinders are tunical-dependent for limiting their expan-

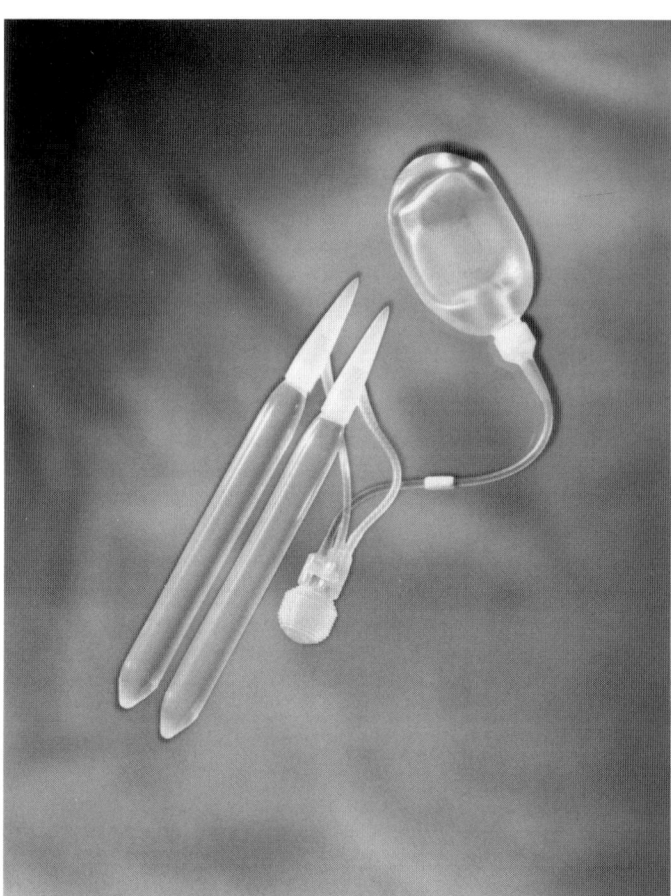

FIGURE 40.4. Mentor Alpha I three piece inflatable penile prosthesis.

sion, and 15 cc will not cause a decent erection over time. This necessitates percutaneous addition of fluid through the scrotal-port maneuver fraught with danger of infection and inadvertent reservoir rupture.

The large hen's egg–sized pump/reservoir can be uncomfortable for a patient with a small scrotum. For this reason the implant is not recommended for slightly built men and may be contraindicated for Asian males. The earlier Mentor two-piece, the Mentor GFS, had problems with excessive periprosthetic capsule formation around the pump/reservoir[13,15] that prevented full deflation. The Mark II has eliminated this complication by incorporation of a textured surface.

## Revisions and Replacement Prostheses

Should revision of the Mentor two-piece become necessary, the surgeon should remember that the cylinders are the same as with the Mentor Alpha I. The usual problems prompting revision are either puncture of the pump/reservoir or patient dissatisfaction. To convert the system to a three-piece inflatable implant, the cylinders can be left in place. Approach the prosthesis through the same incision of the original insertion. Sever the tubing leading to the cylinders. Make a space for the new reservoir in the retroperitoneal space. Place a 75-cc reservoir for cylinder size shorter than 18 cm or a 100-cc reservoir for longer cylinders. Fill the reservoir with an appropriate amount of saline and completely aspirate the cylinders. An Alpha pump can then be attached with three connectors, and a three-piece prosthesis results without the necessity of reopening the corpora cavernosa. Utilizing the existing cylinders avoids potential risk of hemorrhage, dorsal nerve injury, or urethral damage. The Mentor Bioflex cylinders are extremely reliable and rarely develop leaks.[16]

# The AMS Ambicor Two-Piece Prosthesis

Late in 1994, American Medical Systems introduced a new concept in two-piece prostheses to the American market. The implant had already been in use in other parts of the world for about a year. The Ambicor construction is similar to a Dynaflex prosthesis, but with two differences. Instead of having a pump at the end of each cylinder, there is only one tiny pump that is preconnected to the cylinders (Fig. 40.5). As in the Dynaflex, the reservoir is in the base of each cylinder. Deflation is accomplished identically as in the Dynaflex, by flexing the penis for 12 seconds and releasing the flexion, which allows the fluid to flow from the central nondistensible space to the reservoir in the base of the prosthesis. The Ambicor can be inserted through both penoscrotal and infrapubic incisions. Another important difference from the Dynaflex is the availability of 15 cm diameter cylinders in addition to the 11 and 13 cm.

## Pearls, Pitfalls, and Perils

Because of the newness of the prosthesis, there have been virtually no peer review articles that address patient satisfaction and mechanical reliability, but the Ambicor's availability in 15-cm diameter is a positive step that should increase patient satisfaction for it over the Dynaflex. As stated in the section on malleable implantation, the wise implant surgeon always strives for the maximum-girth prosthesis. The tiny pump is a welcome change from the Mentor Mark II that occupies considerable space in the scrotum.

On the negative side, however, is the difficulty of implantation. The manufacturer's instructions require that the tubing from cylinder to pump exit the corporotomy from the base of the cylinder. It is not permissible to run the tubing alongside the cylinder to a more distal corporotomy even though the tubing has protective boots. Implantation of the Ambicor requires a corporotomy deep in the scrotum and placement of closure sutures is laborious, which may markedly increase the degree of difficulty for occasional implanters.

# Multicomponent Inflatables— The Three-Piece Prosthesis

American Medical Systems and Mentor Corporation manufacture similar devices, but with important distinctions among the various models. All three-piece inflatables consist of paired cylinders, a scrotal pump, and an abdominal reservoir. The system can be filled with contrast solution or saline. Reservoir size varies from

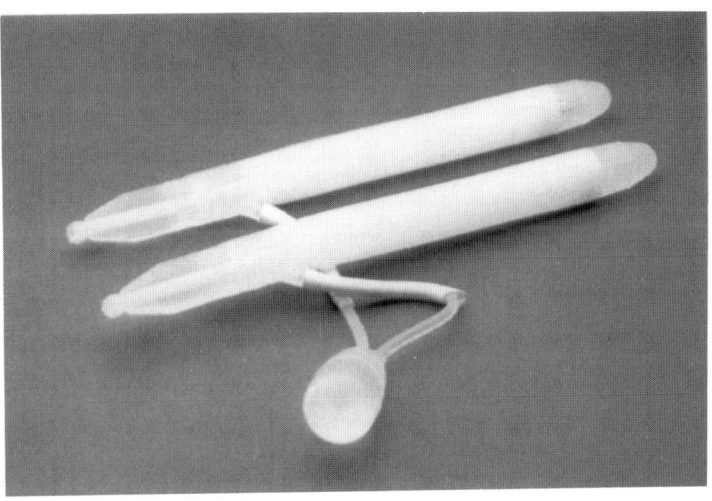

FIGURE 40.5. AMS Ambicor.

50 cc to 125 cc depending on model and cylinder length. Cylinder length varies from 12 cm to 22 cm, and rear tip extenders are available in all models to tailor cylinder length to each individual patient. These are the most expensive of all penile prostheses, and the cost in the United States is presently around $4000 to $4500.

The AMS models are all named the AMS 700. Since the early 1980s the pump and reservoir of the AMS 700 have undergone very little modification. In the late 1980s kink-proof tubing and the "quick-connect" connectors were incorporated, which improved mechanical reliability.[5] Over the years, several types of cylinders were used in this model, accounting for product designations, such as AMS 700 IPP, AMS 700 PPT, AMS 700 PND, and AMS 700 PLX. Presently on the market are the AMS 700 CX, AMS 700 CXM, AMS Ultrex, and the AMS 700 Ultrex Plus. The 700 CX penile prosthesis was first implanted in May 1984 and was commercially introduced in May 1987. The 700 Ultrex penile prosthesis was first implanted in October 1989 and commercially introduced in September 1990.

## The AMS 700 CX and the AMS 700 CXM

The CX cylinders were developed to be used in situations where penile tissue expansion must be controlled—thus the designation for "controlled expansion." The cylinders are of three-ply construction. Two silicone layers are sandwiched around a woven fabric similar to Dacron. Fluid is pumped into the inner silicone chamber, with expansion controlled from 12 mm to 18 mm by the fabric wrap. The outer layer of silicone prevents tissue ingrowth into the fabric layer. A smaller version of this cylinder is also produced as the CXM (controlled expansion, modified). These cylinders have smaller bases and smaller inflatable cylinders. The base of the CXM measures 10 mm versus 12 mm for the standard size CX. The inflatable portion of this three-ply cylinder expands from 9.5 to 14 mm upon inflation. The AMS 700 CXM also features a smaller pump and a 50-cc reservoir.

The CX cylinders have been proven performers since 1987, but with time and wear a device failure may eventually occur. American Medical Systems conducted a multicenter study at the request of the Food and Drug Administration (FDA) to determine device survival. Based on over 500 medical records, the report noted that "82% of men implanted with the 700 CX were free from revision or replacement surgery for five years from the original implant date" (data on file with FDA and reproduced in AMS pamphlet "How Long Can I Expect My Penile Prosthesis To Last?").

## Pearls, Pitfalls, and Perils

### The CX Cylinders

If you were trapped on another planet and restricted to only one prosthesis cylinder, the AMS 700 CX would be the one to choose. Its expansion, although controlled, is adequate for all but the most well-endowed patients. In flaccidity, the silicone cylinders provide the best concealability of all prostheses. Most importantly, the cylinders are ideal for patients having had previous penile surgery and previous implants, as chances for aneurysm formation are significantly decreased.[17] The Mentor Alpha I has advantages in previously unoperated patients, but the CX is the most versatile for use in all types of patients.

### Revisions of AMS 700 CX

The AMS 700 CX and CXM have been associated with a very high degree of patient satisfaction. However, when the prosthesis has failed, contrast medium filling the prosthesis at the time of implantation has not helped diagnose the cause of failure, for radiography has revealed that the contrast had leaked out and had been absorbed by the body. Prepping with normal saline is far easier and more effective.

When the prosthesis has lost fluid and has become nonoperational, the usual culprit is tubing shear by the old suture tie connectors. Product literature from the manufacturer continues to advise suture tie connectors in all revisions. This may be a mistake, as the new "quick connect" connectors are much safer for revisions. If mechanical failure develops in newer prostheses implanted with "quick connect" connectors, the culprit is usually cylinder leak, but it may be cylinder wall wear or breakage of the cylinder-input tubing juncture. The second most common problem of newer 700s has been crease-fold wear of the reservoir wall (Fig. 40.6). The pump itself is virtually free of problems.

### Replacement of CX

Revision operations should be done through the old incision with the electrosurgical unit. Cut down upon the pump and trace out the tubing. Disconnect the reservoir connection and attach a syringe with saline. Pump until the leak is detected. If the implant inflates in a normal fashion, attach the syringe to the reservoir and fill. Reservoir leaks are the size of a pinpoint and may not be detectable. If the cause of the leak is in doubt, remove the entire prosthesis. Nothing is as disappointing to the patient as for the surgeon to presume the prosthesis has been fixed and then to discover that the prosthesis deflates. As a rule of thumb, AMS 700 prostheses over 3 years old should be totally explanted and replaced with a new multicomponent prosthesis. Silicone surfaces of the cylinders and reservoir continue to wear, and single component replacement risks the possibility of another revision all too soon. During revisions involving cylinders, make certain to remove the fabric "boots," which cover the cylinder input tubing where it inserts into the corpora. Because of tissue ingrowth, this can be difficult. Additionally, make certain to remove all rear tip extenders. These are easily extracted by irrigating the proximal corpora with antibiotic irrigant and then placing a Yankov suction tip into the corpora. One final point: Never replace a three-piece prosthesis with a two-piece or a self-contained one. The patient has known the finest erection and the best flaccidity achievable by artificial means. He will be very unhappy with the poorer tumescence and less concealability available from these compromised prostheses.

## Pearls, Pitfalls, and Perils

### The AMS 700 CXM

This downsized version of the traditional 700 prosthesis was developed for the Asian market, where it has found widespread acceptance. The smaller diameter cylinder (Fig. 40.7) is particularly useful in the proximal corpus cavernosum. It is only necessary to dilate the proximal corpora to 10 or 11 mm, whereas the standard size CX requires dilatation to 12 or 13 mm. It is important to stress that the tubing must exit the corporotomy at the base of the cylinder rather than run along the cylinder for a distance and exit in a more distal corporotomy. The narrow proximal corpora found in Asian men will compromise deflation if the tubing is run alongside the cylinder. Many Asian implanters prefer to use the standard CX pump, because the tiny CXM pump is hard to grasp and has a smaller stroke volume.

Western implanters have also found the CXM invaluable in patients with corporal fibrosis. Corporal fibrosis occurs in patients with previously infected implants and in patients with priapism. The spongy erectile tissue is replaced by dense fibrosis, which makes dilatation difficult if not impossible. In these patients, it is sometimes necessary to resect large blocks of corporal tissue to make a space in which the implant can lie. The smaller size of the CXM is very useful, because the remaining corporal tissue can usually be closed over the smaller implant, whereas it would be necessary to use grafting with a synthetic material to cover a standard-size implant.[17,18]

## The AMS 700 Ultrex and Ultrex Plus

The Ultrex cylinder is a modification of the three-ply CX cylinder. The middle fabric layer has been changed to allow some length expansion while controlling girth. The Ultrex cylinder is the only lengthening cylinder commercially available. The cylinders are sized from 12 to 21 cm in 3-cm increments and rear tip extenders are supplied for length adjustment. The pump is identical to the AMS 700 CX. The reservoir is larger and rated at 100-cc fill. The AMS 700 Ultrex Plus is the newest modification of the 700 line. This model features a prefilled pump that has been preconnected to prefilled cylinders. Only the reservoir requires filling and only one connection need be made. Two tubing

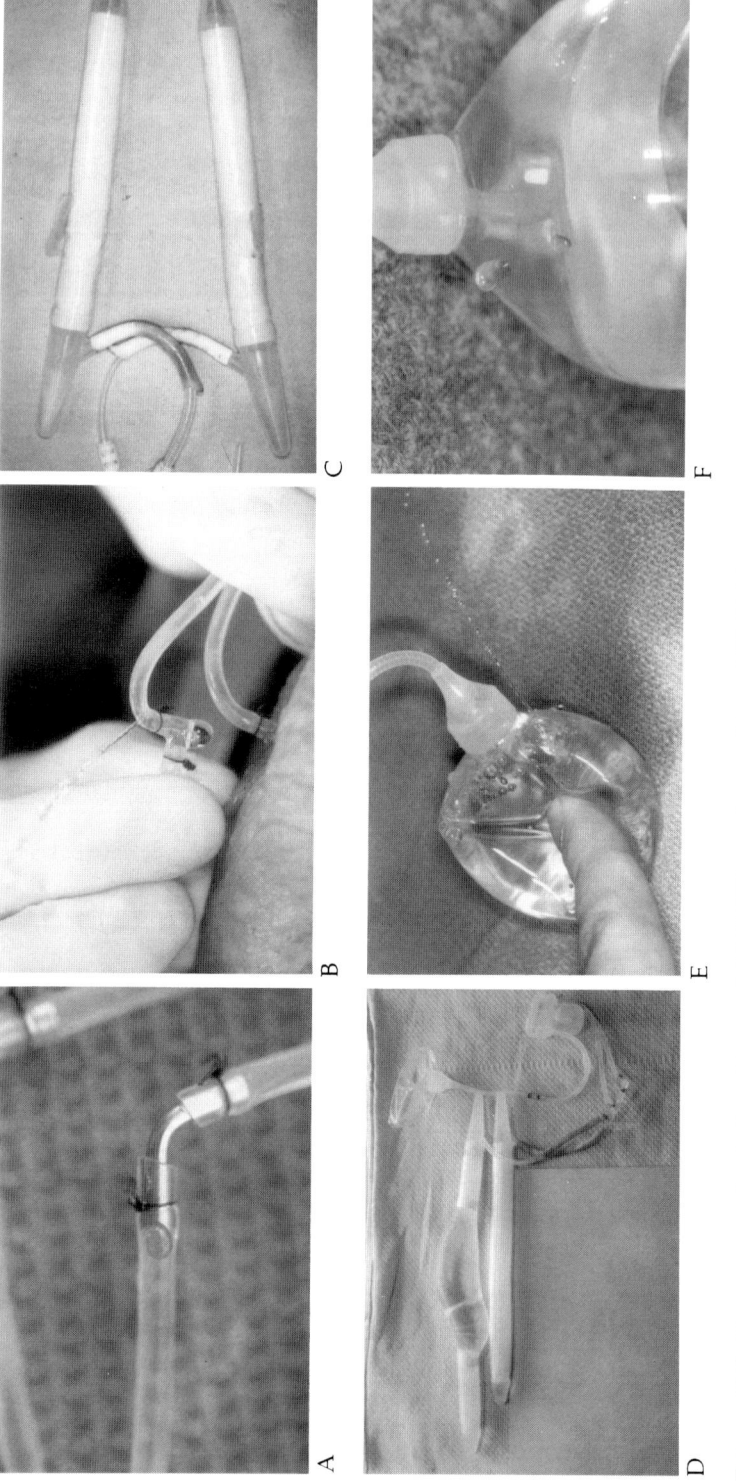

FIGURE 40.6. Common mechanical problems of AMS 700 prostheses. (A and B) Tubing shear by suture tie connectors. (C and D) Silicone cylinder wear. (E and F) Silicone crease-fold wear of reservoir.

FIGURE 40.7. AMS 700 CX and downsized AMS 700 CXM.

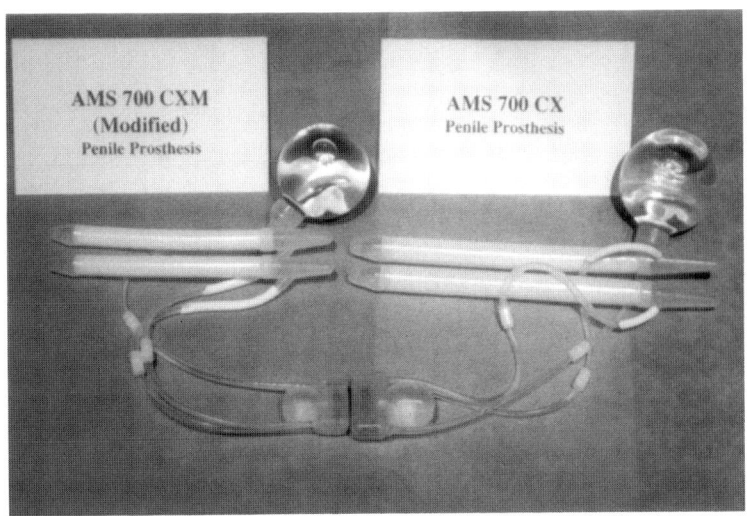

lengths are available, with the shorter length intended for penoscrotal implantation and the longer length for infrapubic insertion. AMS recently published Ultrex survival data collected for the FDA from multiple centers. In analyzing the medical records of 155 patients implanted between August 1990 and December 1991, they noted almost 90% of the patients free from revision or replacement surgery for 2 years following implantation.

## Pearls, Pitfalls, and Perils

### The AMS 700 Ultrex

From clinical research to the final commercial product, the manufacturer steadfastly refused to claim that the lengthening cylinders would lengthen the erect penis. Nevertheless, clinicians and patients alike fervently hoped penile lengthening would occur. The first studies published were meant to document length enhancement but were disappointing in that the erect penis did not lengthen from its preoperative length.[19] Some clinicians believed the Ultrex cylinder advantageous because of lengthening the flaccid penis during inflation;[20] uncontrolled lengthening of the cylinder necessitated a much higher revision rate than with either AMS 700 CX or Mentor Alpha I. Some centers have stopped using this prosthesis cylinder.

### The S-Shaped Deformity

Highly motivated patients sometimes inflate their prosthesis to the maximum for long periods in order to try to achieve greater length. Increase in length of penis does not occur, but the cylinders lengthen at the expense of the corpora, curling up within the erectile body like a snake. This S-shaped deformity severely deteriorates the erection rigidity, is unsightly, and sometimes is so deformed that intercourse is difficult (Fig. 40.8). The S-shaped deformity has occurred more often in patients who inflated their prostheses for long periods, had Peyronie's disease, or in patients whose tunica had been compromised by previous self-contained or rod implantation.[21] In these cases, it is recommended that the Ultrex prosthesis be removed and a CX or Mentor Alpha prosthesis be substituted. The Ultrex S experience has caused some clinicians to determine in a different fashion the size of cylinder to be inserted. Since the days of Dr. F. Brantley Scott, Jr., the inventor of the inflatable penile prosthesis, the recommended method of cylinder sizing had been to measure the intercorporal length with a Furlow inserter and to implant the cylinder size corresponding to the measurement. Montague[22] now recommends downsizing the

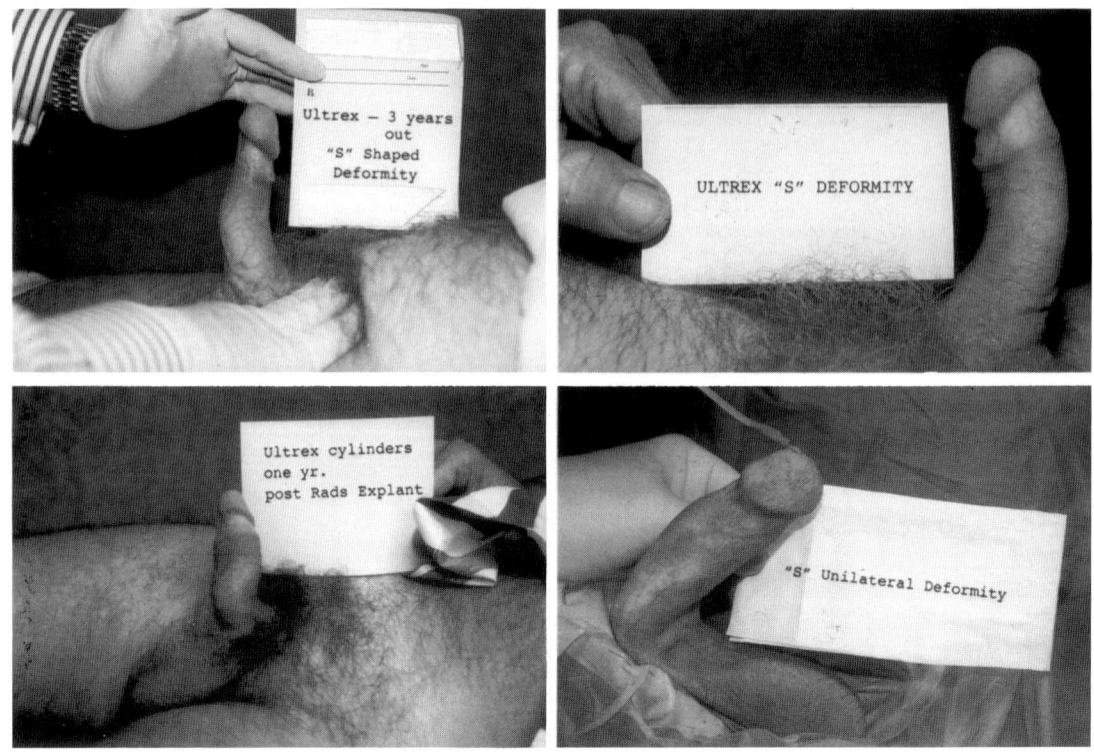

FIGURE 40.8. Examples of the S-shaped deformity in AMS 700 Ultrex.

Ultrex cylinder 3 cm from the traditional method of measuring the size of prosthesis to be implanted. Utilizing this unique (to the Ultrex) method of cylinder sizing, the development of the S deformity may be minimized. However, an alternative is to cease implantation of this device, preferring the dependability of the AMS 700 CX or the better erection rigidity of the Mentor Alpha I.

### Excessive Periprosthetic Capsule Formation

All implanted materials stimulate fibrous capsule formation in the human body. The smooth, spherical silicone reservoir of the AMS 700 is occasionally surrounded by such a tight capsule that full deflation is not possible. The patient complains that his penis is always half erect. Additional deflation may be accomplished by forceful squeezing of the penis while deflating, but the cylinders promptly refill. This excessive capsule formation can be prevented by maxi-

mizing deflation daily for 3 months following implantation. Requesting that the patient deflate the prosthesis several times each day promotes maximum reservoir capacity and, therefore, a larger capsule space. When the space problem is presented to the clinician, it is, of course, too late for preventive medicine. However, not all patients desire correction. Some men enjoy the fullness.[15]

### Capsule Contraction Correction

The repair is simple; it is not necessary to resect the excessive capsule. Merely make a small scrotal incision, locate the connector between pump and reservoir, and disconnect. Place your hand suprapubically and then overdistend the reservoir with up to twice the rated capacity. Although audible evidence ("pop") of capsule splitting frequently occurs with AMS spherical reservoirs, it seldom happens with the Mentor cylindrical reservoir. Palpable rupture always is evident during revision of both prostheses. Re-establish normal reservoir capacity and reconnect the system. If the patient postoperatively maximizes deflation several times daily for 3 months, the problem will not recur. This solution is also effective with Mentor three-piece prostheses, but the cylindrical, textured Bioflex reservoir is significantly less prone to capsule contraction (2%).[15]

## The Mentor Alpha I Prosthesis

Mentor Corporation began manufacturing a three-piece prosthesis in 1983. The design was similar to the original Scott concept featuring paired cylinders, a scrotal pump, and an abdominal reservoir. From inception, the cylinders and reservoir were constructed of Bioflex, a polyurethane polymer. This material has proven to have remarkable longevity. Patients with sets of cylinders and reservoirs that have been in place almost a decade have reported no leaks. Mentor's first model was called the Mentor IPP (inflatable penile prosthesis). It was plagued by tubing shear at the junction of the metal connector. Its current model, Mentor Alpha I, has been commercially available since 1990 and features only one (new design) "Tru-lock" connector between pump and reservoir (Fig. 40.9). Freedom from revision or replacement surgery has been immensely improved over the old models by the very dependable

"Tru-lock" connector. A recent report indicated 15-month device survival at over 95%.[16]

The Mentor Alpha I penile prosthesis is available in cylinder lengths from 12 to 22 cm in 2-cm increments. Unlike the AMS 700 CX or Ultrex, cylinder diameter of the larger prostheses is incrementally wider than the smaller ones. Rear tip extenders of 1 to 3 cm are provided for length adjustment. The Bioflex cylinders are preconnected to a silicone pump. Two tubing lengths are available, with the shorter length designed for penoscrotal incisions and the longer length meant for infrapubic insertion. The cylindrical Bioflex reservoir has a textured surface. Reservoirs are available in 60-, 75-, 100-, and 125-cc capacities.

In April 1996 Mentor introduced a new prosthesis, the Mentor Alpha NB. This prosthesis was intended for placement in patients in whom the Alpha I cylinders were judged to be too large. The cylinders are made of Bioflex, as is the Mentor Alpha I, but the cylinder width is 2 mm narrower in each size than the standard-sized prosthesis. Most importantly, the base is considerably narrower than the standard-size Mentor Alpha I, thus the designation NB for narrow base. To place a Mentor Alpha NB in the proximal corpora requires dilatation to only size 10 Hegar dilators, since the prosthesis with rear tips in place measures only 9 mm in diameter. This Mentor Alpha NB will be a very useful prosthesis for placements

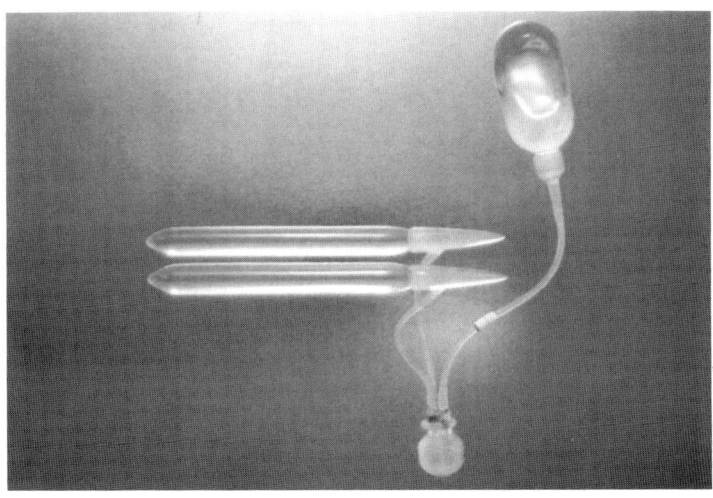

FIGURE 40.9. Mentor Alpha I.

in patients with stenotic corpora secondary to corporal fibrosis because of this narrow-base feature. It should also give better girth expansion than the CXM cylinder since the expansion of the Bioflex is limited only by the tunica albuginea rather than by a fabric wrap, such as with the CXM cylinder.

## The Mentor Alpha I

One of the favorite sayings of the late Dr. Scott was a reflection of what he most liked in life: "faster horses, older whiskey, and younger women." Dr. Scott paraphrased this into a description of the ideal inflatable prosthesis: "larger cylinders, fewer connectors, and a smaller pump." At the present time, the Mentor Alpha I comes closest to the ideal of all prostheses available. Only one connection is needed, and the small spherical pump is very concealable. The Bioflex cylinders are not restricted in girth expansion by a fabric wrap (as in the AMS CX and Ultrex), and the longer cylinders have a larger diameter than do the shorter cylinders. The cylinder configuration permits full expansion until restricted by corporal tissue. This usually ensures the best axial rigidity of any prosthesis. One disadvantage of Bioflex, when compared with AMS cylinder construction, is that folds of this polyurethane polymer are more apparent than with silicone in the flaccid penis. This may lead to patient complaints about palpable "dog ears." The problem can be overcome by encouraging the patient to carry a bit more fluid in his prosthesis and thereby smooth the material crease.

Presently, the Mentor Alpha I is a favored prosthesis for routine implantation in previously unoperated patients. The Alpha's axial rigidity in erection seems subjectively better than other prostheses, and it is particularly useful in a broad penis. Mechanical reliability is acceptable, and Bioflex cylinder longevity is better than the silicone.[23] Teaching the patient to operate the device is very easy and requires less time than with any other self-contained, two-piece, or three-piece prosthesis.

## Pearls, Pitfalls and Perils

The prosthesis should be used with caution in reimplantations and patients with tunical weakening from previous penile surgery. The tunical dependent expansion of this powerful cylinder can cause corporotomy rupture and aneurysms in these complicated cases (Fig. 40.3).

Although the prosthesis has acceptable overall reliability, there may be infrequent but recurrent problems in prostheses implanted via the penoscrotal approach. Tubing fracture with subsequent fluid leak can occur at the junction of the cylinder tubing and the pump. The outside tubing seems more susceptible, but it has also been seen in the inside tubing. The manufacturer has made two separate modifications to reinforce this area (Fig. 40.10), and the problem has decreased markedly. In analyzing a series of over 1000 Alpha implantations, the revision rate for this problem has been 7% overall and has become much less frequent in the reinforced models.[5] It is noteworthy that a large series of 647 Alphas implanted infrapubically had less than 2% incidence of this problem.[24] Virtually no other mechanical problems requiring reoperation developed in either series. Patient satisfaction has been as high as 98.4%.[24]

### Revision of Mentor Alpha I

Present policy on revision of the Mentor Alpha I takes cognizance of the remarkable durability of the Bioflex cylinders and reservoir. The problem necessitating revision is invariably the tubing fracture outlined above. Unlike with the AMS 700, it is only necessary to cut down on the pump through a scrotal incision with the electrosurgical unit. Trace out the tubing until the reservoir connector is located. Sever all three tubings distal to the fracture and remove the pump. Using the cut tubing, aspirate cylinders and reservoir of residual fluid, then purge the system with antibiotic irrigant. After copious irrigation of all components, refill the reservoir and attach a new reinforced pump with

FIGURE 40.10. Mentor Alpha I common mechanical problem: tubing fracture at pump platform.

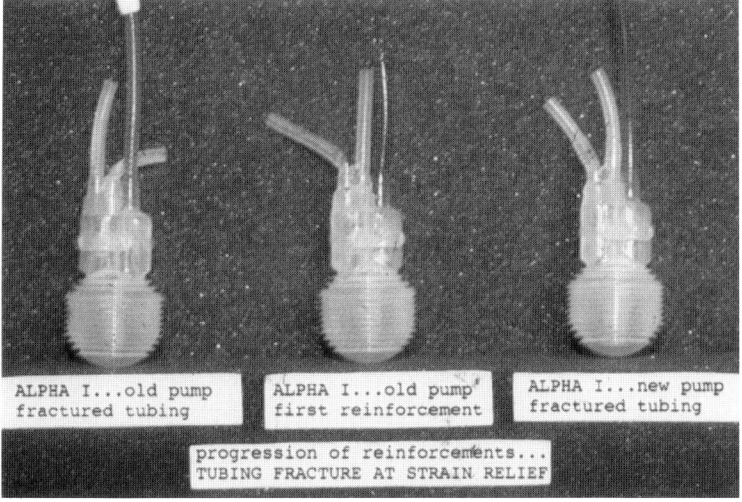

three connectors. This revision is quick and easy on both patient and surgeon and does not risk repeat revision, because of the durability of the rest of the components.

## Implantation of Three-Piece Inflatables

Urologists worldwide seem more familiar with the infrapubic incision and perceive that implantation via this approach is easier than the penoscrotal incision. The penoscrotal incision is, however, actually quicker and easier for the surgeon and associated with less morbidity for the patient. It is particularly recommended for obese patients. Most importantly, the penoscrotal approach minimizes most of the complications of penile implant surgery and avoids the dreaded dorsal nerve injury—the only complication of implant surgery for which there is no cure.

Scott, the inventor of the three-piece inflatable, also developed the penoscrotal approach. He believed the penoscrotal incision lent itself better to outpatient surgery because of less patient discomfort. He was fond of saying that penoscrotal implantation was optimum because the incision was made in the natural scar (scrotal raphe), and the result was completely invisible.

Both implant manufacturers report that 80% of three-piece inflatables are placed through infrapubic incisions. Surgical familiarity with the infrapubic anatomy and fear of the blind reservoir placement are the usual explanations for infrapubic incision preference. However, if the surgical procedure is done properly, implantation can be accomplished in less than 1 hour.

### Pearls, Pitfalls, and Perils

#### The Penoscrotal Incision

The most common infecting organism is the opportunistic staphylococci, e.g., *Staphylococcus epidermidis*. For this reason, give a single dose of vancomycin 500mg IV 1 hour preoperatively. For gram-negative coverage, give a single dose of gentamicin 80mg intravenously. The patient is placed supine, prepped for 10 minutes, and draped. A Foley catheter is inserted to facilitate urethral identification. The Lone Star Medical Products metal retractor (Scott retractor) is placed with the small end surrounding the scrotum and the large end utilized to place the penis on stretch by inserting a hook in the dorsal aspect of the urethral meatus. (It is notable that in the sixth edition of *Campbell's Urology*, the Scott retractor is erroneously used upside down!) The most important aspect of the retractor is a piece of

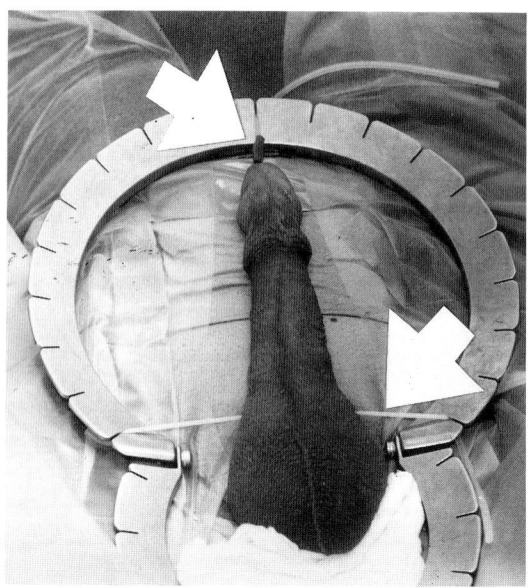

FIGURE 40.11. Proper placement of Lone Star Medical Products (Scott) retractor. Arrows show hook in urethral meatus and polyethylene tubing stretched across middle of retractor to elevate penis.

#15 knife blade is used to make a 2- to 3-cm corporotomy. The corporotomy should be extended proximal enough so that the tubing will exit in the scrotum and not be palpable on the penis. The AMS 700, Mentor Alpha I, or Mentor Mark II can be placed with tubing inside the corpora, running alongside the cylinder until it exits at the corporotomy. Implantation of the AMS Ambicor will require extending the corporotomy deeper in the scrotum until the tubing exits at the base of the cylinder.

### Corporal Dilation

Dilate the corpora with Hegar or Brooks dilators. Do not begin dilatation with a dilator less than size 10 or 11. Smaller dilators are too sharp and are a risk to urethral perforation. The Brooks dilators (Mentor Corp.) are safer than Hegar dilators because their bullet configuration and offset bayonet handle help prevent urethral injury. Proximally the dilators should be advanced until the insertion of the crus on bone is felt. Dilatation should be as large as

polyethylene tubing (cut off some IV tubing) passed from 3 to 9 o'clock on the retractor. This facilitates exposure of the corpora by elevating the base of the penis (Fig. 40.11). Avoid the plastic Scott retractor. It is too light and consequently moves too much during the surgery.

A 3-cm incision is made in the scrotal raphe immediately below the penoscrotal junction. This skin with incision is then moved up on the penis, and the retractor hooks are placed at 1, 5, 7, and 11 o'clock, making certain the hooks hold the incision over the proximal penis—not over the upper scrotum. Finally, two more hooks are placed at 9 and 3 o'clock (Fig. 40.12). If the retractor and hooks are properly placed, the urethra is immediately evident, because it contains a Foley catheter. The urethra is displaced laterally with finger or forceps, and dissection through the tissue overlying the corpora cavernosa is accomplished by spreading with the Metzenbaum scissors. As each layer of overlying tissue is spread, the hooks on that side are lifted and replaced to take the tissue laterally. When the glistening white corporal body is identified, stay sutures are placed, and a

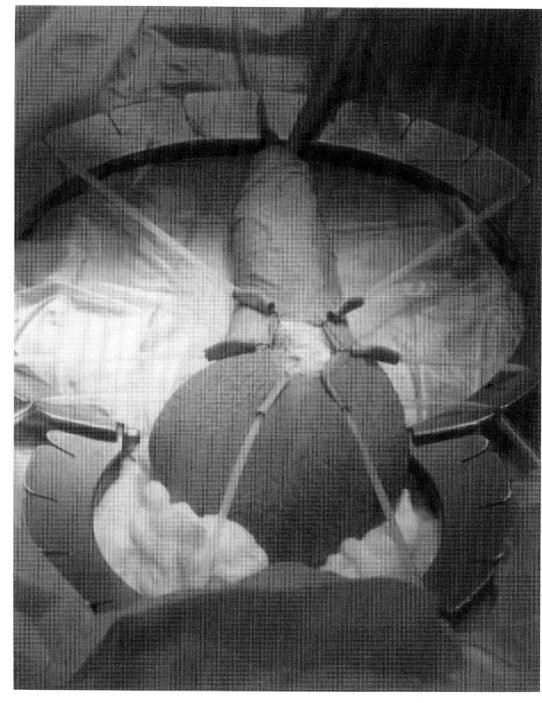

FIGURE 40.12. Correct placement of hooks to facilitate corporal dissection.

possible. Routine dilatation may be to size 14. As mentioned above, dilatation to at least size 12 is necessary for insertion of any of the two- or three-piece prostheses except the AMS 700 CXM and the Mentor Alpha NB.

## Measurements

After dilatation is complete on both sides, the Dilamez inserter or the Furlow inserter is used to measure the total intracorporal length. If measurements are not within 1 cm of each other, something is wrong, and it will be necessary to redilate both sides. A prosthesis of 1 to 3 cm less than the patient's measurement should be requested from the circulating nurse. The surgeon will then create the patient's exact measurement by the addition of rear tip extenders. The prosthesis measurement plus rear tip extender size should exactly match the intracorporal measurement of the patient with his penis mildly stretched by the inserter, if using Mentor Alpha I, Mentor Mark II, AMS 700 CX, or AMS Ambicor. If there is a question about the measurement, place a smaller rather than a longer length. In all models of prosthesis placement, it is always better to err on the short side rather than the long. As mentioned above, the lengthening design of the Ultrex cylinders makes it mandatory to downsize this prosthesis 2 to 3 cm.

The corporal incisions are closed with 00 Vicryl. Copious amounts of antibiotic irrigant should be used throughout the procedure. The most common infecting organisms are common skin bacteria that contaminate the prosthesis through airborne spread or direct contact with the patient's skin. These can be mechanically removed with vigorous irrigation, either with a sterilized plant mister or an asepto syringe.

## Reservoir Insertion

The insertion of the reservoir through the penoscrotal incision is what most surgeons dread. This maneuver should not be frightening, because with a decompressed bladder, there is really no harm that can occur. The operator should pass his finger alongside the penis, medial to the spermatic cord up on to the pubic bone, until the pubic tubercle is felt. Immediately over the tubercle, the external inguinal ring can be palpated. The maneuver is similar to examining a patient for the possibility of hernia. An infant-sized Deaver retractor is used to hook the external inguinal ring, and traction is applied forcefully cephalad. The pubic tubercle is the caudad landmark of the external inguinal ring. If the maneuver is properly done, there is nothing between the surgeon and the space of Retzius except transversalis fascia (the floor of the inguinal canal and the strength layer of the abdomen). This transversalis fascia is a tough structure and cannot be finger-dissected. It will be necessary to forcefully pierce it with a sharp clamp or a Metzenbaum scissors (Fig. 40.13). The operating surgeon must feel a "give," and the piercing instrument can be advanced 6 to 8 cm. Then the instrument is spread until the finger and the Deaver can be inserted through the fascia. Feeling the back of the pubic ramus, the surgeon then palpates the bladder, feeling the Foley balloon with the tip of a finger, and inserts the reservoir into this space.

## Reservoir Insertion in Patients with Previous Pelvic Surgery

It should be noted that the transversalis fascia is thickened in patients with previous radical retropubic prostatectomy and is quite difficult to pierce. Once through the transversalis fascia, the space of Retzius is usually not obliterated. Previous hernia repair does not contraindicate this method of reservoir insertion, but finding the external ring may be impossible, and the surgeon may have to pierce the hernia repair. Previous aorta-femoral bypass surgery or radical cystectomy can obliterate the space of Retzius, but the operator can usually develop a space by careful finger dissection. Rarely is it necessary to make a separate incision for reservoir insertion (Fig. 40.14).

## Reservoir Fill and Cycling the Prosthesis

Fill the reservoir to capacity with saline and make the appropriate connections. It is not nec-

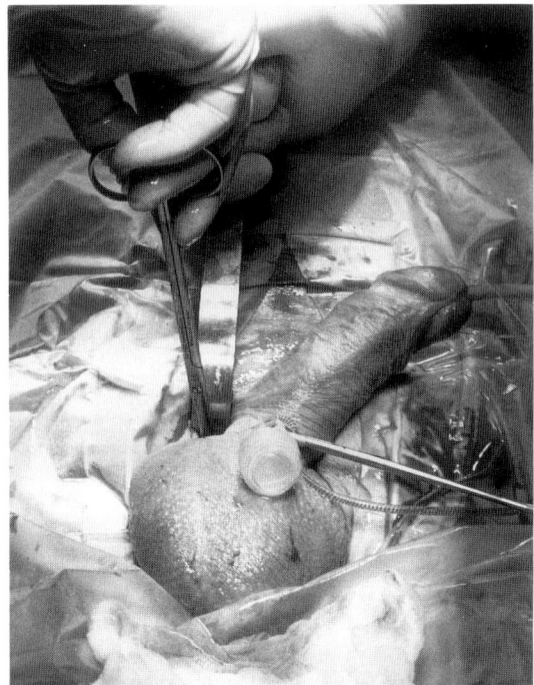

A

B

Figure 40.13. Reservoir placement via penoscrotal incision. (A) The infant-sized Deaver retractor is hooked in the external inguinal ring and traction applied cephalad. The pubic tubercle is used as caudad reference point and the transversalis fascia is pierced with Metzenbaum scissors. (B) Note how deep the scissors are advanced.

essary to waste time trying to remove all the air from the system because it all dissipates within 6 months. A little air is actually good, because it creates an audible turbulence across the pump, making patient instruction easier. Cycle the prosthesis by pumping to the absolute maximum because this is an excellent opportunity to properly seat the cylinders and break down fibrotic areas while the patient is anesthetized. This is the time to ensure a straight erection. Many times, mild curvature will now be noted that was unsuspected preoperatively. This curvature can be "modeled,"[25] resulting in a straightened erection.

## Avoidance of Scrotal Hematoma

After cycling the prosthesis, create a space for the pump by finger dissection of the scrotal septum. The pump should lie in a dependent position of the scrotum between the testicles. It should not be pexed or sutured down in any way. If the pump lies free between the testicles, it can be manipulated by the patient if future malposition should occur. Scrotal hematoma— the most common complication of penoscrotal implantation—can be virtually eliminated by draining with a small silicone drain and partially inflating the prosthesis for 12 to 24 hours. Most scrotal hematomas originate from corporal bleeding, not from a scrotal blood vessel; thus, the need for inflation and drainage. The patient is discharged the same day or the next morning, with 5 days of high-dose ciprofloxacin or ofloxacin.

## After the Implantation

1. Patients should be warned that both AMS and Mentor three-piece inflatables will autoinflate for the first 3 months. Spontaneous cylinder inflation occurs until the reservoir is surrounded by capsule formation. It is important to maximize deflation during this crucial period in order to encourage maximum capsular space. Cylinder capsules can be stretched by forceful inflation, but there is no way to stretch a reservoir capsule once formed. If achieving full deflation becomes a problem, it can be eas-

FIGURE 40.14. Reservoir placed through penoscrotal incision in patient who had previous pelvic exteneration.

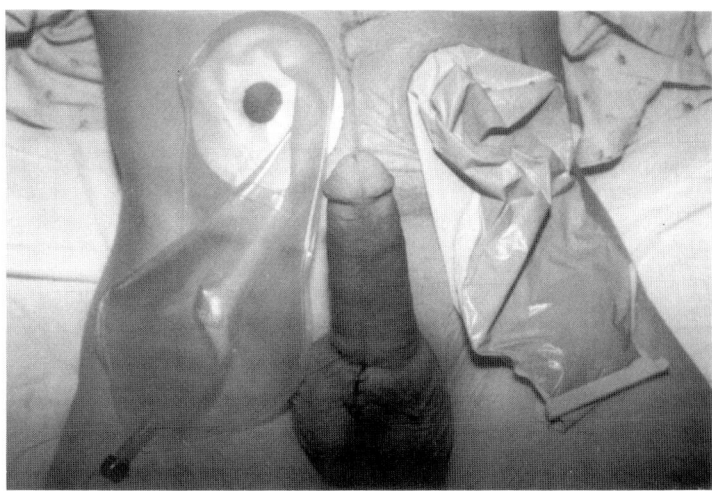

ily corrected by the method outlined earlier in this chapter.

2. The patient should also be warned that his erection may not be as long as a natural erection, because the head of the penis does not swell with an implant.

3. Although achievement of orgasm is unrelated to prosthesis implantation, some patients will complain of difficulty reaching orgasm for months following the implant. This can be overcome by encouraging the patient to spend more time in foreplay and perhaps to enjoy a relaxing glass of wine prior to lovemaking.

4. Pain lasting more than 45 days suggests subclinical opportunistic staph infection, which may be treated with 2 days of IV vancomycin and 30 days of timethoprim/sulfa and/or rifampin.[11]

## Conclusion

Penile prosthetic implantation can be considered a safe, relatively minor surgical procedure. Although the vacuum device and injection erection are considered first-line treatments, prosthesis implantation can be a satisfactory alternative. Device reliability and patient satisfaction combine to make penile prosthesis implantation a popular therapy. The best penile prosthesis will stimulate flaccidity and natural erection to an excellent degree and lend itself nicely to the spontaneity of lovemaking.

## References

1. Morales PA, Suarez JB, Delgado J, et al. Penile implant for erectile impotence. *J Urol* 1973; 109:641–643.
2. Small MP, Carrion HM, Gordon JA. Small-Carrion penile prosthesis: new implant for management of impotence. *Urology* 1975; 5:479–481.
3. Scott FB, Bradley WD, Timm GW. Management of erectile impotence: use of implantable inflatable prosthesis. *Urology* 1973; 2:80–84.
4. Joseph DB, Bruskewitz RC, Benson RC. Long-term evaluation of the inflatable penile prostheses. *J Urol* 1984; 131:1670–1674.
5. Wilson SK, Wahman GE, Lange JL. Eleven years' experience with the inflatable penile prosthesis. *J Urol* 1987; 139:951–952.
6. Wilson SK. Current treatment of impotence with inflatable penile protheses examined. *AUA Today* 1992, Sept; 1–4.
7. Golji H. Experience with penile prostheses in spinal cord injury patients. *J Urol* 1979; 121:288–291.
8. Rossier AB, Fam BA. Indication and results of semirigid penile prostheses in spinal cord injury patients: long term follow up. *J Urol* 1984; 131:59–62.
9. Mulcahy JJ, Krane RJ, Lloyd LK, et al. Duraphase penile prosthesis—results of clinical trials in 63 patients. *J Urol* 1990; 143:518–520.

10. Carson CC. Infections in genitourinary prostheses. *Urol Clin North Am* 1989; 16:139–147.

11. Wilson SK, Delk JR. Inflatable penile implant infection: predisposing factors and treatment suggestions. *J Urol* 1995; 153:659–661.

12. Wilson SK, Cleves M, Delk JR. Long-term results with Hydroflex and Dynaflex penile prostheses: device survival comparison to multicomponent. *J Urol* 1996; 155:1421–1423.

13. Wilson SK, Delk JR. Excessive periprosthetic capsule formation of the penile prosthesis reservoir: incidence in various prostheses and a simple surgical solution. *J Urol* 1995; 153:358A.

14. Baum N, Suarez G, Mobley D. Use of infrapubic incision for insertion of Mentor Mark II inflatable penile prosthesis. *Urology* 1992; 39:436–438.

15. Fallen MJ, Lewis RW. Experience with a two piece inflatable penile prosthesis. *J Urol* 1990; 143:409A.

16. Randrup E, Wilson S, Mobley D, et al. Clinical experience with Mentor Alpha I inflatable penile prosthesis. Report on 333 cases. *Urology* 1992; 42:305–308.

17. Wilson SK, Delk JR, Terry T. Improved implant success in patients with severe corporal fibrosis: a new technique without the necessity of grafting. *J Urol* 1995; 153:359A.

18. Knoll DL, Furlow WL, Benson RC, et al. Management of nondilatable cavernous fibrosis with use of downsized inflatable penile prosthesis. *J Urol* 1995; 153:366–368.

19. Furlow WL, Knoll LD, Benson RC. Penile lengthening and the new AMS 700 Ultrex inflatable penile prosthesis. *Int J Impotence Res* 1992; 4(suppl 2):A124.

20. Montague DK, Lakin MM. Early experience with the controlled girth and length expanding cylinder of the AMS Ultrex penile prosthesis. *J Urol* 1992; 148:1444–1447.

21. Wilson SK, Delk JR. The Ultrex cylinders: problems with uncontrolled lengthening— The S shaped deformity. *J Urol* 1994; 151: 354A.

22. Montague DK. Penile prostheses. In: Bennett AH, ed. *Impotence: Diagnosis and Management of Erectile Dysfunction.* Philadelphia: W.B. Saunders; 1994: 271–295.

23. Long R, Lewis R. Actual outcome of the modern 3-piece inflatable penile prosthesis. *J Urol* 1994; 151:354A.

24. Williams CB. Out-patient implantation of mentor alpha-I inflatable penile prosthesis: results of 647 single surgeon cases. *Int J Impotence Res* 1995; 6(suppl):A59.

25. Wilson SK, Delk JR. A new treatment for Peyronie's disease: modeling the penis over an inflatable penile prosthesis. *J Urol* 1994; 152: 1121–1123.

# 41
# The Complex Penile Prosthesis

John J. Mulcahy

Penile prosthesis placement has remained a predictable and reliable treatment for erectile dysfunction for over two decades. Despite advances in prosthetic design and the use of more durable materials, mechanical problems with these devices may occur. In addition, weakness in the wall of the erectile bodies, the deposition of scar tissue in the penis, problems with blood supply, and the entrance of bacteria into the wound at the time of implant surgery have contributed to a suboptimal result in certain patients. Fortunately, as experience has been gained, the incidence of complications has decreased and the management of problems has become more timely and more gratifying.

Eighty percent of patients are happy with the outcome of prosthesis surgery.[1] In those 20% of patients who are disappointed with the outcome, decrease in size of the penis is by far the most common reason. When prosthesis cylinders are placed, a rim of scar tissue or neocapsule develops around the cylinders as the body's reaction to injury. When the tunica albuginea, the elastic covering of the erectile bodies, fills with blood, the scar tissue does not expand. In addition, scar tissue may contract with time, and when the prosthesis cylinders are inflated, they will be restrained by a nonstretchable wall. If scar tissue is already present, as in Peyronie's disease, postpriapism, or following injury to the penis, a further reduction in the size of the penis may be expected. Scar tissue may also account for asymmetry of the cylinder heads and for some bulging that may be apparent as cylinders are inflated.

Some degree of pain is to be expected following prosthesis placement, and this may be more intense in some patients, especially diabetics, where a neuropathy may be present. This pain is usually more prolonged than in procedures of similar magnitude and may last up to a month. Ejaculation is usually not affected by the placement of a prosthesis. A few patients may note after prosthesis placement a decrease in sensitivity of the penis during sexual activity. In these patients, cutaneous sensation is intact, and the sensitivity will frequently improve with time over a period of months. This is more likely due to changes in the nerve endings than from damage to nerves during the surgical procedure. Why this phenomenon occurs is unknown.

The repair rate with most models of implants is in the range of 5% to 10% within the first 5 years. Beyond that time period, statistics are not available, and there is marked variability among the types of prostheses.

Two key elements guiding a patient in selection of the type of prosthesis to be inserted are manual dexterity and penile size. Although implants are becoming easier to manipulate, some require a modest degree of strength and skill. This consideration is important in patients who have advanced arthritis, Parkinson's disease, multiple sclerosis, quadriplegia, or who are beyond the mid-70s in age. The recommendation of a semirigid rod-type device that requires little or no manual dexterity would be more appropriate for patients in these categories. For the very wide or long penis, a three-piece inflatable device tends to give the best rigidity. The degree of support provided by the cylinders during intercourse depends on the appropriate fit of cylinders in the corporal body with expansion. If the cylinders completely fill the erectile bodies—like a finger in a glove or an inner tube in a bicycle tire—very good support is achieved. If there is room for the prosthesis to shift during inflation in the erectile body, less optimal support will be the result. In addition, with a very large penis, the unitary inflatable or two-piece devices may not give as good flaccidity, as the reservoir capacity is relatively small and less fluid can shift into that cavity. A key to sizing the proper width when selecting cylinders from two or three width sizes is to place two Hegar dilators of the anticipated width into both corporal bodies and then try to touch the thumb to the index finger between the dilators. If wide separation of the dilators is found, a loose fit of the cylinders will be expected. If there is slight separation of the dilators as the thumb touches the index finger, an optimal fit of that size cylinders can be anticipated. If the dilators will not move under these circumstances, there will be a relatively snug fit. In choosing the appropriate cylinder length for hydraulic cylinders, use the same length as the total corporal length measured with the measuring devices. With the nonhydraulic rod-type cylinders, inserting a cylinder $\frac{1}{2}$cm shorter than the measured total corporal length will achieve better bendability and offer less chance of painful pressure at the end of the penis during operation of the device.

## Scarred Corporal Bodies

The presence of scar tissue in the corporal body, or in the tunica albuginea that covers it, will present a challenging situation during the dilation process for placement of prosthesis cylinders, particularly when there has been removal of a previous implant, trauma to the penis, postpriapism, corporal infection, a pharmacologic erection program, or Peyronie's disease.

In the majority of these circumstances, some spongy erectile tissue will remain somewhere in the corporal bodies. The key to selecting a site for corporotomy is to determine where this spongy tissue is located. If an implant has been previously placed and then removed because of an infection through a penoscrotal approach, that area will be scarred and a second attempt at dilating the corporal bodies through this approach would be very difficult. An infrapubic approach in these circumstances would be a better place to start dilation. Upon opening the corporal bodies, spongy tissue will be encountered and the dilation can be accomplished more easily. A midcorporal incision will allow dilation more easily, both proximally and distally, as opposed to a subcoronal incision, which will permit total dilation in only one direction. A Foley catheter placed in the urethra before beginning dilation will provide a reminder as to its location during the dilation process.

Begin the dilation with the points of the Metzenbaum scissors pointed away from the urethra. If resistance is encountered, mild-to-moderate pressure against the resistance will often traverse the scarred area. If great resistance to the passage of the dilating instrument is encountered, make a second incision distally in the region of the glans and dilate backward toward the area of severe scarring. Degloving the foreskin to expose an area of severe scarring and incising into it under direct vision may also prove helpful. Dilate proximally somewhat more aggressively, because the danger of urethral injury in this location is remote. However, take care that aggressive dilation does not result in a proximal perforation.

Once a channel has been opened throughout the length of the corporal body, sequentially larger Hegar dilators can be passed to broaden the caliber of the cavity. Larger dilators will meet with increasing snugness as they are passed in situations of extensive corporal scar tissue. The Otis urethrotome, once used extensively for treating urethral strictures, may prove helpful in this situation. The blade of the urethrotome, opened away from the urethra, may be passed either proximally or distally. Make an incision, and then pass the Hegar dilators once more to ensure that the caliber of the corporal body is adequate. If resistance is still met to passage of larger dilators, a second or third cut may be made with the urethrotome. When cutting a second or third time, rotate the blade 15° or 20° from the previous cut so that the tunica or scar tissue is thinned out rather than completely incised. If a cut is made through the tunica, closure with sutures will be necessary, but rotating the urethrotome blade will avoid this. The Rossello cavernotome (Majorica, Spain), an instrument that resembles a circular wood rasp, has also been of value in increasing the caliber of scarred corporal bodies. It is passed with a twisting motion to make multiple small cuts into the scarred area. In situations where the majority of the corporal body has been replaced with scar tissue, such as in postpriapism, excising much of the scar with sharp dissection will aid in providing an appropriate cavity for cylinder placement.

In some circumstances, placing a single cylinder may give adequate rigidity to the penis for intercourse. This, however, tends to give an asymmetric appearance to the erection, and tilting of the glans to one side or the other may occur. Smaller cylinders, such as the AMS 700 CXM (American Medical Systems, Minneapolis, MN) or Alpha 1 Narrow Base (Mentor Urology, Inc. Santa Barbara, CA), can be placed by dilating the cavity to only 10-mm diameter. These will give equal rigidity to that provided by larger cylinders when extensive scar tissue is present, as they will completely fill the width of the corporal bodies when expanded. If the cylinders can be placed but the edges of the tunica albuginea cannot be approximated over the cylinders, synthetic material can be substituted for the tunica albuginea of the corpora cavernosa. Polytetrafluoroethylene or Dacron, scraps from vascular surgical procedures are useful for this purpose. Fashion a small piece of graft material to cover the defect in the wall of the erectile bodies, and sew in place by using interrupted or running nonabsorbable soft suture. It is advisable to create an adequate cavity for the cylinders rather than to rely on the use of vascular graft material, for this material tends to be bulky within the penis and introduces another foreign body to an already complex procedure. If the proximal corporal bodies are totally scarred and it is impossible to gain access to this area through intracorporal dilation, a proximal crus may be rebuilt by fashioning a synthetic cup of graft material, placing it around the proximal portion of the cylinder, securing the cup to the periosteum of the ischeopubic ramus with permanent soft sutures (Fig. 41.1).

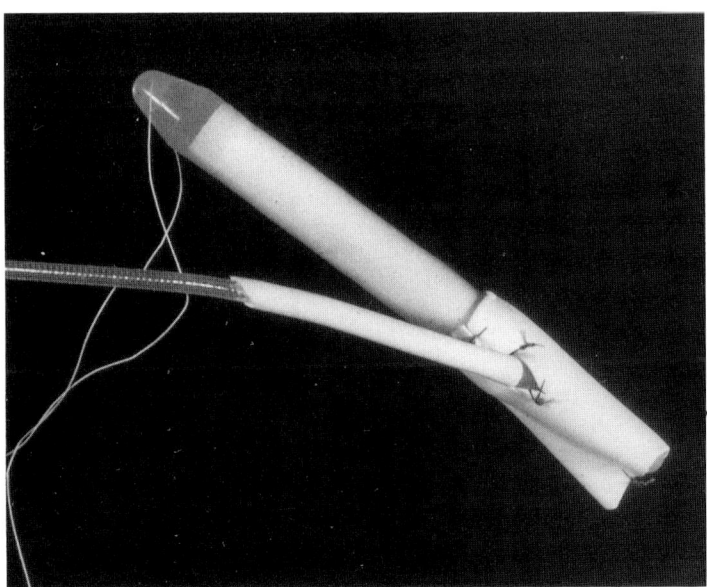

FIGURE 41.1. Cup fashioned from synthetic material (polytetrafluoroethylene) and secured around proximal portion of an inflatable cylinder. The wing of synthetic material is to be secured to the periosteum of the ischeopubic ramus.

# Crural Crossover

Crural crossover occurs when both proximal tips or both distal tips are present in the same corporal body. During dilation, the tips of the dilating scissors should be kept pointing dorsolaterally to avoid urethral entry or septal perforation. Despite good attention to technique, perforation of the septum between the two corporal bodies may occur in up to 25% of procedures and may present in a variety of ways. If cylinders are asymmetrically placed, the penis may take on a lopsided appearance. Alternatively, the tip of one cylinder may be palpable more proximally than that of its mate, and it may be difficult to inflate the cylinders. Similarly, the insertion of the second cylinder may be difficult, whereas the dilation might have proceeded relatively easily. It is better to attend to this problem at the time of surgery when it is easily corrected rather than to have the patient bring it to the attention of the physician during a postoperative visit. When a crossover is suspected, remove both cylinders. Place a Hegar dilator in one of the corporal bodies and place the cylinder in the opposite corporal body by the standard technique. Then remove the Hegar dilator from the first corporal body, and place a cylinder in that corporal body. It may be found that originally the second corporal body had never been adequately dilated.

# Perforation

Perforation of the corporal body may occur proximally or distally at the time of dilation. It occurs more commonly in the proximal location and may be due to misdirected dilation, overaggressive dilation, or weakening of the tunica albuginea. The site of proximal perforation is usually inaccessible surgically from the incisions conventionally used for prosthesis placement. Repositioning the patient and prepping this area for direct surgical repair will be difficult and may predispose to infection. If the perforation was made with a size 8 Hegar dilator, go directly to an 11 or 12. A cylinder may safely be seated under these circumstances. If a 9 Hegar or larger perforates proximally, place a cup fashioned of synthetic material around the proximal crus as a rear tip extender.[2] The sides of the cup material can then be secured to the tunica albuginea of the corpus cavernosum at a convenient location so that the tip of the cylinder is located equal to its mate in the distal corporal body. This technique is applicable to rods or unitary inflatable-type prostheses, but it is not necessary when using cylinders with input tubes, as the polytetrafluoroethylene sleeve surrounding the input tube may be secured to the tunica albuginea of the corpus cavernosum with a permanent stitch and, with time, the perforation will heal by scar formation. If such a defect is left open, the rod or unitary inflatable device would shift forward and backward as the patient manipulated his penis. This would create a ramrod effect, and erosion into the distal penis or buttocks would be inevitable.

A distal perforation may occur through the crus below the glans or into the urethra. In the former situation, open the foreskin and repair the defect primarily. Distal urethral perforations are usually into the fossa navicularis. Surgical access is difficult or impossible without filleting the penis. With such distal perforation, the appropriate maneuver is not to place a cylinder on that side but to return in 2 months or longer for cylinder reinsertion. A Foley catheter should be left in for about 3 days, which allows the perforation site to heal. If a cylinder has already been placed on the opposite side, leave it in place in order to maintain the length of the penis.

# Cylinder Selection

Three-piece inflatable prosthesis cylinders come in two types, those that expand only laterally and those that expand both laterally and distally. AMS markets the CX cylinders as the former type and the Ultrex cylinders as the latter variety. Mentor Corporation (Goleta, CA) distributes the Alpha I cylinders, which expand laterally, and has completed a clinical trial on the Excel cylinders, which expand both laterally and distally. The distally expanding cylinders may accommodate any shortcoming in cylinder sizing, and it has been said that they may slightly lengthen the erect penis.[3] The sheath of scar tissue that will form around these cylinders while in the deflated state will limit their expansion, so that any increase in length or girth achieved by either of these cylinders is not excessive.

Experience with cylinders that expand in both length and girth has been good, but when used in situations where scar tissue is present in the penis, they have tended to exaggerate curvature.[4] These cylinders fill all parts of the corporal body and tend to push against the distal end of the cavity. As the corporal body is tethered by the scar, this excessive pressure distally tends to exaggerate the curve. The cylinders that expand laterally only do not push against the distal end of the cavity but allow it to shift over the end of the cylinder. The cylinders themselves have good intrinsic rigidity and when inflated they tend to straighten the penis (Fig. 41.2). In cases

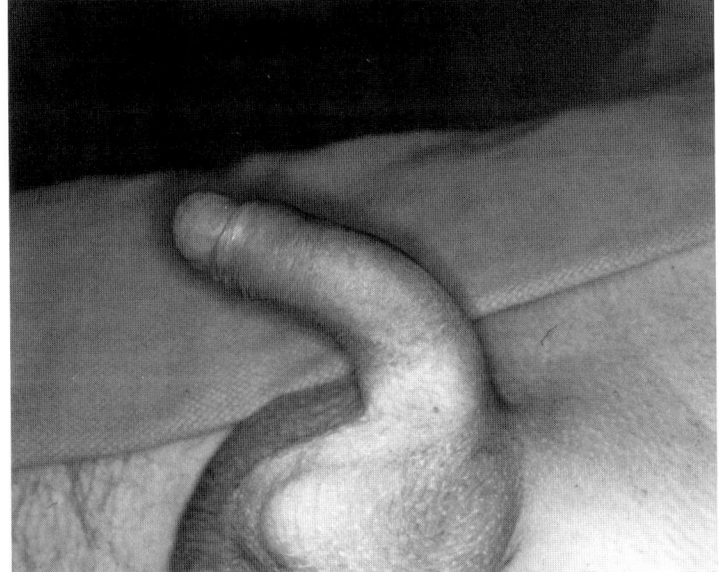

A

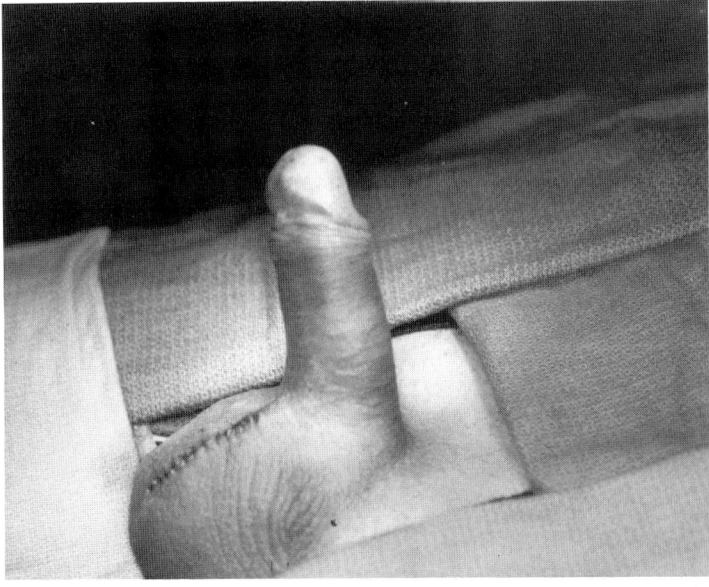

FIGURE 41.2. (A) Curved erection using inflatable cylinders that expand in both length and girth. (B) The same patient after cylinders were changed to the type that expand only in girth.

B

of Peyronie's disease or other situations of injury to the penis, as in removal of a prosthesis associated with infection, excessive scar tissue may be present in the corporal bodies.

Despite using malleable cylinders or appropriate hydraulic cylinders, curvature of the erection may still be present. In this situation two approaches may be used to straighten the penis adequately, but only if the curvature is deemed to be unsuitable for intercourse. Minor curves of 20° or less will usually straighten with modest pressure against the penis during penetration. With the erection in full rigidity and the tubes to the cylinders clamped to avoid excessive back pressure, the penis may be bent (molded) by excessive pressure to the side opposite the curve.[5] A cracking sensation will be noted as the scarred area is fractured. This procedure may adequately straighten the penis, which should be maintained in the semierect position for about 6 weeks postoperatively to allow this scarred area to heal in the straight position.

Another technique that may be helpful is to keep the penis pointed away from the scar during the healing process for the first 6 weeks postoperatively. As scar tissue will be laid down from the corporotomy incisions, this will sometimes afford a modest degree of straightening to the curved penis. For prominent curves that will not respond to molding, take elliptical tucks or wedges from the convex surface of the curve to slightly shorten this area or balance the tethering caused by the original scar and close the defect securely with absorbable suture.[6] Polydioxone synthetic (PDS) or Maxon is recommended for this as well as for the corporotomy closure. This technique was described by Nesbit[7] for congenital ventral curvature, but it tends to slightly shorten the erection. Another approach is to incise the concave surface of the scar directly over the area of tethering, and substitute a graft of synthetic material to close the tunical defect and prevent prosthesis herniation. Before performing a Nesbit-type procedure or incision of scar with graft interposition, elevate the dorsal neurovascular bundle or the corpus

spongiosm to prevent injury to either of these structures.

## Autoinflation

Spontaneous inflation of three-piece hydraulic devices has been noted with activity, such as bending, lifting, or walking. Increased intra-abdominal pressure is transmitted to the reservoir balloon that then pushes a small amount of fluid into the cylinders. If only mild in degree, advise the patients to deflate the device completely during episodes of urination. However, in some cases, this inflation may be embarrassing. The manufacturers attempted to eliminate this problem either by placing a lockout mechanism on the pump or by increasing the tension in the spring in the deflation mechanism, but both of these solutions resulted in a pump that was difficult for patients to operate. To minimize the degree of this autoinflation, ensure that the cavity in which the reservoir is placed is adequate and has minimal surrounding pressure. This is particularly important in patients who have had previous pelvic surgery where scar tissue has replaced the fatty envelope usually surrounding the bladder. If such a cavity cannot be found, the reservoir may be placed in an alternate location, intraperitoneally or in the epigastric area. There should be no pressure in the reservoir pushing fluid into the filling syringe before the balloon tubing is connected to the pump tubing. Putting about 5cc less volume than the maximum intended for the particular balloon will ensure that overfilling of the system will not occur with mild osmotic shifts during overhydration or dehydration. If the patient does not deflate the device frequently during daily activities, the cylinders will stay in the semierect position for extended periods of time and the reservoir will be in the less expanded state. Under these circumstances, a fibrotic capsule will form around the reservoir and prevent complete expansion. This will make complete deflation impossible and will contribute to the autoinflation phenomenon by adding pressure around the outside of the reservoir.

# Aneurysms of the Corporal Body and Cylinders

The prototype inflatable prosthesis was constructed with a single layer of silicone, which eventually would adapt or mold to the interior of the corporal bodies. With increasing pressure from inflation and deflation of the device through daily use, weaknesses in the tunica albuginea of the corpora cavernosa developed. The cylinder aneurysms that formed in these locations exaggerated these areas of weakness by allowing the pressure of the cylinder to be transmitted to them. Unsightly bulges occurred, most commonly at the base of the penis (pear deformity or pyramid deformity). These problems were not seen as commonly with the Mentor-type device made of Bioflex (polyurethane) and more resistant to this internal pressure.

In the mid-1980s American Medical Systems introduced a triple-layered cylinder with a middle layer of Dacron-Lycra to allow expansion without aneurysm formation. In rare cases, the polyurethane does weaken, the Dacron-Lycra covering of the triple layered cylinders may separate, and an aneurysm from either type of cylinder is still possible. More commonly, the wall of the tunica albuginea may weaken in certain locations from the increased pressure that occurs over time from the repeated inflation of the cylinders. A cylinder may completely fill out in these areas, and mild protuberance of the corporal body may be the result. These bulges, usually not unsightly or dysfunctional for intercourse but distasteful to some patients, may easily be attended to by exposing the tunica albuginea over the area of bulge and resecting a small portion of tunica in this location. Close the defect with an absorbable suture, and upon reinflation the tunica should appear flat.

# Erosion

The cylinder heads may wear distally through the tunica albuginea into the subcutaneous tissues over a period of time, especially with increased pressure exerted in this area (Fig. 41.3). The rod heads may become palpable very close to the surface underneath the foreskin, or the ends of the rods may be very close to the tip of the glans penis (Fig. 41.4). Another indication of this occurrence is asymmetry of the cylinder

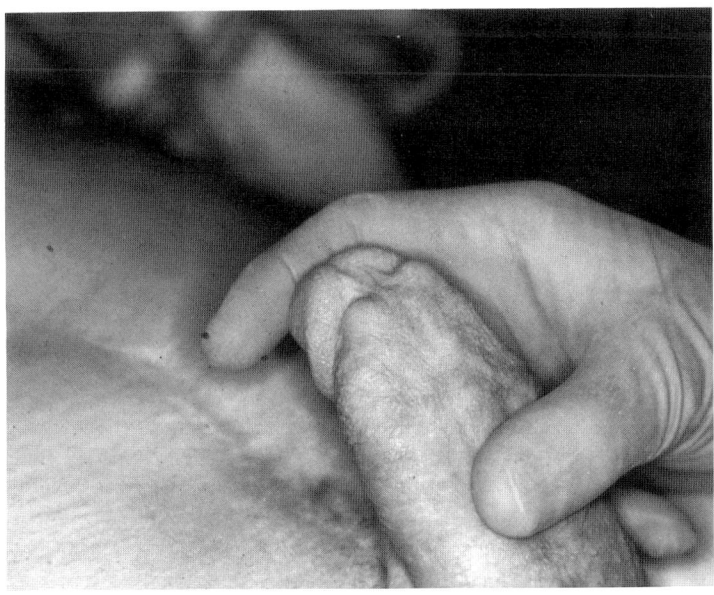

FIGURE 41.3. Mobile glans with rod heads extending through distal tunica albuginea palpable in subcutaneous tissue under foreskin.

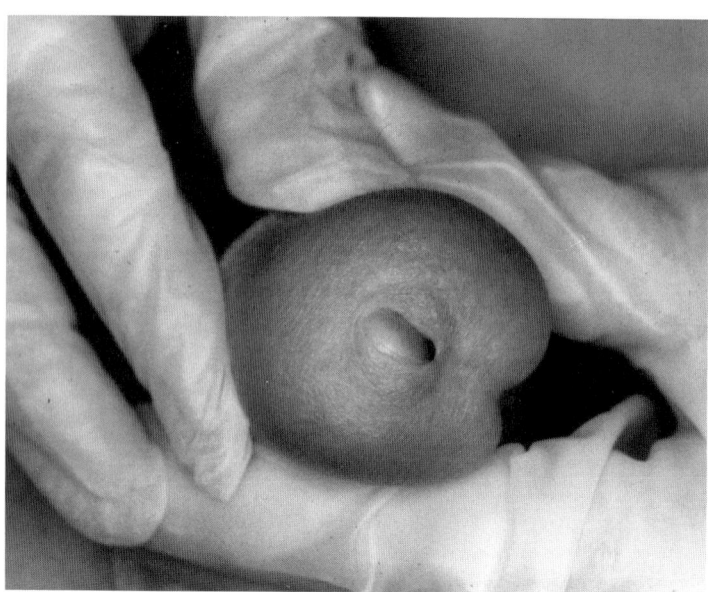

FIGURE 41.4. Tip of cylinder protruding toward skin of glans penis.

heads, with one head becoming more distally placed than the other. This situation is readily managed by exposing the area of erosion, opening the corporal body, and recessing the cylinder in the shaft or removing the cylinder from the shaft of the penis. Tough tunical tissue is then closed distally with nonabsorbable soft suture, and the cylinder is then allowed to reexpand or the rods replaced if a malleable prosthesis was used. This technique of distal corporoplasty is also useful if scar tissue interferes with complete distal filling of the corporal bodies by the cylinder heads or if the cylinder heads are not aligned evenly.

A more difficult problem to manage is erosion of the cylinders into the urethra, usually into the fossa navicularis. This is not an uncommon complication of long-term indwelling catheterization or of patients on intermittent catheterization.[8] It more commonly occurs with the rod-type prosthesis with firm distal tips and constant distal pressure. If patients with prostheses need these forms of catheterization, perineal urethrostomy is recommended. If this is impossible or unacceptable, then a very small catheter and adequate lubrication should be used during the catheterization process.

Others at risk for erosion into the urethra are patients with diminished sensitivity (such as patients with spinal cord injury) who do not appreciate that excessive pressure may be occurring at the ends of the prosthesis. In these patients, use a hydraulic prosthesis, which is soft most of the time and does not exert as much pressure distally. Patients who have had high doses of pelvic irradiation, have been on long-term cortisone therapy, or are having repeated treatments for urethral stricture disease are also at increased risk for this occurrence. If a previous erosion of a prosthesis cylinder into the urethra has occurred and a new prosthesis has been placed, this group of patients would be at greater risk for re-erosion because of the weakened tissue in this area. Symptoms that a distal erosion may have occurred include pain and erythema over the distal portion of the penis or pus appearing at the urethral meatus. This problem may be diagnosed readily by spreading the urethral meatus and observing the prosthesis tips in the fossa navicularis or by performing urethroscopy to visualize this.

When an erosion has occurred, remove the cylinder on that side. During the surgical procedure, cavernoscopy with a flexible cystoscope or palpation along the shaft of the penis with the operating finger will determine whether there is a communication with the cylinder on the opposite side. If this cylinder is communicating with the erosive process, it should be removed and reinserted after 6 months. If the cylinder on the opposite side is not involved, it should be left in place to maintain length of the penis. If a multicomponent prosthesis with input tubing is involved in the erosive process, expose the input tube by a proximal incision, amputate the input tube as it enters the cylinder, and remove the eroded cylinder via the opening in the urethral meatus. If the erosion has been of short duration and is detected shortly after its occurrence, cap the tubing leading from the removed cylinder to the pump with an orthopedic screw or stainless steel mushroom plug.

Infectious organisms present at the site of erosion may migrate up the shaft of the cylinder to the remainder of the prosthesis. If the erosion has been present for a long duration or if there is any question about infection in the remainder of the multicomponent device, the device should be removed and a salvage procedure performed (vide infra). Leave the cylinder on the opposite side, so as to maintain length. If both cylinders are removed and the penis is allowed to heal, with reinsertion at a later date, a 5-cm-shorter erection can be expected. The cylinder should not be reinserted in the side in which an erosion has occurred until the tissue at the site of erosion has been allowed to heal. Proximal erosions of the cylinders into the buttocks region are rare but have been observed in cases where a decubitus ulcer has occurred. Cylinders exposed under these circumstances should be removed. If a partial erosion has occurred, but the cylinders are not exposed, a cup fashioned from synthetic vascular graft material may be used to fix the cylinders in proper position. A visceral erosion in which the balloon reservoir erodes into the bowel or into the bladder is a rare occurrence, and the predisposing factor has been tension on the tubing leading from the reservoir or a small reservoir cavity that exerts pressure on the balloon, pushing it into the viscus (pressure erosion).[9] The treatment under these circumstances is to resect the bowel segment or close the bladder and reposition the reservoir balloon without tension on the tubing in an adequate cavity. If there is any question of infection being present under these circumstances, such as with a urinary tract infection or erosion into the colon, a decision should be made regarding removal or salvage of the remainder of the device.

## Glans Bowing

Excessive tilting of the glans (floppy glans or hypermobile glans) is seen more commonly when there is distal scarring in the cylinder cavities. This may occur in situations of Peyronie's disease or reinsertion of cylinders into a penis after removal of a previous implant following infection. When the cylinders are inflated or placed in position, the distal tunica albuginea does not extend adequately into the glans to give support to the structure. When a patient attempts to penetrate for intercourse, the glans bends and makes proper insertion of the penis difficult or painful. If this is noticed at the time of prosthesis insertion and appears mild in degree, then resist the temptation to fix it at that time. With healing time, the glans may become more securely attached to the corporal bodies before further intercourse is attempted. If, however, it is obvious that there is a major problem with bowing of the glans, correct it simultaneously with placement of the prosthesis cylinders. Make a circumcising or hemicircumcising incision and use sharp dissection to develop the plane between the glans and the distal portion of the tunica albuginea of the corpora cavernosa. Place a nonabsorbable soft suture through the glans substance and through the tunica albuginea adjacent to the cylinder head. When all sutures to be placed are in position, securely tie the sutures dorsally, ventrally, or laterally, wherever the glans needs to be secured over the cylinder heads.[10] Dorsal fixation for ventral bowing is performed by placing a suture on either side of the dorsal neurovascular bundle as described. Ventral fixation performed for dorsal bowing (less common) requires suture placement on either side of the corpus spongiosum. In cases of lateral fixation, only one suture is usually needed. For the very mobile glans, four-quadrant fixation is recommended.

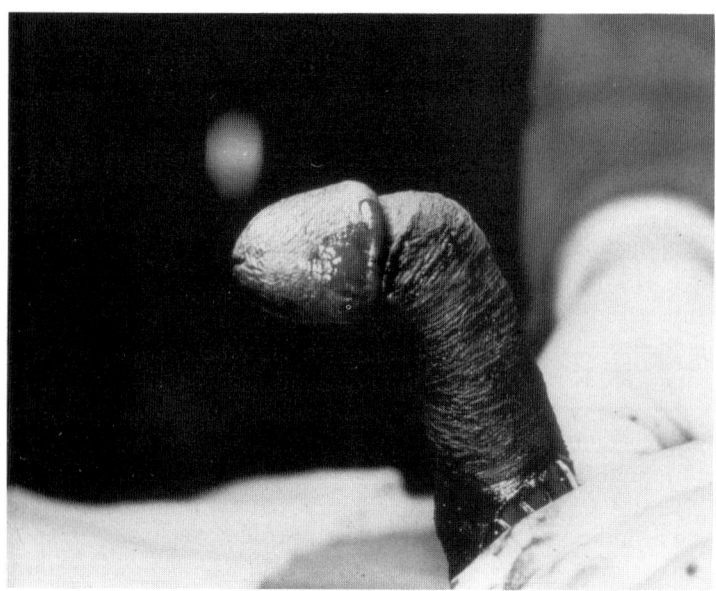

FIGURE 41.5. Bending of distal penis due to inadequate support. Prosthesis rods incompletely fill the length of the corporal bodies.

The floppy glans may be due to use of prosthesis cylinders that are too short for the dimensions of the corporal body (Fig. 41.5). To determine which is the problem, lift the ends of the corporal body off the ends of the cylinder head while the cylinder is inflated. If this is readily done with apparent space left in the corporal body, add rear tip extenders to the cylinder or place longer cylinders.

## Excessive Bleeding

In situations of excessive bleeding postoperatively, the question arises as to when the wound should be explored. An arterial bleeder will usually become manifest by swelling, ecchymosis, and a tensing of the tissues involved (Fig. 41.6). If there is venous oozing, perhaps from the site of the input tube entrance

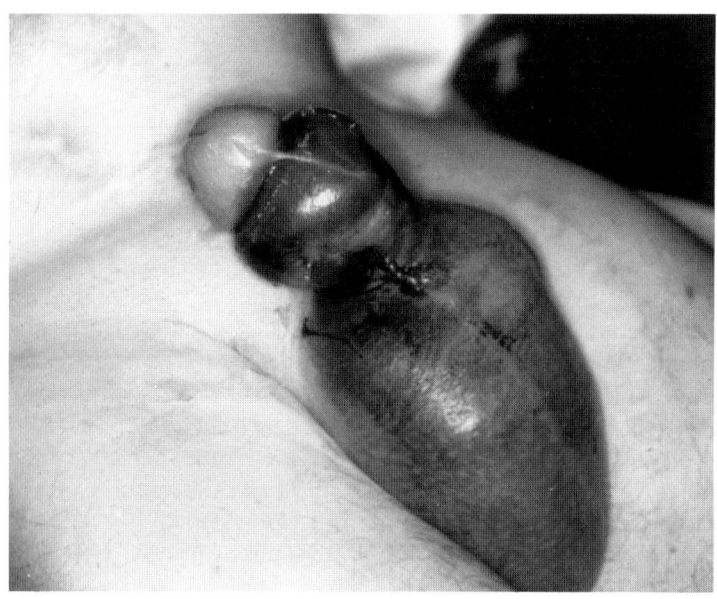

FIGURE 41.6. Tense, swollen, ecchymotic penis 7 hours after surgery. A small bleeding artery was ligated at wound exploration.

into the corporal body, pressure on the subcutaneous tissue will result in swelling with ecchymosis of a relatively soft appearance. In situations of arterial bleeding, the wound should be explored and hemostasis secured appropriately. If the wound remains soft, with swelling and ecchymosis, conservative measures, such as ice packs and perineal pressure dressings, may be applied. Care should be taken not to place pressure dressings on the shaft of the penis, because blood flows to the glans in only one direction. Inflating the prosthesis to a modest degree so as not to interfere with urination may also be helpful.

More appropriate, however, is careful attention to hemostasis prior to wound closure. Areas prone to bleeding are the sites where the input tube exits from the corporal body. These should be inspected thoroughly prior to closure. If the reservoir is placed through a scrotal approach via the inguinal canal, the spermatic cord vessels are also suspects as sites of bleeding. The inferior epigastric artery courses underneath the rectus muscle and may be injured during reservoir placement if dissection is performed *through* the rectus muscle rather than *between* the rectus muscles.

It is rare to have excessive bleeding from the corporal bodies, but this may be seen in very young patients with nerve injuries or in psychogenically impotent patients who have selected prosthesis implantation. If excessive bleeding is occurring during cylinder placement, move rapidly through the surgical procedure to place the cylinders and close the corporotomy as soon as possible.

## Repair of Mechanical Problems

If a unitary hydraulic device or rod-type penile prosthesis becomes defective, both cylinders need to be replaced. If a two-piece hydraulic device develops a mechanical problem, replace the entire device, as both cylinders and pump are part of one continuous system without connectors. If a three-piece inflatable device develops a mechanical problem after 5 to 6 years from the time of installation, replace all parts, because any parts left behind have a diminished life expectancy. If only a brief period of time has elapsed since the date of installation, consider replacing the involved components as needed and leave any parts that seem to be functioning well.

Isolate the connections to the various parts and observe for tubing fractures, particularly where excessive angulation of the tubing is present as it joins to the connector. If fracture is observed, bypass it by connecting intact parts of the tubing.

Test the entire system with an ohmmeter, for more than one part may be defective. The ohmmeter makes use of the fact that both filling solutions and body fluids conduct a current. Place a metal needle on the tubing leading to the part to be tested, fill the part completely with the filling solution, apply one limb of the ohmmeter to the needle, and place the other limb on a retractor in the wound. If there is current conduction indicated by positive deflection of the needle on the ohmmeter dial, this indicates conduction of electrolytes through a defective cover on the part and the part must be replaced. Another method of detecting a defect in that particular component is pressure testing. Fill the particular part with fluid and look for the appearance of fluid in the wound or decreased volume when the filling solution is aspirated from the part. A recent report indicates that ohmmeter testing may not be completely reliable in detecting leaks, possibly because of air traps in the tubing.[11] When in doubt about the integrity of any components of the system, replace at the time of the reparative procedure.

## Infection

Infection associated with placement of penile prosthesis can be a catastrophic event. Fortunately, the incidence of this occurrence is rare—about 1% to 3% in most series.[12-14] Certain procedures are recommended prior to inserting the implant to ensure that the possibility of infection remains remote. Skin lesions, such as comedomes or subaceous cysts, in the area of the surgical field should be eradicated. During the implant procedure, with manipulation of the penis and scrotum, these areas may inadvertently be compressed and thereby seed the wound with pathogenic organisms. Difficulty in retracting the foreskin should be corrected by circumcision as a separate procedure.

The genital area should be thoroughly cleansed with strong soap in the days prior to the surgery. Shave the pubic hair in the operating room just prior to the procedure, then scrub, paint, and spray the skin thoroughly with a strong antiseptic solution, such as povidone iodine. Most urologists believe that use of prophylactic antibiotics in association with prosthesis placement offers added protection against environmental pathogens.[15] Such antibiotics should be started about 1 hour prior to the incision to allow good tissue levels at the time of the procedure and continued for up to 48 hours postoperatively. No benefit is achieved by longer use, as the wound will have sealed by this time.

The organism most commonly isolated from wound infections associated with penile prostheses has been coagulase-negative staphylococcus (*Staphylococcus epidermidis*). Coliform organisms, *Pseudomonas*, *Klebsiella*, *Serratia*, *Proteus*, and other gram negatives have been seen, as well as anaerobes and fungi. Vancomycin 500 mg every 6 hours and gentamicin 80 mg every 8 hours are the most effective combination to use prophylactically against such organisms. Some infectious disease experts, however, have seen no indication for using prophylactic antibacterials during uncomplicated prosthesis placement because the skin is thoroughly cleansed prior to the procedure, and a sterile device is implanted under conditions that should exclude bacteria from the wound.

There has been no controlled study that shows a lower incidence of infection using prophylactic antibacterials as opposed to not using these medications. Washing the wound frequently during the procedure with a sterile solution with or without antibiotics added will certainly aid in eliminating pathogens that may have migrated into the sterile field. A sterile urine at the time of prosthesis placement is a desirable feature, although this may be difficult in certain instances because patients with

indwelling suprapubic tubes or a neurogenic bladder may have infections that are difficult to eradicate. Begin prophylactic antibacterials a few days prior to the procedure in such high risk cases. In addition, when entry into the urethra is more likely, such as in cases of excessive corporal scarring, preoperative urethral washing with dilute povidone iodine solution is advisable.

Despite the best precautions, infection of the prosthesis may develop. Erythema, fever, pain worsening over parts of the prosthesis, fluctuance in the region of prosthesis parts, or fixation of parts to the scrotal wall suggest the presence of an infection. Exposure of any parts of the prosthesis to the outside environment should be treated as an infected situation. Purulent drainage from a portion of the wound may represent a superficial infection, i.e., a stitch abscess; but if compression of part of the prosthesis, such as cylinders or pump, results in an increase in purulent drainage, conclude that the purulent process is in contact with the prosthesis and it should be treated accordingly. When infection of a prosthesis is confirmed or is highly suspect, exploration of the wound is appropriate. The presence of purulent material or slimy exudate around the implant indicates the presence of infection. Take aerobic and anaerobic cultures, and if doubt exists, a Gram stain of the tissue fluid can be done to immediately ascertain the presence of organisms.

If an infection is found, two approaches can be taken. The prosthesis can be removed, the wound cleansed, drains placed, and the infectious process allowed to heal. After 6 months, an attempt to replace the prosthesis may be considered if the patient so wishes. Another approach is to remove the entire prosthesis and all foreign parts and suture material, thoroughly cleanse the wound, and reinsert a new prosthesis at the same sitting, a technique termed a *salvage* or *rescue* procedure. These alternatives should be thoroughly discussed with the patient prior to the exploratory procedure in order that his wishes may be followed. The advantages of salvage are that it maintains the length of the penis, for the most part, and permits an easier insertion of cylinders at the time of the surgery as opposed to 6 months later, at which time shortening of the penis can be expected.

The solutions used in the salvage protocol include saline to which has been added kanamycin and bacitracin, half-strength hydrogen peroxide, and half-strength povidone iodine. The wound is pressure washed with a Water Pik (Simpulse) using 1 g of vancomycin and 80 mg of gentamicin in the 5-liter irrigating fluid bag. A third series of irrigations is performed using the first series of solutions in reverse order, i.e., half-strength povidone iodine, half-strength hydrogen peroxide, and saline containing the antibiotics kanamycin and bacitracin. The success of salvage using this protocol in our series has been 88%, i.e., 14 of 16 cases successfully salvaged (5 to 48 months' follow-up). In two cases of unsuccessful salvage, the contaminating organisms were methicillin-resistant *Staphylococcus aureus* and *Pseudomonas aeruginosa*. Fifty percent of the patients who underwent this salvage procedure had been diagnosed with diabetes mellitus. Fishman et al[16] successfully salvaged infected penile implants in 84% of 44 patients (average follow-up 4 years). Furlow et al[17] saved 16 of 22 cases (73%) of pump erosion by a combination of removing all or part of the prosthesis, cleansing the wound, and reinserting the device. Teloken et al[18] used corporal irrigations of rifamycin for 3 days before reinserting a new prosthesis after an infected device

had been removed. Uniform success in this series was achieved. Salvage is not indicated in cases of urethral erosion, necrotizing infections, or in patients who are very toxic, such as diabetics in ketoacidosis associated with a prosthesis infection.

If the device is removed for a later reinsertion of a new prosthesis, Jackson Pratt drains are placed in the corporal bodies and other cavities in contact with the infectious process.[19] Instill 10 mm of the vancomycin-gentamicin antibiotic solution into the drains every 8 hours, with the drainage tubing left clamped for 20 minutes. The suction grenade is then applied to the drains and the drains are removed in about 5 days. By that time, culture reports will have documented that the organisms present at that time are sensitive to the antibiotics used.

## Penile Necrosis

Necrosis occurs when the blood supply to the glans or the corpus canvernosum is compromised, with resulting death of tissue (Fig. 41.7). This may be seen not only with severe vascular disease but also when vascular disease is not obvious.[20] Use linear, rather than circumferential, incisions on the penis, avoid compression dressings and indwelling urethral catheters, and

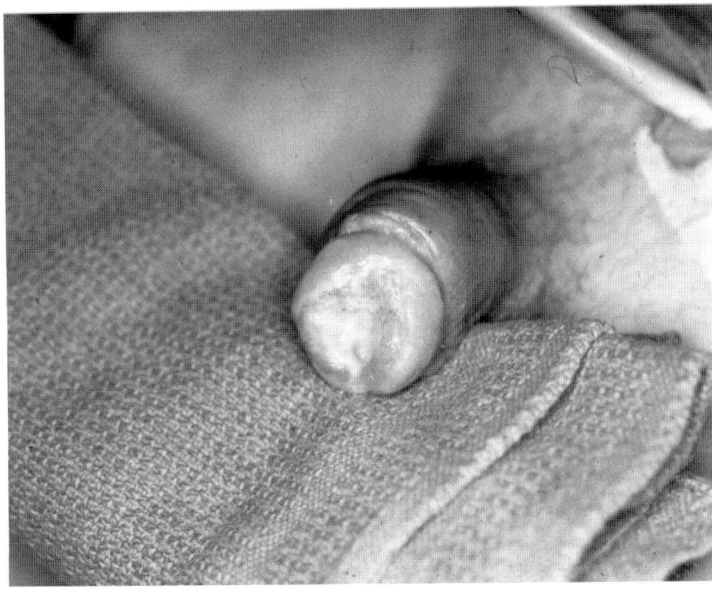

FIGURE 41.7. Necrosis of the central glans associated with a urethral injury during prosthesis placement. The peripheral glans is nourished by blood from the foreskin.

do not attempt extensive penile straightening procedures, corporoplasty, or glans fixation in high-risk patients. When necrosis is present, remove the prosthesis and prescribe antibiotics to cover any concomitant infection. Hyperbaric oxygen has not been found useful, because it does not reconstitute blood supply to the ischemic area. Heat applications and vasodilator medications may be of some benefit. When demarcation of necrotic tissue occurs, perform debridement and save all viable tissue for future reconstruction. Extensive loss of tissue does not occur in many instances and rebuilding portions of the phallus may be warranted. However, it may not be advisable to reinsert another prosthesis in such a patient.

## Conclusion

Attending carefully to details during prosthesis surgery, avoiding factors that could lead to the development of complications, and informing the patient of exactly what a prosthesis does will help to minimize unfortunate results and unrealistic expectations.

## References

1. Fallon B, Ghanem H. Sexual performance and satisfaction with penile prostheses in impotence of various etiologies. *Int J Impotence Res* 1990; 2:35–42.
2. Mulcahy JJ. A technique for maintaining penile prosthesis position to prevent proximal migration. *J Urol* 1987; 17:294–296.
3. Montague DK, Lakin MM. Early experience with the controlled girth and length expanding cylinder of the American Medical Systems Ultrex penile prosthesis. *J Urol* 1992; 148:1444–1446.
4. Wilson SK, Delk JR. The "S" deformity: a complication of AMS 700 ultrex penile prosthesis. *Int J Impotence Res* 1994; 6(suppl 1):D168.
5. Wilson SK, Delk JR. A new treatment for Peyronie's disease: modeling the penis over an inflatable penile prosthesis. *J Urol* 1994; 152: 1121–1123.
6. Mulcahy JJ, Rowland RG. Tunica wedge excision to correct penile curvature associated with the inflatable penile prosthesis. *J Urol* 1987; 138:63–64.
7. Nesbit RM. Congenital curvature of the phallus: report of three cases with description of corrective operation. *J Urol* 1965; 93:230–232.
8. Steidl CS, Mulcahy JJ. Erosion of penile prosthesis: a complication of ureteral catheterization. *J Urol* 1989; 142:736–739.
9. Fitch WP, Roddy T. Erosion of inflatable penile prosthesis reservoir into bladder. *J Urol* 1986; 136:1080.
10. Ball TP. Surgical repair of penile "SST" deformity. *Urology* 1980; 15:603–604.
11. Parulkar BG, Lamb B, Vickers MA Jr. The detection of leakage in inflatable urinary devices (Abstract). *J Urol* 1994; 153:358A(Abstr 519).
12. Kabalin JN, Kessler R. Infectious complications of penile prosthesis surgery. *J Urol* 1988; 139: 953–955.
13. Montague DK. Periprosthetic infections. *J Urol* 1987; 138:68–69.
14. Thomalla JV, Thompson ST, Rowland RG, et al. Infectious complications of penile prosthetic implants. *J Urol* 1987; 138:65–67.
15. Carson CC. Infections in genitourinary prostheses. *Urol Clin North Am* 1989; 16:139–147.
16. Fishman IJ, Scott FB, Selim AM. Rescue procedure. An alternative to complete removal for treatment of infected penile prostheses (Abstract). *J Urol* 1987; 137:202A(Abstr 396).
17. Furlow WL, Goldwasser B. Salvage of the eroded inflatable penile prosthesis: a new concept. *J Urol* 1987; 138:312–314.
18. Teloken C, Souto JC, DaRos C et al. Prosthetic penile infection: rescue procedure with rifamycin. *J Urol* 1992; 148:1905–1906.
19. Moatman TJ, Montague DK. Intracorporeal drainage after removal of infected penile prostheses. *Urology* 1984; 23:184–185.
20. McClellan DS, Masih BK. Gangrene of the penis as a complication of penile prosthesis. *J Urol* 1985; 133:862–863.

# 42
# Management of Patients with Gender Dysphoria

Alexandru E. Benet and Arnold Melman

Gender dysphoria refers to dissatisfaction with one's own anatomical gender and the desire to possess the secondary sexual characteristics of the opposite sex.[1] Persons who express this desire are called transsexuals and represent the extreme of the spectrum of subjective dissatisfaction with assigned anatomy and societally sanctioned gender roles. The term *transsexual* is used to refer to both pre- and postoperative men and women who perceive their identity as incongruous with the anatomical reality and actively seek to resolve the conflict through sex-reassignment surgery. Once surgery is completed, however, and the new sexual identity is achieved, *male* or *female* is the preferred term.

The inner sense of being a female "trapped in a male body" coincident with male chromosomes, male sex organs, and laboratory findings makes it extremely difficult to diagnose and identify gender dysphoria at a very early age. Starting in childhood and intensifying through the years, this inner sense may cause the patients to suffer extreme pain, misunderstanding, and conflict as to gender identity. Degrees of gender dysphoria vary and only persons with the most intense form actually seek sex-reassignment surgery.

The evolving changes in societal attitudes toward human sexuality as well as today's public media have been accompanied by an increased awareness and concern regarding patients with gender dysphoria, leading to increased motivation in research and treatment.

## Historical Notes

Conditions of gender dysphoria (transsexualism) and instances of autocastration and genital mutilation, as the result of a person's intense desire to change his or her sex, have been noted in historical, cultural, anthropological, and literary references to sexual transformation and surgery throughout history.[2-7] Translating the desire for sex-reassignment surgery into a reality, however, required the advances of modern surgical technology and hormonal procedures. Although Abraham[8] reported in 1931 on the first sex-reassignment surgery of two male transvestites, according to Hoyer[9] it was not until publication of Lilly Elbe's autobiography that sex-reassignment surgery became a popular and practical solution for the transsexual's dilemma.

In the United States, the diagnosis and treatment of transsexual patients began with the work of the endocrinologist Dr. Harry Benjamin,[10,11] and the beginning of serious research in the field was initiated with the publication of Benjamin's classic follow-up study[12] of postoperative transsexuals. He classified postsurgical patients into three categories: unsatisfactory, good, and satisfactory. Based on this classification, of 73 men and 20 women who underwent surgery, 85% of the men (N = 62) and 95% of the women (N = 19) showed satisfactory outcomes. Since the sensationalism of the Christine Jorgenson[13] case, large numbers of patients have requested information regarding sex change, and the number of patients going on to request reassignment surgery increases every year.[14,15]

On November 21, 1966, Johns Hopkins Hospital announced its formation of a gender identity clinic, probably the first such clinic in the world. Many enthusiastic supporters were responsible for its establishment, but the main impetus for its creation came from Benjamin,[12] who inspired the concept that was so ably carried out under John Money's imaginative and creative guidance.[16] At the same time, Robert Stoller[17] and colleagues at the University of California at Los Angeles began evaluating transsexuals. His clinic did not have a surgical team, so patients were referred to surgeons who were willing to perform surgical sex-reassignment. Hastings[18] at the University of Minnesota began his program around the same time as the one at Johns Hopkins, but he chose to operate initially on only a limited number of males because his main interest was in the long-term follow-up of operated cases.

In 1968 Pauly[19] reviewed the world literature on 121 cases and concluded that transsexuals who underwent sex-reassignment surgery were 10 times more likely to have a satisfactory outcome, in terms of social and emotional status, than transsexuals who did not.

Throughout the 1970s, increasing numbers of patients sought sex-reassignment surgery. Money and Ehrhardt[16] investigated 17 men and seven woman and compared each patient's preoperative and postoperative adjustment along five dimensions: capacity for a lasting relationship with a partner, adjustment to work, criminality, mental state, and the patient's subjective opinion of the result. The results were very encouraging, as overall satisfaction was noted by 23 of 24 patients.

At Northwestern Medical Center, Arieff[20] studied 14 men and 4 women for 5 years after surgery. The group included three blacks and one Asian. Nine patients (50%) demonstrated better social adjustment; two patients (11%) had better vocational adjustment; five (28%) improved their relationships by getting married; and overall conditions worsened for two patients (11%). Hastings and Markland[21] reported on 25 men who received sex-

reassignment surgery at the University of Minnesota. Using a college grading system (A, B, C, and D), they rated patient outcomes on sexual, economic, and social variables. Twelve patients experienced multiple orgasms; 13 patients were marginally self-supportive; 8 were on welfare; and 10 patients were married, including 6 who had remained with their original spouses. Laub and Fisk[22] reported on 74 patients (50 men and 24 women) who underwent sex-reassignment surgery.

Throughout the mid-1970s, treatment for intense gender dysphoria was made up of hormone treatments and sex-reassignment surgery, with no requirements for psychotherapy or diagnostic evaluation and with little preparation of patients for the absence of expected benefits, for risks, side effects, and limitations.[23,24] The availability of surgery before rational criteria were developed for the comprehensive care of patients motivated members of the Harry Benjamin International Gender Dysphoria Association to pioneer the Standards of Care, a document outlining minimum standards for evaluation and treatment of patients with gender dysphoria.[25]

By 1980, in the United States alone, an estimated 1000 patients had undergone sex-reassignment surgery.[25]

## Epidemiology

As of mid-1978, approximately 40 centers in the Western Hemisphere offered surgical sex reassignment to persons having a multiplicity of behavioral diagnoses applied under a multiplicity of criteria.[24,26,27]

The incidence of male-to-female transsexualism was estimated in 1983 to be 1 in 37,000 in biologic males.[28] Estimates are available about those who seek surgical or psychiatric attention for gender problems, but these are likely to be an underestimation because many individuals with the milder forms of gender identity disorders do not seek medical attention. The incidence may be influenced by the social attitudes in certain countries. In the Netherlands, which has a benevolent climate for transsexuals, the incidence is reported to be 1 in 11,900.[29]

Data from a central registry of all patients seeking sex-reassignment surgery in Sweden[30] have suggested an incidence of 1 in 37,000 males and 0.17 cases per 100,000 persons over age 15. Although most sex reassignments are done in countries of the Western world, the Eastern world also has persons with gender dysphoria. Transsexualism occurs in almost all ethnic groups, including Chinese, Malays, and Indians.[31]

## Etiology

The cause of gender dysphoria is unclear. During the past 20 years, scientific investigations have been made exploring genetic links,[32,33] hormonal effects,[34,35] family dynamics,[34] and psychoanalytic observations.[37] In the majority of cases, gender dysphoria occurs early in childhood during the gender-identity differentiation period. Retrospective studies of transsexuals[38–48] have shown a high incidence of childhood cross-gender behavior. Follow-up studies of children with gender dysphoria have found a high incidence of manifestations continued into adulthood, with a higher incidence of homosexual or bisexual behavior and fantasies than in a control group.[41,42] Additional factors that have been suggested are parents' indifference to or encouragement of opposite-sex behavior; regular cross-dressing as a young boy by a female; lack of male playmates during a boy's first years of socialization; excessive maternal protection, with inhibition of rough-and-tumble play; and absence of or rejection by an older male early in life.[43]

## Differential Diagnosis of Transsexualism

The differential diagnosis of gender dysphoria includes both physical and psychiatric considerations.[44] At one time, transsexualism seemed a relatively straightforward diagnosis if it was based on Stoller's[45] definition that transsexualism is the belief held by biologically normal individuals that they are members of the opposite sex. It was then thought that gender identity was irrevocably fixed by the age of 3 years.[46] In 1980 the *Diagnostic and Statistical Manual of Mental Disorders*, third edition,[47] included a somewhat heterogeneous listing of clinical conditions called discrete psychiatric syndromes that occur in both adults and children. With this recognition came more detailed guidelines that have helped to discriminate among the fine shades of disorders along the spectrum of gender disturbances. Criteria for a diagnosis of transsexualism,[48] the most severe form of gender dysphoria, are (1) persistent discomfort and sense of inappropriateness about one's assigned sex having reached puberty; and (2) persistent preoccupation for 2 or more years with getting rid of one's primary and secondary sex characteristics and acquiring the opposite sex characteristics.

For the vast majority of patients with gender dysphoria, the results of physical examination and laboratory studies are normal with no known organic pathology associated with or responsible for the cross-gender symptoms.[49] The differential diagnosis of patients with gender dysphoric conditions is difficult due to the high prevalence of character pathology[50] and the fact that almost all patients will attempt to convince their evaluator that they are true transsexuals and as such require hormonal and surgical sex reassignment.[51]

# Patient Evaluation Method— Male-to-Female Transsexuals

It is suggested that patients must be 21 years old or older to be considered for sex-reassignment surgery. Patients may be seen by either the surgeon (a urologist) or a psychiatrist for an initial evaluation that includes complete history, physical examination, and laboratory studies of (1) plasma cortisol and triiodothyronine ($T_3$) and thyroxine ($T_4$) uptake, and (2) testosterone and estradiol blood levels. In some cases, additional tests, such as liver-function tests, may be indicated if there is a history of alcoholism or drug abuse, or if the patient has been on estrogen therapy. Patients must be informed of the risks and benefits of the surgical procedure and estrogen therapy. If patients have a clean bill of health (and venereal diseases and endocrine disorders have been ruled out), appointments are made with the various specialists. Each patient must undergo psychotherapy for 1 year with a psychiatrist and a subsequent interview with an additional independent psychiatrist to rule out major psychiatric disorders other than transsexualism and to establish that the patient has truly experienced persistent long-standing discomfort in the male gender role and believes that he is a female. A prerequisite requirement is that the patient must have experienced 2 years of cross-dressing and 1 year of supportive psychological counseling before the operative stage of the transformation is undertaken. (There is some controversy about whether those with very masculine physical traits, such as extreme height, extreme muscularity, or coarse features, should be considered for surgery because some surgeons have found these qualities may foreshadow a poor psychological adjustment after surgery; others, however, have not found them to make any difference.)

If diagnosed as transsexual, each patient is encouraged to go out into society and to live and function in the cross-gender role. Money[46] calls this the "real-life experiment." The length of time patients should live in the cross-gender role prior to undergoing surgical sex-reassignment and whether hormone therapy is indicated are dependent on the psychiatrists' decision. Patients are encouraged to establish their cross-gender identity and to find employment in a compatible role. Some patients may be fortunate enough to obtain employment in their chosen gender role without having to change their previous occupation, for example, hairdresser, salesperson, picture framer, etc.

The major problem for the biologic male in "passing" is the ability to pass convincingly as a woman. A small minority pass exceedingly well as very attractive females (some well enough to work as fashion models), but more transvestite males, in an attempt to look feminine, wear obvious wigs and heavy pancake makeup to cover their beard, and the result is usually a very nonfeminine appearance. Although some clinics run "charm schools" to give direction and advice on how to appear more feminine, each patient has to learn by trial and error how best to present himself when cross-dressed. Patients should be encouraged to allow their own hair to grow, however thin and fine it may be. Natural hair is preferable to wigs that are obviously artificial and draw attention to other indicators of masculinity, such as large hands, thick wrists or neck, and square shoulders. They should also be encouraged not to wear a lot of jewelry, which only attracts attention to their hands and wrists, and to try more flattering colors and a simple style of dress that makes them less noticeable. Almost all biologic males will have to undergo electrolysis of the beard. Some extremely hirsute individuals must also shave or wax their arms, legs, chest, and even back in some exceptional cases.

# Hormone Therapy

Once the patient has successfully established the chosen gender role and has lived and functioned in society in that role for a minimum period of 1 year, hormone therapy may be considered. The first important factor is to ensure that the patient understands the changes that will result from hormone therapy as well as the risks involved and the possible complications that could occur. To safeguard both patient and clinician, the patient is asked to sign an informed consent that outlines the effects of hormone therapy together with the possible complications that could occur.

## Method of Administration of Hormones

A survey of 39 centers in the United States and foreign countries found neither conformity nor standardization among the clinics surveyed in terms of the different hormonal preparations used.[52] In some clinics, estrogen was prescribed in excessively large doses, greater than is necessary for physiologic replacement.[52] Large doses of estrogen tend to increase the risk of complications. In a study of 38 noncastrate, male-to-female transsexuals who were hormonally and physically normal prior to therapy, hormonal levels were measured before or during therapy or at both times using various forms and dosages of hormones. Ethinyl estradiol proved superior to conjugated estrogen in suppression of testosterone and gonadotropins, but both were equal in effecting breast growth. The changes in physical and hormonal characteristics were the same for 0.1 mg daily and 0.5 mg daily of ethinyl estradiol.[49]

All patients should first be referred to an endocrinologist for radioimmunoassay of their hormonal levels prior to commencing treatment. Thereafter, they are similarly assessed at 3- and 6-month intervals, followed by annual checkups as long as they remain on medication. It is important that patients understand they must continue with hormone therapy for the rest of their lives; otherwise, all signs of feminization will disappear within 1 to 6 months. Under the guidance of the endocrinologist, 0.1 mg to 0.5 mg of ethinyl estradiol is administered, one tablet daily. Following sex-reassignment surgery, the dosage of ethinyl estradiol is decreased to 0.05 mg daily. In the biologic male, estrogen therapy will result in a redistribution of body fat around the hips, shoulders, and neck, together with a slight decrease in the growth of facial and body hair with some redistribution in the female contour. In addition, the hairline will stop receding. Mild-to-moderate enlargement of the breasts (gynecomastia) will develop. There will be a decrease in sexual drive, so that the patient may have difficulty in maintaining penile erections and may have decreased orgasmic potential. The sexual pattern varies considerably. Some patients claim they are still able to masturbate or to have a sexual relationship without any erectile or ejaculatory difficulties. Without exception, all patients express a feeling of well-being and contentment not experienced previously, and they are delighted with the feminizing effects and the change in their physical appearance.

The increased risk of thromboembolic disorders due to estrogen therapy is of greater concern in the older biologic male patient who is overweight or who has a family history of diabetes mellitus.[53] This group of men runs a greater risk of coronary or cerebral thrombosis or both. Some reports claim that carcinoma of the breast may develop in male-to-female transsexuals who have been taking estrogens over many years.[54] This risk must be kept in perspective, as 1% of all cases of cancer of the breast occur in men. Unfortunately, some men increase their chance of adverse side effects from hormone treatment by taking unnecessarily large doses of estrogens in the mistaken belief that this will enhance their feminine appearance. However, the body metabolizes the amount of estrogen it requires and excretes the excess. Ingestion of excessive hormones does not enhance femininization, but increases—considerably—the complications of such therapy. It is particularly important that patients be checked annually by an endocrinologist. Liver-function tests are recommended if the physician suspects too much "self-medication" with estrogen.

## Operative Techniques

The aim of the surgical procedure is to create a vagina that resembles that of a natural-looking female sex organ that will also enable the patient to have intercourse. McIndoe[55] described the first such surgical technique used not for sex reassignment but to treat aplasia vaginae in women suffering from the Mayer-Rokitansky-Küster-Houser syndrome. In this technique, the vagina is lined with a split-thickness skin graft. Later techniques used to create a vagina involve the use of penile skin flaps pedicled on the perineum[56] or the abdomen,[57,58] or the use of penile and scrotal skin,[35] the rectosigmoid[26] or other parts of the intestine,[59,60] perineal skin flaps, and free-full thickness penile skin grafts.[61] The most current methods for constructing vaginas are most frequently abdominally pedicled penile skin or less frequently a combination of penile and scrotal skin. The use of rectosigmoid or other parts of the intestine is reserved for cases of failure of the primary construction.[36]

To further improve patients' satisfaction as well as appearance, Malloy et al[62] have used the glans to form a substitute of the uterine cervix. Rubin[63] has used the glans to form a clitoris with the pedicle based on the corpus spongiosum.

# Surgical Procedure

The surgical procedure is made up of two main stages, the creation of the neovaginal space and the creation of the neovaginal lining, the vaginoplasty.

## Preoperative Treatment

Estrogen therapy is discontinued 1 month prior to the operation because of the thrombogenic-promoting properties of estrogen and the need to minimize postoperative tissue swelling. Before the operation, urologic abnormalities must be ruled out by use of urine analysis; blood tests, including blood counts; measurement of electrolytes; and renal and liver functions tests. Cystoscopy is performed if the patient has voiding difficulties. Prior to surgery the bowel is prepared with oral prophylactic broad-spectrum antibiotics.

## Creation of the Neovaginal Space

The surgical procedure is performed under general anesthesia, with the patient in the exaggerated lithotomy position. The technique is identical to Young's[64] approach for radical perineal prostatectomy. The Belt[65] approach beneath the circular rectal sphincter *cannot* be used for this operation. A vertical midline incision is made from the midscrotum to the perineum. The central tendon of the perineum is cut, and the transverse perineal muscles identified and preserved. After division of the levator ani and rectourethralis muscles, a curved Lowsley retractor is inserted into the bladder and by manipulating the retractor the prostate gland is pushed into view. The dissection is advanced on Denonvilliers' fascia, creating a cavity between the rectum, prostate, and bladder to the peritoneal reflection. The cavity is inspected for length and width, bleeding is controlled, and a lap pad is placed in the cavity. To maximize the width, the muscle fibers are transected with electric cautery down to the level of the pelvic wall.

# Vaginoplasty

Three methods of vaginoplasty are commonly employed: (1) the penile inversion technique, in which only a penile skin tube is used to form the lining of the vagina; (2) penile and scrotal skin inversion in which a combination of scrotal and penile skin are sewn together and inverted into the neovaginal cavity so that the anterior vagina is formed by the penile skin and the posterior is formed by the scrotal flap; and (3) colon interposition, which is used if the above two methods fail because of stenosis or shrinkage.[61]

## *Penile Inversion Technique*

A circular incision is made around the coronal sulcus, and tubular dissection of the penile skin superficial to Buck's fascia is performed. The denuded penis is retracted from the surrounding skin into the perineal incision. For those patients undergoing clitoroplasty, the dorsal neurovascular bundle (consisting of the deep dorsal vein, the paired dorsal arteries, and nerves) is identified between the tunica albuginea and Buck's fascia. Two longitudinal incisions are made lateral to the dorsal nerves to free the neurovascular bundle. The dissection is done from the glans penis and the pubic symphysis. The deep dorsal vein is *not* ligated. Great care is taken not to injure the origin of the dorsal arteries. The dissection should be done with magnification. The sensate glans can be trimmed to form the neoclitoris with its intact neurovascular bundle. The corpus spongiosum is dissected from the tunica albuginea distal to the bulbous urethra, and the urethra is clamped and divided at that point. The proximal corpus spongiosum is dissected to the paired crura and separated from it. The corpora are dissected proximally along the ischiopubic rami to their origin, which is clamped with a Kocher clamp and divided. The open end is sutured with a running 2-0 chromic catgut. The abdominal skin is mobilized to allow caudad mobilization of the penile skin so that the origin of the penile tube is positioned more easily over the neovaginal opening. The lower abdominal skin is temporarily sutured to the periosteum of the pubic symphysis with #2 nylon suture. A 60-ml syringe is inserted into the inverted penis and all of the subcutaneous tissue removed from it so that the tube is converted into a full-thickness skin graft. That process allows the tube to stretch and fill and stick to the neovagina. Two small incisions are made in the middorsal portion of the penile skin tube to allow for the passage of the urethra and the neoclitoris. The urethra and the neoclitoris are pulled through the two openings. The penile skin is inverted and pushed into the previously created cavity. The urethra is spatulated and sutured to the penile skin with 4-0 polyglycolic sutures. The glans penis is trimmed to resemble a clitoris and sutured to the same opening. The neurovascular bundle is left under the inverted penile skin. The scrotal skin is used to create the labia majora. The excess scrotal skin is elevated with towel clips and trimmed to create the labia. A stent is placed in the vagina and left there for 7 days. Either a Mentor Corporation silicone vaginal stent is used or a sterile surgical glove packed with vaginal gauze and tied at the end. The glove is safe to use until the skin take occurs. After 7 days, the glove is removed, and the more convenient vaginal stent is inserted.

### Penile and Scrotal Skin Inversion

This method is used less frequently because the disadvantage of hair-bearing scrotal skin at the base of the vagina outweighs several advantages of increased vaginal depth obtained, because the combined scrotal-penile flap can be made longer than the penile flap alone.[35] This method also gives some patients more caudad introitus, which more closely approximates the position in the human female. The penis and scrotum are incised longitudinally along the midline. The remainder of the surgery is the same as the penile inversion method, except that the penile skin is not devascularized. The inverted skin flaps are immobilized for 7 days. Postoperatively, the patient must keep the neovagina patent by dilating it with stents. If these are not inserted correctly, the vaginal cavity will close.

### Colon Interposition

In cases where one of the above two methods fails because of stenosis or shrinkage, a piece of sigmoid colon can be used to augment the vagina. A 15 to 20 cm long segment of sigmoid colon is isolated; its blood supply is reduced to one artery and vein. The distal end is closed, and the proximal end is kept open and brought down to the peritoneal fold. From the stenosed vagina, a tunnel is dissected up to the peritoneal fold. The peritoneum is incised so the isolated sigmoid segment can be brought down to be anastomosed to the vaginal epithelium. This manipulation is necessary because the sigmoid artery is short and does not allow free movement of the sigmoidal segment. To achieve the lowest anastomosis of the sigmoid segment to the vaginal opening, the end-to-end anastomotic (EEA) bowel stapler can be used. Sigmoid segments do not narrow, but fibrous constriction can occur at the sigmoidocutaneous junction if enough tension is placed on the anastomosis so that ischemic fibrosis occurs.

## The Patient with a Small Phallus

The alternatives for the male with the small phallus for whom the eventual overall vaginal depth would prevent satisfactory coitus are the penoscrotal technique, primary skin grafting, or tissue expansion of the penile skin prior to surgery.

Skin grafting has several major disadvantages. The donor skin must be fairly thick, about 20/1000 of an inch, and the donor site either the buttocks or the thighs. Even well-healed donor sites leave unsightly scars, and for a population that is very concerned with appearance the result is not generally satisfactory. The sheets of skin graft are inverted and sutured to one another and to the end of the inverted penile skin tube. The tube is then inserted into the neovagina, and the vaginal stent is used to create opposition to the pelvic sidewall. The latter step is done blindly, and proper placement of the grafted tube cannot be

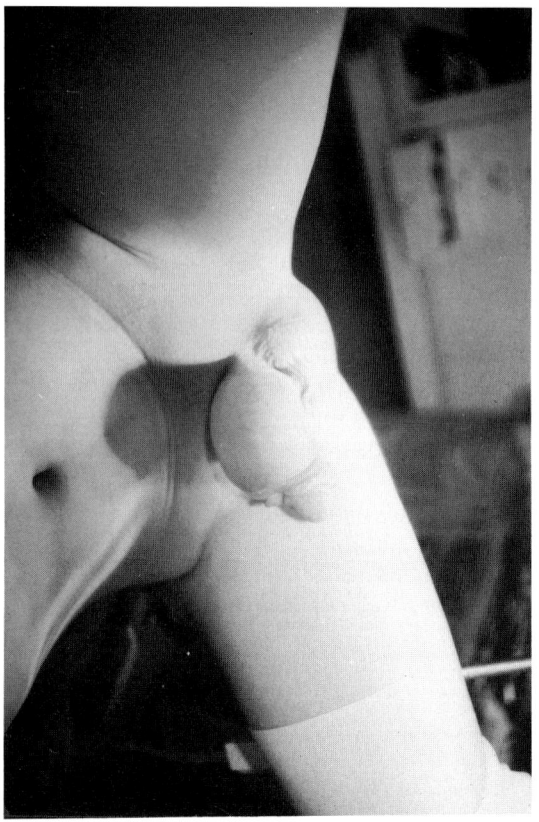

FIGURE 42.1. Patient with penile subcutaneous tissue expander.

assured. Granato[58] has suggested as a primary procedure the use of tissue expansion as a means of bypassing the need for either skin grafts or sigmoid grafts. In patients with marginal or small phalluses, the patient first undergoes insertion of a rectangular tissue expander under Buck's fascia along the entire length of the phallus. The skin is stretched over a 6- to 8-week period and the result is a non–hair-bearing surface of sufficient size to fill the entire neovagina (Fig. 42.1).

## Clitoroplasty

Early methods for constructing a neoclitoris used nonpedicled parts of the corpus cavernosum or corpus spongiosum to create a bud at the upper part of the introitus, but the more recent techniques use a pedicled part of the glans penis, which creates a sensate and erectile clitoris. Although the earlier methods are simpler to perform, they produce a less dramatically sensate clitoris. In 1980 Meyer and Kesselring[66] described their experience using a small bud of corpus cavernosum covered by penile skin. To use the glans penis, the dorsal vessels and nerves supplying the glans are carefully dissected free. The neurovascular bundle is placed subcutaneously in a wide curve in order to avoid kinking. The glans is trimmed and brought through a slit in the neovaginal skin, a couple of centimeters anterior to the urethral meatus. The distal part of the corpus spongiosum can be exposed through the superior aspect of the introitus to resemble a clitoris. In a series of 28 patients who had a clitoroplasty, 6 had a pedicled part of the glans penis as described by Rubin[63] and later modified by Hage et al,[67] and one had a clitoris created from the distal part of the corpus spongiosum.

## Crownplasty

The technique of penile inversion results in the cephalad neolabia as laterally divergent structures. In patients with large labia, obesity, or a profusion of pubic hair, the result may be both cosmetically and functionally satisfactory to the patient. In those thinner or more exacting patients, the appearance is such that a crown or M-plasty is done to correct the problem approximately 6 months after the primary surgery. In those patients, an M-shaped incision is made in the upper labia and the penile skin, thus drawing the labia together into normal anatomic position.

## Postoperative Complications

The most common complaint in transsexual surgery is lack of vaginal depth. This can occur if the patient has not inserted the stent to an adequate depth to keep the vagina patent throughout its entire length, if the tube graft does not fully survive, or if the length of the penis was too short to begin with. Hence, explaining to the patient the need for the constant use of the stent is very important, particularly if the individual is not having regular dilatation of the vagina by coitus.[68] Misplacement of the urethra during its transposition, so that the meatus is sutured in such a position whereby the patient cannot micturate while seated, is also fairly common. However, both problems (lack of depth to the vaginal barrel and urethral misplacement) are relatively simple to correct with a minor surgical procedure. Stenosis of the urethral meatus may occur occasionally. More serious complications are a recto vaginal fistula or a deep-seated infection of the abdominal muscles or of the perineum or both. Unfortunately, concomitant with complications, contracture of the neovagina may also occur and require further surgical intervention.[59,69] The most common complication of male-to-female sexual-reassignment surgery is dyspareunia resulting from a combination of a small male pelvis, a small vagina (usually due to inadequate dilation or small penis size), and retained erectile tissue.[70] Patients return frequently for cosmetic vulvar procedures in order to perfect the appearance of their external genitalia.[71]

Sexual satisfaction following surgical sex-reassignment varies widely, not only depending on the success of the surgical reassignment technique but also on the psychological stability of the patient. Some male-to-female transsexuals claim that they are orgasmic, some even claim multiple orgasms, whereas others report little, if any, sexual arousal, but state that the ability to "contain" a man's penis is sufficient gratification in itself. Some patients who do experience orgasm claim that the sensations they experience postsurgically are different from their previous orgasmic sensations. Instead of an intense propulsive sensation situated at the tip of the penis, there is now a more generalized "warm" feeling, a total body sensation building up gradually to a climax that resolves more slowly. Some patients report ejaculating a small amount of fluid during coitus.

## Follow-up on Operated Male-to-Female Transsexuals

In a series studied, between May 1980 and December 1994, 47 patients underwent sex-reassignment surgery at Montefiore Medical Center. All the patients had been cross-living as females for at least 12 months. They all had received estrogen and progesterone for 6 to 12 months for a sufficient period of time for breast development to occur within normal female sizes and for atrophy of the testes and the prostate. All patients were at least 21 years of age at the time of surgery. Three were married, six divorced, and one widowed. The remaining 37 were single. Prior to surgery, all had a complete and thorough evaluation and had undergone 1 to 2 years or at least 15 sessions of preparation in psychotherapy sessions with psychotherapists who specialized in the field of gender dysphoria. Thus, all patients received some emotional and mental preparation to facilitate the postsurgical process of adjustment.

A questionnaire (Table 42.1) was developed for the purpose of collecting reliable and informative postsurgery data from this population, in order to investigate several very important issues: (1) the kind and degree of personal satisfaction obtained from the surgery; (2) the evaluation of emotional and psychological problems experienced by living in society as females; (3) the evaluation of self-perception as females living among genetic females in society, and the development of interpersonal and sexual relationships with the opposite sex; (4) how the outcome of the surgery impacted on perceptions of the overall quality of life; (5) the level of adjustment required or experienced in places of employment; and (6) the degree of importance given to gynecological and physical examinations and medical follow-up procedures.

Among those patients who were contacted, 28 of the 47 responded willingly and reported high satisfaction in their perceptions of the quality of their lives. Eleven of the 27 who responded were also interviewed on a one-to-one basis to gather more complete data and to verify, validate, and expand some of the detalis provided in their written responses. To maximize accuracy in patients' responses, the personal follow-up interviews were conducted by a physician who was not involved in the original decision for surgery or with the surgery itself. The information obtained by the interviews with 11 patients was far superior to that contained in the written responses (Tables 42.2 and 42.3).

TABLE 42.1. Questionnaire on results of surgery for gender dysphoria.

1) When did you have genital surgery? _____

2) What physical problems have you had as a result of the surgery?

_____

_____

3) What emotional problems have you had as a result of the surgery?

_____

4) Have you been able to follow your surgeon's instructions regarding dilation?

_____

5) Frequency of dilator use (daily frequency/hours)
   First four months after surgery: _____
   Four months later: _____
   The last four months of the first year: _____

6) Have you had a genital examination after your genital surgery? _____

7) Have you been given open-ended prescriptions for hormonal therapy? _____

8) Job history after surgery (please circle one of the following)
   a) Stable, completely self-supporting      b) Mostly self-supporting
   c) Mostly unemployed                       d) Always unemployed

9) Does your present job satisfy you? _____

10) Did you have any suicide thoughts or gestures before or after the surgery?

_____

11) Drugs after surgery (please circle one or more of the following):
    a) No use of drugs
    b) Occasional use (marijuana, alcohol, tranquilizers)
    c) Occasional use of (sleeping pills, amphetamines, cocaine, LSD, crack)
    d) Regular drug use

12) Do you feel that life is easier and more comfortable for you after the surgery?

_____

13) Do you think that the surgery solved your emotional problems?

_____

14) Have you noticed any physical or emotional change in your behavior or attitude to others after the surgery?

_____

15) Are you currently living with:    a) Spouse         b) Male lover      c) Female lover
                                      d) Roommate       e) No partners     f) Parents
                                      g) Your children     Other _____

16) If you become emotionally involved with a partner, do you tell that person about your transsexual past?

_____

17) Sexual partner preference:
    a) Only males      b) Bisexual, mostly males      c) Bisexual, mainly females
    d) Only females    e) No sexual partner

18) Describe your love relationship after the surgery (select one):
    a) Long and stable              c) Usually short-lasting relationship
    b) Recent stable relationship   d) Short-lasting relationship with multiple partners

19) Have friends or family members been:
    a) Very supportive      b) Moderately supportive      c) Not supportive
    How has this affected you?

_____

TABLE 42.1. *Continued*

20) Have you been sexually active since the surgery? _____

21) Is sexual intercourse satisfactory and pleasurable? _____

22) Sexual satisfaction (orgasm):
    a) Consistently orgasmic    b) Usually orgasmic
    c) Infrequently orgasmic    d) Never orgasmic

23) Do you find any change in your ability to have orgasm after the surgery?

24) How important is it to have orgasm?
    a) Very important    b) Somewhat important    c) Not important

25) Do you experience pain during sexual intercourse?
    a) Always    b) Often    c) Infrequently    d) Never

26) Do you need to use lubricants for intercourse?
    a) Always    b) Often    c) Infrequently    d) Never

27) If after the surgery you don't have sexual intercourse, what are the reasons?
(please circle one or more of the following):
    a) No suitable partner found    e) Vaginal stenosis
    b) Too painful    f) Not adequate cosmetic result
    c) Fear to damage the surgical results    g) Other _____
    d) No desire

28) How soon after the surgery have you had sexual intercourse?

29) Surgical decision (please circle one):
    a) No doubts about the surgery
    b) Occasional doubt about surgery, but no doubts about being a woman
    c) Occasional doubt about surgery and about being a woman
    d) Frequent doubts

30) What do you think about the cosmetic result of the surgery?
    a) Excellent    b) Very good    c) Fair    d) Poor

31) How important is the cosmetic result?
    a) Extremely important    b) Very important
    c) Somewhat important    d) Not important

32) Do you regret that you had the surgery?

33) Can you describe how changing your gender through surgery affected the overall quality of your life?

34) How do you perceive the woman's role in the world:
    a) Passive    b) Victim    c) To be taken care of    d) Equal partnership

# Conclusion

Assessment of outcome studies over the past three decades reflects the serious obstacles in measuring the effectiveness of genital surgery. These include lack of long-term follow-up, inadequate patient samples, limited available data,[72] and no large-scale controlled studies.[3,73]

Although few postoperative patients have expressed regret over having had surgery,[70,74] it should be noted that a small percentage of surgeries have produced negative results.[75] Suicides in postoperative sex-change patients are infrequent (0.8% to 2.1%, according to reported follow-up data). A recent 30-year review of sex-reassignment surgery outcomes by Pfafflin and Junge[76] indicated that regrets ex-

TABLE 42.2. Demographic data.

| ID | Age | Marital status | First gender dysphoric thought (Age) | Cross-dressing (Age) | Hormonal therapy (Years) | Previous cosmetic surgery | Orchiectomy prior to surgery | Education | Religion | Occupation | Follow-up (years) |
|----|-----|----------------|------|------|------|------|------|-----------|----------|------------|------|
| 1 | 31 | Divorced | 8 | 29 | 2 | No | No | High school | Catholic | Bank clerk | 3.3 |
| 2 | 59 | Divorced | 9 | 40 | 16 | Yes | No | Dental doctor | Jewish | Dentist | 1.0 |
| 3 | 42 | Single | 6 | 20 | 19 | Yes | No | Elementary | Catholic | Unemployed | 2.2 |
| 4 | 38 | Single | 8 | 31 | 7 | Yes | Yes | Elementary | Catholic | Unemployed | 7.8 |
| 5 | 32 | Single | 11 | 17 | 15 | No | Yes | High School | Buddhist | Unemployed | 5.7 |
| 6 | 32 | Single | 8 | 31 | 1 | No | Yes | College | Jewish | Paralegal | 14.5 |
| 7 | 32 | Single | 5 | 20 | 15 | No | Yes | College | Baptist | Clerk | 6.1 |
| 8 | 42 | Divorced | 6 | 40 | 2 | No | No | College | Catholic | Nurse | 4.0 |
| 9 | 30 | Single | 6 | 23 | 7 | Yes | No | College | Anglo-Saxon Protestant | Computer programmer | 9.9 |
| 10 | 49 | Divorced | 6 | 41 | 10 | No | No | Elementary | Protestant | Superintendent | 4.2 |
| 11 | 41 | Divorced | 6 | 35 | 7 | No | No | College | Catholic | Chemist | 3.4 |
| 12 | 33 | Single | 6 | 18 | 15 | Yes | No | Elementary | Catholic | Hair stylist | 3.7 |
| 13 | 39 | Single | 14 | 29 | 10 | No | No | Elementary | Protestant | Therapist aid | 9.0 |
| 14 | 60 | Divorced | 5 | 57 | 3 | Yes | No | High school | Buddhist | Financier | 1.0 |
| 15 | 51 | Widowed | 8 | 44 | 7 | Yes | No | PhD | Catholic | College mathematics professor | 0.8 |
| 16 | 34 | Single | 5 | 30 | 3 | Yes | No | College | Catholic | Clerk | 6.7 |
| 17 | 33 | Single | 8 | 24 | 10 | Yes | No | Elementary | Catholic | Unemployed | 1.5 |
| 18 | 31 | Married | 10 | 19 | 11 | No | No | College | Catholic | Clerk | 6.0 |
| 19 | 38 | Divorced | 6 | 36 | 2 | No | No | PhD | Anglo-Saxon Protestant | Biology researcher | 0.6 |
| 20 | 24 | Single | 6 | 16 | 7 | No | No | College | Catholic | Manager | 6.3 |
| 21 | 41 | Single | 6 | 37 | 0 | No | Yes | Elementary | Catholic | Bartender | 6.1 |
| 22 | 33 | Single | 6 | 26 | 8 | No | No | College | Jewish | Manager | 3.0 |
| 23 | 37 | Single | 6 | 36 | 2 | No | No | High school | Greek Orthodox | Saleswoman | 4.1 |
| 24 | 37 | Divorced | 9 | 33 | 2 | Yes | No | High school | Protestant | Policewoman | 0.6 |
| 25 | 47 | Single | 7 | 33 | 2 | No | No | High school | Jewish | Nurse | 0.6 |
| 26 | 35 | Single | 5 | 34 | 4 | Yes | No | High school | Anglo-Saxon Protestant | Electronic technician | 1.0 |
| 27 | 37 | Single | 6 | 36 | 2 | Yes | No | College | Catholic | Teacher | 2.0 |
| 28 | 27 | Single | 8 | 22 | 2 | Yes | No | College | Catholic | Teacher | 0.6 |

pressed by less than 1% of female-to-male patients and 1% to 1.5% of male-to-female patients could be attributed to poor differential diagnosis, failure to carry out the true-life test, or, more recently, to lack of adequate and proper patient care.[77] One of the most significant outcomes of this study is the recognition that none of the patients felt any regret whatsoever for having had the surgery or any dissatisfaction with its cosmetic results. However, many of them expressed great dissatisfaction and disappointment in how they subsequently lived their lives. Many realized that although they had entered a hospital with a male organ and had left feeling very pleased with their female genitalia, it takes considerable work and energy beyond surgery or hormone treatments to be able to live their lives as females, even in the most mundane and everyday fashion. Operated male-to-female transsexual patients should be urged to engage in some type of postoperative psychotherapy to relieve some or most of the disappointments inevitable with such a dramatic lifestyle change. The possible benefits of such postoperative psychotherapy (group or individual) would be to help these most unusual and remarkable people to live the life they were surely intended to live, as profoundly and roundly as possible with the female identity. Society raised them to live as men, to accommodate to their genetic selves. The transsexual process must teach them how to claim their true inner gender identity and more of their really female selves.

TABLE 42.3. Surgical outcome and complications.

| NO. | Importance of orgasm for sexual satisfaction | Potential for orgasm | Sexual partners | Intravaginal intercourse | Other sexual outlets | Intercourse frequency | Clitoroplasty | Surgical complications |
|---|---|---|---|---|---|---|---|---|
| 1 | Very important | Yes | Males only | Yes | — | 2/week | No | None |
| 2 | Somewhat important | Yes, infrequently | Females | No | Masturbation, vibrators | N/A | No | None |
| 3 | Very important | No | Males only | No | Masturbation, vibrators, oral | N/A | No | None |
| 4 | Not important important | Yes, infrequently | Males only | Yes | — | 1–2/week | No | None |
| 5 | Very important | Yes | Males only | Yes | — | 2/week | No | None |
| 6 | Very important | No | Males only | Yes | — | N/A | No | Revision of scrotal vaginal flap |
| 7 | Somewhat important | Yes | Males only | No | — | N/A | No | None |
| 8 | Very important | Yes | Males only | Yes | — | N/A | No | None |
| 9 | Somewhat important | Yes, infrequently | Males only | No | Masturbation, vibrators | N/A | No | Colon neovaginoplasty |
| 10 | Not important | Yes | Females | No | Oral, vibrators | N/A | No | None |
| 11 | Very important | Yes | Males only | Yes | — | 2/week | No | None |
| 12 | Very important | Yes | Bisexual | Yes | — | 1/week | No | None |
| 13 | Somewhat important | Yes | Males only | Yes | — | 1/two weeks | No | None |
| 14 | Not important | No | Males only | No | No | N/A | No | None |
| 15 | Very important | No | Males only | No | — | N/A | Yes | None |
| 16 | Somewhat important | Yes, infrequently | Males only | Yes | — | 1/week | No | None |
| 17 | Somewhat important | Yes | Males only | Yes | — | 3/week | No | None |
| 18 | Very important | Yes | Males only | Yes | — | 1/week | No | None |
| 19 | Somewhat important | No | Males only | No | No | N/A | No | None |
| 20 | Not important | Yes | Males only | Yes | — | 2/week | No | None |
| 21 | Somewhat important | Yes, infrequently | Females | No | Masturbation, vibrators, oral | 1/week | No | Sigmoid neovaginoplasty |
| 22 | Very important | Yes, infrequently | Males only | No | Masturbation, vibrators | N/A | No | Sigmoid neovaginoplasty |
| 23 | Very important | Yes | Males only | Yes | — | 1/week | Yes | None |
| 24 | Somewhat important | Yes, infrequently | Bisexual | Yes | — | N/A | Yes | None |
| 25 | Very important | No | Males only | No | — | N/A | Yes | None |
| 26 | Somewhat important | Yes | Bisexual | No | Oral, vibrators | N/A | Yes | None |
| 27 | Very important | Yes | Bisexual | Yes | Masturbation, vibrators | 1/week | Yes | None |
| 28 | Very important | Yes | Males only | Yes | — | N/A | Yes | None |

N/A, not answered.

# References

1. Fisk NM. *Gender Dysphoria Syndrome.* Palo Alto: Stanford University Press; 1973.
2. Green RL. Transsexualism: mythological, historical, and cross cultural aspects. In: Benjamin H, ed. *The Transsexual Phenomenon.* New York: Julian Press; 1966: 173–186.
3. Brown GR. A review of clinical approaches to gender dysphoria [review]. *J Clin Psychiatry* 1990; 51:57–64.
4. Bullough VL. Transsexualism in history. *Arch Sex Behav* 1975; 4:561–571.
5. Forgey D. The institution of bedarche among the North American Plains Indians. *J Sex Res* 1975; 11:1–5.

6. Wames H, Hill G. Gender indentity and the wish to be a woman. *Psychosomatics* 1974; 15:25–29.

7. Money J, DePriest M. Three cases of genital self-surgery and their relationship to transsexualism. *J Sex Res* 1976; 12:283–294.

8. Abraham F. Genitalumwandlung an zwei männlichten transvestiten. *Z Sexualwissenschalft* 1931; 18:223–226.

9. Hoyer N. *Man into Woman.* New York: Dutton; 1993.

10. Benjamin H. Transsexualism and transvestism as psychosomatic and somato-psychic syndromes: symposium. *Am J Psychother* 1954; 8:219–230.

11. Benjamin H. Nature and management of transsexualism with report on 31 operated cases. *West J Surg Obstet Gynecol* 1964; 72:105–111.

12. Benjamin H. *The Transsexual Phenomenon.* New York: Julian Press; 1966.

13. Jorgenson C. *A Personal Autobiography.* New York: Paul E. Ericson; 1967.

14. Hamburger C. Desire for change of sex as shown by personal letters from 465 men and women. *Acta Endocrinol (Copenh)* 1953; 14:361–375.

15. Volkin V. Transsexualism: as examined from the viewpoint of internalized object relations. In: Karasu TB, Socarides CW, eds. *On Sexuality: Psychoanalytic Observations.* New York: International Universities Press; 1979: 189–221.

16. Money J, Ehrhardt AA. [Transsexuals after the change of sex. Experiences and findings in Johns Hopkins Hospital]. [German]. *Beitr Sexualforsch* 1970; 49:70–87.

17. Stoller RJ. A biased view of "sex transformation" operations. An editorial. *J Nerv Ment Dis* 1969; 149:312–317.

18. Hastings D. Inauguration of a research project on transsexualism in a university medical center. In: Green R, Money J, eds. *Transsexualism and Sex Reassignment.* Baltimore: Johns Hopkins University Press; 1969: 243–251.

19. Pauly IB. The current status of the change of sex operation. *J Nerv Ment Dis* 1968; 147:460–471.

20. Arieff A. *Five Year Studies of Transsexuals: Psychiatric, Psychological and Surgical Aspects.* Stanford: University Press; 1973.

21. Hastings D, Markland C. Post-surgical adjustment of twenty-five transsexuals (male-to-female) in the University of Minnesota study. *Arch Sex Behav* 1978; 7:327–336.

22. Laub DR, Fisk N. A rehabilitation program for gender dysphoria syndrome by surgical sex change. *Plast Reconstr Surg* 1974; 53:388–403.

23. Edgerton MT, Knorr NJ, Callison JR. The surgical treatment of transsexual patients. Limita-

tions and indications *Plast Reconstr Surg* 1970; 45:38–46.

24. Edgerton MT. The surgical treatment of male transsexuals [review]. *Clin Plast Surg* 1974; 1:285–323.

25. Berger J, Green R, Laub D, et al. *Standards of Care: The Hormonal and Surgical Reassignment of Gender Sex Dysphoric Persons.* Galveston, TX: University of Texas Medical Branch, Janus Information Center; 1977.

26. Hertoft P, Sorensen T. Transsexuality: some remarks based on clinical experience. *Ciba Found Symp* 1978; 62:165–181.

27. Sorensen T, Hertoft P. Sex modifying operations on transsexuals in Denmark in the period 1950–1977. *Acta Psychiatr Scand* 1980; 61:56–66.

28. Roberto L. Issues in diagnosis and treatment of transsexualism. *Arch Sex Behav* 1983; 12:445–473.

29. Bakker A, van Kesterene PJ, Gooren LJ, et al. The prevalence of transsexualism in The Netherlands. *Acta Psychiatr Scand* 1993; 87:237–238.

30. Ross MJ, Walinder J, Lundstrom B, et al. Cross-cultural approaches to transsexualism: a comparison between Sweden and Australia. *Acta Psychiatr Scand* 1981; 63:75–82.

31. Tsoi WF. The prevalence of transsexualism in Singapore. *Acta Psychiatr Scand* 1988; 78:501–504.

32. Engel H, Pfafflin F, Wiedeking C. H-Y antigen in transsexuality. *Hum Genet* 1980; 55:315–319.

33. Hoening J. Etiological research in transsexualism. *Psychiatr J Univ Ottawa* 1981; 6:184–189.

34. Meyer-Bahlburg HFL, Grisanti GC, Ehrhardt AA. Prenatal effects of sex hormones on human male behavior: medroxyprogesterone acetate (MPA). *Psychoneuroendocrinology* 1977; 2:383–390.

35. Gooren L. The neuroendocrine response of leutinizing hormone to estrogen administration in heterosexual, homosexual, and transsexual subjects. *J Clin Endocrinol Metab* 1986; 63:583–588.

36. Rekers GA, Mead SL, Rosen AC. Family correlates of male childhood gender disturbance. *J Genet Psychol* 1983; 142:31–42.

37. Stoller RJ. *The Transsexual Experiment.* New York: Jason Aronson; 1975.

38. Socarides CW. The desire for sexual transformation: a psychiatric evaluation of transsexualism. *Am J Psychiatry* 1969; 125:1419–1425.

39. Forester BM, Swiller H. Transsexualism: review of syndrome and presentation of possible suc-

cessful therapeutic approach. *Int J Group Psychother* 1972; 22:343–351.

40. Bentler PM. A typology of transsexualism: gender identity theory and data. *Arch Sex Behav* 1976; 5:567–584.

41. Davenport CW. A follow-up study of 10 feminine boys. *Arch Sex Behav* 1986; 15:511–517.

42. Green R. Gender identity in childhood and later sexual orientation: follow-up of 78 males. *Am J Psychiatry* 1985; 142:339–341.

43. Green R. *Sexual Identity Conflict in Children and Adults.* New York: Basic Books; 1974.

44. Brown GR. Bioethical issues in the management of gender dysphoria. *Jefferson J Psychiatry* 1988; 6:23–24.

45. Stoller RM. *On the Development of Masculinity and Femininity.* New York: Science House; 1968.

46. Money J. Sex reassignment as related to hermaphroditism and transsexualism. In: Green R, Money J, eds. *Transsexualism and Sex Reassignment.* Baltimore: Johns Hopkins University Press; 1969: 91–113.

47. American Psychiatric Association. *Diagnostic and Statistical Manual of Mental Disorders.* 3rd ed. Washington, DC: American Psychiatric Association; 1980.

48. American Psychiatric Association. *Diagnostic and Statistical Manual of Mental Disorders.* 3rd ed., revised ed. Washington, DC: American Psychiatric Association; 1987.

49. Meyer WJ, Webb A, Stuart CA. Physical and hormonal evaluation of transsexual patients: a longitudinal study. *Arch Sex Behav* 1986; 15:121–138.

50. Transsexualism and character disorders. 10th International Symposium on Gender Dysphoria, June 9–12, 1987, Amsterdam, the Netherlands.

51. Lothstein LM, Levine SB. Expressive psychotherapy with gender dysphoric patients. *Arch Gen Psychiatry* 1981; 38:924–929.

52. Meyer WJ, Walker PA, Suplee ZR. A survey of transsexual hormonal treatment in twenty gender-treatment centers. *J Sex Res* 1981; 17:344–349.

53. Fortin CJ, Klein T, Messmore HL, et al. Myocardial infarction and severe thromboembolic complications. As seen in an estrogen-dependent transsexual. *Arch Intern Med* 1984; 144:1082–1083.

54. Steiner B. *Gender Dysphoria: Development, Research, Management.* New York: Plenum Press; 1985.

55. McIndoe A. Treatment of congenital absence and obliterative conditions of vagina. *Br J Plast Surg* 1950; 2:254–267.

56. Edgerton MT, Bull J. Surgical construction of the vagina and labia in male transsexuals. *Plast Reconstr Surg* 1970; 46:529–539.

57. Pandya NJ, Stuteville OH. A one-stage technique for constructing female external genitalia in male transsexuals. *Br J Plast Surg* 1973; 26:277–282.

58. Granato RC. Surgical approach to male transsexualism. *Urology* 1974; 3:792–796.

59. Markland C, Hastings D. Vaginal reconstruction using bowel segments in male-to-female transsexual patients. *Arch Sex Behav* 1978; 7:305–307.

60. Goligher JC. The use of pedicled transplants of sigmoid or other parts of the intestine for vaginal construction. *Ann R Coll Surg Engl* 1983; 65: 353–355.

61. Fortunoff S, Lattimer JK, Edson M. Vaginoplasty technique for female pseudohermaphrodites. *Surg Gynecol Obstet* 1964; 118: 545–548.

62. Malloy TR, Noone RB, Morgan AJ. Experience with the 1-stage surgical approach for constructing female genitalia in male transsexuals. *J Urol* 1976; 116:335–337.

63. Rubin SO. A method of preserving the glans penis as a clitoris in sex conversion operations in male transsexuals. *Scand J Urol Nephrol* 1980; 14:215–217.

64. Young HH. Cure of cancer of prostate by radical perineal prostatectomy (prostato seminal vesiculectomy): history, literature and statistics of Young's operation. *J Urol* 1945; 53:188–252.

65. Belt E. Radical perineal prostatectomy in early carcinoma of the prostate. *J Urol* 1942; 48:287–297.

66. Meyer R, Kesselring UK. One-state reconstruction of the vagina with penile skin as an island flap in male transsexuals. *Plast Reconstr Surg* 1980; 66:401–406.

67. Hage JJ, Karim RB, Bloem JJ, et al. Sculpturing the neoclitoris in vaginoplasty for male-to-female transsexuals [review]. *Plast Reconstr Surg* 1994; 93:358–364.

68. Jayaram BN, Stuteville OH, Bush IM. Complications and undesirable results of sex-reassignment surgery in male-to-female transsexuals. *Arch Sex Behav* 1978; 7:337–345.

69. Noe JM, Sato R, Coleman C, et al. Construction of male genitalia: the Stanford experience. *Arch Sex Behav* 1978; 7:297–303.

70. Green R, Fleming D. Transsexual surgery follow-up status in the 1990's. *Annu Revi Sex Res* 1990; 1:163–174.

71. Gregory J, Purcell M. *Transsexualism.* Philadelphia: B.C. Decker; 1987.

72. Meyer JK, Reter DJ. Sex reassignment. Follow-up. *Archi Gen Psychiatry* 1979; 36:1010–1015.

73. Hunt DD, Hampson JL. Transsexualism: a standardized psychological rating format for the evaluation of results of sex reassignemt surgery. *Arch Sex Behav* 1988; 9:255–263.

74. Pfafflin F. Regrets after sex reassignment surgery in gender dysphoria. In: Bockting WO, Coleman E, eds. *Interdisciplinary Approaches in Clinical Management.* Binghamton: Haworth Press; 1992: 69–85.

75. Abramowitz S. Psychosocial outcomes of sex reassignment surgery. *J Consult Clin Psychol* 1986; 4:183–189.

76. Pfafflin F, Junge A. Nachuntersuchungen nach Geschlechusumwandlung: Eine kemmentierte Literatureubersicht 1961–1991 [Follow-up studies after sex-reassignment surgery: a review 1961–1991]. In: Pfafflin F, Junge A, eds. *Geschlechusumwandlung: Abhanddlungen zur Transsexualitat* [Sex change studies on transsexualism]. Stuttgart: Schattauer; 1992: 149–459.

77. Schaefer LC, Wheller CC. Harry Benjamin's first ten cases (1938–1953): a clinical historical note. *Arch Sex Behav* 1995; 24:73–93.

# 43

# Facts and Controversies on the Application of Penile Tumescence and Rigidity: Recording for Erectile Dysfunction

Jeremy P.W. Heaton and Alvaro Morales

In the 1960s, Fisher et al[1] and Karacan et al[2] independently developed a systematic approach to assess nocturnal penile tumescence and rigidity (NPTR) as measurements to use in studying penile erection in sleep. This was the first objective measurement of penile erection with the specific goal of assessing sexual function. In many ways, it opened the field to the possibility of scientific study of human sexuality. Measuring erectile capability has since been used in other applications, such as comparing the efficacy of therapies for erectile dysfunction (drugs or surgery), the effects of disease and drugs, and assessing the parameters of erectile function. With NPTR measurements it is now possible to improve the understanding of the fundamental mechanisms of penile rigidity and the physical properties of the flaccid and erect penis.

## Nocturnal Penile Tumescence and Rigidity

### Historical Perspective

Lue,[3] in his *World Book of Impotence*, quoted Leonardo da Vinci's perceptive writings on the significance of sleep erections: " 'The penis does not obey the order of its master, who tries to erect or shrink it at will, whereas instead the penis erects freely while its own master is asleep. The penis must be said to have its own mind, by any stretch of the imagination.' " The recognition that erections that occur during sleep could be used as a component of the diagnosis of sexual dysfunction came in the mid-20th century.[4] Early measurements of nocturnal penile tumescence (NPT) were made to study dreams and psychological factors.[2] From this point, psychologists and others have developed a substantial body of literature studying sleep and erections, which was thoroughly reviewed up to 1980 by Wasserman et al.[5] Subsequent reviews by Kessler[6] and Karacan[7] have added to the picture. Urologists looking at erectile dysfunction as a primary end point for sleep erection measurement are relative latecomers but have made greater use of its significance.

## Available Methods for Recording NPT

On average, normal men have more than three erections per night, each of duration greater than 10 minutes. Measurement of these phenomena at first sight appears to be a simple matter. However, penile tumescence presents a classical problem of clinical measurement—the more detailed the measurement, the more the measured variable is changed by the process of measurement. Any report of this normal human penile response should be qualified by the conditions of observation and measurement (age of subject, home or laboratory setting, strain gauge or RigiScan measurement device, etc.). The recognition that rigidity, and not merely a change in circumference, is an important aspect of the measurement has brought a further refinement in the equipment available and in corresponding issues of interpretation and norms.

There has been a wide variety of devices used to record NPTR. Common to all devices used at home is the disadvantage of needing to be set up by the patient and of being subjected to conditions out of clinical context. Balancing this is the benefit of the absence of "white-coat" anxiety, that is, anxiety provoked by the presence of medical personnel.[8] On the other hand, any measuring technique not including true measures of sleep (electroencephalogram, electro-oculogram, and electromyogram) risks missing aberrations in sleep itself (e.g., disturbances of rapid eye movement [REM] sleep). This is considered by many researchers to be a major drawback of the simpler methods of NPTR recording. Rigidity measurements are only fully comparable with measurements made by use of similar protocols.

Among the methodologies employed for NPTR recording are the following:

### Observation by the Partner

This method is impractical, subjective, and difficult to quantify.

### Postage Stamps

A simple ring of postage stamps (Fig. 43.1) is wrapped around the subject's penis before he goes to sleep. If the ring of stamps is found to be broken on awakening, the observer assumes that either an erection occurred or movement or bending or some other unknown factor snapped the stamps.[9] This method is unreliable and can be misleading.[10]

### Sliding Bands

This variation on the stamp principle substitutes a paper band that will slide open and remain at its greatest circumference. Thus, only the greatest circumference attained is recorded, but without information about how often or how long an erection occurred, this was found to be unsuitable for diagnostic purposes.[11]

### Strain Gauges

The single paper ring can be replaced by a number of parallel bands of known and increasing strength. Tumescence first breaks one band under tension, then the next band as it comes

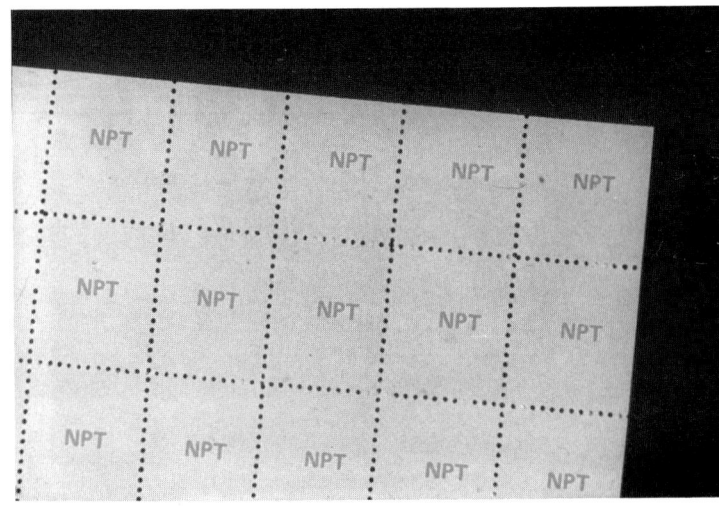

FIGURE 43.1. Photograph of a sheet of NPT stamps is mainly of historical interest, but illustrates what is meant when this method of recording is referred to.

FIGURE 43.2. Photograph of a Dacomed Snap-Gauge in place and demonstrates how easily it could become displaced.

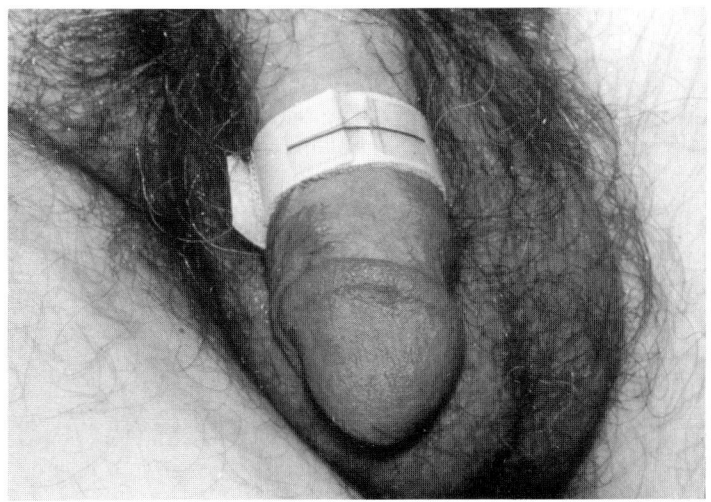

under tension, and the bands fracture sequentially up to a band that has sufficient strength to resist the expansion of the penis. This gives a crude estimate of rigidity during the best erection. This simple method, intended for home use without sleep measurement, is subject to artifact from movement or sabotage and is now regarded as of limited reliability.[12] Snap Gauges (Dacomed Corp., Minneapolis, MN) exemplify this approach (Fig. 43.2).

## Mercury Strain Gauge

This is the first method devised that permits continuous monitoring, and it is still regarded as the standard. The apparatus consists of a rubber tube filled with mercury connected as part of an electrical circuit. The gauge is placed around the penis. The resistance of the gauge increases as it is stretched and lengthened, measuring the dimensional change as a change in electrical property. Although the strain gauge itself can be made accurate far beyond the limitations of clinical interpretation, it can be disturbed by movement, and the elastic force applied circumferentially around the penis changes the initial circumference and thereby biases the percentage change readings, conveying nothing intrinsically about rigidity or about sleep.[13]

## RigiScan (Dacomed Corp., Minneapolis, MN)

This is the first device to offer automation, portable recording, tumescence, and rigidity recording (Fig. 43.3). The fundamentals were reported in the mid-1980s, and although the technology has evolved, the principles remain unchanged.[14] There are many reports based on this technology (40% of the more than 50 papers on NPT in the past 5 years). The patient can use the RigiScan at home, and the data can be examined as a downloaded computer file. A recent paper by Munoz et al[15] provides an excellent summary of the workings of the RigiScan and a description of its flaws. Despite some unexpected variability between devices, it represents the best off-the-shelf technique currently available. As with other techniques, it can be combined with measures of sleep and adapts well to real time recording in an office or laboratory.

## ART-1000 (Surgitek)

This device was targeted to provide information similar to the RigiScan but requires fastidious use of the sensing elements because of their size and method of fixation.[16,17] The technical problems resulted in only slight acceptance of the ART-1000, and it is no longer available.

## Penile Plethysmograph

Lavoisier et al[18] published data on the use of this device that relies for its signal on the pressure change in a sphygmomanometer-type cuff that transmits intracorporal pressure to a mi-

crocomputer or to a portable recording device. The correlation with intracorporal pressure, the essential driving force for rigidity, was good and the measurement was noninvasive and continuous. However, no commercial device using this principle has been made available.

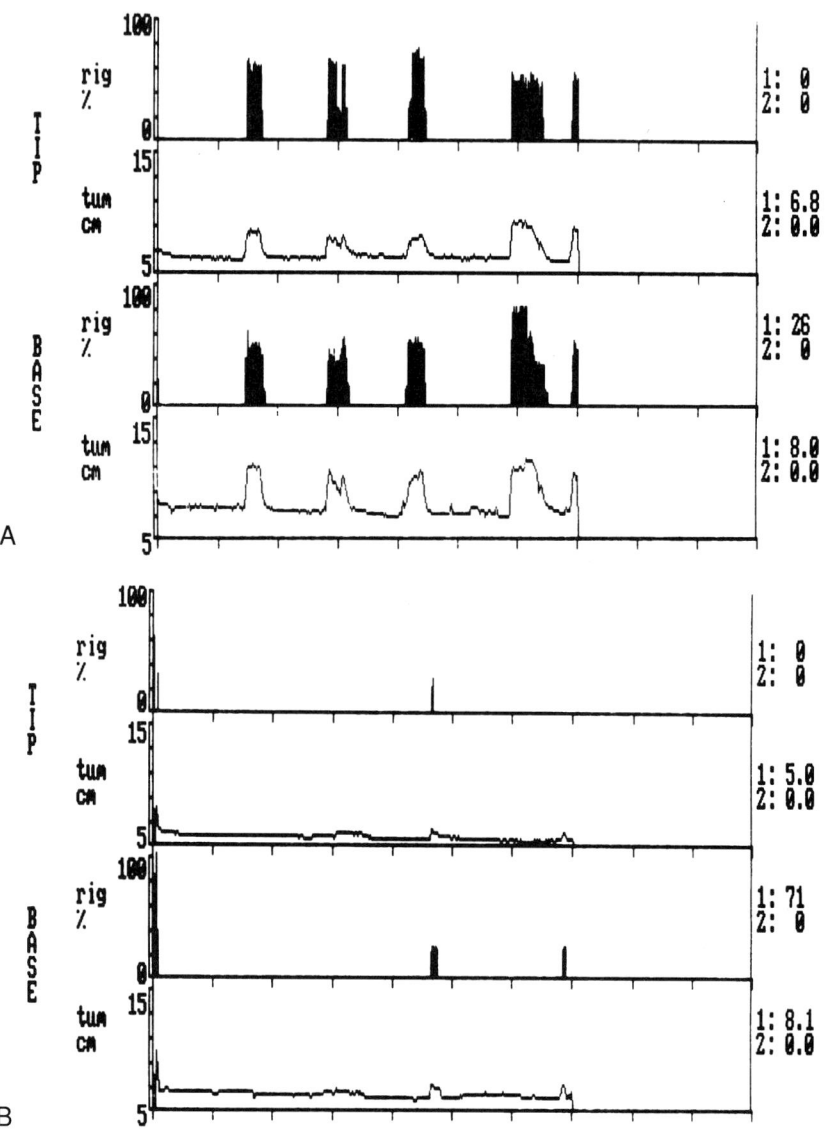

FIGURE 43.3. (A) A tracing of a normal night of spontaneous erections as recorded by a RigiScan device. Time scale units in hours. (B) A full night of NPTR recording using the RigiScan demonstrating the absence of significant erectile activity. Note the two peaks of rigidity that could give an erroneous impression of the maximal response. Time scale units in hours. (C) The use of the RigiScan in recording penile response during a provocative session demonstrating an erection of significant duration in response to an oral erectogenic agent (apomorphine) and audiovisual erotic stimulation. Time scale is 1 hour.

Figure 43.3 *Continued*

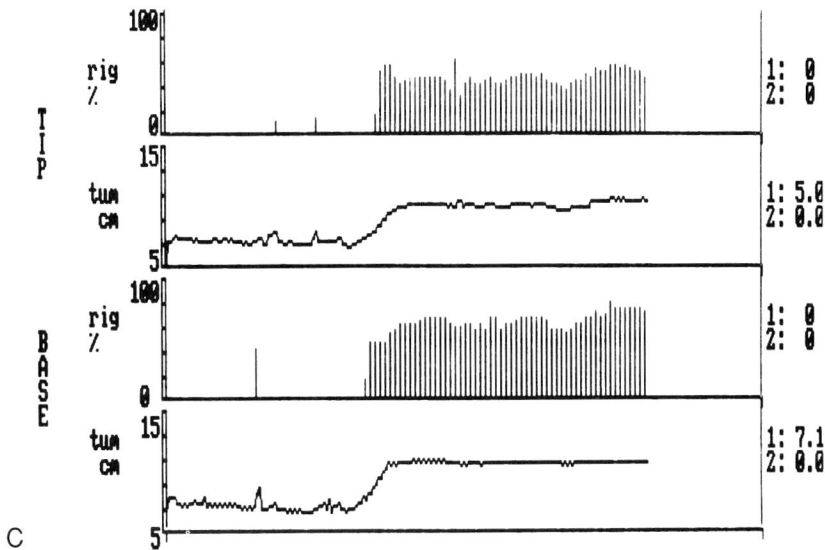

C

## Rigidity Issues

Rigidity, not size (girth and length), permits intromission. Rigidity of the penis is a function of the internal fluid pressure, the arrangement and properties of structural elements, and overall dimensions. A thick, short penis will be more resistant to classic column-type buckling tests than will a long, thin penis with the same internal pressure and structure. The penis is not composed of homogeneous material. Its physical properties vary with the axis of measurement and the time factors during measurement (e.g., fast or slow bending). Goldstein[19] recently emphasized the importance of understanding the mechanical properties of tissues of the penis.

With the intrinsic complexity of analyzing the penis as a structure and the novelty of these concepts, it is not surprising to find some methodologic and interpretational inconsistencies in the definition of rigidity. The penis can be assessed as a problem in mechanical engineering, modeled as a perfect column governed by classic buckling force equations or as an issue of human engineering—measuring in humans the force it takes on average to achieve penetration with an average penis into a normal, well-lubricated vagina of a receptive partner.[20–22] Rigidity can be measured as axial rigidity or as buckling force, whereby there is a measured and increasing force applied to the penis until buckling occurs.[16] The RigiScan measures radial rigidity exclusively.

There is a continuing debate about the reliability of the methods of measurement. There is agreement that rigidities under 60% as measured by RigiScan, under optimal conditions of sleep and normality of other factors, indicate the presence of organic disease and inability for normal sexual intercourse, but there is incomplete agreement as to the meaning of higher rigidity values or variations in conditions.[23–25]

Just as there are issues of repeatability with the RigiScan as an instrument,[15,26] so are there issues with observer and patient variation in measures of buckling strength. In fact, there is said to be significant instability of NPTR in a given individual such that it may give an imprecise indication of awake erectile capacity.[27] However, some longer term studies have found good reproducibility of RigiScan recording.[22]

Criteria for reading RigiScan results have been published, but there are limitations.[15,28–30] A recent article by Licht et al[31] provides two helpful clarifications: the base measurements are more accurate than tip measurements, and use of 70% rigidity as the cutoff point overestimates erectile dysfunction. However, the studies that led to these modifications were done in organically impotent men and therefore may not apply to all patients.

It has been widely advocated that two nights of study are required as a minimum although three nights would be preferable. There are other reports that suggest that a single night can be used reliably, with pharmacologic manipulation to ensure that REM sleep occurs.[23] In the home or in laboratories without considerable experience, the incidence of night-to-night variation and first night effect are probably best addressed by obtaining recordings on a minimum of two nights.

## Sleep Measurement Issues

NPTR with polysomnographic recording (NPT-PSGR) provides the most complete methodology for NPT recording. This cannot be done outside a sleep laboratory because its complexity involves measures of sleep and breathing in addition to measures of tumescence and rigidity. Complete protocols should involve simultaneous recordings of penile physiologic measures, electroencephalogram (Is there sleep?), electro-oculogram (Is there REM?), electromyogram (Are there movement disturbances?), nasal airflow (Is there disordered breathing?), and oxygen saturation (Is there hypoxemia?). In addition, studies may include trained observer assessment of rigidity, buckling pressure determinations, photographs of the erection, and more. It is important for the user of NPTR outside the laboratory to be familiar with factors that can significantly influence the NPTR. To avoid influencing the sleep and the erections any more than needed, these multidimensional assessments should be conducted by experienced laboratories.

## Specific Findings in NPTR

### Puberty and Aging

The characteristics of NPTR change with the onset of puberty. Indeed, NPTR measurements may predict puberty when combined with a knowledge of endocrine status, although this has little clinical relevance.[32] Toward the other end of the scale in healthy aging men, changes in NPT have been documented and found to be related to bioavailable testosterone,[33] but Schiavi et al[34] documented a decline in circumference and rate of increase of circumference in men over 55 years of age. Because sleep patterns change with age, measurement is more complex. However, the sleep parameters of normal men and men with erectile dysfunction in the same age group were found not to differ. This suggests that the changes in NPT are not related to age-based sleep changes.[35]

### Sleep

Measures of NPTR correlate well with episodes of REM sleep.[1,2] The changes in NPTR that can be seen from night to night are those that correlate most closely with REM sleep.[36] In contrast, a dissociation between REM sleep and NPTR has been documented during on-off treatment cycles with a short-acting monoamine oxidase inhibitor (type A).[37]

### Depression

There is wide appreciation of the fact that affective disorders may have a significant impact on erectile function. A recent examination of the link between depression and NPTR demonstrated significant disturbances in tumescence and rigidity in males with clinically significant depression.[38] Interestingly, severe endogenous depression did not correlate with the finding of greatest change in NPTR. The same group of investigators has found that the NPT changes may persist into periods of remission from depression and may not correlate with other measurements of sexual function. In the men studied, it was believed that the NPT changes may have been a part of the depressive trait rather than a simple consequence of active depression.[39] However, other investigators have found a variable response to depression and recovery, in some subjects with subtle changes in NPTR, but in others it was much more pronounced.[40] As a group, the depressed men did not differ from controls, and there were no distinguishing NPTR features, possibly because of a lack of stratification. The intensity of changes in waking affect appear to correlate with the changes in NPTR, only some of which can be accounted for by changes in REM sleep.[41] It is evident that there is need for further study of the effect of depression on erectile function during sleep.

### Testosterone Status

As with other indicators of sexual function, NPTR is markedly affected by hormonal status. Treatment of hypogonadal men with testosterone elevates testosterone levels within hours, and NPTR increases from low or nonexistent to values indistinguishable from normal men over 6 to 12 months.[42] The same response is seen in men with hypopituitarism treated with testosterone or gonadotropin.[43,44] This relationship is not seen when the serum testosterone is only slightly depressed[45]—there is no clear change of NPT as long as the testosterone levels are within the normal range. The decline of NPTR measures in hypogonadal men is one aspect where a distinction is evident between the control of erections in NPT and in audiovisual erotic stimulation; hypogonadal men continue to respond to audiovisual erotic stimulation—a finding reconfirmed recently.[46]

### Antiandrogens and 5α-Reductase Inhibitors

The currently accepted hypothesis that significant changes in serum testosterone will diminish NPTR measures has been shown to hold for treatment with cyproterone acetate.[47] A recent study with the nonsteroidal antiandrogen biclutamide (Casodex) showed that NPTR measures did not decline with this treatment and that serum testosterone increased as expected.[48] Finasteride, a type 2 5α-reductase inhibitor, has been shown not to suppress NPT consistently, although the authors did not rule out a role for dihydrotestosterone in NPTR on this evidence alone.[49] The determining sex hormones for sexual function are not fully defined beyond the significance of large changes in testosterone, the ambiguity of the importance of small abnormalities in testosterone, and the possibility that dihydrotestosterone and other androgens have roles that are currently incompletely understood.

### Disease

Although NPTR is depressed in diabetic men with impotence, NPTR is also abnormal, to the point of meeting some criteria for organicity, in over 70% of diabetic men with normal sexual function.[50] Because another study, in contrast, has shown that at least some of the decrease in NPTR may be due to respiratory changes associated with sleep in persons with diabetes, the issue of the cause of NPTR abnormalities in such individuals is unclear.[51] It is evident, therefore, that an abnormal NPTR recording in a diabetic cannot be taken as prima facie evidence that the patient has organic erectile dysfunction.

NPTR is not a useful discriminant in multiple sclerosis, and normal values may be seen in severely compromised men.[52] In sickle cell disease and after heart transplantation, NPTR brings no new special information to the etiologic diagnosis of erectile dysfunction.[53,54]

### Smoking and Alcohol

Smoking has been studied for its effects on NPTR. Rigidity is adversely affected by chronic smoking in a roughly proportional manner, and heavy smokers experienced the shortest time of erection and detumesced the fastest.[55] Alcohol taken in intoxicating levels, in a single case multinight study, decreased a number of NPTR parameters. The study, however, also suggested caution about overextrapolating from NPT studies, particularly those studies involving drugs to stimulate sexual function.[56]

## Interpretation of NPTR

It is clear that no branch of medicine has the exclusive gift of analysis and insight as far as the study and interpretation of sleep phenomena are concerned. The literature does, however, point to some biases. Urologists are more likely to use the RigiScan, psychologists and psychiatrists are more likely to measure sleep, and it has been said that respirologists seldom look below the belt! The role of NPTR recording as the only objective marker for psychogenicity is undeniable, and as such it carries enormous appeal and legal weight of questionable scientific justification. Several recent discussions specifically dwell on interpretation, although interpretation comes from understanding continually advancing details.[31,57–60] There has been successful use of the RigiScan in family practice oriented to erectile dysfunction,[61,62] and it is clear that access to the technique is now more widespread than ever. NPTR recording will never diminish the understanding of the causes of erectile dysfunction in an individual, but it may present a challenge in integrating it into the scheme of patient assessment.[63]

The analysis of RigiScan data can be standardized better than strain-gauge NPTR-PSGR data because of the essential constraints of the latter method. Even so, there is a vast amount of information in a night's record, and the discussion of tip versus base, tumescence versus rigidity, onset, and detumescence rates can go on for a long time without resolution.[64] New analysis algorithms using area-under-the-curve calculations, tumescence activity units (TAU) and rigidity activity units (RAU),[65,66] may help to standardize reporting, although independent ratification is needed to fully validate the approach.

# NPTR and the Diagnosis of Psychogenic Erectile Dysfunction

Can NPTR alone distinguish psychogenicity from organicity? This question, which may have seemed reasonable 10 years ago, now seems a little faded if not outright naive. Sachs[67] has provided the most comprehensive review of this dichotomy while suggesting a new taxonomy. A simple and reasonable view of the situation may be found in the concept that even the most abstruse feelings have biologic substrates at some point and so even the most "psychogenic" erectile dysfunction may have an organic component, as exemplified by the evolution of the understanding of schizophrenia. Steers[68] has articulated and expanded on this line of reasoning ("With regard to sexual dysfunction, the useful designations of psychogenic or organic impotence have been in some respects misleading since psychogenic

impotence is due to neurogenic mechanisms"), and other authors continue to add more clinical perspectives.[69] Patients in the late twentieth century are unable to benefit fully from such concepts because no matter what label is attached to the psychogenic end of the spectrum of etiologies, there is little in the way of effective etiology-specific therapy. For practical purposes, the pure psychogenic dysfunction has positive NPTR and sexual history, but no organic factors, and treatment should be offered with oral agents (e.g., antidepressants) before invasive approaches are even considered.

When no organicity is found and NPTR is normal (base rigidity >55%),[31] at the very least this indicates integrity of the erectile mechanisms of the penis. The natural corollary of this premise is that treatment should be directed at the systems known to be dysfunctional and cause the minimum damage possible to tissue shown to be competent, i.e., the corpora cavernosa.

How does NPTR complement other tests? As pharmacologic intracavernous injection (ICI) testing gained popularity, efforts were made to evaluate tests as alternatives. The laboratory effect of anxiety[28] and the resulting enhanced inhibition make correlations between NPTR and ICI difficult.[70] Duplex ultrasound has been found to add little to the first-rank diagnostic assignment.[71] A detailed assessment of a similar issue revealed that when a positive NPTR and other positive psychogenic evidence coexisted, the results of duplex ultrasound were unreliable,[21] possibly due to anxiety factors in these men. The other side of the issue can be seen in one report where NPTR data, showing brief episodes of high rigidity, may be used to support a diagnosis of veno-occlusive dysfunction.[72] In brief, sexual history, and tests such as response to intracavernous vasoactive agents, NPTR, and audiovisual erotic stimulation (AVES), have been used to place patients in the traditional diagnostic boxes of organic, psychogenic, or uncertain. These provide complementary but different information about patients.[73]

Does NPTR share the same neural pathways as a sexual erection or an AVES-stimulated erection? Probably not, as the discrepancy between AVES and NPTR in hypogonadal men is one example of a measurable difference. However, the tools presently used to dissect the pathways are very blunt, so the issue carries little clinical relevance at this time.

## Similar Uses for the Measurement Technology— Diurnal Penile Tumescence and Rigidity

NPTR is expensive to perform and intrusive on patient time. REM sleep can occur during morning naps and, when it does, erections can occur (diurnal penile tumescence and rigidity [DPTR]) and be measured using familiar measures of erectile function.[74] As many as 75% of patients or normal men exhibiting positive NPTR have demonstrated positive DPTR.[75,76] It has been recommended that impotent patients scheduled to undergo NPTR reduce sleep time the night before their study. Of interest, successful NPTR studies have been conducted in patients during morning naps.[77]

## Alternative Uses for the Measurement Technology— Response to Therapy

The RigiScan was devised originally with the capability of real-time evaluation, and this functionality is intrinsically available with strain-gauge systems. Use in this situation sets on one side the issues of clinical meaning for NPTR but substitutes all the problems of laboratory effect already mentioned. Whatever technology is used and however the issues of anxiety are handled, the instruments will objectively record what happens to the penis. This makes it an ideal instrument for drug evaluation both at home at night[78] and during daytime laboratory sessions.[79]

In the laboratory, the measurements can be directly interpreted from the recording device or evaluated later. Some global scoring strategies, such as the RigiScan number, that simplify the multiple parameters have been published for awake session use. These appear to have utility but need further validation.[80]

The use of penile tumescence and rigidity (PTR) to document[81] and compare drug effects has great potential. Whenever it is used, there will be issues of anxiety, and protocols that incorporate treatment that modifies the inhibitory factors will have intrinsic advantages over protocols that simply introduce vasodilators. It is critical to control the conditions of the test, because comparisons between studies, although literally accurate in terms of percent of rigidity, may not really express the difference between agents. There are published norms for ICI using RigiScan[82] and excellent comparative studies showing objective superiority of prostaglandin $E_1$ ($PGE_1$) and papaverine alone for ICI.[83]

The concept of complete smooth muscle relaxation, or peak effect, is very important if qualitative comparisons of efficacy are to be made. Peak effect can be achieved through fundamentally different approaches: repeat injection,[84] masturbation,[85] AVES, vibration, simply leaving the patient alone, or having him go home. Much of the uncertainty about the effects of anxiety and inhibition would be improved by the development of validated tools for measurement.

## Audiovisual Erotic Stimulation (AVES)

During laboratory or office assessment, AVES can be introduced to produce or amplify an erectile response while there is some sort of erectile monitoring. AVES is much easier now through the use of video and CD-ROM technology. AVES has been thought to decrease central nervous system inhibitory factors and it certainly diverts attention from the laboratory setting. It is additive with penile vibratory stimulation,[86,87] masturbation, ICI, and pharmacologic manipulation.[80] Habituation to erotic material has been documented,[88] which supports the belief that response to viewing of erotic material can be significantly affected by cultural and societal factors.[89]

AVES has been demonstrated to be one strategy that optimizes or improves the response to ICI during PTR recording.[90–92]

However, this test remains largely invalidated, is difficult to standardize, and requires further study.[89]

AVES has been used to document objective changes in disease states before erectile dysfunction is apparent, as in patients with diabetes and no documented neuropathy who show abnormal responses to AVES when compared with controls.[93] AVES has already been mentioned as contrasting with NPTR with respect to the response rates of hypogonadal men.[46] As many as 25% of castrated men will show a positive response to AVES.[94] Affect[95] and age[96] also can be shown to produce changes in AVES, underscoring that this study parallels NPTR closely even if it does not fully overlap.

## Vibration Stimulation

Penile vibration using oscillating devices has been used as another means of enhancing erectile response,[97] and the enhancement can be monitored by RigiScan or strain-gauge technology. This has been shown to improve submaximal erections after ICI[98] and AVES.[99]

## Indications for Monitoring PTR in the Investigation of Erectile Dysfunction

Indications for monitoring PTR are as follows:

A suspected "psychogenic" etiology
A suspected sleep disorder
An obscure etiology
A male unresponsive to treatment
Planned invasive treatment (major vascular or implant surgery)
A legally sensitive case
Measurement and comparison of drug effects.

NPTR can bring surprises and add information that may have been overlooked by a very comprehensive interview and assessment process. A 28-year-old man was recently seen for a second opinion at the clinic run by the Human Sexuality Group at Queen's University. He had undergone full assessment, including dynamic cavernosometry, had received unsuccessful venous leak surgery, had been reassessed, and had undergone repeat venous surgery. A full dynamic cavernosometry reinvestigation revealed what appeared to be a continuing venous leak. He was asked to do NPTR with a RigiScan in his hotel room. On one night, the RigiScan demonstrated erections of adequate duration with over 55% rigidity, and on the other night he did not sleep at all. A debriefing revealed that he had a previously undisclosed chronic problem with unsatisfactory sleep and waking feeling tired. He was sent for full sleep analysis and dissuaded from further active management of his erectile problems until his sleep issues were resolved. Similarly a man was referred to the Cleveland Clinic after several procedures for venous incompetence. NPTR demonstrated the man to have normal erections, and further assessment disclosed his problem to be premature ejaculation. Treatment of his ejaculatory difficulties restored him to full sexual functioning (Montague DK, personal communication, 1994).

## Conclusion

Objective measures of penile tumescence and rigidity are important because there is so much about sexual and erectile function that can not be easily quantified. We are only just entering an era where validated instruments (questionnaires) are available to characterize erectile and sexual function. These can be compared with existing objective data (e.g., NPTR data) and will enhance the meaning and reproducibility of the evaluation of individuals and new therapies. Interventional techniques, such as cavernosometry or even color duplex scanning, may induce significant artifacts because of the measurements themselves. Although measurements of rigidity are not without their own problems, as already discussed, they provide useful quantitative evidence of penile status that has a vital place in the study of erectile function.

It is still intuitively reasonable to identify that the basic penile mechanisms of erection are intact in a man who has had NPTR recording that is within normal limits. However, it is overly simplistic to say that normal NPTR in a setting of complaints of erectile dysfunction define a clean diagnostic group that can be labeled "psychogenic." Men with nocturnal erections but poor sexual erections may have significant endothelial or respiratory disease, for instance. They may also have the significant problems of anxiety, depression, or partner dissatisfaction that are more traditionally associated with normal NPTR and erectile dysfunction. NPTR measurements, therefore, will not often draw clean diagnostic distinctions but will add materially to the understanding of the erectile status of individuals. In addition, the technology developed to serve the need for NPTR measurements will continue to provide useful objective data during this period of rapid expansion in therapeutic intervention.

## References

1. Fisher C, Gross J, Zuch J. Cycle of penile erection synchronous with dreaming (REM) sleep. *Arch Gen Psychiatry* 1965; 12:29–45.

2. Karacan I, Goodenough DR, Shapiro A, et al. Erection during sleep in relation to dream anxiety. *Arch Gen Psychiatry* 1966; 15:1983–1989.

3. Lue TF, ed. *World Book of Impotence.* London/Nishimura: Niigata-Shi, Smith-Gordon; 1992.

4. Ohlmeyer P, Brilmayer H, Hullstrung H. Periodische Vorgange im Schlaf. *Pflugers Arch* 1944; 248:559–565.

5. Wasserman MD, Pollak CP, Spielman AJ, et al. The differential diagnosis of impotence. *JAMA* 1980; 243:2038–2042.

6. Kessler WD. Nocturnal penile tumescence. *Urol Clin North Am* 1988; 15:81–86.

7. Karacan I. NPT/rigidometry. In: Kirby RS, Carson CC, Webster GD, eds. *Impotence: Diagnosis and Management of Erectile Dysfunction.* Boston: Butterworth, Heinemann; 1991: 62–71.

8. McMahon CG. The reliability of the papaverine test as a screening test for vascular disease in impotence. *Int J Impotence Res* 1990; 2:133–142.

9. Barry JM, Blank B, Boileau M. Nocturnal penile tumescence monitoring with stamps. *Urology* 1980; 15:171.

10. Marshall PG, Morales A, Phillips P, et al. Measuring nocturnal penile tumescence with stamps:

11. Morales A, Marshall PG, Fenemore J. A new device for measuring NPT. *J Urol* 1983; 129:288–291.

12. Condra M, Fenemore J, Reid K, et al. Screening assessment of penile tumescence and rigidity. Clinical test of Snap-Gauge. *Urology* 1987; 29:254–257.

13. Karacan I, Salis PJ, Thornby JI, et al. The ontogeny of nocturnal penile tumescence. *Waking Sleeping* 1976; 1:27–44.

14. Bradley WE, Timm GW, Gallagher JM, et al. New method for continuous measurement of nocturnal penile tumescence and rigidity. *Urology* 1985; 26:4–9.

15. Munoz MM, Bancroft J, Marshall I. The performance of the RigiScan in the measurement of penile tumescence and rigidity. *Int J Impotence Res* 1993; 5:69–76.

16. Rossello BM. The rigidometer. *Arch Esp Urol* 1991; 44:187–188.

17. Kropman RF, Lycklama a Nijeholt AA, Zwartendijk J. Experiences with the Surgitek ART-1000 penile tumescence and rigidity monitor, and comparison with the RigiScan. *J Urol* 1991; 146:43–45.

18. Lavoisier P, Proulx J, Courtois F. Reflex contractions of the ischiocavernosus muscles following electrical and pressure stimulations. *J Urol* 1988; 132:396–399.

19. Goldstein I. Biomechanics of erection. In: *European Society for Impotence Research*, 1995, Proceedings of the 1st Meeting. Thessaloniki; 19–15

20. Saenz de Tejada I, Moroukian P, Tessier J, et al. Trabecular smooth muscle modulates the capacitor function of the penis. Studies on a rat model. *Am J Physiol* 1991; 260:H1590–1595.

21. Karacan I, Moore C, Sahamay S. Measurement of pressure necessary for vaginal penetration. *Sleep Res* 1985; 14:269.

22. Bain CL, Guay AT. Re: classification of sexual dysfunction for management of intracavernous medication-induced erections. *J Urol* 1991; 146:1379.

23. Allen RP, Engel RM, Smolev JK, et al. Comparison of duplex ultrasonography and nocturnal penile tumescence in evaluation of impotence. *J Urol* 1994; 151:1525–1529.

24. Allen RP, Smolev JK, Engel RM, et al. Comparison of RigiScan and formal nocturnal penile tumescence testing in the evaluation of erectile rigidity. *J Urol* 1993; 149:1265–1268.

a comparative study under sleep laboratory conditions. *J Urol* 1988; 130:88–91.

25. Guay AT, Heatley GJ. Re: comparison of RigiScan and formal nocturnal penile tumescence testing in the evaluation of erectile rigidity. *J Urol* 1994; 152:171.

26. Bain CL, Guay AT. Reproducibility in monitoring nocturnal penile tumescence and rigidity. *J Urol* 1992; 148:811–814.

27. Nofzinger EA, Fasiczka AL, Thase ME, et al. Are buckling force measurements reliable in nocturnal penile tumescence studies? *Sleep* 1993; 16:156–162.

28. Sohn MH, Seeger U, Sikora R, et al. Criteria for examiner-independent nocturnal penile tumescence and rigidity monitoring (NPTR): correlations to invasive diagnostic methods. *Int J Impotence Res* 1993; 5:59–68.

29. Kaneko S, Yachiku S, Miyata M, et al. Continuous monitoring of penile rigidity and tumescence in Japanese without erectile dysfunction. *Jpn J Urol* 1991; 82:955–960.

30. Dacomed Corporation, Minneapolis, Minnesota, USA. RigiScan ambulatory rigidity and tumescence system. Selected case studies. Form Number 750 1560486.

31. Licht M, Lewis R, Wollan P, et al. Comparison of RigiScan and sleep laboratory nocturnal penile tumescence in the diagnosis of organic impotence. *J Urol* 1995; 154:1740–1743.

32. Horita H, Kumamoto Y, Aoki M, et al. Clinical significance and usefulness of measuring nocturnal penile tumescence in children. *Jpn J Urol* 1991; 82:1939–1946.

33. Horita H, Kumamoto Y. Study on nocturnal penile tumescence (NPT) in healthy males. Study on age-related changes of NPT. *Jpn J Urol* 1994; 85:1502–1510.

34. Schiavi RC, White D, Mandeli J, et al. Hormones and nocturnal penile tumescence in healthy aging men. *Arch Sex Behav* 1993; 22:207–215.

35. Schiavi RC, Mandeli J, Schreiner-Engel P, et al. Aging, sleep disorders, and male sexual function. *Biol Psychiatry* 1991; 30:15–24.

36. Ware JC, Hirshkowitz M. Characteristics of penile erections during sleep recorded from normal subjects. *J Clin Neurophysiol* 1992; 9:78–87.

37. Steiger A, Benkert O, Holsboer F. Effects of long-term treatment with the MAO-A inhibitor moclobemide on sleep EEG and nocturnal hormonal secretion in normal men. *Neuropsychobiol* 1994; 30:101–105.

38. Thase ME, Reynolds CF, Jennings JR, et al. Diminished nocturnal penile tumescence in depression: a replication study. *Biol Psychiatry* 1992; 31:1136–1142.

39. Nofzinger EA, Thase ME, Reynolds CF, et al. Sexual function in depressed men. Assessment by self-report, behavioral, and nocturnal penile tumescence measures before and after treatment with cognitive behavior therapy. *Arch Gen Psychiatry* 1993; 50:24–30.

40. Steiger A, Holsboer F, Benkert O. Studies of nocturnal penile tumescence and sleep electroencephalogram in patients with major depression and in normal controls. *Acta Psychiatr Scand* 1993; 87:358–363.

41. Nofzinger EA, Schwartz RM, Reynolds CF, et al. Correlation of nocturnal penile tumescence and daytime affect intensity in depressed men. *Psychiatry Res* 1993; 49:139–150.

42. Burris AS, Banks SM, Carter CS, et al. A long-term, prospective study of the physiologic and behavioral effects of hormone replacement in untreated hypogonadal men. *J Androl* 1992; 13:297–304.

43. Clopper RR, Voorhess ML, MacGillivray MH, et al. Psychosexual behavior in hypopituitary men: a controlled comparison of gonadotropin and testosterone replacement. *Psychoneuroendocrinology* 1993; 18:149–161.

44. Horita H, Kumamoto Y. Study on nocturnal penile tumescence (NPT) in healthy males. Study on the relationship between the serum free testosterone level and NPT. *Jpn J Urol* 1994; 85:1511–1520.

45. Buena F, Swerdloff RS, Steiner BS, et al. Sexual function does not change when serum testosterone levels are pharmacologically varied within the normal male range. *Fertil Steril* 1993; 59:1118–1123.

46. Carani C, Bancroft J, Granata A, et al. Testosterone and erectile function, nocturnal penile tumescence and rigidity, and erectile response to visual erotic stimuli in hypogonadal and eugonadal men. *Psychoneuroendocrinology* 1992; 17:647–654.

47. Cooper AJ, Cernovovsky Z. The effects of cyproterone acetate on sleeping and waking penile erections in pedophiles: possible implications for treatment. *Can J Psychiatry* 1992; 37:33–39.

48. Migliari R, Muscas G, Usai E. Effect of Casodex on sleep-related erections in patients with advanced prostate cancer. *J Urol* 1992; 148:338–341.

49. Cunningham GR, Hirshkowitz M. Inhibition of steroid 5 alpha-reductase with finasteride: sleep-related erections, potency, and libido in healthy men. *J Clin Endocrinol Metab* 1995; 80:1934–1940.

50. Nofzinger EA, Reynolds CF, Jennings JR, et al. Results of nocturnal penile tumescence studies are abnormal in sexually functional diabetic men. *Arch Intern Med* 1992; 152:114–118.

51. Schiavi RC, Stimmel BB, Mandeli J, et al. Diabetes, sleep disorders, and male sexual function. *Biol Psychiatry* 1993; 34:171–177.

52. Ghezzi A, Malvestiti GM, Baldini S, et al. Erectile impotence in multiple sclerosis: a neurophysiological study. *J Neurol* 1995; 242:123–126.

53. Burnett AL, Allen RP, Tempany CM, et al. Evaluation of erectile function in men with sickle cell disease. *Urology* 1995; 45:657–663.

54. Livi U, Faggian G, Sorbara C, et al. Use of prostaglandin E$_1$ in the treatment of sexual impotence after heart transplantation: initial clinical experience. *J Heart Lung Transplant* 1993; 12:484–486.

55. Hirshkowitz M, Karacan I, Howell JW, et al. Nocturnal penile tumescence in cigarette smokers with erectile dysfunction. *Urology* 1992; 39:101–107.

56. Cooper AJ. The effects of intoxication levels of ethanol on nocturnal penile tumescence. *J Sex Marital Ther* 1994; 20:14–23.

57. Morales A, Condra M, Heaton JPW. The interpretation of nocturnal penile tumescence monitoring. *Curr Opinion Urol* (in press).

58. Morales A, Condra M, Reid K. The role of nocturnal penile tumescence monitoring in the diagnosis of impotence: a review. *J Urol* 1990; 143:441–446.

59. Morales A, Condra M, Surridge DH, et al. Nocturnal penile tumescence monitoring: is it necessary? In: Lue TF, ed. *World Book of Impotence.* London: Smith-Gordon; 1992: 67–73.

60. Hirshkowitz M, Ware CJ. Studies of nocturnal penile tumescence and rigidity. In: Singer C, Weiner WJ, eds. *Sexual Dysfunction: A Neuro-Medical Approach.* Futura; 1994: 77–99.

61. Shvartzman P. The role of nocturnal penile tumescence and rigidity monitoring in the evaluation of impotence. *J Fam Pract* 1994; 39:279–282.

62. Stoliar L, Shvartzman P, Horenstein I. Nocturnal penile tumescence and rigidity monitor—use in a family practice. *Isr J Med Sci* 1995; 31:359–364.

63. Schiavi RC. The role of the sleep laboratory in the evaluation of male erectile dysfunction. *Mt Sinai J Med* 1994; 61:161–165.

64. Colombo F, Fenice O, Austoni E. NPT: nocturnal penile tumescence test. *Arch Ital Urol Androl* 1994; 66:159–164.

65. Levine LA, Carroll RA. Nocturnal penile tumescence and rigidity in men without complaints of erectile dysfunction using a new quantitative analysis software. *J Urol* 1994; 152:1103–1107.

66. Levine LA, Lenting ER. Use of nocturnal penile tumescence and rigidity in the evaluation of male erectile dysfunction. *Urol Clin North Am* 1995; 22:775.

67. Sachs BD. Placing erection in context: the reflexogenic-psychogenic dichotomy reconsidered. *Neurosci Biobehav Rev* 1995; 19:211–224.

68. Steers W. Current perspectives in the neural control of penile erection. In: Lue TF, ed. *World Book of Impotence.* London/Nishimura: Niigata-Shi, Smith-Gordon; 1992: 23.

69. Van Nueten J, Verheyden B, Van Camp K. Role of penile nocturnal tumescence and rigidity measurement in the diagnosis of erectile impotence. *Eur Urol* 1992; 22:119–122.

70. Montague DK, Lakin MM, VanderBurg Mendendorp S, et al. Infusion pharmacocavernosometry and nocturnal penile tumescence findings in men with erectile dysfunction. *J Urol* 1991; 145:768–771.

71. Gutierrez P, Pye S, Bancroft J. What does duplex ultrasound add to sexual history, nocturnal penile tumescence and intracavernosal injection of smooth muscle relaxant in the diagnosis of erectile dysfunction? *Int J Impotence Res* 1993; 5:123–131.

72. Montorsi F, Ferini-Strambi L, Guazzoni G, et al. Significance of full nocturnal erections with short duration. *Eur Urol* 1994; 25:25–28.

73. Bancroft J, Smith G, Munoz M, et al. Erectile response to visual erotic stimuli before and after intracavernosal papaverine, and its relationship to nocturnal penile tumescence and psychometric assessment. *Br J Urol* 1991; 68:629–638.

74. Gordon CM, Carey MP. Penile tumescence monitoring during morning naps: a pilot investigation of a cost-effective alternative to full night sleep studies in the assessment of male erectile disorder. *Behav Res Ther* 1993; 31:503–506.

75. Morales A, Condra M, Fenemore J, et al. Slumber penile tumescence as an alternative to NPT in the diagnosis of impotence. *J Urol* 1993; 149:343A.

76. Morales A, Condra M, Heaton JP, et al. Diurnal penile tumescence recording in the etiological diagnosis of erectile dysfunction. *J Urol* 1994; 152:1111–1114.

77. Gordon CM, Carey MP. Penile tumescence monitoring during morning naps to assess male erectile functioning: an initial study of healthy men of varied ages. *Arch Sex Behav* 1995; 24:291–307.

78. Saenz de Tejada I, Ware JC, Blanco R, et al. Pathophysiology of prolonged penile erection associated with trazodone use. *J Urol* 1991; 145:60–64.

79. Ogrinc FG, Linet OI. Evaluation of real-time RigiScan monitoring in pharmacological erection. *J Urol* 1995; 154:1356–1359.

80. Heaton JP, Morales A, Adams MA, et al. Recovery of erectile function by the oral administration of apomorphine. *Urology* 1995; 45:200–206.

81. Munoz M, Bancroft J, Turner M. Evaluating the effects of an alpha-2 adrenoceptor antagonist on erectile function in the human male. 1. The erectile response to erotic stimuli in volunteers. *Psychopharmacology* 1994; 115:463–470.

82. Cilurzo P, Canale D, Turchi P, et al. The RigiScan system in the diagnosis of male sexual impotence. *Arch Ital Urol Nefrol Androl* 1992; 64:81–85.

83. Allen RP, Engel RM, Smolev JK, et al. Objective double-blind evaluation of erectile function with intracorporal papaverine in combination with phentolamine and/or prostaglandin $E_1$. *J Urol* 1992; 148:1181–1183.

84. Hatzichristou D, Saenz de Tejada I, Kuppferman S, et al. In-vivo assessment of trabecular smooth muscle tone, its application in pharmaco-cavernosometry and analysis of intracavernous pressure determinants. *J Urol* 1995; 153:1126–1135.

85. Lue TF. Impotence: a patient's goal directed approach to treatment. *World J Urol* 1990; 8:67–74.

86. Janssen E, Everaerd W, Van Lunsen RH, et al. Validation of a psychophysiological waking erectile assessment (WEA) for the diagnosis of male erectile disorder. *Urology* 1994; 43:686–695; discussion 695–696.

87. Janssen E, Everaerd W, Van Lunsen RH, et al. Visual stimulation facilitates penile responses to vibration in men with and without erectile disorder. *J Consult Clin Psychol* 1994; 62:1222–1228.

88. O'Donohue W, Plaud JJ. The long-term habituation of sexual arousal in the human male. *J Behav Ther Exp Psychiatry* 1991; 22:87–96.

89. Condra M, Morales A, Harris C, et al. A call for caution: the use of visual sexual stimulation as a tool for the etiological diagnosis of impotence. *Int J Impotence Res* 1991; 21:203–205.

90. Katlowitz NM, Albano GJ, Morales P, et al. Potentiation of drug-induced erection with audiovisual sexual stimulation. *Urology* 1993; 41:431–434.

91. Katlowitz N, Albano GJ, Patsias G, et al. Effect of multidose intracorporal injection and audiovisual sexual stimulation in vasculogenic impotence. *Urology* 1993; 42:695–697.

92. Lee B, Sikka SC, Randrup ER, et al. Standardization of penile blood flow parameters in normal men using intracavernous prostaglandin $E_1$ and visual sexual stimulation. *J Urol* 1993; 149:49–52.

93. Ali ST, Shaikh RN, Siddiqi NA, et al. Comparative studies of the induction of erectile response to film and fantasy in diabetic men with and without neuropathy. *Arch Androl* 1993; 30:137–145.

94. Greenstein A, Plymate SR, Katz PG. Visually stimulated erection in castrated men. *J Urol* 1995; 153:650–652.

95. Meisler AW, Carey MP. Depressed affect and male sexual arousal. *Arch Sex Behav* 1991; 20:541–554.

96. Rowland DL, Greenleaf WJ, Dorfman LJ, et al. Aging and sexual function in men. *Arch Sex Behav* 1993; 22:545–557.

97. Incrocci L, Slob AK. Visual sexual stimulation and penile vibration in screening men with erectile dysfunction. *Int J Impotence Res* 1994; 6:227–229.

98. Chun S, Fenemore J, Johnston B, et al. Enhancement of erectile responses to vasoactive drugs by a variable amplitude oscillation device. *J Urol* 1994; 151:322A.

99. Rowland DL, den Ouden AH, Slob AK. The use of vibrotactile stimulation for determining sexual potence in the laboratory in men with erectile problems: methodological considerations. *Int J Impotence Res* 1994; 6:153–161.

# Index

593

ISBN 0-387-94859-7

EAN

9 780387 948591 >